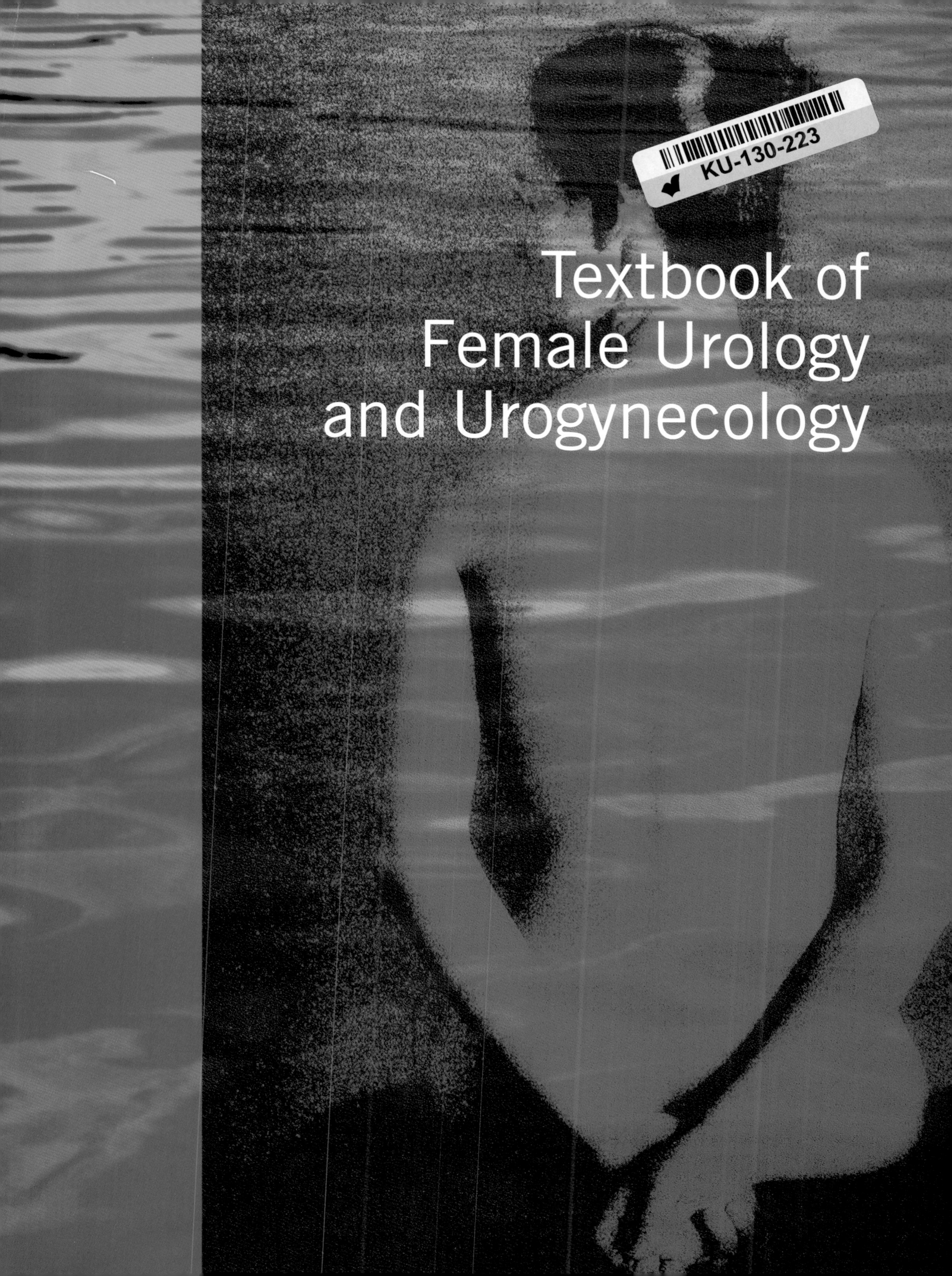
Textbook of
Female Urology
and Urogynecology

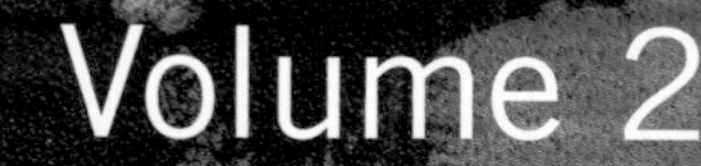

Textbook of Female Urology and Urogynecology

Second edition

Editors-in-Chief

Linda Cardozo MD FRCOG
Professor of Urogynecology, King's College Hospital, London, UK

David Staskin MD
Head, Section of Female Urology, New York Presbyterian Hospital, Cornell
Associate Professor of Urology, Weill-Cornell Medical College,
New York, NY, USA

informa
HEALTHCARE

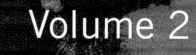

First edition published in the United Kingdom in 2001
by Isis Medical Media Ltd.
Second edition published by Informa Healthcare, an imprint of
Informa UK Ltd, 2 Park Square, Milton Park, Abingdon, Oxon OX14 4RN

Tel: +44 (0)20 7017 6000
Fax: +44 (0)20 7017 6699
Email: info.medicine@tandf.co.uk
Website: www.tandf.co.uk/medicine

A CIP record for this book is available from the British Library.

Library of Congress Cataloging-in-Publication Data
Data available on application

ISBN10: 1-84184-358-X
ISBN13: 978-1-84184-358-2

Distributed in North and South America by

Taylor & Francis
6000 Broken Sound Parkway, NW, (Suite 300)
Boca Raton, FL 33487, USA

Within Continental USA
Tel: 800 272 7737; Fax: 800 374 3401
Outside Continental USA
Tel: 561 994 0555; Fax: 561 361 6018
Email: orders@crcpress.com

Distributed in the rest of the world by
Thomson Publishing Services
Cheriton House
North Way
Andover, Hampshire SP10 5BE, UK
Tel: +44 (0)1264 332424
Email: tps.tandfsalesorder@thomson.com

Composition by Phoenix Photosetting UK
Printed and bound in Singapore by Kyodo Printing Co (S'pore) Pte Ltd

Chapter title image courtesy of Geoffrey W Cundiff MD FACOG
Cover image courtesy of Science Photo Library (photographer: Cristina Pedrazzini)

Contents

VOLUME 1, SECTION 4 – *NON-SURGICAL TREATMENT OF INCONTINENCE, PROLAPSE AND RELATED CONDITIONS*
SECTION EDITOR: ERIC S ROVNER

VOLUME 1, SECTION 5 – *ASSOCIATED DISORDERS*
SECTION EDITOR: PHILIP TOOZS-HOBSON

VOLUME 1, SECTION 6 – *APPENDICES*

VOLUME 2

VOLUME 2, SECTION 7 – *SURGERY FOR URINARY INCONTINENCE*
SECTION EDITOR: ROGER R DMOCHOWSKI

VOLUME 2, SECTION 8 – *SURGERY FOR UROGENITAL PROLAPSE*
SECTION EDITOR: BERNHARD SCHUESSLER

Contributors

Paul Abrams MD FRCS
Professor of Urology, Bristol Urological Institute, Southmead Hospital, Bristol, UK

May Alarab MB ChB MRCOG MRCPI
Department of Obstetrics and Gynecology, University of Toronto, Toronto, ON, Canada

Samih Al-Hayek MD LMSSA LRCP(Lond) LRCS(Eng) MRCS
Bristol Urological Institute, Southmead Hospital, Bristol, UK

Kate Anders RGN BSc
Nurse Specialist in Urogynaecology, Surrey, UK

Karl-Erik Andersson MD PhD
Department of Clinical and Experimental Pharmacology, Lund University Hospital, Lund, Sweden

Rodney A Appell MD FRCS
Professor of Urology and Chief, Division of Voiding Dysfunction and Female Urology, Baylor College of Medicine,
F. Brantley Scott Chair in Urology
St. Luke's Episcopal Hospital, Houston, TX, USA

Walter Artibani MD
Professor of Urology, Chief of Urology Department, University of Padova Via Giustiniani, Padova, Italy

Kaven Baessler MD
Department of Obstetrics and Gynecology, Cantonal Hospital, Lucerne, Switzerland

James Balmforth MRCOG
Department of Urogynaecology, Kings College Hospital, Denmark Hill, London, UK

Vanessa Banz MD
Department of Surgery, Cantonal Hospital, Lucerne, Switzerland

Bary Berghmans PhD MSc RPT
Health Scientist, Epidemiologist, AZM University Hospital Maastricht, The Netherlands

Manuel Besendörfer MD
Chirurgische Klinik mit Poliklinik der Universität Erlangen, Germany

John Bidmead MB BS MRCOG
Research Fellow, Department of Urogynaecology, King's College Hospital, London, UK

Kristie A Blanchard MD
Department of Urology, Ochsner Clinic Foundation, New Orleans, LA, USA

Jerry G Blaivas MD
Clinical Professor of Urology, Cornell Medical Center, UroCenter of New York, New York, NY, USA

Kari Bø PhD
Professor, Norwegian University of Sport and Physical Education, Oslo, Norway

Andrew Browning MB BS MRCOG
Gynecologist, Addis Ababa Fistula Hospital, Ethiopia, Addis Ababa, Ethiopia

Linda P Brubaker MD FACOG FACS
Professor and Director, Section of Urogynecology and Reconstructive Plastic Surgery, Loyola University Medical Center, Maywood, IL, USA

Richard C Bump MD
Eli Lilly and Company Corporate Center, Indianapolis, ID, USA

Kathryn L Burgio PhD
Department of Veterans Affairs Medical Center, Birmingham/Atlanta Geriatric Research, Education and Clinical Center, Birmingham, AL, USA

Antonio Carbone
Associate Professor of Urology, Department of Urology, I.C.O.T. Hospital, Rome, Italy

Linda Cardozo MD FRCOG
Professor of Urogynaecology, Department of Urogynaecology, King's College Hospital, London, UK

Marcus P Carey MB BS FRANZCOG
Director of Urogynaecology, Royal Women's Hospital, Melbourne, Australia

Lesley K Carr MD FRCS
Division of Urology, Sunnybrook and Women's College Health Science Centre, Toronto, ON, Canada

Rufus Cartwright MA MB BS
Department of Urogynaecology, King's College Hospital, London, UK

Maria Angela Cerruto MD
Assistant Professor, Department of Urology, University of Verona, Verona, Italy

David Chaikin MD
Clinical Assistant Professor, Department of Urology, Cornell Medical Center, New York, NY; Associate Attending Urologist, Morristown Memorial Hospital, Morristown, NJ, USA

Charlotte Chaliha MA MB Bchir MRCOG
Sub-specialist trainee in Urogynaecology, St Mary's Hospital, London, UK

Christopher R Chapple BSc MD FRCS
Urology Department, Royal Hallamshire Hospital, Sheffield, UK

Nicholas Christofi MB BS
Fellow in Urogynaecology, St Albans City Hospital, West Hertfordshire Hospitals NHS Trust, St Albans, UK

Calin Ciofu MD
Urology Department, Tenon Hospital, Paris, France

Emily E Cole MD
Fellow, Department of Urology, Vanderbilt University Medical Center, Nashville, TN, USA

Jeffrey Cornella MD
Chair, Pelvic Reconstructive Surgery, Associate Professor, Mayo Medical School Mayo Clinic Scottsdale, Department of Gynecology, Scottsdale, AZ, USA

Sarah M Creighton MD FRCOG
Consultant Gynaecologist, Elizabeth Garrett Anderson Hospital, University College Hospitals, London, UK

Geoffrey W Cundiff MD
Professor, Department of Gynecology and Obstetrics, Johns Hopkins School of Medicine, Baltimore, MD, USA

Alfred Cutner MD MRCOG
Consultant Gynaecologist, University College London Hospitals NHS Foundation Trust, London, UK

Miriam Dambros MD PhD
Urogynaecology Research, Division of Urology, State University of Campinas, UNICAMP, São Paulo, Brazil

Firouz Daneshgari MD
Glickman Urological Institute, The Cleveland Clinic Foundation, Cleveland, OH, USA

Melissa C Davies MRCS
Clinical Research Fellow, Academic Department of Obstetrics & Gynaecology, University College London, London, UK

John O L DeLancey MD
Normal F Miller Professor of Gynecology, Director, Pelvic Floor Research Group
Director, Fellowship in Female Pelvic Medicine and Reconstructive Surgery, Ann Arbor, MI, USA

Hans P Dietz
Associate Professor in Obstetrics and Gynaecology, Western Clinical School, University of Sydney, Penrith, NSW, Australia

Ananias C Diokno MD FACS
Department of Urology, William Beaumont Hospital, Royal Oak, MI, USA

Roger R Dmochowski MD FACS
Professor, Department of Urology, Vanderbilt University Medical Center, Nashville, TN, USA

Richard Dover MB BS
Consultant Obstetrician and Gynaecologist, Royal North Shore Hospital, Sydney, Australia

Harold P Drutz MD
Professor and Head Division of Urogynecology, Department of Obstetrics and Gynecology, University of Toronto, Toronto, ON, Canada

Catherine E DuBeau
Section of Geriatrics, University of Chicago, Chicago, IL, USA

Edmond Edi-Osagie MD MRCOG
Consultant Gynaecologist, St. Mary's Hospital, Manchester, UK

Deborah R Erickson MD
Professor of Surgery, Division of Urology, University of Kentucky College of Medicine, Lexington, KY, USA

Magnus Fall MD PhD
Professor of Urology, Senior Consultant, Department of Urology, Sahgrenska University Hospital, Göteborgs, Sweden

Brigitte Fatton
Gynaecologic Surgeon, Maternité de l'Hotel-Dieu, Centre Hospitalier Universitaire, France

David Fonda MB BS BMed Sci FRACP FAFRM
Associate Professor of Medicine, Monash University, Consultant Geriatrician, Cabrini Medical Centre, Malvern, VIC, Australia

Clare J Fowler MB BS MSc FRCP
Department of Uro-Neurology, National Hospital for Neurology and Neurosurgery, Queen Square, London, UK

Su Foxley RGN Dip NS
Nurse Consultant Incontinence, King's College Hospital, London, UK

Robert M Freeman MD FRCOG
Consultant, Urogynaecology Unit, Directorate of Obstetrics and Gynaecology, Derriford Hospital, Plymouth, UK

Jason P Gilleran MD
Assistant Professor, Division of Urology, 4980 University Hospital Clinics, Columbus, OH, USA

Jason Goh MD
GI Unit, University Hospital Birmingham, UK

Ricardo R Gonzalez MD
Instructor in Urology, Weill Cornell Medical College, New York, NY, USA

James Gray MRCPath
Department of Microbiology, Birmingham Women's Hospital, Birmingham, UK, Department of Urogynaecology, King's College Hospital, London, UK

Jerome Green MD FRCSC
Fellow in Urodynamics, Sunnybrook and Women's College Health Sciences Centre, Toronto, ON, Canada

Derek Griffiths MD
Geriatric Continence Unit, Montefiore Hospital, Pittsburgh, PA, USA

Francois Haab MD
Urology Department, Tenon Hospital, Paris, France

Marie-Andrée Harvey MD Sc(Epi) FRCSC FACLOG
Assistant Professor of Obstetrics, Gynaecology and Urology, Queen's University, Kingston, ON, Canada

Hashim Hashim MB BS MRCS
Urology Research Registrar, Bristol Urological Institute, Southmead Hospital, Bristol, UK

Jeanette Haslam MPhil Grad Dip Phys MCSP
Senior Visiting Fellow, University of East London, Honorary Visiting Lecturer, University of Bradford, Bradford, UK

Sender Herschorn BSc MDCM FRCSC
Division of Urology, Sunnybrook and Women's College Health Sciences Centre, Toronto, ON, Canada

Andrew Hextall MD MRCOG
Consultant Urogynaecologist, West Hertfordshire Hospitals NHS Trust, St Albans, UK

Peta Higgs MB BS FRANZCOG
Urogynaecology Department, Royal Women's Hospital, Melbourne, Australia

Wesley Hilger MD
Fellow, Female Pelvic Medicine and Reconstructive Surgery, Mayo Clinic Scottsdale Department of Gynecology, Scottsdale, AZ, USA

Paul Hilton MD FRCOG
Consultant Gynaecologist, Royal Victoria Infirmary, Newcastle upon Tyne, Senior Lecturer in Urogynaecology, University of Newcastle upon Tyne, UK

Lennox Hoyte MD MSEECS FACOG
Assistant Professor of Obstetrics/Gynecology and Radiology, Harvard Medical School, Director of Clinical Research in the Division of Urogynecology, Dept of Obstetrics/Gynecology,
Senior Clinical Research Scientist, Surgical Planning Laboratory, Dept of Radiology, Brigham and Womens Hospital, Boston, MA, USA

Kenneth C Hsiao MD
Fellow, Female Urology, The Continence Center at Virginia Mason Medical Center, Seattle, WA, USA

Chad Huckabay MD
Fellow, Department of Urology, New York University School of Medicine, New York, NY, USA

Bernard Jacquetin MD
Head, Department of OBGYN, Maternité de l'Hotel-Dieu, Centre Hospitalier Universitaire, France

Mickey M Karram MD
Division of Urogynecology and Pelvic Reconstructive Surgery, Department of Obstetrics and Gynecology, Good Samaritan Hospital, Cincinnati, OH, USA

Rohna Kearney MRCOG MRCPI
Subspecialty Trainee Urogynaecology, University College London Hospitals NHS Foundation Trust, London, UK

Cornelius J Kelleher MD MRCOG
Consultant Physician, Department of Obstetrics and Gynaecology, Guy's and St Thomas's Hospital Trust, London, UK

Christine Kettle SRN SCM Dip Mid PhD
Professor of Women's Health, Academic Unit of Obstetrics & Gynaecology, University Hospital of North Staffordshire & Staffordshire University, UK

Iqbal Khan PhD
GI Unit, University Hospital Birmingham, UK

Vikram Khullar BSC MRCOG
Department of Reproductive Science and Medicine, Division of Paediatrics, Obstetrics and Gynaecology, Mint Wing, St Mary's Campus, Imperial College London, South Kensington Campus, London, UK

Andrew J Kirsch MD FAAP FACS
Clinical Professor of Urology, Emory University School of Medicine, Director Pediatric Urology Fellowship, Georgia Urology, Private Practice

Peter Klarskov MD PhD
Department of Neurology, Glostrup Hospital, Glostrup, Denmark

Kathleen C Kobashi MD
Co-Director, The Continence Center at Virginia Mason Medical Center, Seattle, WA, USA

Heinz Koelbl MD
Department of Obstetrics and Gynecology, Johannes-Gutenberg University, Mainz, Germany

Jenny Lassmann MD
Fellow in Pediatric Urology, The Children's Hospital Philadelphia, Philadelphia, PA, USA

Marie Carmela Lapitan MD
Asia Pacific Continence Advisory Board, Gleneagles Hospital Singapore, Philippine General Hospital, Manila, Philippines

Gary E Lemack MD
Associate Professor and Residency Program Director Holder of the Rose, Mary Haggar Professorship in Urology, University of Texas Southwestern Medical Center, Dallas, TX, USA

Limin Liao MD
Professor of Urology, Chairman of Department of Urology, China Rehabilitation Research Center, Beijing, China

Peter H C Lim AM MB BS MMed DUrol FAMS(UROL) MIUrol (Hon)
Senior Consultant Urological Surgeon, Andrology, Urology and Continence Centre, Gleneagles Hospital, Singapore

Gunnar Lose MD DMSc
Chief Gynecologist, Department of Gynecology, Glostrup Hospital, Glostrup, Denmark

Kevin R Loughlin MD
Division of Urology, Brigham and Women's Hospital, Harvard Medical School, Boston, MA, USA

Karl M Luber MD
Department of Obstetrics and Gynecology, Division of Female Pelvic Medicine and Reconstructive Surgery, Southern California Permanenete Medical Group, San Diego, CA, USA

Adam Magos BSc MD FRCOG
Consultant Gynaecologist, Minimally Invasive Therapy Unit and Endoscopy Training Centre, University Department of Obstetrics and Gynaecology, Royal Free Hospital, London, UK

Christopher Maher FRANZCOG
Royal Women's and Mater Urogynaecology, Brisbane, Queensland, Australia

Amitabha Majumdar MB BS
Research Fellow, Department of Urogynaecology, Birmingham Women's Hospital, Birmingham, UK

Anders Mattiasson MD
Department of Urology, University Hospital, Lund, Sweden

Klaus E Matzel MD
Chirurgische Klinik mit Poliklinik der Universität Erlangen, Erlangen, Germany

Edward J McGuire MD
Professor of Urology, The University of Michigan, Ann Arbor, MI, USA

Jürg Metzger MD
Head of Department Visceral Surgery, Cantonal Hospital of Lucerne, Switzerland

Richard J Millard MB BS FRCS FRACS
Associate Professor and Head, Department of Urology, Prince of Wales Hospital, Randwick, Sydney, NSW, Australia

Jay-James R Miller MD
Evanston Continence Center, Feinberg School of Medicine, Northwestern University Evanston, IL, USA

Ian Milsom MD PhD
Professor of Obstetrics and Gynecology, Department of Obstetrics and Gynecology, Sahlgrenska Academy at Göteborg University and Consultant Gynecologist at Sahlgrenska University Hospital, Göteborg, Sweden

Michelle Y Morrill MD
Senior Fellow, Female Pelvic Medicine and Reconstructive Surgery, University of California, San Diego, USA
Assistant Professor, Division of Urology, University of Pennsylvania Health System, PA, USA

Jacek L Mostwin MD DPhil
Professor of Urology, James Buchanan Brady Urological Institute, Johns Hopkins Medical Institutions, Baltimore, MD, USA

M Louis Moy MD
Attending Surgeon, Division of Urology, Hospital of the University of Pennsylvania, PA, USA

Diane K Newman RNC MSN CRNP FAAN
Co-Director, Penn Center for Continence and Pelvic Health, Division of Urology, University of Pennsylvania Medical Center, Philadelphia, PA, USA

Carl Gustaf Nilsson MD PhD
Department of Obstetrics and Gynecology, Helsinki University Central Hospital, Finland

Victor W Nitti MD
Associate Professor and Vice Chairman, Department of Urology, New York University School of Medicine, New York, NY, USA

Peggy A Norton MD
Professor of Obstetrics and Gynecology, Chief of Urogynecology and Reconstructive Pelvic Surgery, University of Utah School of Medicine, UT, USA

Giacomo Novara MD
University of Padova, Padova, Italy

Ingrid E Nygaard MD
Professor, University of Iowa, Department of Obstetrics and Gynecology, Iowa City, IA, USA

Paulo Palma MD PhD
Head, Division of Urogynaecology, Department of Urology, State University of Campinas, UNICAMP, São Paulo, Brazil

Matthew Parsons MRCOG
Urogynaecology Fellow, King's College Hospital, London, UK

Francesco Pesce MD
Specialist in Urology and Neurology, University of Verona, Italy

Simon Radley MD FRCS
Consultant Surgeon, University Hospital Birmingham, Edgbaston, Birmingham, UK

Stephen Radley MB BS FRCS Ed MRCOG
Senior Registrar in Obstetrics and Gynaecology and Research Fellow in Urogynaecology, Royal Hallamshire Hospital, Urology Research, Sheffield, UK

Katharine H Robb MRCOG
Research Fellow in Urogynaecology, Birmingham Women's Hospital, Birmingham, UK

Jack R Robertson MD
Urogynecologist and Professor Emeritus, University of Nevada Medical School, Reno, NV, USA

Dudley Robinson MRCOG
Department of Microbiology, Birmingham Women's Hospital, Birmingham UK, Department of Urogynaecology, King's College Hospital, London. UK

Peter Rosier MD
Department of Urology, UMC Utrecht, Heidelberglaan, Utrecht, The Netherlands

Eric S Rovner MD
Assistant Professor of Urology, Division of Urology, Department of Surgery, Hospital of the University of Pennsylvania, PA, USA

Brandon S Rubens MD
House Officer in Urology, William Beaumont Hospital, Royal Oak, MI, USA

Stefano Salvatore MD
Divisione di Ginecologia Chirurgica, Ospedale Bassini, Università di Milano, Milan, Italy

Peter K Sand MD
Evanston Continence Center, Feinberg School of Medicine, Northwestern University Evanston, IL, USA

Harriette M Scarpero MD
Assistant Professor, Department of Urology, Vanderbilt University Medical Center, Nashville, TN, USA

Werner Schaefer DI
Associate Professor of Medicine, Director, Continence Research Unit, University of Pittsburgh, Montfiore Hospital, Pittsburgh, PA, USA

Bernhard Schuessler MD
Department of Obstetrics and Gynecology, Cantonal Hospital, Lucerne, Switzerland

Jane A Schulz MD
Urogynecologist and Associate Professor, Department of Obstetrics and Gynecology, University of Alberta, Edmonton, Canada

Bob L Shull MD
Vice-Chairman, Scott & White Women's Health Center, Temple, TX, USA

William A Silva MD
Division of Urogynecology and Pelvic Reconstructive Surgery, Department of Obstetrics and Gynecology, Good Samaritan Hospital, Cincinnati, OH, USA

Mark Slack MMed MRCOG
Simms Black Professor of Gynaecology , Head of Urogynaecology, Addenbrooke's Hospital, Cambridge, UK; Lead Clinician, Department of Urogynaecology, Addenbrooke's Hospital University of Cambridge NHS Foundation Trust, Cambridge, UK

Anthony R B Smith MB ChB FRCOG MD
Consultant Gynaecologist, St Mary's Hospital for Women & Children, Manchester, UK

Howard M Snyder MD
Division of Pediatric Urology, Children's Hospital of Philadelphia, PA, USA, Clinical Professor of Urology, Emory University School of Medicine, Director Pediatric Urology Fellowship Georgia Urology, Private Practice

Anders Spangberg MD PhD
Urologist, Consultant, Department of Urology, University Hospital, Linkoping, Sweden

Jonathan S Starkman MD
Department of Urologic Surgery, Vanderbilt University Medical Center, Nashville, TN, USA

David Staskin MD
Head, Section of Female Urology, New York Presbyterian Hospital, Cornell Associate Professor of Urology, Weill-Cornell Medical College, New York, NY, USA

Ellie Stewart RGN Dip NS
Clinical Nurse Specialist Urogynaecology, Guys and St Thomas NHS Trust, London, UK

Abdul H Sultan MB ChB MD FRCOG
Mayday University Hospital, Croydon, Surrey, UK

Christopher Sutton MD
Professor of Gynaecological Surgery, University of Surrey, Honorary and Emeritus Consultant, Royal Surrey County Hospital, Guildford, Emeritus Consultant, Chelsea and Westminster Hospital, London, UK

Steven Swift MD
Department of Obstetrics and Gynecology, Medical University of South Carolina, Charleston, SC, USA

Alexis E Te MD
Associate Professor of Urology, Weill Cornell Medical College, New York, NY, USA

Ranee Thakar MD MRCOG
Academic Unit of Obstetrics and Gynaecology, University Hospital of North Staffordshire and Staffordshire University, UK

William D Tissot MD
House Officer in Urology. William Beaumont Hospital, Royal Oak, MI, USA

Philip Toozs-Hobson MB BS MRCOG
Consultant Urogynaecologist, Birmingham Women's Hospital, Birmingham, UK

Alberto Trucchi MD FEBU
Assistant Professor of Urology, Department of Urology, Sant'Andrea Hospital, Rome, Italy

Andrea Tubaro MD FEBU
Associate Professor of Urology, Department of Urology, Sant'Andrea Hospital, Rome, Italy

Richard T Turner-Warwick MD
Emeritus Surgeon, The Middlesex Hospital, London, UK

Renuka Tyagi MD
Associate Professor of Urology, Weill Cornell Medical College, New York, NY, USA

Ulf Ulmsten†

Philip van Kerrebroeck MD PhD Fellow EBU
Professor of Urology, University Hospital Maastricht, The Netherlands

Vasiliki Varela MD
Visiting Clinical Fellow, Minimally Invasive Therapy Unit & Endoscopy Training Centre, University Department of Obstetrics and Gynaecology, Royal Free Hospital, London, UK

Maria Vella MRCOG
Clinical Research Fellow, Department of Urogynaecology, King's College Hospital, Denmark Hill, London

Eboo Versi MD PhD
Department of Obstetrics and Gynecology, United Medical and Dental School, New Brunswick, NJ, USA

Arne Victor MD
Medical Product Agency, Uppsala, Sweden

Gopalan Vijaya MRCOG
Specialist Registrar, Department of Obstetrics and Gynaecology, Medway Maritime Hospital, Kent, UK

David B Vodušek MD
Medical Director, Division of Neurology, University Medical Center, Ljubljana, Slovenia

Michael Walker BSc MB ChB MRCS
Specialist Registrar in General Surgery, Department of Surgery, University of Birmingham, Birmingham, UK

Mark D Walters MD
Head, Section of General Gynecology, Urogynecology and Pelvic Reconstructive Surgery, The Cleveland Clinic Foundation, Department of Obstetrics and Gynecology, Cleveland, OH, USA

Alan J Wein MD
Professor and Chief of Urology, Hospital of the University of Pennsylvania, Urology Division, Philadelphia, PA, USA

Ursula Wesselmann MD PhD
Departments of Neurology, Neurological Surgery and Biomedical Engineering, The Johns Hopkins University School of Medicine, Baltimore, MD, USA

Don Wilson MD FRCS FRANZCOG CU
Professor of Obstetrics and Gynaecology, Dunedin School of Medicine, University of Otago, Dunedin, New Zealand

J Christian Winters MD FACS
Department of Urology, Ochsner Clinic Foundation, New Orleans, LA, USA

Brian G Wise MB BS MD MRCOG
Consultant Urogynaecologist, William Harvey Hospital, Ashford, Kent, UK

Jean-Jacques J M Wyndaele MD
Department of Urology and Center for Urological Rehabilitation, University Hospital Antwerp, Belgium

Ilker Yalcin PhD
Eli Lilly and Company Corporate Center, Indianapolis, ID, USA

Stephen A Zderic MD
Professor of Surgery, University of Pennsylvania, School of Medicine, Attending Surgeon, Division of Urology, The Childrens Hospital of Philadelphia, Philadelphia, PA, USA

Philippe Zimmern MD
Department of Urology, University of Texas Southwestern Medical Center, Dallas, TX, USA

Norman R Zinner MD MS FACS
Medical Director, Western Clinical Research Inc, Torrance, CA, USA

Foreword

Female urology / urogynecology is a blooming subspecialty.

We owe our gratitude to the prior outstanding masters from multiple disciplines who have contributed to a solid foundation of practical knowledge from the past. Fortunately, a unique multi-disciplinary culture has flourished over the last decade, and even in the early evolution of this collaborative effort we have embraced a new approach that incorporates the entire 'pelvic floor'. This core approach will continue to be a catalyst from which current and future generations can generate new information and novel techniques based on creativity, innovation, and evidence based analysis of the results.

This new and updated edition of the *Textbook of Female Urology and Urogynecology* continues a tradition from the first volume which is already considered a classic in the field. The text provides the reader with a comprehensive high-quality and inclusive review of the subject of female urology and urogynecology.

This book is a vital and important reflection of the standardised and validated approach put forth for the management of female pelvic floor disorders, following the pathways indicated by the International Continence Society (ICS), the Society of Urodynamics and Female Urology (SUFU), the International Urogynecological Association (IUGA) and the International Consultation on Incontinence (ICI).

This book should be listed as a *must* in the personal library of those interested and involved in female urology and urogynecology. Reading, incorporating and referring to the various chapters of the book will be a pleasure and enrichment both for beginners as well as for experts.

Walter Artibani MD
Chief of Urology Department
University of Padova

Preface

Our decision to produce a second edition of this textbook, a formidable undertaking, is due to the many rapid advances which have occurred in urogynecology/ female urology. The first edition was well received by readers and we had an overwhelmingly favorable response from the contributors to update and where necessary re-write their chapters. In addition, a number of new authors have taken on the task of creating new chapters relating to topics which had not previously been covered and enhancing many areas covered in the previous edition. We are truly grateful to all those whose hard work has resulted in this finished product, of which we can all be very proud.

Our vision was, once again, to assemble an international group of experts as authors, but on this occasion we have been able to recruit the invaluable help of section editors who have guided the authors and prevented too much "overlap" from occurring in the various chapters of the book. Because our authors represent both gynecologists and urologists, as well as some non-medical clinicians, with a true international perspective, we have been able to avoid the polarization of ideas which occurs in many textbooks as a natural product of geography and the training and interests of the contributors. So a *muchísimas gracias - grazie infinite - danke sehr – merci beaucoup* to our section editors, the authors from the first edition and the new authors who have brought fresh ideas and new areas of interest to this textbook.

As previously our mission was to produce a comprehensive textbook which would chronicle past contributions, document the present state of the art, and serve as a foundation, preparing the reader for future developments in the field. The text is arranged in sections enabling the reader to access areas of interest with an extensive bibliography intended to facilitate further study of this fascinating and rapidly changing subject.

The section on surgery has been formatted to serve as both evidence based text and an atlas which should provide information pertaining to the decision making process as well as the technical aspects of the surgical procedures. We do however recognize that as this text goes to press, it is impossible to cover all aspects of female urology and urogynecology comprehensively and that the rapid pace of advances makes it difficult to be completely up to date. We will to try to amend any deficiencies in our 3rd edition!

As editors we are truly grateful to all those authors who have contributed. Researching and writing demands a considerable amount of time and effort and is often a thankless task. We are really grateful to the individuals who sacrificed much of their "quality time and family life" outside of their required hours of clinical and scientific work, to make this project a reality. Once again we would like to thank the publishers for producing a well illustrated book of high quality which should enhance the minds, practices and book shelves of those who own it. Finally, we recognize the contribution from our patients who place their trust in all of us, and without whom this work would be futile. We hope that the textbook contributes to their quality of care and to the ability of those who care for them today and in the future.

Linda Cardozo
David Staskin

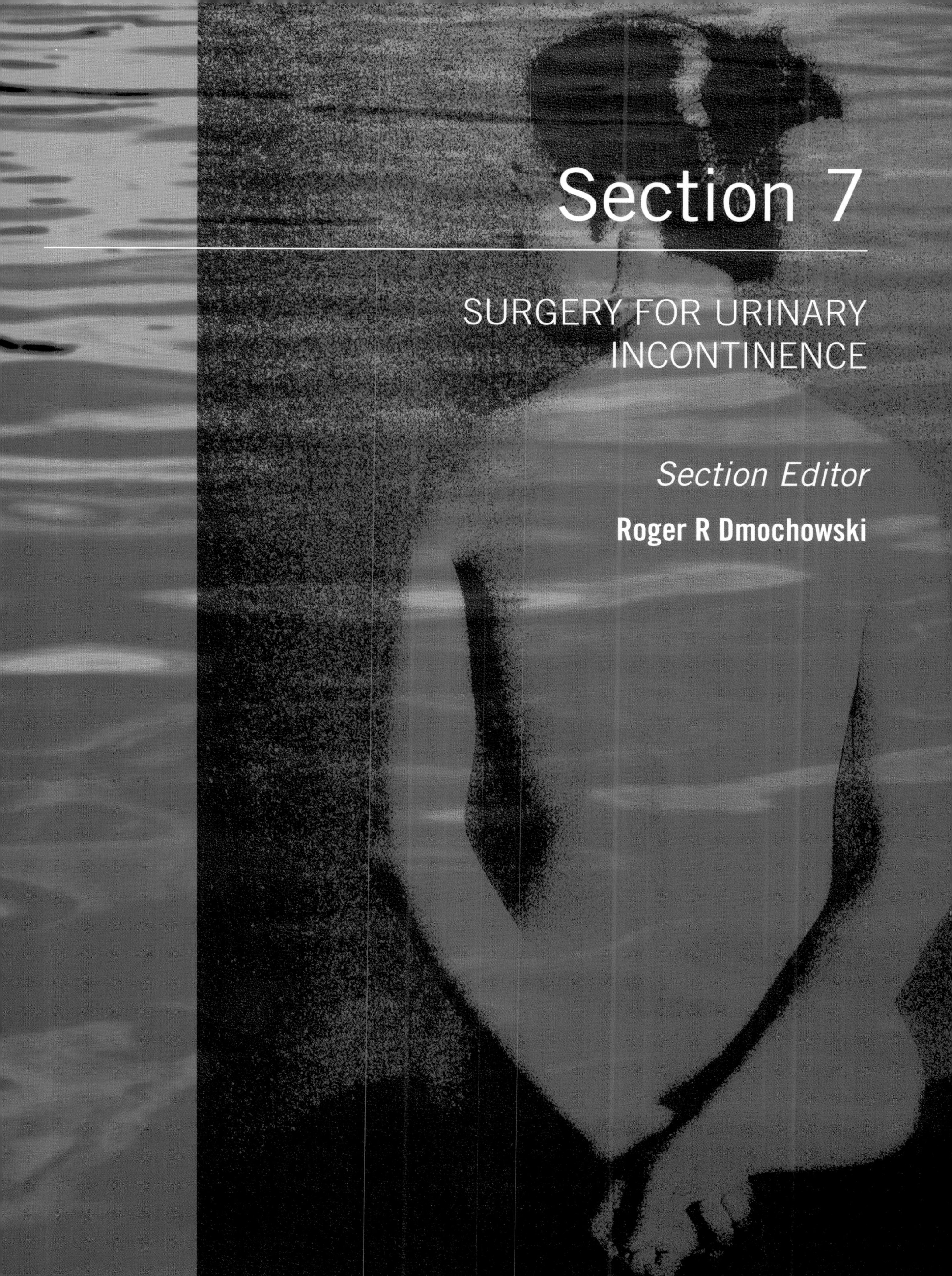
Section 7
SURGERY FOR URINARY INCONTINENCE
Section Editor
Roger R Dmochowski

54

The assessment of outcomes used for incontinence interventions in women

Emily E Cole, Harriette M Scarpero, Roger R Dmochowski

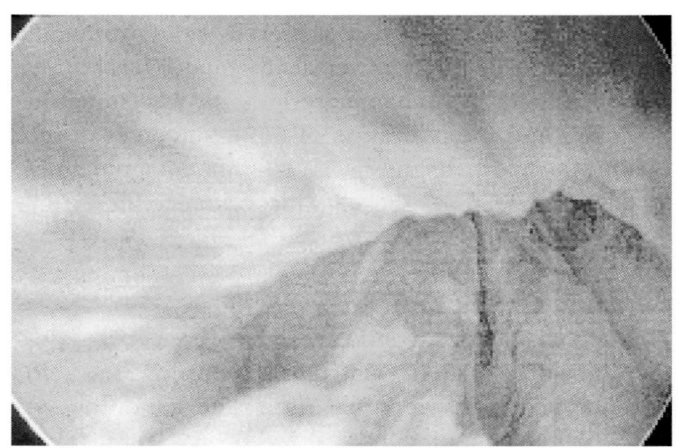

INTRODUCTION

Urinary incontinence is a common condition that affects up to 13–15 million individuals in the United States alone. Urinary incontinence (UI) is described as the involuntary loss of urine. The term incontinence denotes a symptom, a sign, and a condition. The symptom is the patient or caregiver's direct report of involuntary loss of urine, the sign is the objective demonstration of urinary loss on physical examination, and the condition relates to the pathophysiologic reason for urine loss which may be determined via clinical and/or urodynamic testing.

Increased public awareness regarding voiding dysfunction and incontinence has produced heightened interest in the effects of incontinence on the quality of an individual's life. Furthermore, a marked increase in options for the treatment of incontinence has led to the need for accurate assessment as to the impact of any intervention upon the quality of life of the individual. To assess the results of specific therapies for incontinence adequately, outcomes need to be measured and quantified in a standard and consistent manner that permits objective conclusions to be made.

Historically, outcomes assessment for incontinence has been founded on physician-reported results, often established on the basis of patient interview, physician opinion, non-validated surveys, and a variable combination of physical examination, voiding diaries, symptom scores, and urodynamic evaluation. Non-standardized results reporting has prevented critical analysis not only of the overall influence of incontinence on the individual, but also of the success of treatment interventions.

Currently we have objective measures such as urodynamics, pad tests, and physical examination with stress test. Additionally there are the semi-objective measurements of diaries, logs and other tools for assessing voiding frequency, urinary loss, and diurnal variations. Finally, there are the completely subjective (yet validated and psychometrically correct) patient symptom appraisals and quality of life metrics. Various groupings of these modalities have achieved 'standardization' level for reporting, but universal acceptance has not yet been achieved. This chapter reviews the assessment of outcomes and the utilization of these outcomes in the establishment of diagnostic and treatment guidelines for the management of urinary incontinence.

GENERAL CONSIDERATIONS

Whereas the physician and surgeon are concerned with the individual patient, outcomes reporting research is concerned with symptoms, signs, and conditions of entire patient populations and with how specific treatment strategies work with respect to safety, efficacy, and the economic impact on all involved parties. While physicians generate non-quantifiable assessments of UI by patient history, physical examination, laboratory tests, urodynamics and cystoscopy, outcomes reporting must focus on quantifiable variables assessed via validated instruments. Minimal requirements for results reporting include not only certain specified elements with which to assess outcomes, but also longevity of data follow-up and the manner with which data are collected. The elements in question should attempt to capture a blend of subjective and objective outcomes factors so as to present the most comprehensive assessment of the final result for the group of patients under analysis. Outcome instruments must be reliable, valid, and quantifiable.

Reliability

Reliability refers to how reproducible the instrument is over time. Questionnaires that measure the same characteristics should produce similar responses from a subject. Additionally, the same questionnaire should produce similar results for a subject over short intervals of time. Reliability is a quantifiable assessment of these sources of error in measuring devices.[1] There are five measures of reliability: 1) alternate form; 2) test–retest; 3) interobserver; 4) intraobserver; and 5) internal consistency.

- *Alternate form reliability* refers to using two or more alternate wordings of questionnaire items in an attempt to obtain the same information about a specific domain of an instrument. The degree of agreement between the two responses represents alternate form reliability.[2]
- *Test–retest reliability* measures the reproducibility of a response over time. This is evaluated by repeat administration of the questionnaire to subjects over a period of time. Sufficient time should have elapsed for the subjects to forget their responses to the items, but no change in their symptoms should be evident. Correlation coefficients generally used to measure this property include the interclass correlation coefficient, Pearson correlation coefficient, and Spearman rank correlation.[3]
- *Interobserver and intraobserver reliability* addresses the degree of consistency among two or more observations of the same variable by one or more observers, respectively.[2]
- *Internal consistency* measures the similarity of responses among items that are designed to address

the same variable. Because items in a questionnaire query related aspects of the same condition, a relationship should exist between responses to these items. The degree of agreement is measured by Cronbach's coefficient alpha. This statistical tool ranges from 0 to 1, with lower numbers representing lesser degrees of internal consistency.[3]

Validity

Validity refers to how accurately an instrument measures what it intends to measure. There are five methods of assessing validity: 1) content validity; 2) construct validity; 3) concurrent criterion validity; 4) predictive criterion validity; and 5) face validity.

- *Content validity* refers to the relationship of the measuring device to the condition being measured. Questions should cover all of the important aspects of the condition.
- *Content validity* is often established by using focus groups of potential subjects and by asking experts to evaluate the questionnaire.
- *Construct validity* is a theoretic measure of how meaningful the instrument is.
- *Concurrent criterion validity* measures how well an item correlates with a gold standard method of measurement of the same variable.
- *Predictive criterion validity* is a measure of how well a domain of investigation is shown to predict future observations.

Questionnaires

For history taking and patient report of status, the basic element of outcomes assessment has been the questionnaire. In the setting of lower urinary tract symptoms (LUTS), a questionnaire might serve several purposes. It can aid the practitioner in gathering relevant information about the patient's problem, helping to determine the nature of the problem, and the frequency and extent of the symptoms. Questionnaires are useful in assessing the impact the condition has upon the patient's activities and well-being. Ideally, a questionnaire might be able to elucidate the cause of a patient's condition, limiting the need for more costly and/or invasive studies. Following treatment, questionnaires can track the outcomes of treatment strategies, providing more standardized outcome data than informal data retrieval.[4] Specific items used in LUTS questionnaires may vary widely, depending on the purpose and target subjects of the outcomes measurement.[5] To accomplish these tasks, symptom questionnaires must be relevant to clinical practice. Paul Abrams identified four characteristics of a good symptom questionnaire: 1) the questionnaire should be facile; 2) each item of the questionnaire should have a known causal relationship to the condition being measured; 3) the score should help determine appropriate therapeutic options; and 4) use of the questionnaire should directly improve patient management and the effect should be demonstrable.[6]

Questionnaires consist of a series of questions called items. Each item consists of a stem (question or statement) and a response. Responses may be: 1) a categorical response; 2) a Likert response; or 3) a visual analog or 1-item metric:

- A *categorical response* consists of choices that are 'mutually exclusive and collectively exhaustive';
- A *Likert response* is composed of several levels of agreement or disagreement;
- A *visual analog response* utilizes a visual scale usually defined on either end with a word or phrase representing the extreme range of variability.

Outcomes reporting can be divided into primary and secondary outcome measures. Primary outcome measures refer to those variables that directly assess continence including: 1) number of incontinent episodes over a specifically defined time period; 2) the volume of urinary loss; 3) the ease with which the incontinence can be provoked; and 4) the type of incontinence. These variables can be assessed via patient questionnaires, diaries, pad tests, physical examination, and urodynamics. Secondary outcome measures represent factors affecting patient satisfaction and the effect of treatment, including any resulting complication(s) and/or morbidity.[2] In contemporary times, there are many who would assert that – when undertaking an intervention to correct a problem that mostly comprises an effect on a patient's quality of life – patient satisfaction should be considered a primary outcome, if not the most important outcome of all.

In addition to utilizing valid and reliable instruments for measuring signs, symptoms, and specific responses to treatment(s), it is imperative that researchers specify the outcome measures that will be used to define cure, failure, and improvement for each individual study protocol. Outcome after treatment for urinary incontinence should be defined not only in terms of symptoms, signs, and testing, but also in terms of associated symptoms and unwanted side effects resulting from an intervention, after return to baseline activities and medications. Specific definitions of outcomes – such as the

National Institutes of Health Terminology Workshop for Researchers in Female Pelvic Floor Disorders' recommendations for outcomes after treatment for stress urinary incontinence – should be developed to assist in the standardization of outcomes terminology. These recommendations are detailed in Appendix I.[7]

AUA GUIDELINES

The American Urologic Association synthesized an extensive literature review in an attempt to assess the success of interventions for urinary incontinence.[8] The goal of their resultant guidelines was to examine specifically the existing medical literature regarding the surgical treatment of stress urinary incontinence (SUI) in women. The index patient was defined as the otherwise healthy woman, without significant pelvic organ prolapse, who had decided to undergo surgical correction for SUI as either primary or secondary therapy. The panel evaluated the medical literature pertaining to the treatment of SUI from 1950 to 1993: over 5000 articles were identified, of which 457 were selected for data retrieval. Articles were excluded if there was insufficient follow-up (<12 months postoperatively), if more than 50% of the initial cohort of patients was lost to follow-up, or if specific outcome data (number cured or failed) were unstated. The explicit data analysis method was utilized to evaluate abstracted results.

Owing to the large number of individual procedure types reviewed and the lack of significant difference in outcome data between these types, the panel grouped the surgical approaches into four broad categories: retropubic suspensions, slings, transvaginal suspensions, and anterior repairs. The procedural types were evaluated for surgical success (cure of incontinence: dry, improved, failed) as well as outcomes such as postoperative urgency/urge incontinence, urinary retention, urinary outflow obstruction and pelvic prolapse, and complications. Given variations in reporting of surgical complications, six general categories were defined by the panel: general medical complications, intra- and perioperative complications, subjective complications, complications requiring surgery, and transfusions. The data collected by the panel are shown in Appendix II.

Based on the compendium of compiled data, the panel made several recommendations for patient evaluation, citing certain crucial aspects of the preoperative workup: 1) history (including impact of incontinence on the patient's quality of life); 2) physical examination with demonstration of incontinence; 3) urinalysis; 4) diagnostic studies to assess relative contributions of detrusor dysfunction, hypermobility and intrinsic sphincteric deficiency (ISD) to overall presentation; 5) estimation of the severity and frequency of incontinence; and 6) assessment of the patient's expectations for therapeutic outcome.

The panel considered that determination of the patient's quality of life comprised a significant component of pre- and postoperative evaluation. In addition, as above, they addressed the consideration of the patient's understanding of, and expectations for, treatment results. In order to facilitate appropriate decision making by both patient and physician, extensive counseling and communication are necessary during the informed consent process. A specific recommendation concerning choice of procedure was not made by the panel. Difficulties in formulating a true representation of outcomes were encountered due to aberrations in data reporting. The guidelines were criticized for their lack of specific recommendations. However, their assimilation of existing data highlighted the inconsistencies in results reporting and clearly indicated the need for future development of specific outcomes reporting strategies.

RECOMMENDATIONS OF THE URODYNAMIC SOCIETY

The demographics of female voiding dysfunction continue to evolve on the basis of emerging population-based data as extracted from questionnaire-based instruments. Depending on age, it is estimated that as many as 50% of women may experience urinary incontinence at some point in life.[9]

As previously mentioned, incontinence represents a symptom complex, a sign, and a condition. Regarding symptoms, associated aspects of voiding dysfunction include irritative (urgency, frequency) and obstructive (hesitancy, intermittency, incomplete bladder emptying) symptoms, and the complicated component of nocturnal voiding dysfunction. Further confounding the delineation of incontinence is the relatively minor degree of morbidity associated with the symptom complex, except in those women with concomitant recurrent urinary tract infection and related sequelae, or in those patients who have bladder storage abnormalities that compromise renal function.

In 1997, Blaivas et al.[10] introduced minimal standards by which the efficacy of therapy for urinary incontinence may be assessed (Appendix III). These standards were developed by a committee of the Urodynamic Society and were adopted as official recommendations of the American Urologic Association and the Urodynamic Society. They recommended that all clinical trials should include a pre- and post-treatment evaluation that conforms to recommended standards. They mandated that post-treatment evaluation be conducted no less often than 1, 6, and 12 months after treatment and at yearly intervals thereafter, continuing as long as possible. They specified the importance of defining a clear definition of the criteria for success and failure of an intervention and included specific recommendations for pharmacologic studies and studies which examine repetitive therapies (e.g. injection therapy).

RECOMMENDATIONS OF THE INTERNATIONAL CONSULTATION ON INCONTINENCE

The International Consultation on Incontinence (ICI) of 2002 aimed to expand upon the recommendations of the AUA and the Urodynamic Society to improve clinical research design and outcomes reporting. They emphasized that, due to the complexity of incontinence, no single measure can fully express the outcome of an intervention, whether pharmacologic or surgical. They stressed the importance of the correlation of information in the understanding as to why one treatment is better than another, and as to why one treatment works for one patient and not for another. They recommended the collection of detailed data on improvement and deterioration in anatomy, symptoms, lower urinary tract function, complications of the intervention, and the effect on quality of life to help in the understanding of the disease process and how the chosen intervention(s) may benefit. For clarity, they structured their recommendations as follows:[11]

1. Baseline data
2. Observations:
   a. Patient's observation/subjective measures
   b. Clinician's observation/objective measures
3. Tests
   a. Quantification of symptoms – voiding diary/pad tests
   b. Urodynamics
4. Follow-up
5. Quality of life measures

Baseline data/demographics

The ICI recommended that data collection for research purposes should begin with a complete demographic assessment of each subject including age, race, sex, duration of symptoms, prior treatments, medical co-morbidities, medications, etc. Obstetric and gynecologic history is important in women.[7]

Observations – patient

One or more validated symptom instruments should be administered to accurately define baseline symptoms and other areas in which the proposed treatment may produce an effect. There is a variety of validated questionnaires available for the assessment of the incontinent patient. It is important to include instruments that address both specific symptoms and the respondent's overall opinion of the condition. The Urogenital Distress Inventory (UDI) and Incontinence Impact Questionnaire (IIQ) provide a multicomponent quantification of the effects of the symptoms associated with incontinence and bother on the individual's daily activities.[12] Shortened versions of these questionnaires can be easily administered over minimal time intervals and can be used for cross-comparison of results of intervention. Validated questionnaires that assess symptomatic urge and stress incontinence, pad usage and incontinence volume, as well as validated visual analog scales that assess bothersomeness of symptomatic incontinence, are also currently available.[13]

In summary, the ICI recommendations for the reporting of patient observations include the following:

- One or more validated symptom instruments should be chosen at the outset of a clinical trial to accurately define baseline symptoms and other areas in which the treatment may produce an effect;
- The same instruments should be administered after intervention throughout follow-up.[11]

Observations – clinician

According to the ICI, an important and often overlooked element of patient evaluation is the investigation of the possible presence of anatomic changes in the lower urinary tract and its supporting structures. It is paramount to report these observations both before and after any treatment intervention. There are few papers addressing outcomes of stress incontinence surgery that report both functional and anatomic results. These objective measures are particularly important in the explanation of treatment failures. For example, functional results may provide some idea as to the effectiveness of a certain procedure, however, there is no information to explain what happened in cases of failure. Did the treatment fail due to technical factors (e.g. recurrent hypermobility) or due to an inherent limitation of the procedure (e.g. ISD)?

In summary, the ICI recommendations for the reporting of clinicians' observations include the following:

- Clinicians' observations of anatomy should be recorded using standardized, reproducible measurements;
- Pelvic muscle and voluntary sphincter function should be reported using a quantifiable scale;
- These measures should be repeated after intervention and correlated with primary clinical outcome measures.[11]

Tests

Quantification of symptoms

Measures that have been utilized to measure the severity of symptomatic incontinence include standardized diaries and pad-weighing tests. The voiding diary is a self-monitored record of selected lower urinary tract function that is kept for a specific time period. Voiding diaries commonly assess fluid intake, micturition frequency, volume voided, number and degree of incontinence episodes, and pad use.[14] The International Continence Society (ICS) utilizes the largest voided volume recorded in the patient's diary as the definition of functional bladder capacity.[15] Diaries are routinely kept for discrete 24-hour periods and are repeated for 48- to 72-hour periods.[16] Their accuracy is defined by the patient's ability to follow specific directions. The circumstances under which a diary is kept should mimic everyday life and should be similar before and after intervention to allow for meaningful comparisons.

Pad tests provide a semi-objective method for assessing the degree (volume) of urine loss over a specified time period. Several time periods and testing modalities have been described for pad testing, including 1-, 6-, and 24-hour intervals.[15,17,18] Pad weighing quantifies the amount of urine lost over the measured time period. Pad testing can be supplemented with the ingestion of phenazopyridine hydrochloride, which provides a visual corollary to the actual change in weight of the pad. Pad testing is subject to significant variability between and within individuals. This modality is best correlated with the patient's own assessment of urinary loss. Various types of pad test have previously been validated and subjected to testing reliability; however, poor test–retest validation and variability in performance of testing limit widespread usage.[8]

In summary, the ICI recommendations concerning the use of tests include the following:

- Clinical trials of incontinence and LUTS should include bladder diaries as an essential baseline and outcome measure;
- The diary should include measured voided volume (for at least 1 day if a multi-day diary is utilized);
- 24-hour diaries are adequate for most studies;
- Clinical trials of incontinence and LUTS should include a pad test as an essential baseline and outcome measure.[11]

Urodynamics

The ICI also details the recommendations for the usage of urodynamics in clinical research. They caution that due to the lack of universal availability of urodynamic testing and to the lack of 100% sensitivity and/or specificity, subjects should not be stratified into study groups based on urodynamic diagnosis but should be enrolled based on carefully defined symptoms. They call for continued data collection to work towards the determination of the predictive value of urodynamic testing prior to intervention and for the development of new and better tools to improve the sensitivity and specificity of testing.

The ICI recommends the use of urodynamic testing to accurately characterize baseline lower urinary tract function and dysfunction. Preintervention studies can assist in the understanding of the pathophysiology of the disease process. They also recommend that, when possible, post-treatment studies be performed to further clarify the actual effects of the intervention(s).

The problem of interobserver variability is addressed, emphasizing the importance of utilizing standardized techniques at baseline and follow-up. In addition, it is recommended that, when possible, a central blinded reader for urodynamic tracings be assigned in order to reduce investigator bias, particularly in multicenter trials.

In summary, the ICI recommendations for the use of urodynamic testing in clinical research include the following:

- At this time, clinical studies should enroll subjects by carefully defined symptoms, not urodynamic findings;
- To determine the predictive value of urodynamic tests, urodynamics must be performed at baseline but subjects should be enrolled without prejudice of urodynamic test results;
- In the ideal clinical study, urodynamic tests are performed at baseline and at exit to correlate symptom changes with physiologic changes;
- When these ideal conditions cannot be met, urodynamic tests should be performed on a subset of the larger group;
- In all trials, standardized urodynamic protocols (based on ICI recommendations) are defined at the

outset. In multicenter trials, urodynamic tests should be interpreted by a central reader to minimize bias.[11]

Follow-up

The ICI report concurs with the minimal standards for follow-up recommended by Blaivas et al.[10] in the report approved by the Urodynamic Society. As previously described, in addition to standard pre- and post-intervention evaluation, they recommend evaluation of surgical, prosthetic, and implant therapies no less often than 1–3 months and 12 months after treatment, and thereafter at yearly intervals for as long as possible. They recommend the specific definition of the following:

- the method by which data are to be collected;
- the identification of the individual(s) collecting data (e.g. research nurse, clinician);
- the interval between the time of evaluation and the last treatment;
- the identification of the exact type of data collected at each time point in follow-up;
- the specific criteria by which treatment success or failure is to be determined.

In addition, they recommend the mandatory inclusion of the following data at each follow-up interval: 1) the total number of patients treated; 2) the number of subjects actually evaluated in the study; and 3) the total number of subjects lost to follow-up and the reasons why they were lost.

Quality of life measures

The major impact of incontinence is on the sufferer's quality of life and the related physical activity, social, emotional, and psychological limitations. Global assessment of the impact of incontinence implies the necessity for health-related quality of life (HRQOL) measures that reflect the broader impact of this symptom complex. HRQOL is a multidimensional construct that refers to an individual's perceptions of the effect of a health condition and its treatment on quality of life. Primary domains of HRQOL include physical, psychological, and social functioning; overall life satisfaction and well-being; and perceptions of health status. Secondary domains include somatic sensations (symptoms), sleep disturbances, intimacy and sexual functioning, and personal productivity. Considering the complexity of voiding dysfunction and the variety of treatment modalities available, it is important to know not only how well interventions eliminate incontinence, but also how a treatment affects the patient globally.

HRQOL measures can be classified into three broad types: 1) generic – allowing assessment and comparison of quality of life across populations but not reflecting the specifics of the disease or symptom in question; 2) condition specific – providing more critical analysis of the condition under investigation but lacking the capability for cross-population or group comparison; and 3) dimension specific – designed to assess a single component of HRQOL, such as emotional distress. The trend in assessing HRQOL outcomes has been toward the use of a multidimensional generic and/or condition-specific instrument, supplemented with a dimension-specific instrument as needed.[19]

The selection of a HRQOL instrument should be based on the purpose of the study. Descriptive epidemiologic studies should consider the use of both generic and condition-specific instruments. Intervention studies should focus more on condition-specific instruments, with the use of dimension-specific instruments when more detail about a focused subdomain of HRQOL is desired. In the description of study design, a clear description of selected HRQOL measures and of data collection should be presented. Selected instruments should be reliable and sensitive and, if available, information about reliability data should be provided.

Despite the importance of HRQOL measures in defining outcomes, HRQOL should never be used as the sole endpoint of clinical research. The ICI recommends that the focus must always be on the combination of HRQOL with how successfully the target condition or symptom is treated. If a treatment is effective but does not improve HRQOL, possibly due to some adverse event, the treatment can be better. The combination of HRQOL and specific objective postintervention endpoints can add understanding to the reasons behind the success or failure of certain treatment modalities.

In summary, the ICI recommendations concerning the use of HRQOL measures in clinical research include the following:

- Research in incontinence and LUTS should include both generic and condition-specific HRQOL instruments;
- Changes in HRQOL after therapy should be correlated with changes in individual symptoms and with physiologic and anatomic outcome measures to ascertain how that particular therapy is working.[11]

Considerations for specific patient groups

The ICI report also included specific recommendations for certain patient groups (Appendix IV).

They concurred with the recommendations of the ICS report on 'Outcome Measures for Research in Treatment in Adult Males with Symptoms of Lower Urinary Tract Dysfunction' in addressing the factors unique to adult men, the presence of the prostate, and the possible presence of benign prostatic obstruction.[20]

Concerning females, they referenced recommendations from Blaivas et al. and the Urodynamic Society, the ICS, and the Proceedings of the NIH Terminology Workshop for Researchers in Female Pelvic Floor Disorders to define unique factors influencing research on incontinence and LUTS in women including: 1) hormonal effects on the lower urinary tract; 2) obstetric history and the influence of vaginal childbirth on the development of pelvic floor disorders; 3) assessment of pelvic organ prolapse and other measures on physical examination; 4) definitions of outcomes after treatment of lower urinary tract symptoms; and 5) sexual functioning.[7,10,21,22]

The ICI also addressed study design and outcomes in frail older and disabled people, agreeing with recommendations reported in the ICS subcommittee on 'Outcome Measures for Research of Lower Urinary Tract Dysfunction in Frail Older People'.[23]

Concerning children, the ICI referenced the official report from the United States National Institutes of Health (NIH) from 1998, calling for increased and improved pediatric medical research.[24] This report detailed specific responsibilities of each involved party and emphasized the importance of full understanding of the levels of risk and the corresponding nature of assent required for participation.

For investigations involving patients with neuropathic lower urinary tract dysfunction, specific recommendations emphasizing the classification of the neurogenic patient and utilization of objective measures (e.g. urodynamic studies) in assessing baseline and post-treatment outcomes were made.[25]

FUTURE CONSIDERATIONS

At present, the ideal manner with which to report the outcomes of surgical interventions remains unsettled. Although this particular issue is significant for any intervention, for interventions designed to lessen the impact of particular symptoms that are significant for quality of life disruption (e.g. incontinence), this quandary becomes more marked. Without established and generally accepted criteria, the quality of literature outcomes reporting for urinary incontinence will never develop to the level seen for other symptom or disease states (e.g. oncologic outcomes reporting). Currently, efforts are underway to make sense of the multiple factors involved in the evaluation and treatment of incontinence and to provide a workable taxonomy. However, these criteria – such as the above-mentioned ICI recommendations – are inclusive and somewhat cumbersome. Yet these reporting criteria are as important (and in some cases, more so) as isolated efficacy parameters.

There is a paucity of literature addressing the quandary of what to do with those patients who fail to follow-up. Ward et al. reported a prospective trial comparing tension-free vaginal tape and colposuspension for the primary treatment of stress incontinence.[26] They reported outcomes based on several different assumptions and had very different results. By analyzing only data available at 2 years follow-up and ignoring withdrawals, objective cure rates were 81% for TVT and 80% for colposuspension, with no significant difference between the two. If all patients who failed to follow-up were considered successes, the objective cure rates were 85% and 87% for TVT and colposuspension, respectively, again with no statistically significant difference between the two methods. However, if all those who failed to follow-up were considered to be failures, the objective cure rates fell to 63% and 51%, respectively, the difference statistically favoring TVT. Minassian et al. echoed these findings in their comparison of patients with good follow-up versus those with poor follow-up following the TVT procedure.[27] Based on telephone interview of those patients who did not follow-up as scheduled, they found significantly higher subjective and objective cure rates among the patient group with good follow-up. Clearly, how we address the proportion of patients lost to follow-up is important in the assessment of treatment outcomes.

In 1999, Chaikin et al.[28] evaluated 84 women before and after pubovaginal sling. They evaluated the patients pre- and postoperatively with a voiding diary, pad test, symptom questionnaire (administered by a blinded third party), and operating physician evaluation (history and physical examination). At 1 year postoperatively, they compared patient assessment (cured, improved, failure) to the outcome of the pad test, voiding diary, and physician assessment. Agreement was excellent among the four instruments for outcome assessment with respect to cure/improved versus failure, but only good for cured versus improved versus failure. The conclusions from this study confirmed that these four instruments were reliable outcomes measures; however, none was perfect. In response to this and to other studies emphasizing inconsistencies between subjective and objective results, Groutz et al. introduced an incontinence score incorporating several non-invasive outcomes measures to potentially evaluate therapeutic intervention.[29] They evaluated 94 women who underwent pubovaginal sling by the same surgeon, including pre- and postoperative patient questionnaire, 24-hour voiding diary, and 24-hour pad test. Postoperative outcomes were classified twice: once by considering all of the evaluation methods separately, and once by assigning a simple outcomes score based on a combination of responses/results from all methods. The new score was divided into five categories: 1) cure; 2) good response; 3) fair response; 4) poor response; and 5) failure.

Comparison of the two evaluation methods indicated that the outcomes score gave a more accurate measure of postsurgical status. According to the older criteria, 64–69% of patients were classified as cured. Utilizing the newer strict outcomes definition, only 44.7% of patients could be classified as cured, with 26.6% of patients classified as a good response. These findings echoed the consideration that gross classification of results into cured, improved, and failed may not accurately reflect the real clinical status. These results were supported by similar findings in more isolated patient populations such as those with simple stress urinary incontinence and those with mixed urinary incontinence.[30,31] The use of this outcomes score, combining subjective and objective measurement tools, is a step in the positive direction in the movement towards a standardization of results reporting.

There are issues that remain to be addressed by all of the described contemporary recommendations. Although all of the factors detailed in the above discussion have great importance, perhaps what should be asked for is a set study defining primary and secondary outcome variables while honestly reporting the side effects of those complications for the population undergoing the intervention. The concept of a carefully defined therapeutic index, providing a balance between the polar components of outcomes should be a starting point. The blended efficacy analyzes a summation of two, three, or four factors that can then be balanced with the tolerability issues for an ultimate appraisal of the therapy. In addition, the relatively uncharted territory of improvement needs to be better understood and more effectively assessed. It remains clear that the well-informed patient is critical in the overall estimation of procedural outcome. Patients are receptive and happy with improvement and not cure after our interventions, just so long as they are aware that cure is not a universal phenomenon.

It is clear that in the field of urinary incontinence, a standard method of outcome evaluation and reporting is necessary in order to appreciate accurate assessments of treatment efficacy. As is evident in the above discussion, multiple components are paramount in the establishment of a 'result'. In addition to a clear definition of cure, various degrees of improvement, and failure, and a combination of subjective and objective measures need to be utilized to address all aspects of outcome – connecting anatomic and physiologic results with patient assessment of quality of life and satisfaction...*we recommend...*

APPENDIX I
OUTCOMES AFTER TREATMENT FOR STRESS URINARY INCONTINENCE: RECOMMENDATIONS OF THE NIH TERMINOLOGY WORKSHOP FOR RESEARCHERS IN FEMALE PELVIC FLOOR DISORDERS

CURE OF STRESS URINARY INCONTINENCE IS DEFINED AS:

1. Resolution of stress urinary incontinence symptoms;
2. Resolution of the sign (negative full bladder cough stress test, performed under the same conditions as pretreatment). In studies using urodynamics after intervention, absence of genuine stress incontinence should be documented;
3. No new symptoms or side effects. New symptoms or side effects should be specifically described and could include:
   a. new urinary symptoms such as urinary urgency, frequency, urge incontinence, with or without urodynamic changes of detrusor overactivity;
   b. change in sexual function;
   c. development or worsening of pelvic organ prolapse;
   d. adverse effect on bowel function;
   e. onset of urinary tract infections;
   f. surgical complications, such as foreign body reaction to grafts, or development of fistulae or diverticula;
   g. osteitis or osteomyelitis;
   h. neuropathy;
   i. other

FAILURE OF TREATMENT OF STRESS URINARY INCONTINENCE IS DEFINED AS ANY ONE OF:

1. Persistent stress symptoms with the number of incontinent episodes unchanged, or worse, by voiding diary;

2. Positive full bladder cough stress test (performed under the same conditions as pretreatment) or genuine stress incontinence confirmed by urodynamic studies; and
3. Presence or absence of new symptoms or side effects as listed above.

IMPROVEMENT OF STRESS INCONTINENCE INCLUDES:

1. Persistent stress symptoms but with the number of incontinent episodes decreased by voiding diary;
2. Positive full bladder cough stress test (performed under the same conditions as pretreatment) or genuine stress incontinence confirmed by urodynamic studies; and
3. Presence or absence of new symptoms or side effects as listed above.

APPENDIX II OUTCOMES REPORTED BY THE AUA GUIDELINES COMMITTEE

See Tables 54.1–54.7.

APPENDIX III STANDARDS OF EFFICACY FOR EVALUATION OF TREATMENT OUTCOMES IN URINARY INCONTINENCE: RECOMMENDATIONS OF THE URODYNAMIC SOCIETY

GENERAL CONSIDERATIONS

At each post-treatment interval, the following data should be recorded:

- The total number of patients treated during that time interval.
- The total number of patients actually evaluated during that time interval.
- The total number of patients lost to follow-up during that time interval.
- The reasons why patients were lost to follow-up.

PRETREATMENT EVALUATION SHOULD CONSIST OF:

1. Structured micturition history or questionnaire including at least:
   a. number of micturitions/day
   b. number of micturitions/night
   c. number of incontinent episodes/day
   d. number of incontinent episodes/night
   e. type of incontinence (stress, urge, unconscious, continuous)
   f. description of voiding (emptying) symptoms
2. Structured physical examination with full bladder including at least:
   a. Neurourologic examination
      i. Perianal sensation
      ii. Anal sphincter tone and control
      iii. Bulbocavernosus reflex
      iv. Brief screening neurologic examination
   b. (Women) vaginal examination
      i. Demonstration of urinary leakage
         1. spontaneous/continuous
         2. synchronous with stress
         3. after stress
      ii. Presence and degree of
         1. cystocele
         2. urethrocele
         3. uterine prolapse
         4. enterocele
         5. rectocele
   c. (Men) prostate examination
      i. Size and consistency of prostate
      ii. Demonstration of urinary leakage
         1. continuous
         2. synchronous with stress
         3. after stress
3. Micturition diary – self-reported by patient
   a. Time of micturition
   b. Time and type of incontinence
   c. Voided volume
4. Pad test – a quantitative or semi-quantitative pad test should be done to estimate the amount of urinary loss
5. Urodynamics – videourodynamics is the most comprehensive method of evaluation. The minimum evaluation should consist of:
   a. Cystometry (liquid) with simultaneous measurement of vesical and abdominal pressure for determination of detrusor pressure
   b. Synchronous detrusor pressure/uroflow study
   c. Simple uroflow
   d. Assessment of the relative contribution of urethral hypermobility and intrinsic sphincteric deficiency, such as the Q-tip test and leak point pressure
   e. Estimation of post-void residual urine, e.g. by ultrasound or catheterization

Table 54.1. *Comparative outcomes for procedure categories*

Outcomes	Retropubic suspension			Transvaginal suspension			Anterior repair			Sling procedure		
	G/P	Median	CI (2.5–97.5)%	G/P	Median	CI (2.5–97.5)%	G/P	Median	CI (2.5–97.5)%	G/P	Median	CI (2.5–97.5)%
Cure/dry												
12–23 months	15/943	84	(77–89)	13/700	79	(71–86)	6/310	68	(55–80)	5/135	82	(73–89)
24–47 months	23/1870	84	(80–88)	8/424	65	(50–77)	3/113	85	(69–95)	7/34	82	(73–89)
48 months and longer	17/2196	84	(79–88)	4/292	67	(53–79)	5/1088	61	(47–72)	7/473	83	(75–88)
Cure/dry/improved												
12–23 months	16/961	86	(80–90)	13/700	82	(74–87)	6/310	78	(65–88)	5/135	91	(84–96)
24–47 months	24/1941	88	(85–91)	8/424	78	(71–83)	3/113	95	(89–98)	7/344	85	(77–91)
48 months and longer	18/2204	90	(87–92)	4/292	82	(73–89)	6/1101	73	(70–76)	7/473	87	(80–92)
Postoperative urgency												
For patients with urgency and DI preoperatively	6/78	66	(50–79)	6/33	54	(35–73)				4/45	46	(24–68)
For patients with urgency and no DI preoperatively	6/319	36	(22–52)							5/110	34	(13–61)
For patients with no urgency but with DI preoperatively	1/6	4	(0–33)	1/3	7	(0–54)				4/36	20	(5–45)
For patients with no urgency and no DI preoperatively	8/241	11	(8–16)	6/150	5	(3–10)				7/140	7	(3–11)
Retention												
Longer than 4 weeks	5/340	5	(3–7)	6/479	5	(4–8)				7/578	8	(6–11)
Permanent	Less than 5%											
Days in the hospital (panel survery)	From 0 to 5 days											

cont.

Table 54.1. ***Comparative outcomes for procedure categories (cont.)***

Outcomes	Retropubic suspension			Transvaginal suspension			Anterior repair			Sling procedure		
	G/P	Median	CI (2.5–97.5)%	G/P	Median	CI (2.5–97.5)%	G/P	Median	CI (2.5–97.5)%	G/P	Median	CI (2.5–97.5)%
Resumption of normal activities	Typically 6 weeks for all treatment modalities											
Death	Death rate for all procedures presumed to be no different than for other types of elective vaginal/abdominal surgery: approximately 5 out of 10,000											
Transfusion	9/1131	5	(3–8)	10/1083	3	(1–6)	3/857	3	(1–9)	6/279	4	(2–7)
General medical complications												
Significant	21/3136	2	(2–3)	10/805	2	(1–3)	5/1005	2	(1–3	14/1127	4	(2–5)
Not significant	7/1549	2	(1–4)	7/646	4	(1–9)	3/650	8	(2–17)	2/258	6	(3–10)
Intraoperative complications												
Significant	13/1992	2	(1–3)	5/532	2	(1–5)	1/294	1	(0–2)	6/326	3	(1–6)
Not significant	16/2284	3	(1–4)	25/1835	5	(4–8)	1/313	0	(0–1)	19/1077	8	(5–12)
Perioperative complications												
Significant	40/3598	4	(3–5)	40/2814	7	(5–9)	5/970	2	(1–5)	20/1723	7	(5–10)
Not significant	64/6044	14	(14–15)	54/3330	12	(9–15)	13/2322	16	(10–23)	26/1916	12	(8–17)
Subjective complications	13/1001	9	(5–15)	24/1412	11	(8–15)	3/341	2	(1–6)	4/301	6	(2–13)
Complications requiring surgery	15/2718	2	(1–3)	15/1575	2	(1–4)	2/1074	0	(0–1)	11/1119	3	(2–5)

DI, detrusor instability; G, number of groups/treatment arms extracted; P, number of patients in these groups; CI, confidence interval.
Reprinted with permission of the American Urological Association.

Table 54.2. ***Comparative outcomes for procedure categories***

Outcomes	Retropubic suspension			Transvaginal suspension			Anterior repair			Sling procedure		
	G/P	Median	CI (2.5–97.5)%	G/P	Median	CI (2.5–97.5)%	G/P	Median	CI (2.5–97.5)%	G/P	Median	CI (2.5–97.5)%
General medical complications												
Abdominal complication	1/19	6	(1–22)				1/519	0	(0–1)	1/88	1	(0–5)
Cardiovascular	21/3136	3	(2–3)	10/805	2	(1–3)	5/1005	2	(1–3)	14/1127	4	(2–5)
Pulmonary	6/1000	2	(1–3)	5/516	4	(1–11)	3/650	8	(2–17)	2/258	6	(3–10)
Intraoperative complications												
Bladder complication	16/2284	3	(2–4)	25/1835	5	(4–8)	1/313	0	(0–1)	19/1077	8	(5–12)
Ureteral complication	6/730	2	(1–4)	1/255	1	(0–2)						
Urethral complication	5/1003	1	(0–3)	2/128	3	(1–8)				6/326	3	(1–6)
Perioperative complications												
Bleeding	19/1608	5	(3–7)	21/1392	4	(3–5)	3/889	3	(1–6)	4/500	3	(1–6)
UTI	46/4141	13	(12–14)	33/1598	10	(7–13)	11/1743	9	(5–16)	14/984	12	(7–19)
Wound complication	57/5633	7	(5–8)	61/4096	7	(6–8)	7/1806	10	(6–17)	30/2499	9	(6–12)
Subjective complications												
Dysuria	3/175	13	(6–24)	4/119	16	(6–32)				2/178	8	(1–25)
Pain	5/349	6	(3–10)	16/1151	10	(7–14)				1/54	4	(1–11)
Sexual dysfunction	9/766	6	(3–12)	10/609	8	(6–11)	3/341	2	(1–6)	1/69	2	(0–7)
Complications requiring surgery												
Fistula	15/2718	1	(1–2)	14/1568	2	(1–3)	2/1074	1	(0–1)	10/829	3	(1–5)
Stone formation	4/744	2	(1–4)	1/7	16	(2–50)				2/417	3	(1–7)

G, number of groups/treatment arms extracted; P, number of patients in these groups; CI, confidence interval; UTI, urinary tract infection.
Reprinted with permission of the American Urological Association.

Table 54.3. *Comparative outcomes forindividual procedures – cure/dry detail*

	G/P	Median	CI (2.5–97.5)%	G/P	Median	CI (2.5–97.5)%	G/P	Median	CI (2.5–97.5)%
Retropubic suspension									
	Burch			MMK			Lapides		
12–23 months	8/644	85	(78–91)	3/107	72	(55–85)			
24–47 months	9/756	84	(79–88)	10/718	83	(75–89)	2/98	86	(60–98)
48 months and longer	6/529	83	(75–90)	6/1156	83	(76–88)	1/41	44	(30–59)
	Paravaginal			Other					
12–23 months				4/192	85	(70–95)			
24–47 months				5/298	83	(69–93)			
48 months and longer	1/213	88	(83–92)	3/258	90	(83–96)			
Transvaginal suspension									
	Pereyra			Pereyra – modified			Stamey		
12–23 months	1/99	79	(70–86)	5/205	75	(62–86)	2/66	67	(48–83)
24–47 months				2/168	76	(40–97)	3/87	52	(33–70)
48 months and longer				2/196	69	(40–90)	2/96	65	(47–80)
	Raz			Gittes			Other		
12–23 months				2/49	73	(33–96)	3/281	93	(88–96)
24–47 months	1/41	34	(21–49)	1/108	81	(73–88)	1/20	75	(54–90)
48 months and longer									
Anterior repair									
	Kelly plication			Other					
12–23 months	4/270	71	(54–84)	2/40	61	(31–86)			
24–47 months	2/51	94	(83–99)	1/62	74	(62–84)			
48 months and longer	3/1006	60	(41–77)	2/82	62	(38–83)			
Sling procedure									
	Abdominal fascia			Fascia lata			Vaginal wall		
12–23 months				1/10	69	(39–91)			
24–47 months	1/67	82	(72–90)	1/52	98	(92–100)			
48 months and longer	2/98	82	(68–92)				1/82	95	(89–98)
	Homologous			Synthetic			Other		
12–23 months	1/6	96	(67–100)	2/35	86	(68–96)	1/84	82	(73–89)
24–47 months	2/17	61	(18–94)	3/208	82	(70–91)			
48 months and longer				2/91	71	(59–81)	3/202	85	(71–93)

MMK, Marshall–Marchetti–Krantz procedure; G, number of groups/treatment arms extracted; P, number of patients is these groups; CI, confidence interval.

Table 54.4. Comparative outcomes for retropubic suspension procedures: complications details

Outcomes	Retropubic suspension														
	Burch			MMK			Lapides			Paravaginal			Other		
Death	Death rate for all procedures presumed to be no different than for other types of elective vaginal/abdominal surgery: approximately 5 out of 10,000														
	G/P	Median	CI (2.5–97.5)%	G/P	Median	CI (2.5–97.5)%	G/P	Median	CI (2.5–97.5)%	G/P	Median	CI (2.5–97.5)%	G/P	Median	CI (2.5–97.5)%
Transfusion	2/214	3	(1–7)	2/231	8	(4–14)				2/359	2	(0–9)	3/327	5	(1–13)
General medical complications															
Abdominal complication													1/19	6	(1–22)
Cardiovascular	8/916	2	(1–4)	8/1557	3	(1–4)				1/146	2	(1–5)	4/517	3	(1–6)
Pulmonary	1/77	3	(1–8)	3/535	1	(0–3)				1/213	1	(0–2)	1/175	3	(1–6)
Intraoperative complications															
Bladder complication	6/519	5	(2–10)	8/1613	2	(1–3)							2/152	1	(0–4)
Ureteral complication	4/454	2	(1–5)	1/239	0	(0–2)							1/37	3	(0–12)
Urethral complication	1/156	0	(0–2)	4/847	1	(0–4)									
Perioperative complications															
Bleeding	6/702	7	(3–12)	8/400	4	(2–7)							5/506	3	(1–6)
UTI	17/1341	24	(17–33)	19/2036	7	(5–10)	1/63	2	(0–7)	1/146	11	(7–17)	8/555	10	(5–17)
Wound complication	17/1667	6	(4–9)	23/2604	8	(6–11)	2/75	4	(1–12	2/359	2	(0–5)	13/928	7	(4–11)
Subjective complications															
Dysuria				2/75	18	(6–39)							1/100	6	(3–12)
Pain	3/189	6	(2–14)	1/60	2	(0–8)							1/100	6	(3–12)
Sexual dysfunction	7/639	5	(2–10)	2/217	10	(0–49)									
Complications requiring surgery															
Fistula	3/468	2	(0–5)	9/1867	1	(1–2)							3/383	1	(0–3)
Stone formation	1/117	3	(1–7)	1/270	0	(0–2)							2/357	2	(1–4)

MMK, Marshall–Marchetti–Krantz procedure; G, number of groups/treatment arms extracted; P, number of patients in those groups; CI, confidence interval; UTI, urinary tract infection.

Reprinted with permission of the American Urological Association (AUA).

Analysis of individual procedures complications (Tables 54.4–54.7).

Subgroupings of complications for the various individual procedures under each of the four major procedure groupings are displayed in Tables 54.4–54.7. Under the retropubic suspension grouping (Table 54.4), the individual procedures are: Burch, MMK, Lapides, Paravaginal and Other. For transvaginal suspensions (Table 54.5), the individual procedures are Pereyra, Modified Pereyra, Stamey, Raz, Gittes and Other. For the anterior repair grouping (Table 54.6), the Kelly plication and Other are the only procedures listed (because of condiserable variabilty in types of procedures in the Other category). Finally Table 54.7 summarizes sling procedures: Abdominal fascia, Fascia lata, Vaginal wall, Homologous materials, Synthetic materials and Other.

The Other category in each of these tables contains combined procedures as well as a variety of additional procedure modifications. A technical supplement to this report, *Evidence Working Papers* (available from the AUA) contains a full listing of procedures in the Other category.

Rates of complications are generally between the types of retropubic suspensions (Table 54.4), with some exceptions. For example, the Burch procedure appears to have a higher UTI rate (median 24%) than other retropubic procedures. In the panel's opinion, such differences are due to reporting variances between studies and to small overall sample sizes.

For transvaginal suspension procedures (Table 54.5), complication rates are also generally similar. Inconsistencies are due to small numbers of patient groups and/or patients. This is true of the transfusion rate of Pereyra (17%) and of the dysuria rate forStamey (41%).

Complication rates for anterior repairs (Table 54.6) are generally low and reflect differences in reporting and older literature references rather than real differences from the other procedure groupings.

Table 54.7 displays complication rates for sling procedures. Differences in data reported are due to small sample size and older literature.

Table 54.5. ***Comparative outcomes for transvaginal suspension procedures: complications details***

	Transvaginal suspensions								
Outcomes	Pereyra			Pereyra – modified			Stamey		
Death	Death rate for all procedures presumed to be different than for other types of elective vaginal/abdominal surgery: approximately 5 out of 10,000								
	G/P	Median	CI (2.5–97.5)%	G/P	Median	CI (2.5–97.5)%	G/P	Median	CI (2.5–97.5)%
Transfusion	1/95	17	(10–25)	1/93	7	(3–13)	4/457	1	(0–3)
General medical complications									
Abdominal complication									
Cardiovascular	2/285	1	(0–4)	1/30	7	(1–20)	6/465	2	(1–4)
Pulmonary	1/186	1	(0–2)	1/225	1	(0–2)	2/85	5	(0–18)
Intraoperative complications									
Bladder complication	6/565	4	(2–8)	7/539	4	(2–9)	5/189	12	(6–19)
Ureteral complication				1/225	1	(0–2)			
Urethral complication	1/46	3	(0–10)	1/82	1	(0–6)			
Perioperative complications									
Bleeding	3/310	5	(2–9)	3/177	3	(1–7)	7/386	4	(2–6)
UTI	3/306	11	(7–17)	6/216	14	(6–26)	14/684	7	(4–11)
Wound complication	5/614	6	(3–11)	9/611	8	(5–12)	25/1481	12	(8–16)
Subjective complications									
Dysuria				1/30	4	(0–15)	1/44	41	(27–56)
Pain	1/99	27	(19–37)	1/114	2	(0–6)	11/584	12	(9–15)
Sexual dysfunction				1/114	16	(10–23)	2/62	8	(1–23)
Complications requiring surgery									
Fistula	3/420	1	(0–2)	3/393	1	(0–3)	3/147	9	(3–19)
Stone formation							1/7	16	(2–50)

cont.

Table 54.5. ***Comparative outcomes for transvaginal suspension procedures: complications details***

	Transvaginal suspensions								
Outcomes	Raz			Gittes			Other		
Death	Death rate for all procedures presumed to be different than for other types of elective vaginal/abdominal surgery: approximately 5 out of 10,000								
	G/P	Median	CI (2.5–97.5)%	G/P	Median	CI (2.5–97.5)%	G/P	Median	CI (2.5–97.5)%
General medical complications	2/306	1	(0–4)				2/132	6	(1–20)
Abdominal complication									
Cardiovascular							1/25	1	(0–9)
Pulmonary				1/20	35	(17–57)			
Intraoperative complications									
Bladder complications	2/142	6	(1–16)	2/54	8	(2–19)	3/346	1	(0–3)
Ureteral complications									
Urethral complications									
Perioperative complications									
Bleeding	1/17	13	(3–33)	3/177	4	(1–8)	4/325	3	(1–7)
UTI	2/61	15	(4–36)	2/106	6	(1–19)	6/225	4	(7–23)
Wound complication	5/384	7	(3–14)	5/286	6	(3–11)	12/720	9	(6–13)
Subjective complications									
Dysuria							2/45	9	(2–22)
Pain	2/247	5	(2–12)				1/107	3	(1–7)
Sexual dysfunction	2/247	4	(1–12)	2/72	3	(0–12)	3/114	4	(1–10)
Complications requiring surgery									
Fistula	1/206	0	(0–1)				4/402	1	(0–2)
Stone formation									

G, number of groups/treatment arms extracted; P, number of patients is those groups; CI, confidence interval; UTI, urinary treact infection.
Reprinted with permission of the American Urological Association.

Table 54.6 *Comparative outcomes for anterior repair procedures: complications details*

Outcomes	Anterior repairs					
	Kelly plication			Other		
Death	Death rate for all procedures presumed to be no different than for other types of elective vaginal/abdominal surgery: approximately 5 out of 10,000					
	G/P	Median	CI (2.5–97.5)%	G/P	Median	CI (2.5–97.5)%
Transfusion	3/857	3	(1–9)			
General medical complications						
Abdominal complication	1/519	0	(0–1)			
Cardiovascular	4/965	1	(0–3)	1/40	3	(0–11)
Pulmonary	2/610	7	(1–23)	1/40	5	(1–15)
Intraoperative complications						
Bladder complication	1/313	0	(0–1)			
Ureteral complication						
Uretheral complication						
Perioperative complications						
Bleeding	2/849	2	(0–7)	1/40	3	(0–11)
UTI	9/1689	8	(3–15)	2/54	22	(4–55)
Wound complication	5/1706	13	(7–20)	2/100	3	(1–9)
Subjective complications						
Dysuria						
Pain						
Sexual dysfunction	2/319	1	(0–4)	1/22	5	(0–19)
Complications requiring surgery						
Fistula	2/1074	0	(0–1)			
						Stone formation

G, number of groups/treatment arms extracted; P, number of patients in those groups; CI, confidence interval; UTI, urinary tract infection.
Reprinted with permission of the American Urological Association.

Table 54.7. ***Comparative outcomes for sling procedures: complications details***

Outcomes	Sling procedures								
	Abdominal fascia			Fascia lata			Vaginal wall		
Death	Death rate for all procedures presumed to be no different than for other types of elective vaginal/abdominal surgery: approximately 5 out of 10,000								
	G/P	Median	CI (2.5–97.5)%	G/P	Median	CI (2.5–97.5)%	G/P	Median	CI (2.5–97.5)%
Transfusion				1/10	2	(0–22)	1/54	0	(0–5)
General medical complications									
Abdominal complication				1/88	1	(0–5)			
Cardiovascular	2/114	3	(1–9)	4/405	2	(1–5)	1/54	2	(0–8)
Pulmonary				2/258	5	(3–10)			
Intraoperative complications									
Bladder complication	2/77	21	(2–64)	2/147	12	(5–23)	1/82	3	(1–8)
Ureteral complication									
Uretheral complication	3/171	3	(1–7)						
Perioperative complications									
Bleeding				1/170	1	(0–3)			
UTI	2/77	18	(1–67)	2/258	9	(5–14)	1/54	4	(1–11)
Wound complication	3/157	7	(2–17)	4/421	8	(4–14)	1/82	3	(1–8)
Subjective complications									
Dysuria	1/80	1	(0–6)						
Pain							1/54	4	(1–11)
Sexual dysfunction									
Complications requiring surgery									
Fistula				2/93	6	(1–16)			
Stone formation									

cont.

Table 54.7. *Comparative outcomes for sling procedures: complications details (contd.)*

Outcomes	Sling procedures								
	Abdominal fascia			Fascia lata			Vaginal wall		
Death	Death rate for all procedures presumed to be no different than for other types of elective vaginal/abdominal surgery: approximately 5 out of 10,000								
	G/P	Median	CI (2.5–97.5)%	G/P	Median	CI (2.5–97.5)%	G/P	Median	CI (2.5–97.5)%
Transfusion				2/80	5	(1–13)			
General medical complications									
Abdominal complication									
Cardiovascular	1/10	11	(1–38)	4/399	2	(1–5)	2/145	7	(1–21)
Pulmonary									
Intraoperative complications									
Bladder complication	1/10	11	(1–38)	4/339	2	(4–14)	5/422	5	(2–10)
Ureteral complication									
Urethral complication				1/20	6	(1–21)	2/135	2	(0–6)
Perioperative complications									
Bleeding				2/125	7	(1–20)	1/205	1	(0–3)
UTI	1/10	40	(15–70)	7/564	11	(5–19)	1/21	6	(1–20)
Wound complication	1/10	31	(9–61)	13/1038	10	(6–15)	8/791	9	(4–16)
Subjective complications									
Dysuria				1/98	15	(9–23)			
Pain									
Sexual dysfunction				1/69	2	(0–7)			
Complications requiring surgery									
Fistula				7/576	3	(1–5)	1/160	0	(0–2)
Stone formation				2/417	3	(1–7)			

G, number of groups/treatment arms extracted; P, number of patients in those groups; CI, confidence interval; UTI, urinary tract infection.
Reprinted with permission of the American Urological Association.

POST-TREATMENT EVALUATION SHOULD CONSIST OF:

1. Structured micturition history or questionnaire at each follow-up.
2. Structured physical examination with full bladder at least once during follow-up.
3. Micturition diary at each follow-up.
4. Pad test at each follow-up.
5. Uroflow at least once during follow-up.
6. Estimation of post-void residual urine at least once during follow-up.
7. Other urodynamic techniques are optional.

APPENDIX IV RECOMMENDATIONS OF THE INTERNATIONAL CONSULTATION ON INCONTINENCE: CONSIDERATIONS FOR SPECIFIC PATIENT GROUPS

MEN WITH LUTS, INCLUDING INCONTINENCE

- If treatment could change prostate volume, measurements of volume should be performed before and after treatment.
- Consider stratifying patients by prostate volume.
- Whenever feasible, detrusor pressure/uroflow studies should be performed before and after treatment to document the presence and degree of change in bladder outlet obstruction.

WOMEN WITH LUTS AND INCONTINENCE

- Data on hormonal status should be collected on women in all studies of incontinence and LUTS.
- At a minimum, data on vaginal parity should be collected on women in all studies. Additional obstetric history should be obtained as appropriate for individual studies.
- Studies of surgical treatment of incontinence (and other study types as appropriate) should include assessment for pelvic organ prolapse using the ICS staging system, the Pelvic Organ Prolapse Quantification (POP-Q) system.
- Outcomes (cure, failure, improvement) relating to symptoms and signs must be clearly defined at the onset of all studies. Complications and side effects may be included in outcomes but should be reported separately.
- Assessment of sexual function should be included in all studies.

FRAIL OLDER AND DISABLED PEOPLE

- This is a heterogeneous population requiring a detailed study design and careful description of baseline clinical data if results are to be interpretable.
- There is a need for validation of all instruments and procedures used in incontinence research for the population of frail elderly patients.
- 'Clinically significant' outcome measures and relationships of outcome to socioeconomic costs are critically important to establish the utility of treating urinary incontinence in this population.

INCONTINENCE IN CHILDREN

- We support the National Institutes of Health (NIH) statement calling for increased clinical research in children. All investigators that work with children should be aware of the details of the document and particularly the issues surrounding informed consent.
- Long-term follow-up is of critical importance in the pediatric population in order to ascertain the effect of a treatment on normal growth and development.
- Research is needed to develop standardized outcome measures including validated, age-specific symptom and disease-specific quality of life outcome measures.

NEUROPATHIC LOWER URINARY TRACT DYSFUNCTION

- Detailed urodynamic studies are required for classification of neurogenic lower urinary tract disorders in research studies because the nature of the lower urinary tract dysfunction cannot be accurately predicted from clinical data. Videourodynamic studies are preferred but not mandatory.
- Change in detrusor leak point pressure should be reported as an outcome as appropriate, and can be considered a primary outcome in addition to a symptom response.
- An area of high priority for research is the development of a classification system to define neurogenic disturbances. Relevant features would include the underlying diagnosis, the symptoms, and the nature of the urodynamic abnormality.
- It may sometimes by appropriate to group patients with urodynamically similar neurogenic bladder disorders of different etiologies in a clinical trial.

However, great caution must be used if patients with progressive disease (e.g. multiple sclerosis) are grouped with patients having a stable deficit (e.g. traumatic spinal cord injury).

LUTS, lower urinary tract symptoms.

REFERENCES

1. McDowell J, Newell C. Measuring Health: A Guide To Rating Scales And Questionnaires. New York: Oxford University Press, 1996; 10–36.
2. Blaivas JG. Outcome measures for urinary incontinence. Urology 1998;51(Suppl 2A):11–19.
3. Graham CW, Dmochowski RR. Questionnaires for women with urinary symptoms. Neurourol Urodyn 2002;21:473–81.
4. Sirls LT, Keoleian CM, Korman HJ, Kirkemo AK. The effect of study methodology on reported success rates of the modified Pereyra bladder neck suspension. J Urol 1995;85(Suppl 1):1732–5.
5. Donavan J, Naughton M, Gotoh M et al. Symptoms and quality of life assessment. In: Khoury S, Wein A (eds) Incontinence: 1st International Consultation on Incontinence. Plymouth, UK: Health Publication, 1999; 296–331.
6. Abrams P. A critique of scoring systems. Prog Clin Biol Res 1994;386:109–23.
7. Weber AM, Abrams P, Brubaker L et al. The standardization of terminology for researchers in female pelvic floor disorders. Int Urogynecol J Pelvic Floor Dysfunct 2001;12(3):178–86.
8. Leach GE, Dmochowski RR, Appell RA et al. Female stress urinary incontinence clinical guidelines panel. Summary report on the surgical management of female stress urinary incontinence. J Urol 1997;158:875–9.
9. Holroyd-Leduc JM, Straus SE. Management of urinary incontinence in women: clinical applications. JAMA 2004;291:996–9.
10. Blaivas JG, Appell RA, Fantl A et al. Standards of efficacy for evaluation of treatment outcomes in urinary incontinence: recommendations of the Urodynamic Society. Neurourol Urodyn 1997;16:145–7.
11. Payne C, Van Kerrebroeck P, Blaivas J et al. Research methodology in urinary incontinence. In: Wein A (ed) Incontinence: 2nd International Consultation on Incontinence. Plymouth, UK: Health Publication, 2002; 1045–77.
12. Wyman JF, Harkins SC, Choi SC et al. Psychosocial impact of urinary incontinence in women. Obstet Gynecol 1987;70:378–81.
13. Romanzi L, Blaivas JG. Office evaluation of incontinence. In: O'Donnell PD (ed) Urinary Incontinence. St Louis: Mosby, 1997; 475–9.
14. Larsson G, Victor A. Micturition patterns in a healthy female population studied with a frequency/volume chart. Scand J Urol Nephrol 1988;114:53–7.
15. Abrams P, Blaivas JG, Stanton SL et al. The standardization of terminology of lower urinary tract function. Scand J Urol Nephrol 1988;114(Suppl):5–19.
16. Hahn I, Fall M. Objective quantification of stress urinary incontinence: a short, reproducible, provocative pad weighing test. Neurourol Urodyn 1991;10:475–81.
17. Lose G, Gammelgard J, Jorgensen TJ. The one hour pad weighing test: reproducibility and the correlation between the test result, start volume in the bladder and the diuresis. Neurourol Urodyn 1986;5:17–21.
18. Fantl JA, Harkins SW, Wyman JF et al. Urinary incontinence in adults: acute and chronic management. Clinical Practice Guideline. Rockville, MD: United States Department of Health and Human Services, 1996; 1–65.
19. Shumaker SA, Wyman JF, Uebersax JS et al. Health related quality of life measures for women with urinary incontinence: the Incontinence Impact Questionnaire and the Urogenital Distress Inventory. Qual Life Res 1994;3:291–306.
20. Nordling J, Abrams P, Ameda JT et al. Outcome measures for research in treatment of adult males with symptoms of lower urinary tract dysfunction. Neurourol Urodyn 1998;17:263–71.
21. Blaivas JG, Appell RA, Fantl JA. Definition and classification of urinary incontinence: recommendations of the Urodynamic Society. Neurourol Urodyn 1997;16:145–7.
22. Lose G, Fantl JA, Victor A et al. Outcome measures in adult women with symptoms of lower urinary tract dysfunction. Neurourol Urodyn 1998;17:255–62.
23. Fonda D, Resnick NM, Colling J et al. Outcome measures for research of lower urinary tract dysfunction in frail older people. Neurourol Urodyn 1998;17:273–81.
24. National Institutes of Health (NIH) policy and guidelines on the inclusion of children as participants in research involving human subjects, Release Data: March 6, 1998, National Institutes of Health. Online. Available: http://grants.nih.gov/grants/guide/notice-files/not98-024.html.
25. Wein AJ. Pathophysiology and categorization of voiding dysfunction. In: Walsh PC, Retik AB, Vaughan ED Jr, Wein AJ (eds) Campbell's Urology, 7th ed. Philadelphia: WB Saunders, 1998; 917–26.
26. Ward KL, Hilton P. A prospective multicenter randomized trial of tension-free vaginal tape and colposuspension for primary urodynamic stress incontinence: two year follow-up. Am J Obstet Gynecol 2004;190:324–31.
27. Minassian VA, Al-Badr A, Pascali DU et al. Tension-free vaginal tape: do patients who fail to follow-up have the same results as those who do? Neurourol Urodyn 2005;24:35–8.

28. Chaikin DC, Blaivas JG, Rosenthal JE et al. Results of pubovaginal sling for stress incontinence: a prospective comparison of 4 instruments for outcome analysis. J Urol 1999;162:1670–7.

29. Groutz A, Blaivas JG, Rosenthal JE. A simplified urinary incontinence score for the evaluation of treatment outcomes. Neurourol Urodyn 2000;19:127–35.

30. Groutz A, Blaivas JG, Hyman MJ et al. Pubovaginal sling surgery for simple stress urinary incontinence: analysis by an outcome score. J Urol 2001;165:1597–1600.

31. Chou EC, Flisser AJ, Panagopoulos G et al. Effective treatment for mixed urinary incontinence with a pubovaginal sling. J Urol 2003;170(2 Pt 1):494–7.

55

Peri- and postoperative care

Maria Vella, John Bidmead

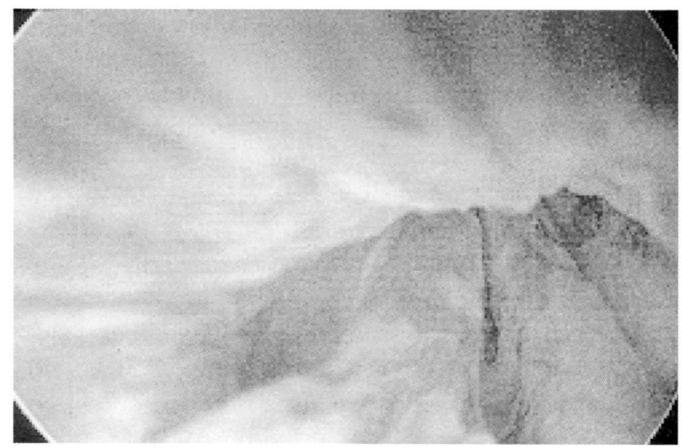

INTRODUCTION

A great deal of a surgeon's attention is naturally focused on the technical performance of an operation. Although surgical technique is a major factor influencing outcome, other factors such as appropriate patient selection, preoperative investigation and preparation, and postoperative care also have a major influence on the results of surgery.

Most urogynecologic surgery is elective. Urinary incontinence and urogenital prolapse, although undeniably distressing, are rarely life threatening. Urogynecologic surgery can therefore be planned in advance and time is available for preparation, which can be used to improve the outcome of surgery.

The elective nature of most urogynecologic surgery means that operative morbidity must be kept to a minimum. Adequate preparation and intervention to reduce surgical and anesthetic complications is mandatory, as is the provision of preoperative counseling.

PREOPERATIVE CONSIDERATIONS

Procedure selection and discussion of alternative therapies

One of the most important factors governing the success of any gynecologic surgery is patient selection. This applies as much to the selection of procedure by the woman herself as it does to the selection of an operation for a patient by the surgeon.

In gynecology, the type of surgery performed may have a profound influence on the emotional, psychological, and sexual well-being of a woman. It is, therefore, vital that, before proceeding to an irreversible surgical procedure, a woman should feel that she has had the opportunity to take part in the decision process. Information on the possible effects of surgery on physical, hormonal, reproductive, and sexual function should be provided. The possible effects of any pathology on these functions also need to be explored, to allow the pros and cons of surgery to be weighed. The full range of therapeutic measures available, both conservative and surgical, should be discussed to allow an informed choice.

It is also important to give a realistic view of any possible complications, their likelihood and possible sequelae. A woman is much more likely to accept slight voiding difficulties after a continence procedure, for example, if this has been explained in advance. Explaining unanticipated difficulties 'after the event' can be fraught and is much more likely to lead to medicolegal action, often with unsatisfactory outcomes for both parties.

Patient selection

It has often been said that the key to successful surgery lies not only with the technical skills of the surgeon but also with the ability to select cases appropriately. This means that the skill and experience of the surgeon should be used during consultation to help guide a woman in making the right choices about treatment.

Use of alternative therapies

Time is also available to permit a number of alternative therapies to be tried before surgical intervention is undertaken.

Recently, alternative conservative treatments for incontinence have become available that offer increased choice for those women unsuitable or unwilling to undergo surgery. Pelvic floor physiotherapy, with or without electrical stimulation, remains the mainstay of conservative management of genuine stress incontinence (GSI). Many studies have shown excellent results, although it is clear that closely monitored therapy by a physiotherapist interested and experienced in this area is necessary. Vague instructions to perform pelvic floor exercises (PFE) are ineffective and may even be counterproductive: fewer than 70% of women are able to perform these exercises correctly without tuition.[1] The use of PFE was first described by Kegel in 1948.[2] In a series of studies Kegel was able to demonstrate an impressive success rate of 84% in women with stress incontinence. More recent studies have confirmed good long-term results.[3,4] Although there are no published data to suggest that prior effective pelvic floor physiotherapy improves the eventual outcome of surgery, this is the impression of many urogynecologists. As the success rate of physiotherapy is good and its influence on surgical outcome may be beneficial, it is recommended that surgical intervention is not resorted to until a woman has had an adequate course of physiotherapy.

A new drug has recently been developed, specifically for the treatment of stress incontinence. Duloxetine is a potent and balanced serotonin and noradrenaline inhibitor (SNRI) that enhances urethral sphincter activity via a centrally mediated pathway.[5] The evidence reported to date suggests that duloxetine offers an effective alternative to surgery and may be complementary to the use of PFEs in the initial management of women with stress incontinence.[6,7] It is given in a 40 mg dose twice daily.

A number of mechanical devices have also become available recently. These may be useful in a number of situations: for example, they may be helpful in the short term, allowing women to regain continence while undergoing physiotherapy or while awaiting surgery.[8] Some women, particularly those with mild GSI only on exercise, may choose to use them as an alternative to surgery (e.g. during aerobics classes or tennis). Lastly, there remains a group of women for whom surgery has failed and where further surgery is inadvisable: women in this group are able to use devices to regain control or manage their incontinence.

Devices vary, as do the women who use them, and so it is often worth trying more than one.

Prosthetic devices for the control of prolapse are also available. Those most commonly used today are a silicon ring pessary which can control vaginal prolapse very effectively if pelvic floor tone is good. Uterovaginal prolapse may be more effectively controlled with a shelf pessary. Although these pessaries may not be suitable for younger women, they can be useful for older women wishing to avoid surgery. Use of such devices/medical therapy while awaiting surgery can improve a woman's quality of life in the short term; they may also be advantageously employed while a woman is undergoing a course of physiotherapy and while coming to a final decision regarding surgery.

Psychological preparation for surgery

Whereas it may be considered desirable to bring any intervention to a satisfactory conclusion as rapidly as possible, the very nature of this surgery allows time for both surgeon and patient to consider all the available options and select the most appropriate. Time is also available to consider factors that may improve the likelihood of a satisfactory outcome and to take measures to reduce the possibility of adverse outcomes. Finally, the effect of surgery on lifestyle can be considered and planning for any period of convalescence initiated.

It is well documented that only 10% of verbal information given during a consultation is remembered by the patient afterwards. This can be substantially increased by the use of written information given to patients during a consultation.[9] Patient information leaflets can be particularly useful if they have been written locally to reflect practice in a particular unit.

Written information leaflets can also be re-read at leisure by women, allowing them time to consider treatment options and think of any questions that may be addressed at subsequent consultations. Although the primary objective of patient information leaflets is not to save the surgeon's time, it would be impractical to discuss all aspects of all the treatment options at a single consultation.

Although not a primary objective, the use of such written information and documentation of this may be particularly useful medicolegally. Many medicolegal disputes arise because patients complain of sequelae about which they feel they were not warned. It is often the case that such problems were discussed but that this was not among the 10% of the consultation remembered by the patient. The documentation of written information being given may be useful in such circumstances.

Use of a nurse counselor

Involvement of nursing staff may be particularly beneficial. Increasingly, a number of units are offering a preoperative counseling service. This is often provided by suitably experienced and trained nursing staff and allows discussion of any anxieties in a more relaxed and leisurely fashion than is possible on a traditional preoperative ward round. It is particularly helpful if a woman has the opportunity to discuss a procedure with an experienced member of the nursing team preoperatively so that she can discuss aspects of surgery that she may have felt unable to discuss with the surgical staff. Nursing staff are also appropriately placed to give information about pre- and postoperative care, catheter regimes, drains, dressings, and ward routine. Ideally, the nurse should be one of the team providing care on the ward.

As previously stated, because most urogynecologic surgery is elective, any investigations can be carried out in advance of any proposed intervention and plans can be modified as a result. There should be no need for a procedure to be performed under conditions of undue stress and there should be no hesitation in deferring an operation until an appropriate time available on a theater list, for example. If a procedure is felt to be inappropriate, further investigations necessary or the patient's condition not optimal, then surgery should be deferred.

Finally, the surgeon has the ultimate sanction and, if it is felt that an intervention is inappropriate or not in a patient's best interest, then (after appropriate explanation) it may be wise to refer back to the general practitioner or suggest a further opinion, or investigations.

Although this may seem to be an extreme measure, it is preferable to continuing on a course of action that may have untoward results for both patient and doctor!

Physical preparation for surgery

Fitness

Before undergoing any surgical procedure it is essential that a woman is as fit, physically, as possible. The elective nature of most urogynecologic procedures allows surgery to be deferred if any intercurrent illness has reduced a woman's fitness. In addition to exercising the pelvic floor muscles, a program of exercise may be beneficial in reducing morbidity and speeding up postoperative recovery. Preoperative exercise will also enhance weight loss if this is a concern. The physiotherapist is in an ideal position to advise a woman on preoperative exercise.

Smoking

In addition to its well known effects on general health, smoking increases the risk of postoperative problems, such as thromboembolism (see 'Thromboembolism and thromboprophylaxis', below). Pulmonary atelectasis and subsequent pneumonia is a particular risk following general anesthesia and this is substantially increased by smoking.

In addition, chronic cough is a factor in development or recurrence of urogenital prolapse. For these reasons it is worth impressing on women the importance of stopping smoking preoperatively.

Weight

It comes as a surprise to many women that obesity is a major cause of surgical difficulty. In addition to the technical difficulties faced by the surgeon, obesity also increases virtually all perioperative risks. For the anesthetist, intravenous access, induction of anesthesia and intubation are all more difficult. Postoperatively, obesity increases the risk of thromboembolism, wound infection, hematoma, and respiratory infection. Although there is little published evidence, it appears that obesity, by raising intra-abdominal pressure, increases the recurrence of urogenital prolapse.

For these reasons the obese woman should be encouraged to lose weight prior to surgery. Rather than giving a general instruction to 'lose some weight', it is more effective to set a reasonable target to be achieved. Referral to a dietitian is often helpful and appetite suppressants may be useful in the short term.

Anemia

Anemia may well be a problem in women presenting for urogynecologic surgery with concomitant menorrhagia. As well as reducing the safe margin for intraoperative blood loss, anemia increases the risk of postoperative wound infection and delays full recovery. Mild-to-moderate anemia may respond to simple oral iron replacement in the form of ferrous sulfate (200 mg daily). Other measures to reduce menstrual loss and allow replenishment of iron stores include the use of mefenamic acid (500 mg three times daily) alone or in combination with tranexamic acid (1 g four times daily).[10]

Gonadotropin-releasing hormone (GnRH) analogs may be useful, with or without 'add-back' hormone replacement therapy (HRT), in extreme cases to suppress menstruation prior to surgery.[11] GnRH analogs have also been shown to be useful in reducing the volume of uterine fibroids prior to hysterectomy or myomectomy, and in reducing blood loss at myomectomy or hysterectomy.[12]

Bowel preparation

It is worth paying attention to preoperative bowel preparation. In women with normal bowel habit undergoing routine surgery, complicated preoperative regimens are unnecessary. However, it is worth ensuring an empty rectum prior to surgery as this may avoid postoperative discomfort and constipation. A single mild aperient such as sodium lauryl sulfoacetate enema given the evening before surgery should suffice.

Women undergoing pelvic reconstructive surgery, such as colposuspension or vaginal repair, may benefit from more thorough bowel preparation (to prevent a loaded rectum interfering with surgery) and a regimen of postoperative laxatives (to reduce postoperative straining that may compromise the repair). A sachet of sodium picosulfate taken the afternoon before surgery will ensure an empty rectum; postoperatively, a stool softener such as lactulose will prevent discomfort and straining due to constipation. Prior to undertaking operations which require complete access to the sacral promontory and where mobilization of the rectum may be required, more thorough bowel preparation is necessary. A full rectum may make the performance of sacrocolpopexy difficult or impossible. A low-residue, low-fiber diet for 48 hours prior to surgery, together with a half-sachet of sodium picosulfate daily, will help to ensure an empty rectum. A disposable phosphate enema can be given preoperatively to women with a history of constipation.

Preoperative investigations

The majority of preoperative investigations should be performed on an outpatient basis with the results available for review prior to admission to allow time for any remedial action to be taken.

An exhaustive list of preoperative investigations is beyond the scope of this chapter and should be tailored to an individual woman's general health and any existing medical problems. Basic preoperative investigations may include hematologic and biochemical investigations, urinalysis, electrocardiography (ECG), and imaging.

Hematologic investigations

Every woman should have a full blood screen performed to include a hemoglobin, hematocrit, white cell count and differential, and hemoglobinopathy screen where appropriate. For all procedures where there is a significant risk of transfusion, typing should be performed and serum retained for cross-matching at short notice.

Biochemical investigations

For the majority of women, no particular biochemical investigations are necessary. However, in women with pre-existing disease such as hypertension or diabetes, biochemical screening may be necessary. Renal function tests should be performed if there is any suspicion of renal failure or ureteric obstruction.

Urinalysis

Simple ward urinalysis is useful to exclude glycosuria and infection. Urine should be tested for beta human chorionic gonadotrophin if there is any possibility of pregnancy.

ECG

ECG traces are not required for most fit women undergoing surgery, but may be required if there is a history of hypertension or cardiac disease. Most anesthetic departments now have guidelines for preoperative ECG testing.

Imaging

The roles of plain and contrast radiology, computed tomography, ultrasonography, and magnetic resonance imaging are discussed in the relevant sections of this book. Routine preoperative chest radiography is now rarely required except in women with cardiac or pulmonary disease. Most anesthetic departments now have guidelines for preoperative chest radiography.

An intravenous urogram should be performed if an anatomic abnormality suggests that the course of the ureters may be aberrant, if malignancy is suspected or in major prolapse where ureteric obstruction is a possibility.

Anesthetic pre-assessment

Preoperative assessment by the anesthetist is essential to ensure the safe and smooth running of the list. It is good practice for the patient to be seen the evening before surgery with the notes and results of investigations available. Where major medical problems exist, or if there have been previous anesthetic problems such as difficult intubation, anesthetic consultation may be carried out prior to admission. The most appropriate type of anesthetic (general, regional or local) should also be selected.

The advice of the relevant specialist should also be sought in the case of significant existing medical conditions. The specialist team will be able to give advice on preoperative preparation and therapy in the immediate postoperative phase.

Informed consent

Before embarking upon any surgical procedure it is imperative that adequate informed consent has been obtained and documented. Increasingly, medicolegal claims involving the issue of consent are being pursued and, as an aspect of good practice as well as risk management, it is important to understand the ethical and legal issues surrounding the concept of informed consent. When considering the issue of informed consent, the British courts use what is known as the Bolam principle. This was developed in the case *Bolam v Friern Hospital Management Committee*, [1957] 1 Wlr 582. This states that 'a Doctor is not negligent when he acts in accordance with a practice accepted as proper by a responsible body of medical men skilled in that particular art'.

Consent is difficult to define succinctly but requires three elements: volition, capacity, and knowledge.

Volition

Volition is based on the principles of self-determination and a respect for individual integrity. This requires that a woman is able to make a decision regarding consent without undue pressure from a third party, either a relative or a member of the medical staff. Legally, a spouse or relative cannot give or withhold consent on a woman's behalf, although it is considered good practice to involve the spouse, particularly where the treatment proposed will affect fertility.

Capacity

Capacity to consent requires that a woman has sufficient intellect to appreciate information discussed prior to giving consent, and the mental capacity to appreciate the risks and the consequences of the operation proposed. This is a particularly difficult area when dealing with women whose mental capacity is limited as a result of either intellectual handicap or psychiatric illness. In these situations it is important to seek additional professional opinion and to seek legal clarification where time allows.

The situation when dealing with minors (in the UK under 16 years of age) is another delicate area. In general, both the parents and child would be involved in giving informed consent. However, in the UK the circumstances of minors giving consent without parental approval or knowledge has recently been clarified in the case of *Gillick v West Norfolk and Wisbech Health Authority*, [1985] 3 All ER 402, in which the House of Lords ruled that parental rights give way to a child's right to make her own decision upon sufficient maturity to understand the nature and consequences of that decision. This has led to the concept of 'Gillick' competency, where a medical practitioner must make a clinical judgment as to whether a minor has sufficient maturity to give informed consent. Although this has clarified the situation in the UK, it is important that practitioners are aware of the law regarding minors in their own country or state.

Knowledge

The third aspect of consent is that of knowledge. This implies that a woman should have sufficient information concerning the diagnosis and prognosis to make a reasoned decision regarding treatment. A woman must also be given sufficient information about alternative treatments and also any reasonably foreseeable adverse effects of the proposed treatment. This is another difficult area, as women's ability to understand the technicalities of a medical condition and its treatment may vary. Similarly, it would be unreasonable to describe in depth every conceivable complication arising from surgery. This area was clarified in the case of *Sidaway v Board of Governors of Bethlem Royal Hospital*, [1985] 1 All ER 643, in which the courts applied the Bolam principle to information about potential risks. In general, the information given should conform to that given by a responsible body of medical opinion. Those risks that are commonly associated with a procedure should certainly be discussed; more uncommon complications need not be. It is left to the medical practitioner to decide on an individual patient's ability or wish to discuss these issues. The need to discuss complications also varies with their potential severity and implications for future health. This means that it is essential to discuss the possibility of a complication that may be relatively remote but which would have a major impact on a woman's life. A good example of this is to perform hysterectomy to control hemorrhage at myomectomy; although this is well reported it is, in fact, a relatively uncommon occurrence. However, as myomectomy is primarily performed to preserve fertility and the loss of the uterus has such major implications for a woman wishing to bear future children, the remote possibility of this should always be discussed and recorded beforehand.

Oophorectomy performed without specific consent has been the subject of a number of recent court actions – both civil cases for negligence and criminal cases for assault. It is essential that the possibility of oophorectomy, either as a technical necessity or for an unforeseen indication, is discussed and documented.

The risks of surgical complications such as bladder trauma requiring catheterization and wound infection should also be discussed, as appropriate.

The issue of informed consent has become clearer in recent years, with some guidance from the cases cited above. The final decision regarding a woman's capacity to give consent and her ability to understand the information given is left to the professional judgment of the surgeon.

Most practitioners will use a standard consent form and record any particular information on this. However, the concept of informed consent embraces more than just a signature and so it is important that good records are kept of any discussion and information given prior to informed consent.

Thromboembolism and thromboprophylaxis

Thromboembolism accounts for around 20% of perioperative hysterectomy deaths.[13] As prophylaxis has been shown to be effective in reducing the risk of thromboembolism, women undergoing gynecologic surgery should be assessed for clinical risk factors and overall risk of thromboembolism, and should receive prophylaxis according to the degree of risk: this is highest for surgery associated with malignancy, less in abdominal hysterectomy, and lowest for vaginal hysterectomy.[14] Other risk factors associated with the disease or surgical procedure include infection, polycythemia, and heart failure. Risk factors associated with the patient are age over 37 years, obesity, previous deep vein thrombosis (DVT), blood group other than O, and the presence of congenital or acquired thrombophilias. Assessment of these risk factors allows categorization into low-, medium- or high-risk categories.

The Royal College of Obstetricians and Gynaecologists (RCOG) has issued guidelines on the use of thromboprophylaxis in gynecologic surgery.[15] Patients deemed at low risk require attention to hydration and early mobilization only. Those at moderate risk should receive specific prophylaxis with either low molecular weight heparin (doses varying depending on the heparin used, for example enoxaparin and tinzaparin) or intermittent pneumatic compression. Patients deemed to be high risk should be given heparin as above and in addition be fitted with graduated compression stockings.

The use of heparin is associated with a small increase in the risk of wound hematoma but no significant fall in postoperative hemoglobin or increase in the need for blood transfusion.

In many units these guidelines are exceeded and heparin, intermittent compression, and compression stockings are used for all but minor day case procedures. In patients who are high risk, a hematologist is actively involved in the management.

Combined oral contraceptive pill

The combined oral contraceptive (COC) pill has been implicated as a risk factor for postoperative thromboembolism. A study by Vessey et al.[16] showed a modest increased risk in users of the COC. Recent RCOG guidelines suggest that the COC should be discontinued at least 4 weeks before major surgery when immobilization is anticipated. Hormonal methods do not need to be discontinued before minor surgery without immobilization. When indicated, the COC should be discontinued at least 4 weeks before surgery and alternative contraception discussed.

Hormone replacement therapy

Recent studies have suggested an increased risk of venous thrombosis in women taking hormone replacement therapy (HRT). There is at present no evidence associating HRT, at physiologic levels, with an increase in postoperative DVT.[17] Therefore there seems little to be gained by stopping HRT prior to surgery and exposing the patient to a recurrence of perimenopausal symptoms. However, routine assessment of risk and appropriate prophylaxis should be undertaken, as many patients in this age group will have other, more significant, risk factors for thrombosis.[18]

Atrophic changes in the vaginal skin can cause difficulty during vaginal reconstructive surgery and compromise postoperative wound healing. Preoperative treatment with topical estrogen for 6 weeks is worthwhile and carries little risk.

Prophylactic antibiotics

Prophylactic antibiotics have been clearly shown to reduce the risk of postoperative wound infection. The use of perioperative antibiotic prophylaxis has been shown, in a systematic review, to reduce markedly the risks of febrile morbidity after elective and emergency cesarean section.[19] A similar reduction in infectious morbidity has been shown with the use of broad spectrum antibiotic prophylaxis in both abdominal and vaginal hysterectomy.[5,6] This reduction was also seen in a study of antibiotic prophylaxis in both general and gynecologic surgery.[7]

Adverse reactions to prophylactic antibiotic regimens are reported rarely, with an incidence of less than 1%. The cost of antibiotic cover is outweighed by the considerable economic savings, most notably the reduction in inpatient stay. The clinical and economic evidence clearly demonstrates the effectiveness of routine perioperative antibiotic prophylaxis.

The choice of antibiotic appears to be between a broad-spectrum penicillin or cephalosporins, either alone or in combination with an aminoglycoside or metronidazole. There appears to be little difference between the penicillins and cephalosporins. The studies showing the greatest reduction in postoperative infection are those when an aminoglycoside was used as part of the combination. As the pattern of microbial resistance varies, the most appropriate combination of agents should be selected after consultation with the local microbial service, and should be reviewed at regular intervals. The development of microbial resistance is a particular concern. Given the clear advantages of routine chemoprophylaxis, it is sensible to continue this; however, to reduce bacterial resistance, short courses should be used with routine 'first line' agents. Newer agents should be reserved for treatment of established antibiotic-resistant infections.

As the aim of chemoprophylaxis is the prevention rather than the treatment of established infection, regimens used should aim to achieve a high tissue concentration of the chosen antibiotics at the time of surgery when inoculation of the wound occurs. However, as this would mean the administration of intravenous antibiotics some hours prior to surgery, a more practical compromise is to give the first dose at the time of induction of anesthesia, with a further two doses in the first 24 hours postoperatively.

POSTOPERATIVE PROBLEMS

Immediate postoperative care

Normal clinical monitoring of postoperative patients with pulse and blood pressure recording is adequate for most gynecologic patients. In high risk cases, the hourly urine output is a sensitive measure of peripheral circulation.

When massive blood loss occurs, which is rare in a urogynecologic setting, a consumptive coagulopathy may develop as all coagulation factors are exhausted. It is therefore important to monitor the coagulation status of the patient repeatedly during resuscitation and if an abnormality develops, expert advice from a hematologist should be sought.

One way of controlling blood loss is the use of tranexamic acid by intravenous infusion. Tranexamic acid impairs fibrin dissolution and is sometimes used in an acute blood loss setting to try to prevent the development of consumption coagulopathy.

Occasionally, embolization of actively bleeding blood vessels using intervention radiology techniques may be an effective alternative to surgery. It requires a skilled team of interventional radiologists who are able to provide an emergency service. This generally avoids very difficult surgery in very sick patients. It is often the more reliable and the faster method of controlling the bleeding. Decision regarding re-exploration may be difficult and the advice and help of the most experienced person should be sought. As a rule of thumb, the sooner after the surgery the bleeding presents, the more likely that re-exploration will identify a single obvious bleeding vessel.

Anticipation of postoperative voiding problems

Voiding difficulties may occur acutely following any pelvic surgery; after continence procedures in particular, voiding difficulties may persist in the medium or long term. The importance of relieving acute urinary retention cannot be overstated. Acute overdistension of the bladder leads to damage of the detrusor syncytium with ischemic damage to the postsynaptic parasympathetic fibers. This may result in insidious deterioration of detrusor function and, later, the onset of voiding dysfunction.[20] A number of factors that increase the risk of acute postoperative retention have been identified, including increased age, long operation time, high doses of opiate analgesia and patient-controlled analgesia, together with large amounts of intravenous fluids.[21] In view of the possible long term sequelae of acute overdistension of the detrusor, it is important that steps are taken to prevent this. Postoperative indwelling urethral catheterization should be used following surgery, although some authors prefer intermittent catheterization.[22] In women judged clinically or urodynamically to be at high risk of retention, suprapubic catheterization may be preferable; this may be performed easily at the time of surgery and avoids the need for repeated urethral catheterization. Following removal of a catheter, close monitoring of fluid balance should be continued to prevent recurrent retention.

As previously stated, voiding difficulties are particularly common following continence procedures initially and may persist for a variable time following surgery. After colposuspension they are particularly common in women with preoperative flow rates of less than 15 ml/s or maximum voiding detrusor pressure below 15 cmH_2O. Between 12 and 25% of women are reported to suffer delayed voiding postoperatively and 11–20% have increased residual volumes and reduced flow rates when measured at 3 months postoperatively.[23] In a study by Smith and Cardozo[24] of 100 women undergoing colposuspension, 21% experienced significant voiding difficulties for up to 6 months following their surgery, although this persisted beyond 6 months in only 2%. Hilton and Stanton[25] performed postoperative urodynamic studies on women 3 months after colposuspension and found highly significant reduced flow rates and increased voiding pressure.

Voiding problems are also common following needle suspension procedures, although published figures vary. Ashken et al.[26] noted no significant changes in flow rate, voiding pressures or urine residual volume in a study of 60 women after successful Stamey procedure; Hilton and Mayne[27] studied 100 women undergoing Stamey procedure and found increased functional urethral length and improved pressure transmission but no significant changes in resting urethral profile or voiding pressure; Mundy[28] found a higher incidence of voiding difficulties and irritative symptoms compared to colposuspension.

Sling procedures are particularly prone to causing voiding difficulty as their mechanism of action is to increase outflow resistance.[25,29]

Whichever continence procedure is to be performed, it is important that women are counseled adequately. The need for suprapubic catheterization, which may occasionally be prolonged, should be carefully explained preoperatively. The occasional need for clean intermittent self-catheterization (CISC) should be discussed. When voiding difficulty is predicted by urodynamic studies, it may be worth teaching CISC prior to surgery. Even though perhaps only a minority of these women will need to self-catheterize, from the psychological standpoint short-term voiding problems are much better dealt with when they have been anticipated.

Enterocele and rectocele formation

The formation of enteroceles and rectoceles is thought to occur as a result of elevation of the anterior vaginal wall creating a posterior defect and causing intra-abdominal pressure to be transmitted directly to the posterior vaginal wall. The incidence of postoperative posterior compartment defects is estimated to be 7–17%.[30] It is important that this is discussed with women preoperatively, together with the potential need for interval posterior vaginal repair.

De novo detrusor instability

It has been shown that detrusor instability (DI) arises de novo in 12–18.5% of women postoperatively,[31] and occurs more commonly following previous continence surgery. It seems likely that a number of cases reflect preexisting DI not detected at cystometry preoperatively. In addition, it has been suggested that damage to the autonomic nerve supply occurs during lateral displacement of the bladder during surgery.[32] The presence of postoperative DI should be excluded with urodynamic investigations. Where DI is present, a trial of anticholinergic therapy should be carried out. This will ensure that symptoms of frequency and urgency can be controlled and that the woman is able to tolerate the side effects of anticholinergic therapy if it is required postoperatively. Such women should be warned that symptoms of frequency and urgency may persist after surgery for stress incontinence and this should be recorded in the case notes.

CONCLUSIONS

Adequate preparation for surgery has an important role in ensuring an optimal outcome and reducing morbidity.

The elective nature of most urogynecologic surgery allows time to ensure that all women are well prepared, both psychologically and physically, before undergoing the chosen operation.

REFERENCES

1. Laycock J. The Investigation and Management of Urinary Incontinence in Women. London: RCOG Press, 1995.
2. Kegel AH. Progressive resistance exercise in the functional restoration of the perineal muscles. Am J Obstet Gynecol 1948;56:238–48.
3. Tapp AJS, Hills B, Cardozo L. Who benefits from physiotherapy? Neurourol Urodyn 1988;7:259–65.
4. Bo K, Talseth T. Five year follow-up of pelvic floor exercise for the treatment of stress urinary incontinence. Neurourol Urodyn 1994;13:374–6.
5. Hemsall DL, Molly C, Heard RA et al. Single dose prophylaxis for vaginal and abdominal hysterectomy. Am J Obstet Gynecol 1987;157:498–501.
6. Duff P, Park RC. Antibiotic prophylaxis in vaginal hysterectomy: a review. Obstet Gynecol 1980;55(Suppl):193–202.
7. Regiori A, Ravera M, Coccozza E et al. Randomised study of antibiotic prophylaxis for general and gynaecological surgery from a single centre in rural Africa. Br J Surg 1996;83:356–9.
8. Choe JM, Staskin DR. Clinical usefulness of urinary insert devices. Int Urogynecol J 1997;8:307–13.
9. Collings LH, Pike LC, Binder A et al. Value of written information in a general practice setting. Br J Gen Pract 1991;41:466–7.
10. Bonnar J, Sheppard BL. Treatment of menorrhagia: a randomized controlled trial of etamysylate, mefenamic acid and tranexamic acid. Br Med J 1996;313:579–82.
11. Thomas EJ, Okuda M, Thomas NM. The combination of a depot GnRH analogue and cyclical HRT for dysfunctional uterine bleeding. Br J Obstet Gynaecol 1991;98:1155–9.
12. Sternquist M. Treatment of uterine fibroids with GnRH analogues prior to hysterectomy. Acta Obstet Gynecol Scand Suppl 1997;194:94–7.
13. Department of Health Report of the National Enquiry into Perioperative Deaths. London: HMSO, 1993.
14. Bergquist D. Postoperative Thromboembolism. London: Springer-Verlag 1983; 106–7.
15. Royal College of Obstetricians and Gynaecologists. Report of RCOG Working party on prophylaxis against thromboembolism in gynaecology and obstetrics. London: RCOG, 1995.
16. Vessey MP, Mant D, Smith A, Yeates D. Oral contraceptives and venous thromboembolism. Br Med J 1986;292:526–31.
17. Carter CJ. Thrombosis in relation to oral contraceptives and hormone replacement therapy. In: Greer IA, Turpie AAG, Forbes CD (eds) Haemostasis and Thrombosis in Obstetrics and Gynaecology. London: Chapman and Hall, 1992; 371–88.
18. Lowe G, Greer I, Cooke T et al. Risk and prophylaxis for venous thromboembolism in hospital patients. Br Med J 1992;305:567–74.
19. Smaill F. Prophylactic antibiotics in caesarean section (all trials). In: Keirse MJNC, Renfrew MJ, Neilson JP, Crowther C (eds) The Cochrane Pregnancy and Childbirth Database, Issue 2. Oxford: Oxford University Press, 1994.
20. Osborne JL. Urodynamics and the Gynaecologist. Alec Bourne Lecture. London: RCOG Press, 1981.
21. Tammela T, Konturri M, Lukkarien O. Postoperative urinary retention 1. Incidence and predisposing factors. Scand J Urol Nephrol 1986;20:197–201.
22. Smith NGK, Murrant JD. Postoperative urinary retention in women: management by intermittent catheterization. Age Ageing 1990;19:337–40.
23. Stanton SL, Cardozo LD, Williams JE et al. Clinical and

urodynamic features of failed incontinence surgery in the female. Obstet Gynecol 1978;51:515–20.

24. Smith RN, Cardozo L. Early voiding difficulties after colposuspension. Br J Urol 1997;160:911–4.

25. Hilton P, Stanton SL. A clinical and urodynamic assessment of the Burch colposuspension for genuine stress incontinence. Br J Obstet Gynaecol 1983;90:934–9.

26. Ashken MH, Abrams PH, Lawrence WT. Stamey endoscopic bladder neck suspension for stress incontinence. Br J Urol 1984;56:629–34.

27. Hilton P, Mayne C. The Stamey endoscopic bladder neck suspension: a clinical and urodynamic investigation including actuarial follow up over four years. Br J Obstet Gynaecol 1991;98:1141–9.

28. Mundy AR. A trial comparing the Stamey bladder neck suspension with colposuspension. Br J Urol 1983;55:687–90.

29. Beck RP, McCormack RN. Treatment of urinary stress incontinence with anterior colporrhaphy. Obstet Gynecol 1982;59:269–74.

30. Burch JC. Coopers ligament urethrovesical suspension for urinary stress incontinence. Am J Obstet Gynecol 1968;100:764–72.

31. Alcalay M, Monga A, Stanton SL. Burch colposuspension: a 10–20 year follow-up. Br J Obstet Gynaecol 1995;102:740–5.

32. Cardozo LD, Stanton SL, Williams JE. Detrusor instability following surgery for GSI. Br J Urol 1979;58:138–42.

56

Synthetic materials for pelvic reconstructive surgery

Mark Slack

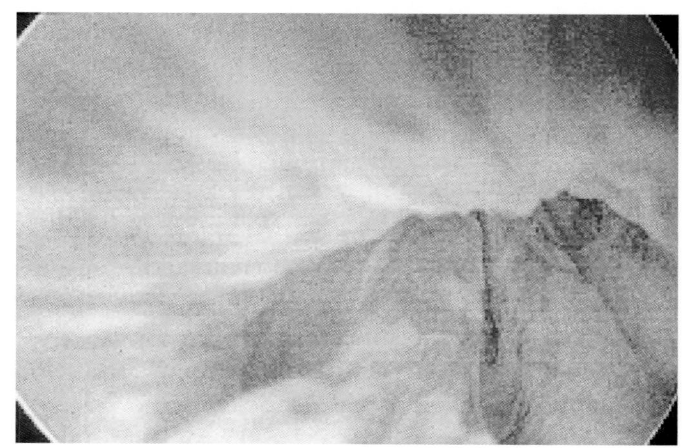

INTRODUCTION

Pelvic organ prolapse and urinary incontinence are common conditions affecting thousands of women worldwide. One study indicated that 11.1% of women aged 20 years will undergo an operation for prolapse or incontinence by the age of 60. Of this group, a staggering 30% will require reoperation for the condition.[1] There are indications that the rates of pelvic organ prolapse (POP) surgery are increasing.[2]

As a result of these figures, together with a perception among the scientific community that the traditional vaginal surgical approach to POP may have limited success, there has been a move to correction with abdominal procedures.[3] Crucial to the success of abdominal procedures has been the utilization of synthetic materials to help with the provision of durable support.

The ideal properties of a synthetic mesh to be placed in the body are that it should be inert, resistant to infection, pliable and biocompatible, and that it should maintain mechanical integrity. Additionally, it must be easily fabricated and sterilizable.

The perfect synthetic material for placement in the body has yet to be discovered. However, significant strides have been made, leading to the increasing availability of materials that match up to the properties described above. There are, however, concerns that the use of synthetic materials in gynecologic surgery could be associated with significant morbidity, especially if surgeons are not familiar with the principles behind their use and the properties of the individual materials.

HISTORY

The use of synthetic mesh in surgery is not new. Some of the earliest descriptions involve the use of a tantalum mesh for the closure of chest wall defects.[4] Although initial results were encouraging, there was fragmentation and disintegration of the mesh, resulting in extrusion of fragments, draining sinuses, and painful wounds.[5]

Teflon (polytetrafluoroethylene, PTFE) was thought to be a promising mesh because it appeared to be covered completely by granulation tissue. It also appeared to withstand infection. However, it proved too weak and developed fraying. To increase its strength it was more tightly woven, and although this did increase tensile strength, it required removal when infected. It was concluded that because of the proximity of the fibers, drainage was prevented and granulation tissue could not grow through the interstices.[6] In a series of animal experiments, Usher and Gannon compared loose and tightly woven Teflon with Marlex (polypropylene) mesh.[7] Little tissue ingrowth was noted with the Teflon mesh as opposed to good fibrous infiltration into and through the Marlex mesh. Adhesions to bowel and omentum were noted. Contemporaneously, the vascular surgery community identified that the ingrowth of tissue is determined by the porosity of the graft material.[8] Surgical mesh made of polypropylene became available from 1962. It was noted to be sterilizable without loss of its properties.[9] Soon after, the makers of Marlex (Ethicon Ltd, Edinburgh) produced a new mesh made of polypropylene (Prolene) and one made of polyester (Mersilene).

Surgeons experienced good results in the surgery for stress urinary incontinence (SUI) using the Aldridge sling.[10] Because of the morbidity associated with graft harvesting, surgeons soon started experimenting with sling operations that utilized a synthetic sling. The first to be described was probably by Bracht in 1951 where a nylon cord was used.[11]

In the United Kingdom, Chassar Moir – on reporting a new operation using Mersilene mesh – encouraged the use of the material in operations for the treatment of SUI.[12] This publication made no mention of the possible complications associated with the use of synthetic materials. The procedures were not without complications, with reported erosion rates of between 2 and 16% and the need to revise or remove the sling in between 2 and 35% of cases.[13] General dissatisfaction with the procedure led to the abandonment of the operation by most surgeons in the UK.

Following the success with the use of synthetic materials in the 'tension-free' surgical management of inguinal hernias, interest in the use of these materials in SUI surgery and POP surgery was renewed.[14]

The publication of articles on the tension-free vaginal tape (TVT) procedure, and the widespread marketing that accompanied the launch, led to the rapid introduction of this operation.[15,16] Subsequent 7-year data on safety are now available for the TVT.[17] Unfortunately, success with this product has led to the development of a range of procedures using a variety of tapes for the treatment of SUI and POP. Most of these new procedures lack any real or substantive data for their safety or success.

SYNTHETIC MESH FOR USE IN HUMAN SURGERY

There are numerous differences in the various mesh materials. These occur as a result of the different ways of creating the mesh and by the substance from which they are created

Artificial materials used for surgical prostheses are divided into whether they are biologic or synthetic (Fig. 56.1). Synthetic meshes are further classified into

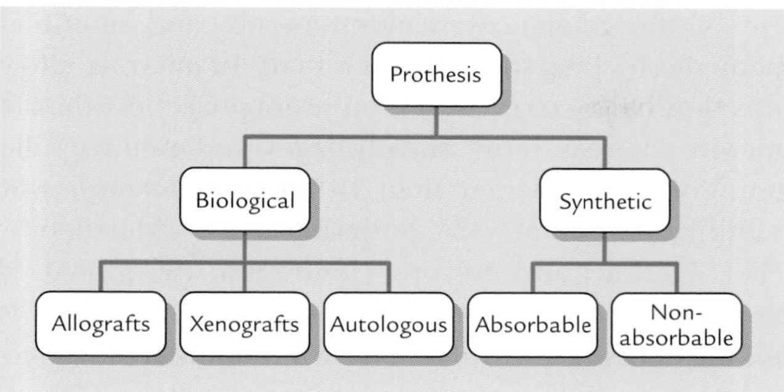

Figure 56.1. *Categorization of surgical prostheses for incontinence and prolapse.*

whether they are absorbable or non-absorbable (Fig. 56.2).

Absorbable mesh

Limited data are available on the use of absorbable mesh in urologic or gynecologic surgery. On first principles it is probably an unsatisfactory prosthesis as it has been demonstrated that adequate fibrous tissue incorporation does not occur before hydrolysis of implanted polyglactin mesh.[18] In this animal model, which compared abdominal wall defect repair with an absorbable mesh versus a non-absorbable mesh, it was demonstrated that after 12 weeks 25% of the animals in the absorbable group had demonstrable gross hernias compared to none in the animals with synthetic repairs. A similar finding was demonstrated by another group.[19]

Two clinical studies have produced conflicting results from randomized trials comparing standard surgery for prolapse with surgery utilizing surgical prostheses: the first study showed an advantage when using mesh,[20] the second study did not.[21]

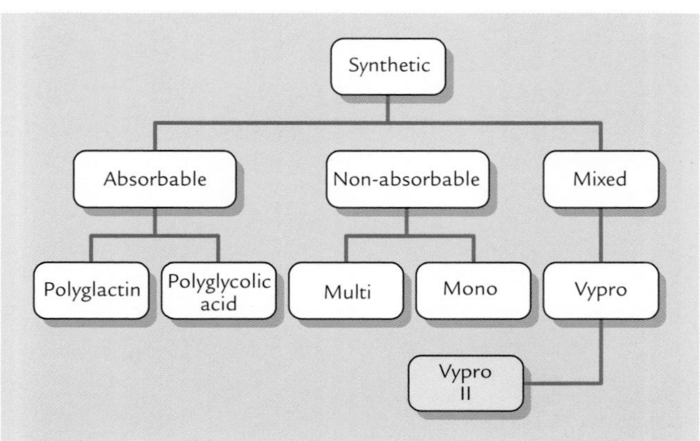

Figure 56.2. *Categorization of synthetic surgical prostheses for the treatment of incontinence and prolapse.*

Corrective surgery for abdominal wall defects has been used as a surrogate for other indications for materials evaluation. Obviously surgery for abdominal wall hernias is very different from prolapse and incontinence work. Although synthetic grafts woven from rapidly hydrolyzed materials such as vicryl may be inadequate, there may be a place for the use of meshes created from materials with a longer life such as polydioxanone (PDS). An absorbable mesh which remains in place long enough for a significant three-dimensional fibrous ingrowth to occur remains an aspirational goal.

With current knowledge the use of absorbable mesh cannot be recommended for reconstructive or incontinence surgery.

Non-absorbable mesh

This represents a complex area dependent on an intricate knowledge of the science behind the technology. This chapter will attempt to give an overview of the science behind the synthetic, non-absorbable mesh materials.

POLYMER TECHNOLOGY

Most of the synthetic meshes are plastics categorized by their chemical nature, the polymerization process that forms them, and their processibility. The manufacture involves procuring the raw materials, synthesizing the basic polymer, compounding the polymer into a useful material for fabrication, and then molding or shaping it into its final form.

Originally, most plastics were made from resins derived from vegetable matter such as cellulose, which is derived from cotton. The initial unit produced is the monomer. The production of nylon was originally based on coal, air and water, although most such products are now derived from petrochemicals. The chemical nature of a plastic is defined by the monomer. This divides them into categories such as acrylics, styrenes, vinyl chloride, polyesters, polyurethanes, polyamides, polyethers, acetals, phenolics, cellulosics, and amino resins.

The first stage in manufacture is polymerization. This is either a condensation reaction (nylon, polyurethane and polyester) or an addition reaction (polyethene, polypropene and polystyrene). Addition polymers have larger molecular weights than the condensation ones. Chemical additives are often used to produce some desired characteristic. In industry antioxidants are used to protect a polymer from chemical degradation by ozone or oxygen. Plasticizers can make it more flexible and pigments can alter the color. Changes to the surface tension can be created by additives. Each company holds the key to its particular formula and will resist any attempts to declare the exact nature of the finished product. It is these additives that impart a degree of individuality to each product. As such, not even mesh derived from the same monomer units is the same.

The final stage employs techniques to shape and finish the polymer. In medicine one of the commonest techniques is that of extrusion. An extruder is a device that pumps plastic through a desired die or shape. Using this technique, long strands of polymer can be produced. These strands can then be woven into mesh. Alternatively, some meshes are made by a bonding process where short strands of polymer are almost stuck together.

Because plastics are relatively inert, the final products do not normally present health hazards. This should not make us complacent as some monomers used in the manufacture of plastics have been shown to have carcinogenic properties.[22]

MESH TECHNOLOGY

Differences in the type and composition of the individual fibers (e.g. weight, mono- or polyfilament, additives) will impart further differences. In addition, the individual characteristics of the mesh such as pore size, porosity, and weave will further determine how it behaves in the body. Differences will occur in relation to foreign body reaction, ability to withstand infection, shrinkage, and erosion. There are also mechanical differences between the various types. Mechanical differences are more likely to be an issue in hernia and other forms of abdominal wall surgery.

Type of filament

It appears that meshes constructed with a monofilament fiber induce a different foreign body reaction when compared with multifilamentous mesh types.[23] This 1996 study compared the foreign body reaction of the monofilament polypropylene mesh (Prolene) and the multifilament Surgipro mesh. Both materials were widely used in hernia work at the time. Mesh was implanted in 12 sites in six pigs. At each of 3, 5 and 12 weeks two animals were sacrificed and the tissue specimens were harvested for histologic examination. The study found that there was a significantly greater foreign body reaction with the multifilamentous mesh than the monofilament insert.

The greater the amount of foreign material, the greater the possibility of harboring or perpetuating infection. This is probably due to the difference in the size of the interstices between mono- and multifilament mesh. Interstices smaller than 10 microns allow infection by bacteria, which on average are less than 1 micron whereas most macrophages and neutrophilic granulocytes are larger than 10 microns. Examples of multifilament mesh are polyester mesh (Mersilene), PTFE (Teflon) and polypropylene mesh (Surgipro). If infections occur in multifilament implants, removal is usually necessary.[24,25] Infection of a monofilament macroporous mesh does not require its removal.

Pore size

The pore size is measured by taking the two longest perpendicular axes of the pore (Fig. 56.3). They can be classified as macroporous (>75 microns) or microporous (<10 microns).

The size of the pore imparts similar properties experienced with mono- and multifilament fibers. As such, it can be seen that microporous mesh types exhibit a greater propensity to infection.[24,25]

Pore size is also implicated in the ingrowth of fibrous tissue. The pore size determines the success of the graft as a scaffold. It has been determined that the optimal pore size is greater than 90 microns but smaller than 5 mm. Pores that are too large incorporate too slowly.[26] The quantity reaches a maximum at 6 weeks without any increase over the next year.[27] This large size is necessary for the rapid ingrowth of vascularized connective tissue. The smaller size does not leave sufficient space for capillary penetration.[28]

There is also evidence that flexibility and stiffness are related to pore size. The larger the pore, the greater the

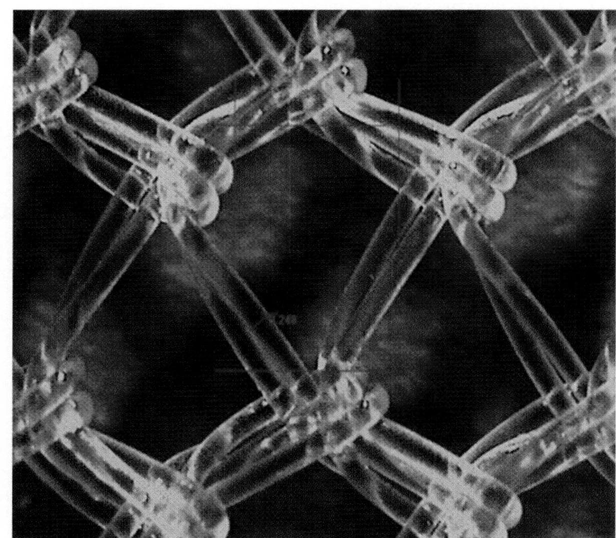

Figure 56.3. *TVT polypropylene type I tape.*

flexibility.[29] The importance of this in the clinical setting has yet to be established.

Pore size is not the only determinant of tissue ingrowth. Teflon mesh has a pore size 157 microns × 67 microns but has less tissue ingrowth than Marlex, which has a pore size of only 68 × 32 microns. It is believed that this can be attributed to the very low critical surface tension of the fibers, which are only 18.5 dynes/cm, making it difficult for fibroblasts to attach to, and spread on, the fibers.[30]

Weight

The density and weight of the mesh are important factors because of their relationship to healing. The extent of chronic inflammation in the tissues adjacent to the mesh is directly related to the amount of foreign material left in the patient.[31] Theoretically, a mesh with a similar pore size to successful mesh materials but with a lower weight might induce an even lower inflammatory response. New materials with a lower weight have demonstrated less of an inflammatory response over time.[32]

Weave

Most articles advocate an open weave as the one that will produce the optimum porosity. Pore size is different from porosity. Porosity, or openness of a fabric, can be defined as the difference between the total fabric area and the area covered by the fabric. Using a sophisticated measuring system combining digitized scanning electron microscope images with custom-built software, this measurement can be calculated accurately. Obviously, the less fabric, the better. This is an alternative method of assessing the nature of the mesh if pore size proves difficult to measure.[33]

Bonded mesh

Bonded mesh is created by fusion welding of the polypropylene fibers (Fig. 56.4). This gives it a very different appearance from mesh made with an open weave. In the experimental setting, it appears to behave in a fashion very similar to type III fibers and therefore should be used with caution until further evidence of clinical safety is established.

Mechanical properties

A range of physical tests can be used to differentiate the mechanical properties of mesh fabrics.

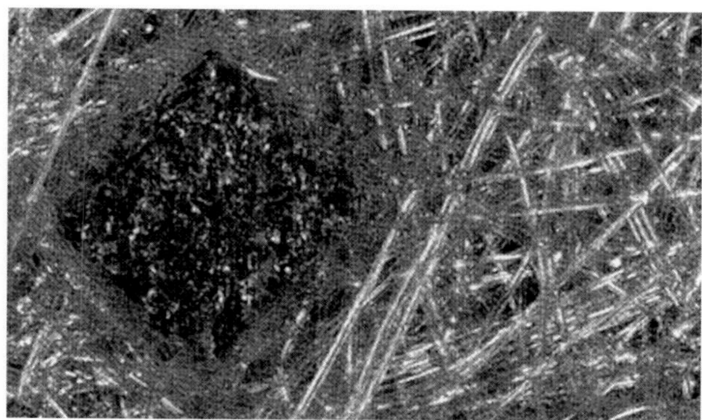

Figure 56.4. *Bonded mesh – Porges Mentor.*

- Tensile breaking strength of woven mesh is assessed by grab, modified grab, and strip tests.
- Bursting strength is used for materials that do not have yarns or where the yarns are not aligned in any given direction (e.g. knits of bonded mesh).
- Flexural rigidity is measured by the cantilever test, the principle of which is based on the level of bend of the specimen under its own weight.
- Wrinkle resistance measures the degree of recovery in a mesh that has undergone controlled creasing.

All of these tests should take place in temperature-controlled environments to ensure that there is uniformity in the test.[29]

Numerous authors have looked at the differences in mechanical properties between the various materials. It is easy to show differences in strength and elasticity in the laboratory but what impact this has on behavior in the body is poorly understood.[34,35] Most of the current materials have the calculated strength to withstand the pressures associated with rises in intra-abdominal pressure. Meshes do not need to withstand much more than 16 N/cm of force. Meshes on the market can usually withstand pressures from 30 to 50 N/cm.[36]

More studies looking at the mechanical properties of explanted materials are required.

Classification of mesh types

Using the above physical characteristics, Amid proposed a classification of mesh types which could help the consumer with choice (Table 56.1).[24]

Based on the experimental work done on mesh, it would appear that type I mesh materials have much lower rates of infection and, if infected, can be treated without removal.[37] The large pore meshes admit macrophages and allow rapid angiogenesis.[38] Type II and type

Table 56.1 *Amid classification of mesh types*

Type	Properties	Pore size	Product
I	Macroporous	>75 microns	Atrium Marlex Prolene Monarc TVT
II	Microporous	<10 microns	Goretex Obtape PTFE
III	Macroporous with multifilamentous filaments	>75 microns	PTFE Mersilene Surgipro
IV*	Submicronic	Not applicable	Silastic

* Type IV mesh is not suitable for gynecologic use as it is a relatively solid sheet and will totally resist incorporation. PTFE, polytetrafluoroethylene; TVT, tension-free vaginal tape.

III mesh materials, however, can harbor bacteria and by so doing can promote growth of the bacteria.[39,40]

These features, added to the better incorporation rates, make type I mesh materials the preferred fabric (Fig. 56.5).[41]

New classification

The Amid classification fails to cover all the categories of mesh types. Considering recent modifications, a more encompassing classification is outlined in Table 56.2. If manufacturers adopted this new classification, researchers would be able to compare the various materials more easily and comparisons would become clinically relevant.

CURRENT CLINICAL PRACTICE

Mesh is used in operations for the treatment of SUI and in the management of POP. This article will not cover a review of the clinical results but will instead try to concentrate on the overall picture and the principles that should be adopted when dealing with mesh. Generally the articles on the various operations are small series with limited follow-up. These are covered in the relevant chapters.

The success of the TVT procedure[42] and the demonstration that the risk of erosion is very small has led to the development of many similar operations. The evidence surrounding the advantages and disadvantages of the types of mesh material is limited, with follow-up of less than a year in most early reports. Some of the operations may differ by the instrumentation, technique, and/or type of sling material. Some of the materials are similar to the loosely knitted 4-0 polypropylene utilized in TVT, but others fall into the type II and III Amid classification.[43] The enthusiasm for these new procedures does not, it appears, reflect any anxiety about the absence of safety data on the different mesh types. It is worth remembering that synthetic sling erosion can create urethral damage requiring reconstructive surgery. This can be associated with postoperative incontinence in 44–83% of women.[44] An infection rate requiring removal in 7.4% of patients who had undergone surgery with multifilament tapes was recently described.[45]

Another series described an erosion rate of 33% in patients treated 3–24 months previously with suburethral polyester slings.[46] The increased erosion rate was attributed to those cases where the vaginal mucosa was closed with a locked suture.

The use of mesh in prolapse surgery has become increasingly more common. Reports demonstrating that the abdominal repair with mesh has a better outcome than vaginal surgery with a sacrospinous fixation[47] have resulted in numerous publications supporting the use of mesh in vaginal surgery. Most of the reported case series described a purely abdominal approach and avoided vaginal surgery. Another surgical trial by Maher and colleagues reached a similar conclusion.[48] Very small rates of erosion were identified in these series. Most of the

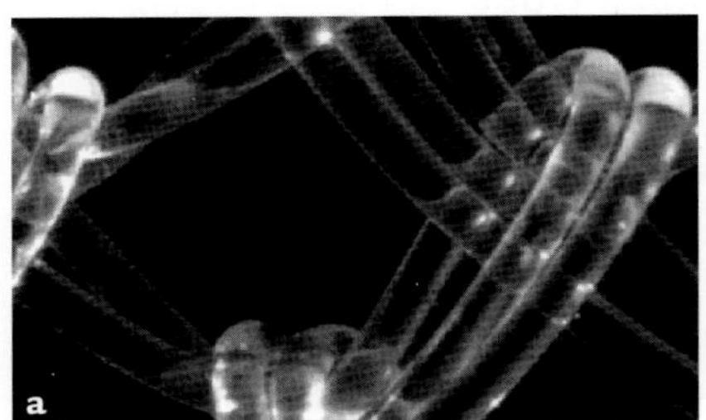

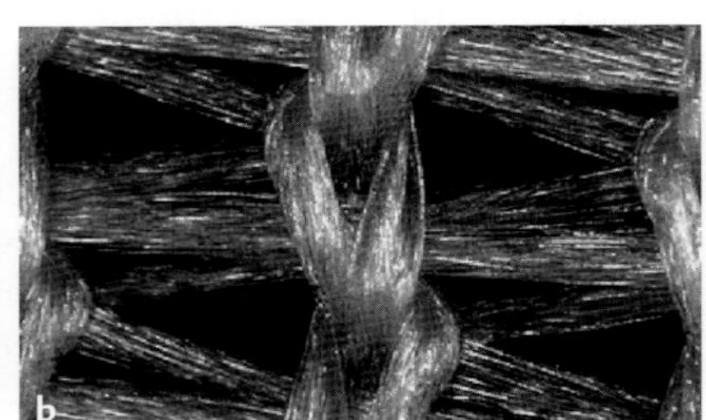

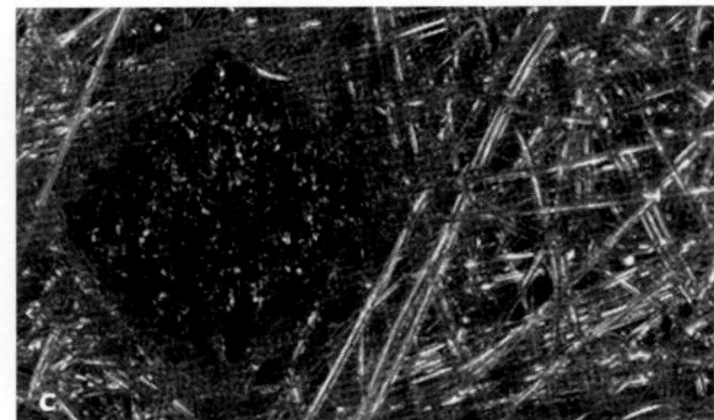

Figure 56.5. *Scanning electron micrographs of (a) type I mesh; (b) type III mesh, and (c) bonded mesh.*

Table 56.2 *Suggested new classification of mesh types*

Type	Properties	Pore size
I	Macroporous	>75 microns
Ia	Lightweight (<5 mg/cm^2)	<5 mg/cm^2
Ib	Heavyweight (>5 mg/cm^2)	>5 mg/cm^2
II	Microporous	<10 microns
III	Macroporous/multifilamentous	>75 microns
IV	Composite mesh (combination of absorbable and non-absorbable)	>75 microns
V	Bonded mesh	<10 microns
VI	Submicronic	Not applicable

studies have concentrated on the surgical technique and outcomes without performing any analysis on the influence of the mesh types.

Visco and colleagues suggested that mesh placed vaginally had a much higher erosion rate (40%) than when placed abdominally (3.2%).[49] The mesh used in this series was Mersilene, which is a type III mesh; vaginal placement of a type I mesh may not create the same problems. It is also not clear which suture types were used to fix the mesh. Defining suture type is essential since erosion is more likely to occur at a suture line than through epithelium that has not previously been incised. The role of intra-operative antibiotic irrigation should also be defined for any mesh type.

A recent paper has described a doubling of dyspareunia rates with the use of mesh for transvaginal repair and a 13% erosion rate.[50] Although not a randomized study, the authors previously demonstrated that an identical surgical technique without mesh had a much lower dyspareunia rate.[51]

The newer operations for prolapse are transvaginal procedures and use a wide variety of mesh materials.[52] The risk and benefit of utilizing a newer material or technique, and the indication for the procedure in the index patient and in subpopulations, should be considered. Each new procedure should declare the properties of the grafts and supply data on erosion and infection rates. Each operation should also supply data on bowel, bladder, and sexual function.

CONCLUSION

The use of mesh in surgery for SUI and POP represents one of the most active areas of clinical and basic research in the science of pelvic reconstruction. Evidence exists to support the use of type I mesh materials in the surgery for SUI. Reporting criteria for any procedure using a new approach and/or material should include the type of mesh employed, technique used, and any special procedural or patient group circumstances. New techniques should also be supported by clinical trial data for the operation that has sufficient follow-up to ensure safety. The use of these materials should only be carried out in controlled trials or under strict audit. A national registry in each country represents an ideal circumstance.

Evidence exists to support the use of synthetic mesh in abdominal surgery for POP. Less evidence exists for the use of the material transvaginally. Furthermore, there is no consensus on the type of suture used to fix the mesh, the vaginal closure technique or the use of antibiotic irrigation to prevent infection.

In summary, it appears that there are multiple reasons that may increase the risk of erosion. These include the route of surgery, the concomitant surgeries performed, the epithelial closure technique, the mesh type, the suture material used to fix the mesh, and the use of prophylactic antibiotics. The prolapse operations employ a much greater volume of mesh than that used in incontinence surgery and this too may be an issue.

One may suggest that stricter governance be employed in the introduction of these techniques. The size of surgical series, the number of cases, and the duration of follow-up are open to standardization. Conversion of all vaginal operations to those employing the use of mesh may be associated with an increase in mesh erosion and clinical morbidities that have been outlined in this chapter, and the risk and benefit of incorporation of mesh into the procedure should be carefully assessed.

REFERENCES

1. Olsen AL, Smith VJ, Bergstrom JO et al. Epidemiology of surgically managed pelvic organ prolapse and urinary incontinence. Obstet Gynecol 1997;89:501–6.
2. Boyles S, Weber A, Meyn L. Procedures for pelvic organ prolapse in the United States, 1979–1997. Am J Obstet Gynecol 2003;188:108–15.
3. Maher CF, Qatawneh AM, Dwyer PL et al. Abdominal sacral colpopexy or vaginal sacrospinous colpopexy for vaginal vault prolapse: a prospective randomized trial. Am J Obstet Gynecol 2004;190:20–6.
4. Morrow AG. The use of tantalum gauze in the closure of a full thickness defect in the chest wall. Surgery 1951;28:1016–21.
5. Effler DB. Prevention of chest wall defects: use of tantalum and steel mesh. J Thorac Surg 1953;26:419–23.
6. Harrison JH. Teflon weave for replacing tissue defects. Surg Gynecol Obstet 1957;104:584–90.

7. Usher FC, Gannon JP. Marlex mesh, a new plastic mesh for replacing tissue defects. I. Experimental studies. AMA Arch Surg 1959;78:131–7.
8. Wesolowski SA, Fries CC, Karlson KE et al. Porosity: primary determinant of ultimate fate of synthetic vascular grafts. Surgery 1961;50:91–6.
9. Usher FC. Hernia repair with knitted polypropylene mesh. Surg Gynecol Obstet 1963;117:239–40.
10. Aldridge AH. Transportation of fascia for relief of urinary incontinence. Am J Obstet Gynecol 1942;44:398–411.
11. Ghoniem GM, Shaaban A. Sub-urethral slings for treatment of stress urinary incontinence. Int Urogynecol J 1994;5:228–39.
12. Chassar Moir J. The gauze hammock operation: a modified Aldridge sling procedure. J Obstet Gynaecol Br Commonw 1968;75:1–9.
13. Jensen JK, Rufford HJ. Sling procedures – artificial. In: Cardozo L, Staskin D (eds) Textbook of Female Urology and Urogynaecology, 1st ed. London: Martin Dunitz, 2001; 544–61.
14. Lichenstein IL, Shulman AG, Amid PK et al. The tension-free hernioplasty. Am J Surg 1989;157:188–93.
15. Ulmsten U, Johnson P, Rezapour M. An ambulatory surgical procedure under local anaesthesia for treatment of female urinary incontinence. Int Urogynecol J 1996;9:81–6.
16. Ulmsten U, Falconer C, Johnson P et al. A multicentre study of tension-free vaginal tape (TVT) or surgical treatment of stress urinary incontinence. Int Urogynecol J 1998;9:210–3.
17. Nilsson CG. Latest advances in TVT tension-free support for urinary incontinence Surg Technol Int 2004;12:171–6.
18. Lamb JP, Vitale T, Kaminski DL. Comparative evaluation of synthetic meshes used for abdominal wall replacement. Surgery 1983;93:643–8.
19. Tyrell J, Silberman H, Chandrasoma P et al. Absorbable versus permanent mesh in abdominal operations. Surg Gynecol Obstet 1989;169:227–32.
20. Sand PK, Koduri S, Lobel RW et al. Prospective randomised trial of polyglactin 910 mesh to prevent recurrence of cystoceles and rectoceles. Am J Obstet Gynecol 2001;184:1357–64.
21. Weber AM, Walters MD, Piedmonte MR et al. Anterior colporrhaphy: a randomised trial of three surgical techniques. Am J Obstet Gynecol 2001;185:1299–1306.
22. Fuller RA, Rosen J. Materials for medicine. Sci Am 1986;255:118–125. In: Szycher M (ed) High Performance Biomaterials: A Comprehensive Guide to Medical and Pharmaceutical Applications. Lancaster, PA: Technomic Publishing; 1991.
23. Beets GL, Peter NY, Go H et al. Foreign body reactions to monofilament and braided polypropylene mesh used as preperitoneal implants in pigs. Eur J Surg 1996;162:823–5.
24. Amid PK. Classification of biomaterials and their related complications in abdominal wall hernia surgery. Hernia 1997;1:15–21.
25. Amid PK, Shulman AG, Lichenstein IL. Selecting synthetic mesh for the repair of groin hernia. Postgrad Gen Surg 1992;4:150–5.
26. Bobyn JD, Wilson GJ, McGregor DC et al. Effect of pore size on peel strength of attachment of fibrous tissue to porous-surfaced implants. J Biomed Mater Res 1975;181:728–34.
27. Rath AM, Zhang J, Amouroux J, Chevrel JP. [Abdominal wall prostheses. Biomechanic and histological study.] Chirurgie 1996;121:253–65.
28. Chavpil H, Holusa R, Kliment K et al. Some chemical and biological characteristics of a new collagen-polymer compound material. J Biomed Mater Res 1969;3:315–22.
29. Chu CC, Welch L. Characterization of morphologic and mechanical properties of surgical mesh fabrics. J Biomed Mater Res 1985;19:903–16.
30. Usher FC, Gannon JP. Marlex mesh, a new plastic mesh for replacing tissue defects. I. Experimental studies. Arch Surg 1959;78:175–7.
31. Bleichrodt RP, Simmermacher RKG, van der Lei B et al. Expanded polytetrafluoroethylene patch versus polypropylene mesh for the repair of contaminated defects of the abdominal wall. Surg Gynecol Obstet 1993;176:18–24.
32. Schumpelick V, Klosterhalfen B, Muller M et al. Minimized polypropylene mesh for preperitoneal net plasty (PNP) of incisional hernias. Chirurg 1999;70:422–30.
33. Pourdeyhimi B. Porosity of surgical mesh fabrics: new technology. J Biomed Res 1989;23:145–52.
34. Dietz HP. Mechanical properties of implant materials used in incontinence surgery. Int Urogynecol J Pelvic Floor Dysfunct 2003;14(4):239–43; discussion 243.
35. Sandhu DR, Staskin D, Slack M. Physical characteristics of suburethral sling material. Int Urogynecol J 2005. (In press).
36. Rosch R. Junge K. Quester R et al. Vypro II mesh in hernia repair: impact of polyglactin on long-term incorporation in rats. Surgical Research 2003;35(5):445–50.
37. Law N, Ellis H. A comparison of polypropylene mesh and expanded PTFE patch for the repair of contaminated abdominal wall defects. Surgery 1991;109:652–6.
38. Arnaud JP, Eloy R, Adloff M et al. Critical evaluation of prosthetic materials in repair of abdominal wall hernias. Am J Surg 1977;133:338–45.
39. Martin RE, Surech S, Classen JN. Polypropylene mesh in 450 hernia repairs: evaluation of wound infection. Contemp Surg 1982;20:46–8.
40. Usher FC, Fries JC, Ochsner JL et al. Marlex mesh: a

new plastic mesh for replacing tissue defects. Arch Surg 1959;78:138–45.

41. Slack MJ, Sandhu S, Staskin DR et al. In vivo comparison of suburethral sling materials. Int Urogynec J Pelvic Floor Dysfunct 2005 Jul 2; [Epub ahead of print].
42. Nilsson CG, Falconer C, Rezapour M. Seven-year follow-up of the tension-free vaginal tape procedure for treatment of urinary incontinence. Obstet Gynecol 2004;104(6):1259–62.
43. deTayrac R, Deffieux X, Droupy S et al. A prospective randomized trial comparing tension-free vaginal tape and transobturator suburethral tape for surgical treatment of stress urinary incontinence. Am J Obstet Gynecol 2004;190:602–8.
44. Blaivas JG, Sandhu J. Urethral reconstruction after erosion of slings in women. Curr Opin Urol 2004;14:335–8.
45. Bafghi A, Benizri E, Trastour C et al. Multifilament polypropylene mesh for urinary incontinence: 10 cases of infection requiring removal of the sling. Br J Obstet Gynaecol 2005;112:376–8.
46. Nemunaitis-Keller J, Alford W, Hopkins M. Experience with polyester fabric grafts when used in suburethral sling operations. J Pelvic Surg 2002;8:78–82.
47. Benson JT, Lucente V, McClellan E. Vaginal versus abdominal colpopexy for the treatment of pelvic support defects: a prospective randomized study with long-term outcome evaluation. Am J Obstet Gynecol 2004;175:1418–21.
48. Maher CF, Qatawneh AM, Dwyer PL et al. Abdominal sacral colpopexy or vaginal sacrospinous colpopexy for vaginal vault prolapse: a prospective randomized trial. Am J Obstet Gynecol 2004;190:20–6.
49. Visco AG, Weidener AC, Barber MD et al. Vaginal mesh erosion after abdominal sacral colpopexy. Am J Obstet Gynecol 2001;184:297–302.
50. Milani R, Salvatore S, Soligo M et al. Functional and anatomical outcome of anterior and posterior vaginal prolapse repair with prolene mesh. Br J Obstet Gynaecol 2005;112:107–11.
51. Milani R, Soligo M, Salvatore S et al. Fascial defect repair for symptomatic rectocele: anatomical and functional outcome. Proceedings of the 33rd Meeting of the International Continence Society: Florence, 5–9 October 2003. 189–90.
52. Hung MJ, Liu FS, Shen PS et al. Factors that affect recurrence after anterior colporrhaphy procedure reinforced with four-corner anchored polypropylene mesh. Int Urogynecol J 2004;15:399–406.

57

Biologic materials for reconstructive surgery

Harriette M Scarpero, Emily E Cole, Roger R Dmochowski

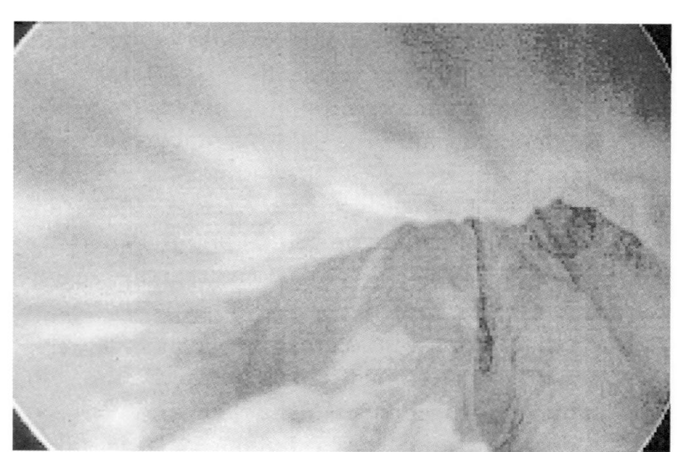

INTRODUCTION

The autologous pubovaginal sling has been used for decades to treat anatomic, functional, and recurrent stress urinary incontinence with excellent and long lasting results. In 1997, the American Urological Association (AUA) Female Stress Incontinence Clinical Guidelines Panel concluded that retropubic suspensions and slings were the most efficacious and durable procedures for stress urinary incontinence (SUI).[1] In their review of the English language peer-reviewed literature, sling success rates were found to be greater than 80% at 48 months follow-up or longer. These results refer to continence achieved with a traditional autologous fascial sling. Whether the same outcome can be expected from another sling material is not clear.

The classic pubovaginal sling requires the harvest of autologous fascia for sling material. Modifications such as alternative sling materials, bone anchor suspension, and midurethral slings have been developed to reduce operating time, surgical morbidity and postoperative complication. The term 'sling procedure' can now mean a variety of procedures that can differ in sling material, sling size, anchoring technique, and placement of sling. Numerous alternative biologic materials are commercially available and obviate the need to harvest autologous fascia. Critical analysis of alternative biologic materials and comparison to standard autologous sling outcomes is hampered by the lack of long-term results and direct prospective randomized comparisons. Use of these tissues poses new questions and concerns regarding biocompatibility, reaction or integration with host tissue, and disease transmission.

Allografts and xenografts are meant to function as scaffolding for the ingrowth of native tissue that ultimately will replace the graft, but recent data question the permanence of some materials. Although there is evidence that such transformation occurs in some orthopedic and ophthalmic applications, its ability to do this in the vaginal environment is not confirmed. Very little is known about biologic responses to allografts and xenografts in comparison to autologous tissue after vaginal implantation. The vaginal microenvironment differs from that of the abdominal wall, orbital cavity, or knee joint in several important ways. First, the histology is different. The vagina is composed of many layers of cells: stratified squamous epithelium and smooth muscle bundles intermixed with collagen bundles. The vagina is highly vascular, richly innervated and is not sterile but maintains a natural flora. The vaginal flora may be altered by hormonal changes, medications or illness. How the graft behaves in the human vagina may alter surgical success, durability, and complication rate. Despite a lack of knowledge about the long-term behavior of alternative biologic materials in vaginal procedures, patient desires for alternatives to self-harvest continue to drive the use of them. This chapter examines currently available biologic sling materials to elucidate their unique characteristics and their role in the correction of SUI.

AUTOLOGOUS MATERIALS

Autologous fascia is an attractive sling material because it is cost-effective, available, and biocompatible by definition. Rectus fascia and fascia lata are the autologous sling materials of choice. The harvest of rectus fascia can be accomplished by extending the suprapubic incision that will be made for passage of the ligature carriers and expanding the dissection over the rectus fascia. If the surgeon is willing to struggle with the reduced exposure provided by a smaller incision, the harvest-site incision does not have to be much larger than the typical suprapubic incision for sling sutures alone. Even in the case of prior abdominal surgery or prior rectus fascial sling surgery, it is commonly possible to harvest more fascia for the sling. Fascia lata is another option that may be chosen first line or when poor or insufficient fascia is encountered abdominally. Unlike the harvest of rectus fascia, the harvest of fascia lata requires patient repositioning, prepping of the patient's thigh, and additional instrumentation to strip the muscle.

Regardless of the material used, the pubovaginal sling attempts to restore sufficient outlet resistance to prevent stress urinary incontinence without compromising normal voiding or producing voiding dysfunction. Historically, the pubovaginal sling was reserved for SUI due to intrinsic sphincteric deficiency (ISD) or prior surgical failure; however, the evolution of our theories of the pathophysiology of SUI has extended the use of pubovaginal slings to all types of SUI. We no longer think of SUI as being purely anatomic or purely functional. Instead, it is felt that all women with SUI and hypermobility also have some degree of ISD since not all women with hypermobility leak. The pubovaginal sling, therefore, may be applied universally in SUI. The choice of what anti-incontinence procedure to perform and by what technique is still based on a variety of factors: patient choice, patient characteristics, and the surgeon's experience and comfort level with a particular technique.

Analysis of success of autologous slings is complicated by the varied definitions of cure and different outcome measures used in studies. It is well identified that results based on retrospective chart review tend to be more favorable than results collected by questionnaire or objective measurements.[1] Numerous studies document the excellent results with autologous materials, even in the long-term. In studies with at least 12 months' follow-up, cure rates vary from 50 to 100% with an average cure rate of 84%[2–42] (Table 57.1). Use of autologous materials provides the security of known efficacy, consistent durability, and lack of immunogenicity. An important part of critical evaluation of any surgical procedure also includes patient satisfaction and improvement in quality of life. Three recent studies have examined patient satisfaction with autologous slings.[14,31,41] Latini et al.[41] retrospectively surveyed 100 women who had undergone an autologous fascia lata sling. At a mean follow-up of 4.4 years, 85% of women stated that they were dry or improved, and 83% felt that it had a positive effect on their life. Similar rates of improvement in quality of life and satisfaction from rectus fascial slings are reported by Richter et al.[31] and Morgan et al.[14]

Complications (Table 57.2) unique to autologous tissues are related to the harvest site such as harvest-site infection, seroma or hematoma formation, herniation, or pain at the site. Transient obstructive symptoms that resolve within a few weeks are quite common. Urinary retention requiring urethrolysis occurs in 1–2% of cases, and rates may be slightly higher in fascia lata slings as compared to rectus fascial slings. No cases of rejection have been reported with autologous materials, and the few reported cases of erosion were likely due to excessive sling tension or overly aggressive periurethral dissection.[43]

Autologous sling materials remain the 'gold standard' against which other sling materials are measured. Success of other available sling materials is judged against our results from autologous slings. While clinical results are solid with autologous materials, some investigators have put available materials to test in an in vivo rabbit model.[44] In an investigation of time-dependent changes in tensile strength, stiffness, shrinkage, and distortion among cadaveric fascia, porcine dermis, porcine small intestine submucosa (SIS), polypropylene mesh, and autologous fascia, only mesh and autologous fascia showed no difference in tensile strength from baseline. Conversely, a significant loss of tensile strength and stiffness occurs in porcine and cadaveric materials within 12 weeks.

ALLOGRAFTS

The term allograft refers to non-autologous material taken from an organism of the same species or cadaveric tissues. The appeal of cadaveric tissue has been to avoid the time and morbidity of fascial harvest, yet maintain a perceived greater biocompatibility and lower risk of erosion compared to synthetics. In the case of sling allografts, the material includes lyophilized dura mater, pericardium, several preparations of fascia lata, and acellular dermis. These tissues have been used for more than 20 years in ophthalmic and orthopedic procedures, but have been used widely in sling surgery only since the mid 1990s. Allografts are commonly used in orthopedic reconstructive surgery for joint arthroplasties, spinal surgery, pediatric, and sports medicine orthopedic procedures. Bone allografts may be used to replace bone and joints lost to metallic implants or the excision of tumors. Orthopedic surgeons cite tissue availability, reduced surgical times, and lack of donor site morbidity as reasons in support of their use. In 2001, approximately 875,000 musculoskeletal allografts were distributed by tissue processors.[45] Remarkably, few cases of disease transmission have been cited with the use of musculoskeletal grafts.

The first use of allografts in sling surgery was reported by Jarvis and Fowlie in 1985.[46] Subsequently, Handa et al. followed with a description of the successful implantation of cadaveric fascia lata (CFL) for genuine stress incontinence which sparked widespread interest in the use of allografts.[47] Success rates with cadaveric allografts from studies with at least 12 months' follow-up vary from 40 to 100% with an average cure rate of 79%.[24,32,33,48–63] Prospective evaluation of subjective outcome, specifically patient satisfaction with CFL allograft sling in 102 patients with a mean time out from surgery of 35 months, found significant improvement in symptoms by validated questionnaire:[54] 80% of patients were better or much better, and 90.2% were somewhat or completely satisfied with their progress. The use of cadaveric tissue sparks several concerns, however: biocompatibility, rejection, disease transmission, and durability.

Lyophilized human dura mater has been used in a variety of urologic procedures in the past, including Peyronie's plaque excision, urethroplasty, and bladder augmentation, and as an interposition material in vesicovaginal fistula repairs. It has been used as a sling material in a few small series, but is a less common allograft for this use. Cure rates with lyophilized dura slings vary from 89 to 92% with follow-up of 6–48 months. No complications from the use of this material have been reported.[64,65] Of considerable concern to any surgeon using this material is a case report of the transmission of Creutzfeldt–Jakob's disease (CJD) in a male patient who received a cadaveric dura graft 12 years earlier for a non-urologic indication.[66] To date there have been no cases of the transmission of infection from the use of lyophilized dura mater in urologic surgery.

Table 57.1. *Results of autologous fascial slings**

Author	Material	No. of patients	Sling length (cm)	Mean F/U (months)	Cure (%)
Kaufman[2]	R	15	15	<48	93.3
Schultz-Lampel et al.[3]	R	11	–	24	63.6
Loughlin[4]	R	22	5	15	72.7
Mason & Roach[5]	R	63	4	12	93.7
Zaragoza[6]	R	60	6–8	25	100
Siegel et al.[7]	R	20	–	185	80
Carr et al.[8]	R	96	11–13	22	97.9
Barbalias et al.[9]	R	32	12	>30	65.6
Chaikin et al.[10]	R	251	15	37	72.9
Maheshkumar et al.[11]	R	43	–	17.4	95.3
Hassouna & Ghoniem[12]	R	82	7	41	89.1
Kane et al.[13]	R	13	5	26	100
Morgan et al.[14]	R	247	6–8	51	82.2
Kochakarn et al.[15]	R	100	–	12.1	94
Groutz et al.[16]	R	67	15	34	67.2
Kuo[17]	R	24	20	24	95.8
Borup & Nielsen[18]	R	31	12	60	96.8
Gormley et al.[19]	R	41	–	>74	95.1
De Rossi[20]	R	27	8	20	100
Lucas et al.[21]	R	156	–	>30	76
Chou et al.[22]	R	98	12	36	95
Pfitzenmaier et al.[23]	R	50	–	60	63.9
Almeida et al.[24]	R	30	–	33	70
Rodrigues et al.[25]	R	126	–	70.3	74.4
Kreder & Austin[26]	R/FL	27	–	22	96.3
Golomb et al.[27]	R/FL	18	15	30.7	88.9
Haab et al.[28]	R/FL	37	12–15	48.2	73
Wright et al.[29]	R/FL	33	13–15	16	93.9
Petrou & Frank[30]	R/FL	14	10	17	50
Richter et al.[31]	R/FL	57	24	42	84
Flynn & Yap[32]	R/FL	71	12	44	90.1
Chien et al.[33]	R/FL	23	10	30.5	94.1
Low[34]	FL	36	>24	>24	94.4
Addison et al.[35]	FL	97	–	12	86.6
Beck et al.[36]	FL	170	>17	>24	98.2
Karram & Bhatia[37]	FL	10	5 × 7	>12	90
Govier et al.[38]	FL	30	>24	14	69.7
Berman & Kreder[39]	FL	14	>17	14.9	71.4
Phelps et al.[40]	FL	27	>20	20	77.8
Latini et al.[41]	FL	63	18–22	53	85
Ellerkmann et al.[42]	FL	39	>24	>24	92.3

* Limited to studies with minimum of 12 months' follow-up. Adapted from ref. 97.
Cure (%), percentage of patients cured; FL, fascia lata; F/U, follow-up period; R, rectus.

Table 57.2. *Complications of autologous slings**

Author	De novo storage symptoms (%)	Voiding dysfunction	Other complications
Kaufman[2]	–	Obstruction 33% Excision 7%	–
Schultz-Lampel et al.[3]	0	–	–
Loughlin[4]	6	Transient retention 23%	–
Mason & Roach[5]	–	Obstruction 3% Excision 2%	DVT 2%
Zaragoza[6]	12	–	–
Siegel et al.[7]	–	Lysis 30%	–
Carr et al.[8]	–	Obstruction 3% Excision 1%	–
Barbalias et al.[9]	0	–	–
Chaikin et al.[10]	8	–	Bladder perforation 1%
Maheshkumar et al.[11]	–	CIC 42% Incision 5%	–
Hassouna & Ghoniem[12]	21	0	Pain 25%
Kane et al.[13]	8	Dilation 8%	Wound infection 15%
Morgan et al.[14]	7	Lysis 2%	–
Kochakarn et al.[15]	5	Mean CIC time = 8.9 wks 39%	Wound infection 1%
Groutz et al.[16]	10	–	–
Kuo[17]	8	Lysis 4%	Subcutaneous hematoma 8%
Borup & Nielsen[18]	13	Obstruction 16% Lysis 3%	Sling erosion 8%
Gormley et al.[19]	–	–	–
De Rossi[20]	7	–	Bladder perforation 14%
Lucas et al.[21]	43	CIC 8%	–
Chou et al.[22]	4	Lysis 1%	–
Pfitzenmaier et al.[23]	–	–	–
Almeida et al.[24]	–	–	–
Rodrigues et al.[25]	–	Obstruction 11%	–
Kreder & Austin[26]	12	Long-term CIC 7%	Thigh hematoma 4%
Golomb et al.[27]	5	Refractory urge 6%	
Haab et al.[28]	27	Refractory urge 24% CIC 3%	–
Wright et al.[29]	10	Lysis 3%	–
Petrou & Frank[30]	0	Long-term CIC 7%	–
Richter et al.[31]	–	High PVR 16% CIC 7%	–
Flynn & Yap[32]	5	Lysis 1%	–
Chien et al.[33]	–	–	–
Low[34]	–	–	UVF 8%

cont.

Table 57.2. ***Complications of autologous slings* (cont.)***

Author	De novo storage symptoms (%)	Voiding dysfunction	Other complications
Addison et al.[35]	–	Obstruction 6%	Bladder perforation 8% Wound infection 2% PE 1%
Beck et al.[36]	–	Lysis 3%	Wound infection 5% FL hematoma 1% Seroma 4% PE 1% DVT %
Karram & Bhatia[37]	–	–	–
Govier et al.[38]	14	Lysis 3%	Leg pain 3%
Berman & Kreder[39]	–	–	Leg hematoma 14%
Phelps et al.[40]	–	Retention/lysis 3% CIC 2%	
Latini et al.[41]	–	–	–
Ellerkmann et al.[42]	–	–	–

* Limited to studies with minimum of 12 months' follow-up. Adapted from ref. 97.
CIC, clean intermittent catheterization; De novo storage symptoms (%), percentage of patients with de novo storage symptoms (i.e. urgency, frequency, urge incontinence); DVT, deep vein thrombosis; FL, fascia lata; Incision, sling incision; Lysis, urethrolysis; PE, pulmonary embolism; PVR, post-void residual; UVF, urethrovaginal fistula.

Cadaveric fascia lata (CFL) debuted as a sling material in the mid 1990s. Not all cadaveric fascia lata is the same. A major source of variability in CFL originates from its technique of processing, either solvent dehydration and gamma irradiation (Tutoplast®) or freeze-drying (tissue banks and FasLata®). Freeze-dried CFL has been implicated as a cause for suture pull-through and immediate failure.[67] Recent studies offer conflicting results regarding whether the method of processing and sterilization structurally weakens tissue. While one study found no statistical difference in tissue thickness or maximum load to failure between freeze-dried CFL, solvent-dehydrated CFL, and acellular cadaveric dermis, another suggested that freeze-dried CFL was less stiff and had a significantly lower maximum load to failure.[68,69] The issue of tissue processing and how it affects tissue strength and longevity is still under investigation, and no consensus exists.

Although many series find results similar to autologous slings in the short-term, newer published allograft sling outcomes suggest an early failure rate (Table 57.3). Fitzgerald et al. reported failure rates as high as 20% within 3 months of surgery with allograft slings.[70] When they reoperated on eight women for persistent or recurrent SUI after allograft sling, the original graft was absent in 14% and degenerated in 6%, suggesting autolysis. Other authors subsequently published failure rates of 28–38% and their observation of similar findings at re-exploration.[59,71,72] Recently, a series of intermediate-term CFL sling failures has been published, prompting significant concern.[73] Freeze-dried CFL was implicated more often than other types of processing. No standardization of processing, sterilization, and packaging of allografts exists. Mechanisms of failure and the factors responsible for early allograft loss are not known, but may include the processing technique leading to destabilization of structural integrity of the material, contamination/infection by vaginal flora, host versus graft reaction, accelerated immunity or autolysis.

Tissue rejection remains a concern with the non-autologous tissues but has not specifically been reported to date. Since inflammation is difficult to distinguish from rejection without the use of specific tissue staining, it is not yet clear whether true rejection after allograft implant occurs. The concern of disease transmission from an allograft sling remains a real threat. DNA has been detected in freeze-dried CFL, solvent-dehydrated CFL, and acellular dermis, but to date there has been no reported cases of disease transmission. All cadaveric tissues undergo serologic screening for human immunodeficiency virus (HIV) and hepatitis B, but false-negative results are possible. The risk of HIV transmission from a frozen allograft has been estimated to be 1 in 8 million, while the risk of developing CJD is approximately 1 in 3.5 million.[44,74] It is not known whether the genetic material found in these allografts is transmissible or poses any long-term health risk. In 1985, HIV was transmitted

Table 57.3. ***Results of allograft slings****

Author	Material	Processing	No. of patients	Sling length (cm)	Mean F/U (months)	Cure (%)
Elliott & Boone[48]	CFL	SD	26	12	15	76.9
Amundsen et al.[49]	CFL	FD	91	15	19.4	62.6
Brown & Govier[50]	CFL	FD	104	24	12	66.3
Vereecken & Lechat[51]	CFL	FD	8	>20	24	100
Walsh et al.[52]	CFL	FD	31	10	13.5	93.5
Flynn & Yap[32]	CFL	FD	63	12	29	87.3
Chien et al.[33]	CFL	–	83	10	27.4	90.1
Bodell & Leach[53]	CFL	SD	186	7	16.4	75.8
Richter et al.[54]	CFL	FD	102	25	35	75
Phelps et al.[40]	CFL	–	36	>20	20	83.3
Hartanto et al.[55]	CFL	–	34	7	12.5	83.3
Almeida et al.[24]	CFL	FD	30	6–8	36	40
Gurdal et al.[56]	CFL	SD	42	4	16	88
Park et al.[57]	CFL	FD	60	20	>36	85
Fitzgerald et al.[58]	CFL	FD	27	–	12	59
Ellerkmann et al.[42]	CFL	SD	32	>24	>24	90.5
Soergel et al.[59†]	CFL	FD	12	10	6	33.3
Crivellaro et al.[60]	CAD	Repliform®	253	4	18	78
Wang et al.[61]	CAD	Repliform®	111	–	36	95
Chung et al.[62]	CAD	–	18	3 × 7	28	89.5
Owens & Winters[63]	CAD	DuraDerm®	24	12	14.8	32

† This study reported 6-month follow-up of the autologous slings, but only short-term follow-up for the allografts. It is noteworthy for its high allograft failure rate within the first 3 months.
Adapted from ref. 97.
CAD, cadaveric dermis; CFL, cadaveric fascia lata; Cure (%), percentage of patients cured; FD, freeze-dried; F/U, follow-up period; SD, solvent-dehydrated.

from a bone allograft from a tissue donor seronegative for HIV.[75,76] More sophisticated donor screening has since been developed and has decreased the risk of seronegative transmission.

Bacterial infections are a rare complication of allografts; however, after the reported death of a 23-year-old male recipient of an allograft contaminated with Clostridim, the Centers for Disease Control investigated and identified 26 other cases of allograft-associated infections.[77] A case of invasive disease with *Streptococcus pyogenes* after reconstructive knee surgery using contaminated allograft tissue was reported in 2003.[78]

Tissue processing and sterilization differs among tissue banks, and clearly there is a need for improved tissue evaluation and processing standards. A questionnaire-based study regarding allograft acquisition in 340 hospitals in the United States revealed that in approximately 85% of the institutions, those responsible for providing surgeons with the allografts had little or no knowledge of the practices of tissue banking and allograft transplantation biology.[79] The surgeon was involved in the selection of the source of allografts in only 15% of hospitals. Given the recognition of the risk of disease transmission, it has become wise, if not imperative, for the surgeons who use allografts to be actively involved in determining the source and processing of the grafts they place in patients.

Cadaveric acellular dermal allografts are an additional biologic alternative to CFL. In this tissue, epidermal and dermal cellular elements are removed, leaving basement membrane behind to act as a framework into which the patient's own cells can grow. Acellular dermis has been shown in animal studies to integrate into tissue consistently without any foreign body reaction. Additionally, it persists up to 6 months after implantation and shows evidence of extensive cellular infiltration and neovascularization. A potential risk of hair follicle and sebaceous gland ingrowth does exist, as does the risk of disease transmission from this material. Several acellular dermal allografts are commercially available as slings: Alloderm™, Repliform®, and Dermal Allograft®. Mechanical load-to-failure testing demonstrates dermal allografts to be strong and to perform in a similar fashion to autologous tissues. To date, there are very few clinical data on the use of cadaveric dermis for sling surgery[60–63] (see Table 57.3).

In a prospective series of 253 patients treated with a human dermal allograft sling and bone anchors, Crivellaro et al. demonstrated a 57% dry rate in type II SUI and a 55% dry rate in type III SUI at 18 months.[60] Overall cured and improved rate was 78%. Wang et al. observed a 95% cured and improved rate in 111 patients treated with a dermal allograft sling at 36 months.[61] In a study examining outcomes of cadaveric dermis for combined cystocele and sling surgery, 16 of 18 patients were cured at 28 months, and one patient experienced graft infection and failure.[62] Conversely, Owens and Winters found disappointing results with dermal allograft slings.[63] At 14.8 months follow-up, only 32% of patients were dry; 24% of the failures occurred within 6–14 months postoperatively. Of the eight failures, one opted to undergo an autologous sling. At the time of her surgery, the graft was almost completely absent without evidence of infection or excessive inflammation. Their finding suggests that the material fails, not because of rejection or infection, but because host infiltration either does not occur or does not occur at a fast enough rate to make the graft permanent.

Complication rates are similar to those seen with other sling materials (Table 57.4). Two recent reports of vaginal erosion after dermal allograft slings are the first with these materials.[80] The cause of the graft erosion in these cases is not clear. Pathologic examination of the graft material was not specific for rejection or inflammation.

Although short-term outcomes have been equivalent to those in autologous slings, newer data call into question the durability of allografts. Outcomes data remain limited, particularly in allografts other than CFL, so it is difficult to draw conclusions, but cadaveric dermal allografts reflect short- and medium-term outcomes similar to cadaveric fascia. The mechanisms of failure with allografts need further elucidation. Host factors may play as big as or a bigger role than tissue processing in failure rates. As Owens and Winters point out in the discussion of their series of intermediate-term dermal

Table 57.4. ***Complications of allograft slings****

Author	De novo storage symptoms (%)	Voiding dysfunction	Other complications
Elliott & Boone[48]	13	–	–
Amundsen et al.[49]	44	Lysis 1%	–
Brown & Gover[50]	–	Long-term retention 2%	–
Vereecken & Lechat[51]	13	Lysis 13%	–
Walsh et al.[52]	–	CIC at 1 year 3%	–
Flynn & Yap[32]	28	Retention 2%	–
Chien et al.[33]	–	–	–
Bodell & Leach[53]	–	–	Osteitis 1%
Richter et al.[54]	–	Impaired emptying 58%	–
Phelps et al.[40]	–	Lysis 3% CIC 2%	–
Hartanto et al.[55]	–	–	–
Almeida et al.[24]	–	–	–
Gurdal et al.[56]	–	CIC for mean of 20 days 12%	–
Park et al.[57]	5	Elevated PVR at 30 days 5% CIC for 1 month 2%	Bladder perforation 2% Blood transfusion 7%
Crivellaro et al.[60]	5.5	Prolonged catheterization 2%	Vaginal infection 1.7%

* Limited to studies with minimum of 12 months' follow-up. Adapted from ref. 97.
CIC, clean intermittent catheterization; De novo storage symptoms (%), percentage of patients with de novo storage symptoms (i.e. urgency, frequency, urge incontinence); PVR, post-void residual.

allograft sling failures,[63] the scarification of the sling into proper position is not the major factor for long-term success with these materials. The apparent rapid degradation of the sling and failure of host remodeling must be explained. As part of informed consent, patients undergoing allograft sling procedures should be told of data suggesting intermediate failures that do not appear to occur with autologous tissues, the lack of long-term data, and the possibility of disease transmission.

The benefits of allograft may only be relevant in a select group of patients unwilling or unable to undergo a fascial harvest, yet not all outcomes are poor. Results of the cadaveric prolapse repair and sling (CAPS), which uses cadaveric fascia lata for the simultaneous repair of a cystocele and placement of a pubovaginal sling by means of a transvaginal approach, continue to show promise.[81] At a maximum of 28 months' follow-up (mean 12.4 months), only 9.8% had recurrent or de novo apical vaginal prolapse. Only 24 of the 132 patients (18.2%) had stress incontinence of any degree.

XENOGRAFTS

The term xenograft refers to the sling material originating from an organism of a different species (non-human). The first animal tissue for urologic use was a porcine corium treated with proteolytic enzymes to remove non-collagenous material. Additional cross-linking of the collagen with glutaraldehyde was needed to reduce antigenicity and then the product was freeze-dried and sterilized with gamma irradiation. Commercially available porcine corium today (DermMatrix™, Pelvicol™, InteXen™) is cross-linked by diisocyanate which is non-toxic and causes no graft mineralization as can occur after cross-linking with glutaraldehyde. Published series of xenograft outcomes are scarce[46,82–86] (Table 57.5). In one study, Nicholson and Brown cured 79% of 24 patients with a porcine dermis sling at a mean follow-up of over 48 months.[83] Thirteen percent of these patients developed urinary retention more than 1 year postoperatively. No cases of sling extrusion or erosion were reported. Porcine dermis has been used at the midurethra with a cure rate of 89% at 12 months.[87] Complications included de novo storage symptoms in 6% and urethral obstruction in 7%. Porcine dermis is the only xenograft with long-term follow-up and randomized comparison to other sling alternatives.[84] In a randomized comparison of Pelvicol™ pubovaginal slings and tension-free vaginal tape (TVT) synthetic midurethral slings in 142 women, results and complication rates were similar at a median follow-up of 12 months. The patient-determined cure rate was 85% in the TVT group and 89% in the Pelvicol™ group. Rates of postoperative voiding dysfunction and de novo urge incontinence were 3.4% and 9% in the TVT group, and 1.4% and 6% in the Pelvicol™ group, respectively.

While rejection has not been reported with porcine dermis, reports of its unpredictable tissue response exist. Cole and colleagues encountered encapsulation of a porcine dermis sling noted at reoperation for retention, 4 months postoperatively.[88] Although the material is meant to act as a scaffold for the ingrowth of native tissue, the encapsulated porcine sling was completely acellular without any host tissue proliferation. Gandhi and colleagues observed a trend toward porcine graft preservation in eight women with persistent urinary retention at up to 42 weeks postoperatively.[89] The histology of the slings removed demonstrated minimal tissue remodeling, and collagen deposition was present only on the periphery of the sling. Inflammation and foreign body reaction were seen in half of the specimens. In women undergoing reoperation for recurrent SUI, the porcine slings were difficult to identify and histologically the graft material was absent. These findings suggest that porcine dermis is in fact immunogenic. Further studies of the long-term tissue characteristics of implanted porcine dermis are needed.

Table 57.5. ***Results of xenograft slings****

Author	Material	No. of patients	Sling length (cm)	Mean F/U (months)	Cure (%)
Jarvis & Fowlie[46]	PD	50	–	21	82
Iosif[82]	PD	53	30	18–48	88.7
Nicholson & Brown[83]	PD	24	–	49	79.2
Arunkalaivanan & Barrington[84]	PD	74	10–12	12	89
Rutner et al.[85]	SIS	115	–	36	94
Pelosi et al.[86]	BP	22	9	20	95

* Limited to studies with minimum of 12 months' follow-up. Adapted from ref. 97.
BP, bovine pericardium; Cure (%), percentage of patients cured; F/U, follow-up period; PD, porcine dermis; SIS, porcine small intestine submucosa.

Porcine SIS is another animal tissue that has recently been marketed for pubovaginal sling use (STRATASIS®). It is harvested from small intestine and the extracellular collagen matrix remains intact. In theory, through the preservation of collagen, growth factors, glycosaminoglycans, proteoglycans, and glycoproteins, host cells may proliferate through the SIS layers, remodeling and replacing these with host connective tissue. SIS has been used in urologic surgery for urethroplasty, Peyronie's plaque excision, and ureteral interposition. The tensile strength of SIS has been challenged by a report of the mean suture pull-through load of freeze-dried SIS being less than that of freeze-dried CFL.[90] Immunogenicity is also a potential concern. Biopsies of SIS slings at reoperation for recurrent SUI found no evidence of inflammation or foreign body reaction at 9, 12, and 17 months, but other investigators have found evidence to the contrary.[91] Two small series of the use of 8-ply SIS tension-free slings describe the development of erythema and inflammation at the suprapubic incisions after implantation.[92,93]

Another xenograft – bovine pericardium – is available in several preparations. The UroPatch™, a purified and detoxified bovine pericardium cross-linked with glutaraldehyde, has shown a 95% cure rate at a mean follow-up of 20 months in a small series of bone anchored slings.[86] A second preparation of the bovine pericardium is a non-cross-linked, propylene oxide-treated, acellular collagen matrix marketed as Veritas™ Collagen Matrix. This tissue is reportedly thinner than freeze-dried or solvent-dehydrated CFL, but possesses greater tensile strength.[94] DNA has been identified within the bovine pericardium, but the amount is less than that found in either freeze-dried or solvent-dehydrated CFL, or cadaveric dermis. As with the other tissues, it is not known whether this DNA is transmissible. Two recent Brazilian studies reported rejections of bovine pericardium in 11 of a combined 15 patients. In all cases, vaginal extrusion and wound dehiscence necessitated sling removal.[95,96]

While all of the available xenografts claim biocompatibility, excellent tensile strength, lack of immunogenicity, and lack of viruses or prions, clinical outcomes suggest that these claims must be strongly scrutinized when considering a xenograft as a sling material. To date, only porcine dermis and 4-ply SIS have shown non-immunogenicity. Porcine dermis is also the only xenograft to have sufficient reports of long-term efficacy.

CONCLUSIONS

Pubovaginal slings remain a reliable surgical procedure for the correction of all forms of SUI, but not all sling materials produce equivalent results. The classic autologous fascial sling can be relied upon to provide a cure rate of 84% or better. Complications related to fascial harvest are possible but acceptable. Outcomes and complications associated with the use of cadaveric and animal tissues are less predictable. Sling surgery with most alternative biologic materials produces short-term success rates comparable to autologous fascia. Rates of postoperative voiding dysfunction and urinary retention also appear similar.

Allografts and xenografts undoubtedly shorten operative times and obviate the morbidity of fascial harvest, but these shortcuts may be costly in the long term. Current literature points to higher risks of early failure and immunogenicity leading to rejection and poor tissue healing. DNA of unclear transmissibility has been isolated in several sling products including CFL, cadaveric dermis, and bovine pericardium.

With so many available sling options, it is imperative that the surgeon be familiar with the nature, behavior, and outcomes of the sling materials as well as the complications of the procedure itself. Patients must be counseled preoperatively and informed consent must include information regarding the sling material to be used.

Further studies into the long-term behavior of allografts and xenografts in the vaginal environment are needed to clarify the efficacy and safety of these materials for the correction of SUI.

REFERENCES

1. Leach GE, Dmochowski RR, Appell RA et al. Female Stress Urinary Incontinence Clinical Guidelines Panel summary report on the surgical management of female stress urinary incontinence. The American Urologic Association. J Urol 1997;158:875–80.
2. Kaufman JM. Fascial sling for stress urinary incontinence. South Med J 1982;75:55–8.
3. Schultz-Lampel D, Fleig P, Hohenfellner M et al. Long term results of surgery for stress urinary incontinence in females: Burch colposuspension and fascial sling procedure. J Urol 1995;153(Suppl):525A [abstract 1185].
4. Loughlin KR. The endoscopic fascial sling for treatment of female urinary stress incontinence. J Urol 1996;155:1265–7.
5. Mason RC, Roach M. Modified pubovaginal sling for treatment of intrinsic sphincteric deficiency. J Urol 1996;156:1991–4.
6. Zaragoza MR. Expanded indications for the pubovaginal sling: treatment of type 2 or 3 stress incontinence. J Urol 1996;156:1620–2.
7. Siegel SB, Allison S, Foster HE. Long term results of

pubovaginal sling for stress urinary incontinence. J Urol 1997;157(Suppl):460A.

8. Carr LK, Walsh PJ, Abraham VE et al. Favorable outcome of pubovaginal slings for geriatric women with stress incontinence. J Urol 1997;157:125–8.
9. Barbalias G, Liatsikos E, Barbalias D. Use of slings made of indigenous and allogenic material (Goretex) in type III urinary incontinence and comparison between them. Eur Urol 1997;31:394–400.
10. Chaikin DC, Rosenthal J, Blaivas JG. Pubovaginal fascial sling for all types of stress urinary incontinence: long-term analysis. J Urol 1998;160:1312–6.
11. Maheshkumar P, Ramsay IN, Conn IG. A randomized trial of 'dynamic' versus 'static' rectus fascial suburethral sling: early results. Br J Urol 1998;81(Suppl 4):65 [abstract 169].
12. Hassouna ME, Ghoniem GM. Long-term outcome and quality of life after modified pubovaginal sling for intrinsic sphincter deficiency. Urology 1999;53:287–91.
13. Kane L, Chung T, Lawrie H et al. The pubofascial anchor sling procedure for recurrent genuine urinary stress incontinence. BJU Int 1999;83:1010–4.
14. Morgan TO, Westney OL, McGuire EJ. Pubovaginal sling: 4-year outcome analysis and quality of life assessment. J Urol 2000;163:1845–8.
15. Kochakarn W, Leenanupunth C, Ratana-Olarn K et al. Pubovaginal sling for the treatment of female stress urinary incontinence: experience of 100 cases at Ramathibodi Hospital. J Med Assoc Thai 2001;84:1412–5.
16. Groutz A, Blaivas JG, Hyman MJ et al. Pubovaginal sling surgery for simple stress urinary incontinence: analysis by an outcome score. J Urol 2001;165:1597–1600.
17. Kuo HC. Comparison of video urodynamic results after the pubovaginal sling procedure using rectus fascia and polypropylene mesh for stress urinary incontinence. J Urol 2001;165:163–8.
18. Borup K, Nielsen JB. Results in 32 women operated on for genuine stress incontinence with the pubovaginal sling procedure ad modum Ed McGuire. Scand J Urol Nephrol 2002;36:128–33.
19. Gormley EA, Latini J, Hanlon L. Long-term effect of pubovaginal sling on quality of life. J Urol 2002;167(Suppl):105 [abstract 418].
20. De Rossi P. Clinical outcome of fascial slings for stress incontinence. Medscape Women's Health 2002;7:1–8.
21. Lucas MG, Giannitsas KL, Warelam K et al. A randomized controlled trial comparing two techniques of tension free autologous fascial sling for surgical treatment of genuine stress incontinence in women. J Urol 2003;169(Suppl):123 [abstract 477].
22. Chou EC, Flisser AJ, Panagopoulos G et al. Effective treatment for mixed urinary incontinence with a pubovaginal sling. J Urol 2003;170:494–7.
23. Pfitzenmaier J, Gilfrich C, Faldum A et al. [Does a combined fascial sling–Burch colposuspension display advantages over a fascial sling alone for treatment of urinary stress incontinence in females?] Akt Urol 2003;34:166–71.
24. Almeida SHM, Gregorio E, Grando JPS et al. Pubovaginal sling using cadaveric allograft fascia for the treatment of female urinary incontinence. Transplant Proc 2004;36:995–6.
25. Rodrigues P, Hering F, Meler A et al. Pubo-fascial versus vaginal sling operation for the treatment of stress urinary incontinence: a prospective study. Neurourol Urodyn 2004;23:627–31.
26. Kreder KJ, Austin CA. Treatment of stress urinary incontinence in women with urethral hypermobility and intrinsic sphincter deficiency. J Urol 1996;156:1995–8.
27. Golomb J, Shenfield O, Shelhav A et al. Suspended pubovaginal fascial sling for the correction of complicated stress urinary incontinence. Eur Urol 1997;32:170–4.
28. Haab F, Trockman BA, Zimmern PE et al. Results of pubovaginal sling for the treatment of intrinsic sphincter deficiency determined by questionnaire analysis. J Urol 1997;158:1738–41.
29. Wright EJ, Iselin CE, Carr LK et al. Pubovaginal sling using cadaveric allograft fascia for the treatment of intrinsic sphincter deficiency. J Urol 1998;160:759–62.
30. Petrou SP, Frank I. Complications and initial continence rates after a repeat pubovaginal sling procedure for recurrent stress urinary incontinence. J Urol 2001;165:1979–81.
31. Richter HE, Varner E, Sanders E et al. Effects of pubovaginal sling procedure on patients with urethral hypermobility and intrinsic sphincter deficiency: Would they do it again? Am J Obstet Gynecol 2001;184:14–9.
32. Flynn BJ, Yap WT. Pubovaginal sling using allograft fascia lata versus autograft fascia for all types of stress urinary incontinence: 2-year minimum follow-up. J Urol 2002;167:608–12.
33. Chien GW, Tawadroas M, Kaptein JS et al. Surgical treatment for stress urinary incontinence with urethral hypermobility. What is the best approach? World J Urol 2002;20:234–9.
34. Low JA. Management of severe anatomic deficiencies of urethral sphincter function by a combined procedure with a fascia lata sling. Am J Obstet Gynecol 1969;105:149–55.
35. Addison WA, Haygood V, Parker RT. Recurrent stress urinary incontinence. Obstet Gynecol Annu 1985;14:254–65.
36. Beck RP, McCormick S, Nordstrom L. The fascia lata sling procedure for treating recurrent genuine stress incontinence of urine. Obstet Gynecol 1988;72:699–703.
37. Karram MM, Bhatia NN. Patch procedure: modified

transvaginal fascia lata sling for recurrent or severe stress urinary incontinence. Obstet Gynecol 1990;75:461–3.

38. Govier FE, Gibbons RP, Correa RJ et al. Pubovaginal slings using fascia lata for the treatment of intrinsic sphincter deficiency. J Urol 1997;157:117–21.

39. Berman CJ, Kreder KJ. Comparative cost analysis of collagen injection and fascia lata sling cystourethropexy for the treatment of type III incontinence in women. J Urol 1997;157:122–4.

40. Phelps J, Lin L, Liu C. Laparoscopic suburethral sling procedure. J Am Assoc Gynecol Laparosc 2003;10:496–500.

41. Latini JM, Lux MM, Kreder KJ. Efficacy and morbidity of autologous fascia lata sling cystourethropexy. J Urol 2004;171:1180–4.

42. Ellerkmann RM, McBride AW, Bent AE et al. Comparison of long-term outcomes of autologous fascia lata slings to Suspend Tutoplast™ fascia lata allograft slings for stress incontinence. J Pelvic Med Surg 2004;10(Suppl 1):S28 [oral poster 38].

43. Webster TM, Gerridzen RG. Urethral erosion following autologous rectus fascial sling. Can J Urol 2003;10:2068–9.

44. Dora CD, Dimarco DS, Zobitz ME et al. Time dependent variations in biomechanical properties of cadaveric fascia, porcine dermis, porcine small intestine submucosa, polypropylene mesh and autologous fascia in the rabbit model: implications for sling surgery. J Urol 2004;171:1970–3.

45. Kainer MA, Linden JV, Whaley DN et al. Clostridium infections associated with musculoskeletal-tissue allografts. N Engl J Med 2004;350:2564–71.

46. Jarvis GJ, Fowlie A. Clinical and urodynamic assessment of the porcine dermis bladder sling in the treatment of genuine stress incontinence. Br J Obstet Gynaecol 1985;92:1189–91.

47. Handa VL, Jensen JK, Germain MM et al. Banked human fascia lata for the suburethral sling procedure: a preliminary report. Obstet Gynecol 1996;88:1045–9.

48. Elliott DS, Boone TB. Is fascia lata allograft material trustworthy for pubovaginal sling repair? Urology 2000;56:772–6.

49. Amundsen CL, Visco AG, Ruiz H et al. Outcome in 104 pubovaginal slings using freeze-dried allograft fascia lata from a single tissue bank. Urology 2000;56(Suppl 6A):2–8.

50. Brown SL, Govier FE. Cadaveric versus autologous fascia lata for the pubovaginal sling: Surgical outcome and patient satisfaction. J Urol 2000;164:1633–7.

51. Vereecken RL, Lechat A. Cadaver fascia lata sling in the treatment of intrinsic sphincter weakness. Urol Int 2001;67:232–4.

52. Walsh IK, Nambirajan T, Donellan SM et al. Cadaveric fascia lata pubovaginal slings: early results on safety, efficacy, and patient satisfaction. BJU Int 2002;90:415–9.

53. Bodell DM, Leach GE. Update on the results of the cadaveric transvaginal sling (CATS). J Urol 2002;167(Suppl):78 [abstract 308].

54. Richter HE, Burgio KL, Holley RL et al. Cadaveric fascia lata sling for stress urinary incontinence: a prospective quality-of-life analysis. Am J Obstet Gynecol 2003;189:1590–6.

55. Hartanto VH, DiPiazza D, Ankem MK et al. Comparison of recovery from postoperative pain utilizing two sling techniques. Can J Urol 2003;10:1759–63.

56. Gurdal M, Tekin A, Huri E et al. Pubovaginal sling using cadaveric allograft fascia for all types of stress urinary incontinence. XIXth European Association of Urology Congress, March 25, 2004; Abstract 317.

57. Park S, Kim S, Choo M et al. Long term follow-up result of pubovaginal sling with cadaveric fascia lata in the management of female stress urinary incontinence. XIXth European Association of Urology Congress, March 25, 2004; Abstract 319.

58. Fitzgerald MP, Edwards SR, Fenner D. Medium-term follow-up on use of freeze-dried, irradiated donor fascia for sacrocolpopexy and sling procedures. Int Urogynecol J Pelvic Floor Dysfunct 2004;15:238–42.

59. Soergel TM, Shott S, Heit M. Poor surgical outcomes after fascia lata allograft slings. Int Urogynecol J 2001;12:247–53.

60. Crivellaro S, Smith JJ, Kocjancic E et al. Transvaginal sling using acellular human dermal allograft: safety and efficacy in 253 patients. J Urol 2004;172:1374–8.

61. Wang D, Bresette JF, Smith JJ. Initial experience with acellular human dermal allograft (Repliform®) pubovaginal sling for stress urinary incontinence. J Pelvic Med Surg 2004;10:23–6.

62. Chung SY, Franks M, Smith CP, Lee JY, Lu SH, Chancellor M. Technique of combined pubovaginal sling and cystocele repair using a single piece of cadaveric dermal graft. Urology 2002;59(4):538–41.

63. Owens DC, Winters JC. Pubovaginal sling using Duraderm graft: intermediate follow-up and patient satisfaction. Neurourol Urodyn 2004;23:115–8.

64. Rottenberg RD, Weil A, Brioschi PA et al. Urodynamic and clinical assessment of the Lyodura sling operation for urinary stress incontinence. Br J Obstet Gynaecol 1985;92:829–34.

65. Enzelsberger H, Helmer H, Schatten C. Comparison of Burch and Lyodura sling procedures for repair of unsuccessful incontinence surgery. Obstet Gynecol 1996;88:251–6.

66. Liscic RM, Brinar V, Miklic P et al. Creutzfeldt–Jakob disease in a patient with a lyophilized dura mater graft. Acta Med Croatica 1999;53:93–6.

67. Chaikin DC, Blaivas JG. Weakened cadaveric fascial sling: an unexpected cause of failure. J Urol 1998;160:2151.

68. Sutaria PM, Staskin D. A comparison of fascial 'pull

through' strength using four different suture fixation techniques. J Urol 1999;161(Suppl 4):79–80.

69. Lemer ML, Chaikin DC, Blaivas JG. Tissue strength analysis of autologous and cadaveric allografts for the pubovaginal sling. Neurourol Urodyn 1999;18:497–503.

70. Fitzgerald MP, Mollenhauer J, Brubaker L. Failure of allograft suburethral slings. BJU Int 1999;84:785–8.

71. Carbone JM, Kavaler E, Hu J et al. Pubovaginal sling using cadaveric fascia and bone anchors: disappointing early results. J Urol 2001;165:1605–11.

72. Huang YH, Lin ATL, Chen KK et al. High failure rate using allograft fascia lata in pubovaginal sling surgery for female stress urinary incontinence. Urology 2001;58:943–6.

73. O'Reilly KJ, Govier FE. Intermediate term failure of pubovaginal slings using cadaveric fascia lata: a case series. J Urol 2002;167:1356–8.

74. Buck BE, Malinin TI. Human bone and tissue allografts: preparation and safety. Clin Orthop 1994;303:8–17.

75. Simonds RJ, Holmberg SD, Hurwitz RL et al. Transmission of human immunodeficiency virus type 1 from a seronegative organ and tissue donor. N Engl J Med 1992;326:726–32.

76. Tomford WW. Transmission of disease through transplantation of musculoskeletal allografts. J Bone Joint Surg 1995;77:1742–54.

77. Update: allograft-associated bacterial infections – United States 2002. MMWR Morb Mortal Wkly Rep 2002;15:207–10.

78. Centers for Disease Control and Prevention (CDC). Invasive Streptococcus pyogenes after allograft implantation – Colorado, 2003. MMWR Morb Mortal Wkly Rep 2003;52:1174–6.

79. Lavernia CJ, Malinin TI, Temple T et al. Bone and tissue allograft use by orthopedic surgeons. J Arthroplasty 2004;19:430–5.

80. Bradley CS, Morgan MA, Arya LA et al. Vaginal erosion after pubovaginal sling procedures using dermal allografts. J Urol 2003;169:286–7.

81. Kobashi KC, Leach GE, Chon J et al. Continued multicenter follow-up of cadaveric prolapse repair with sling. J Urol 2002;168:2063–9.

82. Iosif CS. Porcine corium sling in the treatment of urinary stress incontinence. Arch Gynecol 1987;240:131–6.

83. Nicholson SC, Brown ADG. The long-term success of abdominovaginal sling operations for genuine stress incontinence and a cystocele: a questionnaire-based study. J Obstet Gynaecol 2001;21:162–5.

84. Arunkalaivanan AS, Barrington JW. Randomized trial of porcine dermal sling (Pelvicol™ implant) vs. tension-free vaginal tape (TVT) in the surgical treatment of stress incontinence: a questionnaire-based study. Int Urogynecol J 2003;14:7–23.

85. Rutner AB, Levine SR, Schmaelzle JF. Porcine small intestinal submucosa implanted as a pubovaginal sling in 115 female patients with stress urinary incontinence: A 3 year series evaluated for durability of the results. Society for Urology and Engineering, 17th Annual Meeting, 2002.

86. Pelosi MA II, Pelosi MA III, Pelekanos M. The YAMA Uro-Patch sling for treatment of female stress urinary incontinence: a pilot study. J Lap Adv Surg Tech 2002;12:27–33.

87. Barrington JW, Edwards AS, Arunkalaivanan AS et al. The use of porcine dermal implant in a minimally invasive pubovaginal sling procedure for genuine stress incontinence. BJU Int 2002;90:224–7.

88. Cole E, Gomelsky A, Dmochowski RR. Encapsulation of a porcine dermis pubovaginal sling. J Urol 2003;170:1950.

89. Gandhi S, Kubba LA, Abramov Y et al. Histopathologic changes of porcine dermal implants used for transvaginal suburethral slings. J Pelvic Med Surg 2004;10(Suppl 1): S12 [paper 29].

90. Kubricht WS, Williams BJ, Eastham JA et al. Tensile strength of cadaveric fascia lata compared to small intestinal submucosa using suture pull through analysis. J Urol 2001;165:486–90.

91. Wiedemann A, Otto M. Small intestinal submucosa for pubourethral sling suspension for the treatment of stress incontinence: first histopathological results in humans. J Urol 2004;172:215–8.

92. Ho KLV, Wittie MN, Bird ET. 8-Ply small intestinal submucosa tension-free sling: spectrum of postoperative inflammation. J Urol 2004;171:268–71.

93. Dalota SJ. Small intestinal submucosa tension-free sling. Postoperative inflammatory reactions and additional data. J Urol 2004;172:1349–50.

94. Oray NB, Lambert A, Wonsetler R et al. Physical and biochemical characterization of a novel non-crosslinked, propylene-oxide treated acellular collagen matrix: comparison with solvent-extracted and freeze-dried cadaveric fascia lata. Society for Urology and Engineering, 17th Annual Meeting, 2002.

95. Martucci RC, Ambrogini A, Calada AA et al. Pubovaginal sling with bovine pericardium for treatment of stress urinary incontinence. Braz J Urol 2000;26:208–14.

96. Candido EB, Triginelli SA, Siva FAL. The use of bovine pericardium in the pubovaginal sling for the treatment of stress urinary incontinence. Rev Bras Ginecol Obstet 2003;25:525–8.

97. Gomelsky A, Scarpero HM, Dmochowski RR. Sling surgery for stress urinary incontinence in the female: what surgery, which material? AUA Update Series 2003;XXII(Lesson 34):266–76.

58

Urethral injections for incontinence

Rodney A Appell

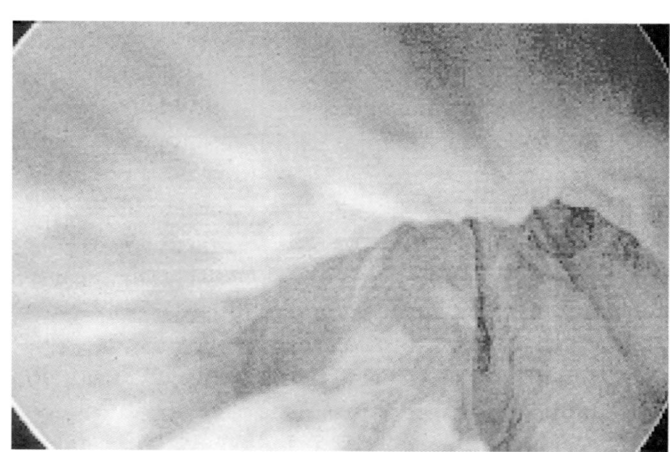

INTRODUCTION

Emphasis on minimally invasive options for the surgical treatment of incontinence (both stress and urge types) has resulted in the development of agents and techniques that improve these conditions substantially towards social continence, but, at this time, suboptimal cure/dry rates. The application of injectable therapy as an office procedure implies the potential for cost-efficient treatment for selected patients with urinary incontinence.

Continuous advancements in materials technology have provided the possibility that multiple new urethral bulking agents will soon be available. Experience continues to accrue in clinical trials for urethral bulking with these agents while parallel utilization for the indication of pediatric vesicourethral reflux has also provided evidence of biologic activity related to these compounds. The agents that are closest to complete analysis are synthetic and represent a variety of material types and characteristics. As these materials evolve, understanding of preferential injection technique is also being gained. Delivery method and site may prove to alter the biologic activity of these compounds substantially.

Both stress urinary incontinence (SUI) and urge incontinence (UI) continue as an increasingly significant health concern for millions of women. According to recent estimates, approximately 180,000 surgical procedures are now performed for genuine stress urinary incontinence (GSUI) alone. The lack of one single, reproducible, permanent and yet minimal risk procedure has led to the development of several minimally invasive options that provide the hope of reasonable efficacy associated with minimal morbidity. Reimbursement trends have also placed an emphasis on interventions that require minimal hospitalization or, more optimally, can be performed entirely in the ambulatory office location without requirements for general or regional anesthesia and attendant recuperative facilities.

Injection therapy has been used sparingly for the management of SUI for nearly two decades, but has been limited by durability and antigenicity issues associated with bovine collagen. Recent Food and Drug Administration (FDA) approval of carbon particulate technology (Durasphere™) has provided another option for bulking, but one that had been somewhat limited by difficulty with the injection (due to carrier extrusion resulting in injection needle obstruction). Due to these concerns, many physicians would only use Durasphere™ in the controlled setting of the operative suite, thus detracting from the financial benefit associated with in-office bulking therapy. This was addressed by the manufacturer and an improved formulation (Durasphere EXP™) was introduced following FDA approval in October 2003, making its injection as easy as collagen. Therefore, the use of bulking therapy had been less than optimal to that date. However, the advent of several new bulking agents, each with unique tissue interaction characteristics and holding the promise of greater durability, with fewer actual injection sessions and no antigenicity, promises to dramatically alter the role of bulking therapy in the overall management schema for SUI. Selection of patients appears crucial to the outcome of the intraurethral injection of bulking agents. The ideal candidate for this procedure is one who has good anatomic support, a compliant stable bladder, and a malfunctioning urethra evidenced by a low leak point pressure.[1] Other subsets of patients who may benefit from the procedure are patients with high leak point pressure and minimal hypermobility, and elderly women with bladder base mobility who are less active and are a poor surgical risk for other interventions.

INJECTABLES FOR SUI

The successful use of periurethral bulking agents is dependent on several factors including the composition of the material, facility of agent use (ease of preparation and implantation), and a receptive host environment (optimized hormonal environment, integrity of urethral anatomic components, and intact periurethral fascia). Three categories of material have been investigated for periurethral bulking: human (autologous or allograft), xenograft, and synthetic.

The optimal attributes for bulking materials are:

- biocompatibility;
- minimal or no immunogenicity (hypoallergenic);
- integrity of the material formulation – there should be little or no separation of agent subcomponents (carrier and particulate solid);
- rheologic (deformation within tissue) characteristics of the agent should also be positively affected by adequate material viscosity, surface tension, and tissue response (wound healing).

These attributes for any specific agent should also be reproducible. Tissue response characteristics should further demonstrate minimal fibrotic ingrowth, little extracapsular inflammatory response (if encapsulation occurs), and agent volume after injection should be retained with minimal resorption. The ideal scenario for any soft tissue-bulking agent would be a single injection with permanent tissue residence of the agent (and partial or total incorporation into the host tissues).

However, the current reality for the available agents is that they do not ideally fulfill the above criteria, either due to isolated or combined agent and host factors (e.g. lack of resorption, agent admixture separation, etc.).

The goal of endoscopic injection therapy for SUI is to provide a minimally invasive, effective, and safe alternative to open surgery. Although the technique has been available for decades, the ideal injectable has yet to be developed. In addition to safety issues by being biocompatible, non-antigenic, non-infectious, and non-carcinogenic, any material must demonstrate 'anatomic integrity'. This implies that the material conserves its volume over time. Despite the safety of using bovine collagen as a material for injection treatment for SUI, it lacks this 'anatomic integrity'. This reduces the ability of collagen to be cost effective. A significant volume is required at each injection session and multiple injection sessions are the rule, not the exception, thus reducing not only the cost effectiveness of this material but also translating into patient inconvenience and, ultimately, to patient dissatisfaction with collagen and (perhaps) injectable therapy in general. Information on the use of collagen in SUI has been well documented.[2]

Durasphere™ pyrolytic carbon-coated zirconium oxide beads

This product was approved by the FDA in 1999. The beads are suspended in a water-soluble β-glucan vehicle. The randomized, multicenter, double-blind study[3] accepted by the FDA compared collagen to Durasphere™ and showed similar outcomes, the original Durasphere™ offering a slight benefit. Durasphere™ is more viscous than collagen and, as mentioned above, its injection was more technically demanding until the introduction of Durasphere-EXP™.

Recently, renewed concern has been expressed about material migration after injection,[4] despite lack of clear evidence demonstrating migration. Microcrystalline components of the bulking agent should be composed of uniform spheroidal particles with sizes above 80 microns (approximate size required to avoid migration, determined in studies involving polytetrafluoroethylene [Teflon]). Migration is clearly influenced by the ability of host macrophages to phagocytize particles, and smaller particle sizes have been shown to migrate to distant locations with Teflon injection. However, direct embolization of material is caused by high pressure injection resulting in material displacement into vascular or lymphatic spaces. Injection technique should therefore rely on larger particle sizes administered with low pressure injection instrumentation. This should not become a problem with Durasphere-EXP™, as its smallest particle is 95 microns with a range up to 200 microns, significantly smaller than the original Durasphere™ (200–550 microns), but still in the size greater than the 80 micron minimum needed for safety.

Ethylene vinyl alcohol co-polymer suspended in dimethyl sulfoxide (DMSO) or Uryx® solution

Approved by the FDA in December 2004, this bulking agent is so new that few data are currently available as it still awaits commercial launch for this indication, although it is considered safe as it has already been in use for neurovascular embolization of arteriovenous malformations and small aneurysms. Upon injection and exposure to solution (blood or extracellular space) at physiologic temperatures, the DMSO diffuses from the co-polymer and causes the ethylene vinyl alcohol to precipitate into a complex spongiform mass. This phase change requires diligent separation of agent and body temperature fluids until implantation occurs. Early experience with this agent suggested that optimal results were obtained with injection in a slightly more distal location within the urethra (approximately 1.5 cm distal to the bladder neck), with a slower rate of injection (at least 30 s/ml/injection site), and without the need to observe visual coaptation at the completion of injection, as the volume injected is limited to 2.5 ml on each side of the urethra. Using these endpoint criteria, results with this agent have been intriguingly good. Again, the interesting difference with this material is that injection consists of this set volume and not an endpoint of coaptation of the urethra/bladder neck at the time of injection. A large scale North American trial incorporated 237 women with GSUI, and used a prospective, randomized (2:1 Uryx® to bovine collagen) schema.[5] All treated patients were followed for 1 year after their last injection. Interestingly, at 12 months, 74% of the Uryx® patients were dry as compared to 40% of the collagen patients. Rates of postimplantation urgency and dysuria were essentially the same between the two arms. This result suggests that, unlike collagen, Uryx® maintains a durability of response not noted with biologic agents and may provide the first synthetic material to do this without substantive complication issues.

Specific agents in development

Calcium hydoxylapatite

Synthetic calcium hydoxylapatite is identical to the same material found in human teeth and bones. The agent is composed of hydroxylapatite spheres (which are extremely uniform in shape, smooth, and 75–125 microns in size) in an aqueous gel composed of sodium carboxylmethylcellulose (trade name, Coaptite®). Plain film radiography or ultrasonography may be used to localize this material and can be useful adjuncts to assessing implantation. In fact, the first FDA approved indication for this material has been obtained, specifically for soft tissue marking (as an adjunct to radiographic focusing for radiotherapeutics). Agent injection is carried out with a small bore (21-gauge needle), with standard cystoscopic instruments.

A large-scale North American pivotal trial has been completed, accruing more than 250 women. In a preliminary report, when 21 women who had received Coaptite® and 18 who had received collagen and had been followed for 1 year since last injection,[6] the average number of injections was 2.0 for Coaptite® and 2.3 for collagen. The total volume injected was 3.7 ml for Coaptite® and 7.4 ml for collagen. Eighty-six percent of Coaptite® patients improved by at least one Stamey grade, 67% improved by two grades, and 38% were completely continent (compared to women who received collagen with 66%, 55%, and 44%, respectively). Overall pad weight reduction in the 1-hour stress pad test was at least 75% in 77% of Coaptite® patients but in only 55% of collagen patients, and a 90% reduction or greater was found in 46% (Coaptite®) and 33% (collagen), respectively. No prolonged retention, urgency, or periurethral erosion or abscess was seen in either group.

This agent has similar injection characteristics to collagen, and thus far appears to require less injected volume for somewhat more durable effect than collagen.

Zuidex™

Zuidex™ – another biologic agent – consists of dextranomer microspheres in a cross-linked hyaluronic acid (HA) vehicle. HA is a water-insoluble, complex glycosaminoglycan composed of disaccharide units, which form molecules of 23 million molecular weight, and is dissolved in normal saline for urethral bulking purposes. This composite gel has significant elasticity and high viscosity. These biologic characteristics have led to the use of hylan gels for soft tissue bulking purposes. It is completely biodegradable and non-immunogenic. Hyaluronic acid functions as the transport compound and is resorbed within 2 weeks after injection. The dextranomer microspheres actually function as the bulking agent, are 80–200 microns in size and do not show fragility with insertion, remaining in the injection site for about 4 years. Injection is performed using standard cystoscopic equipment, with minimal injection pressure. A clinical trial has just begun in the US to evaluate this agent for SUI.

Of interest is that the technique requires no endoscopy. A small device (called the 'Implacer') is inserted into the urethra and the four needles direct the injected material in 0.7 ml aliquots at the midurethra. Substantive data existed for the efficacy and safety of this agent, allowing FDA approval in the US for the indication of vesicoureteral reflux and for pediatric incontinence. It is therefore unlikely that there will be any safety issues in the evaluation of adult incontinence treatment. The incontinence injections are at the bladder neck for the collagen used in this trial whereas the Zuidex™ is placed at the midurethra; it remains to be seen if this affects efficacy.

Results of dextranomer injection for pediatric incontinence show no associated adverse events, and substantial improvement at 12 months postinjection;[7] however, these children were injected at the bladder neck. Sixteen patients (with a variety of underlying etiologies for their incontinence) underwent a mean of 2.3 injections with a mean volume of 2.8 ml with subsequent annual follow up. Seventy-five percent were improved at 6 months and 50% at 12 months as determined by 1-hour pad tests and diary data. Further follow-up at 2 years indicated relative stability of incontinence parameters as compared with the 1-year data. No local injection site complications or immunologic sequelae resulted. Similar durability and safety findings have been identified with this material when used for the reflux indication.

Synthetic agents

Synthetic agents would seem to pose a potential benefit as bulking agents due to their stability (non-biodegradability). Silicone is a hydrogel suspension composed of polyvinylpyrrolidone (povidone) as the carrier (which also acts as a lubricant for the injection system) while the bulking agent is solid polydimethylsiloxane elastomer (vulcanized silicone). The elastomer is a particulate of varying shapes and conformal configurations. Particle size is markedly variable with 25% of particles less than 50 microns in size, and some greater than 400 microns in largest dimension. Silicone delivery also requires high-pressure administration, but, with newer equipment, this material is more easily delivered.

Although well established in Europe, concerns regarding silicone stimulation of the immunologic response have limited evaluation of this agent in the US. However, a clinical trial evaluating this agent (Macroplastique®) for this indication is now in progress in North America. A recent Scandinavian report followed 22 women long term (2 years postinjection) who had received this agent.[8] Subjective and objective criteria showed stability and persistent benefit for those patients. Overall pad test data showed dramatic reduction (147 g mean pretreatment reduced to 9 g post-treatment). No long-term local or systemic complications were noted.

A requirement for FDA trials with these agents is active comparison with bovine collagen. No current head-to-head data exist between these evolving agents for the indication of GSUI. However, a recently completed trial did compare Macroplastique® to dextranomer/hyaluronic acid for the treatment of ureteral reflux in children.[9]

CONCLUSIONS

It is clear that injectable treatment for SUI can be effective and safe; however, it is also clear that durability of the positive results remains a primary concern when implementing this minimally invasive technique. With time and further research, improvements in the use of injectables for SUI are inevitable.

REFERENCES

1. Winters JC, Appell R. Periurethral injection of collagen in the treatment of intrinsic sphincteric deficiency in the female patient. Urol Clin North Am 1995;22:673–8.
2. Kershen RT, Dmochowski RR, Appell RA. Beyond collagen: injectable therapies for the treatment of female stress urinary incontinence in the new millennium. Urol Clin North Am 2002;29:559–74.
3. Lightner D, Calvosa C, Andersen R et al. A new injectable bulking agent for treatment of stress urinary incontinence: results of a multicenter, randomized, controlled, double-blind study of Durasphere. Urology 2001;58:12–5.
4. Ritts RE. Particle migration after transurethral injection of carbon coated beads. J Urol 2002;167:1804–5.
5. Dmochowski RR, Herschorn S, Corcos J et al. Multicenter randomized controlled study to evaluate Uryx urethral bulking agent in treating female stress urinary incontinence. J Urol 2002;167:LB-10 (A).
6. Dmochowski R, Appell RA, Klimberg I et al. Initial clinical results from coaptite injection for stress urinary incontinence, comparative clinical study. In: Program of the International Continence Society, Heidelberg, Germany, August 2002.
7. Caione P, Capozza N. Endoscopic treatment of urinary incontinence in pediatric patients: 2-year experience with dextranomer/hyaluronic acid. J Urol 2002;168:1868–71.
8. Peeker R, Edlund C, Wennberg AL et al. The treatment of sphincter incontinence with periurethral silicone implant (Macroplastique). Scand J Urol Nephrol 2002;36:194–8.
9. Aboutaleb H, Bolduc S, Upadhyay J et al. Subureteral polydimethyl-siloxane injection versus extravesical reimplantation for primary low grade vesicoureteral reflux in children: a comparative study. J Urol 2002;169:313–6.

59

Abdominal and transvaginal colpourethropexies for stress urinary incontinence

Michelle Y Morrill, Karl M Luber

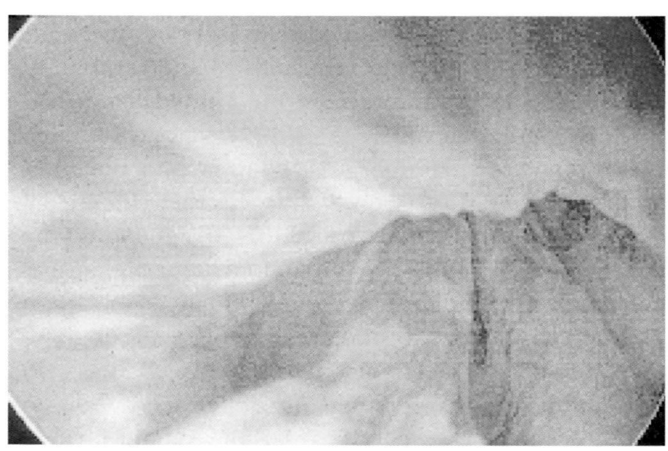

INTRODUCTION

There have been over 100 procedures described for the surgical correction of stress urinary incontinence (SUI), but credit for the first retropubic colposuspension belongs to Marshall, Marchetti and Krantz. In 1949, in an early example of cooperation between pelvic surgeons, this team of two gynecologists and one urologist described their first series of the correction of stress urinary incontinence by simple vesicourethral suspension in a series of 50 patients including 12 men at risk for incontinence following prostatectomy.[1] Others subsequently recognized the value of this approach for women with SUI and, with modifications, it became a gold standard procedure for SUI that has withstood many years of critical review.[2–5] In 1991, Vancaillie and Schuessler introduced a laparoscopic approach to the retropubic space that facilitated a minimally invasive approach to colpourethropexy.[6] The efficacy of this approach has not supported it as a replacement for the open colpourethropexy (CU). Although the role of CU is changing as new, less invasive procedures are introduced, it remains an important technique in the armamentarium of the female pelvic reconstructive surgeon.

Transvaginal needle procedures, originally developed through the pioneering work of Armand Pereyra in the late 1950s, represented a remarkable insight into less invasive surgery.[7] Although transvaginal needle bladder neck suspensions (NBNS) were commonly used for over three decades, recent critical meta-analysis has shown that long-term outcomes compare unfavorably to other available procedures and their use has been largely abandoned.[5,8,9]

INDICATIONS

Before surgery for female SUI is undertaken, it is important that non-surgical care be offered and encouraged.[10] Contemporary non-surgical care has demonstrated good results and exposes women to fewer potential risks.[11] However, even with optimal non-surgical care, there are many women who will elect for surgical intervention. In 1998 nearly 135,000 women in the United States had inpatient surgery for SUI.[12] Four percent of US women responding to a national postal survey said that they had undergone surgery for SUI.[13] With the vast array of surgical options currently available, recommending the optimal surgical procedure for an individual patient has grown more complex but should remain based upon existing methods of evaluation along with ongoing assessment of available outcome data.

Careful evaluation should be undertaken prior to offering a patient surgery for SUI and should include a detailed history of their condition and background medical history to identify other potential contributors such as chronic coughing, limited mobility, etc. A voiding diary is useful to assess storage ability, but must be interpreted in light of the patient's symptoms; for example, a patient may present with small voided volumes and it could easily be assumed that this reflected an overactive bladder. However, further questioning may reveal she has learned to void more frequently to avoid stress loss.

The physical examination should include a directed neurologic evaluation, grading of pelvic floor muscle strength, and assessment of vaginal and urethral support, preferably using the pelvic organ prolapse quantification (POPQ) grading system[14] for prolapse and the Q-tip test for hypermobility.[15] A post-void residual urine volume and stress testing, preferably undertaken in the context of urodynamic testing, are appropriate prior to making any recommendation to surgery. Many surgeons also prefer baseline voiding information to allow for better assessment and care of potential postoperative voiding difficulties.

Once stress incontinence is established and a patient expresses the desire to explore surgical options, consideration must be given to what represents appropriate surgery for that individual. For many years, surgeons have considered women with SUI in three groups based upon two components: support of the urethrovesical junction (UVJ) and the intrinsic function of the urethral closure mechanism. The first group includes women with poor UVJ support, known as urethral hypermobility, who otherwise have good urethral function. The term hypermobile stress incontinence (HSI) is often applied to this group. The second group is composed of women with good urethral support, but poor urethral function. Historically this group has been referred to as Type III incontinence, but is now commonly known as intrinsic sphincter deficiency (ISD).[16] The third group is made up of those women who have both hypermobility (HSI) of the UVJ and poor urethral function (ISD). Recommendations for treatment follow this categorization. HSI is treated primarily by stabilizing the UVJ with a CU, a suburethral sling or, of historical interest, a NBNS. ISD without hypermobility (HM) can be treated with a suburethral sling, often with mobilization of the urethra, or with bulking agents designed to improve urethral coaptation. As women in this group already have good urethral support, a procedure such as CU or NBNS – which functions by improving support – is not likely to provide relief of their symptoms. Therefore, there is no role for CU or NBNS in caring for women with ISD without HM.[17] This leaves debate about the optimal management for that group of women with both hypermobility and poor urethral function (ISD).

Low maximum urethral closure pressure (MUCP; 20 cmH_2O or lower) has been studied as a risk factor for failure of colpourethropexies. McGuire et al. were the first to report that women with HSI who had persistent SUI following colpourethropexy were more likely to have a low preoperative MUCP than women with a successful outcome.[18] They concluded that a low MUCP reflected poor urethral function and that simply stabilizing such a urethra would not correct the SUI. Subsequent investigators confirmed these findings. Sand and colleagues noted that 54% of patients with low urethral pressures continued to have stress incontinence after a Burch procedure compared to only 18% of women with maximum urethral closure pressures of greater than 20 cmH_2O.[19] This led to the broad use of MUCP to identify women with ISD along with HSI and the recommendation to use a sling procedure, rather than a stabilization procedure, to correct their SUI. More recently, both Richardson et al.[20] and Sand et al.[21] have reported clinical series in which women with low MUCP achieved success rates of 78% and 90%, closely approximating those of women with normal MUCP. This issue is made more difficult by the lack of agreement on definition and diagnosis of ISD. Thus, in the absence of a randomized controlled trial, the importance of urethral function to the success of CU is unclear although most thought leaders recommend against CU in patients with evidence of ISD. Current work undertaken by the National Institutes of Health (NIH) sponsored Urinary Incontinence Treatment Network (UITN) is currently investigating this, and the data being generated promises to improve our understanding of this issue.

In the early 1990s, several thought leaders in the surgical care of female SUI began sharing data from clinical series in which suburethral sling procedures were used to treat women with HSI regardless of urethral function.[22] They emphasized that careful sling placement and the absence of tensioning against the urethra reduced the risk of postoperative obstruction to levels comparable to CU. Prior to this, many practitioners felt that the mechanical effect of the graft should be visually confirmed as an indentation on the proximal urethra noted on urethroscopy. As a result, postoperative obstruction rates were troublesomely high. The concept that successful cure of SUI could occur with less obstruction by using a tension-free suburethral sling technique led to a movement away from retropubic urethropexy and needle bladder neck suspension. As this philosophy was adopted, preoperative assessment of urethral function became less critical as the role of CU was reduced and the use of slings was expanded.

Many variables have been examined as risk factors for failure of colpourethropexies, including obesity and previous anti-incontinence surgery. Table 59.1 examines studies of commonly considered risk factors for failure of Burch procedures. Contrary to common recommendations, patients with previous incontinence surgery have outcomes similar to women who have not undergone previous anti-incontinence procedures. Obesity has been identified as a risk factor for SUI[23] and many have taught that it is likewise a risk factor for failure of anti-incontinence surgery. This was not supported in a 5-year follow-up study of incontinence surgery and patient body mass index (BMI) where 87% of the obese patients (BMI >30) were continent.[24] Although obesity may create insurmountable technical difficulties for the surgeon, evidence does not support a reduction in the efficacy of CU in treating women with elevated body mass indices.

In clinical practice, it is common to encounter questions surrounding the route of delivery following surgery for SUI. Unfortunately, there are no studies in the literature designed to answer questions about women who deliver children after surgery for incontinence. Survey studies conducted through the American Urogynecologic Society have revealed that 67% of respondents would recommend performing a cesarean section for a patient after an anti-incontinence procedure rather than allowing subsequent vaginal delivery. Physicians reported outcomes of their patients who delivered after surgery. Forty women delivered vaginally and 22 (55%) were known to be continent. Forty-seven had cesarean sections, after which 35 (74%) were continent.[25] It is not known how many of those women labored before delivering abdominally. The decision to operate on a woman who plans future childbearing mandates a thorough discussion with the patient of the risks and benefits as they relate to subsequent delivery.

Finally, patients anticipating CU or any other form of surgery to correct SUI should be counseled extensively about the risks and benefits. Counseling should include an accurate sense of the long-term correction of SUI along with information about the immediate and long-term risks, especially overactive bladder (OAB) symptoms and voiding dysfunction as outlined in Tables 59.7 and 59.8.

TECHNIQUE

The goal of CU is to create, or more accurately, recreate a backboard against which the hypermobile urethra

Table 59.1. ***Success rates for specific preoperative factors***

Preoperative factor	Objective success (%)	Subjective success (%)	*n*	Follow-up	Reference
Low UCP	46	N/A	41	3 months	Sand et al.[19]
Low UCP HM data not presented	50	N/A	6	1 year	Bergman et al.[58]
Low UCP with HM	78	–	29	–	Richardson et al.[20]
Low UCP, 'poor bladder neck mobility was not a risk factor for failure'	67	90	21	4–36 months (mean 15)	Maher et al.[59]
Low UCP and HM	90	95	19	3 months	Sand et al.[21]
Low UCP and HM	84.6	93	28	33–116 months (mean 72.6)	Culligan et al.[60]
No hypermobility (Q-tip change of <30 degrees)	45	N/A	9	3–12 months	Bergman et al.[17]
Negative Q-tip test	50	N/A	12	1 year	Bergman et al.[58]
Previous incontinence surgery	82.9	N/A	35	5–10 years	Feyereisl et al.[51]
Previous incontinence surgery	81	80% rated surgery highly successful	53	4–72 months (mean 9)	Maher et al.[47]
BMI >30	87	N/A	15	5 years	Zivkovic et al.[24]

BMI, body mass index; HM, hypermobility; *n*, number of subjects in colpourethropexy arm of trial; N/A, not applicable; UCP, urethral closure pressure.

can be compressed during stress. This is done by stabilizing the endopelvic connective tissue that provides the underlying support of the proximal urethra. This underlying support is provided by the anterior vaginal wall and consists of fibromuscular tissue with lateral attachment to the arcus tendineus fascia pelvis.[26] Historically, there has been an emphasis on restoring the urethra to an intra-abdominal location in which the zone of pressure within the abdomen will be equally exerted upon the urethra and the bladder, thus closing the urethra and resisting passage of urine during stress.[27] However, this is not consistent with anatomic observations in cadaver dissections or during surgical procedures, and has given way to the more contemporary explanation above.

Although CUs are commonly undertaken as part of more comprehensive reconstructive surgery, they can be performed as isolated procedures using a laparoscope, a 5–6 cm mini-laparotomy, or a full-sized transverse or midline incision. The cosmetic advantages of laparoscopic surgery and mini-laparotomy are immediately obvious to the patient. The surgical outcomes of open versus laparoscopic CU are discussed later in this chapter.

The original colposuspension was designed to elevate the urethrovesical junction to the pubic symphysis. The initial modification of this was published in 1961[28] when Burch, after becoming frustrated with the inconsistency of support and suture pullout from the midline periosteum, chose to attach them to Cooper's ligament. A meta-analysis of two subsequent trials comparing these two procedures has demonstrated a significant improvement in outcome, with a relative risk of failure for Burch compared to the Marshall–Marchetti–Krantz (MMK) procedure at 1–5 years of 0.38 and a decrease in postoperative retention with the Burch procedure.[29]

Failures following CU can be attributed to several causes. Mechanical failure caused by suture pullout with subsequent loss of urethral support, as well as compromise of urethral function caused by periurethral dissection that can create ISD, can both contribute to failure. Additionally, a subset of women experience successful correction of their SUI only to find that they have developed de novo detrusor overactivity or worsening of pre-existing overactive bladder (OAB) symptoms. It has been observed that development or worsening of urge symptoms is commonly associated with voiding difficulties. This has led many to speculate that new postoperative urge symptoms are the result of a postobstructive phenomenon analogous to urge in the male associated with benign prostatic hyperplasia. By analyzing these failures, we can develop guidelines by which we strive to avoid them.

In his landmark article of 1976,[3] Tanagho outlined technical variations of the Burch procedure that recommended avoiding dissection of the midline neurovascular supply to the urethra to protect against compromising urethral function and creating ISD. Tanagho also suggested that overcorrection of the urethral support not only failed to improve success rates, but was also associated with voiding dysfunction and, often, irritative voiding symptoms. This resulted in the now broadly accepted recommendation that sutures be placed lateral to the urethra and tied in such a way as to support the urethra without excessive elevation and without compression of the urethra against the posterior of the symphysis pubis. The parallel concepts of protecting the midline structures and correcting support while avoiding overcorrection are key to providing the best outcomes for patients.

Mechanical failure of CU is most probably caused by suture pullout from the endopelvic connective tissue of the anterior vaginal wall rather than the sturdier Cooper's ligament. This emphasizes the importance of optimizing the weakest link of the procedure by ensuring that sutures placed into the anterior vaginal wall achieve optimal purchase. This can be accomplished by confident full thickness bites of the endopelvic connective tissue placed with sufficient precision that the operator does not hesitate for fear of injuring adjacent structures, particularly the urinary tract. A triangle of safety can be visualized intraoperatively by creating a line approximately 2 cm from and parallel to the urethra, a second line along the distal aspect of the bladder, and a third along the pelvic sidewall (Fig. 59.1). Within this zone of safety, the surgeon can be confident that deep, elongated bites will provide optimal support without fear of collateral damage to the urinary tract. Longer, full thickness suture placements are also less likely to tear through the venous plexus of the anterior vaginal wall than more tentative bites, making them a hemostatically safer alternative as well.

RESULTS

Outcomes of retropubic colpourethropexy

The long-term goals of reconstructive surgery differ fundamentally from those of extirpative surgery. A procedure designed to create a functional improvement for a patient must stand a different test of cure than an operation intended to remove a mass or a dysfunctional organ. With reconstructive surgery, the adverse effects are weighed against the duration and degree of improvement in the primary symptom. This makes the definition of success a moving target that is difficult to define. When assessing stress incontinence surgery, the successful management of SUI is balanced against intraoperative and long-term functional risks. The potential functional risks of anti-incontinence surgery include voiding difficulties and obstruction, de novo or worsened OAB symptoms, chronic pain, osteitis pubis, and dyspareunia.

Results of colposuspension have been reported using both objective and subjective measures. Objective success rates range from 68 to 95.6% (Table 59.2). The results of colposuspension in the first 5 years after surgery are consistently better than 80%. The 1997 American Urological Association guidelines panel meta-analysis found that success at 48 months averaged 84% with a confidence interval of 79–88%.[5] The Cochrane Review of open retropubic colposuspension focused on randomized controlled trials and found a slow decline in cure to 70% as patients were followed over 5 years.[29] Reports attempting to study women with follow-up of greater than 10 years often lack objective data and suffer from the inevitable drop in follow-up rates. The retrospective studies in Table 59.2 reporting success rates of 90% and 94% at 15 years plus postoperatively are unlikely to be indicative of expected results. Further studies are needed to clarify the longer-term results of colposuspension.

Subjective measures are predictably difficult to meta-analyze because there is great variability in the metrics used to assess outcomes subjectively. However, subjective outcomes are very important. It is essential to understand the effects of surgery on a patient who leaks during an office stress test but states that she does not consider her leakage to be significant or bothersome. The International Continence Society has recognized this by including in the definition of incontinence that it is 'a social or hygienic problem for the patient'.[30] Among studies that provide both subjective and objective outcome data, continence rates can differ by more than 20% (see Table 59.1). Only three of the studies listed in Table 59.2 reported subjective cure rates. Alcalay et al.[31] and Ward and Hilton[32] found subjective cure rates of 73.5% and 62%, respectively. Jarvis' meta-analysis[33] reported a much higher 89.6% subjective cure rate in over 1700 patients. Subjective cure rates in patients evaluated for preoperative risk factors for failure ranged from 80 to 93% (see Table 59.1). Accepting their limitations, subjective measures of success following surgery for SUI remain an important outcome variable that does not always agree with objective data.

Laparoscopic or minimally invasive approaches to colposuspension were developed to speed patient recovery, both in the hospital and after discharge. Descriptions of both extraperitoneal (approaching the space of Retzius without entering the peritoneal cavity) and transperitoneal (incising the peritoneum cephalad to the bladder from a pneumoperitoneum) techniques have been reported. A review published in the Cochrane Database[34]

Table 59.2. ***Success rates of retropubic urethropexy***

Study	*n*	Study design	Cure (objectively dry) (%)	Follow-up 1–5 years	5–10 years	>10 years
Jarvis[33]	1726	Meta-analysis	84.3	≥1 year		
Colombo et al.[61]	40	Prospective randomized	80	2–7 years (mean 3.1)		
Leach et al.[5]	2196	Meta-analysis	84	≥4 years		
Su et al.[62]	46	Prospective randomized	95.6	≥1 year		
Lapitan et al.[29]	2403	Meta-analysis	85–90	1 year		
Ward & Hilton[32]	169	Prospective randomized	80 in 86 who were followed up 68 if LOCF	2 years		
Feyereisl et al.[51]	87	Retrospective cohort	81.6		5–10 years	
Bergman & Elia[36]	33	Prospective randomized	82		5 years	
Lapitan et al.[29]	2403	Meta-analysis	Approx. 70		5 years	
Alcalay et al.[31]	109	Retrospective review	90			10–20 years (mean 13.8)
Langer et al.[63]	127	Retrospective review	94			10–15 years (mean 12.4)

LOCF, last observation carried forward; *n*, number of subjects in colpourethropexy arm of trial.

reported an increased objective failure rate for laparoscopic Burch procedures compared to the open technique (relative risk 2.30). The authors note that one of the three studies had problems with randomization and consistency of suture usage. With that one study removed from the analysis there was no significant difference between laparoscopy and laparotomy up to 18 months after surgery. However, most experts feel that 18 months is not an adequate test of time for an anti-incontinence procedure.[5] Long-term published and unpublished data from Burton were utilized in the Cochrane Database. Burton's data indicate that laparoscopic CU failed to maintain continence as well as open Burch procedures at both 3 and 5 years. In the Cochrane Review, laparoscopy resulted in a shorter hospital stay and shorter time to return to normal activities. The complication rates of voiding dysfunction and de novo urgency were not significantly different.

Clinicians are faced with many surgical choices to treat SUI. Table 59.3 lists studies in which colposuspension has been compared to other procedures. Anterior colporrhaphy (Kelly plication) was one of the first surgeries described to treat SUI in women.[35] Several well-executed randomized controlled trials and carefully performed meta-analyses have shown that anterior colporrhaphy does poorly compared to colposuspension and its use as an anti-incontinence procedure should be considered for historic interest only.[5,36,37] Needle bladder neck suspensions were heralded as a minimally invasive procedure for stress incontinence and underwent innumerable minor modifications over more than 30 years of use. However, like anterior repairs, both clinical trials and meta-analyses revealed the poor longevity of needle bladder neck suspensions and they no longer play a major role in the surgical management of female SUI.[5,33] Midurethral slings, developed in the mid 1990s by Ulmsten and colleagues,[38] have offered a minimally invasive alternative to colpourethropexy. Data from clinical trials have been encouraging and a randomized trial between Burch and one type of midurethral sling – the tension-free transvaginal tape (TVT) – has shown that these two procedures have similar success rates after 2 years.[32]

In a randomized trial between laparoscopic Burch and the TVT procedure, Paraiso et al. determined that there was no statistically significant difference in cure rates between the two procedures, although the study did not have the necessary power to show such a difference.[39] The results tended toward improved outcome for TVT with a 1-year postoperative SUI rate of 3.2% compared to 18.8% in the laparoscopic patients. The TVT procedure was noted to take a significantly shorter length of operative time (mean = 79 versus 132 minutes, p=0.003).

Table 59.3. ***Comparison studies between colpourethropexy and other procedures***

Study	Alternate procedure	Success CU (%) vs. other (%)	*n* CU vs. *n* other	Follow-up
Bergman et al.[58]	Vs. anterior colporrhaphy	89 vs. 63	38 vs. 35	1 year
Bergman et al.[36]		82 vs. 37	33 vs. 30	5 years
Black & Downs[64]		85 vs. 50–70	Meta-analysis	1 year
Leach et al.[5]		84 vs. 61	Meta-analysis	≥4 years
Kammerer-Doak et al.[37]		89 vs. 31	18 vs. 15	1 year
Colombo et al.[54]		74 vs. 42	35 vs. 33	14.2 years vs. 13.9 years
Bergman et al.[58]	Vs. NBNS	89 vs. 65	38 vs. 34	1 year
Bergman et al.[36]		82 vs. 43	33 vs. 30	5 years
Black & Downs[64]		85 vs. 50–70	Meta-analysis	1 year
Leach et al.[5]		84 vs. 67	Meta-analysis	≥4 years
Black & Downs[64]	Vs. sling	Difference not significant	Meta-analysis	1 year
Leach et al.[5]		84 vs. 83	Meta-analysis	≥4 years
Ward & Hilton[32]	Vs. TVT	80 vs. 81 68 vs. 78	108 vs. 137 followed-up 175 vs. 169 LOCF	2 years

CU, colpourethropexy; LOCF, last observation carried forward; *n*, number of subjects in arm of trial; NBNS, needle bladder neck suspensions; TVT, tension-free vaginal tape.

A great deal of emphasis has been placed on urodynamic changes following colpourethropexy in the past. As seen in Table 59.4, there is a significant increase in urethral resistance after Burch colposuspension associated with an alteration in the physiology of micturition and the prevention of leakage in these patients. Changes to flow rates are not consistently significant but a trend can be seen toward slower rates. These are changes which patients may notice and they should be reassured that such changes are common and not worrisome. Maximum capacity and post-void residual volumes do not change significantly in these women. Interestingly, urethral closure pressures do not show significant changes. Of the six studies in Table 59.4, none demonstrated a significant difference in pre- and post-operative urethral closure pressure (UCP). This may be because urethral pressure profiles represent a portion of the urethral sphincter mechanism that is not affected by colposuspension. It is interesting to note that UCP is also unchanged in women who are made continent after periurethral collagen injection.[40]

INTRAOPERATIVE COMPLICATIONS

Operating in the retropubic space or space of Retzius is a delicate procedure that requires specialized training. It is important to be prepared to recognize and manage possible complications that can occur during surgery as listed in Table 59.5. It is equally important to recognize the morbidity associated with functional long-term complications following CU, specifically voiding dysfunction and irritative symptoms.

Hemorrhage and transfusion

The space of Retzius has a robust collection of blood vessels crossing the area dissected for colposuspension. The approach to this area is therefore cautious and it is important to maintain meticulous hemostasis throughout the retropubic space. The proximity of the obturator canal and its neurovascular bundle is another threat that surgeons must be aware of and avoid.[41] The risk of hemorrhage and the possibility of transfusion should be discussed with all patients as part of a complete consent process.

Lower urinary tract trauma

During CU, bladder trauma is possible with dissection, retraction, or suture placement. As the bladder is amenable to repair, it is imperative that this damage is recognized at the time of surgery. Urethropexy sutures passed into the bladder should be removed to avoid stone formation. Their small diameter does not require

Table 59.4. *Urodynamic changes*

Reference	Urodynamic measurement	Preop → postop change	Follow-up	*n*
Bhatia et al.[65]	Urethral resistance (p_{ves}/Q_{max}^2)	0.035 → 0.055	3–12 months	48
Colombo et al.[61]	Urethral resistance (p_{det}/Q_{max}^2)	0.07 → 0.62	3.1 years (range 2–7 years)	40
Su et al.[62]	Urethral resistance (p_{ves}/Q_{max}^2)	0.166 → 0.332	≥1 year	46
Bhatia et al.[45]	Q_{max}	23.2 → 22 (NS)	3–12 months	48
Colombo et al.[61]	Q_{max}	21.6 → 13.0	3.1 years (range 2–7 years)	40
Maher et al.[59]	Q_{max}	38 → 29	15 months (range 4–36 months)	21
Langer et al.[63]	Q_{max}	27.6 → 24.3 (NS)	12.4 years (range 10–15 years)	109
Colombo et al.[61]	Q_{avg}	14.5 → 8.8	3.1 years (range 2–7 years)	40
Maher et al.[47]	Flow rate	27 → 20	9 months (range 4–72 months)	53
Su et al.[62]	MUCP	83.1 → 82.5 (NS)	≥1 year	46
Maher et al.[47]	MUCP	40 → 46 (NS)	9 months (range 4–72 months)	53
Langer et al.[63]	MUCP	46.9 → 43.1 (NS)	12.4 years (range 10–15 years)	109
Langer et al.[63]	MUCP	53.2 → 46.8 (NS)	12.4 years (range 10–15 years)	109
Maher et al.[47]	PVR	5 → 7 (NS)	9 months (range 4–72 months)	53
Maher et al.[59]	PVR	2 → 5 (NS)	15 months (range 4–36 months)	21
Langer et al.[63]	PVR	19.4 → 24.6 (NS)	12.4 years (range 10–15 years)	109
Su et al.[62]	MCC	342 → 335 (NS)	≥1 year	46
Maher et al.[47]	MCC	482 → 500 (NS)	15 months (range 4–36 months)	21
Langer et al.[63]	MCC	486.2 → 459.5 (NS)	12.4 years (range 10–15 years)	109

MCC, maximal cystometric capacity; MUCP, maximal urethral closure pressure; *n*, number of subjects in colpourethropexy arm; NS, change not significant; p_{det}, detrusor pressure at Q_{max}; p_{ves}, 'vesical pressure at voiding'; PVR, post-void residual.

Table 59.5. *Intraoperative complications*

Complication	Reference	Incidence (%)	*n*
Hemorrhage (>1000 ml)	Maher et al.[47]	0	53
	Kenton et al.[66]	2	151
Transfusion	Leach et al.[5]	5 (CI 3–8%)	1131
	Maher et al.[47]	0	53
	Kenton et al.[66]	0.7	151
	Cosson et al.[67]	1.2	82
Cystotomy	Maher et al.[47]	2	53
	Ward & Hilton[68]	2	146
	Kenton et al.[66]	1.3	151
	Cosson et al.[67]	1.2	82
Suture in bladder	Kenton et al.[66]	0.7	151

CI, confidence interval; *n*, number of subjects in colpourethropexy arm.

repair and another suture may be placed, taking care to remain away from the bladder.

Ureteral injury following CU has been reported to be as high as 4/60.[42] Ureteral kinking may occur as the anterior vaginal wall is pulled forward. This is an uncommon complication and if care is taken to remain within the triangle of safety described earlier in this chapter, the ureters should not be at risk. Cystoscopy is recommended after colposuspension[43] and should note efflux from both ureters as well as the absence of suture in the urothelium.

POSTOPERATIVE COMPLICATIONS

Brief urinary retention is common after colposuspension and all patients should be prepared for this (Table 59.6). Retention can be managed with a suprapubic or transurethral catheter or with intermittent self-catheterization. Ideally, these options can be discussed with the patient prior to surgery, allowing the patient to be prepared for whichever technique she finds most comfortable. Most patients will void on their own within 2 weeks,

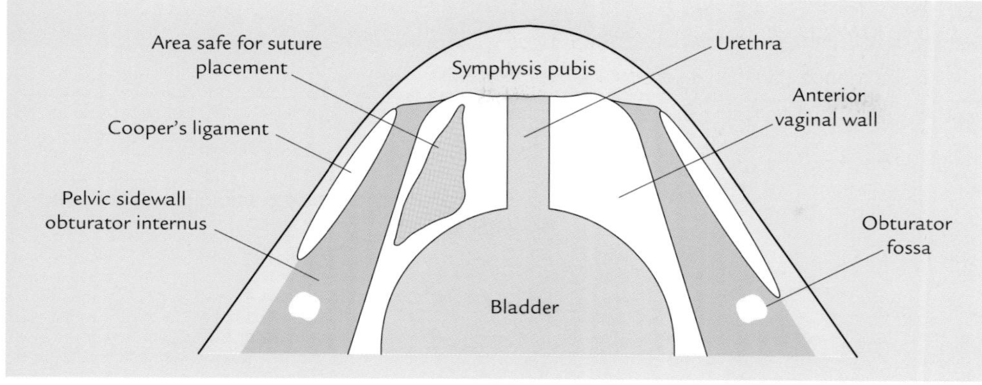

Figure 59.1. *Safe placement of sutures in colpourethropexy.*

although it is estimated that between zero and 21% will experience long-term voiding difficulty as discussed below (Table 59.7).

Prophylactic measures can be taken to decrease some postoperative complications. Confirmation of sterile urine and appropriate perioperative antibiotics for all patients will decrease urinary tract and wound infections.[44,45] Urinary tract infection after catheterization is common and should be anticipated in postcolposuspension patients. A low threshold for testing and treating possible urinary tract infections after pelvic surgery is acceptable. Prophylactic antibiotics in a patient with a suprapubic catheter have been shown to reduce the risk of urinary tract infection and should be administered.[46] Wound complications include infections, seromas, and hernia formation. Infection rates range from 3.5 to 7% after Burch. Attention to the incision site and active management of any signs of infection with antibiotics will minimize this.

Incisional hernias occur in 3–4% of patients.[32,47] Wide bites should be taken in the fascia while closing the wound to reduce the risk of hernia formation.

The risk of deep venous thrombosis (DVT) is present in any pelvic surgery. A DVT rate of 2% has been reported in patients following a Burch procedure and the American College of Obstetricians and Gynecologists quotes a risk of 7–29% in general gynecologic surgery in their guidelines.[48] Sequential compression stockings are recommend for all appropriate patients to reduce the risk of this complication.

Overactive bladder

De novo urgency has been reported following pelvic surgery, particularly after anti-incontinence procedures. The cause is unclear and may involve alteration in the afferent nerves, a shift in the parasympathetic versus sympathetic motor nerves, or a reprogramming of the

Table 59.6. ***Immediate postoperative complications***

Complication	Reference	Incidence (%)	*n*	Notes
Urinary tract infection	Bergman [58]	11	38	>1000 col/ml by SPC
	Maher et al.[47]	8	53	
	Ward & Hilton[68]	32	146	Within 6 weeks after surgery. Note very high catheter use
	Cosson et al.[67]	2.4	82	
Wound infection	Maher et al.[59]	5	21	
	Ward & Hilton[68]	7	146	
	Kenton et al.[66]	3.5	151	
	Cosson et al.[67]	3.7	82	
Retention (1 week–1 month)	Colombo et al.[54]	25	35	Did not resume voiding before discharge from hospital after a mean of 6.7 days
	Ward & Hilton[68]	12	146	

n, number of subjects in colpourethropexy arm; SPC, suprapubic catheter.

Table 59.7. *Long-term complications of colposuspension*

Complication	Reference	Incidence (%)	*n*	Notes
Retention >1 month	Bergman et al.[58]	0	38	SPC
	Leach et al.[5]	5 (CI 3–7%)	Meta-analysis	
	Maher et al.[47]	6	53	One patient had 'voiding difficulties' before and after surgery
	Colombo et al.[54]	0	35	SPC
	Ward & Hilton[68]	21	146	
	Kenton et al.[66]	0.7	151	
Dyspareunia	Wiskind et al.[52]	Decreased from before surgery	131	
	Colombo et al.[54]	8	24	Both with concomitant posterior colporrhaphy
	Langer et al.[63]	3.9	127	
Chronic pain	Galloway et al.[50]	12	50	Postcolposuspension syndrome
	Feyereisl et al.[51]	2.3	87	Postcolposuspension syndrome
	Maher et al.[47]	4	53	'Persistent wound pain'

n, number of subjects in colpourethropexy arm; SPC, suprapubic catheter.

neural control loops secondary to the increase in outflow resistance created by the anti-incontinence procedure. It is possible that a portion of the reported de novo postoperative urgency is persistence of OAB present prior to surgery but less symptomatic because of patients' limited bladder capacity due to SUI; when finally able to hold a larger volume, the patient may pass a threshold volume triggering the sensation of urgency. Table 59.8 lists studies of OAB symptoms following surgery. In a patient with no OAB symptoms, the risk of developing de novo urgency is 5–30%. Paradoxically, resolution of OAB symptoms is reported in 20–73% of women undergoing CU. Because no consistent predictors of outcome of OAB symptoms have been defined, it is appropriate to discuss the possibility of changes in or the development of OAB symptoms with patients considering surgery.

Table 59.8. *Postoperative changes in overactive bladder symptoms*

Postoperative change	Reference	Incidence (%)	*n*	Notes
De novo OAB symptoms	Colombo et al.[61]	5	40	
	Alcalay et al.[31]	15.4	104	
	Su et al.[62]	6.5	46	
	Leach et al.[5]	11 (CI 8–16%)	241	
	Maher et al.[47]	6	53	
	Maher et al.[59]	5	21	
	Klutke & Ramos[69]	30	23	
	Langer et al.[63]	17	102	
	Kenton et al.[66]	8	99	By CMG
Resolution of OAB symptoms	Alcalay et al.[31]	20	5	
	Maher et al.[47]	60	5	In previous surgery patients
	Maher et al.[59]	60	5	In low urethral closure pressure patients
	Langer et al.[63]	52	25	
	Kenton et al.[66]	73	52	By CMG

CMG; cystometrogram; *n*, number of subjects; OAB, overactive bladder.

Urinary retention

There are reports of urinary retention after 1 month ranging from 0.7 to 21% (see Table 59.7). Each of these studies limited the definition of this complication to those women who required catheterization. The wide discrepancy is therefore not explained by a difference in diagnosis. It is possible that this inconsistency is a result of the subjective variation in the tension on the vaginal sutures as they are tied to Cooper's ligament or to differences in the populations studied. Physicians are cautioned to avoid overcorrection when tying sutures. Less frequently reported are the more subtle, but none the less problematic changes in voiding such as double voiding, positional voiding, and prolonged voiding associated with these procedures.

There is debate about the timing of surgical management of postoperative voiding dysfunction. Although it is commonly taught that there is no harm in a watch and wait approach, recent basic science using animal models of obstruction has demonstrated structural changes that occur within the first 4 weeks.[49] Care should be taken to assess obstructive symptoms and early intervention should be considered.

Dyspareunia and chronic pain

Any surgery carries with it the risk of chronic pain. CU can change the axis of the vagina in relation to other organs and supporting structures, causing discomfort. Adhesions and nerve damage can result in pelvic pain. Postcolposuspension syndrome has been described as a pain in the groin that may be relieved by release of the ipsilateral sutures.[50,51]

Dyspareunia, although more commonly attributed to surgery to the posterior vagina, has been reported in 3.9–8% of CU trials. It is notable that in one study there was a decrease in painful coitus after colposuspension.[52]

Pelvic organ prolapse

In 1968, Burch described a high rate of enterocele development after colposuspension, and 'special attention was therefore directed to the cul-de-sac as the most vulnerable part of the repair'.[53] Since then, surgeons have attributed prolapse in various compartments to the colposuspension itself. Colombo et al. demonstrated that the Burch procedure is not an adequate treatment for cystocele and should not be considered a surgery for anterior prolapse.[54] Wiskind et al. published a 26.7% rate of reoperation for prolapse after Burch procedure.[52] However, Olsen et al. estimated that 11.1% of women under 80 will have a prolapse requiring surgery, followed by a reoperation rate nearing 30%.[55] It is believed that the high reoperation rate is due in part to a physiologic predisposition to pelvic floor disorders that necessitated the initial surgery. It is logical that a woman who developed incontinence from a loss of support for the urethra would be at risk of failure of support in other uterovaginal compartments.

A recent large study randomizing women to Burch or TVT found a significantly greater number of women had another surgery for prolapse within 2 years after colposuspension (4.8% versus zero).[32] However, the high urinary retention rate of 21% seen in the Burch arm of that study suggests that the retropubic sutures were tied very tightly and thus could alter the anatomy of the pelvic organs and permit abdominal pressures to create or worsen defects in pelvic floor support. Whether or not colposuspension is a risk factor for prolapse is not yet clear and physicians are well advised to follow Burch's advice to thoroughly evaluate and treat pelvic floor defects at the time of surgery.

Osteitis pubis

Osteitis pubis – an inflammatory condition related to periosteal trauma which causes pain at the symphysis, possibly radiating to the perineum, thighs, and abdomen – has been reported in 2–3% of women undergoing a MMK CU.[56] Pain is aggravated by the use of adjacent musculature such as with ambulation and coughing. There is no literature regarding non-infectious osteitis pubis related to Burch colposuspension. There is one case report of a woman with *pseudomonas* infection causing osteitis pubis following a Burch procedure.[57]

The MMK procedure should be recognized as a significant step forward in the management of SUI but in light of the evidence above, the Burch and its modifications are preferred for colposuspension.

SUMMARY

With the current availability of less invasive surgery, the role of CU in the care of women with SUI has evolved. Although it is routinely offered as a first line therapy for women with surgically managed SUI, women increasingly elect less invasive procedures. In this way, the role of CU has become most important during abdominal reconstruction for pelvic organ prolapse.

The gold standard sacrocolpopexy is often combined with a CU in women with advanced stage pelvic organ prolapse and urodynamic SUI. Recent evidence from the NIH Pelvic Floor Disorders Network indicates that inclusion of a CU may be appropriate for all women undergoing sacrocolpopexy regardless of preoperative testing results. When patients are properly selected and the procedure is performed according to contemporary recommendations, patient and surgeon can anticipate durable results with minimal complications whether the CU is performed as a stand-alone procedure for SUI or as a component of more comprehensive surgery for pelvic organ prolapse.

REFERENCES

1. Marshall VF, Marchetti AA, Krantz KE. The correction of stress incontinence by simple vesicourethral suspension. Surg Gynecol Obstet 1949;88:509–18.
2. Burch JC. Urethrovaginal fixation to Cooper's ligament for correction of stress incontinence, cystocele, and prolapse. Am J Obstet Gynecol 1961;81:281–90.
3. Tanagho EA. Colpocystourethropexy: the way we do it. J Urol 1976;116:751–3.
4. Green TH Jr. Urinary stress incontinence: differential diagnosis, pathophysiology, and management. Am J Obstet Gynecol 1975;122:368–400.
5. Leach GE, Dmochowski RR, Appell RA et al. Female Stress Urinary Incontinence Clinical Guidelines Panel summary report on surgical management of female stress urinary incontinence. The American Urological Association. J Urol 1997;158:875–80.
6. Vancaillie TG, Schuessler W. Laparoscopic bladder neck suspension. J Laparoendosc Surg 1991;1:169–73.
7. Pereyra AJ. A simplified surgical procedure for the correction of stress incontinence in women. West J Surg Obstet Gynecol 1959;67:223–6.
8. Kim HL, Gerber GS, Patel RV et al. Practice patterns in the treatment of female urinary incontinence: a postal and internet survey. Urology 2001;57:45–8.
9. Jha S, Arunkalaivanan AS, Davis J. Surgical management of stress urinary incontinence: a questionnaire based survey. Eur Urol 2005;47:648–52.
10. Fantl JA, Newman DK, Colling J et al. Urinary incontinence in adults: acute and chronic management. Clinical Practice Guideline, No. 2, 1996 Update. Rockville, MD: US Department of Health and Human Services. Public Health Service, Agency for Health Care Policy and Research. AHCPR Publication No. 96-0682. March 1996.
11. Viktrup L, Koke S, Burgio KL et al. Stress urinary incontinence in active elderly women. South Med J 2005;98:79–89.
12. Waetjen LE, Subak LL, Shen H et al. Stress urinary incontinence surgery in the United States. Obstet Gynecol 2003;101:671–6.
13. Diokno AC, Burgio K, Fultz H et al. Prevalence and outcomes of continence surgery in community dwelling women. J Urol 2003;170:507–11.
14. Bump RC, Mattiasson A, Bo K et al. The standardization of terminology of female pelvic organ prolapse and pelvic floor dysfunction. Am J Obstet Gynecol 1996;175:10–7.
15. Karram MM, Bhatia NN. The Q-tip test: standardization of the technique and its interpretation in women with urinary incontinence. Obstet Gynecol 1988;71:807–11.
16. Blaivas JG. Classification of stress urinary incontinence. Neurourol Urodyn 1983;2:103–4.
17. Bergman A, Koonings PP, Ballard CA. Negative Q-tip test as a risk factor for failed incontinence surgery in women. J Reprod Med 1989;34:193–7.
18. McGuire EJ, Lytton B, Pepe V et al. Stress urinary incontinence. Obstet Gynecol 1976;47:255–64.
19. Sand PK, Bowen LW, Panganiban R et al. The low pressure urethra as a factor in failed retropubic urethropexy. Obstet Gynecol 1987;69:399–402.
20. Richardson DA, Ramahi A, Chalas E. Surgical management of stress incontinence in patients with low urethral pressure. Gynecol Obstet Invest 1991;31:106–9.
21. Sand PK, Winkler H, Blackhurst DW et al. A prospective randomized study comparing modified Burch retropubic urethropexy and suburethral sling for treatment of genuine stress incontinence with low-pressure urethra. Am J Obstet Gynecol 2000;182:30–4.
22. Appell RA. Argument for sling surgery to replace bladder suspension for stress urinary incontinence. Urology 2000;56:360–3.
23. Bump RC, Sugerman HJ, Fantl JA et al. Obesity and lower urinary tract function in women: effect of surgically induced weight loss. Am J Obstet Gynecol 1992;167:392–7; discussion 397–9.
24. Zivkovic F, Tamussino K, Pieber D et al. Body mass index and outcome of incontinence surgery. Obstet Gynecol 1999;93:753–6.
25. Dainer M, Hall CD, Choe J et al. Pregnancy following incontinence surgery. Int Urogynecol J Pelvic Floor Dysfunct 1998;9:385–90.
26. DeLancey JO. Structural support of the urethra as it relates to stress urinary incontinence: the hammock hypothesis. Am J Obstet Gynecol 1994;170:1713–20; discussion 1720–3.
27. Germain MM, Ostergard DR. Retropubic Surgical Approach for Correction of Genuine Stress Incontinence in Urogynecology and Urodynamic: Theory and Practice. Baltimore: Williams and Wilkins, 1996.
28. Burch JC. Urethrovaginal fixation to Cooper's ligament for correction of stress incontinence, cystocele, and prolapse. Am J Obstet Gynecol 1961;81:281–90.
29. Lapitan MC, Cody DJ, Grant AM. Open retropubic colposuspension for urinary incontinence in women. Cochrane Database Syst Rev 2003;CD002912.

30. Weber AM, Abrams P, Brubaker L et al. The standardization of terminology for researchers in female pelvic floor disorders. Int Urogynecol J Pelvic Floor Dysfunct 2001;12:178–86.
31. Alcalay M, Monga A, Stanton SL. Burch colposuspension: a 10–20 year follow up. Br J Obstet Gynaecol 1995;102:740–5.
32. Ward KL, Hilton P. A prospective multicenter randomized trial of tension-free vaginal tape and colposuspension for primary urodynamic stress incontinence: two-year follow-up. Am J Obstet Gynecol 2004;190:324–31.
33. Jarvis GJ. Surgery for genuine stress incontinence. Br J Obstet Gynaecol 1994;101:371–4.
34. Moehrer B, Carey M, Wilson D. Laparoscopic colposuspension: a systematic review. BJOG 2003;110:230–5.
35. Kelly HA, Dumm WM. Urinary incontinence in women, without manifest injury to the bladder. Surg Gynecol Obstet 1914;18:444–450.
36. Bergman A, Elia G. Three surgical procedures for genuine stress incontinence: five–year follow-up of a prospective randomized study. Am J Obstet Gynecol 1995;173:66–71.
37. Kammerer-Doak DN, Dorin MH, Rogers RG et al. A randomized trial of Burch retropubic urethropexy and anterior colporrhaphy for stress urinary incontinence. Obstet Gynecol 1999;93:75–8.
38. Ulmsten U, Henriksson L, Johnson P et al. An ambulatory surgical procedure under local anesthesia for treatment of female urinary incontinence. Int Urogynecol J Pelvic Floor Dysfunct 1996;7:81–5; discussion 85–6.
39. Paraiso MF, Walters MD, Karram MM et al. Laparoscopic Burch colposuspension versus tension-free vaginal tape: a randomized trial. Obstet Gynecol 2004;104:1249–58.
40. Monga AK, Stanton SL. Urodynamics: prediction, outcome and analysis of mechanism for cure of stress incontinence by periurethral collagen. Br J Obstet Gynaecol 1997;104:158–62.
41. Shull BL. Anterior paravaginal defects. In: Rock JA, Thompson JD (eds) Te Linde's Operative Gynecology, 8th ed. New York: Lippincott, Williams & Wilkins, 1997: 997–9.
42. Harris RL, Cundiff GW, Theofrastous JP. The value of intraoperative cystoscopy in urogynecologic and reconstructive pelvic surgery. Am J Obstet Gynecol 1997;177:1367–71.
43. Dwyer PL, Carey MP, Rosamilia A. Suture injury to the urinary tract in urethral suspension procedures for stress incontinence. Int Urogynecol J Pelvic Floor Dysfunct 1999;10:15–21.
44. Hamasuna R, Betsunoh H, Sueyoshi T et al. Bacteria of preoperative urinary tract infections contaminate the surgical fields and develop surgical site infections in urological operations. Int J Urol 2004;11:941–7.
45. Bhatia NN, Karram MM, Bergman A. Role of antibiotic prophylaxis in retropubic surgery for stress urinary incontinence. Obstet Gynecol 1989;74(4):637–9.
46. Rogers RG, Kammerer-Doak D, Olsen A et al. A randomized, double-blind, placebo-controlled comparison of the effect of nitrofurantoin monohydrate macrocrystals on the development of urinary tract infections after surgery for pelvic organ prolapse and/or stress urinary incontinence with suprapubic catheterization. Am J Obstet Gynecol 2004;191:182–7.
47. Maher C, Dwyer P, Carey M et al. The Burch colposuspension for recurrent urinary stress incontinence following retropubic continence surgery. Br J Obstet Gynaecol 1999;106:719–24.
48. ACOG Practice Bulletin Number 21, October 2000.
49. Austin JC, Chacko SK, DiSanto M et al. A male murine model of partial bladder outlet obstruction reveals changes in detrusor morphology, contractility and myosin isoform expression. J Urol 2004;172:1524–8.
50. Galloway NT, Davies N, Stephenson TP. The complications of colposuspension. Br J Urol 1987;60:122–4.
51. Feyereisl J, Dreher E, Haenggi W et al. Long-term results after Burch colposuspension. Am J Obstet Gynecol 1994;171:647–52.
52. Wiskind AK, Creighton SM, Stanton SL. The incidence of genital prolapse after the Burch colposuspension. Am J Obstet Gynecol 1992;167:399–404; discussion 404–5.
53. Burch JC. Cooper's ligament urethrovesical suspension for stress incontinence. Nine years' experience – results, complications, technique. Am J Obstet Gynecol 1968;100:764–74.
54. Colombo M, Vitobello D, Proietti F et al. Randomised comparison of Burch colposuspension versus anterior colporrhaphy in women with stress urinary incontinence and anterior vaginal wall prolapse. BJOG 2000;107:544–51.
55. Olsen AL, Smith VJ, Bergstrom JO et al. Epidemiology of surgically managed pelvic organ prolapse and urinary incontinence. Obstet Gynecol 1997;89:501–6.
56. Lentz SS. Osteitis pubis: a review. Obstet Gynecol Surv 1995;50:310–5.
57. Michiels E, Knockaert DC, Vanneste SB. Infectious osteitis pubis. Neth J Med 1990;36:297–300.
58. Bergman A, Ballard CA, Koonings PP. Comparison of three different surgical procedures for genuine stress incontinence: prospective randomized study. Am J Obstet Gynecol 1989;160:1102–6.
59. Maher CF, Dwyer PL, Carey MP et al. Colposuspension or sling for low urethral pressure stress incontinence? Int Urogynecol J Pelvic Floor Dysfunct 1999;10:384–9.
60. Culligan PJ, Goldberg RP, Sand PK. A randomized controlled trial comparing a modified Burch procedure and a suburethral sling: long-term follow-up. Int Urogynecol J Pelvic Floor Dysfunct 2003;14:229–33; discussion 233.

61. Colombo M, Scalambrino S, Maggioni A et al. Burch colposuspension versus modified Marshall–Marchetti–Krantz urethropexy for primary genuine stress urinary incontinence: a prospective, randomized clinical trial. Am J Obstet Gynecol 1994;171:1573–9.
62. Su TH, Wang KG, Hsu CY et al. Prospective comparison of laparoscopic and traditional colposuspensions in the treatment of genuine stress incontinence. Acta Obstet Gynecol Scand 1997;76:576–82.
63. Langer R, Lipshitz Y, Halperin R et al. Long-term (10–15 years) follow-up after Burch colposuspension for urinary stress incontinence. Int Urogynecol J Pelvic Floor Dysfunct 2001;12:323–6; discussion 326–7.
64. Black NA, Downs SH. The effectiveness of surgery for stress incontinence in women: a systematic review. Br J Urol 1996;78:497–510.
65. Bhatia NN, Bergman A, Karram M. Changes in urethral resistance after surgery for stress urinary incontinence. Urology 1989;34:200–4.
66. Kenton K, Oldham L, Brubaker L. Open Burch urethropexy has a low rate of perioperative complications. Am J Obstet Gynecol 2002;187:107–10.
67. Cosson M, Boukerrou M, Narducci F et al. Long-term results of the Burch procedure combined with abdominal sacrocolpopexy for treatment of vault prolapse. Int Urogynecol J Pelvic Floor Dysfunct 2003;14:104–7.
68. Ward K, Hilton P. Prospective multicentre randomised trial of tension-free vaginal tape and colposuspension as primary treatment for stress incontinence. BMJ 2002;325:67–70.
69. Klutke JJ, Ramos S. Urodynamic outcome after surgery for severe prolapse and potential stress incontinence. Am J Obstet Gynecol 2000;182:1378–81.

60

An overview of pubovaginal slings: evolution of technology

Emily E Cole, Harriette M Scarpero, Roger R Dmochowski

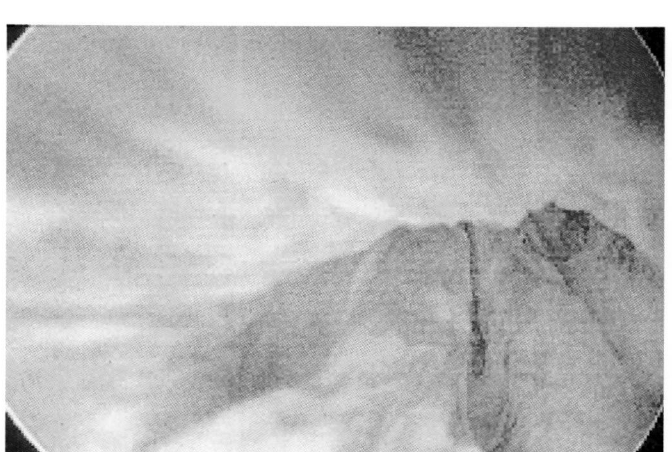

INTRODUCTION

Urinary incontinence has been discussed in the writings of physicians since ancient Egyptian times.[1] During the past century, many corrective procedures have been described showing varying degrees of success. Since the first description of the sling procedure nearly 100 years ago, the popularity of slings has waxed and waned. Initially, the sling was associated with high complication rates and was therefore reserved for the treatment of recurrent or refractory stress urinary incontinence (SUI). In the past 30 years, great strides have been made in the understanding of the pathophysiology of incontinence, leading to a resurgence in the popularity of pubovaginal slings. In 1997, the American Urological Association (AUA) Female Stress Incontinence Clinical Guidelines Panel concluded that suburethral slings, along with retropubic bladder suspensions, were the most efficacious procedures for long-term success in the treatment of SUI.[2] With a greater than 80% probability of *improvement* of symptomatic SUI at 48 months or longer, the pubovaginal sling has become the gold standard for surgical correction of SUI.

Technologic advances resulting in novel methods of suspension, such as the minimally invasive midurethral sling, have contributed to decreased surgical time and shorter postoperative convalescence. At the same time, the glut of technology and the continuous introduction of new suspension techniques have made interpretation of results more difficult. This, combined with controversy surrounding the lack of standardization in outcomes reporting, leads to many questions. Has enthusiasm for new technology been supported by long-term efficacy? Have de novo complications outweighed the utility and efficacy of novel techniques and materials? This chapter will address the current sling techniques and materials available with a systematic evaluation of the contemporary literature. The goal is to discuss the techniques, safety, tolerability, and efficacy of the standard bladder neck sling and the midurethral sling, and potentially identify which procedure is appropriate in certain situations.

PATHOPHYSIOLOGY OF STRESS INCONTINENCE

The popularity of pubovaginal and midurethral slings has mirrored advances in the understanding of the pathophysiology of SUI. In order to understand how a sling prevents SUI, it is first important to appreciate normal pelvic floor adaptation to increases in intra-abdominal pressure. Traditionally, the urethral continence mechanism was considered to be composed of two components: the internal sphincter, which represents a continuation of the detrusor smooth muscle, and the striated external sphincter.[3] From a clinical standpoint, the bladder neck/proximal urethra functions as a sphincteric mechanism in both sexes; however, there is no identifiable anatomic sphincter as such. Rather, a complex interaction of several factors – including smooth and striated muscle, intracellular matrix, and intrinsic mucosal factors – interplay to account for the components of a functional sphincter.[4–6] The principles underlying the function of this complex are: 1) watertight apposition of the urethral lumen; 2) compression of the wall around the lumen; 3) structural support to keep the proximal urethra from moving during increases in pressure; 4) a means of compensating for abdominal pressure changes; and 5) neural control.[7]

While the complex interactions resulting in these functional principles are not completely understood, several factors are known to assist in the maintenance of continence in the neurologically intact female. At rest, a seal composed of richly vascularized submucosal connective tissue compresses mucosal urethral folds to create a watertight closure.[8] This 'mucosal seal' is augmented by heightened wall tension created by luminal secretions from the periurethral glands. In addition, slow-twitch muscle fibers in the paraurethral layer of the external urethral sphincter maintain passive continence by tonic contraction of the urethra.[9,10]

This collective mechanism undergoes several changes in the face of increased intra-abdominal pressure. Reflex contraction of the levator ani musculature and urogenital diaphragm elevates suburethral support tissue, compressing the proximal urethra. These muscle complexes form a broad hammock upon which the pelvic viscera lie. The fascial covering of the levator ani consists of two leaves: the endopelvic fascia (abdominal side) and the pubocervical fascia (vaginal side). The two leaves envelop the proximal urethra and bladder neck medially and fuse laterally to insert along the tendinous arc of the obturator internus.[11] Augmenting the effects of the support network, striated muscle in the urethrovaginal sphincteric mechanism and compressor urethrae aid in compressing the urethra during intra-abdominal pressure transmission. The net result of the interplay of these changes is increased outlet resistance and continence.

Specific aspects of the continence mechanism have led to several theories about the pathophysiology of continence/incontinence. Until the early 1980s the understanding of stress incontinence was mainly based on the Enhorning theory.[12] Enhorning suggested that pressure transmission from the bladder to the urethra occurs because the urethra lies with the bladder within the abdomen. Based on this theory, increases in intra-abdominal pressure were thought to be transmitted directly to the bladder neck and urethra, compressing them and preventing leakage. Stress incontinence was thought to occur due to the descent of the bladder neck, the proximal urethra thereby not residing within the abdomen, and not able to be compressed when subjected to increases in intra-abdominal pressure. Thus, most surgical procedures aimed not only to support but also to elevate the bladder neck and urethra so that they would respond once again to changes in abdominal pressure.[13]

The 1990s witnessed a change in approach stimulated by DeLancey's hammock theory.[14] According to DeLancey, continence was due to tension arising within a subcervical hammock composed of muscle (anterior pubourethral bundle of the levator ani) held by two ligaments (pubourethral and conjunctive) connected to the endopelvic fascia. In the normal continent female, this musculofascial support provides a hammock upon which the urethra is compressed during increases in intra-abdominal pressure. This support mechanism constitutes a hammock under the urethra in its upper and middle portions. The hammock is composed of a segment of the anterior vaginal wall that is attached to the muscles of the pelvic floor and to the arcus tendineus. When either active or passive supports are altered, the urethra and bladder neck are no longer well supported, resulting in a defect in transmission of intra-abdominal pressure to the urethra. Based on the hammock theory, to restore continence the bladder neck and proximal urethra do not have to be elevated, but should be provided with adequate underlying support. This view advocates the placement of slings beneath the bladder neck.

More recently, much attention has been given to a new class of slings placed at the midurethra rather than the bladder neck. The midurethra has previously been found to be the site of maximal intraurethral pressure.[15] With this in mind, Petros and Ulmsten proposed in their 'integral theory' that the midurethra, rather than the bladder neck, may be the key mechanism involved in urinary continence.[16] Their theory is based on the idea that the opening and closure of the urethra and bladder neck are mainly controlled by three anatomical structures: 1) the tension within the pubourethral ligaments; 2) the activity of the pubococcygeus and levator ani muscles; and 3) the condition of the suburethral vaginal hammock. All of these structures are interconnected by connective tissues. Tension in the pubourethral ligaments ensures that the muscular component of support and the hammock provided by the vaginal wall interact correctly. If tension is adequate, three opposing forces result in kinking of the urethra and bladder neck and subsequent continence. The three forces (vectors) that influence the opening and closure of the inner urethra and bladder neck include: 1) forward force resulting from contraction of the pubococcygeus muscle; 2) backward force caused by contraction of the levator ani musculature; and 3) inferior force controlled by the longitudinal muscle of the anus. The midurethral sling was described according to this theory in order to correct the lack of tension in the pubourethral ligaments, to restore the attachment of the urethra to the pubic bone, and to restore the connections of the urogenital structures (Fig. 60.1).

PUBOVAGINAL SLINGS

History

At the beginning of the 20th century, the first slings were performed entirely from an abdominal approach and utilized autologous tissues. Initial attempts to increase outlet resistance using detached or tunneled muscle flaps met with severe complications, such as urethral

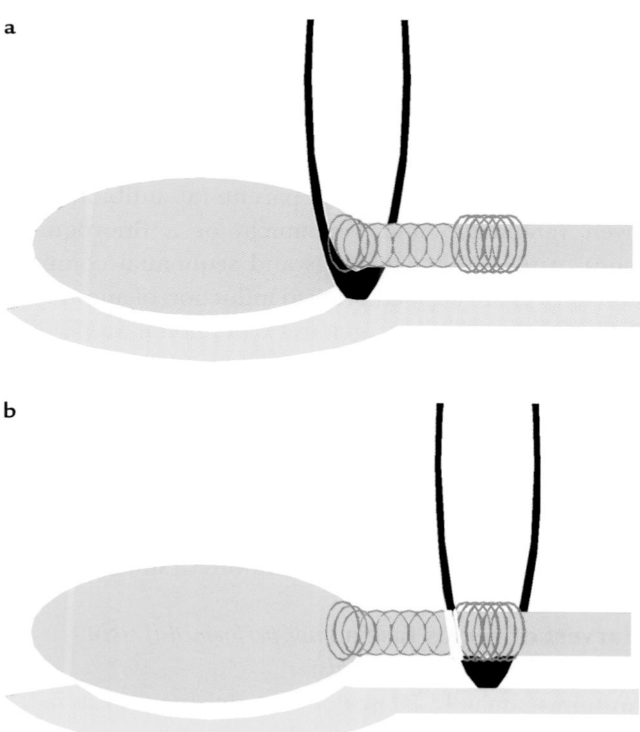

Figure 60.1. *Pressure transmission changes associated with the implantation of bladder neck (a) and midurethral support (b). (Courtesy of Professor D. Staskin, Harvard Medical School, Boston, USA.)*

sloughing, fistula formation, and bladder outlet obstruction. In 1942, Aldridge and colleagues performed the first abdominovaginal sling, proving that careful anatomic dissection revealed an 'almost bloodless plane' on either side of the urethra, permitting minimally traumatic entry into the space of Retzius.[17] Despite reports of long-term success, the complication rate continued to be high, and the popularity of the procedure waned over the following several decades.

As long-term efficacy of needle suspensions began to be questioned in the 1970s, there was a resurgence of interest in the pubovaginal sling. Improving on Aldridge's technique, McGuire and Lytton isolated a strip of rectus fascia and left it attached laterally on one side.[18] The free end of the strip was passed through the body of the rectus muscle, positioned under the urethra and reattached to the rectus fascia on the other side. Blaivas and Jacobs further modified the technique by completely detaching the fascial strip on both ends, and perforating the endopelvic fascia from below.[19]

Operative technique (bladder neck slings)

Preoperative considerations

Informed consent should involve a discussion of the risks, benefits, and options for sling surgery. Risks include, but are not limited to, bleeding, infection, injury to the bladder or urethra, dyspareunia, formation of anterior or apical prolapse, vesico-vaginal fistula formation, urinary retention, and de novo or worsening storage symptoms.

An hour prior to surgery, parenteral antibiotics are given (ampicillin and gentamicin or a fluoroquinolone). Antiembolic stockings and sequential compression devices are applied prior to induction of anesthesia. Following induction of general or regional anesthesia, the patient is carefully placed in a slightly exaggerated dorsal lithotomy position with appropriate pressure points adequately padded. Betadine or Hibiclens preparation solution is used to scrub the surgical field from umbilicus to mid-thigh, including the vagina. The patient is draped in standard surgical fashion, and a urethral catheter is placed for continuous drainage.

Harvest of rectus fascia (*not performed if using alternative biologic materials*)

An approximately 7 cm Pfannenstiel incision is made and carried down through the subcutaneous tissues, exposing the rectus fascia. A strip of rectus fascia approximately 2 × 7 cm is marked and excised using cut electrocautery. The sling is soaked in antibiotic solution while the fascial defect is closed with No. 1 delayed absorbable sutures. The skin is left open to assist in the passage of the sling sutures later in the procedure. Meanwhile, the sling is prepared for placement by securing No. 1 polypropylene sutures at either end. If autologous rectus fascia is not to be utilized, the graft of choice may be placed in antibiotic solution at any time.

Vaginal dissection

The urethral catheter balloon is palpated to confirm the location of the bladder neck. An inverted U is the incision of choice for maximal exposure of the bladder neck. The apex of the U should be based at the midurethra and the ends should extend laterally to the level of the bladder neck. A vertical midline incision from the midurethral to the bladder neck or beyond may be used if concomitant procedures are planned. With either incision, the vaginal mucosa is carefully dissected from the underlying surface of the pubourethral or pubocervical fascia using scissors. Lateral dissection should continue to the inferior edge of the pubic symphysis.

Using an index finger as a guide, the endopelvic fascia is perforated sharply bilaterally. When performing this maneuver, it is recommended that the point of the scissors be oriented towards the ipsilateral shoulder and should remain just under the pubic symphysis. Once this is complete, an index finger can be used to carefully develop the space of Retzius. The openings in the endopelvic fascia should be large enough to accommodate an arm of the fascial sling, allowing the sutured ends of the sling material to reside in the retropubic space.

Suture passage

Ligature carriers are passed into the retropubic space just superior to the pubic symphysis, approximately 2 cm lateral to the midline on each side. Each needle should be guided down along the pubic bone through the opening in the endopelvic fascia using a finger in the retropubic space as a guide. The needle is guided through the fascial opening and out of the lateral aspect of the vaginal incision on each side.

Cystoscopy

Cystourethroscopy should now be performed to ensure the integrity of the bladder, ureters, and urethra. Ureteral integrity can be confirmed with the visualization of efflux from bilateral ureteral orifices. If difficult to assess, indigo carmine can be administered to improve visualization. A 70-degree lens is utilized to check the dome and superolateral aspects of the bladder where penetration with needles is most likely to occur. It is important to visualize the entire path of the needle from the dome to the bladder neck and proximal urethra to rule out injury to these structures. If the bladder has been penetrated, the offending needle should be removed and can be re-passed once the bladder has been completely drained. Cystoscopy should be repeated following each pass to confirm bladder and urethral integrity.

Setting sling tension

The pre-placed sling sutures are fed through the eyes of the passed needles. The needles are then withdrawn, pulling the sling sutures up and out of the abdominal incision. The sling is positioned in the midline at the level of the bladder neck and is fixed to the periurethral fascia bilaterally with 4-0 vicryl sutures. The vaginal incision is closed with 2-0 absorbable sutures.

Sling tension is set in the abdominal incision. Typically, the suture ends are tied together loosely, commonly with two fingers easily able to be inserted under the knot. After two knots have been thrown, a hemostat is used to secure the knot. The urethral catheter is removed and the cystoscope is inserted. If there is no 'road bump' when the cystoscope is passed, this indicates that sling tension is not too great and additional knots can be added to the sutures. If there is a 'road bump', the existing knots should be untied and the sling should be loosened.

The abdominal wound is irrigated and closed in several layers with absorbable sutures. The vagina is packed with premarin-coated gauze. Saline-soaked gauze may be utilized in premenopausal women.

Postoperative course

Patients are usually admitted for overnight observation. The vaginal packing is removed on the following morning and the urethral catheter may or may not be removed. A voiding trial should be performed and if the patient cannot void to completion, the catheter may be replaced or the patient may be discharged with plans for intermittent self-catheterization. If the bladder was penetrated at any time during the procedure, the patient should be discharged with the urethral catheter in place, with plans for an outpatient voiding trial in 2–3 days.

Early ambulation is encouraged, but strenuous exercise and heavy lifting should be avoided. Patients should refrain from sexual intercourse until their vaginal incision is completely healed (approximately 6 weeks). Patients can usually be released to full activity at 6 weeks.

Pubovaginal sling results

Overview

The AUA Female Stress Incontinence Clinical Guidelines Panel investigated the efficacy of different surgical procedures for SUI by conducting a comprehensive review of published results. The panel concluded that suburethral slings, along with retropubic bladder suspensions, are the most efficacious procedures for the treatment of SUI.[2] There was a greater than 80% probability of improvement or cure at 48 months following a suburethral sling. It should be noted that at the time of the panel's report, slings were not yet standard treatment for primary SUI, but were reserved for complicated cases in which prior surgery had failed. It can be extrapolated from this information that if slings were utilized as initial treatment in cases of primary SUI, the success rates would have been even higher. Although medium- to long-term data have only recently been available for the use of slings in the treatment of intrinsic sphincter deficiency (ISD), it was the opinion of the panel that slings would also be an effective treatment for patients with primary ISD.

Since the release of this report, pubovaginal slings have been considered the gold standard for treatment of SUI. With the increased popularity, however, came a desire for improvement of the procedure. Novel sling materials and methods of suspension have decreased operative times and reduced postoperative convalescence. With a rapid influx of new products has come a plethora of short-term results and claims that each procedure is better than the last. There is currently no clear evidence as to which sling material is the best.

Autologous materials

The first autologous tissues used to increase bladder outlet resistance included gracilis muscle,[20] pyrimidalis flaps,[21] and levator ani.[22] Although Aldridge popularized the use of rectus fascia in the 1940s,[17] this material only achieved widespread use nearly 40 years later when its efficacy was confirmed.[18,19] Price[23] introduced the use of fascia lata as a sling material, a practice that has been widely used in the past. Both of these materials are durable, available in most patients, and are not predisposed to rejection. The drawback to the use of this material is that the harvest does require an additional incision and extended convalescence. While the extra incision and dissection associated with the sling harvest does add operating time, in most cases both parts of the procedure can be completed within 1 hour. In our experience, the postoperative convalescence is typically brief and the patient is at full level of activity in less than 6 weeks. The results of autologous slings with rectus fascia are summarized in Table 60.1.

Data supporting the use of autologous materials in sling surgery are abundant. While the subjective and objective cure rates range from 50[53] to 100%,[27,35,42] the

Table 60.1. *Results of rectus fascia and fascia lata slings*

Author	Material	No. of patients	Sling length (cm)	Mean F/U (months)	Cure (%)
Kaufman[24]	R	15	15	<48	93.3
Schultz-Lampel et al.[25]	R	11	–	24	63.6
Loughlin[26]	R	22	5	15	72.7
Mason & Roach[27]	R	63	4	12	93.7
Zaragoza[28]	R	60	6–8	25	100
Siegel et al.[29]	R	20[a]	–	185	80
Carr et al.[30]	R	96	11–13	22	97.9
Barbalias et al.[31]	R	32	12	>30	65.6
Chaikin et al.[32]	R	251	15	37	72.9
Maheshkumar et al.[33]	R	43[b]	–	17.4	95.3
Hassouna & Ghoneim[34]	R	82	7	41	89.1[c]
Kane et al.[35]	R	13	5[d]	26	100
Morgan et al.[36]	R	247	6–8	51	82.2
Kochakarn et al.[37]	R	100	–	12.1	94
Groutz et al.[38]	R	67	15	34	67.2
Kuo[39]	R	24	20	24	95.8
Borup& Nielson[40]	R	31	12	60	96.8
Gormley et al.[41]	R	41	–	>74	95.1
De Rossi[42]	R	27	8	20	100
Lucas et al.[43]	R	156	[e]	>30	76
Chou et al.[44]	R	98	12	36	95[c]
Pfitzenmaier et al.[45]	R	50	–	60[f]	63.9
Guatelli et al.[46]	R	35[g]	>20[h]	26	74.2
Almeida et al.[47]	R	30	–	33	70
Rodrigues et al.[48]	R	126	–	70.3	74.4
Kreder & Austin[49]	R/FL	27	–	22	96.3
Golomb et al.[50]	R/FL	18	15	30.7	88.9
Haab et al.[51]	R/FL	37	12–15	48.2	73
Wright et al.[52]	R/FL	33	13–15	16	93.9
Petrou & Frank[53]	R/FL	14	10	17	50
Richter et al.[54]	R/FL	57[i]	24	42	84
Flynn & Yap[55]	R/FL	71	12	44	90.1
Chien et al.[56]	R/FL	23	10	30.5	94.1[c]
Low[57]	FL	36	>24	>24	94.4
Addison et al.[58]	FL	97	–	12	86.6
Beck et al.[59]	FL	170	>17	>24	98.2
Karram & Bhatia[60]	FL	10	5 × 7	>12	90
Govier et al.[61]	FL	30	>24	14	69.7
Berman & Kreder[62]	FL	14	>17	14.9	71.4
Phelps et al.[63]	FL	27	>20[h]	20	77.8
Latini et al.[64]	FL	63	18–22	53	85[c]
Ellerkmann et al.[65]	FL	39	>24	>24	92.3

[a], includes one non-rectus sling; [b], 18 patients had sling attached to Cooper's ligament; [c], includes cured and improved patients; [d], suprapubic bone anchors; [e], includes full-length and short 'sling on a string'; [f], median follow-up; [g], includes seven porcine dermis slings; [h], attachment point is Cooper's ligament; [i], includes Aldridge-style rectus slings.
Cure (%), percentage of patients cured; FL, fascia lata, F/U, follow-up period; R, rectus,

mean cure rate is nearly 87%, with follow-up exceeding 10 years in some studies. De novo storage symptoms are reported in 0–27% of studies. After many early studies reported long-term voiding dysfunction (refractory urge incontinence, urinary retention requiring clean intermittent catheterization, and sling revision) in up to 33% of patients, more recent reports have quoted these findings in less than 10% of patients. Other reported complications are detailed in Table 60.2.

Both rectus fascia and fascia lata have predictable wound healing characteristics; however, it is our experience that rectus fascia may be stronger than fascia lata due to fiber organization and specimen thickness. In summary, rectus fascia slings are durable and safe and should be considered the 'gold standard' of materials available for sling surgery.

Allograft slings

Cadaveric allograft materials have been widely used in ophthalmic and orthopedic procedures for more than 20 years. The main advantage of allograft materials is the elimination of the need for an additional incision and dissection, causing increased operative time and extended postoperative convalescence. The theoretical advantage includes the use of human tissue with proposed increased biocompatibility and decreased chances of rejection and/or erosion. With any implantation of foreign materials comes concern about potential disease transmission. Although all cadaveric tissues are serologically screened for human immunodeficiency virus (HIV) and hepatitis, and are treated and rendered acellular prior to surgical implantation, false-negative results are possible. The estimated risk for transmission of HIV from a frozen allograft is 1 in 8 million,[67] and the risk of transmission of Creutzfeldt–Jakob disease is 1 in 3.5 million.

There are multiple cadaveric allografts available for implantation. Those utilized in sling surgery have included lyophilized dura mater, cadaveric fascia lata, and acellular dermal grafts. With follow-up ranging from 6 to 150 months, cure rates of lyophilized dura slings have ranged from 86 to 94%.[68–70] While there have been no complications specific to this material reported in the urologic literature, there has been a case of presumed transmission of Creutzfeldt–Jakob disease following implantation of a dural graft, raising concern about the long-term safety of this material.[71]

The use of cadaveric fascia lata (CFL) as a sling material was initially reported in 1996.[72] There are two main processing techniques for CFL materials, both designed to remove cellular materials and preserve integrity: 1) solvent dehydration and gamma irradiation; and 2) freeze drying. Regardless of processing technique, CFL requires 15–30 minutes in saline for rehydration. Results and complications for CFL slings are reported in Tables 60.3 and 60.4, respectively.

Dermal allografts are strong and more pliable than CFL grafts, exhibiting properties similar to autologous tissues in mechanical tests. Acellular dermis has been found to integrate into tissue consistently; however, there is the potential for sebaceous gland and hair follicle ingrowth.

Studies regarding the strength of the available allograft tissues have revealed conflicting results. Sutaria and Staskin found no statistically significant difference in tissue thickness or maximum load to failure between freeze-dried CFL, solvent-dehydrated CFL, and acellular cadaveric dermis.[85] Lemer et al. found that solvent-dehydrated CFL and acellular dermis had a similar load to failure as autologous fascia, whereas freeze-dried CFL was significantly inferior.[86]

The literature has suggested that there is a real risk of early allograft failure (within 3 months of implantation), particularly with the used of freeze-dried CFL.[87–89] Several mechanisms of graft loss have been proposed (autolysis, graft-versus-host reaction, etc.); as of yet, however, there has been no consensus on this subject. Concerning risk for disease transmission, DNA has been detected in freeze-dried CFL, solvent-dehydrated CFL, and acellular dermis.[90,91] These findings have unknown consequences, and raise concern about the potential health risks resulting from the implantation of foreign genetic material.

In summary, the use of allograft materials decreases operative times and potentially reduces postoperative convalescence by eliminating the need for additional dissection. Short- to medium-term cure rates approach those of autologous slings; however, long-term data for a single material is lacking. In addition, the presence of DNA in these materials raises questions about their long-term safety. Additional rigorous long-term surveillance with well-defined outcomes reporting is needed before adequate conclusions can be made about the global use of these materials.

Xenograft slings

Like cadaveric allografts, treated animal tissues have been utilized in surgical reconstructive procedures for many years. More recently, the use of porcine dermis has been popularized in the urologic community. The tissues are initially treated with proteolytic enzymes to remove non-collagenous material, and then are freeze-dried and sterilized with gamma irradiation. These materials are available as either a cross-linked or a non-cross-linked graft. Cross-linking involves treatment with a non-toxic

Table 60.2. *Complications of autologous slings*

Author	De novo storage symptoms (%)	Voiding dysfunction	Other complications
Kaufman[24]	–	Obstruction (33%) Dilation/VIU (27%) Excision (7%)	–
Schultz-Lampel et al.[25]	0	–	–
Loughlin[26]	6	Short-term retention/dilation (23%)	–
Mason & Roach[27]	–	CIC at 3 months (19%), at 6 months (6%) Long-term CIC (3%) Revision (2%)	DVT (2%)
Zaragoza[28]	12	–	–
Siegel et al.[29]	–	Incision (30%)	–
Carr et al.[30]	–	Refractory urinary incontinence (6%) CIC at 3 months (7%) Permanent CIC (3%) Early revision (1%)	–
Barbalias et al.[31]	0	–	–
Chaikin et al.[32]	8	CIC >1 month (2%)	Bladder perforation (1%)
Maheshkumar et al.[33]	–	CIC (42%) Incision (5%)	–
Hassouna & Ghoneim[34]	21	Strain to void (1%)	Pain from procedure (25%)
Kane et al.[35]	8	Dilation/VIU (8%)	Wound (15%)
Morgan et al.[36]	7	Urethrolysis (2%)	Pelvic hematoma (1%) Incisional hernia (1%) DVT (<1%) PE (<1%)
Kochakarn et al.[37]	5	Mean time of CIC = 8.9 weeks (39%)	Wound (1%)
Groutz et al.[38]	10	Weak stream at 3 weeks (22%)	–
Kuo[39]	8	Urethrolysis (4%)	Subcutaneous hematoma (8%) Persistent dysuria (4%)
Borup & Nielson[40]	13	CIC at 6 months (39%) CIC at 1 year (16%) Revision at 1 year (3%)	Sling erosion (8%)
Gormley et al.[41]	–	–	–
De Rossi[42]	7	Weak stream (7%)	Bladder perforation (14%)
Giannitsas et al.[66]	43	CIC (8%) De novo voiding problems (33%)	–
Chou et al.[44]	4	Revision (1%)	–
Pfitzenmaier et al.[45]	–	–	–
Guatelli et al.[46]	6	Obstruction (6%) Incision (3%)	–
Almeida et al.[47]	–	–	–
Rodrigues et al.[48]		Obstruction (11%)	
Kreder & Austin[49]	12	Long-term CIC (7%)	Thigh hematoma (4%) Death from MI (4%)
Golomb et al.[50]	5	Refractory urge (6%)	–

cont.

Table 60.2. *Complications of autologous slings (cont.)*

Author	De novo storage symptoms (%)	Voiding dysfunction	Other complications
Haab et al.[51]	27	Refractory urge (24%) CIC (3%)	–
Wright et al.[52]	10	Urethrolysis (3%)	–
Petrou & Frank[53]	0	Long-term CIC (7%)	–
Richter et al.[54]	–	High PVR (16%) Posture (4%) CIC (7%)	–
Flynn & Yap[55]	5	Retention >45 days (3%) Urethrolysis (1%)	–
Chien et al.[56]	–	–	–
Low[57]	–	–	UVF (8%)
Addison et al.[58]	–	Long-term retention (6%)	Bladder perforation (8%) Wound (2%) PE (1%)
Beck et al.[59]	–	Mean period of voiding dysfunction = 2 months Incision (3%)	Wound (5%) FL hematoma (1%) Seroma (4%) PE (1%) DVT (1%)
Karram & Bhatia[60]	–	Mean time to spontaneous void = 20 days; Maximum = 39 days	–
Govier et al.[61]	14	Mean CIC = 3.3 weeks; CIC at 4 months (3%) Incision (3%)	Leg pain (3%)
Berman & Kreder[62]	–	–	Leg hematoma (14%)
Phelps et al.[63]	–	Retention/incision (3%) CIC (2%)*	–
Latini et al.[64]	–	–	–
Ellerkmann et al.[65]	–	–	–

* Percentages include totals for 27 fascia lata slings and 36 cadaveric fascia lata slings.
CIC, clean intermittent catheterization; De novo storage symptoms (%), percentage of patients with de novo storage symptoms (i.e. urgency, frequency, urge incontinence); Dilation, urethral dilation; DVT, deep vein thrombosis; FL, fascia lata; Incision, sling incision; MI, myocardial infarction; PE, pulmonary embolism; PVR, post-void residual; Revision, sling revision; UVF, urethrovaginal fistula; VIU, visual internal urethrotomy; Wound, wound infection or complication.

substance such as diisocyanate to render them more resistant to degradation by the host. Although cross-linking was initially thought to reduce antigenicity of the graft, cases of encapsulation have raised questions about the remodeling characteristics of tissues treated in this manner.[92] Success rates of porcine dermal slings have been good, but – as with allograft materials – long-term consistent data have been lacking. In one study, Nicholson and Brown reported a cure rate of 79% in 24 patients undergoing porcine dermal sling with a follow-up of more than 48 months. Thirteen percent of their patients developed urinary retention more than a year postoperatively.[93] Cure rates in another study with mean follow-up of 12 months approached 89%, with 7% of patients requiring sling release for obstructive voiding.[94] There have been no reports of sling extrusion or erosion.

Porcine small intestinal submucosa (SIS) has recently been marketed for pubovaginal sling surgery. SIS is harvested from small intestine and the extracellular matrix is maintained intact. The collagen, growth factors, glycosaminoglycans, proteoglycans, and glycoproteins promote host cell proliferation through SIS layers. The SIS ultimately provides a scaffold for tissue remodeling and ingrowth of host connective tissue structures. SIS is currently available for use in pelvic surgery in 1- and

Table 60.3. Results of cadaveric fascia lata slings

Author	Processing	No. of patients	Sling length (cm)	Mean F/U (months)	Cure (%)
Elliott & Boone[73]	SD	26	12	15	76.9
Amundsen et al.[74]	FD	91	15	19.4	62.6
Govier[75,76]	FD	104	24	12	66.3[a]
Vereecken & Lechat[77]	FD	8	>20	24	100
Walsh et al.[78]	FD	31	10	13.5	93.5
Flynn & Yap[55]	FD	63	12	29	87.3
Chien et al.[56]	–	83	10	27.4	90.1[b]
Bodell & Leach[79]	SD	186	7[c]	16.4	75.8[d]
Richter et al.[80]	FD	102	25	35	75[b]
Phelps et al.[63]	–	36	>20	20	83.3
Hartanto et al.[81]	–	34	7[c]	12.5	83.3
Almeida et al.[47]	FD	30	6–8	36	40
Gurdal et al.[82]	SD	42	4	16	88
Park et al.[83]	FD	60	20	>36	85
Fitzgerald et al.[84]	FD	27		12	59
Ellerkmann et al.[65]	SD	32	>24	>24	90.5

[a], updated cure rate with eight additional failures between 4 and 13 months postoperatively[88]; [b], includes cured and improved patients; [c], transvaginal bone anchors; [d], patients reporting >50% improvement and no subjective SUI.
Cure (%), percentage of patients cured; FD, freeze-dried; F/U, follow-up period; SD, solvent-dehydrated.

4-ply sheets for prolapse repairs, and 4- and 8-ply slings. Results for the use of this material in the urologic literature are lacking. Rutner et al. reported results of a SIS sling suspended with bone anchors in 115 adults.[95] At 36 months follow-up, 94% were continent, while only one patient required urethrolysis from excessive sling tension. Palma and colleagues cured 93% of their 28 patients with a mean follow-up of 8 months.[96] The tensile strength of SIS remains questionable. Kubricht et al. found the mean suture pull through load of freeze-dried SIS to be less than freeze-dried CFL.[97] In addition, questions remain about the immunogenicity of SIS. There have been multiple reports of significant inflammatory responses following implantation of SIS slings.[98–100]

Bovine pericardium is currently available in a cross-linked and non-cross linked variety. The material is reportedly thinner than CFL, but may possess greater tensile strength.[101] As with SIS, long-term experience with this material does not yet exist. Pelosi et al. reported a 95% cure rate in 22 patients having undergone use of the YAMA urology patch sling with cross-linked bovine pericardium at a mean follow-up of 20 months.[102] As with other allograft and xenograft materials, immunogenicity is a concern with bovine pericardium. Studies have confirmed the presence of DNA in these materials; however, the amount extracted may be much smaller than either CFL or cadaveric dermis.[103] Additionally, the biocompatibility of bovine pericardium has come into question with recent reports of frequent rejections following implantation.[104,105]

In summary, despite claims that xenograft materials are biocompatible, have excellent tensile strength, are non-immunogenic, and are devoid of viruses and prions, there is insufficient evidence as yet to support these claims. Long-term follow-up is only available for porcine dermis slings, with success and complication rates approaching those of autologous slings. All of the described materials appear to have tensile strength similar to cadaveric allografts; however, claims of biocompatibility and non-immunogenicity should be met with intense scrutiny. Ultimately, ingrowth of native human tissue into a xenograft-derived scaffolding of acellular matrix may offer the ideal material for use in sling operations. Efforts to create these materials are ongoing.

Synthetic slings

In situations when no suitable native tissues were available, experimentation was performed with synthetic materials. In the 1950s, nylon and perlon were used for sling construction.[106] Due to the narrow nature of the

Table 60.4. *Complications of cadaveric fascia lata slings*

Author	De novo storage symptoms (%)	Voiding dysfunction	Other complications
Elliott & Boone[73]	13	–	–
Amundsen et al.[74]	44	Urethrolysis (1%)	–
Govier[75,76]	–	Long-term retention (2%)	–
Vereecken & Lechat[77]	13	Incision (13%)	–
Walsh et al.[78]	–	Posture to void (77%) CIC at 4 months (35%) CIC at 1 year (3%)	–
Flynn & Yap[55]	28	Retention at 56 days (2%)	–
Chien et al.[56]	–	–	
Bodell & Leach[79]	–	–	Osteitis (1%)
Richter et al.[80]	–	Difficulty emptying bladder (58%)	–
Phelps et al.[63]	–	Retention/incision (3%) CIC (2%)*	–
Hartanto et al.[81]	–	–	–
Almeida et al.[47]	–	–	–
Gurdal et al.[82]	–	CIC for mean of 20 days (12%)	–
Park et al.[83]	5	High PVR at 30 days (5%) Suprapubic suture removal (3%) CIC for 1 month (2%)	Bladder perforation (2%) Blood transfusion (7%)
Fitzgerald et al.[84]	–	–	–
Ellerkmann et al.[65]	–	–	–

* Percentages include totals for 27 fascia lata slings and 36 cadaveric fascia lata slings.
CIC, clean intermittent catheterization; De novo storage symptoms (%), percentage of patients with de novo storage symptoms (i.e. urgency, frequency, urge incontinence); Incision, sling incision; PVR, post-void residual.

strips of material, 'strangulation' of the bladder neck commonly resulted in high rates of urethral obstruction. Additionally, high rates of suprapubic abscess and urethrovaginal fistula formation led to several authors condemning synthetics as inappropriate sling materials. Despite the implementation of wider strips and a decrease in complication rates,[107] the interest in synthetic materials waned.

While all synthetic sling materials are strong and non-toxic, they differ in many ways. Almost all are permanent, though experimentation has been performed only with absorbable types. Sling types can also differ in composition (monofilament versus multifilament), pore size, and flexibility. Multifilament meshes contain interstices that are much smaller than standard pores. These small interstices may be large enough to allow bacteria (1 μm) to migrate into the mesh, but may be too small to allow entry of mediators of the body's immune response such as macrophages and lymphocytes (50 μm).[108] In theory, these very small pores may also inhibit the influx of host fibroblasts and deter the ingrowth of new connective tissue, thereby preventing proper sling integration and remodeling.

More recently, there has been a resurgence of the use of synthetic sling materials. Permanent synthetic materials are easily accessible, relatively inexpensive to produce, strong, and non-carcinogenic. All are associated with success rates similar to those of autologous materials. Dense, multifilament meshes such as Gore-Tex and Silastic may not integrate into host tissue well and therefore may be associated with prohibitively high complication rates. Despite larger pore size, high rates of erosion and sinus formation have been seen with other multifilament meshes such as Mersilene. Impregnation with antibiotic protectants has not reduced the complication rates of these materials. Loose monofilament meshes have resulted in greatly reduced complication rates and are clearly the better choice for utilization in sling surgery. Due to the large pore size, monofilament construction, and flexibility, Prolene is currently the synthetic material of choice for use in pelvic reconstructive surgery.

Conclusions

Since the introduction of the pubovaginal sling nearly 100 years ago, there have been countless variations and 'improvements' made to the techniques and materials involved. Only with the introduction of DeLancey's hammock theory did we truly begin to understand why and how the pubovaginal sling has a positive effect in the treatment of SUI. The pubovaginal or bladder neck sling is the support mechanism that was described by DeLancey. The object of the procedure is to provide the necessary backing (i.e. sling) to the bladder neck and proximal urethral to build the framework for adequate closure of the urethra during times of increased abdominal stress. Even in cases with a fixed, open urethra as is seen in the patient with severe ISD, the pubovaginal sling can provide enough of a support backing to ensure continence.

The resurgence of the pubovaginal sling, along with the reduction of the morbidity associated with the procedure, has truly revolutionized surgical treatment of stress urinary incontinence. However, as mentioned previously, the introduction of new technology should always be met with increased scrutiny as to the accuracy of the results reported.

As determined by the AUA panel, autologous rectus fascia pubovaginal slings are viewed as the gold standard in the treatment of SUI. How do the other materials measure up? Are the reductions in operative time and postoperative morbidity worth the possibility for reduced material strength, immunogenicity, and even disease transmission? These questions will remain unanswered until reliable, standardized data are accessible for every new material available.

MIDURETHRAL SLINGS

History

With the above discussion of technologic advances in treatments for SUI, it is natural that what follows is a discussion about midurethral slings. Since its introduction onto the clinical market in 1994–95 by Petros and Ulmsten,[109] the minimally invasive tension-free midurethral sling has achieved widespread acceptance as a first-line treatment for SUI. Initially, this operation was called the 'combined intravaginal sling and tuck operation' and involved minimal dissection at the level of the midurethra and no perforation of the endopelvic fascia. Specialized tunnelers were passed through the urogenital diaphragm from below up through the abdomen, staying just posterior to the pubic symphysis. A 45 cm segment of Mersilene tape was positioned loosely around the midurethra, and the ends were guided up into the abdominal incisions through the tunnelers. The free tape ends were cut and removed entirely 4–8 weeks following the surgery. The authors' initial study reported a cure rate of 82% at 12 months, and 76% at 36 months.[110]

An interesting concept of this procedure was the use of synthetic material in order to reduce the morbidity related to autologous tissue use. Initially, Mersilene was the material of choice, with larger pore sizes and more flexibility than Gore-Tex. However, as more reports of erosion of Mersilene circulated in the literature, and with its ultimate recall in 1999, experimentation was carried out with other materials.[111–113] Ultimately, loosely woven monofilament Prolene mesh was shown to be the best material available for sling construction, and was adopted as the material of choice for midurethral slings.[114]

Why does it work?

The midurethral sling procedure was initially developed to restore the fulcrum-like interaction between the pubourethral ligament and the anterior vaginal wall.

The procedure stemmed from the 'integral theory' previously described by Petros and Ulmsten.[109] Its development was based on the idea that the opening and closure of the proximal urethra and bladder neck are mainly controlled by a direct interaction between the pubourethral ligaments and the suburethral vaginal wall and its muscular support, the levator ani and the pubococcygeus muscles. If the tension in the pubourethral ligaments and the interplay between all involved factors are adequate, then during times of increased intra-abdominal stress the forward contraction of the pubococcygeus muscles and the backward contraction of the levator ani muscles result in kinking of the urethra. Stress incontinence is thought to result when these interactions are interrupted in any way. The midurethral sling was designed to correct the lack of tension in the pubourethral ligaments and to re-establish the connection between the urethra and the pubic bone, thereby re-creating the urethral kinking phenomenon in times of stress, but not affecting the urethra during times of rest.

This concept has been supported by studies such as that of Sarlos et al.[115] that have investigated the effects of a midurethral sling with perineal ultrasound. The positions of the implanted tape, the bladder neck, and the urethra were sonographically documented at rest and with abdominal straining. These images were compared with preoperative examinations. The authors reported dynamic kinking of the urethra in 36 of 40 cases, and movement of the tape against the pubic symphysis, causing compression of the tissue between the tape and the symphysis, in all cases. There was no change in bladder neck position or mobility between pre- and postoperative studies. The authors proposed that even if stress incontinence did not result from defective pubourethral ligaments, the midurethral sling was nonetheless effective by causing urethral kinking and compression during times of intra-abdominal stress. These findings have been echoed by other imaging studies.[116]

Interestingly, studies such as that just described have reported no change in bladder neck and proximal urethral position during straining in those patients who have undergone midurethral sling operation. According to DeLancey's hammock hypothesis, proximal urethral hypermobility would be directly involved in the pathogenesis of genuine stress incontinence, and therefore restoration of vaginal support to the bladder neck and urethra would most effectively cure incontinence. Several studies, however, have demonstrated that the midurethral tape, while curing incontinence, actually has very little clinical effect on the positioning or support of the bladder neck or proximal urethra. Klutke et al.[117] and Lukacz et al.[118] described the results of Q-tip tests both before and after the placement of a midurethral sling. Both centers found some change in the mean straining Q-tip angle; however, in both studies, the majority of patients, despite being cured of their stress incontinence, did have significant postoperative urethral hypermobility. Lo et al.[119] assessed the position and mobility of the bladder neck in 90 women before and after placement of a midurethral tape using ultrasound with the pubic bone as a reference point. Although cure of incontinence occurred in 93%, there were no significant differences in measurements of urethral position and mobility with straining. Halaska et al.[120] reported similar findings determined by dynamic magnetic resonance images. More recently, Atherton et al.[121] compared the effect of midurethral sling and Burch colposuspension on bladder neck mobility using perineal ultrasound, both preoperatively and 4 weeks after surgery. They found that both procedures resulted in more acute resting bladder neck angles and decreased Valsalva angles; however, the Burch procedure produced more dramatic changes than the midurethral sling. These studies raise important questions with their unanimous conclusion that the cure of stress incontinence does not necessarily require correction of urethral hypermobility.

The potential for the reduction in postoperative voiding difficulties has been an important consideration in the development of the midurethral sling. Many authors propose that normal voiding depends on mobility of the proximal urethral for its initiation. It is well accepted that surgical procedures can adversely affect voiding, especially in cases in which they interfere with the proximal urethra. The midurethral sling was designed with this in mind. With minimal vaginal dissection, minimal change in the architecture of the vagina, and minimal effect on the mobility of the proximal urethra, the hypothesis was that incontinence can be corrected with little effect on normal voiding patterns.

Materials available

Since the introduction of the concept of the midurethral sling and its establishment as an acceptable surgical treatment for incontinence, there has been an influx of new procedural methods and surgical tools. Originally, the technique was introduced as the tension-free vaginal tape (TVT), a procedure that involved minimal vaginal dissection, followed by passage of trocars and tape from the vaginal incision, along the pubic bone, and out through two small abdominal stab incisions. Multiple variations of the TVT, including different operative techniques and different tape materials, have been marketed. A transpubic method was introduced in which the trocars are guided much the way as Stamey needles, i.e. from abdominal stab incisions just above the pubic symphysis, along the pubic bone, and into a small vaginal incision. Additionally, a transobturator technique has been introduced involving passage of trocars through the obturator foramen bilaterally. Thus far, there have been no head-to-head trials comparing the different techniques for midurethral tape placement. We would assert that the choice should be made based on surgeon comfort, and that new techniques should be met with skepticism until adequate success and complications data are available.

Operative techniques

Preoperative considerations

As with traditional slings, each patient being considered for midurethral tape placement should be evaluated with a comprehensive history, physical examination, and urodynamic assessment. It is important to characterize the incontinence and to document the presence of urgency, frequency, and/or urge incontinence to assist in preoperative counseling.

Informed consent should involve a discussion of the risks, benefits, and options for sling surgery. Risks include, but are not limited to, bleeding, infection, injury to the bladder or urethra, dyspareunia, formation of anterior or apical prolapse, vesico-vaginal fistula formation, urinary retention, and de novo or worsening storage symptoms.

An hour prior to surgery, parenteral antibiotics are given (ampicillin and gentamicin or a fluoroquinolone). Antiembolic stockings and sequential compression devices are applied prior to induction of anesthesia. Following induction of general or regional anesthesia, the patient is carefully placed in a slightly exaggerated dorsal lithotomy position with appropriate pressure points adequately padded. Betadine or Hibiclens preparation solution is used to scrub the surgical field from umbilicus to mid-thigh, including the vagina. The patient is draped in standard surgical fashion, and a urethral catheter is placed for continuous drainage.

Anesthetic considerations

At the time of the introduction of the TVT, the preference was to perform the procedure under local anesthesia with sedation. Authors suggested that the procedure was less morbid when performed under local anesthesia and they stressed the importance of being able to perform an adequate stress test during the procedure to set adequate, but not excessive, tension on the sling.[122,123] Klutke and Klutke argued that, when properly placed, the local anesthetic does not paralyze the musculature of the pelvic floor, ensuring that biofeedback will be accurate in determining the degree of resistance necessary at the bladder outlet. They also suggested that local anesthetic injected into areas of the pelvis through which the sling would pass will also create tissue 'hydrodissection' that allows easier passage of the trocar. They recommended a long-acting local anesthetic with or without epinephrine.[122]

Some surgeons, however, are uncomfortable performing the procedure under a local anesthetic. More recently, there have been reports that bladder outlet obstruction and urinary retention rates are not influenced by the mode of anesthesia, provided that the tape is positioned loosely.[124] Spinal, general, and local anesthesia have yielded comparable results, but there has yet to be a prospective, randomized study comparing results with specific anesthetic techniques.

Transvaginal midurethral sling

The transvaginal technique has changed little since its first introduction. A midline vaginal incision is made beginning 1.0 cm from the external urethral meatus that encompasses the midurethra and extends 1.5 cm in length. The anterior vaginal epithelium is dissected from the midline incision for a distance of approximately 5 mm on either side. The purpose of this initial sharp dissection is to align the trocar tip in the proper plane and to minimize the risk of vaginal tape exposure later on. After satisfactory initial dissection, the bladder is emptied and a catheter guide is inserted into the urethral catheter. The catheter can then be used as a rigid probe to mobilize the urethra and the bladder neck away from the path of the trocar.

Two suprapubic stab incisions are made approximately one fingerbreadth cephalad and lateral to the pubic tubercles on either side.

The introducer is attached to one trocar, and the tip of the trocar is guided into the lateral aspect of the anterior vaginal wall incision and aimed towards the lateral vaginal sulcus on that side. Once the tip reaches this position, it is directed towards the ipsilateral shoulder in a ventral–lateral direction. The trocar is slowly advanced until a 'give' is felt, indicating that the trocar has breached the endopelvic fascia. Once in the retropubic space, lateral passage stops and the introducer is dropped, rotating the trocar upwards along the inferior pubic ramus and up to the abdominal fascia. The trocar is then guided through the abdominal stab incision. The introducer is removed from the trocar, the urethral catheter is removed, and cystoscopy is performed with the 70-degree lens to ensure bladder integrity. Bladder penetration typically occurs in the upper lateral aspect of the bladder, so it is important to inspect the dome and superior bladder neck. Should bladder penetration occur, the bladder is drained, the cystoscope removed, and the trocar is backed out completely. A second pass may then be attempted. If no penetration occurs, the introducer is removed from the end of the trocar and the trocar with the attached tape is pushed upward vaginally and pulled out through the skin incision. The same sequence is repeated with the other trocar on the opposite side. Once both trocars have been passed, tension of the tape can be adjusted.

Initial tension adjustment is performed using a spacer instrument such as Mayo scissors, a No. 8 Hagar dilator, or a right angle clamp. The plastic sheath around the tape is removed following detachment of the trocars from either end of the tape. The spacing instrument is placed under the tape, and the plastic sheaths are removed by pulling up on each end with hemostats. The free ends of the excess tape are then cut at the level of the skin. The suprapubic stab incisions are closed with 4-0 vicryl and Steri-strips. The vaginal incision is closed with 2-0 vicryl. A vaginal pack can be left at the surgeon's preference.

Transpubic midurethral tape

The transpubic procedure is very much a combination of the transvaginal midurethral sling and the traditional sling techniques. The initial steps are identical. Two suprapubic stab incisions and a 1.5 cm midline vaginal incision are made. Minimal dissection is performed to elevate the vaginal epithelium from the underlying tissue. The trocars, however, are passed in much the same way as Stamey needles are passed during a traditional bladder neck sling. The trocar is introduced into the abdominal incision and the rectus fascia is penetrated. The trocar is guided downwards and slightly medially in very close approximation to the pubic bone. The trocar is then guided through the endopelvic fascia and out of the vaginal incision. This maneuver is repeated on the contralateral side. The urethral catheter is then removed and cystoscopy is performed with the 70-degree lens to ensure bladder and urethral integrity. Once this has been confirmed, the tape ends are connected to the trocar bilaterally, and the trocars are withdrawn through the abdominal incisions, bringing the tape ends out with them. The tape is positioned beneath the midurethra and the trocars are cut off. Tension is adjusted as the plastic sheath is removed in the same manner as that described for the transvaginal approach.

Transobturator midurethral sling

Delorme initially described the transobturator tape technique in 2001.[125] The patient is positioned in an exaggerated dorsal lithotomy position, with the thighs bent back onto the abdomen at an angle of 120 degrees. A vertical midline vaginal incision is made and dissection is performed in the same fashion as that described above. The lateral margin of the ischiopubic ramus is identified between an index finger placed in the lateral vaginal fornix and the thumb placed in front of the obturator foramen. A puncture incision is made 15 mm lateral to the ischiopubic ramus on a horizontal line level with the preputium clitoridis. The tunneler is held in the same hand as the side on which the operator is working. The tunneler is held vertically with the handle downwards. It is introduced through the skin incision and is guided across the obturator membrane. As the membrane is crossed, some resistance should be felt.

The tunneler is then turned to the horizontal position, with the handle pointing medially. The tip of the tunneler is led medially towards the urethra, aiming above the urethral meatus and underneath the symphysis pubis. The safest method is to lead the tunneler around the ischiopubic ramus while remaining in contact with it. A finger is placed in the vaginal incision to ensure that the tunneler is not piercing the vagina and to hold the urethra superiorly, protecting it from the trocar. The finger should make contact with the tunneler laterally underneath the symphysis pubis. The tunneler can then be delivered through the vaginal incision under fingertip guidance. The same procedure is repeated on the opposite side.

Although some authors state that cystoscopy to ensure safe trocar passage is not a necessary step in this procedure,[125,126] bladder perforation has been reported[127] and anecdotal experience confirms this to be a risk of this procedure. We recommend cystourethroscopy following trocar placement to ensure safe passage.

Following confirmation of safe passage, the tape may be secured to the trocar tips and pulled through the lateral stab incisions. Tension can be adjusted as described above for transvaginal and transpubic techniques.

Since this initial description, new Helical tunnelers have been introduced and tailored based on patient anatomy, facilitating the safe passage of the trocars and tape.

More recently, authors have presented an 'inside-out' technique in which the trocars are guided from the vaginal incision out to the thigh folds in the opposite trajectory of that described above.[128] Anatomic studies have detailed that when passed in this manner, the tape avoids the pelvic compartment completely. The proponents of this technique argue that it is more protective against injury to the bladder, urethra, or dorsal nerve of the clitoris.[129]

Postoperative care

Patients are usually discharged home following a brief recovery room stay. The vaginal packing and the urethral catheter are removed prior to discharge. A voiding trial should be performed and if the patient cannot void to completion, the catheter may be replaced or the patient may be discharged with plans for intermittent self-catheterization. If the bladder was penetrated at any time during the procedure, the patient should be discharged with the urethral catheter in place, with plans for an outpatient voiding trial in 2–3 days.

Early ambulation is encouraged, but strenuous exercise and heavy lifting should be avoided. Patients should refrain from sexual intercourse until their vaginal incision is completely healed (approximately 6 weeks). Patients can usually be released to full activity at 6 weeks.

Results

The midurethral sling has become a mainstay of anti-incontinence therapy. TVT has been the most well known product in this market, having been performed in over 200,000 women in Europe. In the original study group from Scandinavia, 91% were cured and 7% were significantly improved at a minimum of 12 months.[130] Nilsson et al. recently published results of 90 women having undergone midurethral sling placement after 7 years of follow-up.[131] They reported subjective and objective cure rates of 81.3% at a mean follow-up of 91 months. De novo urge symptoms were seen in 6.3% of patients, recurrent urinary tract infections were seen in 7.5%, and asymptomatic pelvic organ prolapse was seen in 7.8%. No other long-term adverse effects of the procedure were detected. Medium- and long-term results from several large European and American centers have been published and results of studies with 12 or more months of follow-up are summarized in Table 60.5.

Several studies have reported results comparing the tension-free midurethral tape with other anti-incontinence procedures. Ward and Hilton reported results of a prospective randomized study comparing TVT (175 patients) with open colposuspension (169 patients).[154] They utilized questionnaires, clinical examination, and 1-hour pad tests to assess outcomes with a follow-up of 24 months. When patients who failed to follow-up were considered failures, the cure rates for TVT and colposuspension were 63% and 51%, respectively. Overall per-

Table 60.5. *Results for midurethral slings*

Author	No. of patients	Mean F/U (months)	Cure (%)
Olsson & Kroon[132]	51	36	90
Moran et al.[133]	40	12.3	80
Jacquetin[134]	156	12–36	89
Soulie et al.[135]	120	15.2	87
Haab et al.[124]	62	16.8	87
Wang & Chen[136]	73	27	86
Azam et al.[137]	67	12	81
Nilsson et al.[138]	85	56	85
Meschia et al.[108]	404	21	92
Rezapour & Ulmsten[139]	34	48	91*
Rezapour et al.[140]	49	48	86*
Rezapour & Ulmsten[141]	80	48	89*
Buscant et al.[142]	30	36	84
Liapis et al.[143]	68	24	90
Glavind & Larsen[144]	15	12	93
Kinn[145]	75	24	80
Jeffry et al.[146]	112	25	89
De Val et al.[147]	187	27	90
Lo et al.[148]	45	20	91
Chung & Chung[149]	91	12	100*
Adamiak et al.[150]	103	13	95
Brophy et al.[151]	158	26	86
Sander et al.[152]	45	12	87
Arunkalaivanan & Barrington[94]	68	12	85
Tsivian et al.[153]	55	55	79
Nilsson et al.[131]	80	91	81

* Includes cured and improved patients.
Cure (%), percentage of patients cured; F/U, follow-up period.

ceived health status was better in the TVT group, and enterocele and/or vault prolapse was seen more commonly in the colposuspension group. The discrepancy in these reported results with others in the literature may be due to strict criteria for cure and/or methods of statistical evaluation. The authors felt that, based on their data, they could conclude that TVT 'appears' to be as effective as colposuspension for the treatment of stress urinary incontinence. Their results raise interesting questions concerning outcomes analysis in anti-incontinence surgery, particularly how to address those patients who fail to follow-up.

Paraiso et al.[155] reported a randomized comparison of 36 patients undergoing laparoscopic Burch colposuspension with 36 patients undergoing TVT. They reported a higher rate of urodynamic stress incontinence at 1 year in the colposuspension group (18.8% versus 3.2%). They reported a significant improvement in the number of incontinent episodes per week and in Urogenital Distress Inventory and Incontinence Impact Questionnaire scores in both groups at 1 and 2 years after surgery. However, postoperative subjective symptoms of incontinence were reported significantly more often in the laparoscopic Burch colposuspension group than in the TVT group ($p<0.04$). Another study reported results of a prospective randomized trial comparing porcine dermis pubovaginal sling with TVT with a median follow-up of 36 months.[156] They utilized a questionnaire to measure outcomes. Statistical analysis failed to detect significant differences in cure rates or complications between the two groups. As of yet, there has been no large scale prospective randomized study utilizing objective criteria to compare results of pubovaginal slings with midurethral tape procedures.

Large trials with extended follow-up detailing results and/or complications of the transobturator technique have yet to be published. DeTayrac et al.[157] reported a 1-year cure rate of 84% with the transobturator approach. Delorme et al.[158] recently presented results in 32 patients with a minimum of 1-year follow-up (mean 17 months) following transobturator tape placement with an outside-in technique. They reported that 90.6% of patients were cured and 9.4% of patients were improved. One patient had complete postoperative retention, which resolved following 4 weeks of intermittent catheterization. Five patients had voiding difficulties suggesting outflow obstruction, and two patients developed de novo urge incontinence. De Leval reported initial results following the inside-out technique.[159] He reported a 91% cure and 4% improvement rate in 107 patients with a mean follow-up of 10 months. He reported a 4% incidence of postoperative de novo urge incontinence.

Complications

As with any surgical intervention, strict adherence to standard surgical procedure will minimize the occurrence of complications. The midurethral sling has been demonstrated to be a safe and effective method for the treatment of stress incontinence; however, it is important to be aware of potential complications. A review of currently available complications data is detailed in Table 60.6.

Intraoperative

The majority of intraoperative complications are due to aberrant passage of the trocars. Rates of bladder perforation in smaller series have been reported as high as 61%.[151] However, the incidence of bladder injury seems to be inversely related to experience, as the rate of bladder perforation in studies of over 1000 patients is 3–4%.[160,161] In the majority of cases of inadvertent bladder injury, proper repositioning of the trocar and urethral catheter drainage for 1–2 days is sufficient treatment. In cases of more severe injuries, endoscopic bladder repair has been described.[162]

Ileoinguinal and obturator nerve injury or entrapment may approach 0.1% in large series.[108,133,161,163] Bowel injury from passage of trocars has also been described.[160,164–166]

Vascular complications, including retropubic hematoma and blood loss over 200 cc, may be seen in over 3% of patients.[138] The incidence of major vessel injury approaches 0.1%,[161] and injuries to the external iliac artery have been reported.[167,168] Most commonly, hemorrhagic complications can be managed conservatively;[169] however, as many as 0.5% of patients in large series have required surgery to address the site of hemorrhage.[108,170]

Voiding complications

It is generally accepted that anti-incontinence procedures have an obstructive effect on the urethra that may affect voiding.[171–173] Traditional anti-incontinence procedures carry a risk of permanent voiding dysfunction requiring surgical reversal in 1–20% of cases.[174] Although the midurethral sling is placed without tension at the level of the midurethra, there appear to be significant effects on the voiding phase of micturition. It is well accepted that most obstructive symptoms are transient, requiring only temporary indwelling or intermittent catheterization.[175] However, longer-term urinary retention rates for TVT of between 1.4 and 9% have been reported.[133,160,161,176–178]

Most reported data on postoperative urinary retention has been in the form of case reports and case series. In general, there is a paucity of subjective and/or objective outcomes data that address voiding function

Table 60.6. Complications for midurethral slings

Author	De novo storage symptoms (%)	Voiding dysfunction	Other complications
Moran et al.[133]	3	Retention (5%)	Obturator nerve injury (3%) Periostitis (3%)
Jacquetin[134]	4	–	–
Soulie et al.[135]	–	–	Bladder perforation (10%) Pelvic hematoma (2%)
Haab et al.[124]	6	Voiding dysfunction (8%) Incision (2%)	–
Azam et al.[137]	7	Voiding dysfunction (4%)	Bladder perforation (19%)
Nilsson et al.[138]	8	–	Bladder perforation (1%) Pelvic hematoma (3%) >200 ml blood loss (3%)
Meschia et al.[108]	–	Voiding dysfunction (4%) Incision (0.5%)	Bladder perforation (6%) Pelvic hematoma (1.5%) Vaginal erosion (0.5%) Surgery for bleeding (0.5%) Obturator nerve injury (0.25%)
Rezapour et al.[140]	–	–	Bladder perforation (3%)
Glavind & Larsen[144]	–	–	Urethrovaginal fistula (3%)
Kinn[145]	–	Incision (1%)	Bladder perforation (4%) Vaginal erosion (3%)
Jeffry et al.[146]	26	Voiding dysfunction (12%) Retention (9%)	Bladder perforation (12%) Hemorrhage (2%)
De Val et al.[147]	31	Retention (6%) Incision (2%)	Bladder perforation (10%) Hemorrhage (3%) Pain (1%)
Lo et al.[148]	–	–	Bladder perforation (4%)
Adamiak et al.[150]	6	–	Bladder perforation (9%)
Brophy et al.[151]	–	–	Bladder perforation (61%)
Sander et al.[152]	2	CIC (4%) Urethrolysis (2%)	–
Arunkalaivanan & Barrington[94]	9	Retention 6 weeks (2%) CIC (4%) Dilation (2%) Incision (3%)	Hemorrhage (3%)
Tsivian et al.[153]		Voiding dysfunction (3%)	Bladder perforation (5%) Urethra injury (2%) Erosion (5%)
Nilsson et al.[131]	6	–	–

CIC, clean intermittent catheterization; De novo storage symptoms (%), percentage of patients with de novo storage symptoms (i.e. urgency, frequency, urge incontinence); Dilation, urethral dilation; Incision, sling incision.

after midurethral tape placement. This is compounded by the fact that data from existing series are difficult to compare due to a lack of consensus definitions for obstruction and/or voiding dysfunction. Sander et al.[152] reported a 78% rate of 'voiding difficulty' in 45 patients undergoing TVT procedures. Voiding difficulty was defined as hesitancy, dysuria, and the use of abdominal straining to void, or a sensation of incomplete emptying. Wang et al.[179] utilized objective (post-void residual >100 ml) and subjective (frequency of more than six voids per day and more than two voids per night, and an abnormal stream of urine per patient report) criteria to evaluate 57 patients who had undergone TVT placement. Using this definition, 15 patients (26%) were classified as having voiding dysfunction. Klutke et al.[176] reported a 2.8% rate of urinary retention or symptoms consistent with obstruction lasting more than 1 week from the date of the procedure in their experience with 600 TVT procedures.

Prospective objective voiding data are also limited. Wang[180] described his experience with 79 patients who underwent TVT. Patients were classified as 'dysfunctional voiders' or 'normal voiders' based on symptoms and a urinary free flow ≤12 ml/s and a detrusor pressure at maximum flow of >20 cmH_2O. Both groups were found to have a statistically significant decrease in maximum urinary free flow 1 year postoperatively. Factors highly correlated with postoperative abnormal voiding included abnormal preoperative uroflow, preoperative vaginal vault prolapse or enterocele, concurrent vault suspension procedure, and postoperative urinary tract infection. Lukacz et al. prospectively evaluated 65 patients undergoing TVT placement.[181] Voiding was assessed with patient questionnaires, non-invasive urinary flow rate, and pressure–flow studies both preoperatively and at 1 year postoperatively. Subjective voiding did not change; however, maximum free flow rates decreased from 29 ml/s to 16 ml/s (43% change). Post-void residual measurements revealed no clinically significant increases, changing from a median of 15 to 30 ml postoperatively. Thirty-eight patients (37%) required postoperative catheterization for urinary retention (median duration 4 days). No risk factors could be identified that predicted a requirement for postoperative catheterization. Eight patients (8%) required sling release and were not included in the voiding analysis.

In cases of persistent urinary retention, several treatments have been advocated including stretching of the tape,[152] interposition of mesh,[182] simple transection,[178] and complete urethrolysis.[183]

De novo urge incontinence/overactive bladder

De novo urge incontinence and de novo overactive bladder symptoms are known risks of anti-incontinence procedures. De novo detrusor overactivity (DO) has been reported to occur in 0-30% of patients after anti-incontinence surgery.[184] The incidence of DO following pubovaginal sling procedures has been reported to be between 3 and 24%.[2]

Initial thoughts were that due to the lack of tension at the level of the midurethra, the TVT would result in lower rates of de novo storage symptoms. However, studies have demonstrated that placement of a midurethral tape does have potential to cause new onset storage symptoms in between 0 and 31% of patients (Table 60.6). Conversely, Segal et al.[185] demonstrated resolution of urge incontinence in 63.1% of patients and resolution of overactive bladder symptoms in 57.7% following TVT placement. Further prospective analyses are required prior to formulating consensus recommendations concerning the onset or fate of storage symptoms following midurethral tape placement.

Graft rejection

Reported complications related to the use of synthetic permanent material for tension-free midurethral slings have been relatively rare. In their 2000 review of complications data, Yonneau et al.[186] emphasized the low incidence of vaginal, urethral or bladder erosion with the midurethral tape procedure when performed with Prolene mesh versus other materials. Nilsson and Kuuva,[187] in a study of 161 patients followed for 16 months, found no cases of tape erosion. Ulmsten et al.,[188] in a 3-year follow-up study involving 50 patients, also reported no cases of tape erosion. Karram et al.[189] reviewed their series of 350 TVT procedures and reported poor healing or erosion in three patients. Kuuva and Nilsson,[161] in a nationwide questionnaire-based analysis of complications associated with TVT procedures in 1455 patients, found an incidence of 7/1000 of defective vaginal healing.

Possible reasons for vaginal erosion include inadequate vaginal incision suturing, wound infection, impaired wound healing, or foreign body (tape) rejection. Patients with vaginal erosion may present in a variety of ways. They may complain of vaginal discharge, discomfort reported by their spouse during intercourse, vaginal or pelvic pain, or vaginal bleeding. Most groups recommend removal of the exposed areas of tape to treat vaginal erosions.[190–192] Kobashi and Govier,[193] however, presented four cases of vaginal erosion of polypropylene mesh successfully managed with conservative measures alone.

Urethral or bladder erosion can certainly be caused by technical error during the procedure. Urethral erosion is speculated to be due to excessive tension of the sling on the urethra, or due to technical error during the dissection under the urethra, resulting in compromised thickness of suburethral tissues. A few cases of intravesical erosion have been reported.[162,190,194,195] It is possible that intraoperative bladder perforation had been missed, but theoretically, pressure necrosis with eventual penetration of the tape through the bladder mucosa is a concern. Anecdotal experience with intravesical erosions presenting several years after successful TVT placement raises questions about the significance of the latter theory. Patients with urethral or bladder tape erosions can present with storage and/or voiding symptoms, hematuria, dysuria, pelvic pain, and/or recurrent urinary tract infections. It is well accepted that in cases of urethral or bladder erosion, it is necessary to remove the offending portions of tape.

Specific patient groups

Obese patients

Stress urinary incontinence has been positively associated with obesity in numerous studies.[196–198] Although weight loss may improve stress incontinence in these patients, definitive treatment may be best obtained through surgical intervention.[199]

There have been mixed reports with regard to the success rates of anti-incontinence surgery in obese patients. Some studies have indicated a significantly diminished success rate among patients with a body mass index (BMI) greater than 30 kg/m^2, whereas other data suggest that obesity is not a risk factor for failure of corrective surgery.[200–205] Anecdotally, increased technical difficulty, increased perioperative morbidity, and increased postoperative convalescence are often encountered in obese patients. An effective method for cure of stress incontinence that is technically sound and minimally invasive is an ideal concept in this patient population.

Lovatsis et al.[206] examined the success rate of TVT in 43 patients with a BMI ≥35 kg/m^2, compared to non-obese controls. They reported a success rate of 89% in the obese group versus 91% in the non-obese group, a difference that was not statistically significant. They reported no difference in complication rates between the two groups. These findings were echoed by Mukherjee and Constantine in a non-comparative study.[207]

Some authors propose that good success rates and decreased peri- and postoperative morbidity may make the midurethral sling the ideal surgical modality for correction of stress incontinence in this patient population.

Elderly patients

Large prevalence studies have shown that urinary incontinence in women increases with age. It is estimated that over 35% of community-dwelling elderly women have urinary incontinence.[208] Incontinence has been shown to affect the psychological, occupational, domestic, and sexual lives of 15–30% of women of all ages.[209] Due to comorbidities in the elderly population, injectable therapy has often been the treatment of choice in an attempt to avoid operative morbidity; however, long-term efficacy and durability of this material has in many cases been inadequate.[210] Reports of vaginal and retropubic suspension procedures for stress incontinence in the elderly have suggested a variable rate of success.[211–213]

Much like in the obese patient population, there are anecdotal concerns with performing invasive surgery on elderly patients. Many patients have multiple medical co-morbidities, making them risky surgical candidates. Additionally, postoperative convalescence is expected to be more complicated and longer in this population. A less invasive procedure with reduced postoperative morbidity such as the midurethral sling would be ideal for this patient population.

Walsh et al.[214] reported their evaluation of quality of life outcomes in community-dwelling elderly women compared with younger patients, all of whom underwent TVT for incontinence treatment. They found significantly improved quality of life scores (80% and 91%, respectively) following surgery in both groups; however, the rate of improvement was slightly less in the elderly cohort. Although this study confirms that the midurethral tape procedure is successful in elderly patients, further reports detailing results and complication data are necessary before adequate conclusions should be drawn concerning the use of the midurethral sling as first-line therapy in this population.

Patients with prolapse

Stress urinary incontinence in women is frequently associated with other pelvic floor defects. A vaginal approach to repair is often preferred because anterior, apical, and posterior defects can be addressed by the same approach and without a large abdominal incision. At the present time, pubovaginal sling surgery is advocated as the best choice for treatment of occult incontinence. Recently, interest has piqued about the use of the less invasive midurethral sling during concomitant prolapse repair. Conceptually, there has been concern about the tendency of the midurethral tape to migrate towards the bladder neck if all repairs are done through a common incision. This phenomenon could cause an increased propensity for postoperative urinary retention and/or storage symptoms.

Several studies have investigated the use of the midurethral sling in women with occult stress incontinence undergoing prolapse repair. Reported objective cure rates have been between 85 and 94%, with one exception.[215–221] Pang et al. reported 1-year urodynamic and quality of life outcomes in 45 patients who underwent concomitant TVT insertion during pelvic floor reconstruction surgery.[222] They reported a worse objective cure rate in patients having undergone concomitant cystocele repair when compared with patients at their institution who had undergone TVT alone (38% versus

67%). The discrepancy in results could potentially be due to the stringent outcomes criteria utilized to define cure, a concept that deserves close attention. Rafii et al.[223] reported different findings when they compared cure rates in patients who underwent TVT alone with those who underwent TVT and prolapse repair. No statistical difference was found between the two groups (93.0% versus 93.1%).

Multiple surgical strategies for placement of a midurethral sling during prolapse repair have been described. Pang et al.[222] and Jomaa[216] inserted the TVT needles prior to performing repair of the anterior compartment through an extended anterior vaginal incision. Meschia et al.[217] inserted the vaginal tape prior to anterior repair, but did so through a separate sagittal vaginal incision. In contrast, Lo et al.[215] inserted the tape after coaptation of the paravesical fascia for anterior repair. In all of the above cases, the tension of the TVT tape was adjusted after the necessary prolapse procedures had been completed.

The most common reported perioperative complication in patients undergoing TVT and concurrent prolapse surgery has been transient urinary retention (11–43%).[215–220,222] The mean period of catheterization in these patients was between 3.7 and 5.1 days. Several cases of unresolved urinary retention have been reported. Rafii et al.[223] reported four cases of sling adjustment and three cases of sectioning of the midurethral tape in a series of 186 patients who underwent TVT with or without prolapse repair. Partoll[218] and Meltomaa et al.[224] reported that the time to resolution of retentive voiding was significantly higher in patients who underwent concurrent anterior and/or posterior repair when compared to those who underwent midurethral tape placement alone.

CONCLUSIONS

As can be inferred from the above discussion, a plethora of literature exists that details experiences with various surgical techniques designed to treat stress incontinence. The pubovaginal sling has remained the gold standard; however, with the introduction of minimally invasive techniques – specifically the midurethral tape – questions have been raised as to what is the most appropriate treatment in specific cases. Although no single intervention is optimal for all circumstances, the variety of technologies and procedures currently available provide the surgeon with viable options for most patients. No doubt, continued development will further improve morbidity associated with sling interventions with the hope that greater efficacy can also be achieved.

REFERENCES

1. Balmforth J, Cardozo LD. Trends toward less invasive treatment of female stress urinary incontinence. Urology 2003;62:52–60.
2. Leach GE, Dmochowski RR, Appell RA et al. Female Stress Urinary Incontinence Clinical Guidelines Panel summary report on surgical management of female stress urinary incontinence. The American Urological Association. J Urol 1997;158:875–80.
3. Tanagho EA. Anatomy of the lower urinary tract and mechanical interpretation of storage and voiding. Curr Opin Urol 1992;2:245–7.
4. Zinner NR, Sterling AM, Ritter RC. Role of inner urethral softness and urinary continence. Urology 1980;16:115–7.
5. Oelrich TM. The striated urogenital sphincter muscle in the female. Anat Rec 1983;205:223–32.
6. Myers RP. Male urethral sphincter anatomy and radical prostatectomy. Urol Clin North Am 1991;18:211–27.
7. Blaivas JG, Groutz A. Urinary incontinence: pathophysiology, evaluation, and management overview. In: Walsh PC, Retik AB, Vaughn ED, Wein AJ (eds) Campbell's Urology, 8th ed. Philadelphia: Saunders, 2002; 1027–52.
8. Raz S, Caine M, Zeigler M. The vascular component in the production of intraurethral pressure. J Urol 1972;108:93–6.
9. Versi E, Cardozo LD, Studd J. Distal urethral compensatory mechanisms in women with an incompetent bladder neck who remain continent, and the effect of menopause. Neurourol Urodyn 1990;9:579–90.
10. Gosling J. The structure of the bladder and urethra in relation to function. Urol Clin North Am 1985;12:207–14.
11. Comiter CV, Vasavada SP, Raz S. Anatomy and physiology of stress urinary incontinence and pelvic floor prolapse. In: Resnick MI, Fabrizio MD, Kavoussi LR (eds) Atlas of the Urologic Clinics of North America, vol 8. Philadelphia: Saunders, 2000; 1–22.
12. Enhorning G. Simultaneous recording of the intravesical and intraurethral pressure. Acta Obstet Gynecol Scand 1961;276(Suppl):1–69.
13. Haab F, Traxer O, Ciofu C. Tension-free vaginal tape: why an unusual concept is so successful. Curr Opin Urol 2001;11:293–7.
14. DeLancey JOL. Structural support of the urethra as it relates to stress urinary incontinence: the hammock hypothesis. Am J Obstet Gynecol 1994;170:1713–23.
15. Westby M, Asmussen M, Ulmsten U. Location of maximum intraurethral pressure related to urogenital diaphragm in women studied by simultaneous urethrocystometry and voiding urethrocystography. Am J Obstet Gynecol 1982;144:408–12.

16. Petros PE, Ulmsten U. An integral theory of female urinary incontinence. Acta Obstet Gynecol Scand 1990;69(Suppl 53):7–31.
17. Aldridge A. Transplantation of fascia for relief of urinary stress incontinence. Am J Obstet Gynecol 1942;44:398–411.
18. McGuire EJ, Lytton B. Pubovaginal sling procedure for stress incontinence. J Urol 1978;119:82–4.
19. Blaivas JG, Jacobs BZ. Pubovaginal fascial sling for the treatment of complicated stress urinary incontinence. J Urol 1991;145:1214–8.
20. Hohenfeller R, Petrie E. Sling procedure in surgery. In: Stanton SL, Tanagho EA (eds) Surgery of Female Incontinence, 2nd ed. Berlin: Springer-Verlag, 1986; 105–13.
21. Goebel R. Zur operativen Beseitigung der Angelborenen incontinenz vesicae. Zeitschr Gynakol Urol 1910;2:187–90.
22. Squier JB. Postoperative urinary incontinence. Med Rec 1911;79:868.
23. Price PB. Plastic operation for incontinence of urine and of faeces. Arch Surg 1933;26:1043–53.
24. Kaufman JM. Fascial sling for stress incontinence. South Med J 1982;75:555–8.
25. Schultz-Lampel D, Fleig P, Hohenfellner M et al. Long term results of surgery for stress incontinence in females: Burch colposuspension and fascial sling procedure. J Urol 1995;153(Suppl):525A [abstract 1185].
26. Loughlin KR. The endoscopic fascial sling for treatment of female stress incontinence. J Urol 1996;155:1265–7.
27. Mason RC, Roach M. Modified pubovaginal sling for treatment of intrinsic sphincteric deficiency. J Urol 1996;156:1991–4.
28. Zaragoza MR. Expanded indications for the pubovaginal sling: treatment of type 2 or 3 stress incontinence. J Urol 1996;156:1620–2.
29. Siegel SB, Allison S, Foster HE. Long term results of pubovaginal sling for stress urinary incontinence. J Urol 1997;157(Suppl):460A.
30. Carr LK, Walsh PJ, Abraham VE et al. Favorable outcome of pubovaginal slings for geriatric women with stress incontinence. J Urol 1997;157:125–8.
31. Barbalias G, Liatsikos E, Barbalias D. Use of slings made of indigenous and allogenic material (Goretex) in type III urinary incontinence and comparison between them. Eur Urol 1997;31:394–400.
32. Chaikin DC, Rosenthal J, Blaivas JG. Pubovaginal fascial sling for all types of stress urinary incontinence: long-term analysis. J Urol 1998;160:1312–6.
33. Maheshkumar P, Ramsay IN, Conn IG, A randomized trial of 'dynamic' versus 'static' rectus fascial suburethral sling: early results. Br J Urol 1998;81(Suppl 4):169.
34. Hassouna ME, Ghoniem GM. Long-term outcome and quality of life after modified pubovaginal sling for intrinsic sphincter deficiency. Urology 1999;53:287–91.
35. Kane L, Chung T, Lawrie H et al. The pubofascial anchor sling procedure for recurrent genuine urinary stress incontinence. BJU Int 1999;83:1010–4.
36. Morgan TO, Westney OL, McGuire EJ. Pubovaginal sling: 4-year outcome analysis and quality of life assessment. J Urol 2000;163:1845–8.
37. Kochakarn W, Leenanupunth C, Ratana-Olarn K et al. Pubovaginal sling for the treatment of female stress urinary incontinence: experience of 100 cases at Ramathibodi Hospital. J Med Assoc Thai 2001;84:1412–5.
38. Groutz A, Blaivas JG, Hyman MJ et al. Pubovaginal sling surgery for simple stress urinary incontinence: analysis by an outcome score. J Urol 2001;165:1597–1600.
39. Kuo HC. Comparison of videourodynamic results after the pubovaginal sling procedure using rectus fascia and polypropylene mesh for stress urinary incontinence. J Urol 2001;165:163–8.
40. Borup K, Nielson JB. Results in 32 women operated for genuine stress incontinence with the pubovaginal sling ad modum Ed McGuire. Scand J Urol Nephrol 2002;36:128–33.
41. Gormley EA, Latini J, Hanlon L. Long term effect of pubovaginal sling on quality of life. J Urol 2002;167(Suppl):105.
42. De Rossi P. Clinical outcome of fascial slings for female stress incontinence. Medscape Women's Health 2002;7:1–8.
43. Lucas MG, Giannitsas KL, Warelam K et al. A randomized controlled trial comparing two techniques of tension free autologous fascial sling for surgical treatment of genuine stress incontinence in women. J Urol 2003;169(Suppl):123.
44. Chou EC, Flisser AJ, Panagopoulos G et al. Effective treatment for mixed urinary incontinence with a pubovaginal sling. J Urol 2003;170:494–7.
45. Pfitzenmaier J, Gilfrich C, Faldum A et al. Does a combined fascial sling–Burch colposuspension display advantages over a fascial sling alone for treatment of urinary stress incontinence in females? Akt Urol 2003;34:166–71.
46. Guatelli S, Dall'Oglio B, Schiavon L. Pubovaginal sling. Arch Ital Urol Androl 2004;76:46–8.
47. Almeida SH, Gregorio E, Grando JP et al. Pubovaginal sling using cadaveric allograft fascia for the treatment of female urinary incontinence. Transplant Proc 2004;36:995–6.
48. Rodrigues P, Hering F, Meler A et al. Pubo-fascial versus vaginal sling operation for the treatment of stress urinary incontinence: a prospective study. Neurourol Urodyn 2004;23:627–31.
49. Kreder KJ, Austin CA. Treatment of stress urinary incon-

tinence in women with urethral hypermobility and intrinsic sphincter deficiency. J Urol 1996;156:1995–8.

50. Golomb J, Shenfield O, Shelhav A et al. Suspended pubovaginal fascial sling for the correction of complicated stress urinary incontinence. Eur Urol 1997;32:170–4.

51. Haab F, Trockman BA, Zimmern PE et al. Results of pubovaginal sling for the treatment of intrinsic sphincter deficiency determined by questionnaire analysis. J Urol 1997;158:1738–41.

52. Wright EJ, Iselin CE, Carr LK et al. Pubovaginal sling using cadaveric allograft fascia for the treatment of intrinsic sphincter deficiency. J Urol 1998;160:759–62.

53. Petrou SP, Frank I. Complications and initial continence rates after a repeat pubovaginal sling procedure for recurrent stress urinary incontinence. J Urol 2001;165:1979–81.

54. Richter HE, Varner E, Sanders E et al. Effects of pubovaginal sling procedure on patients with urethral hypermobility and intrinsic sphincter deficiency: Would they do it again? Am J Obstet Gynecol 2001;184:14–9.

55. Flynn BJ, Yap WT. Pubovaginal sling using allograft fascia lata versus autograft fascia for all types of stress urinary incontinence: 2-year minimum follow-up. J Urol 2002;167:608–12.

56. Chien GW, Tawadroas M, Kaptein JS et al. Surgical treatment for stress urinary incontinence with urethral hypermobility. What is the best approach? World J Urol 2002;20:234–9.

57. Low JA. Management of severe anatomic deficiencies of urethral sphincter function by a combined procedure with a fascia lata sling. Am J Obstet Gynecol 1969;105:149–55.

58. Addison WA, Haygood V, Parker RT. Recurrent stress urinary incontinence. Obstet Gynecol Annu 1985;14:254–65.

59. Beck RP, McCormick S, Nordstrom L. The fascia lata sling procedure for treating recurrent genuine stress incontinence of urine. Obstet Gynecol 1988;72:699–703.

60. Karram MM, Bhatia NN. Patch procedure: modified transvaginal fascia lata sling for recurrent or severe stress urinary incontinence. Obstet Gynecol 1990;75:461–3.

61. Govier FE, Gibbons RP, Correa RJ et al. Pubovaginal slings using fascia lata for the treatment of intrinsic sphincter deficiency. J Urol 1997;157:117–21.

62. Berman CJ, Kreder KJ. Comparative cost analysis of collagen injection and fascia lata sling cystourethropexy for the treatment of type III incontinence in women. J Urol 1997;157:122–4.

63. Phelps J, Lin L, Liu C. Laparoscopic suburethral sling procedure. J Am Assoc Gynecol Laparosc 2003;10:496–500.

64. Latini JM, Lux MM, Kreder KJ. Efficacy and morbidity of autologous fascia lata sling cystourethropexy. J Urol 2004;171:1180–4.

65. Ellerkmann RM, McBride AW, Bent AE et al. Comparison of long-term outcomes of autologous fascia lata slings to suspend Tutoplast fascia lata allograft slings for stress incontinence. J Pelvic Med Surg 2004;10(Suppl 1):S28.

66. Giannitsas KL, Emery SJ, Wareham K et al. The impact of urge syndrome and voiding problems, before and after sling surgery, in women with genuine stress incontinence. J Urol 2003;169(Suppl):124.

67. Buck BE, Malinin TI. Human bone and tissue allografts: preparation and safety. Clin Orthop 1994;303:8–17.

68. Iosif CS, Results of various operations for urinary stress incontinence. Arch Gynecol 1983;233:93–100.

69. Rottenberg RD, Weil A, Broschi PA et al. Urodynamic and clinical assessment of the Lyodura sling operation for urinary stress incontinence. Br J Obstet Gynaecol 1985;92:829–34.

70. Enzelsberger H, Helmer H, Schatten C. Comparison of Burch and Lyodura sling procedures for repair of unsuccessful incontinence surgery. Obstet Gynecol 1996;88:251–6.

71. Liscic RM, Brinar V, Miklic P et al. Creutzfeldt–Jakob disease in a patient with a lyophilized dura mater graft. Acta Med Croatica 1999;53:93–6.

72. Handa VL, Jensen K, Germain MM et al. Banked human fascia for the suburethral sling procedure: a preliminary report. Obstet Gynecol 1996;88:1045–9.

73. Elliott DS, Boone TB. Is fascia lata allograft material trustworthy for pubovaginal sling repair? Urology 2000;56:772–6.

74. Amundsen CL, Visco AG, Ruiz H et al. Outcome in 104 pubovaginal slings using freeze-dried allograft fascia lata from a single tissue bank. Urology 2000;56(Suppl 6A):2–8.

75. Brown SL, Govier FE. Cadaveric versus autologous fascia lata for the pubovaginal sling: Surgical outcome and patient satisfaction. J Urol 2000;164:1633–7.

76. O'Reilly KJ, Govier FE. Intermediate term failure of pubovaginal slings using cadaveric fascia lata: a case series. J Urol 2002;167:1356–8.

77. Vereecken RL, Lechat A. Cadaver fascia lata sling in the treatment of intrinsic sphincter weakness. Urol Int 2001;67:232–4.

78. Walsh IK, Nambirajan T, Donellan SM et al. Cadaveric fascia lata pubovaginal slings: early results on safety, efficacy and patient satisfaction. BJU Int 2002;90:415–9.

79. Bodell DM, Leach GE. Update on the results of the cadaveric transvaginal sling (CATS). J Urol 2002;167(Suppl):78.

80. Richter HE, Burgio KL, Holley RL et al. Cadaveric fascia lata sling for stress urinary incontinence: a pro-

spective quality of life analysis. Am J Obstet Gynecol 2003;189:1590–6.

81. Hartano VH, DiPiazza D, Ankem MK et al. Comparison of recovery from postoperative pain utilizing two sling techniques. Can J Urol 2003;10:1759–63.

82. Gurdal M, Tekin A, Huri E et al. Pubovaginal sling using cadaveric allograft fascia for all types of stress urinary incontinence. XIXth European Association of Urology Congress, March 25, 2004; Abstract 317.

83. Park S, Kim S, Choo M et al. Long term follow-up result of pubovaginal sling with cadaveric fascia lata in the management of female stress urinary incontinence. XIXth European Association of Urology Congress, March 25, 2004; Abstract 319.

84. Fitzgerald MP, Edwards SR, Fenner D. Medium-term follow-up on use of freeze-dried, irradiated donor fascia for sacrocolpopexy and sling procedures. Int Urogynecol J Pelvic Floor Dysfunct 2004;15:238–42.

85. Sutaria PM, Staskin DR. A comparison of fascial 'pull-through' strength using four different suture fixation techniques. J Urol 1999;161:79–80.

86. Lemer ML, Chaikin DC, Blaivas JG. Tissue strength analysis of autologous and cadaveric allografts for the pubovaginal sling. Neurourol Urodyn 1999;18:497–503.

87. Chaikin DC, Blaivas JG. Weakened cadaveric fascial sling: an unexpected cause of failure. J Urol 1998;160:2151.

88. Fitzgerald MP, Mollenhauer J, Bitterman P et al. Functional failure of fascia lata allografts. Am J Obstet Gynecol 1999;181:1339–46.

89. Fitzgerald MP, Mollenhauer J, Brubaker L. Failure of allograft suburethral slings. BJU Int 1999;84:785–8.

90. Choe JM, Bell T. Genetic material is present in cadaveric dermis and cadaveric fascia lata. J Urol 2001;166:122–4.

91. Hathaway JK, Choe JM. Intact genetic material is present in commercially processed cadaver allografts used for pubovaginal slings. J Urol 2002;168:1040–43.

92. Cole EE, Gomelsky A, Dmochowski R. Encapsulation of a porcine dermis pubovaginal sling. J Urol 2003;170:1950.

93. Nicholson SC, Brown ADG. The long-term success of abdominovaginal sling operations for genuine stress incontinence and cystocele: a questionnaire-based study. J Obstet Gynecol 2001;21:162–5.

94. Arunkalaivanan AS, Barrington JW. Randomized trial of porcine dermal sling (Pelvicol implant) vs. tension-free vaginal tape (TVT) in the surgical treatment of stress incontinence: a questionnaire-based study. Int Urogynecol J 2003;14:17–23.

95. Rutner AB, Levine SR, Schmaelzle JF. Porcine small intestinal submucosa implanted as a pubovaginal sling in 115 female patients with stress urinary incontinence: a 3-year series evaluated for durability of the results. Society for Urology and Engineering, 17th Annual Meeting, 2002.

96. Palma PC, Dambros M, Riccetto CL. Pubovaginal sling using the porcine small intestinal submucosa for stress urinary incontinence. Braz J Urol 2001;27:483–8.

97. Kubricht WS, Williams BJ, Eastham JA et al. Tensile strength of cadaveric fascia compared to small intestinal submucosa using suture pull-through analysis. J Urol 2001;165:486–90.

98. Konig JE, Pannek J, Martin W et al. Severe post-operative inflammation following implantation of a Stratasis sling. Urologe A 2004;43:1541–3.

99. Ho KL, Witte MN, Bird ET. 8-ply small intestinal submucosa tension-free sling: spectrum of post-operative inflammation. J Urol 2004;171:268–71.

100. Dalota SJ. Small intestinal submucosa tension-free sling: post-operative inflammatory reactions and additional data. J Urol 2004;172:1349–50.

101. Oray NB, Lambert A, Wonsetler R et al. Physical and biochemical characterization of a novel non-crosslinked, propylene-oxide treated acellular collagen matrix: comparison with solvent-extracted and freeze-dried cadaveric fascia lata. Society for Urology and Engineering, 17th Annual Meeting, 2002.

102. Pelosi MA II, Pelosi MA III, Pelekanos M. The YAMA Uro-Patch sling for treatment of female stress urinary incontinence: a pilot study. J Lap Adv Surg Tech 2002;12:27–33.

103. Mooradian DL, Lambert A, Wonsetler R et al. Residual DNA in biological sling materials: a comparison between PO-treated bovine pericardium, human dermis, solvent-extracted and freeze-dried cadaveric fascia lata. Society for Urology and Engineering, 17th Annual Meeting, 2002.

104. Martucci RC, Ambrogini A, Calada AA et al. Pubovaginal sling with bovine pericardium for treatment of stress urinary incontinence. Braz J Urol 2000;26:208–14.

105. Candido EB, Triginelli SA, Silva Filho AL et al. The use of bovine pericardium in the pubovaginal sling for the treatment of stress urinary incontinence. Rev Bras Ginecol Obstet 2003;25:525–8.

106. Hohenfellner R, Petrie E. Sling procedure in surgery. In: Stanton SL, Tanagho E (eds) Surgery of Female Incontinence, 2nd ed. Berlin: Springer-Verlag, 1986; 105–13.

107. Moir JC. The gauze hammock operation: a modified Aldridge sling procedure. J Obstet Gynaecol Br Commonw 1968;75:1–9.

108. Meschia M, Pifarotti P, Bernasconi F et al. Tension-free vaginal tape: analysis of outcomes and complications in 404 stress incontinent women. Int Urogynecol J 2001;2(Suppl 2):S24–7.

109. Petros PE, Ulmsten UI. The combined intravaginal sling and tuck operation: an ambulatory procedure for cure of stress and urge incontinence. Acta Obstet Gynecol Scand 1990;69(Suppl 153):53–9.

110. Petros PE, Ulmsten U. An integral theory and its method

for the diagnosis and management of female urinary incontinence. Scand J Urol Nephrol 1993;153:1–93.

111. Melnick I, Lee RE. Delayed transection of urethra by Mersilene tape. Urology 1976;8:580–1.

112. Smith DN, Rackley RR, Fralick R et al. Biocompatibility analysis of Meadox material for sling formation. J Urol 1997;157(Suppl):459A.

113. Kobashi KC, Dmochowski RR, Mee SL. Erosion of woven polyester pubovaginal sling. J Urol 1999;162:2070–2.

114. Ulmsten U. An introduction to tension-free vaginal tape (TVT) – a new surgical procedure for treatment of female urinary incontinence. Int Urogynecol J 2001;12(Suppl 2):S3–S4.

115. Sarlos D, Kuronen M, Schaer GN. How does tension-free vaginal tape correct stress incontinence? Investigation by perineal ultrasound. Int Urogynecol J 2003;14:395–8.

116. Masata J, Martan A, Kasikova E et al. Ultrasound study of effect of TVT operation on the mobility of the whole urethra. Neurourol Urodyn 2002;21:286–8.

117. Klutke JJ, Carlin BI, Klutke CG. The tension-free vaginal tape procedure: correction of stress incontinence with minimal alteration in proximal urethral mobility. Urology 2000;55:512–4.

118. Lukacz ES, Luber KM, Nager CW. The effects of the tension-free vaginal tape on proximal urethral position: a prospective longitudinal evaluation. Int Urogynecol J Pelvic Floor Dysfunct 2003;14(3):179–84; discussion 184.

119. Lo TS, Wang AC, Horng SG et al. Ultrasonographic and urodynamic evaluation after tension-free vaginal tape procedure (TVT). Acta Obstet Gynecol Scand 2001;80:65–70.

120. Halaska M, Otcenasek M, Havel R et al. Suspension of the lower third of the urethra in out-patient practice – minimally invasive treatment of stress urinary incontinence of urine: technique and initial experience. Ces Gynek 2000;1:4–9.

121. Atherton MJ, Stanton SL. A comparison of the bladder neck movement and elevation after TVT and colposuspension. Br J Obstet Gynaecol 2000;107:1366–70.

122. Klutke JJ, Klutke CG. Tension-free vaginal tape procedure. AUA Update Series 2003;XXII:Lesson 10.

123. Ulmsten U. The basic understanding and clinical results of tension-free vaginal tape for stress urinary incontinence. Urologe A 2001;40:269–73.

124. Haab F, Sananes S, Amarenco G et al. Results of the tension-free vaginal tape procedure for the treatment of type II stress urinary incontinence at a minimum follow-up of 1 year. J Urol 2001;165:159–62.

125. Delorme E. La bandelette transobturatrice: un procede mini-invasif pour traiter l'incontinence urinaire de la femme. Prog Urol 2001;11:1306–13.

126. Dargent D, Bretones P, George P et al. Insertion of a suburethral sling through the obturator membrane for treatment of female urinary incontinence. Gynecol Obstet Fertil 2002;30:576–82.

127. Minaglia S, Ozel B, Klutke C et al. Bladder injury during transobturator sling. Urology 2004;64:376–7.

128. De Leval J. Novel surgical technique for the treatment of female stress urinary incontinence: transobturator vaginal tape inside-out. Eur Urol 2003;44:724–30.

129. Bonnet P, Waltregny D, Reul O et al. Transobturator vaginal tape inside out for the surgical treatment of female stress urinary incontinence: anatomical considerations. J Urol 2005;173:1223–8.

130. Ulmsten U, Falconer C, Johnson P et al. A multicenter study of tension-free vaginal tape (TVT) for surgical treatment of stress urinary incontinence. Int Urogynecol J 1998;9:210–3.

131. Nilsson CG, Falconer C, Rezapour M. Seven-year follow-up of the tension-free vaginal tape procedure for treatment of urinary incontinence. Obstet Gynecol 2004;104:1259–62.

132. Olsson I, Kroon U. A three-year post-operative evaluation of tension-free vaginal tape. Gynecol Obstet Invest 1999;48:267–9.

133. Moran PA, Ward KL, Johnson D et al. Tension-free vaginal tape for primary genuine stress incontinence: a two-centre follow-up study. BJU Int 2000;86:39–42.

134. Jacquetin B. [Use of 'TVT' in surgery for female urinary incontinence.] J Gynecol Obstet Biol Reprod (Paris) 2000;29:242–7.

135. Soulie M, Delbert-Juhes F, Cuvillier X et al. [Repair of female urinary incontinence with prolene 'TVT': preliminary results of a multicenter and prospective survey.] Prog Urol 2000;10:622–8.

136. Wang AC, Chen MC. Randomized comparison of local versus epidural anesthesia for tension-free vaginal tape operation. J Urol 2001;165:1177–80.

137. Azam U, Frazer MI, Kozman EL et al. The tension-free vaginal tape procedure in women with previous failed stress incontinence surgery. J Urol 2001;166:554–6.

138. Nilsson GG, Kuuva N, Falconer C et al. Long-term results of the tension-free vaginal tape (TVT) procedure for surgical treatment of female stress urinary incontinence. Int Urogynecol J 2001;12(Suppl 2):S5–S8.

139. Rezapour M, Ulmsten U. Tension-free vaginal tape (TVT) in women with recurrent stress urinary incontinence – a long-term follow-up. Int Urogynecol J 2001;12(Suppl 2):S9–S11.

140. Rezapour M, Falconer C, Ulmsten U. Tension-free vaginal tape (TVT) in stress incontinent women with intrinsic sphincter deficiency (ISD) – a long-term follow-up. Int Urogynecol J 2001;12(Suppl 2):S12–S14.

141. Rezapour M, Ulmsten U. Tension-free vaginal tape (TVT) in women with mixed urinary incontinence – a long-term follow-up. Int Urogynecol J 2001;12(Suppl 2):S15–S18.

142. Buscant F, Roumeguere T, Anaf V et al. [A new approach in techniques to treat urinary incontinence: TVT (tension free vaginal tape).] Rev Med Brux 2001;22:166–9.

143. Liapis A, Bakas P, Creatsas G. Management of stress urinary incontinence in women with the use of tension free vaginal tape. Eur Urol 2001;40:548–51.

144. Glavind K, Larsen EH. Results and complications of tension-free vaginal tape (TVT) for surgical treatment of female stress urinary incontinence. Int Urogynecol J 2001;12:370–2.

145. Kinn AC. Tension-free vaginal tape evaluated using patient self-reports and urodynamic testing: a two year follow-up. Scand J Urol Nephrol 2001;35:484–90.

146. Jeffry L, Deval B, Birsan A et al. Objective and subjective cure rates after tension-free vaginal tape for treatment of urinary incontinence. Urology 2001;58:702–6.

147. De Val B, Jeffry L, Al Najjar F et al. Determinants of patient dissatisfaction after a tension-free vaginal tape procedure for urinary incontinence. J Urol 2002;167:2093–7.

148. Lo TS, Huang HJ, Chang C.L et al. Use of intravenous anesthesia for tension-free vaginal tape in elderly women with genuine stress incontinence. Urology 2002;59:349–53.

149. Chung MK, Chung RP. Comparison of laparoscopic Burch and tension-free vaginal tape in treating stress urinary incontinence in obese women. JSLS 2002;6:17–21.

150. Adamiak A, Milart P, Skorupski P et al. The efficacy and safety of the tension-free vaginal tape procedure do not depend on the method of analgesia. Eur Urol 2002;42:29–33.

151. Brophy MM, Klutke JJ, Klutke GG. Urethral function testing prior to tension-free vaginal tape: does valsalva leak point pressure make a difference? J Urol 2002;167(Suppl):104.

152. Sander P, Moller LM, Rudnicki PM et al. Does the tension-free vaginal tape procedure affect the voiding phase? Pressure–flow studies before and one year after surgery. BJU Int 2002;89:694–8.

153. Tsivian A, Mogutin B, Kessler O et al. Tension-free vaginal tape procedure for the treatment of female stress urinary incontinence: long-term results. J Urol 2004;172:998–1000.

154. Ward KL, Hilton P. A prospective multicenter randomized trial of tension-free vaginal tape and colposuspension for primary urodynamic stress incontinence: two-year follow-up. Am J Obstet Gynecol 2004;190:324–31.

155. Paraiso MF, Walters MD, Karram MM et al. Laparoscopic BURCH colposuspension versus tension-free vaginal tape: a randomized trial. Obstet Gynecol 2004;104:1249–58.

156. Abdel-Fattah M, Barrington JW, Arunkalaivanan AS. Pelvicol pubovaginal sling versus tension-free vaginal tape for treatment of urodynamic stress incontinence. Eur Urol 2004;46:629–35.

157. DeTayrac R, Deffieux X, Droupy S et al. A prospective randomized trial comparing tension-free vaginal tape and transobturator suburethral tape for surgical treatment of stress urinary incontinence. Am J Obstet Gynecol 2004;190:602–8.

158. Delorme E, Droupy S, deTayrac R et al. Transobturator tape (Uratape): a new minimally-invasive procedure to treat female urinary incontinence. Eur Urol 2004;45:203–7.

159. De Leval J. Reply to V. Delmas: Letter to the editor. Eur Urol 2004;46:134–6.

160. Tamussino KF, Hanzal E, Kolle D et al. Tension-free vaginal tape operation: results of the Austrian registry. Obstet Gynecol 2001;98:732–6.

161. Kuuva N, Nilsson CG. A nationwide analysis of complications associated with the tension-free vaginal tape (TVT) procedure. Acta Obstet Gynecol Scand 2002;81:72–7.

162. Jorion JL. Endoscopic treatment of bladder perforation after tension-free vaginal tape procedure. J Urol 2002;168:197.

163. Geis K, Dietl J. Ileoinguinal nerve entrapment after tension-free vaginal tape (TVT). Int Urogynecol J 2002;13:136–8.

164. Brink DM. Bowel injury following insertion of tension-free vaginal tape. S Afr Med J 2000;90:450–2.

165. Peyrat L, Boutin JM, Bruyere F et al. Intestinal perforation as a complication of tension-free vaginal tape procedure for urinary incontinence. Eur Urol 2001;39:603–5.

166. Meschia M, Busacca M, Pifarotti P et al. Bowel perforation during insertion of tension-free vaginal tape (TVT). Int Urogynecol J Pelvic Floor Dysfunct 2002;13:263–5.

167. Zilbert AW, Farrell SA. External iliac artery laceration during tension-free vaginal tape procedure. Int Urogynecol J 2002;12:141–3.

168. Primicerio M, De Matteis G, Montanino OM et al. Use of the TVT (tension-free vaginal tape) in the treatment of female urinary stress incontinence: preliminary results. Minerva Ginecol 1999;51:355–8.

169. Walters MD, Tulikangas PK, LaSala C et al. Vascular injury during tension-free vaginal tape procedure for stress urinary incontinence. Obstet Gynecol 2001;98:957–9.

170. Vierhout ME. Severe hemorrhage complicating tension-free vaginal tape (TVT): a case report. Int Urogynecol J 2001;12:139–40.

171. Wall LL, Hewitt JK. Voiding function after Burch colposuspension for stress incontinence. J Reprod Med 1996;41:161–5.

172. Klutke JJ, Klutke CG, Bergman J. Bladder neck suspen-

sion for stress urinary incontinence: how does it work? Neurourol Urodyn 1999;18:623–7.

173. Bhatia NN, Ostergard DR. Urodynamic effects of retropubic urethropexy in genuine stress incontinence. Am J Obstet Gynecol 1981;140:936–41.

174. Goldman HB, Rackley RR, Appell RA. The efficacy of urethrolysis without resuspension for iatrogenic urethral obstruction. J Urol 1999;161:196–8.

175. Cross CA, Cespedes RD, English SF et al. Transvaginal urethrolysis for urethral obstruction after anti-incontinence surgery. J Urol 1998;159:1199–201.

176. Klutke C, Siegel S, Carlin B et al. Urinary retention after tension-free vaginal tape procedure: incidence and treatment. Urology 2001;58:697–701.

177. Niemczyk P, Klutke JJ, Carlin BJ et al. United States experience with tension-free vaginal tape procedure for urinary stress incontinence: assessment of safety and tolerability. Tech Urol 2001;7:261–5.

178. Rardin CR, Rosenblatt PL, Kohli N et al. Release of tension-free vaginal tape for the treatment of refractory postoperative voiding dysfunction. Obstet Gynecol 2002;100:898–902.

179. Wang KH, Neimark M, Davilla GW. Voiding dysfunction following TVT procedure. Int Urogynecol J 2002;13:353–8.

180. Wang AC. The correlation between preoperative voiding mechanism and surgical outcome of the tension-free vaginal tape procedure, with reference to quality of life. BJU Int 2003;91:502–6.

181. Lukacz ES, Luber KM, Nager CW. The effects of the tension-free vaginal tape on voiding function: a prospective evaluation. Int Urogynecol J 2004;15:32–8.

182. Kolle D, Stenzl A, Koelbl H et al. Treatment of postoperative urinary retention by elongation of tension-free vaginal tape. Am J Obstet Gynecol 2001;185:250–1.

183. Romanzi LJ, Blaivas JG. Protracted urinary retention necessitating urethrolysis following tension–free vaginal tape surgery. J Urol 2000;164:2022–3.

184. Kershen RT, Appell RA. De novo urge syndrome and detrusor instability after anti-incontinence surgery: current concepts, evaluation and treatment. Curr Urol Rep 2002;3:345–53.

185. Segal JL, Vassallo B, Kleeman S et al. Prevalence of persistent and de novo overactive bladder symptoms after the tension-free vaginal tape. Obstet Gynecol 2004;104:1263–9.

186. Yonneau L, Chartier-Kastler E, Bohin D et al. Materials used for treatment of stress urinary incontinence with suburethral sling. Prog Urol 2000;10:1238–44.

187. Nilsson CG, Kuuva N. The tension-free vaginal tape procedure is successful in the majority of women with indications for surgical treatment of urinary stress incontinence. Br J Obstet Gynaecol 2001;108:414–9.

188. Ulmsten U, Johnson P, Rezapour M. A three-year follow-up of tension free vaginal tape for surgical treatment of female stress urinary incontinence. Br J Obstet Gynaecol 1999;106:345–50.

189. Karram MM, Segal JL, Vassallo BJ et al. Complications and untoward effects of the tension-free vaginal tape procedure. Obstet Gynecol 2003;101:929–32.

190. Volkmer BG, Nesslauer T, Rinnab L et al. Surgical intervention for complications of the tension-free vaginal tape procedure. J Urol 2003;169:570–2.

191. Boublil LJ, Blaivas JG. Complications of urethral sling procedures. Curr Opin Obstet Gynecol 2002;14:515–8.

192. Clemens JQ, DeLancey JO, Faerber GJ et al. Urinary tract erosions after synthetic pubovaginal slings: diagnosis and management strategy. Urology 2000;56:589–92.

193. Kobashi KC, Govier FE. Management of vaginal erosion of polypropylene mesh slings. J Urol 2003;169:2242–3.

194. Sweat SD, Itano NB, Clemens JQ et al. Polypropylene mesh tape for stress urinary incontinence: complications of urethral erosion and outlet obstruction. J Urol 2002;168:144–6.

195. Wyczolkowski M, Klima W, Piasecki Z. Reoperation after complicated tension-free vaginal tape procedure. J Urol 2001;166:1004–6.

196. Mommsen S, Foldspang A. Body mass index and adult female urinary incontinence. World J Urogynecol 1994;12:319–22.

197. Dwyer PL, Lee ET, Hay DM. Obesity and urinary incontinence in women. Br J Obstet Gynaecol 1988;95:91–6.

198. Yarnell JW, Voyle GJ, Sweetnam PM et al. Factors associated with urinary incontinence in women. J Epidemiol Community Health 1982;36:58–63.

199. Cummings JM, Rodning CB. Urinary stress incontinence among obese women: review of pathophysiology therapy. Int Urogynecol J 2000;11:41–4.

200. Stanton SL, Cardozo L, Williams JE et al. Clinical and urodynamic features of failed incontinence surgery in the female. Obstet Gynecol 1978;51:515–20.

201. Zivkovic F, Tamussino K, Pieber D. Body mass index and outcome of incontinence surgery. Obstet Gynecol 1999;3:753–6.

202. Brieger G, Korda A. The effect of obesity on the outcome of successful surgery for genuine stress incontinence. Aus N Z J Obstet Gynaecol 1992;32:71–2.

203. Gillon G, Engelstein D, Servadio C. Risk factors and their effect on the results of Burch colposuspension for urinary stress incontinence. Isr J Med Sci 1992;28:354–6.

204. Hutchings A, Griffiths J, Black NA. Surgery for stress incontinence: factors associated with a successful outcome. Br J Urol 1998;82:634–41.

205. Cummings JM, Boullier JA, Parra RO. Surgical correction of incontinence in the morbidly obese woman. J Urol 1998;160:754–5.

206. Lovatsis D, Gupta C, Dean E et al. Tension-free vaginal tape procedure is an ideal treatment for obese patients. Am J Obstet Gynecol 2003;189:1601–4.

207. Mukherjee K, Constantine G. Urinary stress incontinence in obese women: tension-free vaginal tape is the answer. BJU Int 2001;12(Suppl):881–3.

208. Diokno AC, Brock BM, Brown MB et al. Prevalence of urinary incontinence and other urological symptoms in the noninstitutionalized elderly. J Urol 1986;136:1022–5.

209. Thomas TM, Plymat KR, Blannin J et al. Prevalence of urinary incontinence. Br Med J 1980;281:1243–5.

210. Groutz A, Blaivas JG, Kesler SS et al. Outcome results of transurethral collagen injection for female stress incontinence: assessment by urinary incontinence score. J Urol 2000;164:2006–9.

211. Gillon G, Stanton SL. Long-term follow-up of surgery for urinary incontinence in elderly women. Br J Urol 1984;56:478–80.

212. Schmidbauer CP, Chiang H, Raz S. Surgical treatment for female geriatric incontinence. Clin Geriatr Med 1986;2:759–63.

213. Couillard DR, Deckard-Janatpour K, Stone AR. The vaginal wall sling: a compressive suspension procedure for recurrent incontinence in elderly patients. Urology 1994;43:203–8.

214. Walsh K, Generao SE, White MJ. The influence of age on quality of life outcome in women following a tension-free vaginal tape procedure. J Urol 2004;171:1185–8.

215. Lo TS, Chang TC, Chao AS et al. Tension-free vaginal tape (TVT) procedure on genuine stress incontinent women with coexisting genital prolapse. Acta Obstet Gynecol Scand 2003;82:1049–53.

216. Jomaa M. Combined tension-free vaginal tape and prolapse repair under local anesthesia in patients with symptoms of both urinary incontinence and prolapse. Gynecol Obstet Invest 2001;51:184–6.

217. Meschia M, Pifarotti P, Spennacchio M et al. A randomized comparison of tension-free vaginal tape and endopelvic fascia plication in women with genital prolapse and occult stress urinary incontinence. Am J Obstet Gynecol 2004;190:609–13.

218. Partoll LM. Efficacy of tension-free vaginal tape with other pelvic reconstructive surgery. Am J Obstet Gynecol 2002;186:1292–5.

219. Huang KH, Kung FT, Liang HM et al. Concomitant surgery with tension-free vaginal tape. Acta Obstet Gynecol Scand 2003;82:948–53.

220. Gordon D, Gold RS, Pauzner D et al. Combined genitourinary prolapse repair and prophylactic tension-free vaginal tape in women with severe prolapse and occult stress urinary incontinence: preliminary results. Urology 2001;58:547–50.

221. Darai E, Jeffry L, Deval B et al. Results of tension-free vaginal tape in patients with or without vaginal hysterectomy. Eur J Obstet Gynecol Reprod Biol 2002;103:163–7.

222. Pang MW, Chan LW, Yip SK. One-year urodynamic outcome and quality of life in patients with concomitant tension-free vaginal tape during pelvic floor reconstruction surgery for genitourinary prolapse and urodynamic stress incontinence. Int Urogynecol J Pelvic Floor Dysfunct 2003;14:256–60.

223. Rafii A, Paoletti X, Haab F et al. Tension-free vaginal tape and associated procedures: a case-control study. Eur Urol 2004;45:356–61.

224. Meltomaa S, Backman T, Haarla M. Concomitant vaginal surgery did not affect outcome of the tension-free vaginal tape operation during a prospective 3-year follow-up study. J Urol 2004;172:222–6.

61

Pubovaginal fascial sling for the treatment of all types of stress urinary incontinence: surgical technique and long-term outcome

Jerry G Blaivas, David Chaikin

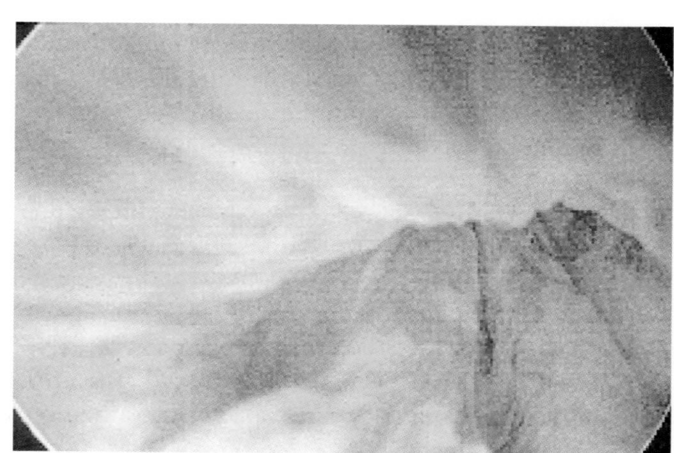

INTRODUCTION

Although a plethora of surgical techniques has been devised for the treatment of stress urinary incontinence, over the last decade two have emerged as the gold standards – the Burch colposuspension and the pubovaginal sling. Historically, pubovaginal sling had been reserved for women with complicated, severe and/or recurrent sphincteric incontinence; however, recently it has been advocated for almost all types of sphincteric incontinence – simple and complicated. Fueled by a stampede of commercial innovations in sling materials, allograft and synthetic sling operations have become the most common operations performed for sphincteric incontinence in women.[1] Over the last few years, many surgeons have paid increasing attention to synthetic and allograft materials to replace autologous tissue for slings in order to decrease operative time and perhaps to decrease operative morbidity. As more synthetics are used for sling surgery, hopefully there will be sufficient studies using validated outcome instruments to show that they compare favorably to autologous slings with respect to efficacy and morbidity.

The objective of this chapter is to provide the reader with an update on surgical technique and long-term outcome of the full-length autologous rectus fascial sling for sphincteric incontinence in women and to describe their role in the armamentarium of the pelvic surgeon.

OPERATIVE TECHNIQUE

The procedure is performed in the dorsal lithotomy position. For most patients a short (6–8 cm) transverse incision is made just above the pubis below the pubic hairline (Fig. 61.1). In obese patients a larger incision is usually necessary. The incision is carried down to the surface of the rectus fascia which is dissected free of subcutaneous tissue. Two parallel horizontal incisions, 2 cm apart, are made in the midline of the rectus fascia, approximately 2 cm above the pubis (Fig. 61.2). Using Mayo scissors, the incisions are extended superolaterally towards the iliac crest following the direction of the fascial fibers. The wound edges are retracted laterally on either side to permit a sling of approximately 16 cm to be obtained. The undersurface of the fascia is freed from muscle and scar and each end of the fascia is secured with a 2-0 delayed absorbable monofilament suture using a running horizontal mattress placed at right angles to the direction of the fascial fibers (Fig. 61.3). The fascial strip is excised (Fig. 61.4) and placed in a basin of saline. The wound is temporarily packed with saline-soaked sponges and attention turned to the vagina.

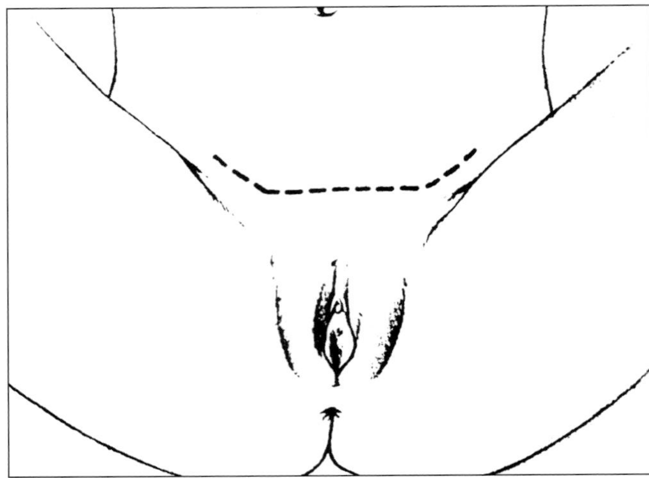

Figure 61.1. *Abdominal incision. For most patients a short (6–8 cm) transverse incision is made just above the pubis below the pubic hairline (the horizontal portion of the incision). In obese patients, a larger incision may be necessary (the incision as shown).*

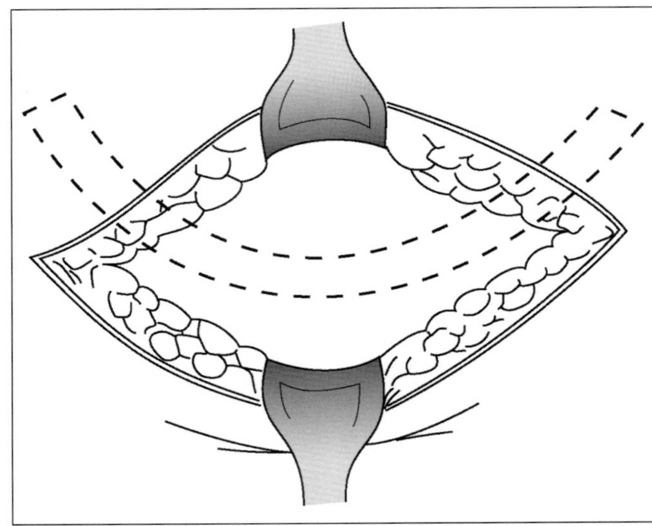

Figure 61.2. *A 2 cm wide graft is outlined, keeping the incision parallel to the direction of the fascial fibers.*

A weighted vaginal retractor is placed in the vagina and a Foley catheter inserted into the urethra. The labia are retracted with sutures. The vesical neck is identified by placing gentle traction on the Foley catheter and palpating the balloon, and a gently curved horizontal incision is made in the anterior vaginal wall with the apex of the curve over the vesical neck, approximately 2 cm proximal to the palpable distal edge of the balloon (Fig. 61.5). It is important that this incision is made superficial to the pubocervical fascia. This is accomplished by the technique outlined in Figures 61.6–61.12.

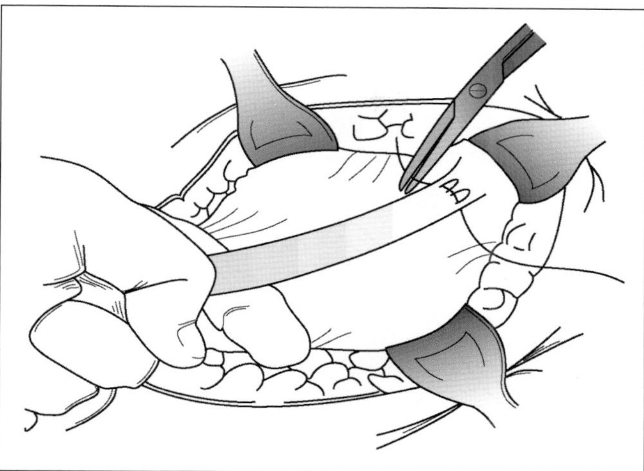

Figure 61.3. *A plane is created between the fascia and rectus muscle with Mayo scissors and an index finger places traction on the fascia as the incision is extended superolaterally to the point where the rectus fascia divides to pass around the external oblique muscle. If further length is needed, the incision is extended superiorly. At this point, it is important to avoid the underlying peritoneum. A No. 2-0 non-absorbable running horizontal mattress suture is placed across the lateral-most portion of the graft and the ends are left long.*

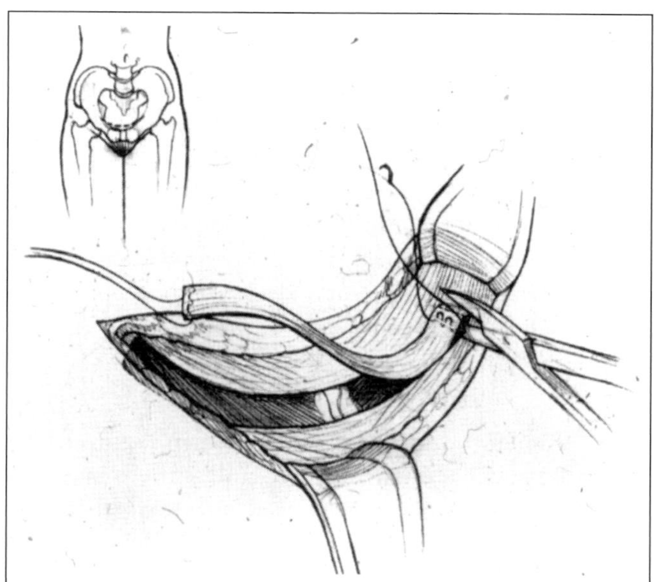

Figure 61.4. *Each end of the fascial graft is transected approximately 0.5 cm lateral to the mattress suture.*

Five ml of indigo carmine are given intravenously and cystoscopy performed to ensure that there has been no damage to the urethra, vesical neck, bladder or ureters. The sling is put on tension by pulling up on the sutures and the position of the sling is noted by observing where

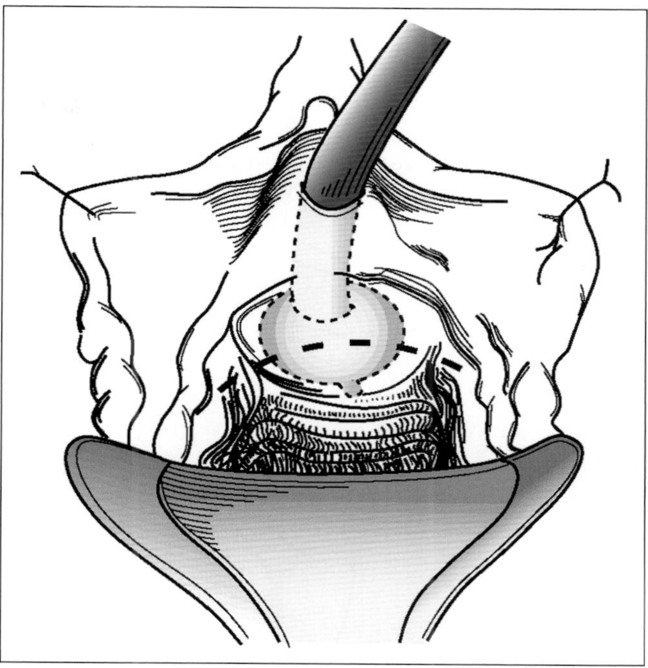

Figure 61.5. *A 4 cm transverse or slightly curved incision is made in the anterior vaginal wall about 2 cm proximal to the proximal edge of the Foley catheter balloon. This is the approximate site of the vesical neck. The depth of this incision extends just superficial to the pubocervical fascia.*

the urethra coapts. Historically, the sling has been intentionally placed at the bladder neck and we continue to place it there, but if cystoscopy shows that the sling is distal to the bladder neck, we do not attempt to reposition it. This is not the proper forum to discuss whether it is better to place the sling at the midurethra or vesical neck. Suffice it to say that the results presented herein are based on placing the sling at the vesical neck, not the midurethra. However, if cystoscopy shows that the sling is inadvertently placed proximal to the vesical neck, it is removed and a new tunnel created more distally. We generally place a trocar 14 Fr suprapubic tube percutaneously into the bladder and its position is visually inspected to ensure that it is well away from the trigone. While this is not necessary in all patients, we find that it facilitates the postoperative voiding trial.

The sutures attached to the sling are pulled through the separate stab wounds in the inferior leaf of the rectus fascia on either side (not pictured here) and the rectus fascia is closed with a continuous 2-0 delayed absorbable monofilament suture. The long sutures attached to the ends of the fascial graft are tied to one another in the midline, securing the sling in place without tension (see Fig. 61.12). In order to ensure that excessive tension is not placed on the sling, we utilize several techniques.

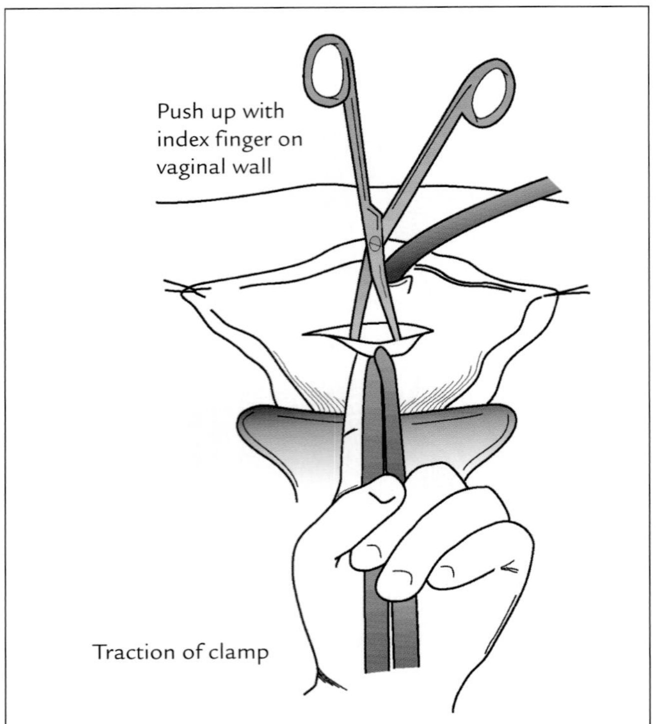

Figure 61.6. *An Allis clamp is placed on the cranial edge of the vaginal incision in the midline. The clamp is grasped by the left hand of the surgeon and caudad traction is applied while, at the same time, the left index finger pushes upward. A plane is created superficial to the pubocervical fascia by dissecting with Metzenbaum scissors at an angle of 60–90 degrees to the undersurface of the vaginal incision. The proper plane is identified by noting the characteristic shiny white appearance of the undersurface of the anterior vaginal wall. A small posterior vaginal flap is made for a distance of about 2 cm, just wide enough to accept the sling.*

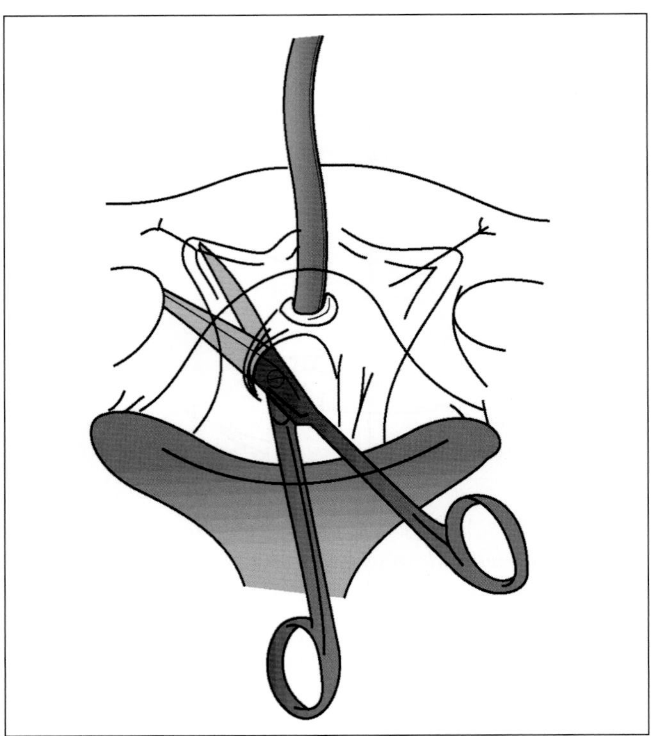

Figure 61.7. *The lateral edges of the wound are grasped with Allis clamps and retracted laterally (not pictured here). The dissection continues just beneath the vaginal epithelium with Metzenbaum scissors pointed in the direction of the patient's ipsilateral shoulder until the periosteum of the pubis is palpable. During this part of the dissection, it is important to stay as far lateral as possible to ensure that the urethra, bladder and ureters are not injured. This is accomplished by dissecting with the concavity of the scissors pointing laterally and exerting constant lateral pressure with the tips of the scissors against the undersurface of the vaginal epithelium. Once the periosteum is reached, the endopelvic fascia is perforated and the retropubic space entered.*

- With the cystoscope in the bladder, the sutures on each end of the fascial strip are grasped and gently pulled upward while downward pressure is applied to the cystoscope. This depresses the vesical neck and puts the sling on stretch.
- The sutures are then released, removing the excess tension from the sling.
- Next, the cystoscope is removed and a well-lubricated Q-tip is placed in the urethra. With the table exactly parallel to the floor, the urethral angle is measured. If the angle is negative, downward pressure is placed on the Q-tip at the bladder neck until the angle is 0° or greater.
- The sutures attached to the sling are then tied over the rectus fascia with no added tension. It is usually possible to place two fingers comfortably between the sutures and the rectus fascia.

The completed procedure is depicted in Figure 61.13. A vaginal pack is usually not left, unless there has been excessive bleeding. If one is used, it is soaked in sterile lubricating jelly to facilitate its painless removal postoperatively.

POSTOPERATIVE MANAGEMENT

If a vaginal pack was used it is removed the day after surgery. Voiding trials are begun as soon as the patient is comfortable, usually on the first or second postoperative day. If the patient is unable to void by the time she is to be discharged, she is taught intermittent self-catheterization.

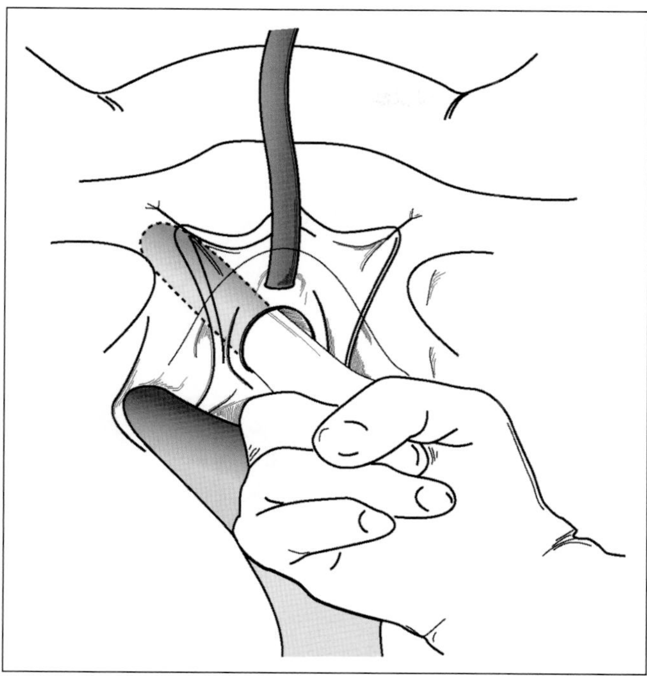

Figure 61.8. *Alternatively, the endopelvic fascia is perforated with the index finger and the retropubic space entered. The bladder neck and proximal urethra are bluntly dissected free of their vaginal and pelvic wall attachments.*

Over 90% of patients void well enough by 1 week so that intermittent catheterization is not necessary and over 99% are catheter-free by 1 month. Permanent intermittent catheterization or urethral obstruction requiring surgery is necessary in less than 1% of patients.

RESULTS

Our own results have been published in four reports over the last 15 years and are summarized below.[2–5]

Since 1988, all women who undergo pubovaginal sling have been evaluated by structured history and physical examination, voiding diary, pad test, videourodynamics and cystoscopy. Postoperatively, the diaries, pad tests, uroflow and post-void residual urine are repeated at each follow-up visit. Other outcome instruments – including questionnaires, symptom scores and patient satisfaction indices – have been added over the years. The most accurate tool, in our estimation, is the simplified urinary outcome score (SUIOS).[5] The SUIOS is comprised of three components: a 24-hour voiding diary, 24-hour pad test and a patient outcome questionnaire, each with a range of scores from 0 to 2 (Table 61.1). Cure is defined as 0 points, consisting of the patient's statement that she is cured, a dry pad test and no incontinence episodes on a voiding diary. Scores of 2–5 are considered improvement and 6 is failure (Table 61.2). For the purposes of outcome analysis, we divided patients into two groups: simple and complex incontinence. Complex incontinence was defined as sphincteric incontinence with one or more of the following conditions: urge incontinence, 'pipe stem urethra' (a fixed scarred urethra), urethral or vesicovaginal fistula, urethral diverticulum, grade 3

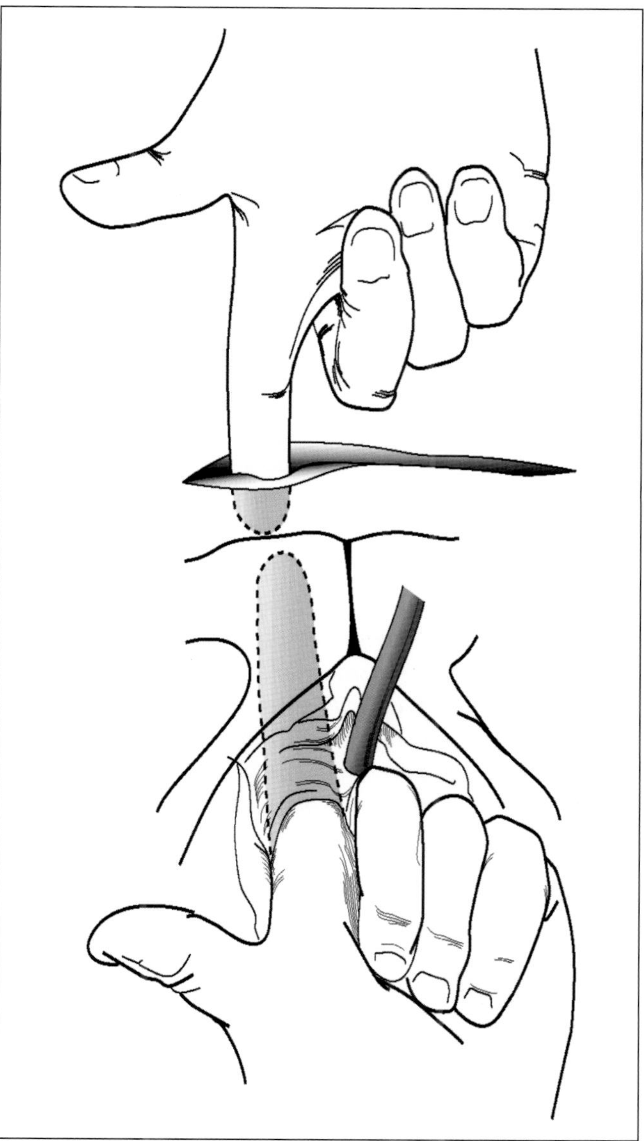

Figure 61.9. *A Kocher clamp is placed on the inferior edge of the rectus fascia in the midline and the fascia pulled upward (not pictured). The left index finger is reinserted into the vaginal wound, retracting the vesical neck and bladder medially. The tip of the finger palpates the right index finger, which is inserted just beneath the inferior leaf of the rectus fascia and guided along the undersurface of the pubis until it meets the left index finger from the vaginal wound.*

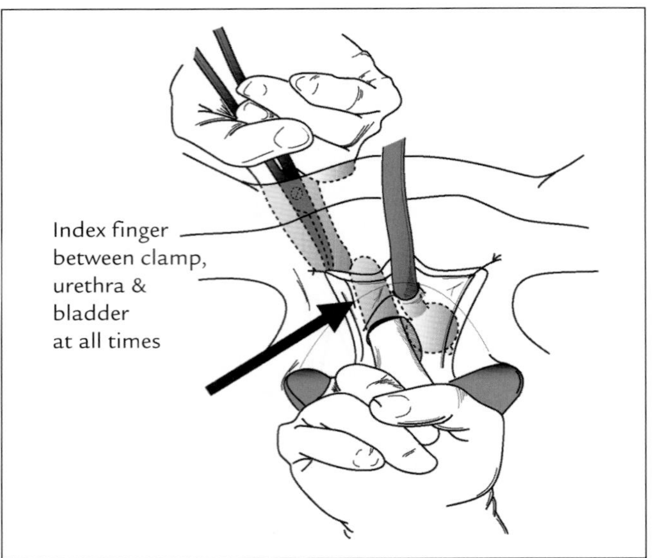

Figure 61.10. *A long curved clamp (DeBakey) is inserted into the incision and directed to the undersurface of the pubis. The tip of the clamp is pressed against the periosteum and directed toward the left index finger, which retracts the vesical neck and bladder medially. At all times, the left index finger is kept between the tip of the clamp and the bladder and urethra, protecting these structures from injury. In this fashion, the clamp is guided into the vaginal wound.*

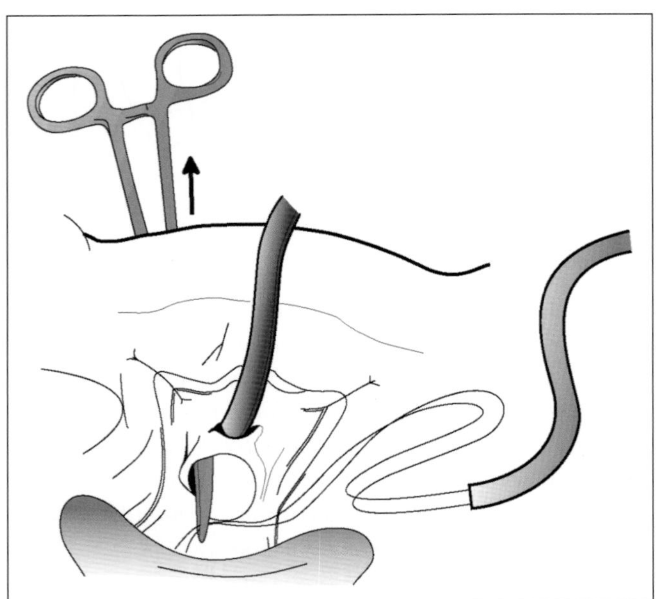

Figure 61.11. *When the tip of the clamp is visible in the vaginal wound, the long suture attached to the fascial graft is grasped and pulled into the abdominal wound. The procedure is repeated on the other side. The fascial sling is now positioned from the abdominal wall on one side around the undersurface of the vesical neck and back to the abdominal wall on the other side.*

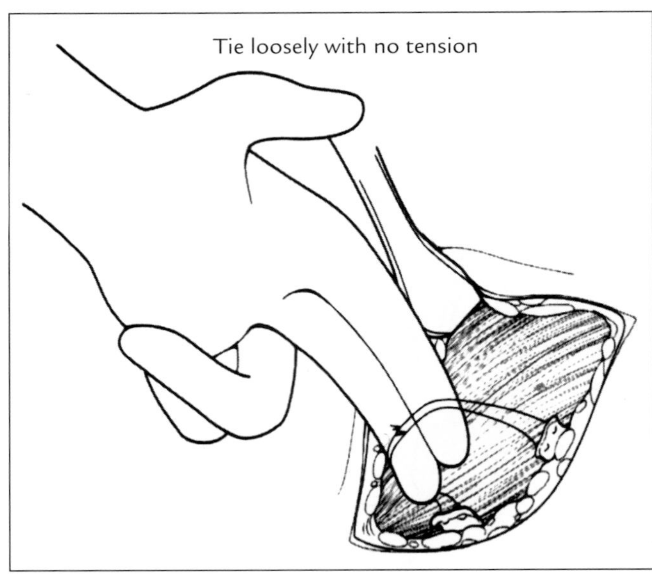

Figure 61.12. *Two small stab wounds are made in the rectus fascia, just above the pubis (not pictured). The ends of the sutures attached to the sling are pulled through the stab wounds on either side and the rectus fascia closed with a 2-0 continuous delayed absorbable monofilament suture. The sutures attached to the ends of the fascial graft are tied to one another in the midline, securing the sling in place without tension, and the wound is closed.*

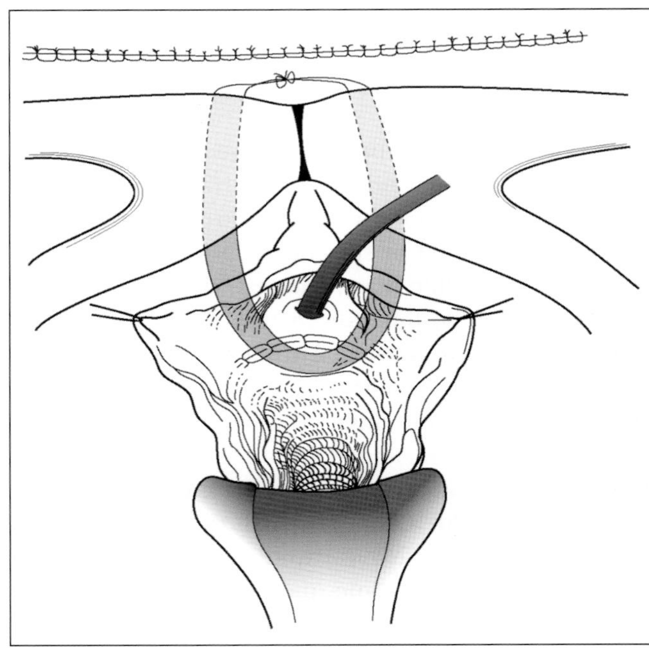

Figure 61.13. *Anatomic drawing of the completed procedure.*

Table 61.1. *Urinary incontinence instruments*

	Score		
Instrument	0	1	2
24-hour incontinence episodes	0	1–2	≥3
24-hour pad test (weight gain in grams)	≤8	9–20	≥21
Patient questionnaire, subjective assessment	Cure	Improve	Fail

Table 61.2. *Urinary incontinence outcome score*

Outcome	Total score
Cure	0
Good response	1–2
Fair response	3–4
Poor response	5
Failure	6

or 4 cystocele, or neurogenic bladder. In the absence of any of these, the incontinence was considered to be simple.

Overall, with a mean follow-up of 4 years, the cure/improve versus fail rate for 325 simple and complicated patients was 93% and 7%, respectively (Table 61.3); for 67 patients with uncomplicated incontinence it was 100% cure/improve (Table 61.4).[3] It should be noted, however, that, from an objective perspective, patients with scores of 5 and 6 might well be considered as failures, but are included as improved because, despite persistent incontinence, the patients themselves stated that they were improved. Further, we have had two short-term failures that were not included in these reports because they occurred after the end of the study period, and two patients who were initial successes failed because of recurrent stress incontinence 9 years postoperatively.

In a separate analysis of 98 women, no difference was found in the cure/improve versus fail rate in those with stress (97%) versus mixed (93%) incontinence (p=0.33) using a SUIOS = 4 as the cut-off between cure/improve and fail.[6] In that study patients were also analyzed in two groups: cured versus not cured.[4] For the patients with mixed incontinence, there was no difference between cured and not cured with respect to age, surgery, menopausal status, bladder capacity, leak point pressure, pad weight or type of overactive bladder. However, patients who failed had more daily preoperative urgency (5.6 versus 4.1) and urge incontinence episodes (5.1 versus 3) than those who were cured, and they voided much more frequently (12 versus 8). This suggests that the more severe the overactive bladder, the less likely the patient is to respond favorably to surgery.

Table 61.3. *Urinary incontinence outcome score after pubovaginal sling in patients with simple and complex sphincteric incontinence*

Outcome	Total score	
Cure	0	45%
Good response	1–2	27%
Fair response	3–4	14%
Poor response	5	7%
Failure	6	7%

Table 61.4. *Urinary incontinence outcome score after pubovaginal sling in patients with simple sphincteric incontinence*

Outcome	Total score	
Cure	0	67%
Good response	1–2	21%
Fair response	3–4	9%
Poor response	5	3%
Failure	6	0%

In our combined series, most failures occurred either within the first 6 months or after 9 years, and the most common cause of failure was persistent urge incontinence, not stress incontinence. De novo urge incontinence occurred in about 3% of our series.

Over the years, significant complications have been uncommon. There was one death in over 500 patients (<0.2%) due to a cardiac arrhythmia in an 80-year-old woman. Other complications included wound infections (1%), incisional hernia (1%) and unexpected long-term urethral obstruction requiring surgery or intermittent catheterization (1%). It was not possible to identify any preoperative prognostic factors associated with urinary retention, in no small part due to the fact that it was so uncommon that it would take an enormous number of patients to power a study sufficiently to detect differences. Empirically, however, there are two causes: grades 3 and 4 pelvic organ prolapse and placing the sling under too much tension. Adjusting tension comes in large part from experience; there has been no long-term urethral obstruction requiring surgery or long-term catheterization in our last 300 pubovaginal slings.

DISCUSSION

In a meta-analysis of the peer review English literature, the AUA Female Stress Urinary Incontinence Clinical Guidelines Panel concluded that, with a short (1 year) and medium term (4 years) success rate of over 80%, pubovaginal sling and retropubic suspension are the most efficacious procedures for stress incontinence.[7] Although there was insufficient data to study subpopulations, it was felt that slings are likely to be more effective for intrinsic sphincter deficiency than retropubic procedures.

In that same study, the authors decried the paucity of scientifically valid outcome studies and recommended that better outcome instruments be developed and used in prospective trials. Since that report, a number of outcome instruments have been developed, including the SUIOS, and we are hopeful that future studies will be better.

Many peer review studies have corroborated the guideline panel's conclusions (albeit with the same scientific pitfalls), reporting persistent urge incontinence rates of 11–57% and de novo urge incontinence rates of zero to 30%.[2–6,8–24] Urethral obstruction requiring surgery or long-term intermittent catheterization was reported in 1–7%. A new AUA guidelines panel is currently reviewing the literature and their report is expected within the next few years.

Traditionally, patients were classified on an anatomic (types 0–3) or functional basis (urethral hypermobility or intrinsic sphincter deficiency), and the type of surgery was based in part on such classification.[25] We no longer use either of these classification systems, but characterize incontinence by two parameters: leak point pressure and degree of urethral mobility (Q-tip angle). No matter what the type, we and others advocate autologous fascial pubovaginal sling.[3,16,25]

CURRENT AND FUTURE ROLE OF AUTOLOGOUS TISSUE FOR SLINGS

In our judgment, autologous fascial pubovaginal sling remains the gold standard against which other surgeries for sphincteric incontinence should be compared. We have demonstrated that it can be performed in a reproducible fashion with minimal morbidity. Using a validated objective, semi-objective and subjective outcome instrument, cure/improve rates of over 90% have been documented. Urinary retention following the procedure should be minimal, as the sling is not tied with excessive tension. Persistent and de novo urge incontinence remain a vexing problem about which the patient should be counseled preoperatively.

While we believe that some form of synthetic or allograft sling will be shown to have equal or better efficacy and less morbidity in the future, none has yet achieved that status.

When and if allograft and synthetic slings are shown to be as safe and efficacious as autologous tissue, there will be little need for the latter except in certain specific circumstances. Before describing those circumstances in more detail, it is important to state emphatically that that time has not yet come; none of these new materials has met the test of time – the future is not now! There is mounting evidence (largely unpublished except in abstract form) that, by 3 years postoperatively, both allograft and xenograft slings have an unacceptably high failure rate, approaching 40%, and there is some evidence that synthetics placed by a transobturator technique may not be as efficacious for intrinsic sphincter deficiency as an autologous fascial bladder neck sling.[26–28] Whether the retropubic techniques for passing synthetics will fare as well is unknown. The time saved may come with a price in the long term.

At the present time, we believe that, because of the likelihood that allograft and xenograft slings have an unacceptably high failure rate, autologous fascia should be used whenever synthetic slings are relatively contraindicated: 1) after urethral erosion of a prior synthetic sling; 2) at the time of urethral reconstruction; 3) in patients at high risk for wound infection (e.g. chronic steroid use); 4) in patients with intrinsic sphincter deficiency who have failed prior sling surgery; and 5) in patients for whom planned intermittent catheterization is necessary.

REFERENCES

1. Appell RA. Primary slings for everyone with genuine stress incontinence? The argument for. Int Urogynecol J 1998;9:249–51.
2. Blaivas JG, Jacobs BZ. Pubovaginal fascial sling for the treatment of complicated stress incontinence. J Urol 1991;145:1214–8.
3. Chaikin DC, Rosenthal J, Blaivas JG. Pubovaginal fascial sling for all types of stress urinary incontinence: long-term analysis. J Urol 1998;160:1312–6.
4. Chou EC, Flisser AJ, Panagopopous G, Blaivas J. Effective treatment of mixed urinary incontinence with a pubovaginal sling. J Urol 2003;170:494–7.
5. Groutz A, Blaivas JG, Hyman MJ, Chaikin DC. Pubovaginal sling surgery for simple stress urinary incontinence: analysis by an outcome score. J Urol 2001;165:1597–600.
6. Barrington JW, Fulford S, Bales G, Stephenson TP. The

modified rectus fascial sling for the treatment of genuine stress incontinence. J Obstet Gynaecol 1998;18:61–2.

7. Leach GE, Dmochowski RR, Appell RA et al. Female Stress Urinary Incontinence Clinical Guidelines Panel summary report on surgical management of female stress urinary incontinence. J Urol 1997;158:875–80.
8. Cross CA, Cespedes RD, McGuire EJ. Our experience with pubovaginal slings in patients with stress urinary incontinence. J Urol 1998;159:1195–8.
9. Fulford SCV, Flynn R, Barrington J, Appanna T, Stephenson TP. An assessment of the surgical outcome and urodynamic effects of the pubovaginal sling for stress incontinence and the associated urge syndrome. J Urol 1999;162:135–7.
10. Hassouna ME, Ghoniem GM. Long-term outcome and quality of life after modified pubovaginal sling for intrinsic sphincter deficiency. Urology 1999;53:287–91.
11. Kochakarn W, Leenanupunth C, Ratana-Olarn K, Roongreungsilp U, Siripornpinyo N. Pubovaginal sling for the treatment of female stress urinary incontinence: experience of 100 cases at Ramathibodi Hospital. J Med Assoc Thai 2001;84:1412–5.
12. McGuire EJ, Lytton B. Pubovaginal sling procedure for stress incontinence. J Urol 1978;119:82–4.
13. McGuire EJ, Bennet CJ, Konnak JA, Sonda LP, Savastano JA. Experience with pubovaginal slings for urinary incontinence at the University of Michigan. J Urol 1987;138:525–6.
14. McGuire EJ, Lytton B, Pepe V et al. Value of urodynamic testing in stress urinary incontinence. J Urol 1980;124:256–8.
15. Morgan TO, Westney OL, McGuire EJ. Pubovaginal sling: 4-year outcome analysis and quality of life assessment. J Urol 2000;163:1845–8.
16. Zaragoza MR. Expanded indications for the pubovaginal sling: treatment of type 2 or 3 stress incontinence. J Urol 1996;156:1620–2.
17. Siegel SB, Allison S, Foster HE. Long term results of pubovaginal sling for stress urinary incontinence. American Urological Association Annual Meeting, New Orleans, LA, 1997. Abstract 1798.
18. Borup K, Nielsen JB. Results in 32 women operated for genuine stress incontinence with the pubovaginal sling procedure ad modum Ed McGuire. Scand J Urol Nephrol 2002;36(2):128–33.
19. Gormley EA, Latini J, Hanlon L. Long-term effect of pubovaginal sling on quality of life. American Urological Association Annual Meeting, Orlando, FL, 2002. Abstract 418.
20. Rodrigues P, Hering F, Meler A, Campagnari JC, D'Imperio M. Pubo-fascial versus vaginal sling operation for the treatment of stress urinary incontinence: a prospective study. Neurourol Urodyn 2004;23(7):627–31.
21. Beck RP, McCormick S, Nordstrom L. The fascia lata sling procedure for treating recurrent genuine stress incontinence of urine. Obstet Gynecol 1988;72(5):699–703.
22. Karram MM, Bhatia NN. Patch procedure: modified transvaginal fascia lata sling for recurrent or severe stress urinary incontinence. Obstet Gynecol 1990;75(3 Part 1):461–3.
23. Govier FE, Gibbons RP, Correa RJ, Weissman RM, Pritchett TR, Hefty TR. Pubovaginal slings using fascia lata for the treatment of intrinsic sphincter deficiency. J Urol 1997;157(1):117–21.
24. Latini JM, Lux MM, Kreder KJ. Efficacy and morbidity of autologous fascia lata sling cystourethropexy. J Urol 2004;171(3):1180–4.
25. Blaivas JG, Olsson CA. Stress incontinence: classification and surgical approach. J Urol 1988;139:727–31.
26. Colvert JR III, Kropp BP, Cheng EY et al. The use of small intestinal submucosa as an off-the-shelf urethral sling material for pediatric urinary incontinence. J Urol 2002;168(4 Part 2):1875–6.
27. Palma PCR, Dambros M, Riccetto CLZ, Herrmann V, Netto NR Jr. Pubovaginal sling using the porcine small intestinal submucosa for stress urinary incontinence. Braz J Urol 2001;27(5):483–8.
28. Rutner AB, Levine SR, Schmaelzle JF. Porcine small intestinal submucosa implanted as a pubovaginal sling in 115 female patients with stress urinary incontinence: a 3 year series evaluated for durability of the results. Society for Urology and Engineering, 17th Annual Meeting, Orlando, FL, 2002.

62

Tension-free vaginal tape procedure for treatment of female urinary stress incontinence

Carl Gustaf Nilsson

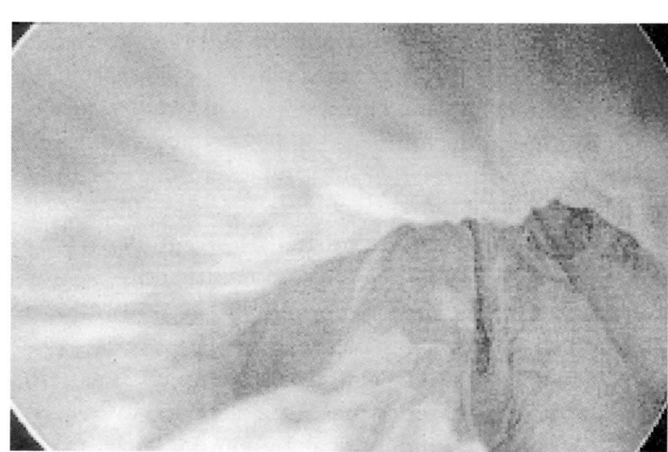

INTRODUCTION

The tension-free vaginal tape (TVT) procedure for treatment of female urinary stress incontinence is a sling operation. For over a century sling operations have been developed and performed with a satisfactory degree of success in terms of achieved dryness. The classic sling operations as described by Goebbel,[1] Frangenheim,[2] Stoeckel,[3] and Aldridge[4] are all major invasive surgical procedures, with the inevitable risk of complications, postoperative morbidity and voiding difficulties. Slings of many different materials – allografts, xenografts, and synthetics – have been used. Classic slings are placed at the bladder neck in order to correct hypermobility and to enhance transmission of intra-abdominal pressure provoked by straining. This mechanism of action is consistent with the most popular theories of the past century describing the causes of urinary incontinence.[5]

Growing awareness of the magnitude of the urinary incontinence problem in the aging population of the developed world has regenerated increasing interest in finding more effective, less invasive, and more affordable methods of curing incontinence. As hypermobility of the bladder neck correlates poorly with symptoms of incontinence and severity of leakage,[6] a shift of interest from correcting anatomic changes to an attempt to restore function of the urethral closure mechanism has occurred. Many findings through the years have identified the midurethra as the focus of interest when dealing with female stress incontinence, with anatomic, physiologic, and histologic investigations consistently supporting the concept of the midurethra as being important in maintaining urinary continence in the female.

Pubourethral ligaments, inserting at the midurethra, were identified by Zaccharin in the 1960s,[7] and further demonstrated by DeLancey in the 1990s.[8] Histologic evaluation of the female urethra by Huisman revealed prominent vascularization specifically at the midurethra.[9]

The early urodynamic investigations by Asmussen and Ulmsten[10] further strengthened the impression of the more distal parts of the urethra playing a major role in the closure mechanism. The maximal closure pressure is located at the midurethra and in fertile women pulsatility can be demonstrated at the same location, indicating strong vascular support.[10]

Ingelman-Sundberg found that the ventral parts of the pubococcygeal muscles inserted into the anterior vaginal wall at the site of the midurethra and utilized this finding in his sling plasty.[11] Furthermore, Westby and colleagues showed elegantly in radiographic experiments how, in continent women, the urethra closes at its middle section on holding urination and that the maximal closure pressure is situated at the same level of the urethra.[12]

By combining these findings, a new theory for describing the causes of female urinary incontinence was presented by Petros and Ulmsten – the 'midurethra theory' (in early literature the 'integral theory').[13] According to this theory, damage to the pubourethral ligaments supporting the urethra, impaired support of the anterior vaginal wall to the midurethra, and weakened function of the part of the pubococcygeal muscles that inserts adjacent to the urethra are responsible for causing stress urinary incontinence. Connective tissue is an important element of the involved structures since the quality of this tissue has an influence on continence.[14]

THE TVT PROCEDURE

Development of the procedure

The TVT procedure was developed based on the elements of the midurethra theory. The goal was to create a minimally invasive operation that would reinforce the pubourethral ligaments, strengthen the support of the urethra by the anterior vaginal wall, and achieve conditions that would favor ingrowth of fresh connective tissue into the region. The procedure was performed under local infiltration anesthesia from the very beginning in order to facilitate early same day discharge from hospital.

Several different sling materials were evaluated. The one finally chosen is a synthetic polypropylene monofilamentous mesh, with a pore size between 75 and 150 microns, which is optimal for ingrowth of fibrous tissue and allows leukocytes and macrophages to enter into the mesh, thus avoiding colonization of bacteria. The special weave of this type I mesh has favorable properties in terms of elasticity and strength.[15]

An effort was made to standardize the operation in order to facilitate training of doctors to perform the procedure in a manner that includes certain in-built safety features and makes good clinical results possible. The use of local anesthesia – prilocaine (2.5 mg/ml) with epinephrine (2 mcg/ml), diluted with saline to 0.25% – causes vasoconstriction in the operating region, thus decreasing the risk of intraoperative bleeding and hematoma formation. The recommended anesthetic volume of 75–100 ml results in hydrodissection of tissues at the operation site and facilitates passage of the specially designed instrument, with the attached polypropylene tape, through the correct layers of tissue, thus avoiding complications such as bladder injury.

If the local anesthesia is placed only in the region where the tape should be positioned, deviation by the instruments from this safe sector during performance of the operation causes the patient to react and, thereby, guides the surgeon to correct his performance. Local anesthesia interferes least with the function of the pelvic floor and allows intraoperative testing of optimal tension-free placement of the tape by a cough test in order to avoid postoperative voiding difficulties.

Operation technique

The TVT device consists of an 11 mm wide × 40 cm long tape of polypropylene, both ends of which are attached to stainless steel, specially curved, 5 mm diameter insertion needles. The tape is covered by plastic sheets to protect it from contamination and to facilitate its passage through the tissues. A reusable handle fits to the needles and is used to insert the needles. A rigid catheter guide is placed into an 18 Fr Foley catheter and helps to deflect the bladder away from the path of needle insertion.

The patient is placed in a lithotomy position, avoiding more than 70 degrees of flexion of the thighs. After premedication with, for example, 0.5 mg midazolam, the local anesthetics are placed. The operation requires three small incisions: two 1-cm wide suprapubic skin incisions at the upper rim of the pubic bone, each 2–2.5 cm lateral to the midline, and a vaginal midline incision not more than 1.5 cm wide starting 0.5 cm from the external meatus of the urethra.

Five cc of anesthetics are placed under the skin at the site of the planned skin incisions. Another 20 cc are placed on each side retropubically, closely following the posterior surface of the pubic bone down to the urogenital diaphragm. Vaginal infiltration of the anesthetics includes 10 cc on each side paraurethrally up to the urogenital diaphragm and another 5 cc under the vaginal mucosa at the site of the midurethra.

The skin incisions facilitate passing of the needles through the skin. After the vaginal incision is made, careful minimal blunt dissection, using Metzenbaum scissors, should be undertaken paraurethrally between the vaginal mucosa and the pubocervical fascia to a depth of not more than 2 cm. The TVT needle is placed in its starting position within the dissected paraurethral tunnel with the needle tip between the index finger of the surgeon's hand in the vagina and the lower rim of the pubic ramus. With slow controlled pressure, the needle is brought through the urogenital diaphragm, the space of Retzius, and the rectus muscle fascia using the skin incision as a point of direction. It is important to keep the needle in close contact with the dorsal surface of the pubic bone at all times in order to avoid bladder perforation or entrance into the abdominal cavity. The same procedure is repeated on the other side.

After passing each needle to the extent that the needle tip is visible at the skin incision, cystoscopy, using a 70-degree optic, is performed to confirm bladder integrity. If bladder perforation is noted, the needle is withdrawn and passed once more, ensuring that it stays close to the pubic bone and within the safe sector. Once bladder integrity is confirmed, both needles and the tape are brought through and the final adjustment of the tape can take place. The recommendation is to fill the bladder with 300 cc of saline and perform a cough test. The patient is asked to cough vigorously while the tape is adjusted to a point when leakage is only a drop of saline at the urethral meatus. This procedure will ensure tension-free placement of the tape and minimize risks of postoperative voiding problems.

After the final adjustment of the tape has been made, the plastic sheets are taken off. At this point it is important to make sure that no further tightening of the tape occurs by placing Metzenbaum scissors between the urethra and the tape when removing the plastic sheets. No fixation of the tape is required.

Clinical performance

The results of the first clinical trial of the TVT operation were encouraging, with an objective cure rate of 80%.[16] Surgeons at six different centers were given personal hands-on training in the TVT technique, after which a multicenter, two-country, prospective clinical trial was initiated. The aim of this study was to investigate the performance of the procedure in a normal clinical setting. A total of 131 carefully selected primary cases of genuine stress incontinence were enrolled. The 1-year follow-up results revealed an objective cure rate of 91%, with a further 7% of patients being significantly improved. Only 2% were regarded as failures. The complication rate was low, and included one case of bladder injury and one wound infection. Three patients had short-term (≤3 days) voiding problems and only one patient experienced retention symptoms for 12 days.[17] These promising results prompted further studies in unselected groups of women with indications for surgical treatment of their urinary incontinence. In a prospective clinical trial of 161 consecutive TVT operations, which included 28% with prior failed incontinence surgery, 37% with mixed incontinence and 11% with intrinsic sphincter deficiency (ISD), the overall objective cure rate at 16 months of follow-up was 87%, 7% were significantly improved and only 5% were classified as failures.[18] No serious complications occurred. The bladder perforation rate was 3.7%, and 4.3% of the women experienced short-term voiding difficulties. De novo urge symptoms were noted in 3% of the women, while as many as 80% of those women who preoperatively complained of urge symptoms were relieved of these symptoms at their 16-month follow-up visit.

The next step was to study the effectiveness of the TVT procedure in special groups of patients. Table 62.1 shows the objective cure rates found in patients with prior failed incontinence surgery, patients with mixed incontinence, and patients with ISD. From the results it can be concluded that the performance of the TVT procedure is as good in recurrent and mixed incontinence cases as it is in primary cases of urinary incontinence. The cure rates found in patients with ISD appear to be somewhat lower than in other forms of incontinence, a finding also encountered with other types of incontinence operation.

Long-term results

Table 62.2 shows the objective cure rates in the long-term follow-up trials published to date. Some of the problems of evaluating long-term results of incontinence surgery include the growing number of patients lost to follow-up, and the fact that, in many of these often elderly patients, new illnesses appear that might affect bladder function and thus complicate estimation of long-term effectiveness and safety of an anti-incontinence surgical intervention.

Table 62.1. ***Objective cure rate and time of follow-up in recurrent, mixed and intrinsic sphincter deficiency (ISD) cases of incontinence***

	n	Follow-up	Cure rate (%)
Recurrent			
Kuuva & Nilsson[19]	51	24 months	89.6
Lo et al.[20]	41	12 months	82.9
Rezapour & Ulmsten[21]	34	3–5 years	82.0
Liapis et al.[22]	33	20 months	70/90*
Mixed			
Nilsson & Kuuva[18]	59	16 months	81.4
Rezapour & Ulmsten[23]	80	3–5 years	85.0
ISD			
Nilsson & Kuuva[18]	18	16 months	77.8
Rezapour & Ulmsten[24]	49	3-5 years	74.0

* 70% with fixed urethra, 90% with mobile urethra.

Table 62.2. ***Objective cure rate during long-term follow-up***

	n	Follow-up	Cure rate (%)
Olsson & Kroon[25]	51	3 years	90
Ulmsten et al.[26]	50	3 years	86
Nilsson et al.[27]	90	5 years	84.7
Nilsson et al.[28]	90	7 years	81.3

The rate of loss to follow-up in the long-term reports, the results of which are presented in Table 62.2, ranges between zero and 11%. This low rate demonstrates a reliable picture of the actual performance of the TVT operation over time. The cure rates at 7 years after surgery are in line with those reported in the initial early trials, suggesting minimal decline in effectiveness over the years. Attempts to predict the risk of failure or declining effectiveness of the TVT procedure have been described in many reports; however, it has not been possible to identify any single significant factor. A tendency towards higher failure rates appears to be associated with older age at the time of operation and the presence of a low pressure urethra.

An important finding of long-term follow-up is the absence of signs of rejection or adverse tissue reaction to the polypropylene tape material. No erosion of the tape into the urethra or the bladder was seen.

Randomized clinical trials

A randomized clinical trial is the preferred method of comparing new treatment methods with established ones. Colposuspension has, for decades, been regarded as the 'gold standard' of incontinence operations. Colposuspension is performed either as an open laparotomy procedure or as a laparoscopic operation. Four randomized clinical trials comparing the TVT operation with colposuspension have been published. The largest one by Ward and Hilton compared TVT with open colposuspension in a 14-center study in the UK and Ireland.[29] Valpas et al. compared TVT with laparoscopic colposuspension using mesh in a six-center trial,[30] while Persson et al. (single center study)[32] and Paraiso et al. (two-center study)[31] used four Gore-Tex and four polyester sutures, respectively, in their laparoscopic colposuspension operations. Table 62.3 shows the results of these trials. There was no difference in cure rate between the TVT procedure and open colposuspension, but there was a significantly more rapid recovery after surgery in the TVT group and significantly more patients in the colposuspension group needed later surgery for uro-

Table 62.3. ***Cure rates in randomized clinical trials comparing tension-free vaginal tape (TVT) with colposuspension (Colpo)***

	n (TVT/Colpo)	Follow-up	Cure rate (%) (TVT/Colpo)
Ward & Hilton[29]	175/169	24 months	63/51
Valpas et al.[30]	70/51	12 months	86/57
Paraiso et al.[31]	36/36	18 months	97/81
Persson et al.[32]	37/31	12 months	94/100

genital prolapse. The cure rate in the TVT group in the trials of Valpas et al. and Paraiso et al. was significantly higher than in the colposuspension group. No difference in cure rates between the groups in the Persson et al. study could be detected.

Complications

Quality of life has become an important concept when discussing the outcome of incontinence surgery. Quality of life for the incontinent woman is governed not only by the absence of urinary leakage, but also by the absence of voiding difficulties, urinary tract infections and other adverse symptoms caused by complications associated with the surgical procedure. Minimal invasiveness and standardization of a surgical intervention is a means of bringing down the rate of complications. Systematic prospective registering of complications is the only way to get an accurate picture of the risk and the rate of specific complications. Fortunately, two such registers have been established and published. The one from Finland is unique, as it comprises every single TVT procedure performed in the country as it was introduced to the clinics within a systematic hands-on training program.[33] The Finnish material also includes the learning curve of all the surgeons involved. The other registry is from Austria and includes nearly 3000 cases, but does not involve all the clinics of the country.[34]

A few other more comprehensive studies focusing on complication rates have been published. The rates of the most common complications associated with incontinence surgery in these studies and the two registries are shown in Table 62.4. It is interesting to note that the rate of bladder injury is fairly consistent in these reports, being around 4% on average. The definition of voiding difficulties varies between the reports but mostly refers to the need for short-term intermittent catheterization within the first two postoperative days. In the report by Abouassaly et al. (which has the highest rate of voiding difficulties), only one patient needed an indwelling catheter for more than 48 hours.[37] The risk of postoperative urinary tract infection (UTI) also varies somewhat, with the highest rate being reported in the Austrian material. This may be the result of adhering to a policy of using an indwelling catheter postoperatively (63% of the cases). The recommendation is to perform the TVT operation under local anesthesia, a situation that does not necessitate the use of a postoperative catheter in the bladder. In a report by Bodelsson et al. it was found that the risk of bladder perforation was three times higher if the TVT operation was performed under spinal anesthesia compared to local anesthesia.[38]

The TVT operation has been found to be effective in the treatment of women with stress incontinence complicated by the simultaneous existence of urge symptoms or/and urge incontinence. The cure rates reported in these cases of mixed incontinence are more than 80%.[18,23]

Table 63.4. ***Rate of complications (%) associated with the TVT procedure***

	Kuuva & Nilsson[33]	Tamussino et al.[34]	Karram et al.[35]	Levin et al.[36]	Abouassaly et al.[37]	Nilsson & Kuuva[18]
	n: 1455	*n*: 2795	*n*: 350	*n*: 313	*n*: 241	*n*: 161
Bladder injury	3.8	2.7	4.9	5.1	5.8	3.7
Bleeding	1.9	2.3	0.9	nr	2.5	1.8
Voiding difficulties	7.6	nr	4.9	2.5	19.7	4.3
Hematoma	2.4	nr	1.7	nr	1.9	1.2
Wound infection	0.8	nr	nr	nr	0.4	1.8
Urinary tract infection	4.1	17	10	nr	nr	6.2
Defect healing	0.7	nr	0.9	1.3	0.4	nr
De novo urge	0.2	nr	12	8.3	15	3.1

nr, not reported.

Pre-existing urge symptoms resolve in 50–80% of cases.[18,39] Occurrence of de novo urge symptoms varies between 0.2 and 15% (Table 62.4). Seven years of follow-up suggest that there is no risk of the number of cases with de novo urge problems increasing over time, the rate of these symptoms being 6% at 7 years postoperatively.[28]

Although the TVT operation is a partly blind procedure, the risk of excessive (>200 ml) intraoperative bleeding and retropubic hematoma formation is rare. Excessive bleeding occurs on average in 2% of cases (Table 62.4) and is mostly managed by manual compression and tamponade. In a systematic evaluation of the occurrence of postoperative retropubic hematoma formation, Flock et al. reported a rate of 4.1% among 249 consecutive cases, with only four cases exceeding 300 ml and requiring surgical intervention.[40]

The potential for more serious vascular complications exists with a partly blind procedure; however, the incidence of such has been very low. The rate of serious vascular complications in the Finnish registry report was 0.07%, with the Austrian registry reporting bowel perforation in 0.04%.

SUMMARY

Available data obtained from published clinical reports show that the TVT operation is effective in curing stress incontinence. In prospective trials where strict criteria for cure and significant improvement have been used, approximately 95% of women having a TVT operation are found to be cured or significantly improved of their stress incontinence. Furthermore, the TVT procedure appears to perform well in all categories of patients for whom incontinence surgery is traditionally recommended, i.e. in primary cases of stress incontinence, cases of prior failed incontinence surgery, and in cases with mixed incontinence and in those with ISD. The risk of intraoperative and short-term postoperative complications is low if proper training is provided and the operation is performed in a standardized way. No long-term adverse effects of the procedure have been reported.

In a cost-utility analysis by Manca et al., the TVT operation was found to be cost saving compared with open colposuspension.[41]

REFERENCES

1. Goebbel R. Zur operativen Beseitigung der angeborenen Incontinentia vesicae. Ztschr f Gynäk u Urol 1910;2:187–91.
2. Frangenheim P. Zur operativen behandlung der inkontinenz der männlichen hahnröre. Verhandl d Deutsch Gesellsch f Chir 1914;43:149–54.
3. Stoeckel W. Uber die verwendung der musculi pyramidales bei der operativen behandlung der incontinentia urinae. Zentralbl f Gynäk 1917;41:11–9.
4. Aldridge HA. Transplantation of fascia for relief of urinary stress incontinence. Am J Obstet Gynecol 1942;44:398–411.
5. Enhörning G. Simultaneous recording of intravesical and intraurethral pressure. Acta Chir Scand 1961;276(Suppl):1–68.
6. Peschers UM, Fanger G, Schaer GN et al. Bladder neck mobility in continent nulliparous women. BJOG 2001;108:320–4.
7. Zaccharin RF. The anatomic supports of the female urethra. Obstet Gynecol 1968;21:754–9.
8. DeLancey JOL. Structural support of the urethra as it relates to stress urinary incontinence: the hammock hypothesis. Am J Obstet Gynecol 1994;170:1713–23.
9. Huisman AB. Aspects on the anatomy of the female urethra with special relation to urinary continence. Contrib Gynecol Obstet 1983;10:1–31.
10. Asmussen M, Ulmsten U. On the physiology of continence and pathophysiology of stress incontinence in the female. Contrib Gynecol Obstet 1983;10:32–50.
11. Ingelman-Sundberg A. Urinary incontinence in women, excluding fistulas. Acta Obstet Gynecol Scand 1953;31:266–95.
12. Westby M, Asmussen M, Ulmsten U. Location of maximal intraurethral pressure related to urogenital diaphragm in the female subject as studied by simultaneous urethrocystometry and voiding urethrocystography. Am J Obstet Gynecol 1982;144:408–12.
13. Petros P, Ulmsten U. An integral theory of female urinary incontinence. Experimental and clinical considerations. Acta Obstet Gynecol Scand 1990;153(Suppl):7–31.
14. Ulmsten U, Ekman G, Giertz G et al. Different biochemical composition of connective tissue in continent and stress incontinent women. Acta Obstet Gynecol Scand 1987;66:455–7.
15. Dietz HP, Vancaille P, Svehla M et al. Mechanical properties of implant materials used in incontinence surgery. Proceedings of the International Continence Society 31st Annual Meeting, Seoul, Korea, September 18–21, 2001.
16. Ulmsten U, Henriksson L, Johnson P et al. An ambulatory surgical procedure under local anesthesia for treatment of female urinary incontinence. Int Urogynecol J 1996;7:81–6.
17. Ulmsten U, Falconer C, Johnson P et al. A multicenter study of tension-free vaginal tape (TVT) for surgical treatment of stress urinary incontinence. Int Urogynecol J 1998;9:210–3.

18. Nilsson CG, Kuuva N. The tension-free vaginal tape procedure is successful in the majority of women with indications for surgical treatment of urinary stress incontinence. BJOG 2001;108:414–9.
19. Kuuva N, Nilsson CG. Tension-free vaginal tape procedure: an effective minimally invasive operation for treatment of recurrent stress urinary incontinence. Gynecol Obstet Invest 2003;56:93–8.
20. Lo TS, Hornig SG, Chang CL et al. Tension-free vaginal tape procedure after previous failure in incontinence surgery. Urology 2002;60:57–61.
21. Rezapour M, Ulmsten U. Tension-free vaginal tape (TVT) procedure in women with recurrent stress urinary incontinence – a long-term follow up. Int Urogynecol J 2001;12(Suppl 2):9–11.
22. Liapis A, Bakas P, Lazaris D et al. Tension-free vaginal tape in the management of recurrent stress incontinence. Arch Gynecol Obstet 2004;269:205–7.
23. Rezapour M, Ulmsten U. Tension-free vaginal tape (TVT) in women with mixed urinary incontinence – a long term follow up. Int Urogynekol J 2001;12(Suppl 2):15–8.
24. Rezapour M, Ulmsten U. Tension-free vaginal tape (TVT) in stress incontinent women with intrinsic sphincter deficiency (ISD) – a long term follow up. Int Urogynecol J 2001;12(Suppl 2):12–4.
25. Olsson I, Kroon UB. A three-year postoperative evaluation of tension-free vaginal tape. Gynecol Obstet Invest 1999;48:267–9.
26. Ulmsten U, Johnson P, Rezapour M. A three-year follow up of tension free vaginal tape for surgical treatment of female stress urinary incontinence. BJOG 1999;106:345–50.
27. Nilsson CG, Kuuva N, Falconer C et al. Long-term results of the tension-free vaginal tape (TVT) procedure for surgical treatment of female stress urinary incontinence. Int Urogynecol J 2001;12(Suppl 2):5–8.
28. Nilsson CG, Falconer C, Rezapour M. Seven-year follow up of the tension-free vaginal tape procedure for treatment of urinary incontinence. Obstet Gynecol 2004;104:1259–62.
29. Ward KL, Hilton P. A prospective multicenter randomized trial of tension-free vaginal tape and colposuspension for primary stress incontinence. Two-year follow-up. Am J Obstet Gynecol 2004;190:324–31.
30. Valpas A, Kivelä A, Penttinen J et al. Tension-free vaginal tape and laparoscopic mesh colposuspension for stress urinary incontinence. Obstet Gynecol 2004;104:42–8.
31. Paraiso M, Walters M, Karram M et al. Laparoscopic Burch colposuspension versus tension-free vaginal tape: a randomized trial. Obstet Gynecol 2004;104:1249–58.
32. Persson J, Teleman P, Eten-Bergqvist C et al. Cost-analyses based on a prospective, randomized study comparing laparoscopic colposuspension with tension-free vaginal tape procedure. Acta Obstet Gynecol Scand 2002;81:1066–73.
33. Kuuva N, Nilsson CG. A nationwide analysis of complications associated with the tension-free vaginal tape (TVT) procedure. Acta Obstet Gynecol Scand 2002;81:72–7.
34. Tamussino K, Hanzal E, Kölle D et al. Tension-free vaginal tape operation: results of the Austrian registry. Obstet Gynecol 2001;98:732–6.
35. Karram M, Segal JL, Vassallo BJ et al. Complications and untoward effects of the tension-free vaginal tape procedure. Obstet Gynecol 2003;101:929–32.
36. Levin I, Groutz A, Gold R et al. Surgical complications and medium-term outcome results of tension-free vaginal tape: a prospective study of 313 consecutive patients. Neurourol Urodyn 2004;23:7–9.
37. Abouassaly R, Steinberg JR, Lemieux M et al. Complications of tension-free vaginal tape surgery: a multi-institutional review. BJU Int 2004;94:110–3.
38. Bodelsson G, Henriksson L, Osser S et al. Short term complications of the tension-free vaginal tape operation for stress urinary incontinence in women. BJOG 2002;109:566–9.
39. Segal JL, Vassallo B, Kleeman S et al. Prevalence of persistent de novo overactive bladder symptoms after the tension-free vaginal tape. Obstet Gynecol 2004;104:1263–9.
40. Flock F, Reich A, Muche R et al. Hemorrhagic complications associated with tension-free vaginal tape procedure. Obstet Gynecol 2004;104:989–94.
41. Manca A, Sculpher MJ, Ward K et al. A cost–utility analysis of tension-free vaginal tape versus colposuspension for primary urodynamic stress incontinence. BJOG 2003;110:255–62.

63

SPARC – midurethral sling suspension system

David Staskin, Renuka Tyagi

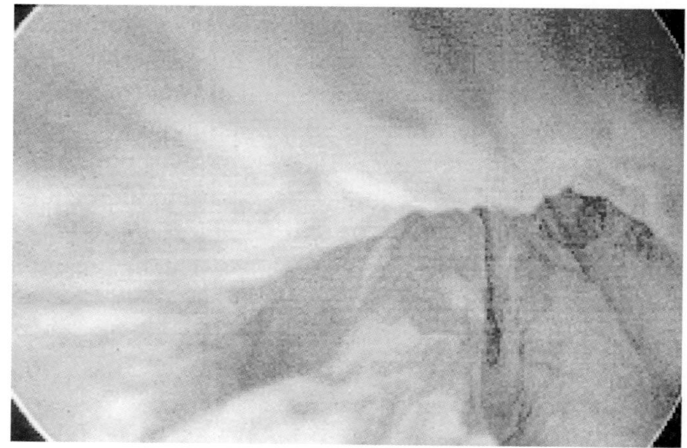

INTRODUCTION

Minimally invasive slings placed at the level of the mid- to distal urethra have simplified the treatment of genuine stress urinary incontinence (GSI)[1] with minimal morbidity. Variations in surgical technique, materials, and shape of the slings used have resulted from the drive to decrease surgical morbidity associated with autologous fascia harvesting without affecting long-term surgical outcomes.[2–9] The effective and long-term treatment of stress incontinence due to urethral hypermobility and intrinsic sphincter deficiency has been documented following placement of Burch urethropexy and classic pubovaginal slings.[10–13] In addition, similar cure rates between midurethral slings and the Burch colposuspension have been documented in prospective randomized studies.[14,15]

The SPARC sling system is a minimally invasive sling procedure using a loosely knitted, self-fixating, 1 cm wide, 4-0 polypropylene mesh, which is placed at the level of the midurethra by passing the suspension needle via a suprapubic to vaginal approach.[16–18]

MECHANISM OF ACTION

Continence is dependent upon multiple factors: resting urethral tone, active sphincter contraction, external compression, pressure transmission, and integrity of anatomic configuration. The success of midurethral sling techniques has prompted a re-evaluation of the pathophysiology of GSI and the paradigm for its surgical correction. The mechanism of action for midurethral slings is presumed to be mimicking of the support provided by the pubourethral ligaments and suburethral fascial support.[19]

The importance of urethral stabilization from rotational motion has generally been accepted and has been introduced as the 'integral theory' from data collected during radiologic evaluation of micturition.[20] This correlated with structures documented on anatomic dissection and dubbed an anatomic hammock.[21] The importance of urethral configuration suggests that midurethral support prevents the separation of the posterior urethral wall from anterior urethral wall during rotational motion around the inferior portion of the pubic ramus, which appears integral to continence.[22] Suburethral support and stability in conjunction with urethral coaptation appear to be the critical factors in the restoration of continence, and elevation of the bladder neck may no longer be a prerequisite.

DEVICE DESIGN

The SPARC sling system is illustrated in Figure 63.1.

SURGICAL TECHNIQUE

Anesthesia

Anesthesia may be selected as per patient and surgeon preference and include general, spinal or epidural, or local anesthesia with/without intravenous sedation. If a local anesthetic is selected, it should be noted that the primary source of discomfort for the patient is contact with the periosteum of the pubic bone during needle passage. Local injections should include two approaches: 1) the abdominal surface with the local anesthetic of the abdominal skin, rectus fascia and muscle; and 2) a paravaginal approach to anesthetize the inferior border of the pubic ramus.

Positioning

A standard or modified lithotomy position may be selected based on surgical preference and concomitant procedures, with a supine, pelvis-inclined (Trendelenburg) position recommended. Adequate distal vaginal exposure for a 1.5 cm midurethral incision is required; however, vaginal retraction sutures or complex retractor is usually not required for sling placement alone. A weighted speculum and placement of a Foley catheter (14–18 Fr) per urethra to drain the bladder completely is preferred.

Incisions

Two parallel 15-blade stab incisions are made over the pubic symphysis 1.5 cm from the midline (3 cm apart). The surgeon should avoid incisions lateral to this area to avoid impingement of the ilioinguinal nerve exiting from the external ring (Fig. 63.2).

Next, the bladder neck should be identified; the submeatal fold may be elevated using an Allis clamp, and a midline incision performed through the vaginal mucosa over the midurethra. This incision, centered over the midurethra, may vary between 1.5 and 3 cm as per surgeon preference (Fig. 63.3). If the procedure is performed without local anesthetic, a saline injection at the level of the midurethra, extending laterally, may be elected to aid in development of the plane of dissection between the vaginal epithelium and the periurethral fascia. Submucosal dissection is performed bilaterally with Metzenbaum scissors, creating a tunnel to the inferior border of the pubic ramus at the level of the midurethra. The tunnel may be small enough (1.5 cm) for only the needle and dilator–connector to traverse the distance, or wide enough (3 cm) for the fingertip to

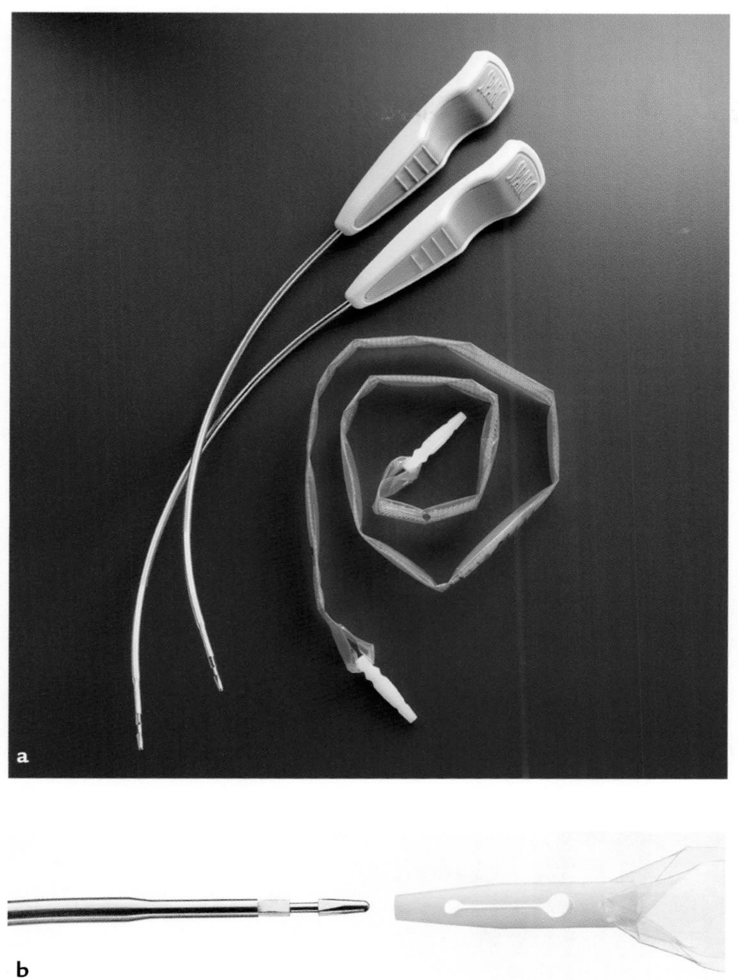

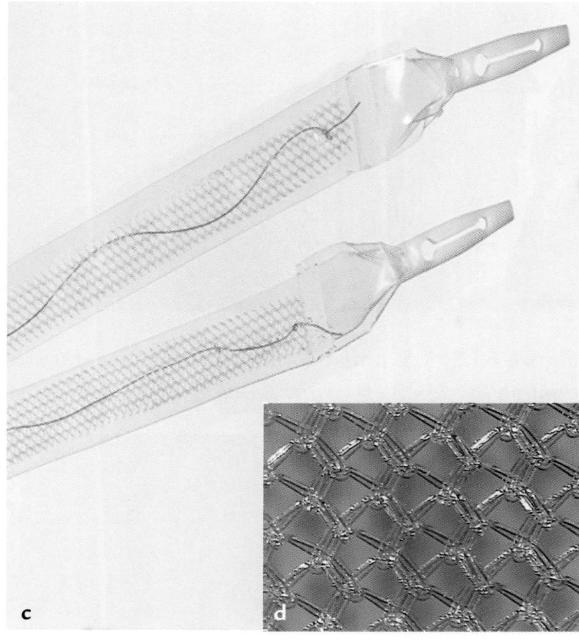

Figure 63.1. *SPARC sling system: (a) Suspension needles: disposable ergonomic, 0.118 in. diameter, 8.2 in. long, and non-cutting. (b) Dilator–connectors: create the sling tract and enable the suspension needles to be of small diameter and minimizing trauma, do not require sling attachment and tract formation until the needle position is confirmed, and permit untwisting of the mesh after attachment. (c) Plastic sheath: permits smooth placement of self-fixating mesh. Absorbable tensioning suture: placed within the mesh sling and knotted at various intervals; this absorbable suture prevents 'pre-tensioning' of the mesh sling during the removal of the plastic sheath and permits intra- and postoperative sling adjustment. (d) Mesh sling: biocompatible 4-0 loosely knitted polypropylene.*

be inserted. The 'small tunnel' approach involves placement of the fingertip in the paravaginal fornix outside of the incision in order to palpate needle perforation through the endopelvic fascia (recommended). The 'large tunnel' approach allows the surgeon to palpate the perforation point of the periurethral fascia from within the incision and to guide the needle under direct fingertip control.

Needle passage

Effective needle passage is divided into two phases with entrance into and traversing of the retropubic space first, followed by perforation of the endopelvic and periurethral fasciae. Needle passage may be described in five substeps:

1. *Needle passage to the superior surface of pubic symphysis:* Holding the needle itself with the fingertips of both hands, the needle is passed through the stab incisions above the pubic symphysis directly down to the bone. During this maneuver the needle handle is pointed toward the surgeon (Fig. 63.4).
2. *Rotation around the superior surface of the pubic symphysis:* The needle tip is guided along the superior surface of the bone and then directed downward to perforate the rectus fascia and muscle. Grasping the needle itself near the end with the

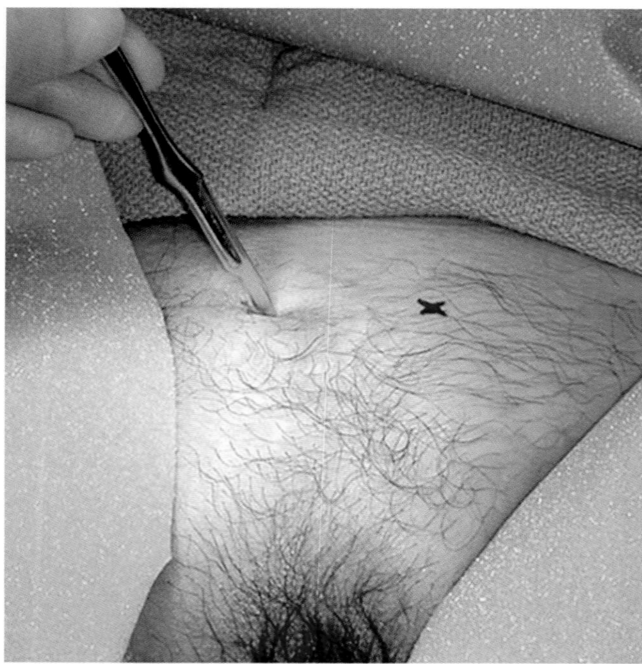

Figure 63.2. *Suprapubic skin incisions. Stab incisions through the skin 3 cm apart, flanking the abdominal midline.*

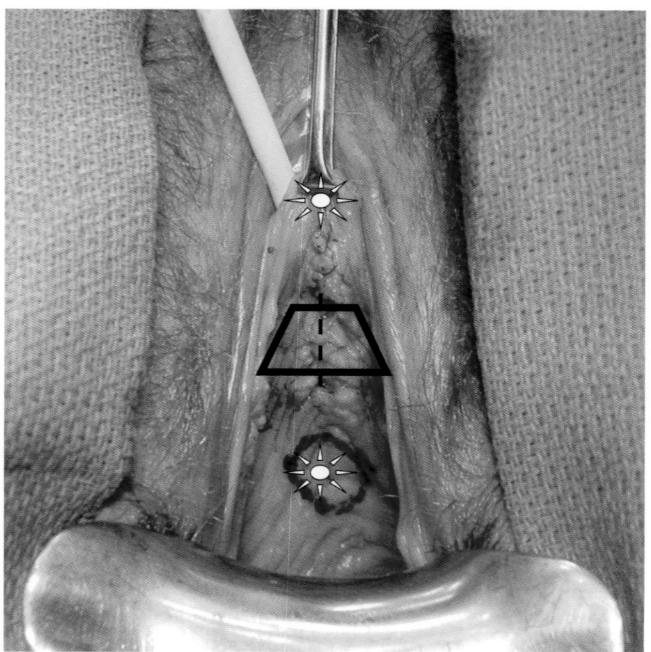

Figure 63.3. *Midline vaginal incision, 1.5–2.0 cm in length.*

fingertips rather than the handle permits more control of the straight portion of the curved needle. After fascial perforation, the needle handle should rotate to 90 degrees (up to the ceiling) as the needle is advanced to keep the tip of the needle on the posterior surface of the pubic bone (Fig. 63.5).

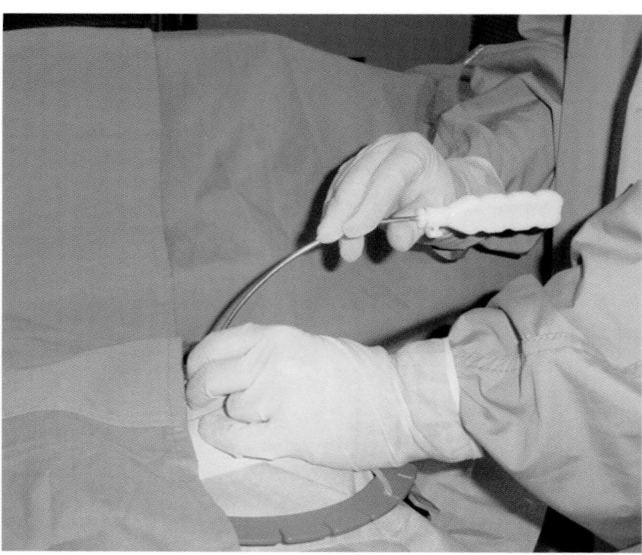

Figure 63.4. *Needle passage along the superior surface of pubic symphysis.*

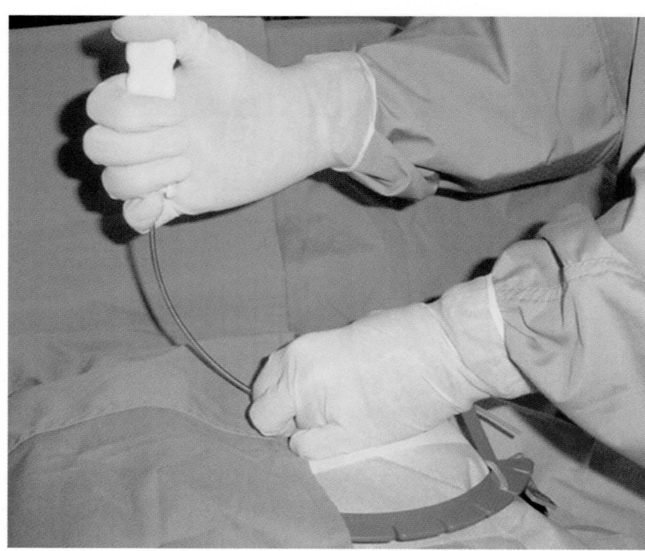

Figure 63.5. *Rotation of needles around the superior pubic symphysis onto the posterior (retropubic) surface.*

3. *Traversing the retropubic space*: The needle is guided inferiorly, with the handle rotated 10 degrees medially – 'walked downward along the bone' – again with the fingertips, until the endopelvic fascia is encountered (Fig. 63.6).
4. *Placement of the needle tip at the perforation point*: Grasping the handle of the needle, the needle tip is palpated with the alternate index finger beneath the vaginal wall and is guided to the desired point of perforation. Remember: 'Find the needle point beneath the vaginal wall with the finger' and guide it to the perforation point, rather than 'Find the finger

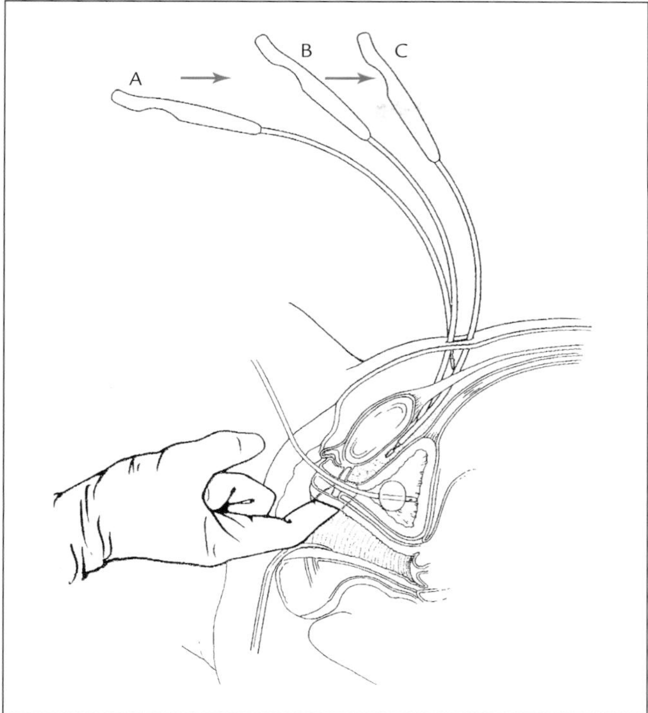

Figure 63.6. *Needle traverses the retropubic space on the posterior surface of the pubic symphysis.*

placed at the perforation point' with the needle. The perforation point is as lateral as possible against the inferior border of the pubic ramus, at the level of the midurethra (Fig. 63.7).

5. *Perforation of the endopelvic/periurethral fascia and directing the needle through the vaginal incision*: Perforation of the fascia can be performed by pushing the needle through the endopelvic and periurethral fasciae without placing a finger within the vaginal incision (recommended) or by placing a finger in the incision (preferred for less experienced surgeons). A finger placed outside of the incision against the bone within the fornix is most effective. Once the needle perforates the fasciae and can be felt *only* beneath the epithelial layer, it can be guided through the dissected tunnel with or without a finger placed within the vaginal incision. Be sure the needle has perforated the fasciae before directing it medially. If necessary, allow needle-point perforation of the vaginal epithelium, withdraw the needle and then guide it out of the incision. Failure to perforate the fasciae completely before medial direction of the needle out of the incision decreases the distance between the perforation point and the urethra (Fig. 63.8).

The following guidelines are suggested to avoid intraoperative 'misadventures' during needle passage.

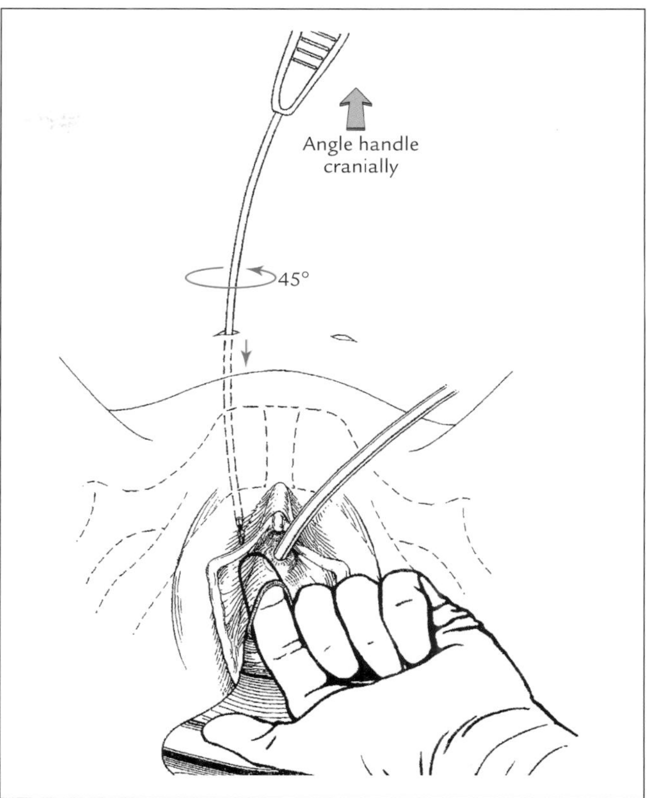

Figure 63.7. *Placement of the needle tip at the point of endopelvic fascia perforation.*

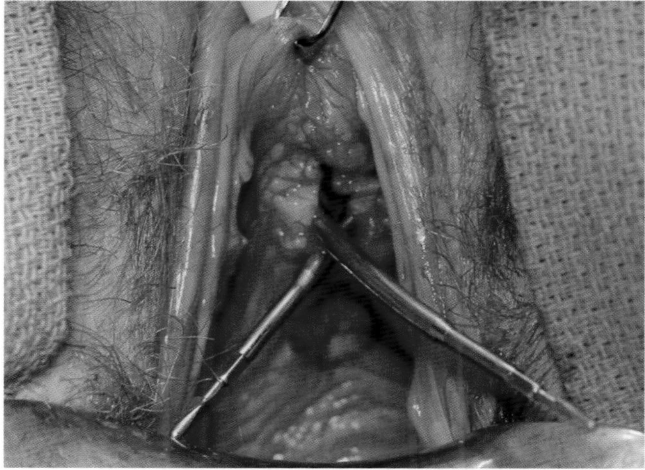

Figure 63.8. *Perforation of the endopelvic/periurethral fascia and maneuvering the needle tip through the vaginal incision.*

- To avoid perforation of the bladder during needle passage, keep the tip of the needle on the superior then posterior portion of the symphysis pubis at *all* times.

- To avoid urethral trauma, pass the needle directly against the surface of the inferior portion of the pubic ramus at the level of the midurethra onto the tip of the index finger, while deviating the urethral catheter medially with the superior surface of the finger.
- Major vessel injury and bowel injury should be avoided by adhering to the surface of the pubic bone. The inferior epigastric artery and vein and the endopelvic veins are subject to inadvertent trauma with any needle passage. The iliac and obturator veins are not in the direct surgical field and are not in the direction of needle passage or the force vector of perforation with suprapubic needle passage, as distinct from periurethral or endopelvic fascia perforation from the vaginal approach. Small and large bowel should not be adherent to the pubic bone except in the case of prior abdominal surgery that entered the retropubic space, or the presence of a lower abdominal incisional or inguinal hernia.

Cystoscopy

After passage of both needles, cystoscopy is performed with a minimum of 350 cc in the bladder to ensure that the needles are not in a bladder fold or 'mucosal pinch'. Needle perforation, if present, is often noted at 10 or 2 o'clock near the bladder neck, and additional care should be taken to view the urethra on scope insertion and/or removal. The bladder is left distended upon scope removal.

Sling attachment and transfer

1. The plastic sheath containing the sling material may be irrigated with sterile saline or water prior to attachment to aid in smooth removal of the plastic.
2. The sling is positioned for attachment to the needles by placing the markings in the center facing the surgeon.
3. The connectors are attached to the needle tips using gentle pressure until a 'snap' is felt and a 'click' is heard. The center of the sling is clearly marked with arrow radiating from the center (Fig. 63.9).
4. The surgeon confirms that the sling is correctly positioned flat and with the markings on the outside of the mesh. The connectors can be twisted on the needle tips to adjust the sling position.
5. The needles are directed to the retropubic space by placing the index finger at the tip of the connector and pushing the connector/needle back into the retropubic space. This 'pushing' maneuver minimizes disruption of the periurethral and endopelvic fasciae. The surgeon should avoid pulling the handle of the needle until the white connector has been 'pushed' back into the retropubic space through the periurethral fascia.
6. The needle and needle handle are utilized to complete retrograde removal of the suspension needle. Gentle traction on the needle at the level of the skin permits complete needle removal with minimal dilation at the skin level. The sling is pulled through the skin incision for several centimeters on each side.
7. Before adjusting sling tension, the plastic sheath should be re-examined at the vaginal incision for leakage from the bladder. If there is any suspicion of leakage, a repeat cystoscopy should be performed. If the sling is identified within the bladder, it should be cut closely below the white dilator–connector, withdrawn within the plastic sheath, and repositioned with an alternative 'free suspension needle' by suturing the plastic to the needle tip. The Foley catheter is now replaced for drainage of the bladder.

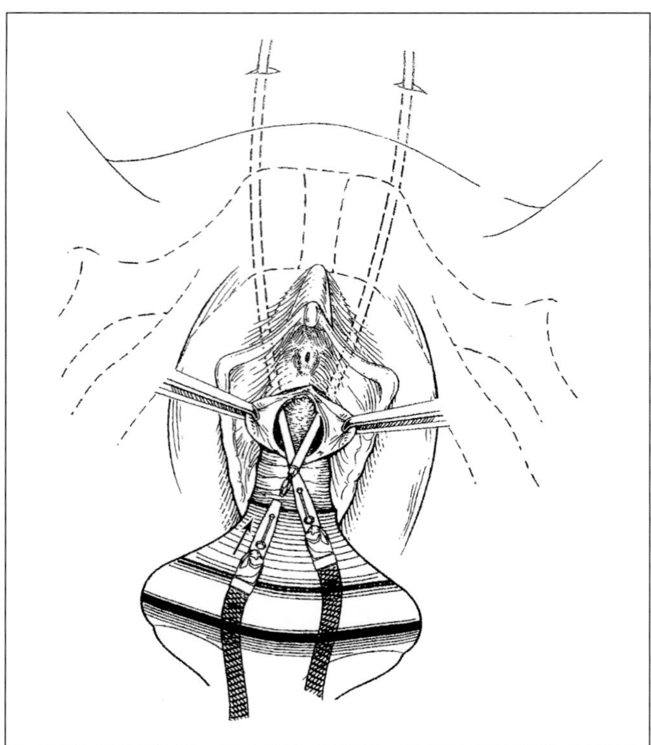

Figure 63.9. *Sling with connector positioned for attachment to the needle tip. Note the marked arrow radiating from the center of the sling.*

Sling tensioning and fixation

To adjust the sling tension, the sling is pulled up through the suprapubic incisions against a spacer placed in the vaginal loop; individual surgeon preference may be a scissor (large) or dilator (No. 8 Hagar preferred). Optimal sling tension is demonstrated when slight movement of the instrument within the mesh loop initially occurs.

The sling and plastic sheath are cut at the level of the 'blue dots' below the dilator–connectors (Fig. 63.10). Hemostats are placed on each of the cut plastic sheaths using care to avoid the mesh. The suburethral spacer is stabilized with one hand as the plastic sheath on each side is removed with the other. The mesh is then cut below the skin level, with gentle traction on the ends to allow retraction of the mesh beneath the skin level (Fig. 63.11).

Closure

Steri-strips are applied to the suprapubic incisions and the vaginal incision is closed using a running 2-0 absorbable suture.

CONCOMITANT PROCEDURES

If additional pelvic organ prolapse repair procedures are planned, apical and anterior vaginal repairs may be completed prior to placement of the SPARC sling. In particular, if a cystocele repaired is planned, the cystocele repair should be performed with repair of the bladder base but *not* the bladder neck area. A Kelly repair is not recommended as it may elevate bladder neck support, and may disrupt the pressure transmission to the midurethra by altering bladder neck motion with reference to the sling. In addition, utilizing a separate incision, if possible, for placement of the SPARC sling avoids extension of a hematoma or drainage from the cystocele repair and prevents resultant disruption of the incision over the sling.

POSTOPERATIVE CARE

The patient is sent to the recovery room with a Foley catheter in place. It is important, especially after epidural or spinal anesthesia, that the patient be fully ambulatory and free of any residual anesthetic prior to the voiding trial (Table 63.1) to avoid iatrogenic–anesthetic retention.

Managing postoperative retention

The SPARC procedure results in placement of the sling below the midurethra with no tension and minimal disruption of normal proximal urethral mobility. This change in sling placement has resulted in a substantial

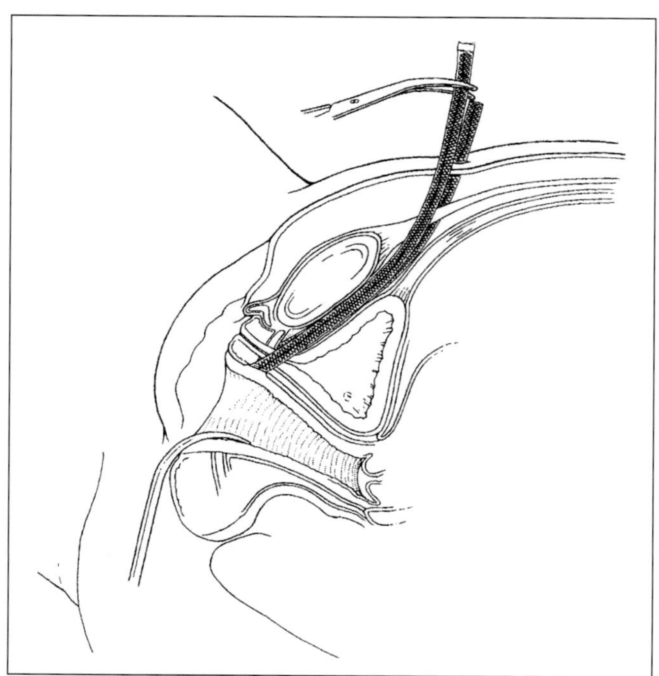

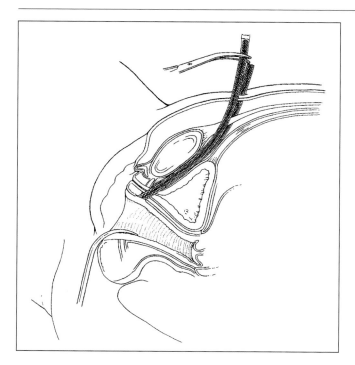

Figure 63.10. *Removal of the needles and connectors. The sling and plastic sheath are cut at the level of the 'blue dots'.*

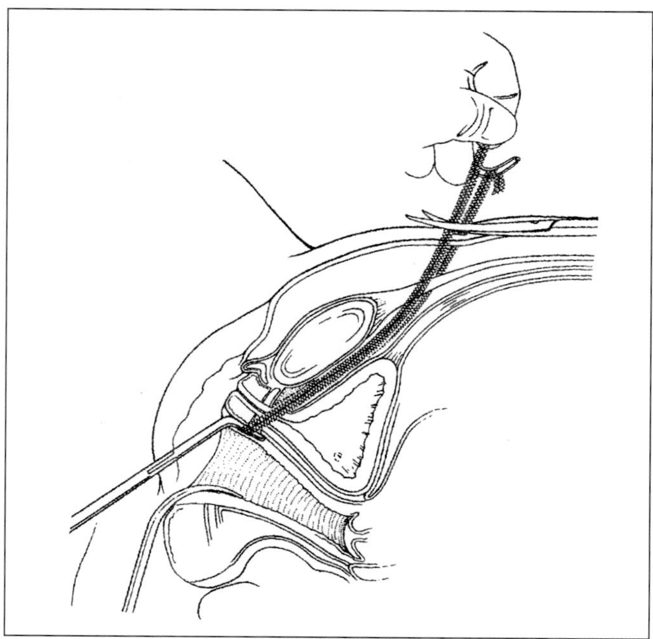

Figure 63.11. *Excess mesh is cut at the abdominal incision. Note gentle traction is placed on the mesh end to allow retraction of the mesh below the skin incision.*

Table 63.1. *Voiding trial*

1. Fill the bladder via the Foley catheter to 300 cc or until full.
2. Remove the catheter and commence the voiding trial.
3. Measure the void: a void of >200 cc (two-thirds of capacity) or a residual measured by ultrasound of <100 cc (one-third of capacity) is considered adequate for discharge.
4. If the residual is >100 cc, the patient is rechecked following an additional void. The patient may elect to be discharged with a leg bag and repeat the voiding trial in the office the following day.

decrease in urinary retention, and is similar to other minimally invasive pubovaginal slings.[18]

Loosening of the SPARC sling may be initiated intraoperatively if the sling is tensioned too tightly during removal of the plastic sheath, or postoperatively if the patient presents with urinary retention or symptomatic impaired voiding. The tensioning suture within the sling mesh provides a restraint to sling stretching during loosening of the sling tension. The sling can be loosened by placement of a right angle beneath the sling, and then pulling the sling down with a right angle clamp or with a No. 1 Prolene suture that has been placed around the sling. The timing of postoperative sling adjustment should be within 2–3 weeks following implantation, as local tissue ingrowth and biodegradation of the tensioning suture begin to affect the ability to 'move' the sling. Pulling on the sling will result in a 'pop' and slight patient discomfort at the suprapubic site, indicating that the sling has moved at the rectus fascia layer.

Late postoperative retention that does not improve with conservative management or early adjustment of sling tensioning may be addressed with urethrolysis. A midline urethrolysis may be performed if there is no significant tissue ingrowth into the sling. If significant ingrowth exists, a lateral approach is recommended to avoid urethral injury. Following identification of the sling, a nerve hook or right angle clamp may be used to mobilize the sling and hold it on tension. The sling may then be transected with scissors and sling tension adjusted.

Managing postoperative sling extrusion

The disadvantages of synthetic mesh graft include the risk of infection, rejection, extrusion, and erosion. Erosion should refer to the entrance (or placement) of the sling within the urinary tract (the bladder or urethra), whereas extrusion refers to the migration or exposure of the sling material into the vagina. Extrusion of sling mesh into the vagina can be managed immediately in the postoperative period by thorough antibiotic irrigation and wound closure. Delayed closure may involve mobilization of the vaginal edges. Observation and conservative management until the vaginal wall completely heals over the sling mesh may be elected for late extrusion. If the vaginal wall heals 'through the mesh', the exposed portion of the mesh should be excised. The vaginal wall can be closed primarily or may be left to heal secondarily.

Complication rates with artificial materials may be underreported since erosion can occur relatively late, at 1–4 years postoperatively. In fact, the American Urological Association Female Stress Urinary Incontinence Clinical Guidelines Panel recommends 5-year follow-up as a true test of time for such continence procedures. Initial success with a novel graft material must therefore be judged cautiously until long-term results are available. Given the fact that the midurethral polypropylene slings are made of loosely knitted mesh, and are placed under no tension, the incidence of significant problems appears to be lower than previously anticipated, in the region of 1–6%.[17,23,24]

REFERENCES

1. Leach GE, Dmochowski RR, Appell RA. Female stress urinary incontinence clinical guidelines (AUA). J Urol 1997;158:875–80.
2. Beck RP, McCormick S, Nordstrom L. The fascia lata sling procedure. Obstet Gynecol 1988;72:699–703.
3. Hilton P. A clinical and urodynamic study comparing the Stamey bladder neck suspension and suburethral sling procedures in the treatment of genuine stress incontinence. Br J Obstet Gynecol 1989;96:213–20.
4. Niknejad K, Plzak LS 3rd, Staskin DR, Loughlin KR. Autologous and synthetic urethral slings for female incontinence. Urol Clin North Am 2002;29(3):597–611.
5. Staskin DR, Plzak L. Synthetic slings: pros and cons. Curr Urol Rep 2002;3(5):414–7.
6. Ghoniem GM, Shaaban A. Sub-urethral slings for treatment of stress urinary incontinence. Int Urogynecol J 1994;5:228–39.
7. Morgan JE, Heritz DM, Stewart FE, Connolly JC, Farrow GA: The polypropylene pubovaginal sling. J Urol 1995;154:1013–5.
8. Jarvis GJ. Surgery for genuine stress incontinence. Br J Obstet Gynaecol 1994;101:371–4.
9. Kersey J. The gauze hammock sling operation in the treatment of stress incontinence. Br J Obstet Gynaecol 1983;90:945–9.
10. Bergman A, Elia G. Three surgical procedures for

genuine stress incontinence: five-year follow-up of a prospective randomized study. Am J Obstet Gynecol 1995;173(1):66–71.

11. El-Toukhy T, Mahadevan S, Angharad E et al. Burch colposuspension: a 10 to 12 years follow up. J Obstet Gynaecol 2000;20(2):178–9.
12. Maher CF, Dwyer PL, Carey MP, Moran PA. Colposuspension or sling for low urethral pressure stress incontinence? Int Urogynecol J Pelvic Floor Dysfunct 1999;10(6):384–9.
13. Bidmead J, Cardozo L, McLellan A, Khullar V, Kelleher C. A comparison of the objective and subjective outcomes of colposuspension for stress incontinence in women. BJOG 2001;108(4):408–13.
14. Ward KL, Hilton P. UK and Ireland TVT Trial Group. A prospective multicenter randomized trial of tension-free vaginal tape and colposuspension for primary urodynamic stress incontinence: two-year follow-up. Am J Obstet Gynecol 2004;190(2):324–31.
15. Ward K, Hilton P. Prospective multicentre randomized trial of tension-free vaginal tape and colposuspension as primary treatment for stress incontinence. BMJ 2002;325:67–70.
16. SPARC Sling System. Patent 6,612,977, Appl. No. 917443. Minnetonka (MN): American Medical Systems Inc, September 2, 2003.
17. Deval B, Levardon M, Samain E et al. A French multicenter clinical trial of SPARC for stress urinary incontinence. Eur Urol 2003;44:254–9.
18. Staskin DR, Tyagi R. The SPARC sling system. Atlas Urol Clin 2004;12:185–95.
19. Papa Petros PE, Ulmsten U. An anatomical classification – a new paradigm for management of urinary dysfunction in the female. Int Urogynecol J Pelvic Floor Dysfunct 1999;10(1):29–35.
20. Petros P, Ulmsten U. An integral theory on female urinary incontinence. Acta Obstet Gynecol Scand 1990;153(Suppl):7–31.
21. DeLancey JOL. Structural support of the urethra as it relates to stress incontinence: the hammock hypothesis. Am J Obstet Gynecol 1994;170:1713–20.
22. Plzak L, Staskin D. Genuine stress incontinence: theories of etiology and surgical correction. Urol Clin North Am 2002,29:527–35.
23. Tseng LH, Wang AC, Lin YH, Li SJ, Ko YJ. Randomized comparison of the suprapubic arc sling procedure vs tension-free vaginal taping for stress incontinent women. Int Urogynecol J Pelvic Floor Dysfunct 2005;16(3):230–5.
24. Kobashi KC, Govier FE. Perioperative complications: the first 140 polypropylene pubovaginal slings. J Urol 2003;170(5):1918–21.

64

Other sling variants

Kristie A Blanchard, J Christian Winters

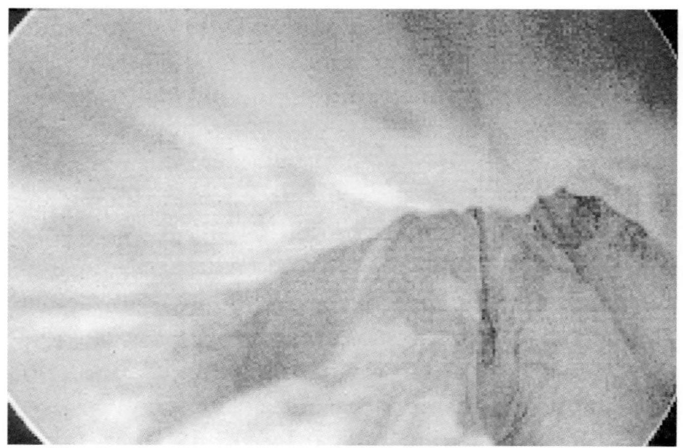

INTRODUCTION

As the evidence becomes clearer that pubovaginal sling procedures are most efficacious in the surgical management of stress urinary incontinence, innovation and technology have merged to create pubovaginal sling procedures that strive to obtain the clinical efficacy of autologous fascia slings while minimizing morbidity. Many novel concepts were designed to eliminate the need for an abdominal incision, improve sling fixation, and promote the preservation of normal postoperative voiding. Transvaginal placement of bone anchors eliminated the need for an abdominal incision, and provided stabilization of the suburethral sling. The use of the vaginal wall in a variety of sling techniques eliminated the need for an additional fascial harvest. New generation self-fixating slings provide the advantages of minimally invasive tension-free midurethral sling placement combined with biologic materials which decrease the potential for erosion. These procedures can be utilized in place of the conventional autologous fascia sling in special circumstances, and have been documented to achieve acceptable levels of efficacy while decreasing morbidity. In this chapter we will profile these procedures, and how they may be utilized by pelvic surgeons.

BONE-ANCHOR SLINGS

Bone anchors in incontinence surgery: historical perspective

Benderev[1] introduced a novel procedure with the use of a bone anchor and a variation of suture placement that essentially facilitated transvaginal bladder neck stabilization.[2] The Vesica™ procedure introduced many urologists to the principles of bone anchor insertion. Although initial results with this procedure were encouraging,[3] subsequent data revealed a lack of long-term efficacy.[4]

Bone anchor technology was also utilized in pubovaginal sling surgery. Appell introduced the in-situ vaginal wall sling performed with suprapubic bone anchor implantation and preservation of the endopelvic fascia.[5] Favorable results were achieved with minimal complications in patients without significant intrinsic sphincteric deficiency. Hom et al. used a synthetic graft and suprapubic bone anchors to perform a pubovaginal sling,[6] and Nativ et al.[7] utilized an entirely transvaginal approach to perform cystourethropexy. Bone anchors were inserted by a transvaginal route, and the sutures from the bone anchor were utilized to complete fixation of the sling to the undersurface of the pubic bone. The operative time was only 28 minutes, and at 1 year follow-up 82% of the patients were dry. Important findings in these patients were the minimal need for narcotics and early ambulation. Subsequently, many surgeons have utilized transvaginal bone anchor placement with biologic allografts to perform a pubovaginal sling.[8,9] These procedures are presently the most widely utilized operations for stress incontinence employing bone anchor technology.

The transvaginal anchor sling procedures were coupled with repair of anterior compartment defects to provide a stable point of fixation, augmenting the prolapse repair. Leach and colleagues reported on a cadaveric prolapse repair and sling (CaPS) procedure utilizing a large patch of cadaveric fascia.[10] Distally the patch was fashioned as a sling anchored to the pubic bone, and the proximal extension of the patch extended to the vaginal apex to reinforce the anterior repair. Shah et al. described a repair of complete vaginal prolapse utilizing transvaginally placed bone anchors combined with mesh fixation to the sacrospinous ligament.[11] Both series have reported excellent reduction of prolapse and correction of stress urinary incontinence.

Transvaginal bone anchor slings

Technique

After positioning in the dorsal lithotomy position, the operation commences with an anterior vaginal wall incision. An inverted 'U' incision is created unless an anterior repair is performed. In this instance, a midline incision is chosen. The dissection proceeds laterally to the level of the endopelvic fascia, which is perforated. The retropubic space is entered, and the tissue is swept off the pubic bone to facilitate placement of the transvaginal bone anchor insertion tool. However, it is not necessary to perforate the endopelvic fascia, but to develop just enough space behind the pubic bone to insert the anchor insertion tool.

The anchor insertion tool is introduced through the vaginal incision and positioned behind the pubic bone. The device should be placed perpendicular to the bone, and the tool should be felt firmly against the bone. This is done by gently 'scraping' the tool behind the bone to test for position. (Fig. 64.1) The anchor is placed into the bone positioned on the undersurface of the pubic bone approximately 2–3 cm from the urethra on each side. The suspension sutures are removed through the insertion tool, and the strength of fixation to the undersurface of the pubic bone can be verified by pulling on these sutures (Fig. 64.2). The wound is liberally irrigated with antibiotic solution.

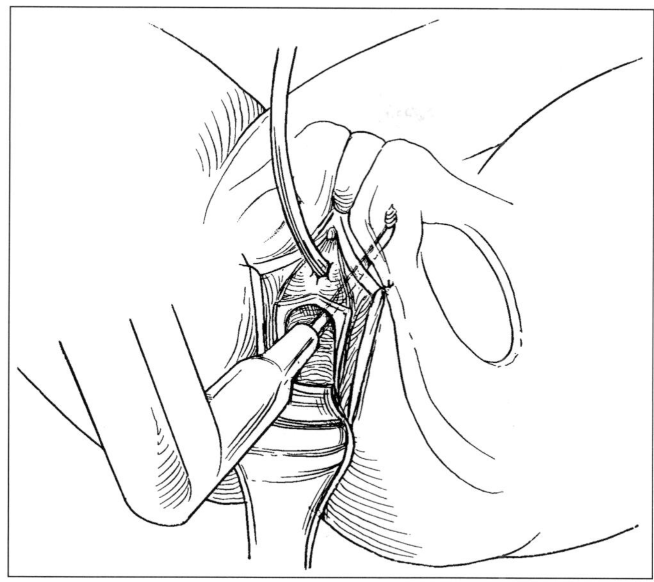

Figure 64.1. *Placement of anchors into pubic bone via transvaginal approach.*

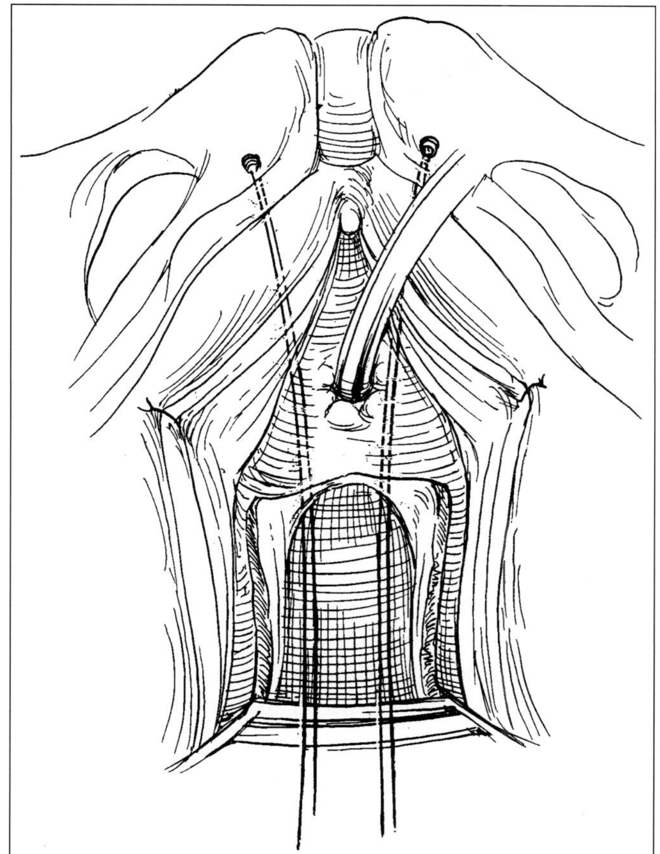

Figure 64.2. *Anchors utilized to secure permanent sutures to pubic bone. These two sutures will be used to secure the sling.*

Biologic graft material is most commonly utilized as sling material, but autologous or synthetic material may be used. A 2 × 5–7 cm segment is chosen. A tacking suture is then placed to position the sling in its proximal location, which is determined by palpation of the Foley balloon. The proximal suture is placed just beyond the bladder neck in the midline to ensure that the sling supports the bladder neck and proximal urethra. The suspension sutures from the anchors are then threaded through the edges of the sling by placing the sutures though a hollow core needle passed through the sling. Tension is adjusted by placing a large right-angle clamp between the urethra and the sling. One side of the sling is secured to its attachment. The second side of the sling is then tied loosely with the clamp still in place between the sling and the urethra, thus preventing the sling from being tied too tightly. Using the previously placed proximal suture, the sling is then fastened at the level of the bladder neck with 3-0 absorbable suture. An additional suture is then placed distally in the midline to extend the sling across the proximal urethra. Additional sutures are placed as needed to spread out the sling and prevent it from rolling over (Fig. 64.3). Liberal antibiotic irrigation of the wound follows. Cystoscopy is performed to verify lower urinary tract integrity. Vaginal closure is then completed with 2-0 absorbable suture.

Results

When interpreting the results of the transvaginal anchor-based slings, it should be noted that the follow-up is limited by a small number of studies and short follow-up duration. Elias and associates reported a 92.5% rate of

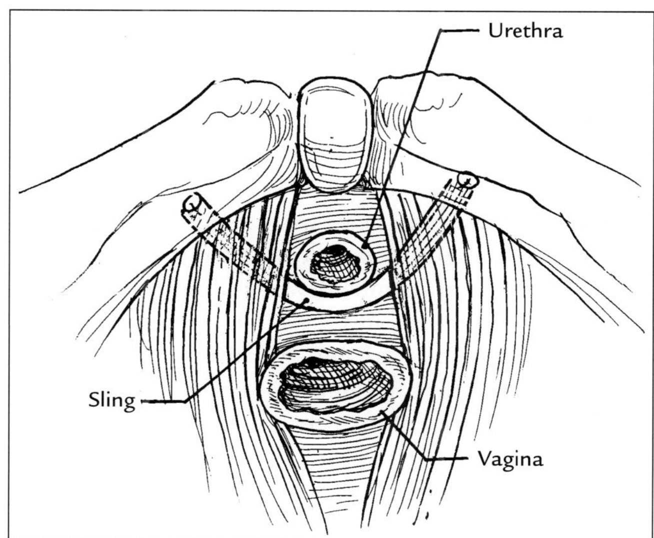

Figure 64.3. *Final suburethral sling position utilizing transvaginal bone anchors.*

'complete cure' in 40 patients followed for an average of 6.5 months.[12] In 15 patients undergoing an isolated transvaginally anchor-based sling, Payne noted that 14 were discharged on the same day.[13] Overall, he utilized this procedure in 54 patients with minor complications; two early sling failures were encountered in patients with low leak point pressures (<50 cmH_2O). More recently, however, success rates have been reported to be less than 80%, with Franco et al. reporting a success rate of 71% in 65 patients after 30 months.[14] After 18 months, 78% of 234 patients experienced success with 53% totally dry.[15] Carbone et al. reported a disappointing success rate of only 62% in 154 patients observed for an average of 10.9 months.[16] When the patients underwent repeat surgery following failed transvaginal anchor sling, all anchors were properly positioned. The cadaveric grafts appeared to be fragmented, attenuated or absent in all cases. Utilizing the CaPS procedure[10] in the correction of urinary stress incontinence and cystocele, 82% of the patients had no stress incontinence and only 12.9% had recurrence of cystocele at a mean follow-up of 12.4 months.[17]

Complications

Most authors report low complication rates from transvaginal bone anchor sling procedures. Bladder perforation was the most common intraoperative complication, ranging from 2.1 to 4.5%.[15,16] Almost all series report a low incidence of prolonged urinary retention. Dyspareunia is seen in 8.5–13% of patients following transvaginal sling, with 4–6% complaining of significant pelvic or suprapubic pain. Although most report the incidence of de novo bladder instability to be less than 10%, Franco et al. reported that 16 out of 30 patients (53%) developed de novo postoperative urge incontinence.[14]

Infection is perhaps the most feared complication involving bone anchor procedures. Osteomyelitis is an infectious condition which is progressive until adequate treatment is rendered. Pain and wound drainage are common complaints.[18] In its early stages, it is often very difficult to distinguish osteomyelitis from osteitis pubis, a non-infectious inflammatory condition involving the pubic bone. Osteomyelitis results in progressive bone loss until adequately treated, usually requiring surgical debridement with removal of the bone anchors and 4–6 weeks of culture-specific antibiotics. Graham and Dmochowski published nine cases of osteomyelitis; only three patients were continent and pain-free following treatment.[18] Although severe, osteomyelitis after transvaginal bone anchor placement is rare, with a reported incidence of less than 1% in bone anchor procedures.[19,20] Appell reported osteomyelitis in two women after suprapubic placement of bone anchors, both of whom were taking steroids.[21] Leach reported only five cases of osteomyelitis in 7000 bone anchor procedures.[22]

Surgical removal of bone anchors has also been necessary in patients who developed severe pain and vaginal granulomas.[23,24] Additionally, there are reports of anchors becoming dislodged from the pubic bone. Tsivian et al. identified 12 anchors becoming detached in eight patients:[25] two required cystoscopic removal from the bladder, and three were spontaneously expelled through the vagina; the other seven anchors were detected in the retropubic space on x-ray.

VAGINAL WALL SLINGS

The vaginal wall sling was originally described by Raz et al.[26] to provide compression and coaptation to the urethra, utilizing midline vaginal mucosa and underlying periurethral support structures to form the sling. The anterior vaginal wall is ideally located and allows the sling to be easily tailored to the length and width necessary to provide an even distribution of pressure over a long urethral segment. It also requires no extravaginal harvesting incision which minimizes morbidity and postoperative pain. The major limiting factor of this procedure is the fact that long-term durability relies on the integrity of the periurethral tissue which may be weak or attenuated and potentially stretch over time. Additionally, sutures may become dislodged or pull through points of fixation. Relative contraindications to this procedure include sexually active women with short vaginal lengths and women with atrophic vaginitis who have thin attenuated vaginal walls.

Technique

An inverted 'U' incision is made with the apex about 1 cm proximal to the urethral meatus and the base several centimeters proximal to the bladder neck. Lateral dissection and perforation of the endopelvic fascia is performed bilaterally. A transverse incision is then made at the level of the bladder neck to create a rectangular island of vaginal wall that will function as the sling. The vaginal wall proximal to the sling is undermined to form a flap, which will be advanced to cover the sling (Fig. 64.4). Non-absorbable sutures are placed at the four corners of the rectangle, including all layers of the underlying fascial supportive tissues (Fig. 64.5) The sutures are transferred through a small suprapubic incision using a double-pronged ligature carrier and then tied to the rectus fascia. Cystoscopy is performed to confirm bladder integrity and ureteral patency. The proximal vagi-

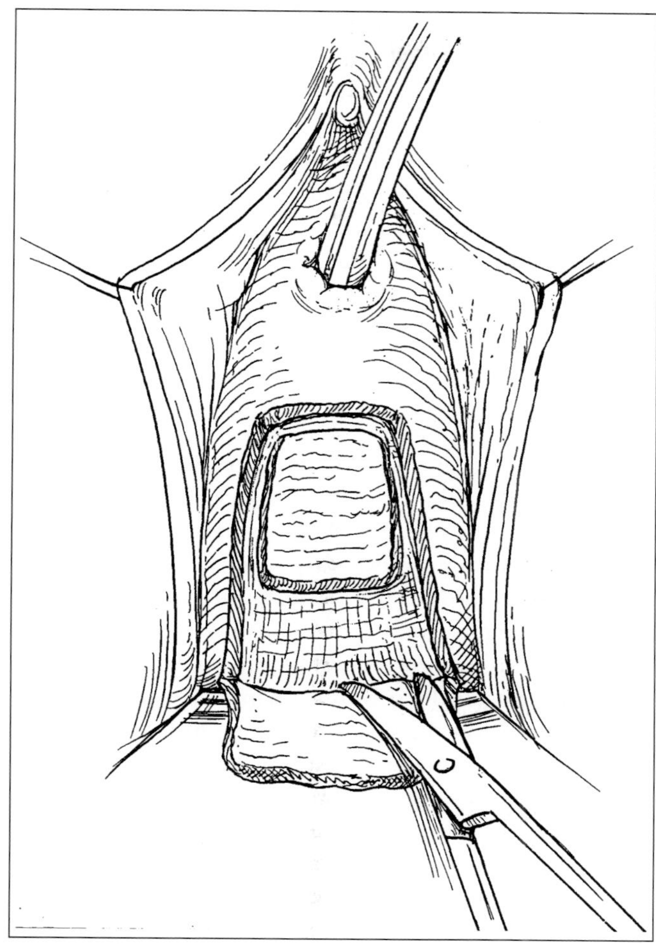

Figure 64.4. *Isolation of anterior vaginal wall segment to be used for sling.*

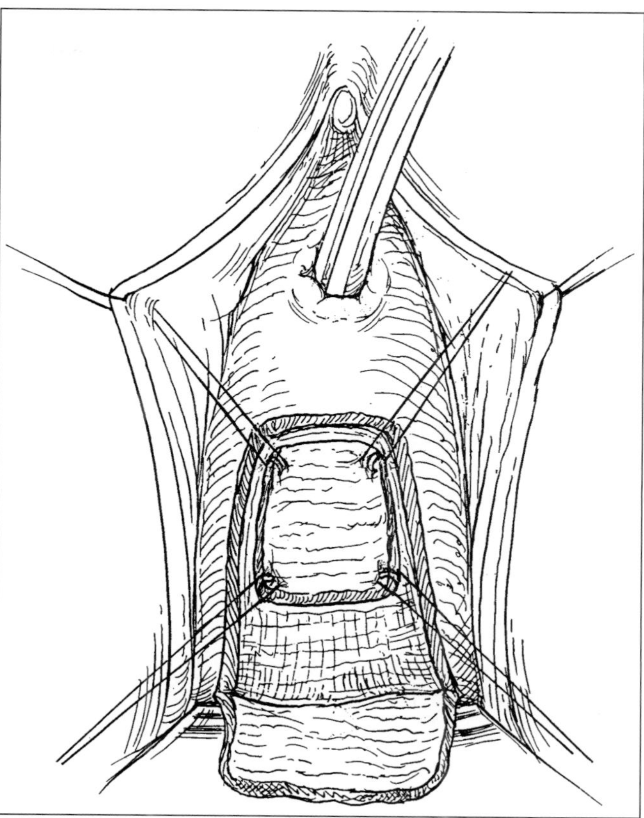

Figure 64.5. *Placement of helical permanent sutures into four corners of isolated vaginal segment.*

nal wall flap is then advanced over the sling to provide an epithelial covering and restore the integrity of the vagina (Fig. 64.6).

Appell[27] modified this technique using bone anchors placed in each pubic tubercle to secure the sling and leaving the endopelvic fascia intact. The sutures from the bone anchor are then transferred via needle under finger guidance into the vaginal lumen. A horizontal mattress suture is performed by placement of the suture onto a free Mayo-type needle and beginning the pass of the suture from behind the sling to incorporate the pubocervical fascia, after which the suture is passed back out of the sling proximally. The suture is then transferred to the abdominal wound and the procedure repeated on the opposite side. After cystoscopy confirms urinary tract integrity, the sling sutures are tied without excessive tension using a suture spacer over the pubic tubercle. This procedure was devised to utilize the advantages of the vaginal wall as a sling, and a minimally invasive route of fixation.

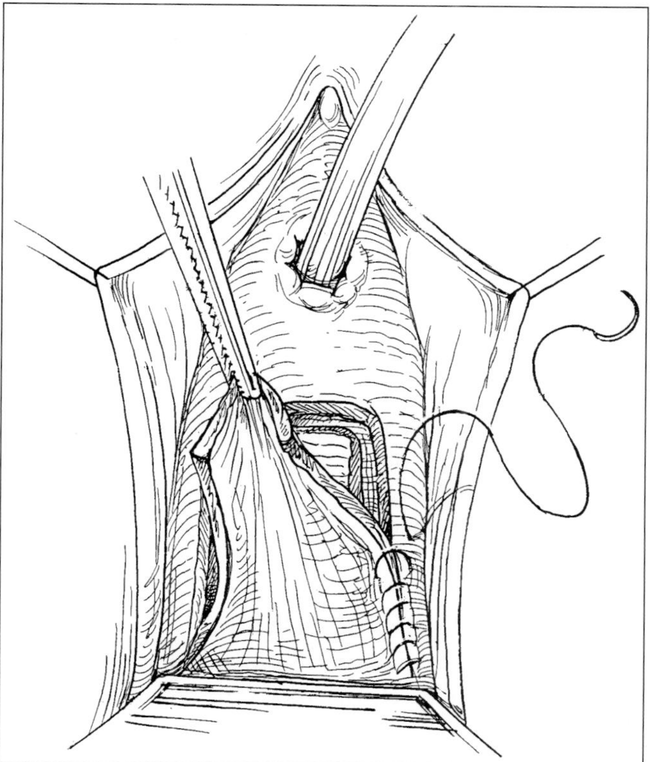

Figure 64.6. *Advancement of vaginal wall flap to cover vaginal wall sling.*

Results

Raz et al. noted that urinary continence was achieved in 29 of 32 patients undergoing the vaginal wall sling procedure.[26] Juma et al. published the results of this procedure in 54 patients with an average follow-up of 24 months.[28] Results were excellent in 90.7% and good in 3.7% for an overall success rate of 94.4%. Kaplan et al.[29] retrospectively compared outcomes in patients undergoing autologous rectus fascia pubovaginal slings and those undergoing vaginal wall slings: 89% of patients following fascial slings and 94% of patients following vaginal wall slings were satisfied with the surgical outcome. In addition, the vaginal wall sling patients had significantly less morbidity. These findings led the authors to conclude that vaginal wall slings should be the preferred method of surgical treatment of intrinsic sphincter deficiency (ISD), although the follow-up in the patients undergoing fascial slings was longer.

The efficacy of the vaginal wall sling in the treatment of stress urinary incontinence was documented at 18 months in 18 elderly patients. All patients were completely dry and 17/18 were voiding freely.[30] In another study, using the in-situ sling technique, 20 patients were followed for at least 24 months, and a success rate of 95% was reported. Two patients developed de novo detrusor instability, which resolved after 2 months.[31] Several authors have noted that the anterior vaginal wall procedures are more successful in cases of genuine stress urinary incontinence than for those patients with ISD;[32] in fact, in one of these reports the success rate of vaginal wall sling was only 42% when the leak point pressure was less than 50 cmH_2O.[33]

Complications

A major advantage of this procedure is that there appear to be few associated complications. Complications reported include suture abscesses, dyspareunia, persistent suprapubic pain, and de novo instability in 9–15% of patients.[28,32,34] The most bothersome and persistent complication has been detrusor instability. There has also been a report of an epithelial inclusion cyst formation requiring surgical incision;[35] this occurrence is probably underreported.

'HYBRID' MIDURETHRAL SLINGS

There has been an explosion in the number of midurethral tension-free tape procedures for the surgical management of stress urinary incontinence. The hallmark of these procedures is the minimal morbidity and excellent results obtained via these methods. These procedures utilize a polypropylene mesh material to restore the ability to maintain continence at the level of the midurethra. Despite encouraging results, there are several situations in which placing mesh below the urethra may be problematic. Thus, in these patients, alternate choices of sling placement should be considered. In this population, a 'hybrid' biologic or biodegradable midurethral sling may be advantageous. These sling procedures combine the minimally invasive nature of the tension-free midurethral synthetic slings with the lower risk of erosion from biologic tissue.

BioArc™

The BioArc™ (Fig. 64.7) is a version of the SPARC™ procedure that allows the surgeon to interpose any type of sling graft into a SPARC™ delivery system. Essentially, the long continuous mesh strips are equipped with two clamps that allow the surgeon to suture the biologic tissue of choice into the system. This leaves two self-fixating mesh arms to secure the sling, with a central biologic material acting as the suburethral graft. Positioned without tension below the urethra, there is little worry about retention. Additionally, the suburethral portion of the sling is not a mesh, but a biologic or autologous graft which may be less likely to erode. Future applications of this sling may be placement by a transobturator tape (TOT) approach, and to facilitate prolapse reconstruction by incorporating a larger graft in the sling, augmenting anterior compartment repairs.

Technique

This is essentially the same as described for the SPARC™ procedure. Prior to placement, the material chosen to comprise the suburethral component of the sling must

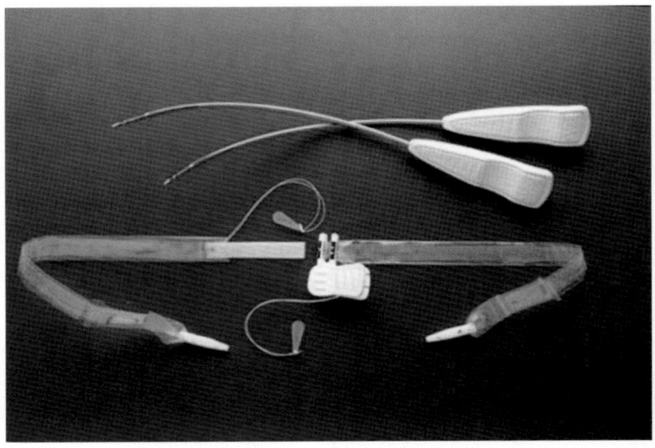

Figure 64.7. *BioArc™ sling system. (Courtesy of American Medical Systems, Minneapolis, MN.)*

be incorporated. A length of approximately 7–8 cm is preferable, and the edges of this material should be trimmed to the same width as the mesh in order to facilitate the tunneling process. The surgeon may choose to have the central portion of the sling material slightly wider (approximately 2 cm) by tapering the edges or have a 1 cm graft throughout. The material is incorporated into the mesh by placing it into the clamps that are pre-attached to the mesh. A permanent suture is utilized to attach the graft to the mesh. Following this, the clamps are removed, and the tape sleeves are advanced over the suture. The sling is inserted and tensioned in a manner similar to the SPARC™ procedure (Fig. 64.8).

Other hybrid midurethral slings

The basic premise of these sling variants is to place a non-synthetic material below the urethra via a minimally invasive approach. This can be accomplished by using a degradable material that will dissolve over time, or by fashioning a biologic sling material in such a way as to facilitate self-fixation. Examples of these sling variants are the T-Sling with Centrasorb™ which contains a central portion of absorbable suture and the Sabre™ which is a completely biodegradable sling system. The Stratasis TF™ (Fig. 64.9) sling can be applied by an antegrade or retrograde retropubic approach. This sling is a completely biologic natural biomaterial (small intestinal submucosa) that reportedly remodels with host tissue. Fashioned in a manner to promote self-fixation, this sling is placed in a fashion similar to SPARC™ or TVT™ techniques.

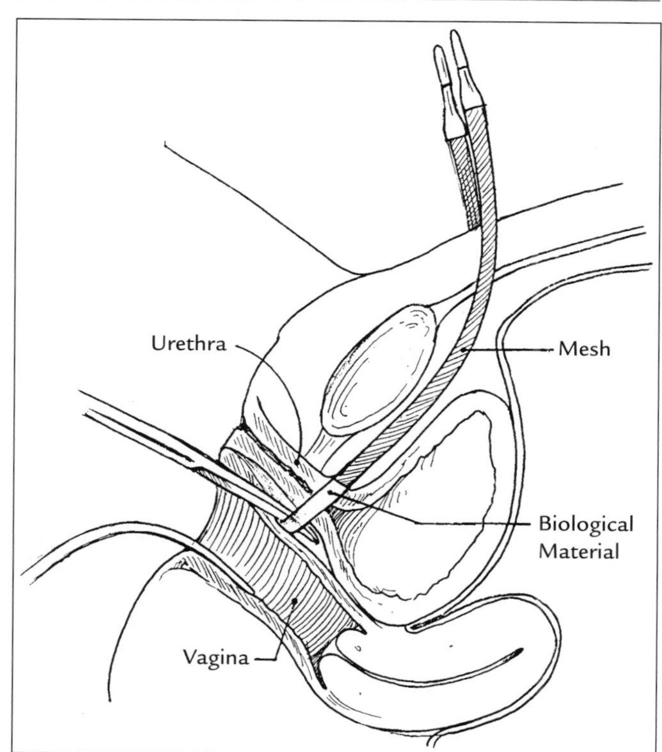

Figure 64.8. *Final placement of BioArc™ sling system. Note: Biologic material in suburethral position.*

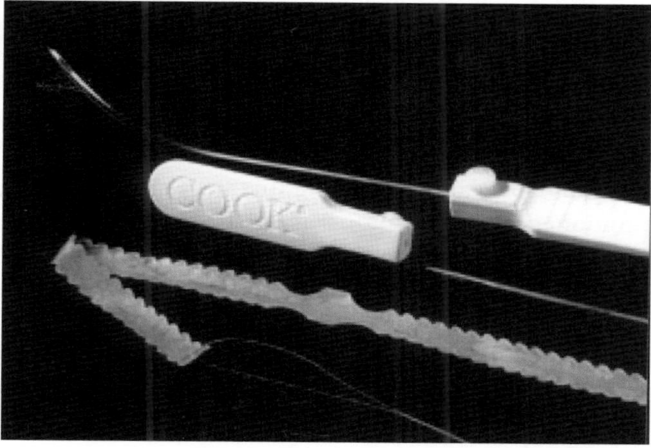

Figure 64.9. *Stratasis TF™ sling system. (Courtesy of Cook Urological, Spencer, IN.)*

Results

Clinical data with these sling variants are scarce. Much of the data are on feasibility and ease of use. Anger et al.[36] noted that BioArc™ was an effective alternative in the surgical correction of stress urinary incontinence in women with more severe SUI requiring a more coaptive sling to provide continence. Eisenberg and Badlani[37] demonstrated the versatility of the BioArc™ system in women with SUI and pelvic organ prolapse.

Although the clinical follow-up is too short to offer meaningful conclusions regarding efficacy, the use of these sling systems appears safe and offers the surgeon more flexibility to tailor the procedure to meet the needs of the patient. Ho et al.[38] reported a series of inflammatory reactions utilizing small intestinal submucosa.

POLYPROPYLENE SLING/'PVT'

The most widely used tension-free midurethral slings utilize insertion kits that 'tunnel' the sling into the retropubic or transobturator position. These procedures have made many surgeons more at ease with the use of synthetic material as a sling graft. Based on this, Rodriguez et al.[39] reported on their experience using a modified polypropylene sling for the treatment of stress urinary incontinence. Based on the principles of traditional pubovaginal sling placement, the authors described a procedure that achieves placement of a thinly woven polypropylene mesh under the distal urethra without tension. This is accomplished via two small lateral incisions in the anterior vagina, perforation of the endopelvic fascia, and tunneling under the anterior vagina. The mesh is positioned without tension utilizing two Allis-type clamps to ensure that the graft is properly positioned when the sutures are tied.

This procedure has also been described by Rackley and colleagues[40] who coined the term 'PVT', or percutaneous vaginal tape. They concluded that the PVT procedure is reproducible, and achieves excellent results.

Both groups note the significant cost advantage when this approach to midurethral polypropylene sling is performed.

Results

Rodriguez and Raz[41] reported that following polypropylene sling only 2.3% of 301 patients required treatment for persistent stress urinary incontinence. In 92 patients with at least 12 months follow-up, the objective cure rate was 92% and the subjective cure rate was 89%. These authors also concluded that Valsalva leak point pressure (LPP) was of minimal benefit in predicting outcome after polypropylene sling, as patients did well following this procedure regardless of LPP.[42] Complication rates following these procedures appear minimal.

CONCLUSIONS

The success and exponential rise in the use of the tension-free midurethral sling procedures (TVT™, SPARC™, TOT) have dramatically altered the approach to the surgical management of stress urinary incontinence in women. Bone anchor slings, vaginal wall slings, and bladder neck slings incorporating biologic graft materials are being utilized much less frequently, and these procedures have almost assumed a role of historical interest. However, there are occasions when the use of mesh may be precarious, or the type of stress urinary incontinence requires tighter compression of the bladder neck. It is in these situations, coupled with other factors (age, prolapse, vaginal wall integrity, and detrusor overactivity), that the pelvic surgeon may consider any of the procedures described in this chapter.

Utilizing the techniques described above, excellent early and intermediate results are reported with few complications. This leads one to question whether the less frequent utilization of these sling variants has occurred because they are not as efficacious, or because the newer generation of slings achieves similar results more quickly and with less morbidity.

REFERENCES

1. Benderev T. Anchor fixation and other modifications of endoscopic bladder neck suspension. Urology 1992;40:409–18.
2. Marshall V, Marchetti A, Krantz K. The correction of stress urinary incontinence by simple vesicourethral suspension. Surg Gynecol Obstet 1949;88:509–18.
3. Appell R, Rackley R, Dmochowski R. Vesica percutaneous bladder neck stabilization. J Endourol 1996;10:221–5.
4. Schultheiss D, Hofner K, Oelke M, Grunewald V, Jonas U. Does bone anchor fixation improve the outcome of percutaneous bladder neck suspension in female stress urinary incontinence? Br J Urol 1998;82:192–5.
5. Appell R. The use of bone anchoring in the surgical management of female stress urinary incontinence. World J Urol 1997;15:300–5.
6. Hom D, Desautel M, Lumerman J, Feraren R, Badlani G. Pubovaginal sling using polypropylene mesh and Vesica bone anchors. Urology 1988;51:708–13.
7. Nativ O, Levine S, Madjar S, Issaq E, Moskovitz B, Beyar M. Incisionless per vaginal bone anchor cystourethropexy for the treatment of female stress incontinence: experience with the first 50 patients. J Urol 1997;158:1742–4.
8. Payne C. A transvaginal sling procedure with bone anchor fixation. Urol Clin North Am 1999;26:423–30.
9. Kovac S, Cruikshank S. Pubic bone suburethral stabilization sling for recurrent urinary incontinence. Obstet Gynecol 1997;89:624–7.
10. Kobashi KC, Mee SL, Leach GE. A new technique for cystocele repair and transvaginal sling: the cadaveric prolapse repair and sling (CAPS). Urology 2000;56(6 Suppl 1):9–14.
11. Shah DK, Paul EM, Rastinehad AR, Eisenberg ER, Badlani GH. Short-term outcome analysis of total pelvic reconstruction with mesh: the vaginal approach. J Urol 2004;171:261–3.
12. Elias I, Schahar M, Alex C et al. Per vaginal pubovaginal sling procedure using a bone anchor device and synthetic sling for the treatment of stress urinary incontinence. J Urol 1999;161:912A.
13. Payne C. A transvaginal sling procedure with bone anchor fixation. Urol Clin North Am 1999;26:423–30.
14. Franco N, Shobeiri S, Echols K. Medium-term follow-up of transvaginal suburethral slings: variance in outcome success using two different evaluation methods. Urology 2002;60:607–11.
15. Crivellaro S, Smith J, Kocjancic E, Bresette J. Transvaginal sling using acellular human dermal allograft: safety and efficacy in 253 patients. J Urol 2004;172:1374–8.
16. Carbone J, Kavaler E, Hu J, Raz S. Pubovaginal sling using cadaveric fascia and bone anchors: disappointing early results. J Urol 2001;165:1605–11.

17. Kobashi K, Leach G, Chon J, Govier G. Continued multicenter followup of the cadaveric prolapse repair with sling. J Urol 2002;168:2063–8.

18. Graham C, Dmochowski R. Pubic osteomyelitis following bladder neck surgery using bone anchors: a report of 9 cases. J Urol 2002;168:2055–8.

19. Fredrick R, Carey J, Leach G. Osseous complications after transvaginal bone anchor fixation in female pelvic reconstructive surgery: report from single largest prospective series and literature review. Urology 2004;64:669–74.

20. Rackley R, Abdelmalak J, Madjar S et al. Bone anchor infections in female pelvic reconstructive procedures: a literature review of series and case reports. J Urol 2001;165:1975–8.

21. Appell R. The use of bone anchoring in the surgical management of female stress urinary incontinence. World J Urol 1997;15:300–5.

22. Leach G. Local anesthesia for urologic procedures. Urology 1996;48:284–8.

23. Fialkow M, Lentz G, Miller E et al. Complications from transvaginal pubovaginal slings using bone anchor fixation. Urology 2004;64:1127–32.

24. Schultheiss D, Hofner K, Oelke M et al. Does bone anchor fixation improve the outcome of percutaneous bladder neck suspension in female stress urinary incontinence? Br J Urol 1998;82:192–5.

25. Tsivian A, Shtricker A, Levin S et al. Bone anchor 4-corner cystourethropexy: long-term results. J Urol 2003;169:2244–5.

26. Raz S, Siegel A, Short J et al. Vaginal wall sling. J Urol 1989;141:43–6.

27. Appell R. In situ vaginal wall sling. Urology 2000;56:499–503.

28. Juma S, Little N, Raz S. Vaginal wall sling: four years later. Urology 1992;39:424–8.

29. Kaplan S, Santarosa P, Te A. Comparison of fascial and vaginal wall slings in the management of intrinsic sphincteric deficiency. Urology 1996;47:885–9.

30. Couillard D, Deckard-Janatpour K, Stone A. The vaginal wall sling: a compressive suspension procedure for recurrent incontinence in elderly patients. Urology 1989;43:203–8.

31. Vasavada S, Rackley R, Appell R. In situ vaginal wall sling formation with preservation of the endopelvic fascia for the treatment of stress urinary incontinence. Int Urogynecol J 1988;9:379–84.

32. Litwiller S, Nelson R, Fone P et al. Vaginal wall sling: long-term outcome analysis of factors contributing to patient satisfaction and surgical success. J Urol 1997;157:1279–82.

33. Goldman HB, Rackley RR, Appell RA. The in situ anterior vaginal wall sling: predictors of success. J Urol 2001;166:2259–62.

34. Raz S, Stothers L, Young G et al. Vaginal wall sling for anatomic incontinence and intrinsic sphincter dysfunction: efficacy and outcome analysis. J Urol 1996;156:166–70.

35. Baldwin DD, Hadley HR. Epithelial inclusion cyst formation after free vaginal wall sling procedure for stress urinary incontinence. J Urol 1997;157:952.

36. Anger J, Amundsen C, Webster G. The use of a polypropylene mesh sling with suburethral insert of biologic material: a minimally invasive approach to treating intrinsic sphincteric deficiency with minimal urethral mobility. J Urol 2004;171(Suppl 4):1240A.

37. Eisenberg E, Badlani G. BioArc™: a versatile and minimally invasive sling system for stress urinary incontinence and pelvic prolapse. J Urol 2004;171(Suppl 4):V936.

38. Ho K, Witte M, Bird E. 8-ply small intestinal submucosa tension-free sling: spectrum of postoperative inflammation. J Urol 2004;171:268–71.

39. Rodriguez L, Berman J, Raz S. Polypropylene sling for treatment of stress urinary incontinence as an alternative to tension-free vaginal tape. Tech Urol 2001;7:87–9.

40. Rackley R, Abdelmalak J, Tchetgen M, Madjar S, Jones S, Noble M. Tension-free vaginal tape and percutaneous vaginal tape sling procedures. Tech Urol 2001;7:90–100.

41. Rodriguez L, Raz S. Prospective analysis of patients treated with a distal urethral polypropylene sling for symptoms of stress urinary incontinence: surgical outcome and satisfaction determined by patient driven questionnaires. J Urol 2003;170:857–63.

42. Rodriguez L, de Almeida F, Dorey F, Raz S. Does Valsalva leak point pressure predict outcome after the distal polypropylene sling? Role of urodynamics in the sling era. J Urol 2004;172:210–4.

65a

Transobturator midurethral sling technique for stress urinary incontinence

Jonathan S Starkman, Harriette M Scarpero, Roger R Dmochowski

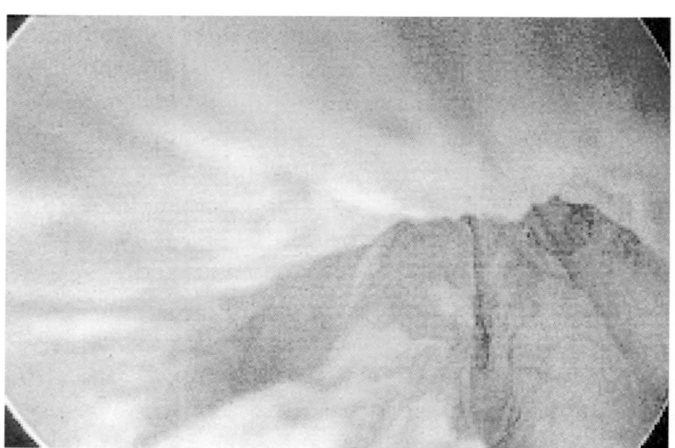

INTRODUCTION

Over the past decade there have been a number of new minimally invasive surgical procedures for the treatment of stress urinary incontinence. The introduction of the tension-free vaginal tape (TVT) procedure by Ulmsten in 1996 revolutionized the field and has gained widespread acceptance due to its systematic and prospective evaluation.[1,2] In a recent review of the surgical techniques used to correct stress urinary incontinence in European hospitals, 83.9% of all procedures were midurethral synthetic slings.[3] Of the synthetic slings, the transobturator approach was used in 26.9% of the procedures. As the number and variety of transobturator slings continue to expand, the overall number of procedures is anticipated to increase.

A successful minimally invasive surgical procedure should at the very least provide acceptable long-term efficacy, as well as a low incidence of short- and long-term complications. Retropubic midurethral sling procedures (i.e. TVT, SPARC, etc.) have shown efficacy in a variety of clinical situations including: 1) primary stress incontinence; 2) recurrent stress incontinence; 3) mixed urinary incontinence; and 4) intrinsic sphincter deficiency.[4–6] In 2001, Delorme[7] described the placement of a synthetic polypropylene mesh via a novel transobturator route. The procedure was simple to perform, eliminated complications typically seen with retropubic needle passage, and did not require routine cystoscopy. Currently there is a wide variety of transobturator slings available, all of which are variations on a common theme.

In this chapter we review the pathophysiology, relevant anatomy, variations of technique and sling materials, potential complications, and results in the literature of the transobturator midurethral slings.

PATHOPHYSIOLOGY OF MIDURETHRAL SLINGS FOR SUI

A common anatomic abnormality found in women with stress urinary incontinence is urethral hypermobility. Procedures including retropubic and transvaginal suspension have attempted to correct the stress urinary incontinence associated with urethral hypermobility by fixing the proximal urethra and bladder neck in a high retropubic position. In 1994, DeLancey[8] suggested that increased urethral closure pressure is achieved by the urethra being compressed against a hammock-like supportive layer consisting of the anterior vaginal wall, endopelvic fascia, and the arcus tendineus fascia pelvis (ATFP). Along similar lines, Petros and Ulmsten[9] proposed that laxity in vaginal and ligamentous support were responsible for the symptoms of stress urinary incontinence and served as a basis for the ultimate success of the TVT procedure. These anatomic observations and the high success rates associated with tension-free midurethral sling procedures have made it apparent that providing suburethral support, rather than correcting hypermobility, is the critical factor in the resolution of stress incontinence.[1,10,11]

Much of our understanding of the mechanism of action for transobturator platform slings is extrapolated from studies investigating the mechanical forces involved in successful TVT procedures. Studies utilizing perineal ultrasonography show that, in patients cured of stress incontinence with TVT, a functional kinking of the urethra during stress occurs when the tape is placed at the midurethra.[12] In a 3-year follow-up study by the same group, 92% of patients with the tape identified at the midurethra had sonographic evidence of functional urethral kinking, which they refer to as the 'urethral knee angle'. Placement of the tape at the proximal urethra in their series only resulted in three of five patients being continent (60%), most likely due to the lack of a fulcrum effect by the tape.[13]

A study by Minaglia et al.[14] utilizing ObTape® showed no difference in resting urethral angles after placement of the tape. Although there was a statistical difference in the urethral angle with straining, urethral hypermobility was maintained in most women, and the authors concluded that correction of urethral hypermobility is not necessary to achieve continence. In fact, continence was seen in 90.4% of their patients with documented hypermobility and in only 50% of patients without urethral mobility. Despite the fact that a subanalysis of their patients was not performed to ascertain which factors predicted failure, the study concluded that a persistent positive Q-tip test was predictive of a successful outcome. Concomitant prolapse surgery or previous anti-incontinence surgery did not predict outcomes in their series.

It appears that minimally invasive midurethral slings, including the transobturator approach, restore the supportive hammock as described by DeLancey. This creates a backboard of support with increases in abdominal pressure that enhances urethral compression to restore continence.

SURGICAL ANATOMY OF THE TRANSOBTURATOR APPROACH (Fig. 65a.1)

Successful results achieved with transobturator midurethral slings depend on a detailed understanding of the surgical anatomy of the obturator foramen, adductor

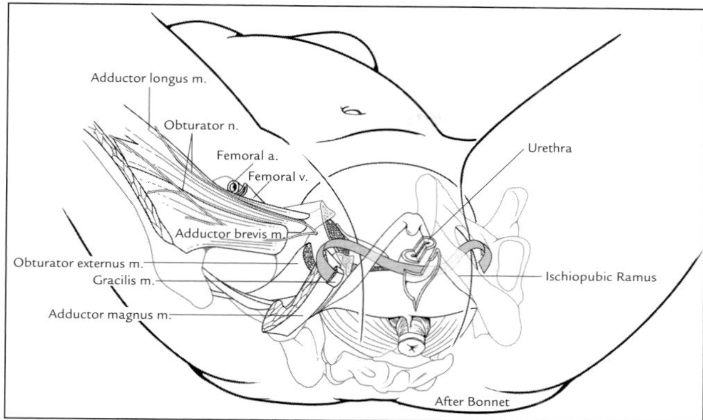

Figure 65a.1 *Illustration of the anatomic postion of a transobturator midurethral sling within the pelvis and its relationship to other pelvic structures (Adapted from Bonnet et al*[15]*).*

musculature, and relevant neurovascular structures, as well as the pertinent pelvic and perineal anatomic relationships. This is of critical importance to optimize efficacy and minimize potential complications. An outstanding illustrative review was performed by Bonnet et al.[15] defining the relevant anatomy in cadaveric dissections using the 'inside-out' transobturator technique as described by Jean de Leval.

The tension-free vaginal tape-obturator (TVT-O) technique was performed in 13 cadavers and anatomic dissections were performed to determine the path of the tape and its relationship to nearby neurovascular structures and organs. Cadaveric dissection was started at Scarpa's femoral triangle and extended medially through the adductor and obturator externus muscle toward the inferior pubic ramus. The perineal space was entered by removing the obturator internus membrane and muscle and sectioning the inferior ramus and pubic bone. This was followed by dissection of the superficial anterior perineum and pelvis.

Important points observed during the dissections are summarized further.

Stage 1 dissection (region of Scarpa's femoral triangle)

1. The tape never penetrated the adductor longus muscle (since this is the medial boundary of the femoral triangle, there was sufficient distance from major neurovascular structures);
2. The tape constantly traversed the adductor magnus and gracilis, and adductor brevis in 70% of the cases;
3. No adductor tendinous structure was perforated by the tape

Stage 2 dissection (obturator region)

1. At the level of the obturator region the tape penetrated the obturator externus muscle, the obturator membrane, and the obturator internus muscle;
2. The shortest distance between the tape and obturator nerve was 22 mm (range 22–30 mm), with a mean distance of 26.2 mm ± 2 mm at the level of the obturator membrane;
3. The rotational trajectory of the helical passer, as well as positioning the patient with thighs in hyperflexion, contributes to divergence of the obturator nerve from the track of the tape;
4. The anterior branch of the obturator artery is protected from injury by the bony architecture of the inferior pubic ramus.

Stage 3 dissection (sectioning of inferior pubic ramus)

1. Tape location corresponds to the most anterior compartment of the ischiorectal fossa;
2. This corresponded to a triangular avascular region bounded by the levator ani (medial and cranial), perineal membrane (caudal), and the obturator internus muscle (lateral);
3. Tape topography was always outside the pelvic space. The tape did not traverse the levator ani muscles.

Stage 4 dissection (pelvis)

1. Complete pelvic dissection never revealed the presence of the synthetic mesh, confirming that the levator musculature was never compromised;
2. The anterior perineal pathway showed consistent tape placement above the perineal membrane;
3. The dorsal nerve of the clitoris is consistently caudal to the perineal membrane.

These key observations confirmed the highly reproducible anatomic relationships associated with passage of the synthetic mesh via an 'inside-out' approach.

Cadaveric dissections performed by Delmas et al.[16] utilizing the 'outside-in' approach on 10 female cadavers have also provided pertinent information and anatomic detail relevant to this minimally invasive technique. Femoral dissection verified that the tape follows a path consistently 4 cm opposite and caudal to the obturator canal, confirming that injury to major neurovascular structures is minimal. The tape is in a plane between the perineal membrane and levator ani musculature above the pudendal pedicle (the pudendal pedicle is protected by the bony architecture of the inferior pubic ramus). In pelvic dissections, the tape courses posterior to Santorini's plexus. Thus, these authors conclude that passage of the tunneler too far anteriorly risks injury to the bladder, while passage in an exaggerated posterior direction risks vaginal perforation.

In a separate study by Whiteside and Walters[17] involving six female cadaveric dissections of the obturator region, the following anatomic observations were made:

- The synthetic mesh passed on average 2.4 cm inferomedial to the obturator canal;
- The anterior and posterior divisions of the obturator nerve are 3.4 and 2.8 cm from the pathway of the transobturator tunneler, respectively;
- The tunneling device passed on average 1.1 cm away from the most medial branch of the obturator vessels.

Given that the tunneling device and tape are within 1–3 cm of neurovascular structures, the authors emphasize that risk of injury is not negligible.

Description of the operative technique

An in-depth description of the surgical technique is beyond the scope of this review. The critical points are reviewed in the following section and the reader is referred for a more extensive discussion.[7,10,18]

Transobturator outside-in

ObTape®, UraTape®, Aris™ TOT, Monarc™, BioArc™ TO, Uretex® TO, ObTryx™, I STOP®

- The patient is placed in the lithotomy position in 120-degree hyperflexion.
- A vertical midline incision is made at the level of the midurethra and the dissection is carried laterally toward the ischiopubic ramus with Metzenbaum scissors.
- A puncture incision is made 15 mm lateral to the ischiopubic ramus at the level of the clitoris.
- Using the 'Hook' or 'Helical' tunneler, the obturator membrane is perforated, at which point a specific resistance is noted by the surgeon.
- With the index finger in the incision palpating the ischiopubic ramus and obturator internus muscle, the tunneler is turned medially, advanced on the tip of the index finger, and brought out the vaginal incision.
- At this point, inspect the vaginal fornix and urethra to ensure that perforation of these structures has not occurred.
- The tape is then loaded onto the tunneler and brought out the inner thigh stab incision and the procedure repeated on the contralateral side.
- It is important to ensure that the tape exerts no tension by allowing a clamp to pass easily between the tape and the urethra.
- The excess tape is cut flush with the skin at the inner thigh and the incisions are closed with absorbable suture.

Transobturator inside-out

TVT-O™

There are three specific surgical instruments unique to TVT-O:

1. a stainless steel *helical passer*;
2. polyethylene *plastic tubes*;
3. a stainless steel *introducer*.

- The initial vaginal portion of the procedure is essentially identical to the 'outside-in' technique.
- 5 mm stab incisions are made 2 cm superior to a horizontal line level with the urethra and 2 cm lateral to the thigh folds. This is the exit point of the helical passer.
- Once the upper part of the ischiopubic ramus is reached, the obturator membrane is perforated sharply with scissors.
- The introducer is passed at 45 degrees relative to the urethral sagittal plane until it reaches and perforates the obturator membrane with the open side facing the surgeon.
- The distal end of the tubing is mounted on the spiral segment of the helical passer and slipped along the open gutter of the introducer.
- Once aligned parallel to the sagittal axis, the passer is rotated so the pointed tip of the tubing exits the inner thigh stab incision.
- The tubing is pulled from the supporting passer until the first few centimeters of the tape become externalized. The procedure is repeated on the contralateral side.
- The plastic sheaths are removed simultaneously from both ends of the tape and the tape is centered at the midurethra without tension.

Results with transobturator approach

Since the original description of the transobturator midurethral sling in 2001 by Delorme,[7] excellent continence results have been noted with relatively short-term follow-up (Table 65a.1). Continence outcomes range from 80.5 to 96% using various objective and subjective tools such as the cough stress test, uroflowmetry, and questionnaire/quality of life instruments. These studies include a variety of patients with mixed incontinence, those who have failed previous anti-incontinence procedures, and patients who had concomitant prolapse repairs. In the studies by Delorme et al.[19] and Mellier et al.[20] 15.6% and 28% of patients had intrinsic sphincter deficiency, respectively. High success rates were consistently reported despite a relatively diverse patient population. These studies, however, failed to perform a subanalysis of their patient outcomes based upon preoperative clinical and urodynamic parameters. Therefore, we do not know which variables are predictive of success and failure with the transobturator sling. Does intrinsic sphincter deficiency (ISD), coinciding prolapse repair or mixed incontinence have a negative impact on the durability and efficacy of this technique? These questions should be answered with further prospective studies and longer follow-up, as in the TVT literature.

Two non-randomized studies compared the transobturator tape (TOT) to the TVT procedure and found no statistical difference in terms of continence outcomes, postoperative obstructive symptoms, and complications.[11,20] There were more bladder injuries (10% versus 0%) and hemorrhage (10% versus 2%) with TVT than with TOT, but this did not reach statistical significance. It is anticipated that the long-term results of the transobturator procedure will parallel the excellent long-term results experienced in the TVT and SPARC literature.[1,21]

Synthetic sling procedures may be differentiated by technique, anatomic position of the sling, and the conformation of the mesh/tape. The major difference between the different transobturator slings, aside from subtle modifications to the tunneling device and ancillary equipment, is the composition of the synthetic sling material. The properties of the mesh have a profound influence upon the local inflammatory response, ingrowth of collagen and fibrous tissue, and integration of the tape into the surrounding host tissues (Table 65a.2). These properties may have important consequences with regard to infection, erosion, and rejection. In a study by Slack et al.,[22] in vivo studies comparing three different polypropylene meshes confirmed similar inflammatory responses, while the amount of fibrous collagen, capillary ingrowth and tissue integration was superior for the larger pore, open knit polypropylene meshes. These in vivo observations have been supported by similar data in the general surgical literature.[23] Although data from in vivo studies support the utilization of open knit, large diameter monofilament mesh for implantation, further clinical correlation is needed to guide surgical preferences.

- The ObTape and UraTape polypropylene meshes comprise small pore, non-knitted, thermally bonded mesh with a 15 mm silicone suburethral component. The Mentor Corporation has recently developed a second generation transobturator tape called the Aris™ TOT which has a larger 200 micron pore size to allow improved tissue ingrowth with less encapsulation.
- ObTryx, TVT-Obturator, Monarc, I STOP, and Uretex-TO are large pore (macropore), open knit polypropylene meshes.
- BioArc is unique in that it allows the surgeon to suture a biological graft material to the polypropylene tape which is placed in a suburethral position.

COMPLICATIONS OF THE TRANSOBTURATOR APPROACH

Although the transobturator approach is minimally invasive, a number of peri- and postoperative complications have been described in the literature (Table 65a.3).

Bladder perforation

Bladder perforation is the most common complication observed with midurethral sling procedures via the retropubic approach, with an incidence of 2–11% in the reported literature.[11,24,25] With the initial description of the transobturator technique it was felt that the risk of cystotomy during tunneler passage was negligible.[7] However, with greater experience, a number of surgical series have shown that the risk of bladder injury should be considered with the technique.

Minaglia et al.[14] reported three cases of intraoperative bladder injury while performing the transobturator technique. All injuries were recognized intraoperatively, as cystoscopy is performed routinely at their institution. The procedure was completed with placement of the sling followed by catheter drainage for 7 days postoperatively. There were no further sequelae or complications from their management.

Table 65a.1. ***Outcomes***

Study	*n*	Follow-up	Cured/improved/ failed	Assessment of outcome	Patient age (years)	Pure SUI	Mixed UI	ISD	Previous anti-incontinence surgery	Previous hysterectomy	Concomitant prolapse repair
Delorme et al.[19]	150 (32 with 1-year f/u)	17 months (13–29)	90.6%; 9.4%; 0	Cough stress test; Uroflow	64 (50–81)	14 (44%)	18 (56%)	5 (15.6%)	5 (15.6%)	5 (15.6%)	0
Costa et al.[27]	183	7 months (1–21)	80.5%; 7.5%; 12%	Cough stress test/ questionnaire	56 (29–87)	53%	27.3%	10 (5.4%) (MUCP <20 cm)	14.2%	25.7%	26 (14.2%)
de Tayrac & Madelenat[3]	30	12 months	90%; 3.3%; 6.7%	Cough stress test/ questionnaire	54.7	27	3	4	4	2 (4 previous prolapse symptoms)	None
Cindolo et al.[26]	80	4 months (1–8)	92% objective cure; 97% subjective; 96% overall satisfaction	Questionnaire/ quality of life instrument	56 (39–79)	62 with +Q-tip test (78%)	22 (28%)	Not applicable	16 (20%)	Not applicable	None
Mellier et al.[20]	94	12.8 months (2–20)	95%; 4%; 1%	Telephone-based questionnaire	58.1 (± 9.3)	94 (100%) defined on 3 grade scale	12 (13%) preoperative urgency	26 (28%) (MUCP <30 cm)	28 (30%)	17 (18%)	None
Queimadelos et al.[40]	47	18 months	45/47 (96%)	Questionnaire	55 (40–69)	47	0	3	Not applicable	Not applicable	0
Krauth et al.[36]	604 (140 with 1-year f/u)	1–3 months in 572; 1 year in 140	85.5% satisfied at 1 year	Subjective questioning	57	47.3%	52.7%	Not reported	Not reported	Not reported	8%

f/u, follow-up; ISD, intrinsic sphincter deficiency; MUCP, maximum urethral closure pressure; SUI, stress urinary incontinence; UI, urinary incontinence.

Table 65a.2. *Mesh characteristics*

Company	Brand name	Mesh material	Pore size
Mentor	ObTape	Prolene, 15 mm silicone	50 micron
	UraTape	Prolene, 15 mm silicone	50 micron
	Aris	Polypropylene	200 micron
AMS	Monarc	Knitted polypropylene	Large, open knit
	BioArc	Polypropylene with biologic suburethral component	Large, open knit
GyneCare	TVT-Obturator	Polypropylene	Large, open knit
Bard	Uretex-TO	Polypropylene	Large pore
Boston Scientific	ObTryx	Polypropylene with detangled suburethral segment	Large pore, >100 microns
CL Medical, France	I STOP	Monofilament Prolene	>75 microns, low weight/area weave

Table 65a.3. *Adverse events*

Study	*n*	Adverse events
Delorme et al.[19]	32	None reported
de Leval[18]	107	1 superficial vein thrombosis with abscess; ?(27/107) 15.9% transient thigh pain
Domingo et al.[30]	65	9 vaginal mesh erosions
Costa et al.[27]	183	3 vaginal erosions; 2 urethral erosions; 1 bladder perforation; 1 vaginal perforation; 2 urethral perforations
de Tayrac & Madelenat[3]	30	6 uncomplicated UTI; 1 obturator hematoma
Cindolo et al.[26]	80	1 vaginal erosion with inguinal abscess
Mellier et al.[20]	94	2% intraoperative hemorrhage (300 cc); 1 urethral perforation
Queimadelos et al.[40]	47	None reported
Krauth et al.[36]	604 (140 with 1-year follow-up)	0.3% vaginal erosion; 2.5% UTI; 0.5% bladder perforation; 0.33% vaginal perforation; 2.3% perineal pain

UTI, urinary tract infection.

Cindolo et al.[26] and Costa et al.[27] also reported a single bladder laceration in their series which was recognized and managed intraoperatively.

Furthermore, anatomic studies have shown that with tunneler passage via the 'outside-in' transobturator approach, the needle passes through the retropubic space and true pelvis, which can result in cystotomy.[17,28]

Based on the published literature, there have been no published cases of bladder injury when performing the TOT via an 'inside-out' approach using the TVT-O.

In our opinion, cystoscopy should continue to be performed in select cases.

Vaginal tape erosion

Since the introduction of synthetic mesh as a sling material for the correction of stress urinary incontinence, mesh erosion has been observed with varying frequency. A 1997 meta-analysis of synthetic slings quoted a vaginal erosion rate of 0.7% and a rate of urethral erosion greater than 2.7%.[29] This complication is thought to be due to the intrinsic characteristics of the mesh utilized in the reconstruction. Although the mechanism of erosion is unclear, subclinical infection and mechanical friction between the sling and host tissues may predispose to this phenomenon.30,31

Recently, Domingo et al.[30] reported a relatively high incidence of vaginal erosion (13.8%) in their series utilizing UraTape and ObTape. They hypothesized that the characteristics of the polypropylene mesh (fusion welded, thermally bonded, non-woven, non-knitted) reduced the pore size to 50 microns. These characteristics of the tape led to encapsulation and poor tissue ingrowth, which contributed to the higher vaginal erosion rate. They concluded that a synthetic mesh with larger pore size facilitates vascular and tissue ingrowth, optimizing mesh integration with the host tissues.[23,30]

Successful management of this complication includes complete removal of the tape via a transvaginal approach and, if indicated, a combined transobturator approach. Despite tape removal, continence status was good at 78% in their series.[30]

An alternative to complete tape removal was suggested by Kobashi and Govier[32] who managed vaginal tape erosion conservatively after SPARC and observed excellent results due to the exceptional tissue ingrowth and granulation tissue associated with this polypropylene mesh. Since most obturator tapes utilize a macropore, open-knit polypropylene mesh, it seems reasonable to conclude that they may behave in a similar fashion.

Postoperative voiding dysfunction

Midurethral slings can be complicated by postoperative bladder outlet obstruction, manifesting as urinary retention, high post-void residual urine, de novo urgency, and worsening of preoperative urgency. De novo urgency has been reported to occur in zero to 20.6% of patients following TVT.[33] The incidence following TOT procedures has been between 2.1 and 6.7% in the reported literature (Table 65.6).

Two non-randomized studies comparing TVT and TOT showed no statistical differences with regard to efficacy and postoperative voiding dysfunction, including bladder outlet obstruction and urinary retention.[11,34] The rate of obstructive voiding after the transobturator midurethral sling can be seen in 1.5–15.6% of patients (Table 65.6). This is usually a transient problem with exceedingly few patients requiring clean intermittent catheterization or a tape release procedure. Long-term retention after TVT is a rare complication (0.6–3.8%) and can be expected to be equally infrequent in the TOT population based on a similar pathophysiologic mechanism of action, namely recreating DeLancey's supportive hammock.

Patients with refractory voiding dysfunction after TOT can be managed successfully with release of the tape, which in most cases will improve the patient's symptoms without compromising continence status.[11] In patients presenting with early voiding symptoms suggestive of obstruction, downward displacement on the tape to reduce tension under local anesthesia has been shown to provide symptomatic relief.[35]

The risk of postoperative voiding dysfunction after transobturator sling placement is low and, if recognized in a timely fashion, active intervention can provide symptomatic relief.

OTHER COMPLICATIONS

One interesting complication with this approach is the finding of postoperative leg pain. In de Leval's series,[18] 15.9% of patients had temporary groin pain which abated by the second postoperative day. In the series by Krauth et al.,36 14 patients (2.3%) had postoperative perineal/groin pain. The pain was transient in all but one case, responding to non-steroidal anti-inflammatory medications.

The etiology of the pain is unclear and may be related to subclinical hematoma or transient neuropathic pain. Although the pain reported by these investigators was transient in nature, case reports have shown that isolated leg pain may be the first manifestation of an occult erosion.[37] Therefore, persistent leg pain that does not

Table 65.6. *Voiding dysfunction*

Study	*n*	Urinary retention	De novo urgency
Delorme et al.[19]	32	5 (15.6%) with obstructive voiding (Q_{max} <15/PVR >20%); 1 with urinary retention CIC × 4 weeks	2 (6.25%)
de Leval[18]	107	3 required tape release	Not reported
Costa et al.[27]	183	7 (3.3%); 3 required tape release; 2 on CIC (PVR >100 cc) at 1 year	4 (2.1%)
de Tayrac & Madelenat[3]	30	PVR >100 cc (4 POD 1 [13.3%]; 3 POD 2; 1 after day 2)	2 (6.7%)
Cindolo et al.[26]	80	None	2 (2.5%)
Mellier et al.[20]	94	7% PVR >100 cc on POD 1; no patients on long-term CIC	4 (4.2%)
Queimadelos et al.[40]	47	None	None
Krauth et al.[36]	604 (140)	9 (1.5%) transient retention; no CIC; 1 required tape release	5.2% at 3 months; 1.5% at 1 year

CIC, clean intermittent catheterization; POD, postoperative day; PVR, post-void residual.

respond to conservative measures should prompt an appropriate investigation to identify mechanical causes for the pain.

Other less common complications have been described anecdotally and include thigh abscess requiring drainage and infected obturator hematoma requiring bilateral transobturator exploration.[18,38,39]

CONCLUSION

The transobturator suburethral sling has excellent short-term continence results. Pathophysiologically, efficacy appears to relate to a platform of suburethral support at the midurethra as described by DeLancey's hammock hypothesis. The technique is easy to learn and master, has short operative time, and acceptable complication rate. Moreover, major vascular and bowel complications have not been reported as the retropubic space is not violated. Initial retrospective comparisons with TVT have shown no statistically significant differences in outcomes. Prospective, randomized studies with longer follow-up are needed to confirm the initial good results.

REFERENCES

1. Nilsson CG, Falconer C, Rezapour M. Seven-year follow-up of the tension-free vaginal tape procedure for treatment of urinary incontinence. Obstet Gynecol 2004;104:1259–61.
2. Ulmsten U, Henriksson L, Johnson P et al. An ambulatory surgical procedure under local anesthesia for treatment of female urinary incontinence. Int Urogynecol J Pelvic Floor Dysfunct 1996;7:81–6.
3. de Tayrac R, Madelenat P. [Evolution of surgical routes in female stress urinary incontinence]. Gynecol Obstet Fertil 2004;32:1031–8.
4. Kuuva N, Nilsson CG. Tension-free vaginal tape procedure: an effective minimally invasive operation for the treatment of recurrent stress urinary incontinence? Gynecol Obstet Invest 2003;56:93–8.
5. Rezapour M, Falconer C, Ulmsten U. Tension-free vaginal tape (TVT) in stress incontinent women with intrinsic sphincter deficiency (ISD) – a long-term follow-up. Int Urogynecol J Pelvic Floor Dysfunct 2001;12(Suppl 2):S12.
6. Ulmsten U, Falconer C, Johnson P et al. A multicenter study of tension-free vaginal tape (TVT) for surgical treatment of stress urinary incontinence. Int Urogynecol J Pelvic Floor Dysfunct 1998;9:210–3.
7. Delorme E. [Transobturator urethral suspension: mini-invasive procedure in the treatment of stress urinary incontinence in women.] Prog Urol 2001;11:1306–13.
8. DeLancey JO. Structural support of the urethra as it relates to stress urinary incontinence: the hammock hypothesis. Am J Obstet Gynecol 1994;170:1713–20.
9. Petros PE, Ulmsten UI. An integral theory and its method for the diagnosis and management of female urinary incontinence. Scand J Urol Nephrol Suppl 1993;153:1–93.
10. Delorme E, Droupy S, de Tayrac, R et al. [Transobturator tape (UraTape). A new minimally invasive method in the treatment of urinary incontinence in women.] Prog Urol 2003;13:656–9.
11. de Tayrac R, Deffieux X, Droupy S et al. A prospective randomized trial comparing tension-free vaginal tape and transobturator suburethral tape for surgical treatment of stress urinary incontinence. Am J Obstet Gynecol 2004;190:602–8.
12. Lo TS, Wang AC, Horng SG et al. Ultrasonographic and urodynamic evaluation after tension free vaginal tape procedure (TVT). Acta Obstet Gynecol Scand 2001;80:65–70.
13. Lo TS, Horng SG, Liang CC, Lee SJ, Soong YK. Ultrasound assessment of midurethra tape at three-year follow up after tension free vaginal tape procedure. Urology 2003;63:671–5.
14. Minaglia S, Ozel B, Klutke C et al. Bladder injury during transobturator sling. Urology 2004;64:376–7.
15. Bonnet P, Waltregny D, Reul O et al. Transobturator vaginal tape inside out for the surgical treatment of female stress urinary incontinence: anatomical considerations. J Urol 2005;173:1223–8.
16. Delmas V, Hermieu J, Dompeyre P et al. The UraTape transobturator sling in the treatment of female stress urinary incontinence: mechanism of action. Eur Urol Supplement 2003;2:196.
17. Whiteside JL, Walters MD. Anatomy of the obturator region: relations to a trans-obturator sling. Int Urogynecol J Pelvic Floor Dysfunct 2004;15:223–6.
18. de Leval J. Novel surgical technique for the treatment of female stress urinary incontinence: transobturator vaginal tape inside-out. Eur Urol 2003;44:724–30.
19. Delorme E, Droupy S, de Tayrac R et al. Transobturator tape (UraTape): a new minimally invasive procedure to treat female urinary incontinence. Eur Urol 2004;45:203–7.
20. Mellier G, Benayed B, Bretones S et al. Suburethral tape via the obturator route: is the TOT a simplification of the TVT? Int Urogynecol J Pelvic Floor Dysfunct 2004;15:227–32.
21. Tseng LH, Wang AC, Lin YH et al. Randomized comparison of the suprapubic arc sling procedure vs. tension-free vaginal taping for stress incontinent women. Int Urogynecol J Pelvic Floor Dysfunct 2005;16(3):230–5.
22. Slack M, Sandhu JS, Staskin DR et al. In vivo comparison of suburethral sling materials. Int Urogynecol J Pelvic Floor Dysfunct 2005 Jul 2; [Epub ahead of print].

23. Amid PK, Lichtenstein IL. [Current assessment of Lichtenstein tension-free hernia repair.] Chirurg 1997;68:965–9.
24. Olsson I, Kroon U. A three-year postoperative evaluation of tension-free vaginal tape. Gynecol Obstet Invest 1999;48:267–9.
25. Kobashi KC, Govier FE. Perioperative complications: the first 140 polypropylene pubovaginal slings. J Urol 2003;170:1918–21.
26. Cindolo L, Salzano L, Rota G et al. Tension-free transobturator approach for female stress urinary incontinence. Minerva Urol Nefrol 2004;56:89–98.
27. Costa P, Grise P, Droupy S et al. Surgical treatment of female stress urinary incontinence with a trans-obturator-tape (T.O.T.) Uratape: short term results of a prospective multicentric study. Eur Urol 2004;46:102–6; discussion 106–7.
28. Hermieu JF, Messas A, Delmas V et al. [Bladder injury after TVT transobturator.] Prog Urol 2003;13:115–7.
29. Leach GE, Dmochowski RR, Appell RA et al. Female Stress Urinary Incontinence Clinical Guidelines Panel summary report on surgical management of female stress urinary incontinence. American Urological Association. J Urol 1997;158:875–80.
30. Domingo S, Alama P, Ruiz N et al. Diagnosis, management and prognosis of vaginal erosion after transobturator suburethral tape procedure using a nonwoven thermally bonded polypropylene mesh. J Urol 2005;173:1627–30.
31. Kobashi KC, Dmochowski R, Mee SL et al. Erosion of woven polyester pubovaginal sling. J Urol 1999;162:2070–2.
32. Kobashi KC, Govier FE. Management of vaginal erosion of polypropylene mesh slings. J Urol 2003;169:2242–3.
33. Peschers UM, Tunn R, Buczkowski M et al. Tension-free vaginal tape for the treatment of stress urinary incontinence. Clin Obstet Gynecol 2000;43:670–5.
34. Mansoor A, Védrine N, Darcq C. Surgery of female urinary incontinence using trans-obturator tape (TOT): a prospective randomised comparative study with TVT. Neurourol Urodyn 2003;22:526.
35. Ozel B, Minaglia S, Hurtado E et al. Treatment of voiding dysfunction after transobturator tape procedure. Urology 2004;64:1030.
36. Krauth JS, Rasoamiaramanana H, Barletta H et al. Suburethral tape treatment of female urinary incontinence – morbidity assessment of the trans-obturator route and a new tape (I-STOP): a multi-centre experiment involving 604 cases. Eur Urol 2005;47:102–6; discussion 106–7.
37. Mahajan ST, Kenton K, Bova DA et al. Transobturator tape erosion associated with leg pain. Int Urogynecol J Pelvic Floor Dysfunct 2005 Jun 18; [Epub ahead of print].
38. Game X, Mouzin M, Vaessen C et al. Obturator infected hematoma and urethral erosion following transobturator tape implantation. J Urol 2004;171:1629.
39. Goldman HB. Large thigh abscess after placement of synthetic transobturator sling. Int Urogynecol J Pelvic Floor Dysfunct 2005 Jun 29; [Epub ahead of print].
40. Queimadelos MA, Cimadevilla GA, Lema GJ, Rodrigues NH, Perez FD, Lamas CP. Monarc transobturator suburethral sling: eighteen months' experience. ICS/IUGA, France, 2004; Abstract 559.

65b

Transobturator approach

Calin Ciofu, Francois Haab

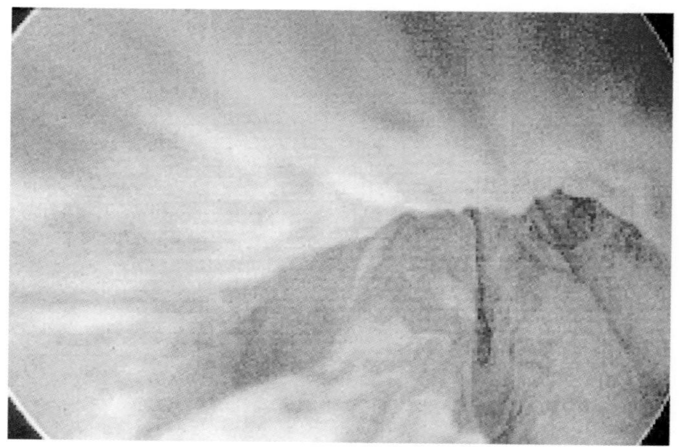

INTRODUCTION

Since 2001, when Delorme first published the transobturator insertion of a suburethral sling for the treatment of stress urinary incontinence,[1] few articles have been published on the technique, despite the principle of the technique being considered both interesting and promising. The technique was developed in order to avoid the risk of urethral, bladder, and bowel injury.

The paucity of articles in the literature permits only expert opinion-based and no evidence-based considerations. The former were limited to retrospective case controls, classifying the technique as having a grade B of recommendation. Nevertheless, based on DeLancey's anatomic studies, the technique – comprising insertion and passage of the suburethral tape from one foramen obturator to the other (transobturator tape, or TOT) – appears to restore the physiologic support more effectively and, therefore, continence (Fig. 65b.1).

THE ANATOMIC RATIONALE FOR TRANSOBTURATOR TAPE

The mechanism of continence is still controversial. Many authors correlate incontinence with urethral hypermobility. DeLancey's hammock theory suggests that urinary continence is due to muscular, ligamentous and fascial support of the urethra. In order to correct incontinence, the surgical procedure has to restore urethral support. Tension-free vaginal tape (TVT) and TVT-like procedures restore this support, replacing the muscular structures with a polypropylene U-shaped tape.[2]

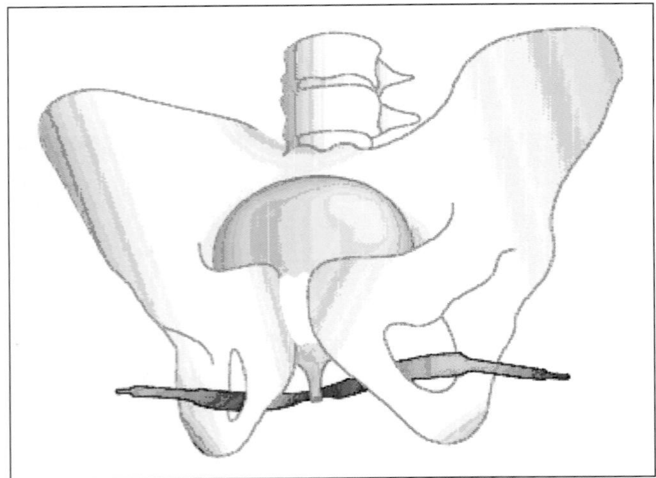

Figure 65b.1. *Tape position once inserted through the foramen obturator.*

The two main concerns of the TVT technique (obstruction and bleeding) can be avoided by the anatomic specificity of TOT.

In the TOT technique, the polypropylene tape inserted through the lower part of the foramen obturator is closer to the physiologic shape of the hammock. Between the left and the right part of the tape there is a very large open angle. Anatomic studies showed that the direction of the tape keeps the same transverse orientation as the muscular fibers of the hammock.[3] This implies, at least from a theoretical point of view, that it is difficult to obstruct the urethra.

On the other hand, anatomic studies showed that the tape passes through spaces where vascular and neurologic structures are very scarce (although not completely absent). Perineal dissection showed that the tape passes between the perineal membrane and the muscular levator ani; pelvic dissection showed that the tape is situated far behind the pubovesical and pubourethral venous plexus (Santorini). Perforation of the obturator membrane is performed in its lowest part, far below the vascular structures and nerves. In its lateral progress from the foramen obturator to the mediofemoral region, the tape crosses the adductor muscles and, here again, there are no important vessels or nerves.[4] This makes hemorrhage and nerve injury less probable, although not entirely impossible.

THE OPERATIVE TECHNIQUE

The procedure can be performed under either spinal or general anesthesia; however, local anesthesia is not excluded.

The patient is placed in the lithotomy position, with the thighs in hyperflexion on the abdomen and the buttocks at the edge of the table. A 16 Fr Foley catheter is inserted in the bladder and retained throughout the entire operation in order to facilitate the identification and protection of the urethra.

Several specifically designed devices are needed for the procedure (Fig. 65b.2):

- An 'introducer', a several centimeters long stainless steel gutter.
- Two 'passers', sometimes improperly named 'needles', also made of stainless steel. Each is composed of a handle and a curved needle. The curve describes a 90-degree angle with the handle. One passer has a curve designed to fit the right side; the other, the left.
- The tape, which is of polypropylene, has both ends fixed in a polyethylene tube. This plastic tube has

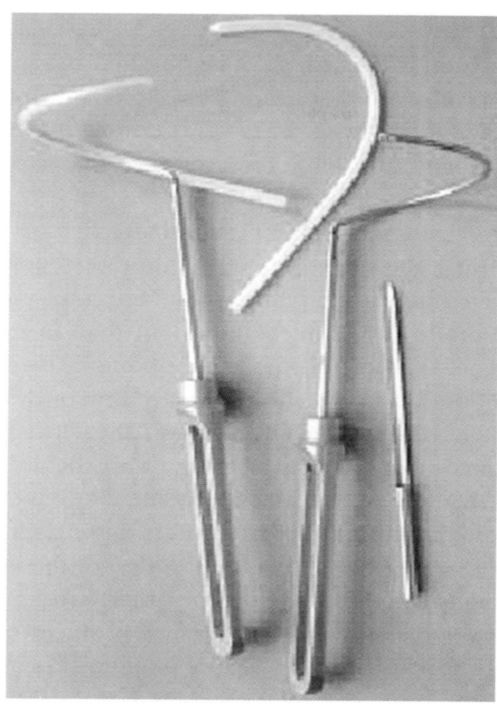

Figure 65b.2. *Devices necessary for the transobturator tape procedure. Right: the introducer; central and left: the passer. The curved part of the needle is protected by a plastic sheath that has been removed from the central device.*

a lateral opening through which the curve of the passer is guided up to its end.

The mid-third of the urethra is identified and the vaginal mucosa incised for 1–2 cm, along the median line, between two Allis clamps. The incision must penetrate the thickness of the vaginal wall.

The dissection is continued, with fine dissection scissors, starting from the incision and directed laterally and horizontally towards the upper part of the ischiopubic ramus. The dissection can be helped by earlier hydrodissection, performed before incising the vagina. The dissection should be done with care in order not to perforate the vaginal wall or vestibular mucosa.

Once bone contact is perceived, the dissection is stopped. The introducer is inserted, with the hollow part of the gutter facing the operator and keeping contact with the upper margin of the ischiopubic ramus. The obturator membrane is then perforated and the introducer's progression stopped.

The future cutaneous exit point is then located by a 0.5 cm vertical incision of the skin several millimeters above the line of the urethral meatus, 2 cm outside the thigh folds.

The passer within the polyethylene tube is then guided through the hollow part of the introducer until its distal end reaches the foramen obturator (Fig. 65b.3). The introducer is removed and the passer pulled further with a rotational movement in order to reach and exit through the previously made skin incision (Fig. 65b.4). The top of the plastic tube is then grasped with a clamp and the introducer removed. The same technique is applied to the opposite side. The two tubes are then extracted on both sides. Traction is exerted simultaneously on both sides in order to adjust the position of the tape. The top of the Mayo scissors should be kept between the tape and the urethra until the final position is found in order to avoid excessive tension. Once the correct tension is applied to the tape, its plastic sheath is removed. The tape ends are then cut at the subcutaneous layer. The femoral skin and vaginal mucosal incisions are closed with resorbable sutures.

The indwelling bladder catheter is retained for 24 hours. The absence of post-voiding residue should be

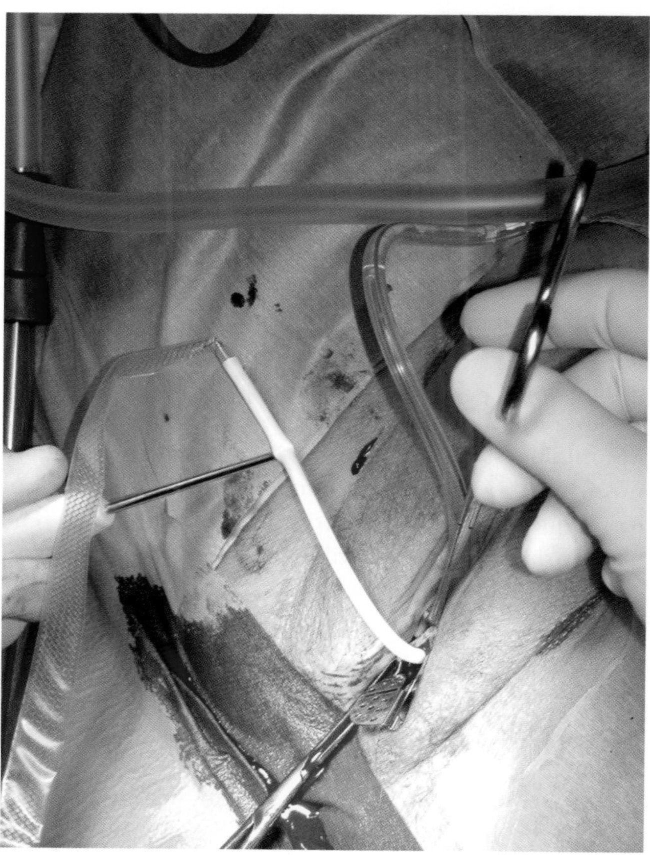

Figure 65b.3. *The passer takes a circular direction, perforating the obturator membrane.*

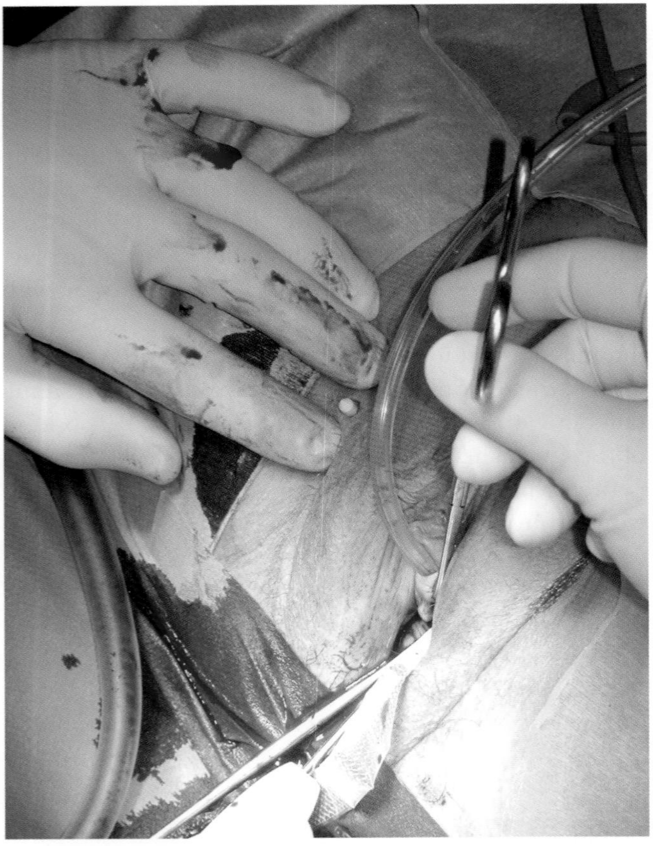

Figure 65b.4. *The passer exits through the skin incision at the thigh.*

checked after catheter ablation. If voiding is incomplete, intermittent self-catheterization for several days can be suggested. An indwelling catheter is sometimes necessary but should never be retained for more than 1 week.

The duration of the operation is approximately 15 minutes (14–16 minutes) and hospitalization does not usually exceed 48 hours.

Several variations of the technique are mentioned. It was initially suggested that the tape be passed through, not from the vagina to the femoral region (inside-out technique), but inversely (outside-in technique). The main variation of the technique concerns the shape and curves of the passer.

RESULTS

In the few retrospective series published to date, cure and improvement rates with TOT at 1 year appear to be similar to those of TVT. Cure rate is 90–95% and improvement rate 3–9%; however, the follow-up period is still very short (Table 65b.1).

Complications are few. Perioperative hemorrhage is exceptional and not important. One case report notes an infected hematoma with urethral erosion.[8]

The urethral risk is less important than in the TVT technique. It is perhaps more important in the outside-in technique, but protection of the urethra by the operator's finger can easily avoid any lesion, thus obviating the need for cystoscopy as is necessary with the TVT technique. In addition, the bladder is situated more cranial to the direction of the passer and is therefore difficult to injure. Nevertheless, bladder erosion of the tape has been highlighted[9] by several operators. Erosion is less a postoperative consequence than a problem of graft-versus-host reaction,[10,11] indicating that erosion may also occur with the TOT operation.

Prolonged retention (2.8%) and pain have been recognized as complications of the TOT procedure. Pain usually lasts for 1–3 days and can be treated with non-opioid analgesics (Table 65b.2).

DISCUSSION

Transobturator insertion of suburethral tape is a new technique and current follow-up does not exceed 1 year. It is probable that in the following years more complications will be identified. The results at 1-year follow-up appear to be as good as those with the TVT technique although these results are conclusions of retrospective non-randomized series. Prospective randomized series are necessary to confirm these initial results.

If DeLancey's hammock theory is correct, the transobturator tape appears to restore suburethral support most closely to the physiologic aspect. This led Delorme et al.[13] to suggest that there should be no reason for patients to develop de novo bladder hyperactivity. We only partially agree with this opinion because the

Table 65b.1. *The results of treatment with the transobturator tape procedure as reflected by the literature*

Authors	No. of patients	Method of evaluation	Follow-up (months)	Cure (%)	Improvement (%)	Failure (%)
Delorme et al.[5]	150	Clinical assessment by independent investigator: cough test	17	90.6	9.4	0
Mellier et al.[6]	94	Telephone questionnaire	3	95.0	4.0	1
Cindolo et al.[7]	80	Questionnaire	4	94.0	3.0	3

Table 65b.2. *Peri- and postoperative complications of the transobturator tape procedure as reflected by the literature*

Authors	De Leval[12]	Delorme et al.[5]	Mellier et al.[6]	Cindolo et al.[7]
No. of patients	107	150	94	80
Perioperative complications	None	None	Hemorrhage <200 ml (2 patients)	Bladder neck laceration (1 patient)
Pain (%)	15.9	0	?	?
Erosion	0	0	0	Vaginal + inguinal abscess (1 patient)
Superficial venous thrombosis (%)	0.8	–	–	–
De novo bladder hyperactivity (%)	–	1.33	4.1	2.5
Postoperative retention (%)	2.8	0	1.0	–
Voiding dysfunction (%)	–	3.33 (Q_{max} <15 ml/s)	25 ('some difficulty to void')	–

natural hammock is a muscular structure, physiologically able to contract, whereas the artificial tape is not able actively to obstruct the urethra during stress. On the other hand, the TOT procedure respects the orientation of muscle fibers better than the TVT operation, and the dissection is less extensive, making tape migration less likely to occur.

From the anatomic point of view one could be tempted to add that voiding difficulty should be less frequent than with TVT series. This appears to be confirmed by two studies comparing TVT and TOT retrospectively, not simultaneously, and non-randomized.[6,14] Postoperative retention appears to be less frequent with TOT. These data need confirmation with prospective randomized series.

CONCLUSIONS

There are several proven advantages concerning the feasibility of the TOT technique compared to the TVT procedure:

- the short duration of the operation;
- the low risk of urethral and bladder lesion, making cystoscopy redundant;
- the absence of risk of bowel lesion;
- the low risk of hemorrhage.

Initial results appear to suggest a cure rate similar to that of the TVT procedure but these data need confirmation and longer follow-up.

REFERENCES

1. Delorme E. [Transobturator urethral suspension: mini-invasive procedure in the treatment of stress urinary incontinence in women.] Prog Urol 2001;11:1306–13.
2. Haab F, Traxer O, Ciofu C. Tension-free vaginal tape: why an unusual concept is so successful. Curr Opin Urol 2001;11:293–7.
3. Delmas V, Hermieu J, Dompeyre P et al. The Uratape transobturator sling in the treatment of female stress urinary incontinence: mechanism of action. Eur Urol (Suppl) 2003;2:776.
4. Delmas V, Hermieu JF, Dompeyre P et al. The transobturator slingtape Uratape: anatomical dangers. Eur Urol (Suppl) 2003;2:777.
5. Delorme E, Droupy S, de Tayrac R, Delmas V. Transobturator tape (Uratape): a new minimally-invasive procedure to treat female urinary incontinence. Eur Urol 2004;45(2):203–7.
6. Mellier G, Benayed B, Bretones S, Pasquier JC. Suburethral tape via the obturator route: is the TOT a simplification of the TVT? Int Urogynecol J Pelvic Floor Dysfunct 2004;15:227–32.
7. Cindolo L, Salzano L, Rota G, Bellini S, D'Afiero A. Tension-free transobturator approach for female stress urinary incontinence. Minerva Urol Nefrol 2004;56(1):89–98.
8. Game X, Mouzin M, Vaessen C, Malavaud B, Sarramon JP, Rischmann P. Obturator infected hematoma and urethral erosion following transobturator tape implantation. J Urol 2004;171:1629.
9. Hermieu JF, Messas A, Delmas V, Ravery V, Dumonceau O, Boccon-Gibod L. Plaie vésicale après bandelette transobturatrice. Prog Urol 2003;13:115–7.
10. Boublil V, Ciofu C, Traxer O, Sebe P, Haab F. Complications of urethral sling procedures. Curr Opin Obstet Gynecol 2002;14:515–20.
11. Dietz HP, Vancaillie P, Svehla M, Walsh W, Steensma AB, Vancaillie TG. Mechanical properties of urogynecologic implant materials. Int Urogynecol J Pelvic Floor Dysfunct 2003;14:239–43.

12. de Leval J. Novel surgical technique for the treatment of female stress urinary incontinence: transobturator vaginal tape inside-out. Eur Urol 2003;44(6):724–30.
13. Delorme E, Droupy S, de Tayrac R, Delmas V. [Transobturator tape (Uratape). A new minimally invasive method in the treatment of urinary incontinence in women.] Prog Urol 2003;13:656–9.
14. Ansquer Y, Marcollet A, Yazbeck C et al. The suburethral sling for female stress urinary incontinence: a retropubic or obturator approach? J Am Assoc Gynecol Laparosc 2004;11:353–8.

66

The artificial urinary sphincter for treatment of stress urinary incontinence in women

Emily E Cole, Harriette M Scarpero, Roger R Dmochowski

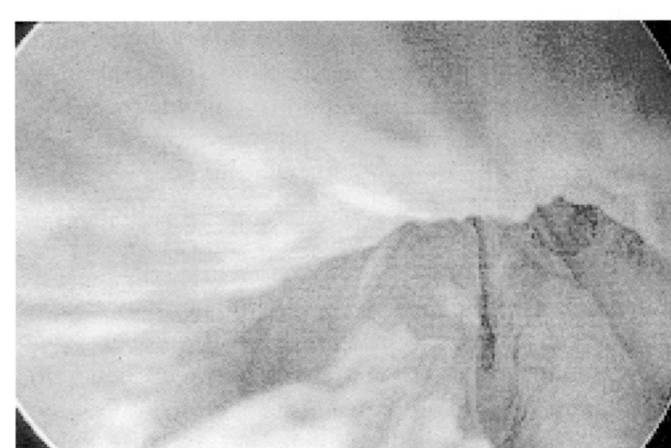

INTRODUCTION

The artificial urinary sphincter (AUS) is an effective alternative to pubovaginal and/or midurethral slings and periurethral injection therapy in the management of urinary incontinence, particularly in those patients in whom the above-mentioned procedures have failed. Historically, the AUS has been reserved for treatment of incontinence due to primary urethral sphincter deficiency – type III stress urinary incontinence, or intrinsic sphincter deficiency (ISD).[1–3] The primary pathophysiology of ISD is characterized by an inability of the urethra to function as a sphincter, either at rest or in response to minimal stress activity. ISD may be the result of urethral scarring related to prior anti-incontinence procedures, neurologic disorders (myelomeningocele, peripheral neuropathy), radical pelvic operations, pelvic radiation therapy, and, in some cases, the effects of aging and estrogen deficiency on the urethra and anterior vaginal wall. Current thinking denotes the pubovaginal sling to be the gold standard for the treatment of ISD; however, it is clear that not all patients will have adequate results despite several attempts.[4] A patient in this situation with documented urethral weakness and good anterior vaginal wall support may benefit from treatment with an AUS. The AUS allows for higher intraurethral pressures by increasing pressure evenly around the urethra, thereby preventing incontinence due to the transmission of intra-abdominal forces.

The placement of an AUS may be accomplished via either a transabdominal or a transvaginal approach. The device is composed of three parts: the inflatable cuff, the pressure-regulating balloon, and the pump. The cuff is placed circumferentially around the bladder neck, the pressure-regulating balloon is positioned in the prevesical space, and the pump is placed in the labium majus. When the pump is compressed, fluid within the system is transferred from the cuff into the regulating balloon. This decompression opens the bladder neck, allowing the patient to void. After 1–2 minutes, the pressure-regulating balloon promotes cuff refilling by transfer of fluid through a resistor in the pump, re-establishing urethral compression, coaptation, and continence. The American Medical System AMS 800 is the only AUS currently available for implantation (Fig. 66.1).

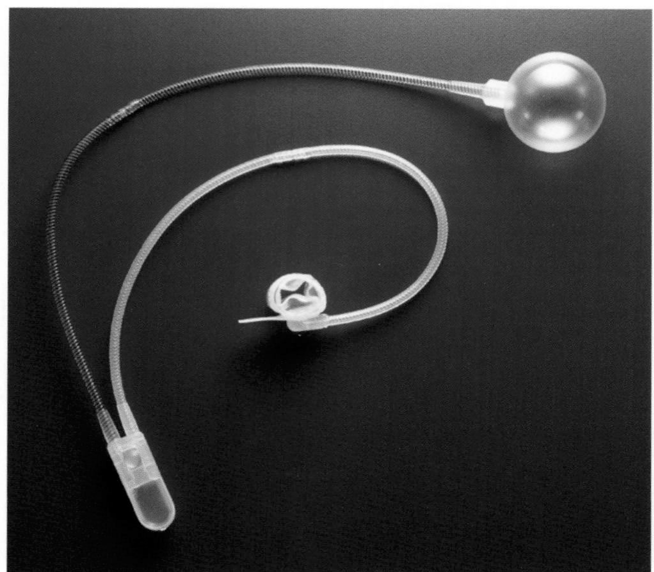

Figure 66.1. *Single Cuff AMS 800™ Urinary Control System. (Courtesy of American Medical Systems, Inc., Minnetonka, MN.)*

EVALUATION

Patients undergoing a workup for stress urinary incontinence (SUI) who may be considered as candidates for implantation of an AUS require a detailed evaluation including a focused urologic history and physical examination. The patient with genuine SUI due to primary urethral sphincter deficiency will typically report a significant loss of urine with abdominal straining. However, particular attention should be paid to the characterization of incontinence as purely stress, associated with urgency, spontaneous, or mixed, to rule out coexistence of detrusor overactivity. In addition, the degree of incontinence and resultant bother should be quantified to counsel the patient accurately about options.

A detailed past surgical history should be obtained. A history of prior anti-incontinence surgery may affect the vascularity and thickness of the periurethral tissue and anterior wall of the vagina, thereby making dissection in the bladder neck and periurethral areas difficult. The history should also assess the patient for any neurologic or orthopedic disorders that may affect the patient's abilities to manipulate the labial pump mechanism.

A complete physical examination should be performed, paying special attention to the vaginal and lower abdominal components. Examination may confirm previous surgical procedures in many cases. Findings such as a weakened pelvic floor, anterior and/or posterior compartment defect(s) or atrophic vaginitis are identified and considered when future surgical options are discussed. Urethral hypermobility should be assessed by direct examination or the Q-tip test. A hypermobile bladder neck or urethra may respond more appropriately to a standard suspension or sling procedure. The size of the vaginal vault and basic anatomic structures should be assessed. Objective demonstration of stress urinary incontinence in the supine or upright position is recommended.

Besides a urine sample for analysis and culture, the patient should undergo at least a simple urodynamic evaluation to assess bladder function. Urine storage at low intravesical pressures is critical before proceeding with increasing urethral resistance with the AUS. A cystometrogram (CMG) determines filling pressures and whether there is adequate bladder capacity. High-pressure urinary storage is a contraindication to AUS placement. The CMG is also helpful in the detection of detrusor overactivity, which may be treated with anticholinergic medications. Measurement of abdominal leak point pressure (LPP) is necessary to assess sphincteric competency and to confirm a diagnosis of ISD. Some authors recommend the utilization of urethral pressure profilometry to confirm low urethral closure pressures (<25 cmH_2O).[5] Uroflowmetry and measurement of post-void residual urine reflect bladder emptying. Incomplete emptying may indicate the necessity for intermittent catheterization postoperatively.

Radiographic evaluation should include a voiding cystourethrogram (VCUG) with resting and straining views. A well-supported urethra with an open bladder neck at rest is consistent with ISD. The VCUG will also confirm the absence of fistulae and vesicoureteral reflux.

PATIENT SELECTION

The AUS is indicated for those patients who suffer from intrinsic sphincter deficiency who demonstrate low-pressure urinary storage. As in all cases, conservative measures should be considered prior to operative intervention. Non-invasive measures such as timed voiding, fluid restriction, pelvic floor exercises, vaginal estrogen therapy, and anticholinergic medications to address any urge component may be considered. If these measures are not sufficient, or if the degree of incontinence is as such, operative intervention may be considered.

Patients who demonstrate elevated intravesical storage pressures are subject to upper tract deterioration when outlet resistance is increased. These patients should demonstrate a urodynamically confirmed response to anticholinergic therapy prior to AUS implantation. Simultaneous or staged augmentation cystoplasty should be considered in those patients who demonstrate persistently high pressures despite maximal pharmacologic therapy.

Patients with incomplete emptying and high preoperative post-void residuals may be considered for AUS implantation. These patients may require intermittent self-catheterization following the procedure, and should be adequately counseled preoperatively. Those who are unwilling or unable to perform intermittent catheterization but can operate the labial pump may be considered for AUS implantation. When compared to the pubovaginal sling, the AUS is less likely to cause permanent urinary retention. Following decompression of the cuff, the bladder may be emptied by Credé maneuvers. These patients should be carefully selected, demonstrating preoperatively a clear ability to empty via abdominal strain.

Women of childbearing age are eligible for sphincter implantation. Many investigators believe that if the patient becomes pregnant, the device should be deactivated in the third trimester to diminish excessive pressure on the cuff and bladder neck. If the situation will not allow for deactivation throughout the third trimester, it should be deactivated during labor and delivery to permit bladder emptying. There is no contraindication to cesarean section as the components are within the retropubic space.[6]

TRANSVAGINAL IMPLANTATION

The advantage inherent in the transvaginal approach for AUS cuff placement, compared with a purely abdominal approach, is the accessibility of the poorly defined urethrovaginal plane. The dissection of this plane is even more difficult following one or more anti-incontinence procedures, and direct visualization during the procedure can be helpful. A controlled surgical entrance and optimal closure of the anterior vaginal wall eliminates the need for dissection of this difficult plane from within the retropubic space, eliminating the risk for an inadvertent and potentially unrecognized injury to the vaginal wall.[7,8]

The patient is admitted to the hospital on the day of the operation. Preoperative broad-spectrum antibiotics are administered parenterally at least 1 hour prior to surgery. Following the administration of regional or general anesthesia, the patient is placed in the dorsal lithotomy position. The lower abdomen and vagina are shaved and prepared with a 10-minute scrub with povidone-iodine (Betadine) or Hibiclens solution. A posterior-weighted vaginal retractor is placed for exposure of the anterior vaginal wall. Lateral labial retraction sutures or a Lone-Star retraction system can be utilized for retraction of the labia. A 14 Fr Foley catheter is inserted in sterile fashion and the bladder is drained.

A midline incision is made in the anterior vaginal wall. The incision should extend from a point midway between the bladder neck and urethral meatus to the proximal bladder neck (Fig. 66.2). With sharp dissection, a plane under the vaginal wall is created on each

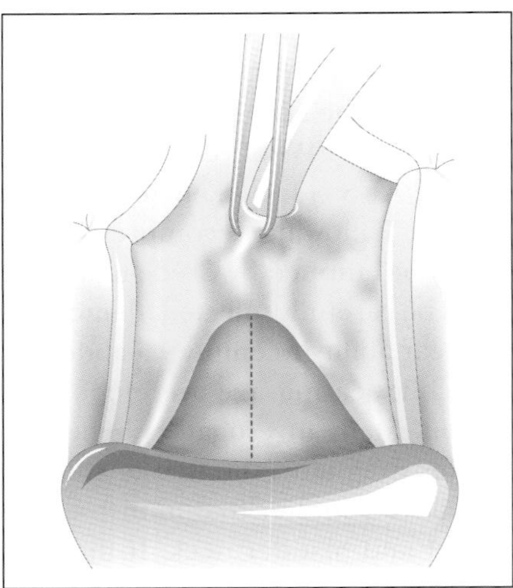

Figure 66.2. *With the patient in the dorsal lithotomy position, a midline vaginal incision is performed.*

side of the incision. Sufficiently thick vaginal flaps are created in anticipation of closure of the vagina over the AUS cuff. If the patient has not had a prior procedure involving dissection around the bladder neck, blunt finger dissection may be used to separate the endopelvic fascia from its lateral attachments to the pubic rim. The fascia should be swept from lateral to medial, creating a window into the retropubic space (Fig. 66.3). In cases of prior operations, the retropubic space should be entered sharply, using Metzenbaum scissors positioned against the pubic symphysis pointed in the direction of the ipsilateral shoulder. Once the retropubic space is entered bilaterally, the urethra and bladder neck can be separated posteriorly and laterally from the vagina and pelvic sidewall utilizing a combination of sharp and blunt dissection.

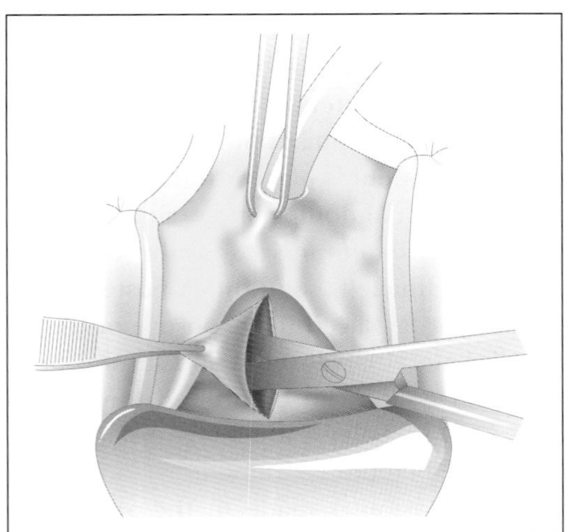

Figure 66.3. *Using a combination of sharp and blunt dissection, the vaginal mucosa is dissected off the underlying tissues and the retropubic space is entered bilaterally.*

Attention should then be directed to the anterior aspect of the proximal urethra and bladder neck to free the attachments from the pubic symphysis. If possible, blunt finger dissection through the vaginal incision should be used to perform this part of the procedure. In the patient who has had a previous retropubic operation, dense scarring may be encountered in this area, making this dissection particularly difficult. To facilitate exposure of the dorsal urethra, a separate suprameatal incision (1–2 cm) may be used (Fig. 66.4a).[9] Through this incision, sharp dissection can be performed in the midline below the pubic symphysis (Fig. 66.4b). After the bladder neck and urethra are separated from the pubic symphysis, lateral blunt dissection can be performed to complete the dissection to the retropubic space previously opened through the initial vaginal incision. Overly aggressive dissection during this stage of the procedure may lead to unintentional bladder or urethral tear. If

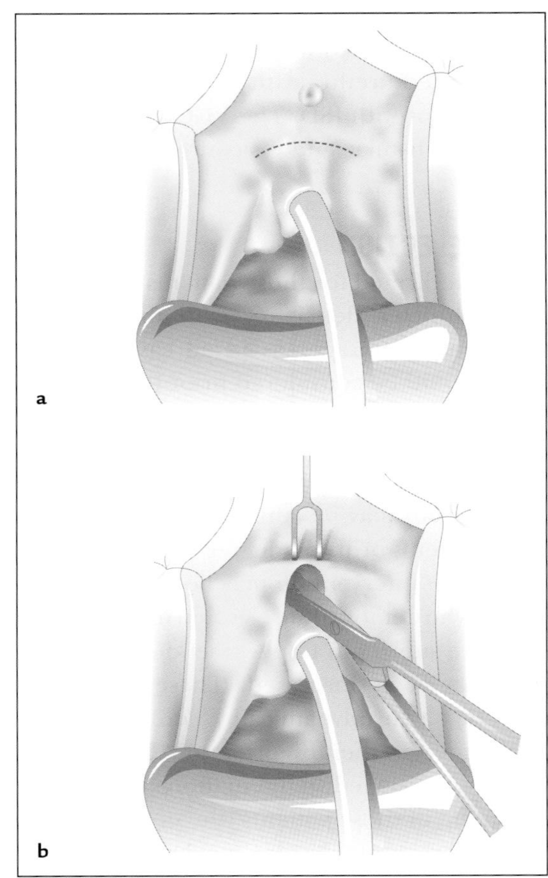

Figure 66.4. *(a) If dense scarring is encountered anterior to the urethra, a separate incision can be made above the urethral meatus. (b) The suprameatal dissection is performed in the midline, just below the pubic symphysis.*

this occurs, conventional wisdom may dictate that the procedure be abandoned. However, Salisz and Diokno reported on successful repair of this type of injury with subsequent successful implantation of the device.[10]

After the proximal urethra and bladder neck have been freed circumferentially, a right-angle clamp is passed around the urethra from left to right. The cuff measuring tape is grasped and passed around the bladder neck and the circumference of the bladder neck is measured. If the circumference is equivocal, it is best to err in favor of a slightly larger cuff size. Using a right-angle clamp, the appropriate sized cuff is placed around the bladder neck (Fig. 66.5). If the AUS pump is to be placed into the right labum majus, the cuff should be drawn from right to left, and vice-versa. The cuff is then locked in place and rotated 180 degrees so that the locking button of the cuff lies anteriorly, away from the anterior vaginal wall (Fig. 66.6).

On the side on which the pressure-regulating balloon and pump mechanism are to be implanted, a transverse suprapubic incision (approximately 4 cm) is made. A straight clamp is passed under fingertip guidance from the suprapubic incision lateral to the midline down to the ipsilateral side of the vaginal incision. The cuff tubing is grasped and the clamp is withdrawn, pulling the tubing up into the suprapubic incision. Shods (rubber sleeves) should be utilized during this phase of the procedure to ensure that the end of the tubing is not open to the field. The anterior rectus sheath is then incised vertically and the retropubic space is developed adjacent to the bladder. The pressure-regulating balloon is inserted into this space. The reservoir may be selected to be in the 50–70 cm H_2O pressure range, and may contain 22–25 cm H_2O. The choice of apropos pressure and volume is dependent on surgeon preference and patient specific factors (such as degree of urethral atrophy and history of pelvic radiation etc.)

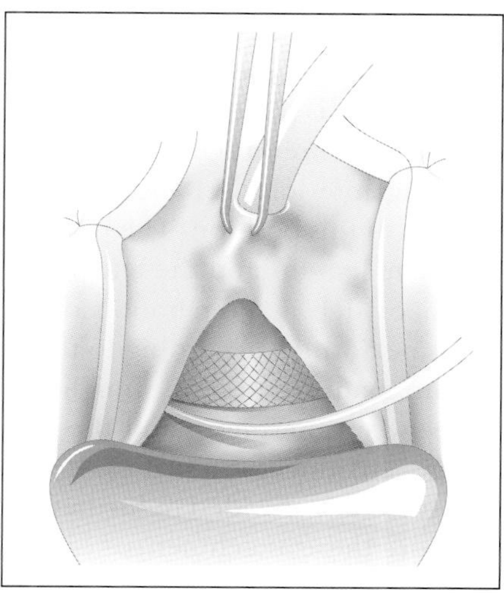

Figure 66.6. *The cuff is rotated 180 degrees clockwise so that the locking button lies anterior to the urethra, away from the anterior vaginal wall.*

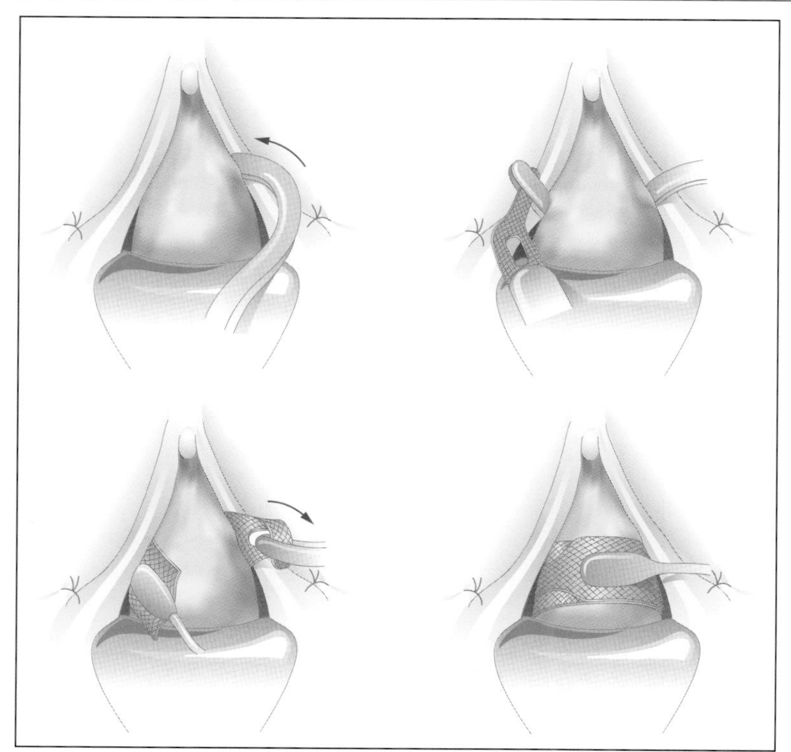

Figure 66.5. *The cuff of the artificial urinary sphincter is passed around the bladder neck and locked into place.*

From the suprapubic incision, a subcutaneous tunnel into the labium majus is created with blunt and sharp dissection. The pump is passed into the labium majus to rest at the level of the urethral meatus with the deactivation button facing anteriorly. A Babcock clamp is used to secure the pump in this position. The tubing is trimmed to the appropriate lengths and the ends are irrigated to remove any air or debris. Preparation of the cuff and the reservoir is performed according to the instructions specified by the manufacturer. A straight connector is then placed between the pump and the balloon reservoir. A right-angle connector attaches the pump to the cuff. Quick connectors provided in the implantation kits are used to secure these attachments.

The suprapubic and vaginal incisions are irrigated copiously with antibiotic solution. The wounds are then closed in several layers with absorbable sutures to ensure coverage of implanted materials with healthy tissue. If the integrity of the anterior vaginal wall is in question, the interposition of a vascularized flap (e.g. Martius flap) should be considered. Following closure, vaginal packing is placed. Prior to awakening the patient, deactivation of the AUS cuff should be ensured.

The vaginal packing and Foley catheter can be removed on the first postoperative day. The cuff should be left in the deactivated position for a period of 6 weeks.

TRANSABDOMINAL IMPLANTATION

Some centers favor the transabdominal approach for its easy access to the retropubic space and lack of an anterior vaginal wall incision.[11] As in the transvaginal approach, the patient should be admitted to hospital on the day of the procedure and should receive parenteral broad-spectrum antibiotics 1 hour prior to the start of the operation. Following induction of anesthesia, the patient should be placed in the dorsal lithotomy position allowing access to both the abdomen and vagina. The abdominal wall and vagina should be shaved and a 10-minute skin preparatory scrub should be performed. A 14 Fr Foley catheter is placed and the bladder drained.

A lower midline or Pfannenstiel incision should be made to allow appropriate access to the retropubic space. The incision is carried down through the fascial layers, and the retropubic space is developed using a combination of sharp and blunt dissection. This dissection can be complicated in those patients who have had prior pelvic procedures. In cases where the space does not develop easily, the dissection should follow the posterior face of the pubic bone, trying not to injure the anterior bladder wall. Repair of any cystotomy should be performed with absorbable sutures.

As the dissection approaches the bladder neck, it should proceed laterally and may be facilitated by a finger or sponge stick in the vagina (Fig. 66.7). The bladder neck is located by palpation of the Foley catheter balloon and the endopelvic fascia is entered approximately 2 cm on either side of the bladder neck. The dissection of the vesicovaginal plane is continued through the periurethral fascia until the vagina is completely visible. The bladder neck is then dissected from the vagina below the periurethral fascia in both directions at the level of the catheter balloon. Extreme caution must be taken during these steps to avoid perforation of the vaginal wall. In extremely difficult cases, an intentional anterior cystotomy may aid in identification of the bladder neck and facilitate separation within the vesicovaginal plane. To verify the integrity of the bladder, it can be filled with sterile water dyed with methylene blue. Any inadvertent cystotomies may be repaired (preferably in multiple layers) with absorbable sutures. Any accidental perforations of the vaginal wall should be repaired directly. In cases of extensive injury, it may be advisable to convert to a pubovaginal sling. If AUS is determined to be the only option,

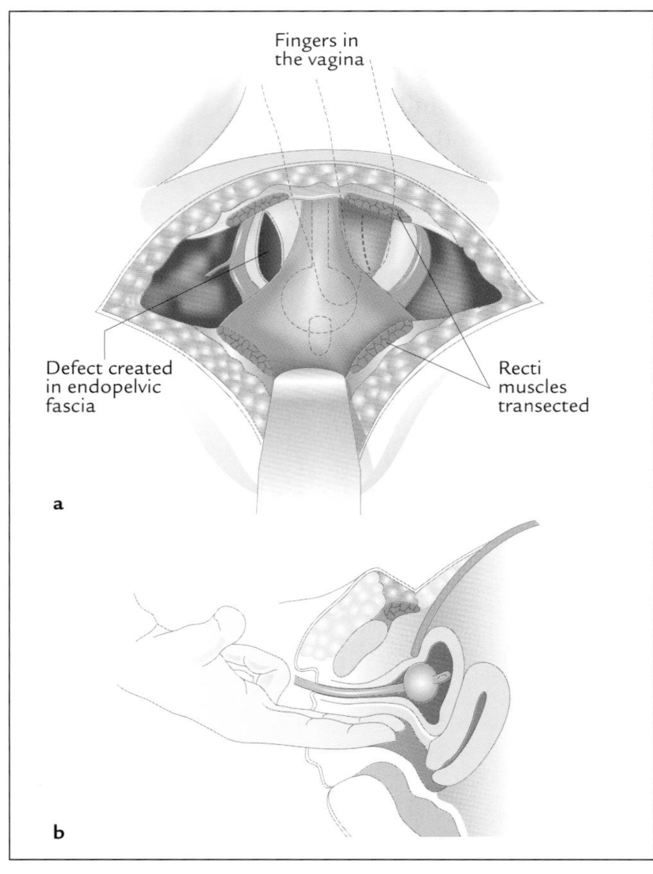

Figure 66.7. *Aiding the dissection with an intravaginal finger: (a) frontal view; (b) lateral view.*

it is preferable to implant the cuff and close the vaginal wall following the interposition of a Martius flap.

When the bladder neck has been freed circumferentially, the cuff sizer is used, again taking care to choose the larger size in cases of intermediate measurement. The appropriate sized cuff is drawn around the bladder neck with a right-angle clamp and positioned so that the locking button lies on the opposite side from the labium majus in which the pump is to be placed (Fig. 66.8).

The appropriate pressure-regulating reservoir is chosen as previously described. The balloon is placed on the same side as the labium majus where the pump will be placed. The system is primed and filled as previously described. A subcutaneous tunnel is created from the suprapubic incision down into the labium majus using sharp and blunt dissection. The pump is placed in the labium majus to rest at the level of the urethral meatus with the deactivation button facing anteriorly. A Babcock clamp is utilized to hold the pump in place. An absorbable suture can be placed within the tunnel to prevent migration.

The tubing is then connected as described previously. The cuff is deflated and the device is deactivated. Following inspection for adequate hemostasis, the wound is copiously irrigated with antibiotic solution. The abdominal incision is then closed without drainage. Figure 66.9 illustrates the device in place.

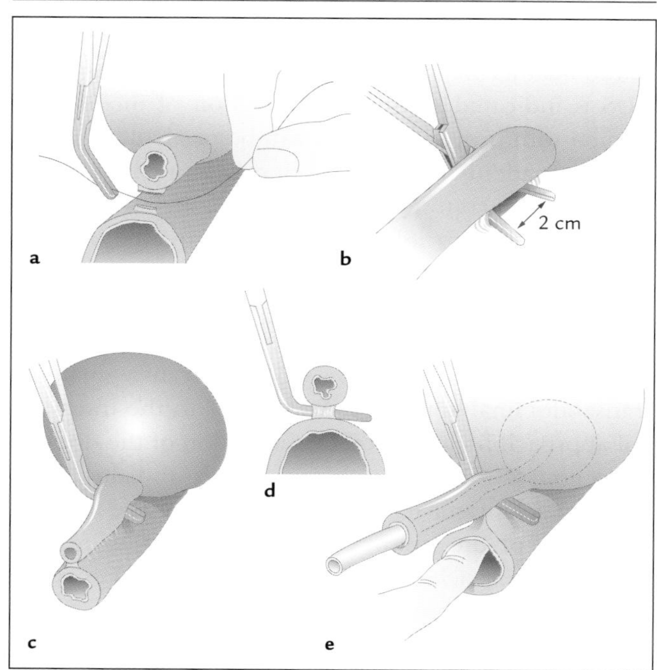

Figure 66.8. *(a, b) Insertion of right-angle clamp; (c, d) right-angle clamp in place; (e) clamp, catheter and finger in position.*

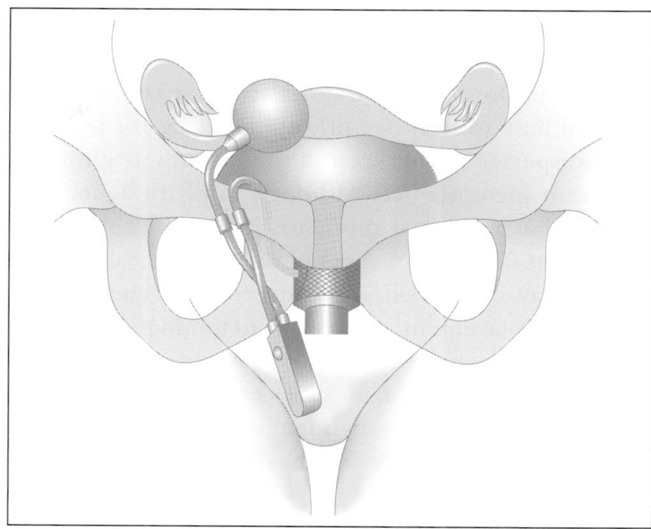

Figure 66.9. *Artificial urinary sphincter in place.*

The Foley catheter can be withdrawn on the first postoperative day. In cases of accidental or intentional cystotomy, a longer period of catheter drainage is preferred. The device is left in a deactivated position for a period of 6 weeks.

COMPLICATIONS

Complications associated with AUS implantation include intraoperative injury to the bladder, urethra or vaginal wall, device failure, erosion, and infection.

When a number of risk factors for explantation were compared, including patient age, type and number of prior procedures, time lapsed between last procedure and AUS implantation, and perioperative injury, Costa et al. found the only significant factor to be perioperative injury. Of 49 patients who had perioperative injuries, eight explantations resulted, compared with only four in the 155 cases that did not have injuries.[12] Major intraoperative complications can be minimized with meticulous surgical technique. Recognized injuries should be repaired primarily under direct visualization with the interposition of well-vascularized tissues if necessary. In many cases, inadvertent injury to the bladder, urethra, or vaginal wall should not preclude implantation of the device. Good surgical judgment should be utilized to determine the safety of completing the procedure.

With improvements in the design and manufacture of the device, AUS malfunctions have decreased significantly. Potential pitfalls included fluid loss secondary to tubing fracture at connection sites, cuff leakage at stress points, and kinking of the tubing. Some problems have resulted from the cuff mechanism itself. Atrophy of the periurethral tissues decreases the compressive bulk within the cuff, not allowing for pressure to be dispersed evenly around the urethra, resulting in recurrent incontinence. Although newly designed cuff backing has addressed this issue, it must be considered in cases of failure.[13] In cases of mechanical failure, the device may be revised. The surgeon's judgment concerning replacement of a malfunctioning portion of the device rather than the whole device is critical. Clear indications for complete replacement of the device include fluid leakage, which may allow foreign material into the system, or a device that has been in place for more than 3 years.[14]

Device erosion has decreased since the introduction of modified cuffs; however, it remains a concern with any foreign body implantation. Significant risk factors for erosions include perioperative injury, incorrect implantation technique, history of prior procedures, and infection.[12] Erosion of the sphincter cuff into the urethra is commonly associated with recurrent incontinence, although urinary tract infection may be the first and only symptom. Erosion of the cuff through the vaginal wall is associated with vaginal bleeding and discharge. Erosion of the pressure-regulating reservoir into the bladder is rare, and may present as a urinary tract infection or infection of the device. Pump erosion through the labium majus is diagnosed by direct examination.

Infection or erosion should be treated with explantation of the entire device in the majority of cases. Reimplantation may be considered after 4–6 months. In cases of cuff erosion into the urethra, the placement of an omental flap between the cuff and urethra is recommended at reoperation.

Experience with penile prosthesis implantation raises questions about the appropriateness of salvage procedures. In cases of erosion of the cuff into the urinary tract, salvage of the AUS is not recommended. In the isolated case of erosion of the sphincter tubing through the abdominal skin, or erosion of the pump through the labium, aggressive irrigation and debridement of the tissues may make replacement of certain AUS components and wound closure a possibility. When replacement of the pump is necessary, it should be moved to the opposite labium. The device with cuff erosion into the vaginal wall may be salvaged utilizing a Martius flap and vaginal wall closure. Before all salvage attempts, the patient should be counseled as to the high risk of eventual necessity for removal of the complete device.

RESULTS

Published data on success rates for implantation of the AUS in female patients are shown in Table 66.1. The average success rate ranges from 68% in a series of 31 women by Donovan et al.[15] to 100% in smaller series by Appell[1] and Abbassian.[9] In the largest series involving 207 patients, Costa et al. reported success rates of 88.7% and 81.8% in patients with non-neurogenic and neurogenic bladder, respectively.[12] A study comparing AUS and pubovaginal sling in 77 patients with confirmed ISD revealed favorable results for both procedures (84% versus 91%, respectively).[16]

Table 66.1 also includes the published complications from the same series. Infection was seen in 3–7% of cases. Erosions represented the most common complications, occurring in 7–29% of cases. Reoperation for cuff malfunction or tubing problems has been as high as 21% in earlier series;[17] however, there is a clear trend towards reduced numbers of device failures due to technologic advancements made over the years.

Long-term follow-up data for the AUS in women are sparse. Existing reports indicate that revision of the AUS is likely to be necessary 10 years after implantation for either mechanical or non-mechanical reasons.[3]

CONCLUSION

The use of the AUS in women is still rare compared to its use to treat male incontinence. The purpose of the AUS is to provide uniform circumferential compression of the bladder neck, without changing its position. The AUS is indicated in the subpopulation of incontinent women with proven ISD, and can be particularly useful in those patients who have undergone previous unsuccessful anti-incontinence procedures. In addition, in those women with ISD and a hypocontractile bladder, the AUS may be the initial treatment of choice over the sling due to its lower incidence of prolonged postoperative urinary retention.

The AUS may be placed via either a transvaginal or a transabdominal approach. Advantages to the transvaginal approach include direct visualization of the difficult dissection of the urethrovaginal plane, and the ability to make a suprameatal incision to assist in the anterior dissection of the urethra. Advantages of the transabdominal approach include lack of a vaginal incision and improved exposure to the endopelvic fascia and anterior bladder neck dissection. Additionally, transabdominal exposure allows the opportunity to perform a deliberate cystotomy to assist in a particularly difficult dissection. Regardless of operative approach, emphasis should be placed on meticulous surgical approach as

Table 66.1. *Success rates for implantation of the artificial urinary sphincter*

Author	No. of patients	Success	Complications	Revisions
Scott[18]	139	84%	3 infxn (3%) 4 erosions (4%)	
Light & Scott[19]	39	87% dry 5% 2–3 ppd	1 infxn (2.5%) 3 erosions (7%)	21 revisions (11 cuff malf)
Donovan[15]	31	68%	9 erosions (29%) 1 abuse (3%)	
Diokno et al.[17]	32	94% dry 3% improved	1 dehiscence (3%) 1 abscess (3%)	7 revisions (4 cuff malf)
Abbassian[9]	4	100% dry	0	0
Appell[1]	34	100% dry	0	3 revisions (2 cuff malf)
Duncan et al.[20]	29	52% improved	8 erosions (28%) 1 infxn (3.5%)	1 revision
Webster et al.[2]	25	92% dry 8% 1–2 ppd	1 postoperative death (4%)	4 revisions (3 cuff malf)
Costa et al.[21]	54	93% improved	3 erosions (6%) 1 infxn (2%)	
Hadley et al.[14]	18	89% dry	2 erosions (11%)	
Stone et al.[22]	54	84% dry 12% improved	4 lost to follow-up 3 erosions (6%) 2 unable to use (4%)	11 revisions
Costa et al.[12]	190	88% dry 8% improved	12 explants (5.9%)	

infxn, infection; malf, malfunction; ppd, pads per day.

intraoperative complications place the patient at risk for postoperative problems such as infection and erosion with eventual device explantation.

The success of the AUS compares well to the success of more traditional procedures for urinary incontinence. The data suggest that placement of the AUS is a safe and effective treatment option for the carefully selected patient with ISD.

REFERENCES

1. Appell RA. Techniques and results in the implantation of the artificial urinary sphincter in women with type III stress urinary incontinence by a vaginal approach. Neurourol Urodyn 1988;7:613–9.
2. Webster GD, Perez LM, Khoury JM et al. Management of type III stress urinary incontinence using artificial urinary sphincter. Urology 1992;39:499–503.
3. Fulford SC, Sutton C, Bales G et al. The fate of the 'modern' artificial urinary sphincter with a follow-up of more than 10 years. Br J Urol 1997;79:713–6.
4. Wilson TS, Lemack GE, Zimmern PE. Management of intrinsic sphincteric deficiency in women. J Urol 2003;169(5):1662–9.
5. Appell RA. Sphincter insufficiency: testing and treatment. Curr Opin Urol 1997;7:197–204.
6. Fishman IJ, Scott FB. Pregnancy in patients with the artificial urinary sphincter. J Urol 1993;150:340–1.
7. Wang Y, Hadley HR. Artificial sphincter: transvaginal approach. In: Raz S (ed) Female Urology, vol. 1, 2nd ed. Philadelphia: Saunders, 1996; 428–34.
8. Hadley R. Transvaginal placement of the artificial urinary sphincter in women. Neurourol Urodyn 1988;7:292–3.
9. Abbassian A. A new operation for insertion of the artificial urinary sphincter. J Urol 1988;140:512–3.
10. Salisz JA, Diokno AC. The management of injuries to the urethra, bladder or vagina encountered during difficult placement of the artificial urinary sphincter in the female patient. J Urol 1992;148:1528–30.
11. Long RL, Barrett DM. Artificial sphincter: abdominal approach. In: Raz S (ed) Female Urology, vol. 1, 2nd ed. Philadelphia: Saunders, 1996; 419–27.

12. Costa P, Mottet N, Rabut B et al. The use of an artificial urinary sphincter in women with type III incontinence and a negative Marshall test. J Urol 2001;165(4):1172–6.

13. Kowalczyk JJ, Mulcahy JJ. Use of the artificial urinary sphincter in women. Int Urogynecol J 2000;11:176–9.

14. Hadley R, Loisides P, Dickinson M. Long-term follow-up (2–5 years) of transvaginally placed artificial urinary sphincters by an experienced surgeon. J Urol 1995;153:432A [abstract 812].

15. Donovan MG, Barrett DM, Furlow WL. Use of the artificial urinary sphincter in the management of severe incontinence in females. Surg Gynecol Obstet 1985;161: 17–20.

16. Mark SD, Webster GD. Stress urinary incontinence due primarily to intrinsic sphincteric deficiency: experience with artificial urinary sphincter and sling cystourethropexy. J Urol 1994;151(Suppl);420A [abstract 769].

17. Diokno AC, Hollander JB, Alderson TP. Artificial urinary sphincter for recurrent female urinary incontinence: indications and results. J Urol 1987;138:778–80.

18. Scott FB. The use of the artificial urinary sphincter in the treatment of urinary incontinence in the female patient. Urol Clin North Am 1985;12:305–15.

19. Light JK, Scott FB. Management of urinary incontinence in women with the artificial urinary sphincter. J Urol 1985;134:476–8.

20. Duncan HJ, Nurse DE, Mundy AR. Role of the artificial urinary sphincter in the treatment of stress incontinence in women. Br J Urol 1992;69:141–3.

21. Costa P, Mottet N, Le Pellec L et al. Artificial urinary sphincter AMS 800 in operated and unoperated women with type III incontinence. J Urol 1994;151(Part 2):477A [abstract 1000].

22. Stone KT, Diokno AC, Mitchell BA. Just how effective is the AMS 800 artificial urinary sphincter? Results of long-term follow-up in females. J Urol 1995;153(Part 2):433A [abstract 817].

67

New technologies for stress urinary incontinence

Jay-James R Miller, Peter K Sand

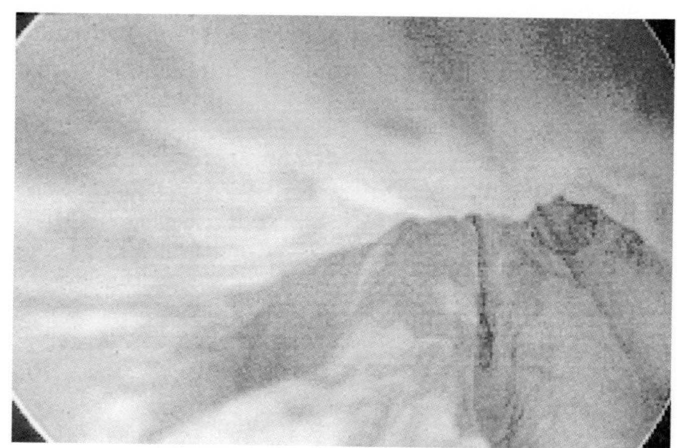

INTRODUCTION

New technologies in the treatment of stress urinary incontinence can be divided into two categories: revolutionary novel approaches and evolutionary improvements on existing therapies. Some evolutionary therapies are new bulking agents for periurethral injections, the prepubic tension-free vaginal tape, and the Remeex device; novel approaches include radiofrequency therapy and duloxetine pharmacotherapy.

EVOLUTIONARY THERAPIES

Some longstanding treatments for stress urinary incontinence – urethral bulking and suburethral slings – are increasing in popularity with technologic advances. These advances have improved efficacy while simultaneously decreasing known complications. Recent evolutionary examples include carbon coated zirconium beads (Durasphere) and the transobturator tape procedures. Presented here are the newest evolutions in stress urinary incontinence treatment.

Urethral bulking materials

Periurethral bulking to treat urinary incontinence is not new. It was first described more than 60 years ago to treat urinary incontinence. Current United States Medicare guidelines limit bulking agents to patients with intrinsic sphincter dysfunction (ISD). The ideal periurethral bulking agent would be non-reactive, permanent, non-migratory, and treat incontinence with a single injection without complication. The search for such an ideal bulking agent continues. There are several urethral bulking materials currently under investigation with the aim of providing an effective, durable, biocompatible, and safe agent. These new agents include calcium hydroxylapatite, autologous chondrocytes, autologous stem cells, ethylene vinyl alcohol co-polymer, and dextranomer/hyaluronic acid co-polymer.

Perhaps the best-studied agent is calcium hydroxylapatite. It is a normal constituent in bone and remains pliable after its injection into soft tissues.[1] It is easily injected, radiopaque, non-immunogenic, and non-inflammatory.[2] In an early study of 10 women with ISD who were treated with injection of 3.9 ml of calcium hydroxylapatite, three were cured and four were significantly improved at 1 year.[3]

Sand et al.[2] recently reported on a multicenter prospective randomized trial comparing calcium hydroxylapatite to bovine collagen. The interim analysis showed that calcium hydroxylapatite was as easy to inject as bovine collagen, did not require antigenicity testing and provided greater improvement in Stamey grades, pad weight reduction, and leakage reduction (Table 67.1). Durability of treatment with calcium hydroxylapatite as compared to bovine collagen was demonstrated by the maintenance of the outcomes when the 6-month data were compared to the 12-month data. Long-term follow-up showed no evidence of ossification or interference with subsequent surgery, if required, with calcium hydroxylapatite.

Autologous chondrocytes, harvested from ear cartilage, can be readily grown in cell culture and have been injected for childhood ureterovesical reflux with preliminary success and a favorable risk profile.[4] Bent et al.[5] used autologous chondrocytes harvested from auricular cartilage in the treatment of 32 women with type III incontinence. All patients received a single injection distal to the bladder neck. Incontinence severity grading indicated that 16 women were dry and 10 improved at 12 months postinjection. Eighty-one percent of the women were dry or improved. There was also significant improvement in pad weight tests and quality of life scores after treatment. In women who were dry post-treatment, the mean pad weight decreased from 22.4 to 0.1 g (p<0.001). The Urogenital Distress Inventory declined for all categories except bladder emptying and lower abdominal pain. One woman had prolonged urinary retention requiring self-catheterization for 4 weeks but there were no serious adverse events. Periurethral injection of autologous chondrocytes appears to be safe, effective, and durable

Table 67.1. *Calcium hydroxylapatite versus collagen at 6 and 12 months after injection*

	Improvement (%) (1 Stamey grade)	Improvement (%) (to Stamey grade 0)	No wet pads (%)	*n*
CaHA (6 months)	81*	49	49	45
Collagen (6 months)	62	48	48	43
CaHA (12 months)	80†	63	41	32
Collagen (12 months)	57	39	31	29

* p=0.0447; † p=0.0281; CaHA, calcium hydroxylapatite.

with 50% of the patients dry at 12 months after one injection.

Frauscher et al.[6] recently treated five female patients who had stress urinary incontinence with ultrasound-guided injections of autologous myoblasts and fibroblasts. Skeletal muscle biopsies were taken from the left arm to obtain cultures of autologous myoblasts and fibroblasts. Both transurethral and three-dimensional ultrasound were used to investigate the lower urinary tract and direct the injections. The fibroblasts were mixed with collagen as a carrier for the cells and injected into the urethral submucosa to treat atrophy of the urothelium, while the myoblasts were injected directly into the striated urethral rhabdosphincter to reconstruct the muscle. Urinary incontinence was cured in all five patients 1 year after injection of autologous stem cells and quality of life was significantly improved postoperatively. Transurethral ultrasound showed a significantly increased thickness of the urethra and rhabdosphincter. Contractility of the rhabdosphincter was also improved as measured by electromyography after therapy.

Uryx is an injectable solution of ethylene vinyl alcohol (EVOH) dissolved in dimethyl sulfoxide (DMSO). Upon contact with an aqueous environment the DMSO dissipates and the EVOH solidifies as a soft spongy mass which can be utilized as a bulking agent. The injected volume remains fixed and is equivalent to the final volume. The intraurethral bulking volume does not migrate or otherwise change with time. In one study,[7] Uryx made more subjects continent than Contigen while injecting a lower mean volume (Table 67.2). There were no unanticipated or unique complications associated with EVOH injection. The three most prevalent complications in both treatment groups were delayed voiding, dysuria, and frequency. The majority of complications occurred early and resolved rapidly.

Stenberg et al.[8] originally reported on dextranomer/hyaluronic acid co-polymer as a biocompatible material for urethral injection in 1998. These authors subsequently reported 5-year follow-up data[9] and now this material is being used in the novel Zuidex system (Fig. 67.1). This system allows for placement of the bulking agent without endoscopic guidance at four sites in the proximal urethra. Long-term follow-up was available for 16 of the 20 patients included in the original study (four were deceased from causes unrelated to the procedure). Three (15%) failed to respond to treatment and four (25%) others experienced recurrence of incontinence. A sustained response was noted

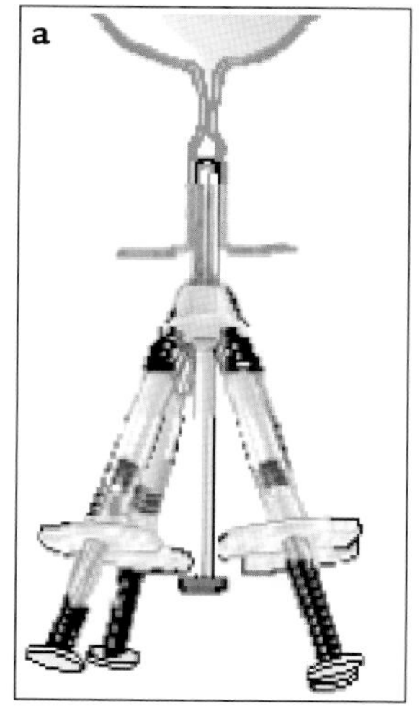

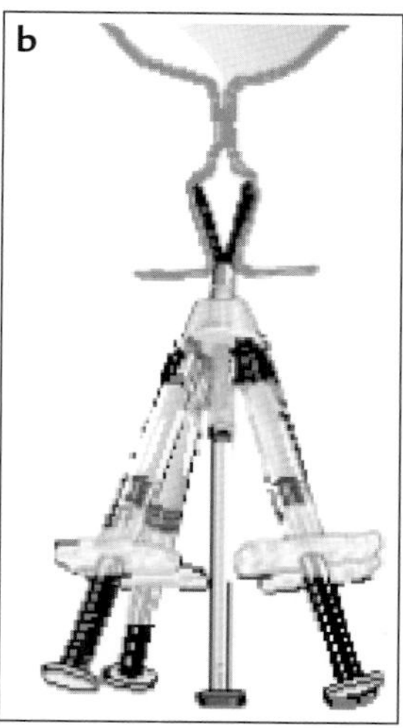

Figure 67.1. *Zuidex system. (a) The patient is prepared as for cystoscopy and appropriate analgesia is administered. The length of the urethra is measured before introducing the implacer (with the tube covering the needles) so that top of tube is located at the level of the midurethra. The tube should not move backward during insertion, so pressure must be applied on rear end of the tube during insertion. (b) The tube is pulled back to release the needles within the urethra. A firm grip on the handpiece is maintained as one syringe is retracted 5–10 mm and then pushed forward to its bottom position in order to penetrate the mucosa. The contents of syringe are injected and the emptied syringe is left in place. The maneuver is repeated clockwise with the three remaining syringes. The syringes with needles are removed one by one and finally the implacer is removed. (Courtesy of Q-Med, Uppsala, Sweden.)*

Table 67.2. *Uryx versus Contigen at 12 months after injection*

	Improvement (%) (to Stamey grade 0)	Improvement (%) (>50% I-QoL scores)	Dry pad weights (%)
Uryx (all patients)	34	32	68
Contigen (all patients)	33	20	44
Uryx (1–2 injections)	45	–	72
Contigen (1–2 injections)	27	–	36

in nine patients (57%), five (32%) of whom remained dry.[9]

Prepubic tension-free vaginal tape procedure

Although the tension-free vaginal tape (TVT) procedure is a relatively safe and straightforward procedure, it is not without risk; for example, during the blind passage of the needle in the retropubic space, perforation of the bladder, vessels, nerves, or intestine may occur. Patients who have been operated on previously may have adhesions that increase the risk of visceral perforation. In an effort to avoid these potential complications the transobturator systems have been developed. A prepubic TVT alternative has also been developed[10] in which the conventional TVT needles are placed superficial to the pubic bone (Fig. 67.2).

After placing the needles, the procedure for tensioning the tape is slightly different from that used in conventional TVT operations. The plastic sheath covering the polypropylene mesh is first removed only on one side. Scissors or forceps are then placed between the urethra and the tape. The tape is then adjusted by pulling on the side where the plastic sheath has not been removed. It takes greater force to adjust the tape than with a conventional TVT operation because the axis of the tape is

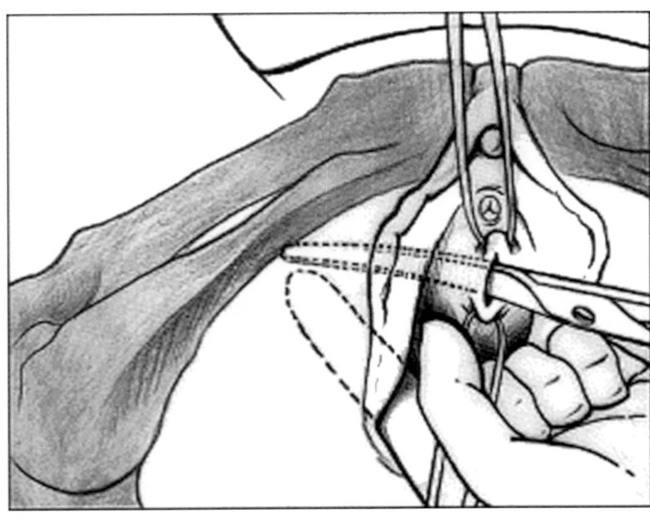

a

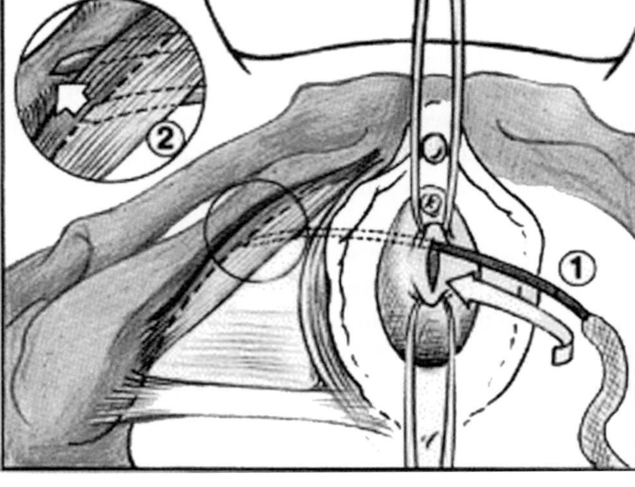

b

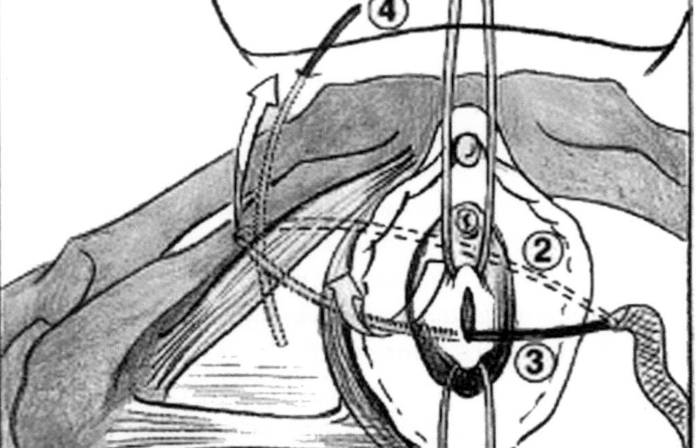

c

Figure 67.2. *Prepubic sling. The surgical procedure is carried out under local, spinal or general anesthesia. The technique uses the conventional tension-free vaginal tape (TVT) kit, except that the handle is not attached to the TVT needles (i.e. it is hand-held). (a) The vaginal incision is made 0.5–1 cm more proximal to the midurethra than with the conventional TVT procedure. The paraurethral space is developed as with the conventional TVT, but then the dissection is directed more laterally toward the mid-ischiopubic bone. (b) When the bone is reached, the TVT trocar is introduced into the dissected periurethral space* a. *With the trocar tip aiming laterally, the ischiocavernosus muscle is perforated together with the superficial perineal fascia. This is done with the trocar tip in close contact with the pubic bone (see insert* b*). (c) When the muscle has been perforated, the trocar tip is angled straight up and the needle is passed under the vulva to the ipsilateral skin incision* c. *The suprapubic incision is the same as with the conventional TVT. The other trocar is then passed on the contralateral side of the urethra* d. *The ends of the tape are cut just as with the conventional TVT procedure. (Reproduced from ref. 10 with permission.)*

more horizontal and anterior. The final tension under the midurethra should be the same as the conventional TVT operation. The remaining plastic sheath can now be removed and the tape ends cut in the subcutaneous layer. The vaginal and abdominal incisions are then closed. Since the bladder cannot be perforated, cystoscopy is not necessary with the prepubic TVT procedure. The mean operative time is 18 minutes.[10] The postoperative instructions are the same as those given to patients after a conventional TVT procedure.

Daher and colleagues recently published their experience with 74 consecutive patients who underwent prepubic TVT.[10] The mean postoperative follow-up was 5 months. Sixty (81%) of the patients were cured of stress urinary incontinence and another 10 patients (13%) were improved. There were four (6%) failures. Subjects who failed the procedure were incontinent within 2 months of surgery and there were no late recurrences. Postoperative retention was defined as post-void residual greater than 100 ml and was observed in three subjects. No patient suffered from de novo detrusor overactivity or had significant intraoperative bleeding defined as greater than 200 ml. Eleven patients complained of discomfort when sitting immediately after the procedure, but this symptom abated in all eleven within 7 days postoperatively. Some ecchymoses were noted in nine subjects after the procedure. The vaginal epithelium was perforated twice when introducing the needle tip lateral to the pubic bone. Both times it was noticed intraoperatively and the trocars were reinserted without any postoperative healing problems.[10]

Externally readjustable sling

Some researchers have attempted to develop a device that would allow for adjustment of the suburethral tension of a sling with the aim of reducing postoperative urinary retention without decreasing its ability to treat stress urinary incontinence effectively. A Spanish group reported on a device and method that permits readjustment of sling tension, both intraoperatively and during the postoperative period.[11] The method uses a device called Remeex, taken from the Spanish initials for mechanical external regulation – REgulación MEcánica EXterna (Fig. 67.3).

The suburethral support is placed through a vaginal incision and the traction threads are guided through into the retropubic space where they are first passed through the varitensor. The sutures are passed through a previously made 4 cm suprapubic incision and are finally wound up by turning the manipulator clockwise. Tension-free placement is assured by placing two fingertips between the rectus fascia and the varitensor. The external manipulator is left protruding from the suprapubic incision as it is closed.

After the operation, the device is tensioned by rotating the external manipulator until urinary leakage with increased intra-abdominal pressure disappears in the patient with a full bladder. The patient is then asked to urinate. If she has more than 100 ml of residual volume, then the external manipulator is rotated counterclockwise while simultaneously applying pressure to the suburethral support with either a urethral dilator or cystoscopy sheath. Suburethral pressure readjustment is repeated until the patient is able to void easily without urinary leakage. When stress urinary incontinence has disappeared and the post-void residual is less than 100 ml, a 'disconnector' is placed inside the external manipulator. Rotating the disconnector counterclockwise separates the external manipulator from the varitensor, and both the disconnector and the external manipulator can be removed. If either stress urinary incontinence or urinary retention reappears, then the external manipulator can be reattached to the varitensor under local anesthetic and the tension readjusted.

The 113 subjects were followed for an average of 22 months after the Remeex procedure. Of these, 108 (95.5%) were objectively cured of their stress urinary incontinence. Fourteen subjects (12.3%) had either persistent or de novo urge urinary incontinence. Postoperative readjustment was required in 22 (19.4%) of the women: 15 (13.2%) because of slight persistence of stress urinary incontinence and seven (6.2%) because of voiding difficulty.[11]

Complications consisted of 15 women (13.2%) with bladder perforations, seven (6.1%) had wound seromas, four (3.5%) had wound infections, and one (0.8%) had a vaginal erosion. Five (4.4%) varitensors were removed in this series: four from the women with wound infections and one from an extremely thin patient who complained of suprapubic discomfort. In all of these cases the traction threads were tied one to the other. One (0.8%) suburethral component was removed for a vaginal erosion. There were no device malfunctions.[11]

Mantovani et al. reported a cure rate of 97% (31 of 32 subjects). Three subjects (9%) needed readjustment and one device (3%) was removed for infection.[12]

Early experience with the Remeex device has demonstrated success rates comparable to other synthetic slings but with a lower rate of urinary retention. The disadvantages are the complications of the varitensor: specifically, wound infection, seroma, and discomfort in thin subjects.

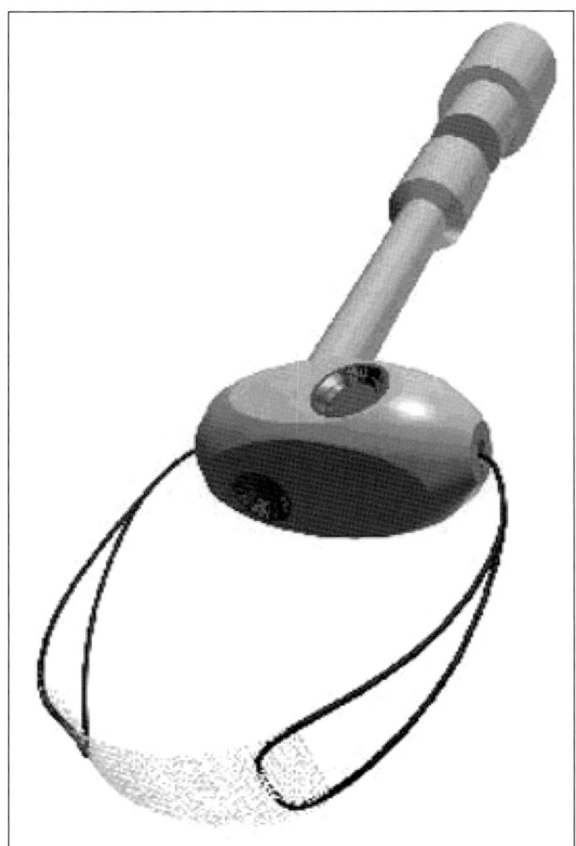

Figure 67.3. *Remeex system. The device is made up of two parts: a mechanical regulation unit and a urethral support sling. The mechanical regulation component is a subcutaneous permanent implant with a 'varitensor' that permits adjustment of sling support from outside the body by means of an 'external manipulator', a disposable part of the set that is removed once the desired continence level is achieved. The urethral support portion of the device is made of a short (3 × 1.5 cm) suburethral polypropylene monofilament sling attached to two non-resorbable polypropylene monofilament traction threads used to elevate or lower the sling support. (Courtesy of Neomedic International, Barcelona, Spain.)*

NOVEL APPROACHES

Improving existing treatments is important for medicine, but every once in a while there comes along a treatment that not only improves existing technology but also changes the face of a disease. The most recent of these advances to gain wide acceptance for the treatment of stress urinary incontinence is the TVT midurethral sling. This procedure was more than an evolution of the traditional sling. It not only introduced a tension-free and minimally invasive approach but also changed the sling position from the bladder neck to the midurethra. These departures from the traditional sling clearly made the TVT procedure a novel approach to treating stress urinary incontinence. Other treatment modalities as unique as the TVT are radiofrequency therapy and a new medication. Further research and greater clinical experience will be needed before it is known whether either treatment should be as widely accepted as the TVT.

Radiofrequency therapy

Radiofrequency energy is a form of electromagnetic energy that is reliable and highly controllable. This thermal therapy can produce well-defined areas of tissue heating. The technology has been used extensively in dermatologic and orthopedic surgery for tissue shrinkage and ablation. Radiofrequency thermal therapy is now being applied to the endopelvic connective tissue at the bladder neck and urethra for treating urethral hypermobility in patients with stress urinary incontinence with the Food and Drug Administration (FDA) approved SURx system. The mechanism of action is believed to be shrinkage of the collagenated tissue that supports the bladder neck and proximal urethra.

Fulmer and coworkers[13] reported using the SURx system via laparoscopy. The radiofrequency electrothermal probe is placed through a laparoscopic working trocar and positioned on the periurethral portion of the endopelvic connective tissue. Precisely controlled radiofrequency energy is applied to the endopelvic connective tissue, from an external generator, on either side of the urethra to heat and shrink the tissue. The average operative time was less than 60 minutes and 98% of the women were discharged home from the recovery room. Treatment surface area decreased an average of 17% in length and 21% in width. Preoperatively 41.2% of subjects reported using one pad or less daily, while at 1, 3, 6 and 12 months postoperatively 85.6%, 90.4%, 87.2%, and 86.9%, respectively, required one pad or less daily. Urodynamic evaluation at 12 months showed no leakage during the Valsalva maneuver in 78% of cases. There were no major postoperative complications and the minor complication rate was 5.3%.[13]

Dmochowski et al[14] reported on transvaginal radiofrequency treatment as a new outpatient modality for genuine stress incontinence with urethral hypermobility. The SURx transvaginal system (Fig. 67.4) was used to apply radiofrequency energy to the endopelvic connective tissue to induce its shrinkage, thereby stabilizing the proximal urethra and bladder neck. In 120 subjects with more than 1-year follow-up at 10 institutions, the average operative time was less than 30 minutes and all women were treated as outpatients.[14] Preoperatively 101 subjects (84%) averaged one or more episodes of urinary incon-

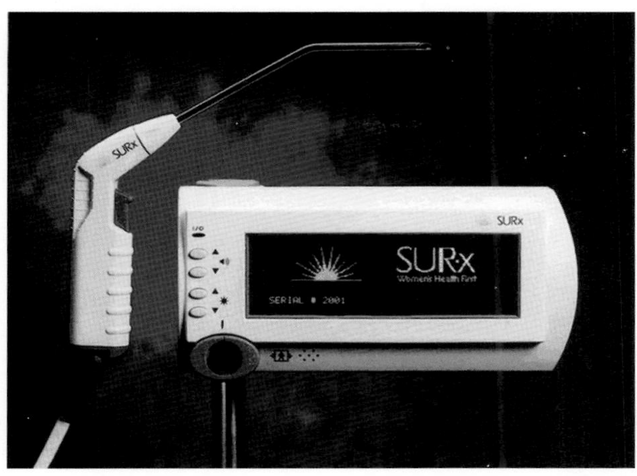

Figure 67.4. *Transvaginal SURx system. This system is composed of a small bipolar radiofrequency generator and a sterile, single-use disposable bipolar applicator that allows application of radiofrequency energy to the tissue. The applicator has a handle, trigger and a 270-degree rotational tip with microbipolar electrodes and a saline drip at the distal end of the probe to cool the tissue. There is a thermistor located between the electrodes for accurate monitoring of the treatment tissue temperatures. An electrode data collection device is used to collect automatically real-time device performance on 26 different treatment parameters during each procedure. Application of radiofrequency energy is accomplished by drawing the radiofrequency applicator tip over the connective tissue in a slow sweeping manner along the longitudinal axis, ensuring that both tines of the applicator tip are equally in contact with the connective tissue until all of the endopelvic connective tissue is treated. (Reproduced from ref. 14 with permission from Lippincott, Williams & Wilkins.)*

tinence per day. At 3, 6, and 12 months postoperatively 57%, 66%, and 59% of patients, respectively, averaged one or no daily episodes of incontinence. At 12 months, 79 of 109 (73%) women reported being continent or improved. A total of 30 cases were classified as failures and 11 women were lost to follow-up.[14] There were no intraoperative complications, three (4%) minor postoperative complications occurred which resolved, and no device-related complications were reported.[14]

Another more minimally invasive application of radiofrequency technology is in the Novasys micro-remodeling system which is a non-incisional, transurethral application of radiofrequency technology. The device is placed in the urethra similar to the placement of a Foley catheter and requires no visualization of the treatment site (Fig. 67.5). The Novasys system utilizes microscopic suburothelial radiofrequency energy to heat submucosal tissue to collagen remodeling temperatures (as opposed to higher ablation temperatures, which produce gross tissue shrinkage and cell destruction). Remodeling temperatures cause microscopic regions of the patient's own submucosal collagen to denature without significant associated necrosis or small vessel thrombosis. Upon cooling and healing, these minute regions of collagen renature in a significantly more compact, less compliant architectural pattern. Creation of a limited number of these microscopic collagen remodeling sites in a helical pattern around the proximal urethra and bladder neck results in reduced dynamic compliance so there is less bladder neck and proximal urethral mobility in the face of increased intra-abdominal pressure. Since the remodeling is so limited, there is no gross luminal narrowing or significant effect on static compliance. Proven safe and effective for the treatment of fecal incontinence,[15] anal fistula,[16] and gastroesophageal reflux disease,[17] radiofrequency tissue remodeling within the lower urinary tract may improve stress urinary incontinence.

A 12-month pilot study was performed to demonstrate the safety, effect on quality of life, effectiveness, and durability of a Novasys treatment.[18] The study enrolled 52 women with mild, moderate, or severe stress urinary incontinence and urethral hypermobility. There were no serious adverse events, no woman required catheterization at discharge, and recovery was rapid. At 6 and 12 months postoperatively, I-QoL scores had improved 78–82% and 70–82%, respectively, compared to baseline values. The proportion of 'dry' women at 12 months ranged from 22 to 67% in the different treatment groups.[18] The results suggest that radiofrequency tissue remodeling may safely improve the quality of life for women with mild, moderate, and severe stress urinary incontinence, and may offer physicians and stress urinary incontinence patients a safe, rapid, and effective therapeutic option. Because this simple procedure does not require cystoscopic assistance, it may allow a larger number of physicians to provide treatment for this common disorder.

Medication for stress urinary incontinence

New agents for the treatment of stress urinary incontinence are being sought worldwide. Most of the attention has focused on α-agonists with a high specificity for the urethral smooth muscle and selective serotonin–norepinephrine reuptake inhibitors. The serotonin–norepinephrine reuptake inhibitor class of antidepressants, and specifically duloxetine, have been shown to be beneficial in mild to moderate stress urinary incontinence when compared to placebo (Table 67.3).

Cardozo and colleagues[19] published a study showing duloxetine was superior to placebo for the treatment of

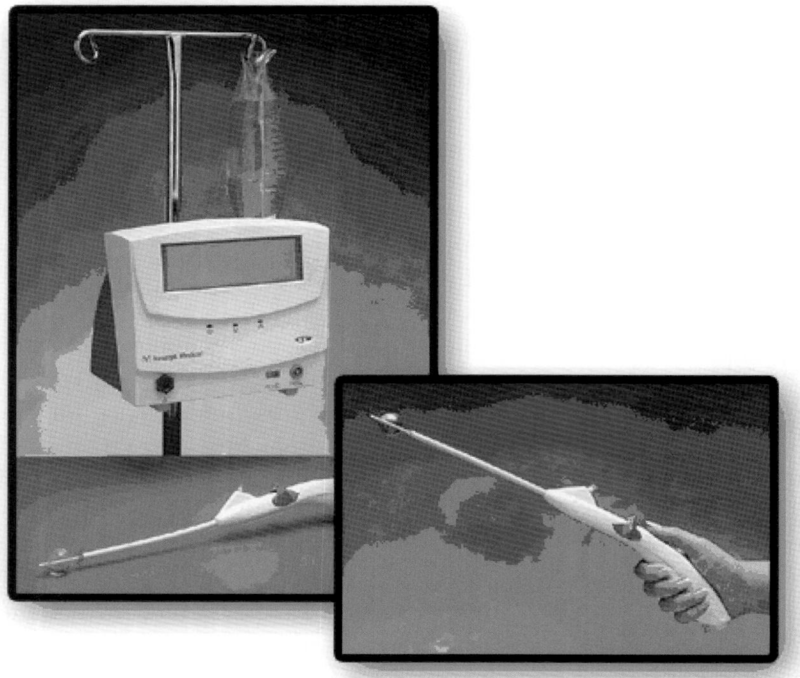

a

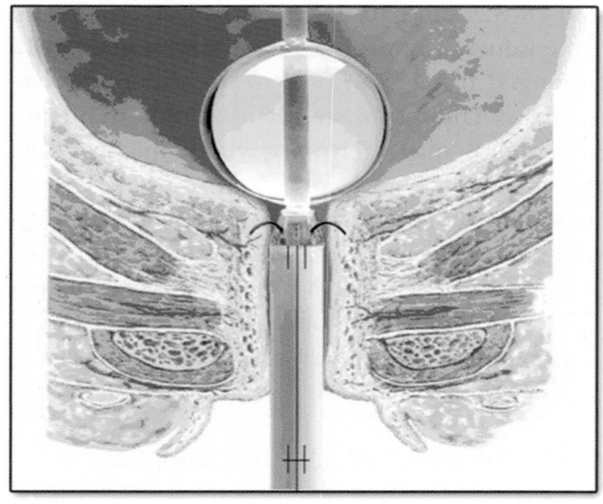

b

Figure 67.5. *Novasys Micro-Remodeling System. This catheter-based system uses radiofrequency energy to increase bladder outlet resistance without the need for surgery. (Courtesy of Novasys Medical, Inc., Newark, CA.)*

severe stress incontinence in women with pure urodynamic stress incontinence between the ages of 35 and 75 who were scheduled to have surgery.[19] At the conclusion of the 8-week study, ten women (22%) in the duloxetine group no longer wanted surgery, compared with none in the placebo group. Perhaps the most interesting finding was that duloxetine was equally effective in women both with and without a low-pressure urethra.[19]

The effectiveness of duloxetine in the treatment of stress urinary incontinence in women both with and without a low-pressure urethra is linked to its mechanism of action. It inhibits the presynaptic reuptake of

Table 67.3. *Median incontinence episode frequency decrease in duloxetine versus placebo*

Study	Duloxetine		Placebo		
	n	IEF (%)	*n*	IEF (%)	*p*-value
Millard et al.[24]	227	54	231	40	0.05
van Kerrebroeck et al.[23]	247	50	247	29	0.002
Cardozo et al.[19]	46	60	52	27	0.001
Dmochowski et al.[22]	344	50	339	27.5	0.001
Norton et al.[21]	137	59	138	41	0.002

IEF, median incontinence episode frequency decrease.

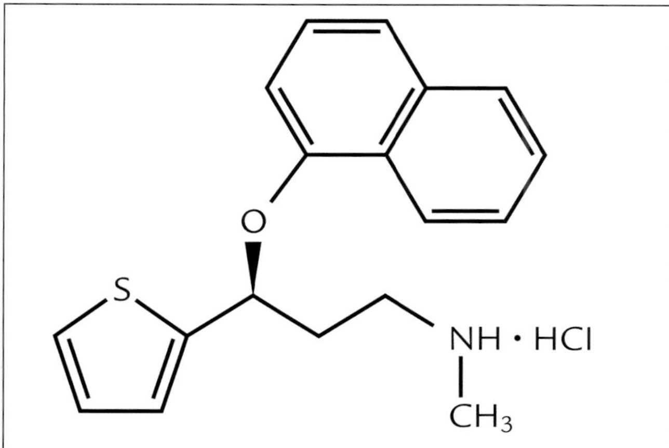

Figure 67.6. *Molecular structure of duloxetine.*

serotonin and norepinephrine in the motor neurons of the pudendal nerve, thereby increasing the amount of these neurotransmitters in the synapse. Since these synapses are in the sacral spinal cord (Onuf's nucleus), the effect is on the central nervous system. Animal studies have shown that increasing the serotonin and norepinephrine in the synapse led to increased pudendal stimulation of the urethral striated sphincter muscle.[20] These studies measured an eight-fold increase in electromyographic activity during bladder storage. Human female subjects with stress urinary incontinence probably benefit from a similar mechanism. In addition to stimulating the striated urethral sphincter, animal studies have shown that duloxetine most likely decreases bladder overactivity.[20]

The most commonly reported adverse events with duloxetine use were nausea, fatigue, dry mouth, insomnia, constipation, dizziness, and somnolence. After 4 weeks of treatment the incidence of side effects was similar to that of placebo.[21–24]

CONCLUSION

As the science of medicine continues to advance, so do the treatments for stress urinary incontinence. Some of these advancements will be major leaps like the TVT. Most, however, will be improvements like the transobturator tapes and Durasphere. It is important to study all of the new technologies presented in this chapter regardless of the long-term success of any because it is as important to be familiar with the failures as it is to know about the successes. Armed with this knowledge researchers will be less likely to revisit past mistakes and more likely to innovate successfully.

REFERENCES

1. Pettis GY, Kaban LB, Glowacki J. Tissue response to composite ceramic hydroxyapatite/demineralized bone implants. J Oral Maxillofac Surg 1990;48:1068–74.
2. Sand PK, Appell RA, Goldberg RP et al. Prospective randomized trial of calcium hydroxylapatite vs. bovine collagen for treatment of type III incontinence [abstract]. American Urogynecologic Society/Society of Gynecologic Surgeons Joint Scientific Meeting, San Diego, California, July 29–31, 2004.
3. Mayer R, Lightfoot M, Jung I. Preliminary evaluation of calcium hydroxylapatite as a transurethral bulking agent for stress urinary incontinence. Urology 2001;57:434–8.
4. Diamond DA, Caldamone AA. Endoscopic correction of vesicoureteral reflux in children using autologous ear chondrocytes: preliminary results. J Urol 1999;162: 1185–8.
5. Bent AE, Tutrone RT, McLennan MT et al. Treatment of intrinsic sphincter deficiency using autologous ear chondrocytes as a bulking agent. Neurourol Urodyn 2001;20:157–65.
6. Frauscher F, Klauser A, Zur Nedden D et al. Ultrasound-guided transurethral injection of adult stem cells for treatment of urinary incontinence: first clinical results [abstract]. 90th Scientific Assembly and Annual Meeting

of The Radiological Society of North America, Chicago, Illinois, November 28–December 3, 2004.

7. Dmochowski RR, Herschorn S, Corcos J et al. Multicenter randomized controlled study to evaluate Uryx urethral bulking agent in treating female stress urinary incontinence [abstract]. 98th Annual Meeting of the American Urological Association, Chicago, Illinois, April 26–May 1, 2003.
8. Stenberg A, Larsson G, Johnson P et al. DiHA dextran copolymer, a new biocompatible material for endoscopic treatment of stress incontinent women: short term results. Acta Obstet Gynecol Scand 1999;78:436–42.
9. Stenberg A, Larsson G, Johnson P. Urethral injection for stress urinary incontinence: long-term results with dextranomer/hyaluronic acid copolymer. Int Urogynecol J Pelvic Floor Dysfunct 2003;14:335–8.
10. Daher N, Boulanger JC, Ulmsten U et al. Pre-pubic TVT: an alternative to classic TVT in selected patients with urinary incontinence. Eur J Obstet Gynecol Reprod Biol 2003;107:205–7.
11. Sousa-Escandon A, Lema-Grille J, Rodriguez-Gomez JI et al. Externally readjustable device to regulate sling tension in stress urinary incontinence: preliminary results. J Endourol 2003;17:515–21.
12. Mantovani F, Castelnuovo C, Bernardini P et al. ReMeEx device (External Mechanical Regulator) for incontinence implantation and regulation procedure, complications and results: 3 years follow up. Arch Ital Urol Androl 2004;76:49–50.
13. Fulmer BR, Sakamoto K, Turk TM et al. Acute and long-term outcomes of radio frequency bladder neck suspension. J Urol 2002;167:141–5.
14. Dmochowski RR, Avon M, Ross J et al. Transvaginal radio frequency treatment of the endopelvic fascia: a prospective evaluation for the treatment of genuine stress urinary incontinence. J Urol 2003;169:1028–32.
15. Takahashi T, Garcia-Osogobio S, Valdovinos MA et al. Extended two-year results of radio-frequency energy delivery for the treatment of fecal incontinence (the Secca procedure). Dis Colon Rectum 2003;46:711–5.
16. Filingeri V, Gravante G, Baldessari E et al. Radiofrequency fistulectomy vs. diathermic fistulotomy for submucosal fistulas: a randomized trial. Eur Rev Med Pharmacol Sci 2004;8:111–6.
17. Bergman JJ. Gastroesophageal reflux disease and Barrett's esophagus. Endoscopy 2005;37:8–18.
18. Sotomayor M, Feria-Bernal G. Non-surgical, palpation-based outpatient treatment for stress urinary incontinence [abstract]. 33rd Annual Meeting of the International Continence Society, Florence, Italy, October 5–9, 2003.
19. Cardozo L, Drutz HP, Baygani SK et al. Pharmacological treatment of women awaiting surgery for stress urinary incontinence. Obstet Gynecol 2004;104:511–9.
20. Thor KB, Katofiasc MA. Effects of duloxetine, a combined serotonin and norepinephrine reuptake inhibitor, on central neural control of lower urinary tract function in the chloralose-anesthetized female cat. J Pharmacol Exp Ther 1995;274:1014–24.
21. Norton PA, Zinner NR, Yalcin I et al. Duloxetine versus placebo in the treatment of stress urinary incontinence. Am J Obstet Gynecol 2002;187:40–8.
22. Dmochowski RR, Miklos JR, Norton PA et al. Duloxetine versus placebo in the treatment of North American women with stress urinary incontinence. J Urol 2003;170:1259–63.
23. van Kerrebroeck PE, Abrams P, Lange R et al. Duloxetine versus placebo in the treatment of European and Canadian women with stress urinary incontinence. BJOG 2004;111:249–57.
24. Millard RJ, Moore K, Reneken R et al. Duloxetine versus placebo in the treatment of stress urinary incontinence: a four-continent randomized clinical trial. BJU Int 2004;93:311–8.

68

Diagnosis and treatment of obstruction following incontinence surgery – urethrolysis and other techniques

Chad Huckabay, Victor W Nitti

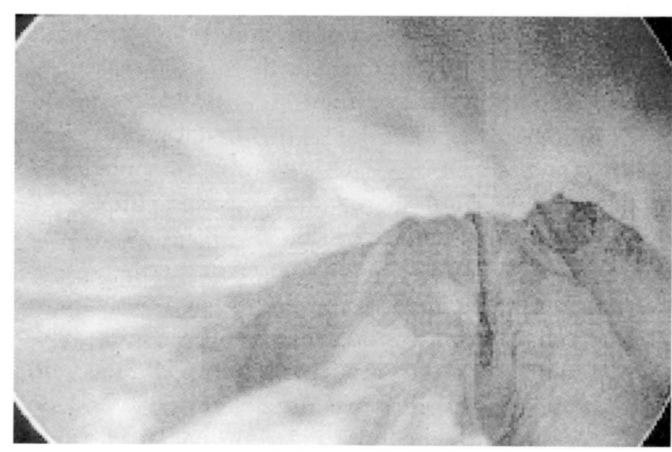

INTRODUCTION

The increasing use of incontinence procedures to treat stress urinary incontinence (SUI) will lead to a rise in the number of patients having postoperative voiding problems. The physician treating incontinence and performing interventions will need to recognize voiding dysfunction and difficulties promptly. Furthermore, an expedient diagnosis must be made in some circumstances, especially now that synthetic slings such as the tension-free vaginal tape (TVT) are commonplace. The management alternatives for problems after TVT are unique from historical management options for pubovaginal slings, and retropubic and transvaginal suspension procedures. The most important factor in reducing obstruction has probably been the appreciation that operations for SUI work by restoring support, not by changing the position of the urethra. Obstruction will unavoidably occur in 1–2% of patients even with the most practiced surgeons.

In this chapter we will explore the frequency of voiding dysfunction after incontinence surgery. The methods of diagnosis are delineated, but patient history remains the key. We will discuss diverse surgical techniques including urethrolysis by a variety of approaches, sling incision, and new less invasive methodologies applicable to midurethral synthetic slings.

INCIDENCE OF OBSTRUCTION AND VOIDING DYSFUNCTION AFTER STRESS INCONTINENCE SURGERY

The true incidence of voiding dysfunction and iatrogenic obstruction after incontinence surgery is unknown and likely underestimated. Estimates of 2.5–24% have been reported for various procedures.[1–5] In a 1997 review, the incidence of postoperative urgency for patients with no urgency and no detrusor overactivity before incontinence surgery was 8–16% (median CI: 11%) for retropubic suspensions, 3–10% (median CI: 5%) for transvaginal suspensions, and 3–11% (median CI: 7%) for sling procedures. For the same procedures, urinary retention longer than 4 weeks occurred in 3–7% (median CI: 5%), 4–8% (median CI: 5%), and 6–11% (median CI: 8%), respectively. The incidence of permanent retention for all three procedures was thought to be less than 5%.[6] Chaikin et al. found postoperative de novo urge incontinence in 3%, persistent urge incontinence in 23%, and unexpected permanent urinary retention in 2% of patients undergoing pubovaginal sling.[7] For the same procedure, Morgan and colleagues reported de novo urgency in 23% and de novo urge incontinence in 7%; five women had retention after 3 months requiring urethrolysis. Interestingly, they reported a 74% resolution of urge incontinence (although concomitant anterior colporrhaphy may have contributed, p=0.07) and return to normal voiding in 92% at 1 month postoperatively.[8] Reported rates of urinary retention after TVT have ranged from 1.4 to 9%.[9–15] Others have described rates of voiding dysfunction after TVT as being 2–4%.[16]

Dunn et al. recently performed an extensive literature review to determine the incidence of 'voiding dysfunction' after incontinence procedures.[17] They searched the Medline database from 1966 to 2001 for various procedures. All available data were retrospective collections, case reports or case cohort series. Rates of voiding dysfunction varied from 4 to 22% following Burch colposuspension, 5 to 20% following Marshall–Marchetti–Krantz (MMK) urethropexy, 4 to 10% following pubovaginal sling, 5 to 7% after needle suspension, and 2 to 4% following TVT. While it cannot be said that all patients with voiding dysfunction in these series were obstructed, it can be inferred that a number were.

Postoperative urgency occurs more frequently in patients with pre-existing urgency symptoms. The large review sponsored by the American Urological Association in 1997 suggested postoperative urgency occurred in 36–66% of these patients after retropubic suspensions, 54% after transvaginal procedures, and 34–46% after slings.[6]

ETIOLOGY

In general, voiding dysfunction after incontinence surgery is related to obstruction, detrusor overactivity, or impaired detrusor contractility. The risk of iatrogenic obstruction is usually related to technical factors. In a retropubic urethropexy, sutures placed too medial, close to the urethra, can cause urethral deviation or periurethral scarring. Sutures placed too distally can cause kinking with obstruction and an inadequately supported bladder neck/proximal urethra with potentially continued stress incontinence. If retropubic sutures are tied too tight, elevating the bladder neck toward the pubic bone excessively, this may result in overcorrection of the urethrovesical angle or 'hypersuspension'. With suburethral sling procedures, excessive tension on the sling around or under the urethra is usually responsible for obstruction. Less commonly, displacement of the sling from its intended position may result in obstruction. The same holds true for bladder neck and midurethral slings. We have noticed that excessive tension on a midurethral synthetic sling can result in the rolling of the sling into a tight band.

Kinking or angulation of the urethra, as well as external compression, may occur secondary to vaginal prolapse. This can result from prolapse that was not corrected (undiagnosed or ignored) at the time of incontinence surgery or from prolapse that occurred after (or as a result of) incontinence surgery. It is essential to examine and rule out apical, anterior or posterior prolapse as an etiology of urethral obstruction.

Occasionally, postoperative voiding dysfunction is caused by a learned voiding dysfunction (also termed dysfunctional voiding) or failure of relaxation of the striated urethral sphincter.[18] In these cases, patient education and sometimes biofeedback can be helpful. When the problem persists, botulinum A toxin injection into the urethral sphincter has been reported to be successful.[19] Finally, impaired detrusor contractility may be responsible for a 'relative obstruction' after incontinence surgery. Sometimes this can be diagnosed preoperatively and the patient may be warned of the possibility of voiding dysfunction after surgery.

PRESENTATION

The most obvious symptom/sign of obstruction is complete/partial urinary retention, and the inability to void continuously or the presence of a slow stream with or without intermittency. However, many women will present with predominate storage symptoms of frequency, urgency and urge incontinence, with or without voiding symptoms. The prevalence of various symptoms varies greatly according to different authors. While some authors report on cohorts with predominately obstructive symptoms or retention, others have shown the true variable nature by which obstruction presents. Carr and Webster reviewed the presenting symptoms in 51 women subsequently undergoing urethrolysis and found storage (irritative) symptoms (75%), voiding (obstructive) symptoms (61%), de novo urge incontinence (55%), need for intermittent catheterization (40%), persistent retention (24%), recurrent urinary tract infections (8%), and painful voiding (8%).[20] Suffice to say that in any case of de novo voiding and/or storage symptoms, the diagnosis of obstruction should at least be entertained.

IDENTIFYING RISKS FOR POSTOPERATIVE VOIDING DYSFUNCTION

Ideally, the surgeon would like to know who is at risk for postoperative voiding dysfunction. As with other aspects of voiding dysfunction following incontinence surgery, this problem has no definitive answer. Urodynamic studies have been investigated to determine any factors that may be predictive. Miller et al. noted that women undergoing allograft pubovaginal sling who voided with no or minimal detrusor pressure had a significantly increased risk of postoperative retention. Of 21 women with no or minimal detrusor contraction, four developed retention whereas no patient with a detrusor contraction developed retention postoperatively. The presence of Valsalva voiding in this study did not affect the incidence of postoperative retention.[21] Similarly, Weinberger and Ostergard in a study of 108 women undergoing synthetic suburethral slings found that the absence of detrusor contractions predicted delayed return to normal voiding. Valsalva voiding had no association with voiding dysfunction.[22] Bhatia and Bergman, reporting on a series of Burch cystourethropexies, cited patients who void with Valsalva maneuver (intra-abdominal pressures greater than 10 cmH_2O during voiding and detrusor pressures less than 15 cmH_2O) being at 12 times greater risk of needing prolonged catheterization.[23] Others have found that patients with preoperative Valsalva voiding or detrusor hypocontractility are more likely to report de novo urgency.[24] Wang and Chen noted that patients with preoperative dysfunctional voiding – defined as maximum free flow (NIQ_{max}) less than 12 ml/s and detrusor pressure at maximum flow ($p_{det}Q_{max}$) of ≥20 cmH_2O – were more likely to have a lower objective cure rate and lower quality of life scores after TVT than those with normal pressure–flow voiding dynamics.[25] The association of low voiding detrusor pressures and Valsalva voiding with subsequent voiding dysfunction has not been found in several other studies.[26,27] Pressure–flow studies are helpful in understanding the voiding dynamics of incontinent women; however, findings of low detrusor pressures or Valsalva voiding should not per se exclude patients from an anti-incontinence procedure.

DIAGNOSTIC EVALUATION

Transient voiding dysfunction and urinary retention are frequent and expected after many types of anti-incontinence surgery. This is the rationale behind concomitant placement of suprapubic tubes or teaching clean intermittent catheterization preoperatively. TVT and transobturator slings are an exception to this as retention and obstruction should not persist beyond a few days. After traditional pubovaginal sling (and variants) or colposuspension, most women will begin voiding sufficiently on their own within a few days to weeks while others may take longer to resume normal voiding. Storage symptoms such as urgency, frequency, and urge incontinence are often more refractory than retention because they can be related to bladder changes. Such symptoms can sometimes take months to resolve.

It has been common practice to delay evaluation of the patient with urinary retention or severe storage symptoms after pubovaginal sling, colposuspension or needle suspension for approximately 3 months postoperatively. Although this time frame is arbitrary, most data found in the literature are based on a waiting period of at least 3 months to allow adequate time for obstruction/ retention to resolve and to minimize the risk of recurrent stress incontinence. After 3 months, there is a very low probability that any persistent retention will resolve without intervention. More recently, some surgeons (including ourselves) have advocated earlier intervention in cases of complete retention; however, little data on outcomes and recurrence of stress incontinence are available. Few studies have focused on outcomes with respect to waiting a longer period before intervention. While it seems intuitive that longstanding symptoms (especially detrusor overactivity) will be less likely to respond to relief of obstruction the longer the patient is obstructed, this has not been proven conclusively. Leng et al. recently conducted a retrospective review of 15 women who underwent urethrolysis and found that patients with persistent symptoms postoperatively (n=8) had a significantly longer time from surgery to intervention than those who had no symptoms (n=7).[28] Mean time to urethrolysis was 31.25 ± 21.94 months versus 9 ± 10.1 months respectively. The large overlap, small sample size, and the fact that more patients in the successful group had urinary retention (5/7 versus 3/8) make it difficult to come to definitive conclusions. We have not excluded obstructed patients from intervention based on duration of obstruction.

The waiting period advocated for obstruction and retention for more traditional anti-incontinence procedures has been largely abandoned for TVT and TVT-like procedures. In theses cases quicker intervention is suggested when obstruction is suspected.[9,11,29,30] Due to the immobility of the polypropylene mesh and the tremendous ingrowth of fibroblastic tissue at 1–2 weeks, patients with severe symptoms or urinary retention are less likely to improve after this time period.

History and physical examination

The diagnostic evaluation of the patient with voiding dysfunction after incontinence surgery begins with a focused history and physical examination. Key points in the history are the patient's preoperative voiding status and symptoms, and the temporal relationship of the lower urinary tract symptoms to the surgery. The type of procedure performed and the number and type of other procedures done are also important. Urodynamic data such as uroflow and pressure–flow studies from before incontinence surgery are useful if available. If patients are straining to void (perhaps by habit), they should be instructed to stop this behavior, as incontinence procedures are designed to prevent the flow of urine with abdominal straining. Finally, it is important to determine if the symptom of stress incontinence persists.

The most obvious presenting symptom of obstruction after incontinence surgery is inability to void or intermittent retention. Patients may also experience voiding (obstructive) symptoms including slow or interrupted stream and straining to void. Storage (irritative) symptoms of urinary frequency, urgency, and urge incontinence which persist after surgery may also be a sign of obstruction, even if emptying is complete.

Physical examination may show overcorrection or hypersuspension where the urethra and urethral meatus appear to be pulled up toward the pubic bone and 'fixed'. The angle of the urethra becomes more vertical than is normal. When severe, this is usually quite obvious, but can be confirmed by a Q-tip test. However, not all obstructed patients will appear to be overcorrected. It is important to assess for cystocele and other forms of prolapse which may cause obstruction (due to a kinking of the urethra). The patient should also be examined for persistent urethral hypermobility and stress incontinence.

Urodynamics

Recent interest in female bladder outlet obstruction (BOO) has resulted in the publication of several unique proposals of urodynamic criteria for the diagnosis of female BOO. Chassagne et al. used the cut-off values of detrusor pressure at maximum flow rate ($p_{det}Q_{max}$) of ≥20 cmH_2O and maximum flow rate (Q_{max}) of <15 ml/s to define obstruction.[31] In 2000, Lemack and Zimmern revised these values to a cut-off of Q_{max} of ≤11 ml/s and $p_{det}Q_{max}$ of ≥21 cmH_2O.[32] As a third update from this same group, new criteria were published in 2004, for the first time using a small group of asymptomatic controls, thus elevating the $p_{det}Q_{max}$ cut-off to 25 cmH_2O.[33]

Nitti et al. used videourodynamic criteria, with less emphasis on pressure–flow dynamics, to diagnose BOO.[34] In this study, obstruction was defined as radiographic evidence of an obstruction between the bladder neck and distal urethra in the presence of a sustained detrusor contraction of any magnitude during voiding. Blaivas and Groutz, realizing the possibility of test-induced catheter obstruction, designed a nomogram based on the maximum non-invasive flow rate (free Q_{max}) and the maximum detrusor pressure during voiding (p_{detmax}).[35] Although each urodynamic definition for obstruction has merit, further investigation should provide a better understanding of when to use which criteria.

The diagnosis of obstruction in women after incontinence surgery can be particularly difficult to make urodynamically. In cases of urinary retention and incomplete emptying, urodynamic studies may not be necessary before intervention, particularly if preoperative contractility and emptying are known to be normal. However, in cases of de novo or worsened storage symptoms, including urge incontinence without a significantly elevated post-void residual, a formal urodynamic evaluation is preferred. Classic high pressure, low flow voiding dynamics (or obstruction by any of the above criteria) will confirm the diagnosis of obstruction, but its absence does not always rule out obstruction. Many women with suspected obstruction after incontinence surgery do not generate a significant contraction on urodynamic studies but are obstructed nevertheless. Outcomes of surgical intervention in such cases are identical to those in women with classic high pressure, low flow dynamics.

There appear to be no consistent preoperative parameters, urodynamic or otherwise, which predict success or failure of urethrolysis. For example, Foster and McGuire found that patients with detrusor overactivity had a higher rate of failure, but a later study, as well as others, found this not to be the case.[36] Nitti and Raz found that, as the post-void residual increased, so did the rate of failure, but others have not confirmed this correlation.[37] Carr and Webster found that the only parameter predictive of success was no prior urethrolysis.[20] It is well established that urodynamics may fail to diagnose obstruction in a significant number of women obstructed as a result of anti-incontinence procedures. Additionally, patients with non-diagnostic urodynamic studies or who failed to produce a detrusor contraction have the same outcomes as those with urodynamic findings classic for obstruction, namely high pressure, low flow voiding. In the study by Nitti and Raz, four women who failed to generate a contraction during urodynamic testing had a successful urethrolysis.[37] They also reported that the urodynamic findings in patients considered to be failures after transvaginal urethrolysis failed to elucidate the reason for their continued voiding dysfunction. Due to the limitations of urodynamics in these patients, the temporal relationship of the surgery to the onset of voiding and storage symptoms is relied upon as an indicator of obstruction. Likewise, if the patient fails to resume preoperative voiding or improve significantly, then continued obstruction is suspected.

Classic high pressure, low flow voiding dynamics do confirm the diagnosis of obstruction, but are a far from consistent finding. Urodynamics can also yield important information regarding instability, impaired compliance, bladder capacity, and voiding characteristics. Based on our experience, videourodynamics offers an advantage over simple urodynamics in this patient population, because of the ability to simultaneously image the bladder outlet.

The utility of urodynamics may be considered as follows:

- For the patient in retention, urodynamics can provide valuable information (e.g. detrusor overactivity or significantly impaired compliance, the latter being an absolute indication for intervention) and can confirm a diagnosis of obstruction, but should not exclude the patient from urethrolysis, even if there is no contraction or impaired contractility. Urodynamics may also identify learned voiding dysfunction.
- For the patient with storage symptoms with normal emptying, urodynamics can diagnose obstruction and – equally as important – rule out obstruction. It can help to provide a specific diagnosis that is useful in directing therapy, especially if obstruction can be excluded.

Endoscopy and imaging

Endoscopic evaluation of the urethra may show scarring, narrowing, occlusion, kinking, or deviation of the urethra. These finding are especially helpful in cases where urodynamics are equivocal. The urethra and bladder should be carefully inspected for eroded sutures or sling material and the presence of a fistula. This is facilitated by the use of a rigid scope with a zero to 30-degree lens and little or no beak to allow for complete distension of the urethra. In cases where intervention is anticipated, endoscopy should be done routinely, either before surgery or at the time of surgery prior to incision.

Radiographic imaging may be done independent of videourodynamics. A standing cystogram in the anteroposterior, oblique and lateral positions, with and without straining, assesses the degree of bladder and urethral prolapse and displacement or distortion of the bladder. A voiding cystourethrogram can assess the bladder, bladder neck, and urethra during voiding to determine narrowing, kinking or deviation (Fig. 68.1). While not mandatory, imaging can be extremely useful in equivocal cases.

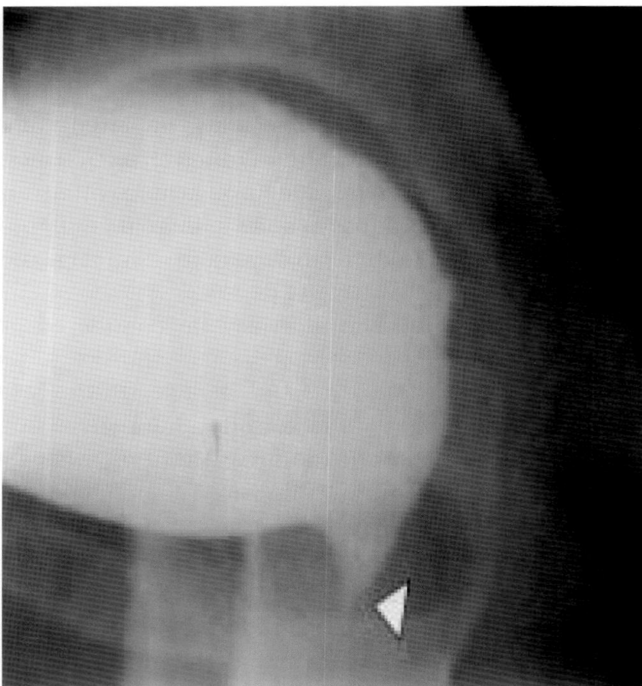

Figure 68.1. *Obstruction at the midurethra by midurethral sling with proximal urethral and bladder neck dilation.*

Summary

In summary, the diagnosis of obstruction is made on the basis of clinical presentation (type and onset of symptoms), physical examination, and testing such as urodynamics, imaging or endoscopy, depending on the circumstances. A temporal relationship between surgery and the onset of symptoms is the most critical factor in diagnosis. Patients with normal emptying before incontinence surgery (especially if preoperative urodynamics showed normal voiding) who have significant retention or obstructive voiding symptoms after incontinence surgery, need little in the way of a diagnostic workup.

MANAGEMENT OF IATROGENIC OBSTRUCTION

Conservative treatment

Treatment of obstruction and its timing are usually dictated by the degree of bother of symptoms. In some cases an obstructed patient will opt for conservative management including clean intermittent catheterization (CIC) if necessary. In the woman who is not very bothered by catheterization and prefers this option to repeat surgery and a risk of recurrent stress urinary incontinence, CIC is a reasonable treatment plan. Although most women ultimately choose definitive treatment, chronic CIC is an option in select cases. Patients who are emptying well but have significant storage symptoms secondary to iatrogenic obstruction may be treated initially with pharmacotherapy (anticholinergics) or pelvic floor physiotherapy. In our experience these measures are not usually successful when obstruction exists, but can be considered before surgery.

The role for urethral dilation in cases of iatrogenic obstruction secondary to pubovaginal sling and colposuspension is not clear. While many practitioners report anecdotal success, no peer reviewed literature exists. It is our opinion that urethral dilation is of limited utility in these cases. Karram et al. reported an 82% cure or improved rate with urethral dilation using a Walther sound when performed within 2–6 weeks of TVT insertion for varying levels of voiding dysfunction in 28 women.[29] There are concerns about the potentially traumatic nature of dilation which could induce scarring of the urethra. The cutting of suspension or sling sutures above the rectus has been described anecdotally with variable success.

When conservative measures in a symptomatic patient fail, definitive surgical therapy by either formal urethrolysis (transvaginal or retropubic) or sling incision may be required. In addition, there is a limited but growing experience with manipulation of midurethral synthetic slings in the early postoperative period.

Surgical intervention

When voiding dysfunction secondary to obstruction exists beyond a proper waiting period (see 'Diagnostic evaluation', above), surgical intervention is indicated. Success rates for various procedures range from 67 to 100% (Table 68.1) and appear to be independent of the particular procedure chosen, i.e. in general, one procedure is not superior to another, except perhaps under certain circumstances.

To date, no consistent predictors for success have been identified. Individual series have cited certain factors which were associated with success or failure, but different series have not identified the same factors. For example, Carr and Webster found that the only predictors of success were no prior urethrolysis and omental interposition.[20] Nitti and Raz found that as the post-void residual increased, so did the risk of failure.[37] Foster and McGuire noted that patients with detrusor overactivity had a higher rate of failure.[36] Others have not confirmed these findings.[38] Certainly, high pressure, low flow voiding on urodynamics confirms obstruction; however, urodynamics often may be equivocal or non-specific.

Table 68.1. ***Summary of series on urethrolysis and sling incision/loosening for the treatment of obstruction after incontinence surgery***

	n	Type of urethrolysis	Success*	Recurrent SUI†
Zimmern et al.[49]	13	Transvaginal	92%	N/A
Foster & McGuire[36]	48	Transvaginal	53%	0
Nitti & Raz[37]	42	Transvaginal	71%	0
Cross et al.[38]	39	Transvaginal	72%	3%
Goldman et al.[40]	32	Transvaginal	84%	19%
Carey et al.[47]	23	Transvaginal with Martius flap	87%	16%
Petrou et al.[48]	32	Suprameatal	67%	3%
Webster & Kreder[39]	15	Retropubic	93%	13%
Petrou & Young[50]	12	Retropubic	83%	25%
Carr & Webster[20]	54	Mixed	78%	14%
Amundsen et al.[43]	32	Transvaginal and sling incision	94% retention 67% urge symptoms	9%
Nitti et al.[44]	19	Sling incision	84%	17%
Goldman[45]	14	Sling incision	93%	21%
Klutke et al.[9]	17	TVT incision and/or loosening	100%	6%
Rardin et al.[11]	23	TVT incision	100% retention 30% urge symptoms cured 70% urge symptoms improved	39% (two-thirds less SUI than pre-TVT)

* Success is usually defined as cure or significant improvement in presenting symptoms (resumption of normal bladder emptying for patients in retention, and resolution of symptoms for patients with obstructive symptoms or frequency, urgency or urge incontinence). In some series success for specific symptoms is noted.
† Recurrent stress urinary incontinence (SUI) is defined as percentage of patients without SUI before urethrolysis who experienced SUI after urethrolysis.

Several studies failed to show any correlation between urodynamic findings and the likelihood of successful voiding after urethrolysis.[36,37,39] Furthermore, outcomes of urethrolysis in women without a demonstrable detrusor contraction on urodynamics (who voided normally prior to incontinence surgery) are equivalent to those women with classic findings of obstruction.

With all surgical interventions for obstruction there is an inherent risk of recurrent stress incontinence. In general, this risk is approximately 15%, but reported rates vary from zero to 39% (see Table 68.1). While some have recommended concomitant anti-incontinence procedures at the same time as the procedure to relieve obstruction (e.g. urethrolysis and transvaginal needle suspension or sling), no significant benefit has been shown by others, and we do not routinely perform a repeat anti-incontinence procedure.[36,37,40] In the majority of cases, patients are so disturbed by the symptoms caused by obstruction, that relieving them must be the primary goal. If stress incontinence does recur, it can be treated separately with a urethral bulking agent or even a repeat surgical procedure in the future.

Surgical techniques are usually tailored toward individual scenarios and previous surgeries. For example, in certain cases where the incontinence procedure causing obstruction was a retropubic suspension, a retropubic urethrolysis approach may be used to cut sutures and free retropubic adhesions. For transvaginal sling procedures, transvaginal sling lysis alone or formal urethrolysis can usually be performed successfully with less patient morbidity and quicker convalescence. Some have advocated a transvaginal suprameatal approach; however, we rarely perform this operation. With the much more common use of the TVT or synthetic midurethral slings, sling loosening techniques, urethral dilation, and sling incision alone are commonly performed in the clinic setting with local anesthesia within a shorter postoperative period before significant scarring occurs.

In this section we will describe surgical techniques for the treatment of iatrogenic obstruction in order of invasiveness. This is not to imply that one technique should be chosen first over another; that decision depends upon multiple factors including the incontinence procedure performed, associated complications, surgeon comfort, and other factors.

Midurethral sling loosening or incision

In women with postoperative urinary retention after midurethral synthetic sling procedures, some surgeons, including ourselves, advocate early intervention within 7–14 days. With midurethral synthetic slings, unlike traditional pubovaginal slings, the vast majority of patients are able to empty fairly normally within 72 hours. Early intervention allows one to perform a minimally invasive procedure, under local anesthesia in an office setting if preferred. The anterior vaginal wall is infiltrated with local anesthetic and the suture used to close the vaginal wall is opened. The synthetic sling is usually easily visualized. The sling is hooked with a right-angle clamp (or alternatively a Metzenbaum scissors or Hegar dilator). Spreading of the right-angle clamp or downward traction on the tape will usually loosen it (1–2 cm).[9] This is usually possible if intervention is done by 10 days. Thereafter, tissue ingrowth may prevent loosening of the sling, in which case we recommend cutting it in the midline. The incision is suture closed, and the patient is allowed to attempt to void.

Loosening or cutting of TVT has excellent results.[9,11,29,30] In the two largest series of 17 and 23 patients, restoration of normal voiding and emptying occurred in all patients,[9,11] storage symptoms were partially relieved in 70%, and completely relieved in 30%.[11] Klutke et al. reported resolution of obstruction in all 17 patients while recurrent stress incontinence occurred in one patient.[9] Rardin et al. found that impaired bladder emptying resolved in 100% of 23 patients, with 61% remaining continent, 26% with partial recurrence, and 13% with complete recurrence of stress incontinence.[11]

In cases of voiding difficulty or dysfunction beyond 4–6 weeks, the lysis of the TVT sling is better performed in the operating theatre. Scarring and patient discomfort are factors to consider as more extensive dissection may be needed to identify and cut the sling. The technique described below for sling incision is applicable to midurethral synthetic slings.

Transvaginal sling incision

The transvaginal incision of the pubovaginal sling (autologous, allograft, xenograft or synthetic) rather than formal urethrolysis may limit morbidity, potential soft tissue and nerve injury, and fibrosis from surgical dissection. Notably, sling incision alone may effectively eliminate obstruction with results similar to formal urethrolysis. In 1995, Ghoniem and Elgamasy described a technique of incising the sling in the midline and using a free vaginal epithelial interposition graft sutured to each cut end of the pubovaginal sling, keeping it intact to theoretically reduce the risk of postoperative stress incontinence.[41] Over time, the technique has evolved and interposition is no longer routinely used.[42–45]

Our technique starts with cystoscopy to assess the urethra and rule out erosion or urethral injury, followed by an inverted U or midline incision to expose the area of the bladder neck and proximal urethra.[44] As the vaginal flap is dissected off, the sling should be identified above the periurethral fascia. The sling may be encased in scar tissue and thus require careful dissection of the scar to identify the sling. If the sling has significant tension on it, it may be especially difficult to identify. Insertion of a cystoscope or sound into the urethra with upward retraction, may help to expose the bladder neck and isolate the sling. Once the sling is isolated it should be separated from the underlying periurethral fascia with sharp or blunt dissection. The dissection may be facilitated by grasping the sling with an Allis clamp on either side of the midline and exerting downward pressure. Care should be taken to avoid injury to the bladder and urethra by beginning the dissection distally, identifying normal urethra then proceeding more proximally until the plane between the sling and urethra is identified. A right-angle clamp can be placed between the urethra and periurethral fascia and the sling, lifting the sling. The sling is then cut in the midline (Fig. 68.2a). Alternatively, if scarring is dense and the plane between the sling and periurethral fascia cannot be developed easily, the sling can be isolated lateral to the midline, off of the urethra. The edges of the sling are mobilized off the periurethral fascia to, but not through, the endopelvic fascia (Fig. 68.2b). In cases of extreme tension, the ends of the sling may retract back into the retropubic space after incision, but more often the sling stays secure to allow this mobilization. Lateral support is preserved because the retropubic space is not entered, and the urethra is not freed from the undersurface of the pubic bone. The ends of the sling can be left in situ or excised. We typically excise synthetic material and leave autografts and allografts in place. If there is any concern about urethral injury, cystourethroscopy should be carried out. In cases of autologous or biologic materials, if the sling cannot be clearly identified, then formal transvaginal urethrolysis (see below) should be performed.

TVT and other midurethral synthetic slings can be isolated and incised in a similar manner. Unlike autologous and biologic slings, it is imperative to identify the sling and cut it. Conversion to urethrolysis without specifically cutting the sling may fail to relieve obstruction.

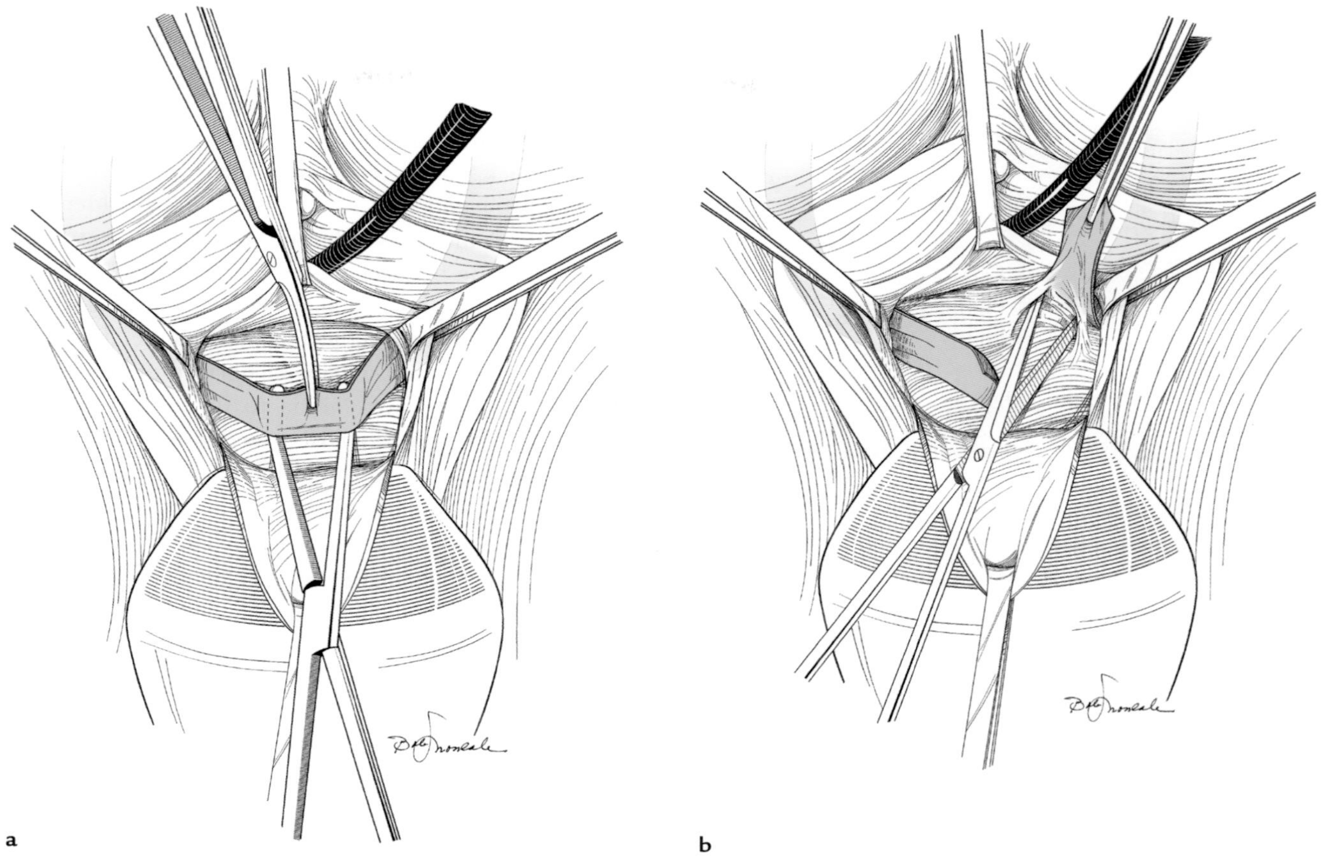

Figure 68.2. *(a) After an inverted U or midline incision, the sling is isolated in the midline and incised. A right-angle clamp may be placed between the sling and the periurethral fascia to avoid injury to the urethra. (b) The sling is freed from the undersurface of the urethra toward the endopelvic fascia. Ends may be excised or left in situ. (Reproduced from ref. 44 with permission.)*

Usually the sling is easily found, and identification can be aided by palpation of the sling (Fig. 68.3). However, sometimes this can be quite difficult, especially in cases where the sling has rolled onto itself and created a tight narrow band (Fig. 68.4). In such cases, patient and careful dissection to isolate the sling is required. In many cases after the midurethral sling is cut it retracts away from the urethra. At the surgeon's discretion segmental resection of the suburethral portion of the sling may be performed. Our experience with sling incision has shown results equivalent to formal urethrolysis. The success rate for this procedure ranges from 84 to 93.5% with a 9–21% recurrent stress incontinence rate.[43–45] If sling incision is not successful in relieving obstruction, formal urethrolysis may be carried out.

Transvaginal urethrolysis

Formal urethrolysis may be accomplished through a retropubic or a transvaginal approach. Both methods have shown equivalent success rates and rates of recurrent stress urinary incontinence, although most of these series include patients who are obstructed as a result of a number of different anti-incontinence surgeries. The type of urethrolysis chosen will depend on several factors including patient presentation, type of incontinence procedure performed, failed prior urethrolysis, and surgeon preference. It has been our practice to perform transvaginal urethrolysis as a primary operation, and retropubic urethrolysis as a secondary operation (e.g. after failed transvaginal urethrolysis). We prefer the transvaginal technique because of its ease and the reduced morbidity and recovery time afforded by avoiding an abdominal procedure. However, there are times when a retropubic approach may be the best primary procedure, for example: when vaginal anatomy precludes a transvaginal approach; in cases where original incontinence surgery was associated with bladder perforation, fistula or other operative complication; when there is a synthetic sling which must be removed; or in cases where the patient wishes to avoid a vaginal incision.

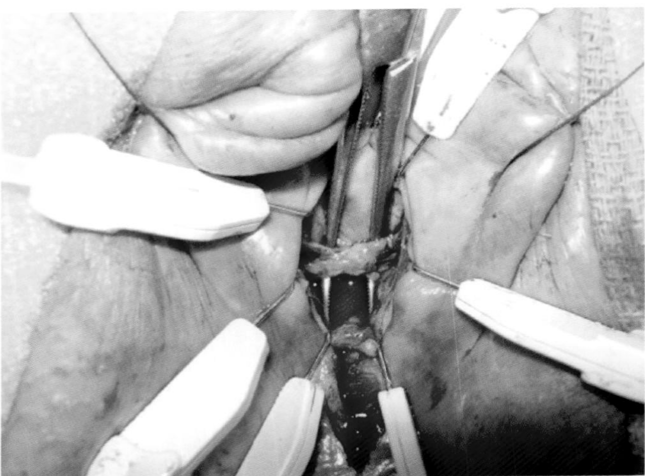

Figure 68.3. *Isolated midurethral polypropylene sling causing obstruction 1 year after implantation. Note the ingrowth of tissue between the mesh (blue).*

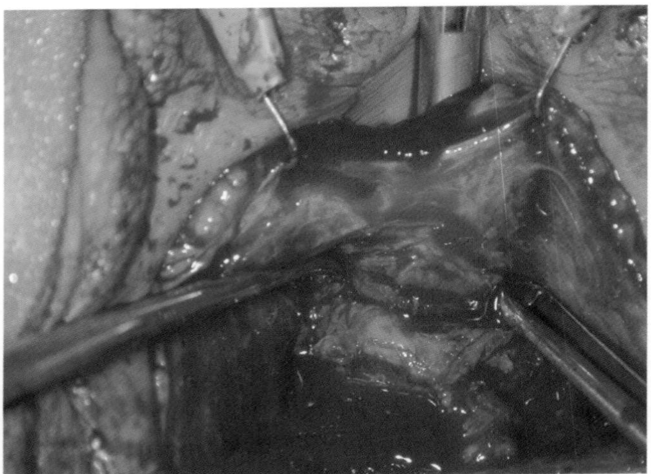

Figure 68.4. *Obstructing midurethral polypropylene sling which has twisted into a 2 mm band. A right-angle clamp can be placed between the tension-free transvaginal tape (TVT) and the periurethral fascia and the TVT can be isolated and cut.*

All urethrolysis procedures begin with a thorough endoscopic examination of urethra, bladder neck, and bladder. Urethroscopy may show scarring, narrowing, occlusion, kinking or deviation of the urethra. Eroded sutures or sling material or evidence of a fistula should be excluded. A rigid scope with a zero to 30-degree lens and little or no beak to allow for complete distension of the urethra is ideal for female urethroscopy. It is common to find that the urethra and/or urethrovesical function are fixed and there is lack of mobility when moving the cystoscope up and down. After urethrolysis, mobility should be restored.

The most commonly used transvaginal technique was originally described by Leach and Raz.[46] A midline or inverted U incision approximately 3 cm long is made in the anterior vaginal wall. A midline incision should extend from the midurethra to 1–2 cm proximal to the bladder neck. In the case of an inverted U, the apex should be located half way between the bladder neck and urethral meatus, with the lateral wing extending proximal to the bladder neck. With either incision, lateral dissection is performed along the glistening surface of the periurethral fascia to the pubic bone. The retropubic space is entered sharply by perforating the attachment of the endopelvic fascia to the obturator fascia (Fig. 68.5a). The urethra is dissected bluntly and sharply off the undersurface of the pubic bone and completely freed proximally to the bladder neck. Sharp dissection is usually required here (Fig. 68.5b). The urethra should be completely freed proximally to the bladder neck so that the index finger can be placed between the urethra and the symphysis pubis. Attachments to the undersurface of the pubic bone are sharply incised or swept down with the index finger retropubically. After initial mobilization, a right-angle clamp can be placed between the pubic bone and the urethra and a Penrose drain placed around the urethra. Downward traction on the Penrose drain further aids visualization and sharp dissection of all retropubic attachments (Fig. 68.6). The index finger may then be placed completely around the urethra between the pubic bone. When urethrolysis is complete there should be full mobility of the urethra which can be tested with up and down movement of an intraurethral sound or cystoscope. Once this is achieved, the vaginal wall is closed with absorbable sutures. Prior to closure, endoscopic examination is performed to rule out urethral or bladder injury. In cases of extensive urethrolysis it is good practice to assess ureteral integrity by giving intravenous indigo carmine prior to endoscopy and assessing ureteral efflux. Success rates with transvaginal urethrolysis vary from 53 to 93% (see Table 68.1).

Carey et al. reported the use of a Martius labial fat pad flap with transvaginal urethrolysis with success in 87% of patients.[47] The Martius flap may decrease the risk of recurrent fibrosis, provide some urethral support, and with any future surgery a sling may be placed outside the fat pad, thus decreasing the risk of urethral injury. We reserve it for select cases (e.g. repeat urethrolysis, extensive fibrosis) and usually divide the robust fat pad flap midway along its longitudinal axis and wrap the flap around the urethra, effectively supporting the undersurface and retropubic surface of the urethra.

In select cases (e.g. extensive mobilization or stress incontinence coexisting with obstruction) it may be desir-

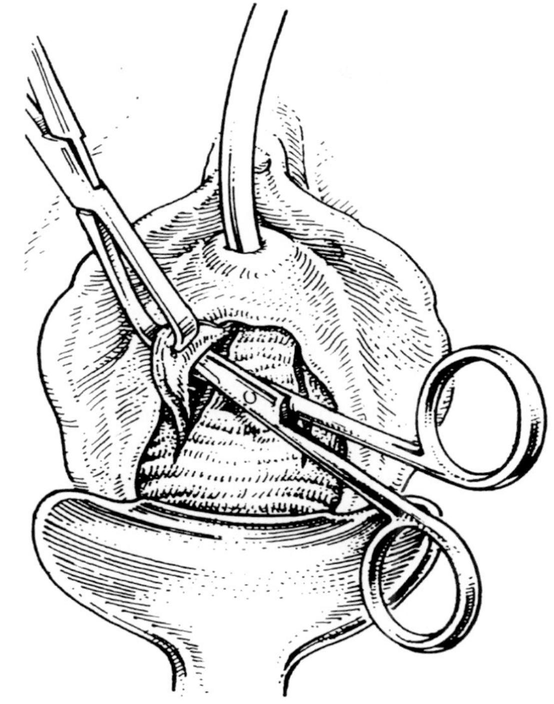

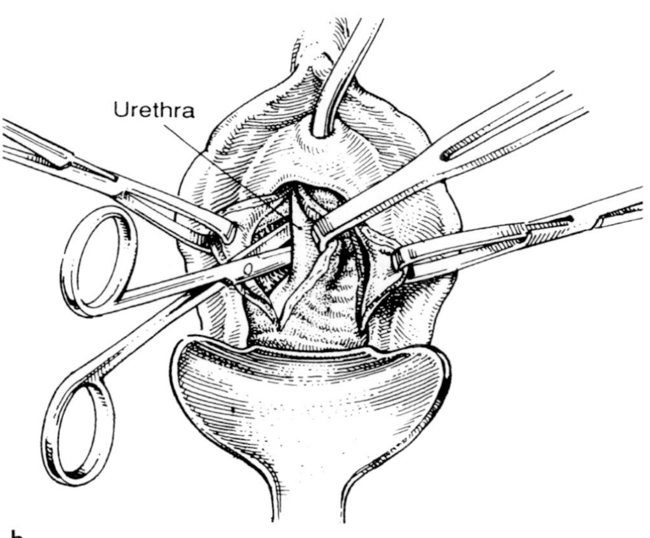

Figure 68.5. *Transvaginal urethrolysis. (a) An inverted U incision in the anterior vaginal wall and entrance into the retropubic space. (b) The urethra is sharply dissected off the undersurface of the pubic bone. The endopelvic fascia, periurethral fascia, and vaginal wall are retracted medially to expose the urethra in the retropubic space. (Reproduced from ref. 37 with permission.)*

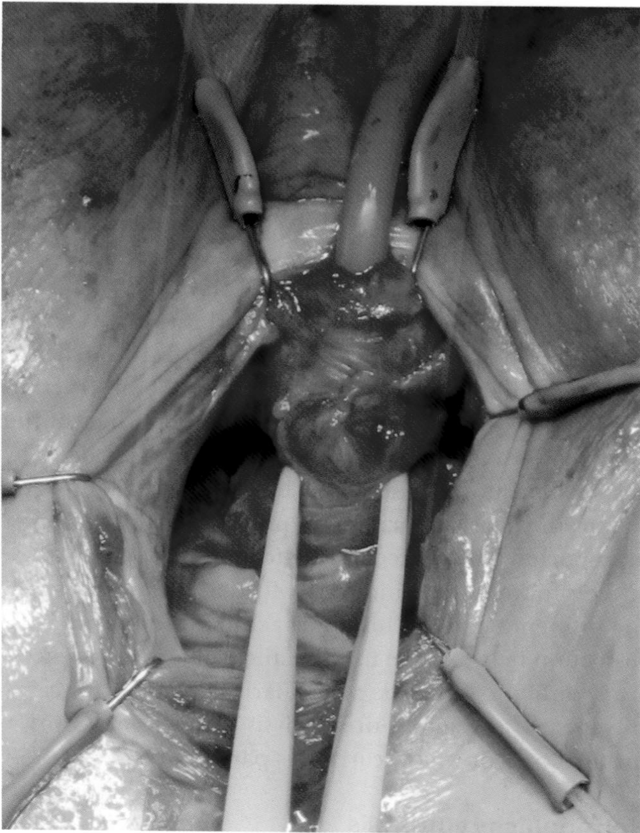

Figure 68.6. *Intraoperative photo after completed urethrolysis. A Penrose drain has been placed around the urethra, isolating it from the pubic bone.*

able to resupport the urethra at the time of urethrolysis. Resuspension or pubovaginal sling may be carried out. Currently our practice is to consider a resuspension or sling only if the patient has stress incontinence prior to urethrolysis or if support structures are severely compromised during urethrolysis. Resuspension does increase the risk of persistent obstruction and since most patients are distraught about obstruction, we feel it is best to take care of that problem and deal with recurrent SUI at a later time should it occur. Rates of recurrent SUI after resuspension vary between zero and 19%.[20,36,38,40,47] Many of these patients may be salvaged with transurethral collagen injections should stress incontinence recur. Goldman et al. reported a 66% response rate to collagen in women with recurrent stress incontinence after transvaginal urethrolysis.[40] In addition, the option for repeat surgery for SUI at a later date is preserved. It is important to discuss the pros and cons of resuspension and the treatment of recurrent stress incontinence with patients preoperatively, as this could affect the decision on whether or not to resuspend.

A variant of transvaginal urethrolysis is the suprameatal approach described by Petrou et al.[48] We have found this to have quite limited applicability. A theoretical advantage of this technique is that lateral perforation of the urethropelvic ligament is not required, minimizing the chance of recurrent urethral hypermobility and subsequent incontinence. An inverted U incision is made around the top of the urethral meatus (approximately 1 cm away) between the 3 and 9 o'clock positions. Using sharp dissection, a plane is developed above the urethra. Then, with a combination of sharp and blunt dissection, the urethra, vesical neck and bladder are freed from the pubic and pelvic attachments anteriorly and laterally. The index finger may then be passed into the retropubic space and, with a sweeping motion from medial to lateral, further freeing may be performed. If obstruction is caused by a pubovaginal sling, the lateral wings of the sling may be cut. Likewise, if the obstruction is caused by suspension sutures, these may be cut. As with transvaginal urethrolysis, a Martius flap may be placed. Petrou et al. reported a 65% success rate for retention and a 67% success for urgency symptoms, with a 3% recurrent stress incontinence rate.[48] This approach may be beneficial if dissection between the urethra and pubic bone is excessively difficult. It may be particularly applicable for cases of repeat transvaginal urethrolysis (after a failed prior urethrolysis) or when scarring is particularly dense.

Retropubic urethrolysis

Retropubic approaches to urethrolysis may be the preferred method under circumstances which include surgeon experience/familiarity with vaginal anatomy, inadequate vaginal access, original incontinence surgery or urethrolysis associated with bladder perforation, fistula, synthetic sling removal (Fig. 68.7), and when the patient desires to avoid another vaginal incision. Complicated cases that have failed prior extensive transvaginal urethrolysis may also be performed retropubically. Previous retropubic surgery such as the MMK still may be managed transvaginally as shown by Zimmern et al.[49]

The technique of retropubic urethrolysis has been described by Webster and Kreder (Fig. 68.7).[39] It may be accomplished through a Pfannensteil or low midline incision. The rectus fascia and muscle are opened in midline to the level of the pubic symphysis. After exposing the retropubic space, all prevesical and retropubic adhesions are sharply incised. Complications can be avoided by keeping the tips of the scissors against the pubic symphysis during sharp dissection. The objective is to restore complete mobility to the anterior vaginal wall allowing free movement of the vesicourethral unit.

The urethra and urethrovesical junction are dissected off the pubic bone, without separating them from the anterior vaginal wall. The boundaries of the vagina in relation to the urethrovesical junction are identified by placement of the index finger of the surgeon's nondominant hand into the vagina. Alternatively, a sponge stick or similar instrument may be used. Some degree of sharp dissection lateral to the urethra is usually required. In cases of severe scarring, it may be necessary to mobilize laterally as far as the ischial tuberosities. This often results in a paravaginal defect. In cases where a paravaginal defect is created as a consequence of urethral mobilization, the defect should be repaired by reapproximating the paravaginal fascia to the fascia of the obturator internus along the arcus tendineus. The paravaginal repair sutures are left untied. Finally, the peritoneum is opened with a small incision and an omental flap is mobilized. The flap is then placed

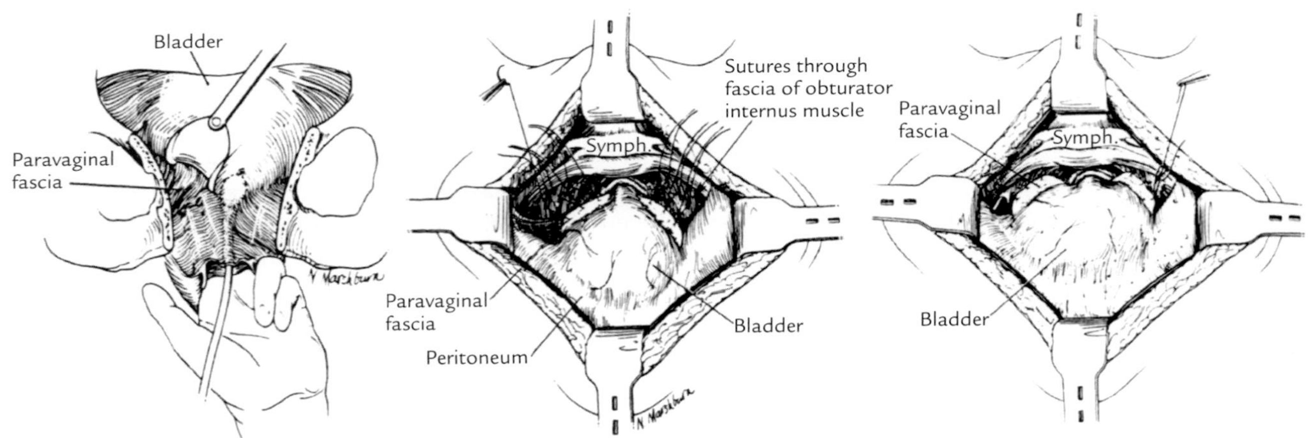

Figure 68.7. *Retropubic urethrolysis. The urethra and urethrovesical junction are dissected off the pubic bone, without separating them from the anterior vaginal wall. with sharp dissection. A paravaginal defect repair is then performed. Symph, symphysis pubis. (Reproduced from ref. 39 with permission.)*

between the pubic bone and the urethra and secured to the underside of the pubic bone with a 2-0 polyglycolic acid (PGA) suture. The omentum fills the dead space and helps to prevent recurrent adhesion.[20] The paravaginal repair sutures are then tied and the abdomen is closed. Cystoscopy is performed to rule out urethral injury and confirm efflux of indigo carmine from the ureteral orifices.

Webster and Kreder reported a successful outcome in 93% of 15 women undergoing retropubic urethrolysis and obturator shelf repair.[39] In another series of 12 women, Petrou and Young reported resolution of obstruction in 10 patients, with new onset stress incontinence in 2 of 11 patients (18%).[50] Carr and Webster reported complete or significant resolution of symptoms in 86% of patients with retropubic urethrolysis.[20]

Failed urethrolysis

Failure of urethrolysis may be due to persistent or recurrent obstruction, detrusor overactivity, impaired detrusor contractility or learned voiding dysfunction. Recurrent obstruction may result from periurethral fibrosis and scarring, or intrinsic damage to the urethra that has occurred as a consequence of the urethrolysis surgery. We believe that inadequate dissection and lysis of the urethra probably represents the most common reason for failure of initial urethrolysis. When obstruction persists it is reasonable to attempt a repeat urethrolysis. We have found this to be effective in relieving urinary retention, but not as effective in treating persistent storage symptoms. We recently reported on the efficacy of repeat urethrolysis in 24 women who failed initial urethrolysis and remained in urinary retention.[51] Both transvaginal and retropubic approaches were chosen depending on the clinical situation. Obstruction was cured in 92%, but storage symptoms completely resolved in only 12% and were improved and required medication in 69%. SUI recurred in 18%.

These data clearly support aggressive repeat urethrolysis in the face of initial failure, at least for retention and incomplete emptying. In general, if an aggressive transvaginal urethrolysis fails, then a retropubic approach may be considered. In cases where the aggressiveness of the initial transvaginal procedure is unknown, or if only a sling incision was performed, then a repeat transvaginal approach may be appropriate.

CONCLUSION

It is indeed a challenging prospect to treat the patient with significant irritative and obstructive features after performing an operation for incontinence. While keeping in mind the patient's symptoms and goals, the physician must use careful decision making when assessing, diagnosing, and treating obstruction. Fortunately, the various urethrolysis techniques are highly successful for restoring efficient voiding. We still seek improved methods of identifying those at risk for obstruction, diagnosing obstruction, and treating troublesome irritative voiding symptoms.

REFERENCES

1. Juma S, Sdrales L. Etiology of urinary retention after bladder neck suspension [abstract]. J Urol 1993;149:400A.
2. Spencer JR, O'Conor VJ Jr, Schaeffer AJ. A comparison of endoscopic suspension of the vesical neck with suprapubic vesicourethropexy for treatment of stress urinary incontinence. J Urol 1987;137:411–5.
3. Rost A, Fiedler U, Fester C. Comparative analysis of the results of suspension-urethroplasty according to Marshall–Marchetti–Krantz and of urethrovesicopexy with adhesive. Urol Int 1979;34:167–75.
4. Mundy AR. A trial comparing the Stamey bladder neck suspension procedure with colposuspension for the treatment of stress incontinence. Br J Urol 1983;55:687–90.
5. Cardozo LD, Stanton SL, Williams JE. Detrusor instability following surgery for genuine stress incontinence. Br J Urol 1979;51:204–7.
6. Leach GE, Dmochowski RR, Appell RA et al. Female Stress Urinary Incontinence Clinical Guidelines Panel summary report on surgical management of female stress urinary incontinence. The American Urological Association. J Urol 1997;158:875–80.
7. Chaikin DC, Rosenthal J, Blaivas JG. Pubovaginal fascial sling for all types of stress urinary incontinence: long-term analysis. J Urol 1998;160:1312–6.
8. Morgan TO Jr, Westney OL, McGuire EJ. Pubovaginal sling: 4-year outcome analysis and quality of life assessment. J Urol 2000;163:1845–8.
9. Klutke C, Siegel S, Carlin B, Paszkiewicz E, Kirkemo A, Klutke J. Urinary retention after tension-free vaginal tape procedure: incidence and treatment. Urology 2001;58:697–701.
10. Niemczyk P, Klutke JJ, Carlin BI, Klutke CG. United States experience with tension-free vaginal tape procedure for urinary stress incontinence: assessment of safety and tolerability. Tech Urol 2001;7:261–5.
11. Rardin CR, Rosenblatt PL, Kohli N, Miklos JR, Heit M, Lucente VR. Release of tension-free vaginal tape for the treatment of refractory postoperative voiding dysfunction. Obstet Gynecol 2002;100:898–902.
12. Sander P, Moller LM, Rudnicki PM, Lose G. Does the tension-free vaginal tape procedure affect the voiding phase?

Pressure–flow studies before and 1 year after surgery. BJU Int 2002;89:694–8.

13. Tamussino K, Hanzal E, Kolle D, Ralph G, Riss P. The Austrian tension-free vaginal tape registry. Int Urogynecol J Pelvic Floor Dysfunct 2001;12 (Suppl 2):S28–9.

14. Kuuva N, Nilsson CG. A nationwide analysis of complications associated with the tension-free vaginal tape (TVT) procedure. Acta Obstet Gynecol Scand 2002;81:72–7.

15. Moran PA, Ward KL, Johnson D, Smirni WE, Hilton P, Bibby J. Tension-free vaginal tape for primary genuine stress incontinence: a two-centre follow-up study. BJU Int 2000;86:39–42.

16. Rackley RR, Abdelmalak JB, Tchetgen MB, Madjar S, Jones S Noble M. Tension-free vaginal tape and percutaneous vaginal tape sling procedures. Tech Urol 2001;7:90–100.

17. Dunn JS, Bent AE, Ellerkman RM, Nihira MA, Melick CF. Voiding dysfunction after surgery for stress incontinence: literature and survey results. Int Urogynecol J 2004;15:25–31.

18. FitzGerald MP, Brubaker L. The etiology of urinary retention after surgery for genuine stress incontinence. Neurourol Urodyn 2001;20:13–21.

19. Smith CP, O'Leary M, Erickson J, Somogyi GT, Chancellor MB. Botulinum toxin urethral sphincter injection resolves urinary retention after pubovaginal sling operation. Int Urogynecol J Pelvic Floor Dysfunct 2002;13:185–6.

20. Carr LK, Webster GD. Voiding dysfunction following incontinence surgery: diagnosis and treatment with retropubic or vaginal urethrolysis. J Urol 1997;157:821–3.

21. Miller EA, Amundsen CL, Toh KL, Flynn BJ, Webster GD. Preoperative urodynamic evaluation may predict voiding dysfunction in women undergoing pubovaginal sling. J Urol 2003;169:2234–7.

22. Weinberger MW, Ostergard DR. Postoperative catheterization, urinary retention, and permanent voiding dysfunction after polytetrafluoroethylene suburethral sling placement. Obstet Gynecol 1996;87:50–4.

23. Bhatia NN, Bergman A. Urodynamic predictability of voiding following incontinence surgery. Obstet Gynecol 1984;63:85–91.

24. Gateau T, Faramarzi-Roques R, Le Normand L, Glemain P, Buzelin JM, Ballanger P. Clinical and urodynamic repercussions after TVT procedure and how to diminish patient complaints. Eur Urol 2003;44:372–6; discussion 376.

25. Wang AC, Chen MC. The correlation between preoperative voiding mechanism and surgical outcome of the tension-free vaginal tape procedure, with reference to quality of life. BJU Int 2003;91:502–6.

26. Kobak WH, Walters MD, Piedmonte MR. Determinants of voiding after three types of incontinence surgery: a multivariable analysis. Obstet Gynecol 2001;97:86–91.

27. McLennan MT, Melick CF, Bent AE. Clinical and urodynamic predictors of delayed voiding after fascia lata suburethral sling. Obstet Gynecol 1998;92:608–12.

28. Leng WW, Davies BJ, Tarin T et al. Delayed treatment of bladder outlet obstruction after sling surgery: association with irreversible bladder dysfunction. J Urol 2004;172:1379–81.

29. Karram MM, Segal JL, Vassallo BJ, Kleeman SD. Complications and untoward effects of the tension-free vaginal tape procedure. Obstet Gynecol 2003;101:929–32.

30. Croak AJ, Schulte V, Peron S, Klingele C, Gebhart J, Lee R. Transvaginal tape lysis for urinary obstruction after tension-free vaginal tape placement. J Urol 2003;169:2238–41.

31. Chassagne S, Bernier PA, Haab F, Roehrborn CG, Reisch JS, Zimmern PE. Proposed cutoff values to define bladder outlet obstruction in women. Urology 1998;51:408–11.

32. Lemack GE, Zimmern PE. Pressure–flow analysis may aid in identifying women with outflow obstruction. J Urol 2000;163:1823–8.

33. Defreitas GA, Zimmern PE, Lemack GE, Shariat SF. Refining diagnosis of anatomic female bladder outlet obstruction: comparison of pressure–flow study parameters in clinically obstructed women with those of normal controls. Urology 2004;64:675–9; discussion 679–81.

34. Nitti VW, Tu LM, Gitlin J. Diagnosing bladder outlet obstruction in women. J Urol 1999;161:1535–40.

35. Blaivas JG, Groutz A. Bladder outlet obstruction nomogram for women with lower urinary tract symptomatology. Neurourol Urodyn 2000;19:553–64.

36. Foster HE, McGuire EJ. Management of urethral obstruction with transvaginal urethrolysis. J Urol 1993;150:1448–51.

37. Nitti VW, Raz S. Obstruction following anti-incontinence procedures: diagnosis and treatment with transvaginal urethrolysis. J Urol 1994;152:93–8.

38. Cross CA, Cespedes RD, English SF, McGuire EJ. Transvaginal urethrolysis for urethral obstruction after anti-incontinence surgery. J Urol 1998;159:1199–201.

39. Webster GD, Kreder KJ. Voiding dysfunction following cystourethropexy: its evaluation and management. J Urol 1990;144:670–3.

40. Goldman HB, Rackley RR, Appell RA. The efficacy of urethrolysis without re-suspension for iatrogenic urethral obstruction. J Urol 1999;161:196–8; discussion 198–9.

41. Ghoniem GM, Elgamasy AN. Simplified surgical approach to bladder outlet obstruction following pubovaginal sling. J Urol 1995;154:181–3.

42. Kusuda L. Simple release of pubovaginal sling. Urology 2001;57:358–9.

43. Amundsen CL, Guralnick ML, Webster GD. Variations in strategy for the treatment of urethral obstruction after a pubovaginal sling procedure. J Urol 2000;164:434–7.

44. Nitti VW, Carlson KV, Blaivas JG, Dmochowski RR. Early results of pubovaginal sling lysis by midline sling incision. Urology 2002;59:47–51; discussion 51–2.

45. Goldman HB. Simple sling incision for the treatment of iatrogenic urethral obstruction. Urology 2003;62:714–8.

46. Leach GE, Raz S. Modified Pereyra bladder neck suspension after previously failed anti-incontinence surgery. Surgical technique and results with long-term follow-up. Urology 1984;23:359–62.

47. Carey JM, Chon JK, Leach GE. Urethrolysis with Martius labial fat pad graft for iatrogenic bladder outlet obstruction. Urology 2003;61:21–5.

48. Petrou SP, Brown JA, Blaivas JG. Suprameatal transvaginal urethrolysis. J Urol 1999;161:1268–71.

49. Zimmern PE, Hadley HR, Leach GE, Raz S. Female urethral obstruction after Marshall–Marchetti–Krantz operation. J Urol 1987;138:517–20.

50. Petrou SP, Young PR. Rate of recurrent stress urinary incontinence after retropubic urethrolysis. J Urol 2002;167:613–5.

51. Scarpero HM, Dmochowski RR, Nitti VW. Repeat urethrolysis after failed urethrolysis for iatrogenic obstruction. J Urol 2003;169:1013–6.

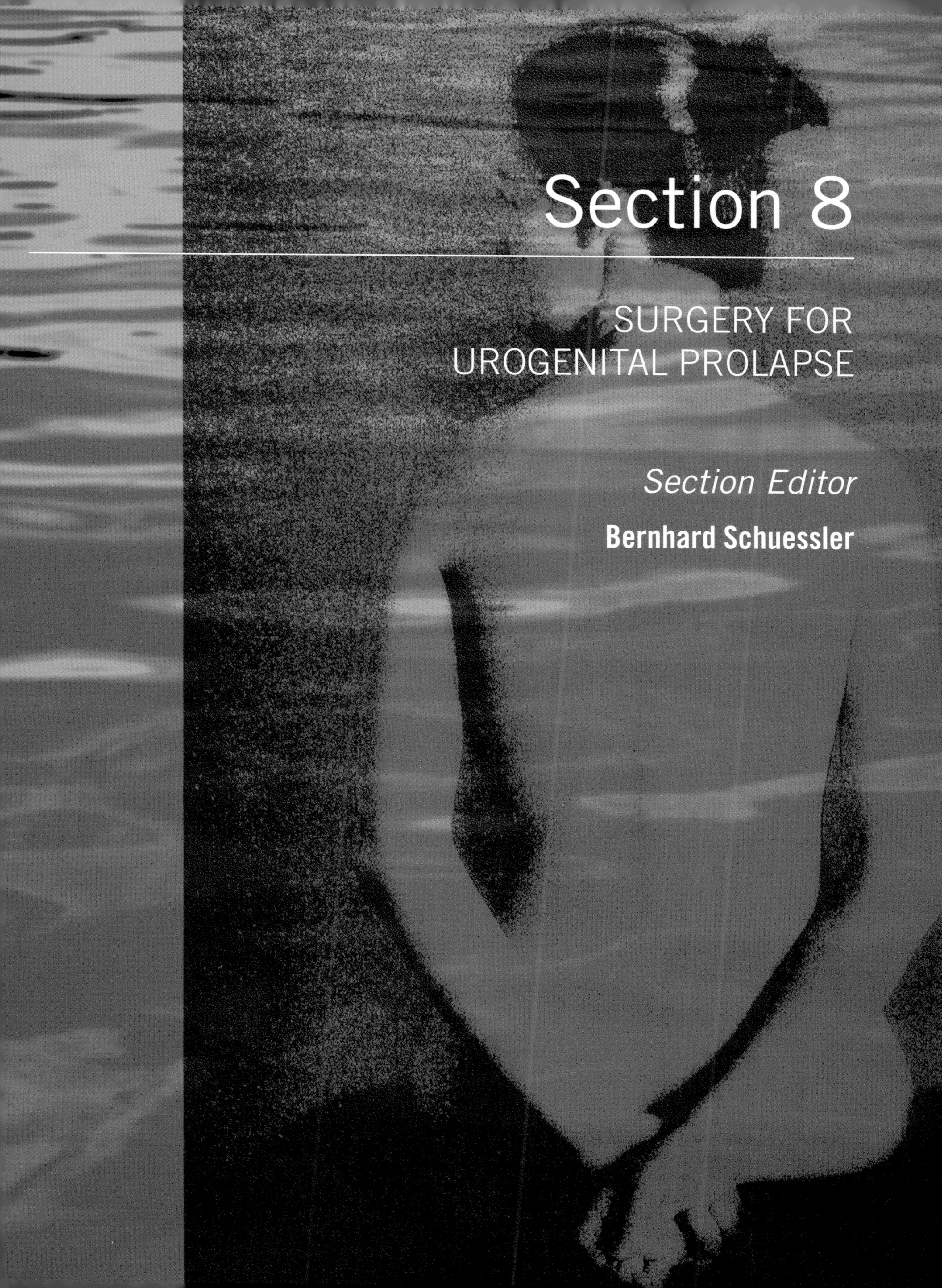

Section 8

SURGERY FOR UROGENITAL PROLAPSE

Section Editor

Bernhard Schuessler

69

Classification and epidemiology of pelvic organ prolapse

Steven Swift

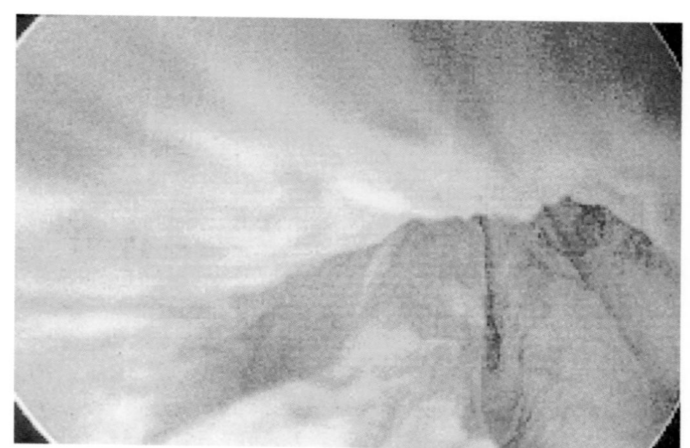

INTRODUCTION

The study of pelvic organ prolapse is one area of medicine that seems so intuitive but in actuality is replete with anecdotal evidence, case series, and very little hard science. Most of this stems from the lack of a scientifically validated and universally agreed upon definition of the disease state of 'pelvic organ prolapse'. A classification system to codify pelvic organ support has been defined and has gained international recognition. However, while it accurately describes the degree or stage of pelvic organ support, it does not classify it into normal versus abnormal or 'prolapse'. This is akin to having a blood pressure cuff to measure blood pressure but no definition as to what represents normal versus hypertension. Until we can define the disease, we cannot properly identify its etiology or make any statements regarding therapy, prognosis or natural history. Therefore, all of the scientific literature regarding pelvic organ prolapse should be viewed with caution, paying particular attention to how pelvic organ prolapse is described and defined. Despite the current state of affairs, studies into the classification and epidemiology of pelvic organ prolapse are moving forward as the scientific community has recognized the problems and is addressing them via research protocols.

CLASSIFICATION OF PELVIC ORGAN SUPPORT

The above title specifically does not use the term 'prolapse' but instead uses 'support' as none of the current pelvic organ prolapse classification systems attempts to define 'prolapse'. Instead, they only address where the vaginal walls or structures extend anatomically without making any reference as to what is normal versus abnormal or 'prolapsed'.

The history of classification systems for pelvic organ support extends back into the 19th century, with a new system appearing every generation or so, but with no system ever attaining widespread acceptance as the 'gold standard'.[1–7] Several of these systems are diagramed in Figure 69.1. Over the last decade, the pelvic organ prolapse quantification (POPQ) system has gained international recognition as the 'gold standard' for classifying pelvic organ support and it is the first and only system to gain recognition by most of the major societies that study pelvic organ support defects: the International Continence Society (ICS), the American Urogynecologic Society (AUGS), and the Society of Gynecologic Surgeons (SGS).[8] It is also the only system to be extensively studied with several reports in the literature documenting excellent inter- and intraexaminer reliability.[9–11] The only other system that has gained some widespread notoriety is the Baden and Walker

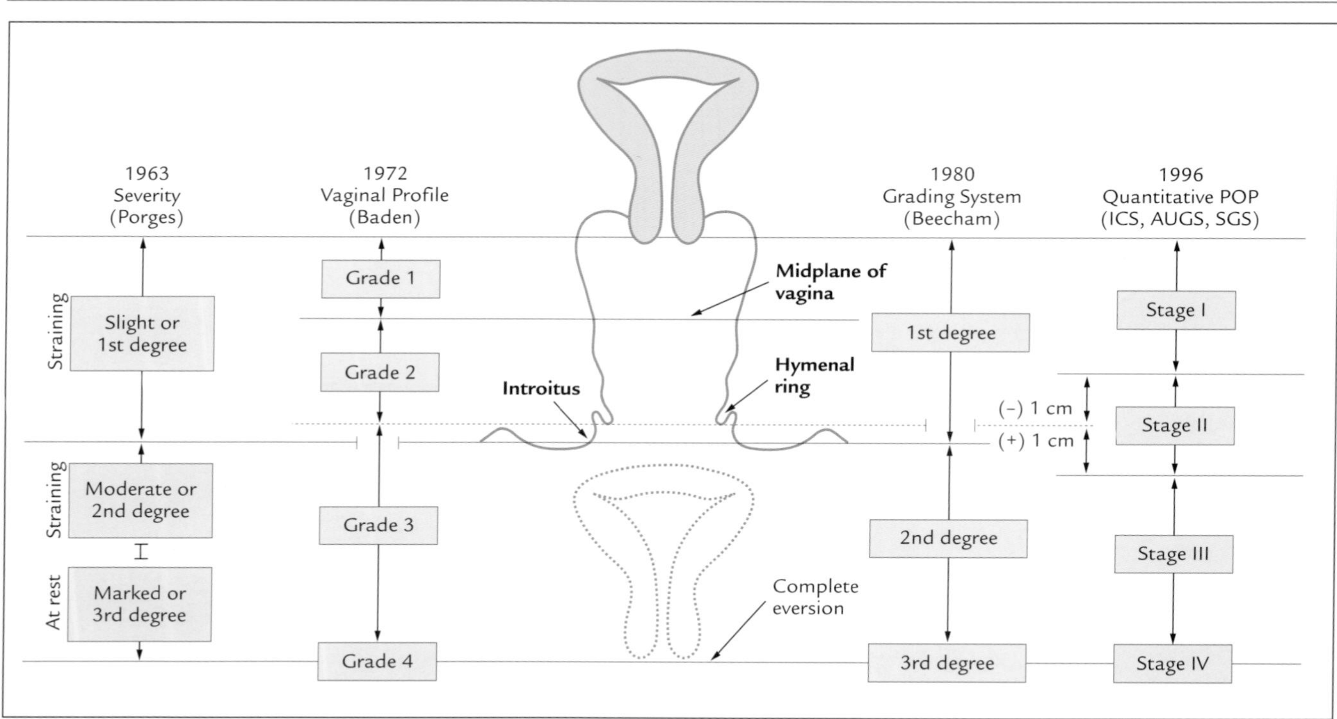

Figure 69.1. *Comparison of the four most commonly used pelvic organ prolapse (POP) grading systems. AUGS, American Urogynecologic Society; ICS, International Continence Society; SGS, Society of Gynecologic Surgeons.*

'half-way' system. In a recent survey of the literature on pelvic organ prolapse, it was the second most commonly employed classification system (with the POPQ being the first), and it is the only other system to be studied for interexaminer reliability.[10,12]

Currently, there is only one internationally recognized classification system for codifying pelvic organ support – the POPQ. It has proven itself to be a reliable system and it is the system that should be employed in research regarding pelvic organ support. The Baden and Walker 'half-way' system remains a common system in clinical practice and this may stem from its ease of use; however, it should not continue to supplant the POPQ in research studies and the scientific literature.[10]

THE PELVIC ORGAN PROLAPSE QUANTIFICATION SYSTEM

While the POPQ system is recognized as the standard for describing pelvic organ support, it has not resolved all of the questions regarding pelvic organ prolapse. First, while it is a good system for codifying pelvic organ support, like its predecessors it does not establish any diagnostic criteria for pelvic organ prolapse. In addition, while it is the only universally recognized system, it has yet to gain universal acceptance in research or clinical practice. Despite being initially described and published in 1996, as of 2003, it still only appeared in about 30% of the literature regarding pelvic organ support defects, and, as of 2006, is only used clinically by about 40% of the members of the societies (ICS, AUGS) that acknowledge it as the recognized scientific standard for describing pelvic organ support.[12,13]

There are many reasons why the POPQ system has not gained widespread clinical use, but the most commonly cited reasons are: 1) not used by colleagues; 2) too time consuming; and 3) too confusing.[13] There is some validity to these concerns, but there are also some misconceptions. If only 40% of the members of the ICS and AUGS use it their clinical practice, it would be surprising to find that other healthcare providers outside of these societies had embraced the POPQ in their clinical practice. While there is no literature on how the system is used outside of the field of urogynecology there is a study of 54 obstetrics and gynecology house officers and students who were trained to use the system. When specifically queried, only one of 54 reported seeing or using the system outside of their urogynecology rotation.[14] Concerns about taking too much time to complete are unwarranted as it only takes 2–3 minutes to complete the examination, even in neophytes.[9]

Finally, while it may seem difficult to understand at first, when tested, obstetrics and gynecology house officers and medical students improved greatly on written understanding of the POPQ system after minimal instruction.[14] Therefore, for all the concerns about the POPQ, only clinical use appears valid. Despite these barriers to its routine clinical use, it remains the only universally recognized pelvic organ prolapse classification system.

Performing the POPQ examination

The POPQ examination takes nine measures of the position of midline vaginal structures (Table 69.1). All of the measurements are in centimeters relative to the hymeneal ring. The remnant of the hymeneal ring is used as the reference point because it is a fixed and easily identified landmark, as opposed to the introitus, which is a non-standardized anatomic structure (it is defined

Table 69.1. *Sites measure in the quantitative pelvic organ prolapse examination*

Point	Description
A anterior (Aa)	A point on the anterior vaginal wall 3 cm above the hymeneal ring
B anterior (Ba)	Most dependent or distal point on the anterior vaginal wall segment between A anterior and point C or the cuff if subject is status posthysterectomy
C	Anterior lip of the cervix or the cuff if subject is status posthysterectomy
A posterior (Ap)	A point on the posterior vaginal wall 3 cm above the hymeneal ring
B posterior (Bp)	Most dependent or distal point on the posterior vaginal wall segment between A posterior and point D or the cuff if subject is status posthysterectomy
D	Posterior fornix (this space is left blank in the subject who is status posthysterectomy)
Genital hiatus (gh)	Middle of external urethral meatus to posterior hymeneal remnant
Perineal body (pb)	Posterior hymen to middle of anal opening
Total vaginal length (tvl)	Hymeneal ring to vaginal apex

as 'entrance into the vagina'). All of the points recorded during the examination, with the exception of total vaginal length, are measured with the subject performing a Valsalva maneuver or a deep cough. Structures that lie above the hymeneal ring are recorded as negative, whereas structures that prolapse beyond the hymeneal ring are recorded as positive (both recordings in centimeters) (Fig. 69.2). Any structure that descends to the level of the hymeneal ring is recorded as zero centimeters. Nine measurements are taken during the examination: two from the anterior vaginal wall, two from the apex of the vagina, two from the posterior vaginal wall, and one each recording the genital hiatus, perineal body, and the total vaginal length at rest (see Table 69.1). These points are depicted diagrammatically in Figure 69.2; note also the two diagrams representing a large anterior segment defect with some apical descent (Profile A) and a large posterior defect (Profile B). The nine points may be recorded in a convenient manner using a three-by-three grid as noted in the figure. Any rigid measuring device – such as a marked wooden Pap smear spatula, ruler or engraved instrument – may be used.

For descriptive purposes, an ordinal staging system is used whereby the prolapse stage is defined by the vaginal

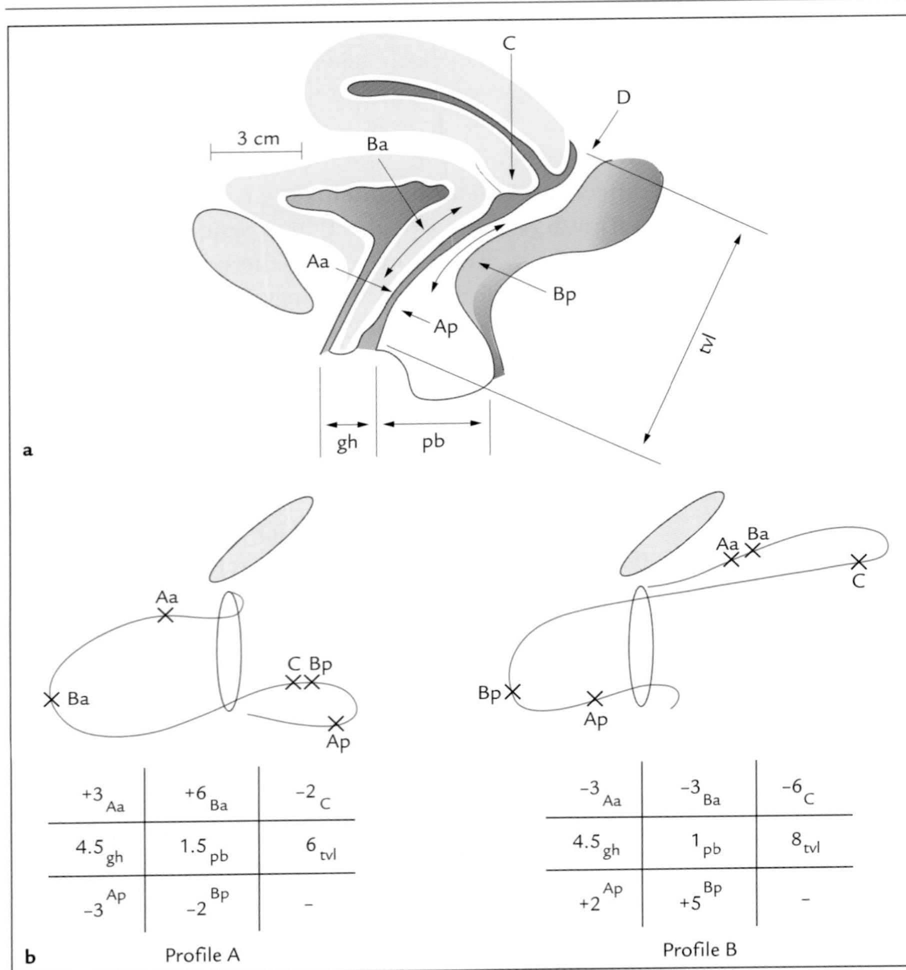

Figure 69.2. *(a) The nine points recorded for the pelvic organ prolapse classification system. Terms are defined in Table 69.1. (b) Profile A represents a large anterior wall defect with some apical descent; Profile B represents a large posterior defect. Note the grid system used for recording the nine points.*

Table 69.2. ***Staging of pelvic organ prolapse***

Stage	Description
0	No descensus of pelvic structures during straining
I	The leading surface of the prolapse does not descend below 1 cm above the hymeneal ring
II	The leading edge of the prolapse does not extend from 1 cm above the hymen to 1 cm through the hymeneal ring
III	The prolapse extends more than 1 cm beyond the hymeneal ring, but there is not complete vaginal eversion
IV	The vagina is completely everted

structure that demonstrates the greatest degree of prolapse (Table 69.2). An easy method of remembering this staging system involves understanding stage II. Any vaginal structure that descends such that the leading edge is at or between 1 cm above and 1 cm past the hymeneal ring is stage II. If the vaginal structure or leading edge has some movement but remains above –1 cm it is stage I, and any structure or leading edge that descends beyond +1 cm is stage III up to complete eversion, which is stage IV. Stage 0 is no descent of any vaginal segment.

At a practical level, an efficient method of performing the examination consists of placing a bivalved speculum in the vagina and measuring apical descent, using the posterior blade of the speculum to measure anterior and then posterior structures, and then measuring the perineal structures. Further information regarding the performance of the POPQ examination, including a videotape, is available at the AUGS website (www.augs.org).

One aspect of this system that may be awkward, or even anathema, to adherents of prior systems is the strict avoidance of terms such as cystocele, rectocele or enterocele. The rationale behind this seemingly dogmatic practice is to avoid erroneous assumptions regarding the prolapsing organs. Since the vagina is relatively opaque it is not possible to identify which organ is on the other side of the epithelium. It is often difficult even for experienced observers to discriminate between a high rectocele and a pulsion enterocele. Furthermore, patients who have had prior reconstructive pelvic surgery may have gross alterations in their vaginal axis, which result in unusual patterns of prolapse (e.g. anterior enterocele after sacrospinous ligament suspension). Another change from previous systems is the avoidance of staging the individual vaginal segments, i.e. a patient having a stage II cystocele and stage III rectocele. Instead, the patient is given one overall stage; for example, the previously noted patient would be described as having a POPQ stage III examination.

DEFINING PELVIC ORGAN PROLAPSE

A recent National Institutes of Health (NIH) consensus conference recognized that without a standard validated definition of pelvic organ prolapse there could be little progress in studying the disease and its treatment. They noted that currently there are no clinically or scientifically validated definitions and felt that any proposed definition should take into account both a subject's anatomy as well as their symptoms.[15] Developing a knowledge base regarding the normal distribution of pelvic organ support in the female population and determining how symptoms relate to various degrees of support is paramount to defining the disease of pelvic organ prolapse.

Currently there are several studies examining the distribution of pelvic organ support in various general female populations. These studies are being undertaken to determine the normal distribution of pelvic organ support.[16–23] However, only three studies have looked at general populations of a significant age range employing the POPQ system.[16–18] From the distribution of these three studies as plotted in Figure 69.3, it can be seen that POPQ stage II support represents between 30 and 50% of the populations studied. However, it is doubtful that pelvic organ prolapse is this prevalent; therefore the NIH definition may be too broad. Only 2–11% of subjects in these studies have stage 3 and 4 examinations, which is more consistent with current estimates on the percent of subjects undergoing surgical treatment for this condition. There is an 11% lifetime risk of undergoing surgical correction of pelvic organ prolapse and the incidence of surgery for pelvic organ prolapse is 22.7 per 10,000.[24,25]

Pelvic organ prolapse is a disease with essentially no mortality and only minimal morbidity; however, it is a condition that impacts greatly on quality of life. Therefore, symptoms play a central role in defining at what point a patient goes from 'normal' pelvic organ support to 'abnormal' pelvic organ prolapse. Despite the concerns involving a lack of data on symptoms and how they relate to anatomy, the NIH consensus conference did propose a definition of pelvic organ prolapse.[15] They suggested that all POPQ stage II or greater pelvic organ support be considered 'pelvic organ prolapse', but felt that this definition would required scientific validation before it could be recommended as a clinical or research standard.

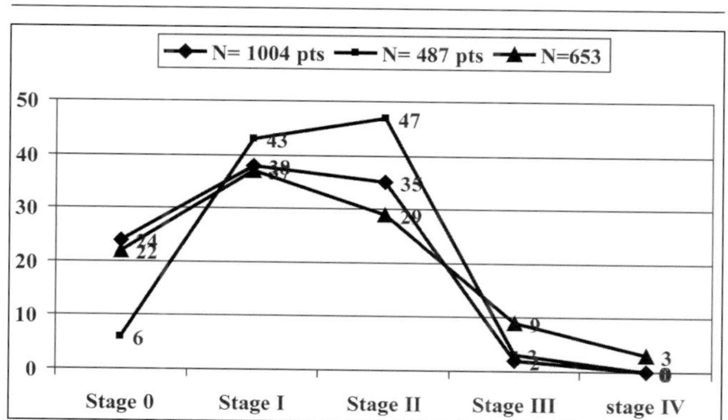

Figure 69.3. *Percent of subjects in each POPQ stage in three studies of general female populations. n, the number of subjects examined in each study.*

There are currently several studies investigating the correlation between symptoms and pelvic organ support. Most demonstrate that there is a very weak (if any) correlation between symptoms and advancing degrees of pelvic organ prolapse with the exception of the symptom of a bothersome vaginal bulge.[26–30] In the few studies that correlated POPQ stage with symptoms it appears that symptoms begin to significantly increase once the leading edge of the vaginal wall extends to or just beyond the hymen.[17,25] Therefore, a reasonable definition of pelvic organ prolapse may be protrusion of any vaginal segment to or beyond the hymen in symptomatic patients; however, this definition needs further study to document its validity.

EPIDEMIOLOGY OF PELVIC ORGAN PROLAPSE

As previously noted, there is no currently accepted definition of pelvic organ prolapse; therefore each study into its epidemiology is left to employ its own definition. Generally, the literature defines prolapse in one of two ways – either anatomically by examination or by surgical admission for corrective surgery. The concern regarding surgical admissions is that they miss those patients that manage their prolapse conservatively; the concern regarding anatomic descriptions is that no two studies use the same anatomic cutoffs.[17,19,21,23,24,31–35] A list of the major epidemiologic studies and their definitions is provided in Table 69.3. This plethora of definitions makes it difficult to evaluate trends in the literature into the various etiologies and can lead to conflicting results. This portion of the chapter will examine the various proposed etiologies of pelvic organ prolapse, bearing in mind that the frequently conflicting results stem from the various definitions employed in each study.

The only universally accepted risk factor for pelvic organ prolapse is increasing age. Regardless of the definition used, this factor is always identified as an etiology and most estimates suggest that there is roughly a doubling in the risk of prolapse with every completed decade of life.[16,17,23,31] The other proposed etiologies for pelvic organ prolapse are many but for the most part involve two types of insult: either the acute damage that occurs with pregnancy or the chronic insults from conditions that lead to continuous intermittent increases in intra-abdominal pressure. In addition, other areas that have been investigated include prior pelvic surgery and genetic factors.

Effect of pregnancy

The relationship between pregnancy and pelvic organ prolapse has been extensively studied and is mentioned in almost every treatise on this subject. It is assumed that as the fetal vertex passes through the birth canal there is direct damage to the nerves, fascia, and muscle that leads to eventual relaxation of the pelvic floor musculature and pelvic organ prolapse. While it is generally recognized that any parity is associated with an increased risk of prolapse, what role the delivery mode plays is more controversial.[16–19,21,30–32,34] Specifically, can one delivery mode (i.e. cesarean section) provide protection against prolapse? The majority of the literature supports the notion that increasing parity increases the risk of pelvic organ prolapse.[16,17,19,30,32] Studies suggest that anywhere from a four- to an 11-fold increase in the risk of prolapse is dependent on parity, with increasing parity imparting greater risk.[17,19,31]

However, the literature on the mode of delivery is mixed. When women who delivered only by cesarean section were compared to women who had any vaginal

Table 69.3. *Definitions of pelvic organ prolapse from the various epidemiologic studies*

Author	Definition
Jorgensen et al.[35]	Surgical admission for surgery to correct prolapse
Olsen et al.[24]	Surgical admission for surgery to correct prolapse
Mant et al.[19]	Surgical admission for surgery to correct prolapse
Chiaffarino et al.[32]	Baden and Walker stage 2 and greater
Marchionni et al.[33]	Baden and Walker stage 2 and greater
Samuelsson et al.[21]	Presence of any cystocele, rectocele, uterine descent, or absence of the urethrovesical crease
Gruel & Gruel[34]	Any vaginal relaxation to the introitus (roughly equivalent to Baden and Walker stage 2 and greater)
Swift et al.[31]	POPQ stage 3 prolapse
Hendrix et al.[23]	Stage 1 or greater prolapse by a unique system defined for this study (stage 1 is defined as in the vagina)
Swift et al.[17]	Leading edge at –0.5 cm above the introitus or greater (some POPQ stage 2 and all stage 3 and 4)

delivery, the data are inconclusive and do not suggest a protective effect.[17] The data on instrumented vaginal delivery are sparse and in one study forceps delivery was not identified as a risk factor for the development of prolapse.[32] In addition, there is one study suggesting that episiotomy protects against prolapse.[33]

The data regarding infant weight are more consistent, with most studies demonstrating an increase in prolapse with increasing fetal weight; delivery of a macrosomic infant carries the greatest risk.[17,21,31,32]

Pregnancy and macrosomia are consistently identified as risk factors for pelvic organ prolapse, but whether cesarean delivery or avoidance of an operative vaginal delivery can protect against pelvic organ prolapse remains a topic of debate with no clear evidence to support or refute this supposition.

Modifiable lifestyle risk factors

There are several opinions regarding how to counsel patients in ways to prevent pelvic organ prolapse. Factors such as occupations that require a lot of lifting, together with obesity and smoking, all contribute to pelvic organ prolapse, and modifying or removing these insults will reduce the risk.

The data on occupation as a risk for prolapse stem from an article published in 1994 on nursing assistants in Denmark. The investigators noted a 60% increased risk of surgery to correct pelvic organ prolapse and herniated lumbar disks in nursing assistants over the general population,[35] and felt this was due to the excess heavy lifting of patients inherent in their job description. Since then, two large studies have incorporated job description into their data collection.[17,32] Both found that manual workers and housewives had a slightly increased risk of prolapse over women who classified themselves as professionals.

Obesity is another risk factor commonly quoted for pelvic organ prolapse. It is felt that the increasing weight from abdominal adipose tissue increases the pressure on the intra-abdominal organs, leading to pelvic floor weakness and prolapse. Here the literature is divided, with several studies suggesting it as a risk factor[17,19,23,24,33] and several studies finding no association.[21,31,33]

Smoking is the final modifiable risk factor often associated with pelvic organ prolapse. Again the data are mixed, with several studies suggesting that current smokers are at risk,[19,23,24] two showing no relationship,[21,32] and one study suggesting smoking has some protection against pelvic organ prolapse.[17]

Among the lifestyle or modifiable etiologies, the only factor that demonstrates a consistent relationship with an increased risk of pelvic organ prolapse is job description, with those individuals engaged in more manual labor having a greater risk of prolapse.

Medical illnesses

Other areas that are commonly discussed and implicated as being etiologies of pelvic organ prolapse are chronic medical or congenital illnesses that result either in increased intra-abdominal pressure or in microvascular disease and poor quality collagen. The relationship between chronic illness and prolapse has been investigated in large epidemiologic studies with mixed results. It would seem intuitive that those illnesses associated with chronic recurrent increases in intra-abdominal pressure, constipation, and chronic obstructive pulmonary disease (COPD) would increase the risk of pelvic organ prolapse. Constipation is an illness that can be difficult to define; however – when evaluated – it appears consistently related to an increase in prolapse.[23,36]

Two studies evaluated COPD and neither noted it as a risk for prolapse.[24,31] In one of these studies the number of subjects with COPD was very small and in the other the pelvic organ prolapse was defined by surgical admission so the data could be questioned. However, when taken with data on smoking, there does not appear to be a strong relationship between pulmonary disease and prolapse.

Medical illnesses that lead to long-term damage to the microvasculature and peripheral neuropathies, such as hypertension and diabetes mellitus, have been suggested as a potential cause of pelvic organ prolapse. However, as with many etiologic studies, the results are mixed. In one large study the presence of any chronic illness was not associated with an increased incidence of prolapse;[17] in another study, only hypertension was identified as a risk factor.[31]

There are also a few studies in women with collagen vascular diseases, such as Marfan and Ehlers–Danlos syndrome, which suggest that these patients are at an increased risk of prolapse.[37,38] However, again the data are somewhat conflicting and this may stem from the lack of any definition of prolapse in these studies.

Race

There is a long history of observational data to suggest that women of certain racial groups are at a greater or lesser risk of pelvic organ prolapse. There are early anecdotal reports of African–American and 'Chinese' women having a very low risk of pelvic organ prolapse in comparison to Caucasian women.[39–41] While it can be difficult to classify women into race (with the Tiger Woods phenomenon), it appears that African–American women having a slightly decreased risk of prolapse when compared to their Caucasian counterparts, and Hispanic women have an increased risk over Caucasian women.[17,23,31] The data on Asian women in these trials are too sparse to draw any conclusions.

Menopausal status and hormone replacement therapy

The association between menopausal status, hormonal therapy and pelvic organ prolapse is a very complicated issue. First, women who are menopausal tend to be older than their premenopausal counterparts and, as pointed out earlier, increasing age is probably the greatest risk factor for pelvic organ prolapse. In addition, women who take hormone replacement therapy (HRT) may not have taken it consistently since menopause and can be on any of a myriad of dosing schedules, further complicating any comparative studies. The majority of the studies suggest that postmenopausal women are at greater risk; however, when a multiple logistic regression analysis takes age into account, menopausal status becomes non-significant, suggesting that it may be the age factor more than the decreased estrogen levels that places the woman at risk for prolapse.[17,23,31,32]

In these same studies, when the role of HRT was evaluated in menopausal women, the results are even less clear. One study suggested that past use decreases risk but not current use, another suggested no difference between ever and never using HRT, and one suggested that postmenopausal women with current use had a risk equal to that of premenopausal women. It should be noted that, while HRT may not protect menopausal women from developing prolapse, it has never demonstrated a negative effect.

Prior pelvic surgery

This is another area where it is difficult to determine if there are any significant relationships. First, it is known that up to 30% of women who undergo surgery for pelvic organ prolapse will require a second procedure to correct recurrent prolapse.[24] Therefore, subjects who have had prior prolapse surgery have many of the underlying conditions that put them at risk for prolapse, and using this as a risk factor is similar to noting the increased risk of cancer in patients undergoing treatment for cancer. Conversely, many patients who have undergone a hysterectomy had it done to correct pelvic organ prolapse, as pelvic relaxation is the third most common indication for hysterectomy in the US.[42] Therefore, many of these patients have already been treated for prolapse and many will have been treated successfully. However, when hysterectomy is evaluated, most studies suggest that it does expose patients to an increased risk of pelvic organ prolapse.[19,21,31,33] When the hysterectomy was done specifically for prolapse it increases the risk even more.[33] The mechanism behind this phenomenon may be the disruption of the normal apical supports of the vagina in subjects with otherwise good support. This emphasizes the need to be ever mindful of providing strong attachment of the cardinal and uterosacral ligament complex to the vaginal cuff at the time of hysterectomy. In subjects who have undergone prior prolapse surgery there appears to be upwards of a five-fold increase in their risk of developing pelvic organ prolapse.[31]

Family history

This is one area where we have almost no data; however, this may be of central importance when we counsel patients about other modifiable risk factors. There is one study where subjects who had undergone surgery for prolapse were asked about any family history of other relatives undergoing similar surgery.[32] The authors noted that there was an increased risk of pelvic organ prolapse surgery if a patient's mother or sister had undergone prolapse surgery.

SUMMARY

While we are still in the infancy of understanding pelvic organ prolapse, we are moving forward. There is now a growing body of literature regarding the classification and epidemiology of pelvic organ prolapse incorporating the POPQ and well-described definitions of pelvic organ prolapse that are beginning to help us understand this complex disease.

Currently, it is difficult to evaluate the various etiologies of pelvic organ prolapse because of the lack of a standard definition. This makes the plethora of emerging data difficult to interpret because often we are comparing apples and oranges. There are a few consistencies, with age and pregnancy being acknowledged risk factors for pelvic organ prolapse. Other factors that probably play a role include obesity, a job with a greater proportion of manual labor and lifting, lack of HRT, hysterectomy, and family history. However, before recommendations can be made regarding preventive strategies, more studies using a consistent definition are required.

REFERENCES

1. Scanzoni FW. Senkung und Vorfall des uterus und der scheide. In: Scanzoni FW (ed) Lehrbuch der Krankheiten der Weiblichen Geschlechstorgane, 5th ed. Vienna: Braumueller, 1875; 654–64.
2. Kelly HA. Operative Gynecology. New York: Appleton & Co., 1898.
3. Kuestner O. Prolapsus uteri et vaginea. In: Kuestner O, Bumm E, Doederlein A, Kroenig B, Menge C (eds) Kurzes Lehrbuch der Gynaekologie. Jena: G Fischers, 1912; 159–81.
4. Baden WF, Walker TA. Genesis of the vaginal profile: a correlated classification of vaginal relaxation. Clin Obstet Gynecol 1972;15:1048–54.
5. Baden WF, Walker TA. Physical diagnosis in the evaluation of vaginal relaxation. Clin Obstet Gynecol 1972;15:1055–69.
6. Beechum CT. Classification of vaginal relaxation. Am J Obstet Gynecol 1980;136:957–8.
7. Porges RF. A practical system of diagnosis and classification of pelvic relaxations. Surg Gynecol Obstet 1963;117:761–73.
8. Bump RC, Mattiasson A, Bo K et al. The standardization of terminology of female pelvic floor dysfunction. Am J Obstet Gynecol 1996;175:10–7.
9. Hall AF, Theofrastous JP, Cundiff GC, Harris RL, Hamilton LF, Swift SE, Bump RC. Interobserver and intraobserver reliability of the proposed International Continence Society, Society of Gynecologic Surgeons, and American Urogynecologic Society pelvic organ prolapse classification system. Am J Obstet Gynecol 1996;175:1467–71.
10. Kobak WH, Rosenberger K, Walters MD. Interobserver variation in the assessment of pelvic organ prolapse. Int J Urogynecol Pelvic Floor Dysfunct 1996;7:121–4.
11. Prien-Larsen J, Mouritsen L. Pelvic organ prolapse: is ICS-grading without POP-Q measurement reliable? [abstract]. Int Urogynecol J 2001;12(Suppl 3):S45.
12. Muir T, Stepp K, Barber M. Adoption of the pelvic organ prolapse quantification system in peer-reviewed literature. Am J Obstet Gynecol 2003;189:1632–6.
13. Auwad W, Freeman R, Swift S. Is the pelvic organ prolapse quantification system (POPQ) being used? A survey of the members of the International Continence Society (ICS) and the American Urogynecology Society (AUGS). Int Urogynecol J 2004;15:324–7.
14. Steele A, Mallipeddi P, Welgloss J, Soled S, Kohli N, Karram M. Teaching the pelvic organ prolapse quantification system. Am J Obstet Gynecol 1998;179:1458–64.
15. Weber AM, Abrams P, Brubaker L et al. The standardization of terminology for researchers in female pelvic floor disorders. Int Urogynecol J 2001;12:178–86.
16. Swift SE. The distribution of pelvic organ support in a population of female subjects seen for routine gynecologic health care. Am J Obstet Gynecol 2000;183:277–85.
17. Swift SE, Woodman P, O'Boyle A et al. Pelvic Organ Support Study (POSST): the distribution, clinical definition and epidemiology of pelvic organ support defects. Am J Obstet Gynecol 2005 (in press).
18. Slieker-ten HMCP, Vierhout M, Bloembergen H, Schoenmaker G. Distribution of pelvic organ prolapse in a general population: prevalence, severity, etiology and relation with the function of pelvic floor muscles. Abstract presented at the Joint meeting of the ICS and IUGA, August 25–27, 2004, Paris, France.
19. Mant J, Painter R, Vessey M. Epidemiology of genital prolapse: observations from the Oxford Family Planning Association study. Br J Obstet Gynaecol 1997;104:579–85.
20. Bland DR, Earle BB, Vitolins MZ, Burke G. Use of the pelvic organ prolapse staging system of the International Continence Society, American Urogynecologic Society, and the Society of Gynecologic Surgeons in perimenopausal women. Am J Obstet Gynecol 1999;181:1324–8.
21. Samuelsson EU, Victor FTA, Tibblin G, Svardsudd KF. Signs of genital prolapse in a Swedish population of women 20 to 59 years of age and possible related factors. Am J Obstet Gynecol 1999;180:299–305.
22. Versi E, Harvey M-A, Cardozo L, Brincat M, Studd WW. Urogenital prolapse and atrophy at menopause: a prevalence study. Int Urogynecol J 2001;12:107–10.
23. Hendrix SL, Clark A, Nygaard I, Aragki A, Barnabei V, McTiernan A. Pelvic organ prolapse in the Women's Health Initiative. Am J Obstet Gynecol 2002;186:1160–6.
24. Olsen AL, Smith VJ, Bergstrom VO, Colling JC, Clark AL. Epidemiology of surgically managed pelvic organ prolapse and urinary incontinence. Obstet Gynecol 1997;89:501–6.
25. Rown JS, Waetjen LE, Subak LL, Thom DH, Van Den Eeden S, Vittinghoff E. Pelvic organ prolapse surgery in the United States, 1997. Am J Obstet Gynecol 2002;186:712–6.
26. Swift SE, Tate SB, Nichols J. Correlation of symptomatology with degree of pelvic organ support in a general population of women: what is pelvic organ prolapse? Am J Obstet Gynecol 2003;189:372–9.
27. Barber M, Walters M, Bump R. Association of the magnitude of pelvic organ prolapse and presence and severity of symptoms. Abstract presented at the 24th annual scientific meeting of the American Urgynecologic Society, September 11–13, 2003, Hollywood, FL.
28. Elkerman RM, Cundiff GW, Melik CF, Nihira M, Leffler K, Bent AE. Correlation of symptoms with location and severity of pelvic organ prolapse. Am J Obstet Gynecol 2001;185:1332–8.
29. Heit M, Culligan P, Rosenquist C, Shott S. Is pelvic organ prolapse a cause of pelvic or low back pain? Obstet Gynecol 2002;99:22–8.

30. Burrows LJ, Meyn LA, Walters MD, Weber AM. Pelvic symptoms in women with pelvic organ prolapse. Am J Obstet Gynecol 2004;104:982–8.

31. Swift SE, Pound T, Dias JK. Case-control study of etiologic risk factors in the development of severe pelvic organ prolapse. Int Urogynecol J 2001;12:187–92.

32. Chiaffarino F, Chatenoud L, Dindelli M et al. Reproductive factors, family history, occupation and risk of urogenital prolapse. Eur J Obstet Gynecol Reprod Biol 1999;82:63–7.

33. Marchionni M, Luca Braco G, Checcucci V et al. True incidence of vaginal vault prolapse: thirteen years' experience. J Reprod Med 1999;44:679–84.

34. Gruel H, Gruel SA. Pelvic relaxation and associated risk factors: the results of logistic regression analysis. Acta Obstet Gynecol Scand 1999;78:290–3.

35. Jorgensen S, Hein HO, Gyntelberg F. Heavy lifting at work and risk of genital prolapse and herniated lumbar disc in assistant nurses. Occup Med 1994;44:47–9.

36. Spence-Jones C, Kamm MA, Henery MM, Hudson CN. Bowel dysfunction: a pathologic factor in uterovaginal prolapse and urinary stress incontinence. Br J Obstet Gynaecol 1994;101:147–52.

37. Carley ME, Schaffer J. Urinary incontinence and pelvic organ prolapse in women with Marfan and Ehlers–Danlos syndrome. Am J Obstet Gynecol 2000;182:1021–3.

38. McIntosh LJ, Stanitski DF, Mallett VT, Frahm JD, Richardson DA, Evans MI. Ehlers–Danlos syndrome: relationship between joint hypermobility, urinary incontinence and pelvic floor prolapse. Gynecol Obstet Invest 1996;41:135–9.

39. van Dongen L. The anatomy of genital prolapse. S Afr Med J 1981;60:357–9.

40. Zacharin RF. 'A Chinese anatomy' – the pelvic supporting tissues of the Chinese and Occidental female compared and contrasted. Aust N Z J Obstet Gynecol 1977;17:1–11.

41. Cox PSV, Webster D. Genital prolapse amongst the Pokot. East Afr Med J 1975;52:694–9.

42. Wilcox LS, Koonin LM, Pokras R, Struass LT, Xia Z, Peterson HB. Hysterectomy in the United States, 1988–1990. Obstet Gynecol 1994;83:549–55.

70

Anterior vaginal wall prolapse

Mark D Walters

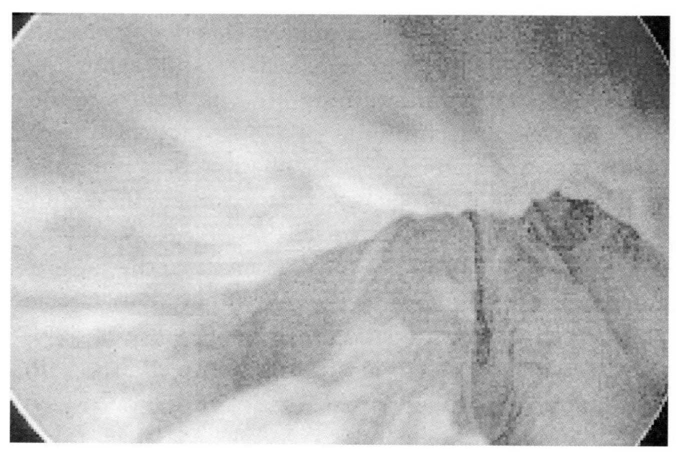

INTRODUCTION

Anterior vaginal prolapse occurs commonly and may coexist with disorders of micturition. Mild anterior vaginal prolapse often occurs in parous women but usually presents few problems. As the prolapse progresses, symptoms may develop and worsen, and treatment becomes indicated. This chapter reviews the anatomy and pathology of anterior vaginal prolapse, with and without stress incontinence, and describes methods of vaginal repair.

ANATOMY AND PATHOLOGY

Anterior vaginal prolapse (cystocele) is defined as pathologic descent of the anterior vaginal wall and overlying bladder base. According to the International Continence Society (ICS) standardized terminology for prolapse grading,[1] the term 'anterior vaginal prolapse' is preferred to 'cystocele'. This is because information obtained at the physical examination does not allow the exact identification of structures behind the anterior vaginal wall, although it usually is, in fact, the bladder. The ICS grading system for prolapse is discussed in detail in Chapter 69.

The etiology of anterior vaginal prolapse is not completely understood, but it is probably multifactorial, with different factors implicated in prolapse in individual patients. Normal support for the vagina and adjacent pelvic organs is provided by the interaction of the pelvic muscles and connective tissue.[2] The upper vagina rests on the levator plate and is stabilized by superior and lateral connective tissue attachments; the midvagina is attached to the arcus tendineus fasciae pelvis (white line) on each side.[3] Pathologic loss of that support may occur with damage to the pelvic muscles, connective tissue attachments, or both.

Nichols and Randall described two types of anterior vaginal prolapse: distension and displacement.[4] Distension was thought to result from overstretching and attenuation of the anterior vaginal wall, caused by overdistension of the vagina associated with vaginal delivery or atrophic changes associated with aging and menopause. The distinguishing physical feature of this type was described as diminished or absent rugal folds of the anterior vaginal epithelium caused by thinning or loss of midline vaginal fascia. The other type of anterior vaginal prolapse – displacement – was attributed to pathologic detachment or elongation of the anterolateral vaginal supports to the arcus tendineus fasciae pelvis. It may occur unilaterally or bilaterally and often coexists with some degree of distension cystocele, with urethral hypermobility, or with apical prolapse. Rugal folds may or may not be preserved.

Another theory ascribes most cases of anterior vaginal prolapse to disruption or detachment of the lateral connective tissue attachments at the arcus tendineus fasciae pelvis, resulting in a paravaginal defect and corresponding to the displacement type discussed earlier. This was first described by White in 1909[5] and 1912,[6] but disregarded until reported by Richardson in 1976.[7] Richardson described transverse defects, midline defects, and defects involving isolated loss of integrity of pubourethral ligaments. Transverse defects were said to occur when the 'pubocervical' fascia separated from its insertion around the cervix, whereas midline defects represented an anteroposterior separation of the fascia between the bladder and vagina. A contemporary conceptual representation of vaginal and paravaginal defects is shown in Figure 70.1.[8]

There have been few systematic or comprehensive descriptions of anterior vaginal prolapse based on physical findings and correlated with findings at surgery to provide objective evidence for any of these theories of pathologic anatomy. In a study of 71 women with anterior vaginal wall prolapse and stress incontinence who underwent retropubic operations, DeLancey[9] described

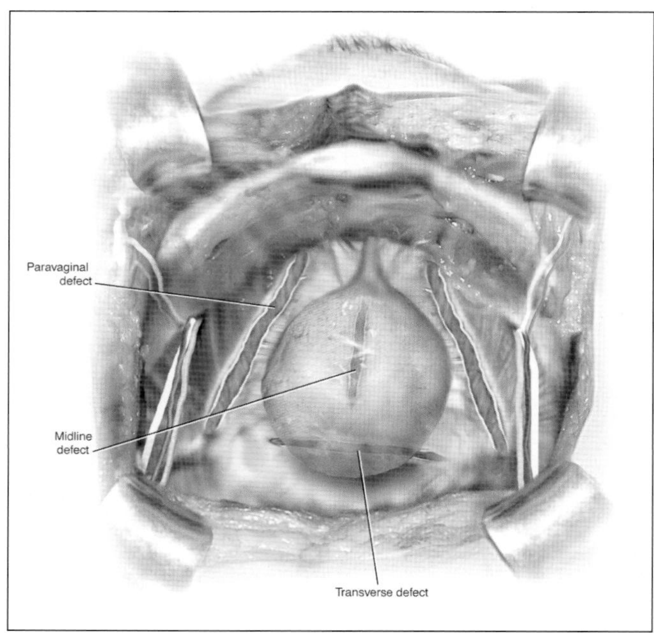

Figure 70.1. *Three different defects can result in anterior vaginal wall prolapse. Lateral or paravaginal defects occur when there is a separation of the pubocervical fascia from the arcus tendineus fasciae pelvis, midline defects occur secondary to attenuation of fascia supporting the bladder base, and transverse defects occur when the pubocervical fascia separates from the vaginal cuff or uterosacral ligaments. (Reproduced from ref. 8 with permission.)*

paravaginal defects in 87% on the left and 89% on the right. The arcus tendineus fasciae pelvis were usually attached to the pubic bone but detached from the ischial spine for a variable distance. The pubococcygeal muscle was visibly abnormal with localized or generalized atrophy in over half of the women.

Recent improvements in pelvic imaging are leading to a greater understanding of normal pelvic anatomy and the structural and functional abnormalities associated with prolapse. Magnetic resonance imaging (MRI) holds great promise, with its excellent ability to differentiate soft tissues and its capacity for multiplanar imaging. Further work is needed to correlate the different images with anatomy and histology under normal conditions and with pelvic support abnormalities.

The pelvic organs, pelvic muscles, and connective tissues can be identified easily with MRI. Various measurements can be made that may be associated with anterior vaginal prolapse or urinary incontinence, such as the urethrovesical angle, descent of the bladder base, the quality of the levator muscles, and the relationship between the vagina and its lateral connective tissue attachments. Aronson et al.[10] used an endoluminal surface coil placed in the vagina to image pelvic anatomy with MRI, and compared four continent nulliparous women with four incontinent women with anterior vaginal prolapse. Lateral vaginal attachments were identified in all continent women. In Figure 70.2, the 'posterior pubourethral ligaments' (bilateral attachment of arcus tendineus fasciae pelvis to posterior aspect of the pubic symphyses) are clearly seen. In the two subjects with clinically apparent paravaginal defects, lateral detachments were evident (Fig. 70.3). Although this study involved only a small number of subjects, it provides the basis for further work in describing the anatomic abnormalities that accompany anterior vaginal prolapse and other abnormalities of pelvic support. This may ultimately guide the choice of surgical repair.

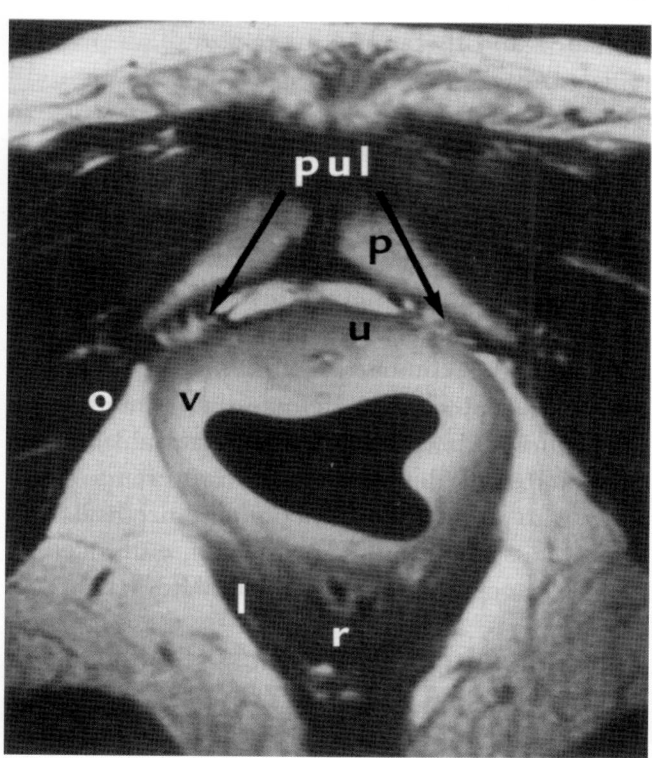

Figure 70.2. *Axial T1-weighted image from a continent 38-year-old nulliparous woman, showing the connection of the anterior vaginal wall (v) to the posterior pubic symphysis (p) by the pubourethral ligaments (pul). The anterior vaginal wall and endopelvic fascia function as a sling or hammock for support of the urethra (u). o, Obturator internus muscle; r, rectum; l, levator ani musculature. (Reproduced from ref. 10 with permission.)*

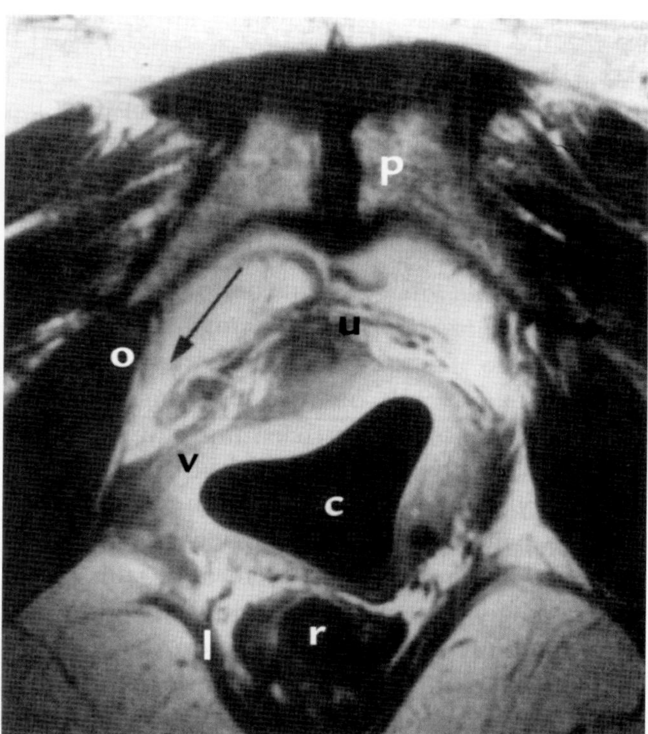

Figure 70.3. *Axial T1-weighted image from a 57-year-old woman, para 5, with stress urinary incontinence. The paravaginal detachment (arrow) is seen at the level of the urethrovesical junction. v, anterior vaginal wall; p, posterior pubic symphysis; u, urethra; o, obturator internus muscle; c, endovaginal coil; r, rectum; l, levator ani musculature. (Reproduced from ref. 10 with permission.)*

Anterior vaginal prolapse commonly coexists with urodynamic stress incontinence. Some features of pathophysiology may overlap, such as loss of anterior vaginal support with bladder-base descent and urethral hypermobility; other features, such as sphincteric dysfunction, may occur independent of vaginal and urethral support. The pathophysiology of stress incontinence is covered more fully in Chapter 11.

EVALUATION

History

When evaluating women with pelvic organ prolapse or urinary or fecal incontinence, attention should be paid to all aspects of pelvic organ support. The reconstructive surgeon must determine the specific sites of damage for each patient, with the ultimate goal of restoring both anatomy and function.

Patients with anterior vaginal prolapse complain of symptoms directly related to vaginal protrusion or of associated symptoms such as urinary incontinence or voiding difficulty. Symptoms related to prolapse may include the sensation of a vaginal mass or bulge, pelvic pressure, low back pain, and sexual difficulty. Stress urinary incontinence commonly occurs in association with anterior vaginal prolapse. Voiding difficulty may result from advanced prolapse. Women may require vaginal pressure or manual replacement of the prolapse in order to accomplish voiding. Women may relate a history of urinary incontinence that has since resolved with worsening of their prolapse. This can occur with urethral kinking and obstruction to urinary flow; women in this situation are at risk for incomplete bladder emptying and recurrent or persistent urinary tract infections and for the development of de novo stress incontinence after the prolapse is repaired.

Physical examination

The physical examination should be conducted with the patient in the lithotomy position, as for a routine pelvic examination. The examination is first performed with the patient supine. If physical findings do not correspond to symptoms or if the maximum extent of the prolapse cannot be confirmed, the woman is re-examined in the standing position.

The genitalia are inspected, and if no displacement is apparent, the labia are gently spread to expose the vestibule and hymen. The integrity of the perineal body is evaluated, and the approximate size of all prolapsed parts is assessed. A retractor or Sims speculum can be used to depress the posterior vagina to aid in visualizing the anterior vagina. After the resting examination, the patient is instructed to strain down forcefully or to cough vigorously. During this maneuver, the order of descent of the pelvic organs is noted, as is the relationship of the pelvic organs at the peak of straining.

It may be possible to differentiate lateral defects, identified as detachment or effacement of the lateral vaginal sulci, from central defects, seen as midline protrusion but with preservation of the lateral sulci, by using a curved forcep placed in the anterolateral vaginal sulci directed towards the ischial spine. Bulging of the anterior vaginal wall in the midline between the forcep blades implies a midline defect; blunting or descent of the vaginal fornices on either side with straining suggest lateral paravaginal defects. Studies have shown that the physical examination technique to detect paravaginal defects is not particularly reliable or accurate. In a study by Barber et al.[11] of 117 women with prolapse, the sensitivity of clinical examination to detect paravaginal defects was good (92%), yet the specificity was poor (52%) and, despite an unexpectly high prevalence of paravaginal defects, the positive predictive value was poor (61%). Less than two-thirds of women believed to have a paravaginal defect on physical examination were confirmed to possess the same at surgery. Another study by Whiteside et al.[12] demonstrated poor reproducibility of clinical examination to detect anterior vaginal wall defects. Thus, the clinical value of determining the location of midline, apical, and lateral paravaginal defects remains unknown.

Anterior vaginal wall descent usually represents bladder descent with or without concomitant urethral hypermobility. In 1.6% of women with anterior vaginal prolapse, an anterior enterocele mimics a cystocele on physical examination.[13]

Diagnostic tests

After a careful history and physical examination, few diagnostic tests are needed to evaluate patients with anterior vaginal prolapse. A urinalysis should be performed to evaluate for urinary tract infection if the patient complains of any lower urinary tract dysfunction. If the patient's estrogen status is unclear, a vaginal cytologic smear can be obtained to assess maturation index. Hydronephrosis occurs in a small proportion of women with prolapse; however, even if identified, it usually does not change management in women for whom surgical repair is planned.[14] Therefore, routine imaging of the kidneys and ureters is not necessary.

If urinary incontinence is present, further diagnostic testing is indicated to determine the cause of the incontinence. Urodynamic (simple or complex), endoscopic or radiologic assessments of filling and voiding function are generally indicated only when symptoms of incontinence or voiding dysfunction are present. Even if no urologic symptoms are noted, voiding function should be assessed to evaluate for completeness of bladder emptying. This procedure usually involves a timed, measured void, followed by urethral catheterization or bladder ultrasound to measure residual urine volume.

In women with severe prolapse, it is important to check urethral function after the prolapse is repositioned. As demonstrated by Bump et al.,[15] women with severe prolapse may be continent because of urethral kinking; when the prolapse is reduced, urethral dysfunction may be unmasked with occurrence of incontinence. A pessary, vaginal retractor or vaginal packing can be used to reduce the prolapse before office bladder filling or electronic urodynamic testing. If urinary leaking occurs with coughing or Valsalva maneuvers after reduction of the prolapse, the urethral sphincter is probably incompetent, even if the patient is normally continent. This is reported to occur in 17–69% of women with stage III or IV prolapse.[15,16] In this situation, the surgeon should choose an anti-incontinence procedure in conjunction with anterior vaginal prolapse repair.[16] If sphincteric incompetence is not present even after reduction of the prolapse, an anti-incontinence procedure is not indicated.

SURGICAL REPAIR TECHNIQUES

Anterior colporrhaphy

The objective of anterior colporrhaphy is to plicate the layers of vaginal muscularis and adventitia overlying the bladder ('pubocervical fascia') or to plicate and reattach the paravaginal tissue in such a way as to reduce the protrusion of the bladder and vagina. Modifications of the technique depend on how lateral the dissection is carried, where the plicating sutures are placed, and whether additional layers (natural or synthetic) are placed in the anterior vagina for extra support.

The operative procedure begins with the patient supine, with the legs elevated and abducted and the buttocks placed just past the edge of the operating table. The chosen anesthetic has been administered, and one perioperative intravenous dose of an appropriate antibiotic may be given as prophylaxis against infection. The abdomen, vagina, and perineum are sterilely prepped and draped, and a 16 Fr Foley catheter with a 5 ml balloon is inserted for easy identification of the bladder neck. If indicated, a suprapubic catheter is placed into the bladder.

A weighted speculum is placed into the vagina. If a vaginal hysterectomy has been performed, the incised apex of the anterior vaginal wall is grasped transversely with two Allis clamps and elevated. Otherwise, a transverse or diamond-shaped incision is made in the vaginal mucosa near the apex. A third Allis clamp is placed about 1 cm below the posterior margin of the urethral meatus and pulled up. Additional Allis clamps may be placed in the midline between the urethra and apex. Hemostatic solutions (such as 0.5% lidocaine with 1:200,000 epinephrine) or saline may be injected submucosally, along the midline of the anterior vaginal wall, to decrease bleeding and to aid in dissection. The points of a pair of curved Mayo scissors are inserted between the vaginal epithelium and the vaginal muscularis, or between the layers of the vaginal muscularis, and gently forced upward while being kept half-opened/half-closed (Fig. 70.4). Countertraction during this maneuver is important to minimize the likelihood of perforation of the bladder.

The vagina is then incised in the midline, and the incision is continued to the level of the midurethra. Alternatively, a scalpel can be used to make a midline anterior vaginal incision. As the vagina is incised, the edges are grasped with Allis or T-clamps and drawn laterally for further mobilization. Dissection of the vaginal flaps is then accomplished by turning the clamps back across the forefinger and incising the vaginal muscularis with a scalpel or Metzenbaum scissors, as shown in Figure 70.4c. An assistant maintains constant traction medially on the remaining vaginal muscularis and underlying vesicovaginal adventitia. This procedure is performed bilaterally until the entire extent of the anterior vaginal prolapse has been dissected; in general, the dissection should be carried further laterally with more advanced prolapse. The spaces lateral to the urethrovesical junction are sharply dissected toward the ischiopubic rami. It is also important to use sharp dissection to mobilize the bladder base from the vaginal apex as shown in Figure 70.5.

In most cases, even if the patient does not suffer from urinary incontinence, plicating sutures at the urethrovesical junction should be placed to augment posterior urethral support and to ensure that stress incontinence, if not present at the time of operation, does not develop postoperatively. Vesical neck plication can also be used to treat mild stress urinary incontinence, but this is

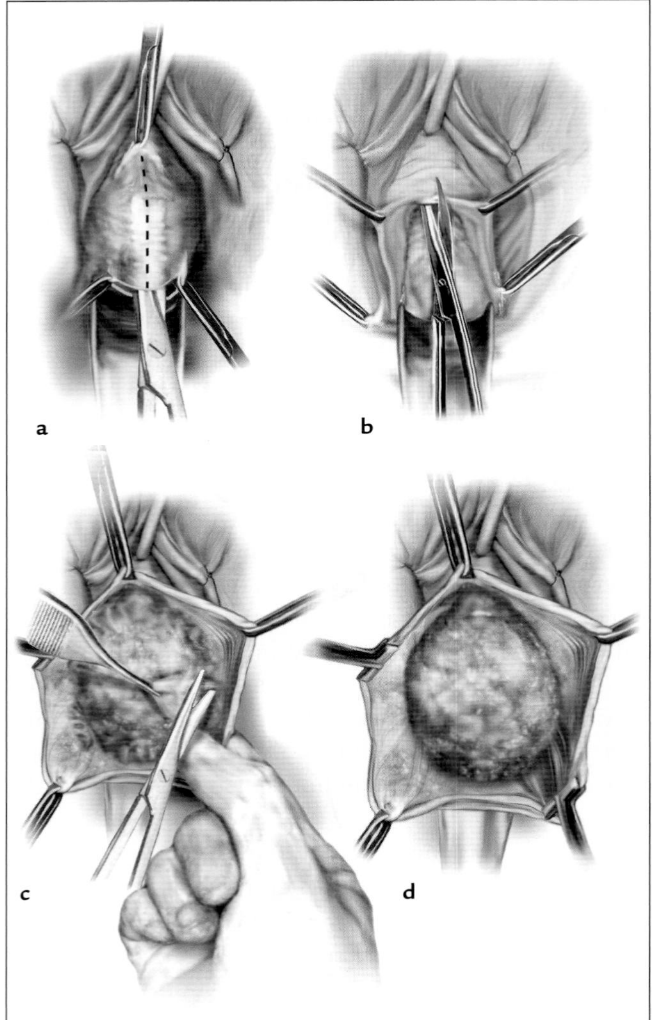

Figure 70.4. *Cystocele repair: (a) initial midline anterior vaginal wall incision; (b) the incision is extended to the level of the proximal urethra; (c) sharp dissection and traction on the bladder facilitate dissection of the bladder off the vaginal wall; (d) mobilization of the cystocele off the vaginal wall is completed. (Reproduced from ref. 8 with permission.)*

probably only indicated in select women with very mild symptoms.

Once the vaginal flaps have been completely developed, the urethrovesical junction can be identified visually or by pulling the Foley catheter downward until the bulb obstructs the vesical neck. Repair should begin at the urethrovesical junction, using No. 0 delayed absorbable or non-absorbable suture. The first plicating stitch is placed into the periurethral endopelvic fascia and tied (Fig. 70.6a). One or two additional stitches are placed to support the length of the urethra and urethrovesical junction.

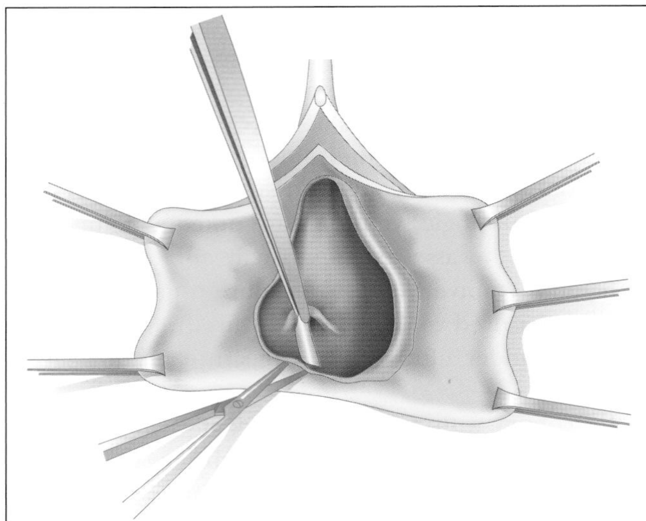

Figure 70.5. *Cystocele repair. Sharp dissection is used to mobilize the bladder base from the vaginal apex during anterior colporrhaphy.*

After the stitches for vesical neck plication have been placed and tied, attention is turned to the anterior vaginal prolapse repair. In a standard anterior colporrhaphy, stitches using No. 2-0 or 0 delayed absorbable or non-absorbable sutures are placed in the vaginal tissue (muscularis and adventitia) medial to the vaginal flaps and plicated in the midline without tension. Depending on the severity of the prolapse, one or two rows of plication sutures or a purse-string suture followed by plication sutures are placed (Fig. 70.6b). The vaginal epithelium is then trimmed from the flaps bilaterally, and the remaining anterior vaginal wall is closed with a running No. 3-0 subcuticular or locking suture.

One modification of the standard repair is to extend the dissection and mobilization of the vaginal flaps laterally to the ischiopubic rami on each side. After the vesical neck plication has been performed, stitches are then placed laterally in the paravaginal tissue (lateral to the vaginal muscularis and adventitial layers, but not including the epithelium of the vaginal flaps). The paravaginal connective tissue is plicated in the midline under tension using No. 0 delayed absorbable or non-absorbable sutures. This produces a firm bridge of tissue across the anterior vaginal space, but it also results in narrowing of the anterior vagina, which must be considered when planning a concomitant posterior colporrhaphy. The vaginal flaps are trimmed and closed as usual.

Another modification involves the use of a prosthetic material to provide support in the anterior vagina. This can be done in several ways and the surgical techniques

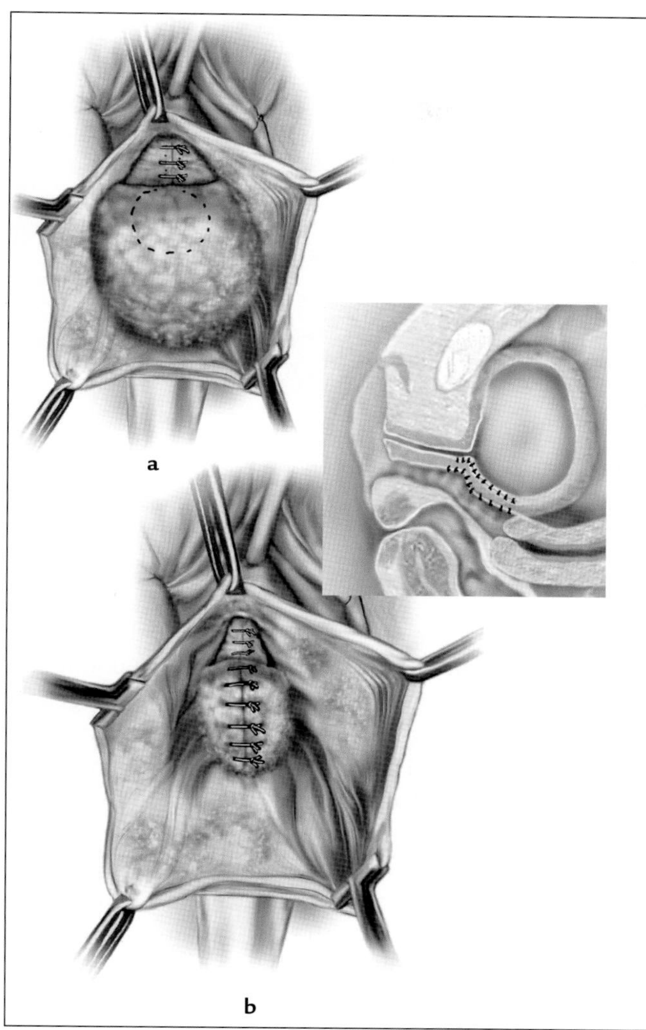

Figure 70.6. *Cystocele repair. (a) Kelly plication sutures have been placed and tied, plicating the pubocervical fascia across the midline at the level of the bladder neck. (b) The bladder base has been plicated. Inset: Preferential support of the bladder neck when compared to the bladder base. (Reproduced from ref. 8 with permission.)*

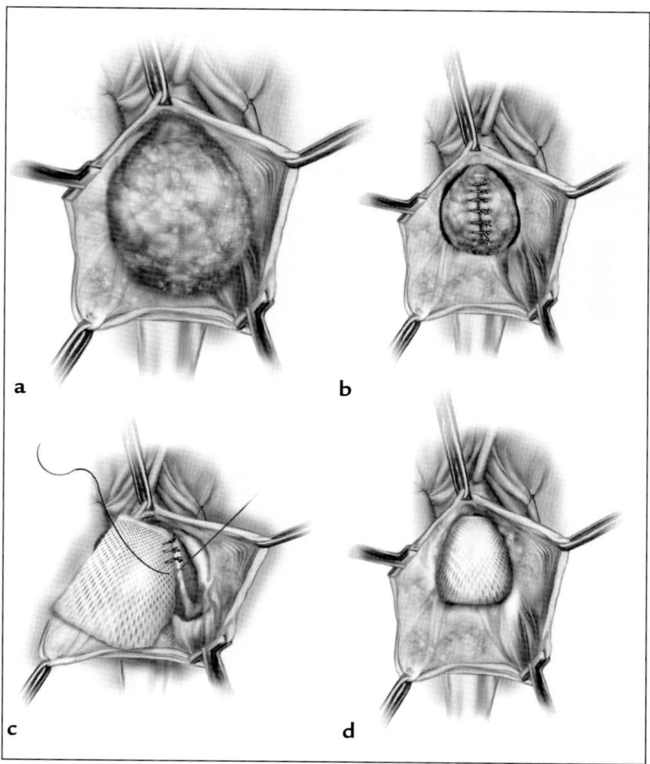

Figure 70.7. *Cystocele repair with mesh: (a) the bladder is dissected bilaterally and off the vaginal apex; (b) midline plication is completed; (c) after entering the left paravaginal space and exposing the arcus tendineus fasciae pelvis (white line), the prosthetic mesh is sewn to it; (d) the mesh is attached bilaterally and all sutures are tied, supporting the bladder.*

continue to evolve. One modification is to place a piece of polyglactin 910 mesh into the fold of the imbricated bladder wall below the trigone and the apical portion of the anterior colporrhaphy. In a second modification, after the plication sutures have been placed and tied, the prosthetic layer is placed over the stitches and anchored in place at the lateral limit of the previous dissection, using interrupted stitches of No. 2-0 absorbable or non-absorbable suture. The anchor points are usually at or near the arcus tendineus fasciae pelvis or obturator fascia bilaterally, as shown in vure 70.7. Biologic materials that have been used include segments of rectus fascia, fascia lata, cadaveric fascia or other allograft or xenograft materials. Permanent (usually polypropylene) mesh may be used, although non-absorbable material carries a risk of infection or erosion, with need for subsequent revision or removal in 2–12% of cases (Table 70.1). A more recent innovative approach is to anchor an allograft, xenograft or polypropylene mesh without tension via strips placed through the obturator foramen with a special device (Perigee, American Medical Systems, Minneapolis, MN). This latter technique awaits study of safety and efficacy.

Anti-incontinence operations are often performed at the same time as anterior vaginal prolapse repair to treat coexistent stress incontinence; sling placement may also improve the cure rate of the prolapse. Bladder neck suspension procedures (sling procedures or retropubic colposuspension) effectively treat mild anterior vaginal prolapse associated with urethral hypermobility and stress incontinence. More advanced anterior vaginal prolapse will not be treated adequately and, in these cases, anterior colporrhaphy should be performed, usually in conjunction with a midurethral sling. Surgical

Table 70.1. *Literature review of anterior vaginal wall prolapse repair with non-absorbable mesh**

Author (year)	Mesh	*n*	Follow-up (months)	Success rate (%)	Vaginal erosion
Nicita (1998)[25]	Polypropylene	44	14	93.2	1 (2.3%)
Flood et al. (1998)[23]	Marlex	142	36	94.4	2 (2.1%)
Julian (1996)[26]	Marlex	12	24	100	1 (8.3%)
Mage (1999)[27]	Mersuture	46	26	100	1 (2.2%)
Migliari & Usai (1999)[28]	Mixed fiber†	15	23.4	93	0
Migliari et al. (2001)[29]	Polypropylene	12	20.5	75	0
Hardiman et al. (2000)[30]	Polypropylene	18	1.5	100	2 (11.1%)
Salvatore et al. (2002)[24]	Polypropylene	32	17	87	4 (13%)
De Tayrac et al. (2005)[31]	Polypropylene	87	24	91.6	7 (8.3%)

* Definitions of success and surgical techniques vary.
† 60% polyglactin 910 and 40% polyester.

judgment is required to perform the bladder plication tightly enough to reduce the anterior vaginal prolapse sufficiently, yet preserve enough mobility of the anterior vagina to allow adequate urethral suspension. If anterior colporrhaphy is combined with a sling procedure (midurethral or bladder neck), the cystocele should be repaired before the final tension is set for the sling. A midurethral sling, such as a tension-free vaginal tape (TVT) or transobturator sling, is best done through a separate midurethral incision after the cystocele repair is complete.

Vaginal paravaginal repair

The aim of paravaginal defect repair for anterior vaginal prolapse is to reattach the detached lateral vagina to its normal place of attachment at the level of the arcus tendineus fasciae pelvis.[17] This can be accomplished using a vaginal or retropubic approach. Retropubic paravaginal defect repair is discussed in Chapter 68, along with other retropubic procedures such as the Burch colposuspension.

The preparation for vaginal paravaginal repair begins as for an anterior colporrhaphy. Marking sutures are placed on the anterior vaginal wall on each side of the urethrovesical junction, identified by the location of the Foley balloon after gentle traction is placed on the catheter (Fig. 70.8a). In patients who have had a hysterectomy, marking sutures are also placed at the vaginal apex. If a culdeplasty is being performed, the stitches are placed but not tied until completion of the paravaginal repair and closure of the anterior vaginal wall. As for anterior colporrhaphy, vaginal flaps are developed by incising the vagina in the midline and dissecting the vaginal muscularis laterally. The dissection is performed bilaterally until a space is developed between the vaginal wall and retropubic space. Blunt dissection using the surgeon's index finger is used to extend the space anteriorly along the ischiopubic rami, medially to the pubic symphysis, and laterally toward the ischial spine. If the defect is present and dissection is occurring in the appropriate plane, one should easily enter the retropubic space, visualizing retropubic adipose tissue. The ischial spine can then be palpated on each side. The arcus tendineus fasciae pelvis coming off the spine can be followed to the back of the symphysis pubis (Fig. 70.8b). After dissection is complete, midline plication of vaginal muscularis can be performed, either at this point or after placement and tying of the paravaginal sutures.

On the lateral pelvic sidewall, the obturator internus muscle and the arcus tendineus fasciae pelvis are identified by palpation and then visualization. Retraction of the bladder and urethra medially is best accomplished with a Breisky–Navratil retractor, and posterior retraction is provided with a lighted right-angle retractor. Using No. 0 non-absorbable suture, the first stitch is placed around the tissue of the white line just anterior to the ischial spine. A Capio device works well to facilitate suture placement. If the white line is detached from the pelvic sidewall or clinically not felt to be durable, then the attachment should be to the fascia overlying the obturator internus muscle. The placement of subsequent sutures is aided by placing tension on the first suture. A series of four to six stitches are placed and held, working anteriorly along the white line from the ischial spine to the level of the urethrovesical junction (Fig. 70.8c). Starting with the most anterior stitch, the surgeon picks up the edge of the periurethral tissue (vaginal muscularis or pubocervical fascia) at the level of the urethrovesical junction and then tissue from the undersurface of the vaginal flap at the previously marked sites. Subsequent stitches move posteriorly until the last stitch closest to the ischial spine is attached to the vagina nearest the apex, again using the previously placed marking sutures for guidance. Stitches in the vaginal wall must be placed carefully to allow adequate tissue for subsequent midline vaginal closure. After all the stitches are placed on one side, the same procedure

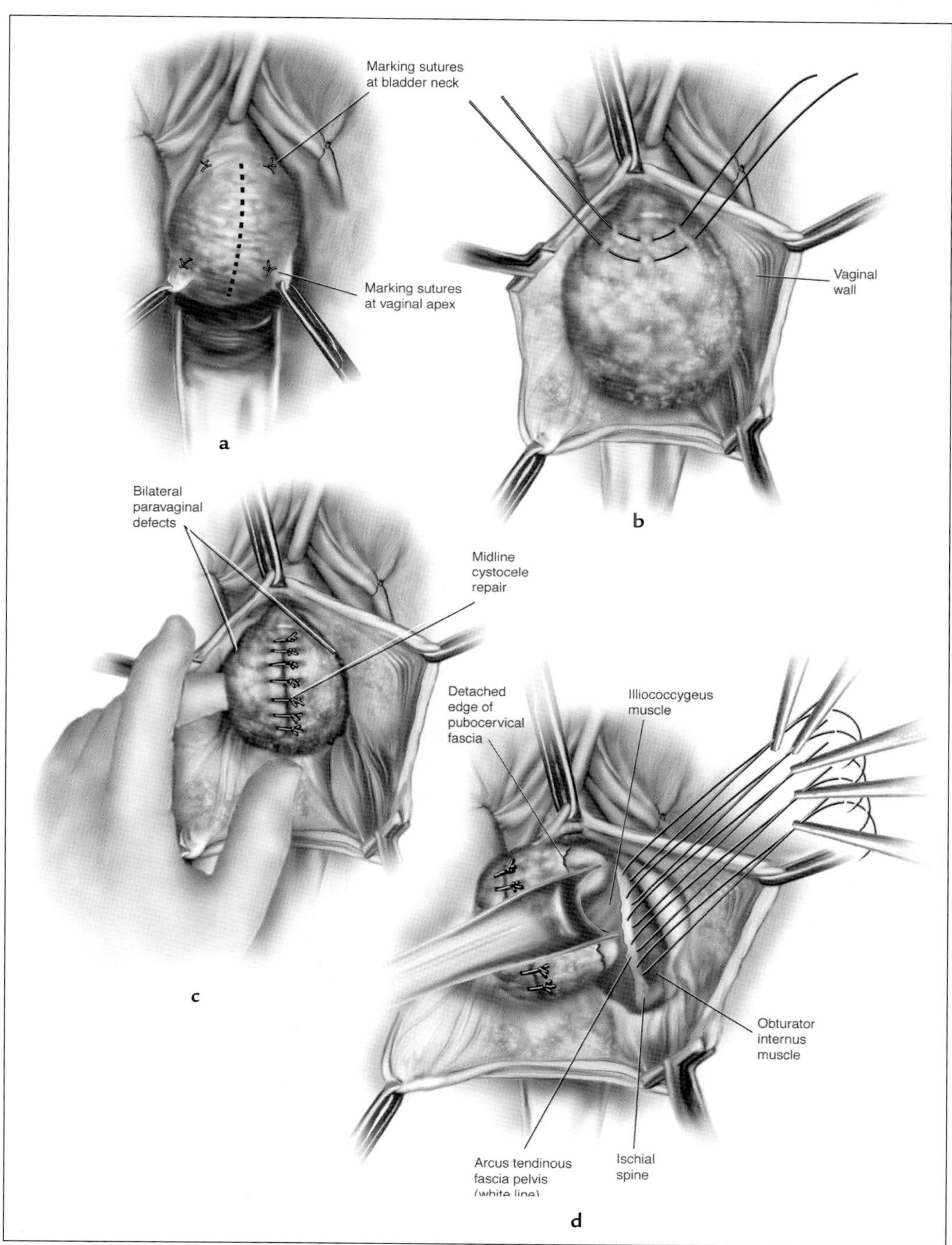

Figure 70.8. *Technique of vaginal paravaginal repair. (a) Marking sutures are placed at the bladder neck and vaginal apex. A midline anterior vaginal wall incision is made. (b) The bladder is dissected bilaterally and off the vaginal apex. Midline plication is performed. (c) Midline plication is completed; obvious bilateral paravaginal defects are present. (d) The bladder is retracted medially and numerous sutures are passed through the arcus tendineus fasciae pelvis (white line).*

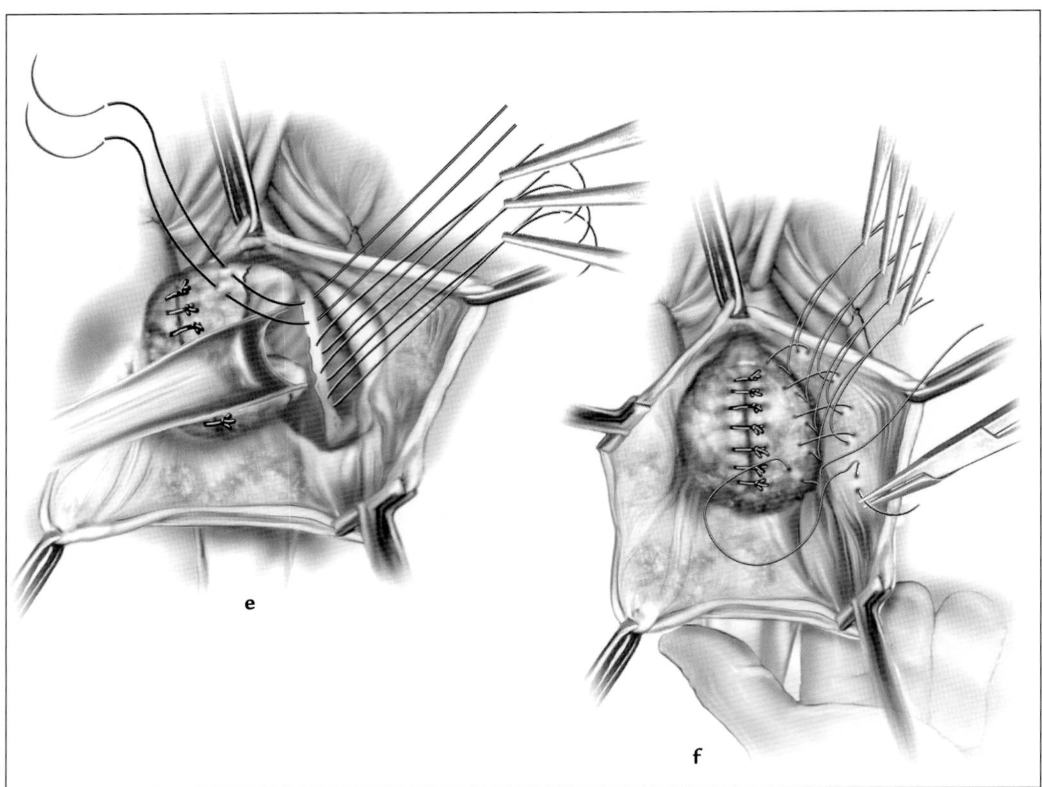

Figure 70.8. *(e) Sutures are then passed through the detached pubocervical or endopelvic fascia. (f) Sutures are passed through the inside of the vaginal wall, thus completing the three-point closure. (Reproduced from ref. 8 with permission.)*

is carried out on the other side. The stitches are then tied in order from the urethra to the apex, alternating from one side to the other. This repair is a three-point closure involving the vaginal epithelium, vaginal muscularis and endopelvic fascia (pubocervical fascia), and lateral pelvic sidewall at the level of the arcus tendineus fasciae pelvis (Fig. 70.8d). There must be tissue-to-tissue approximation between these structures. Suture bridges must be avoided by careful planning of suture placement. Vaginal tissue should not be trimmed until all the stitches are tied. As previously stated, if not already performed, vaginal muscularis can then be plicated in the midline with several interrupted stitches using No. 0 delayed absorbable suture. The vaginal flaps are trimmed and closed with a running subcuticular or interlocking delayed absorbable suture.

Abdominal cystocele repair

Abdominal repair of mild anterior vaginal prolapse can be accomplished at the time of abdominal hysterectomy.[18] After the cervix has been amputated from the vagina, the bladder is dissected off the anterior vaginal wall, nearly to the level of the ureters. A full-thickness midline wedge of anterior vaginal wall is excised, and the vagina is closed with running delayed absorbable suture. The vaginal cuff is then repaired according to the surgeon's preference. This procedure has no effect on the bladder neck or urethral support, and care should be taken not to unmask latent stress incontinence by treating anterior vaginal prolapse without simultaneous urethral suspension.

Cystoscopy

Cystoscopy is usually performed after cystocele repair, especially if slings or apical suspension procedures are also being performed. The purpose is to ensure that no sutures or mesh have been placed in the bladder and to verify patency of both ureters.

RESULTS

The main indication for surgical repair of anterior vaginal prolapse is to relieve symptoms when they exist, or as part of a comprehensive pelvic reconstructive procedure for multiple sites of pelvic organ prolapse with or without urinary incontinence. Few studies have addressed the long-term success of surgical treatments for anterior vaginal prolapse. Most published studies are uncontrolled series. Definitions of recurrence vary and sometimes are not stated, and loss to follow-up is often not declared. In our review of surgical techniques for the correction of anterior vaginal prolapse,[2] reported failure rates ranged from zero to 20% for anterior colporrhaphy and from 3 to 14% for paravaginal repair.

Weber et al.[19] studied three variations of anterior colporrhaphy using a prospective randomized study design and a very strict definition of success (Aa and Ba points at –3 or –2 cm; Stage 0 or I). Standard anterior colporrhaphy resulted in 30% of patients with a optimal or satisfactory anatomic result; anterior colporrhaphy with polyglactin 910 mesh overlay had 42% optimal or satisfactory result, and ultralateral plication under tension a 46% optimal or satisfactory result. No difference was seen in anatomic or functional outcomes and most patients reported satisfaction with their symptom improvement. In another randomized controlled trial using a different staging system, Sand et al.[20] noted fewer recurrent cystoceles when polyglactin 910 mesh was incorporated into the imbrication of the repair.

Prosthetic augmentation of cystocele repair is a promising though evolving innovation. There are many variations in techniques and materials used but there are few quality studies to date; one technique variation is shown in Figure 70.7. Biologic prosthetic materials placed over a midline cystocele plication as a simple overlay and anchored laterally has been carried out but does not appear to offer significant lasting improvement over standard repair.[21] However, anchoring the mesh to the obturator fascia, the addition of suburethral slings,[22] and anchoring of the prosthesis to the apical portion of the repair may significantly improve long-term results.

Placement of non-absorbable mesh into an anterior vaginal prolapse repair is a promising, though more controversial, variation. Polypropylene mesh has limited foreign body reaction in general and is probably the best choice. Technique variations include mesh overlays, modified four-corner attachments, transobturator attachments, and anterior flaps as part of an apical mesh procedure. Cure rates appear high (see Table 70.1) but comparative trials with more traditional sutured repairs have not been undertaken. Vaginal mesh erosions continue to be a problem; they occur in 2.1–13% of cases,[23,24] a significant number of which require re-operation for mesh removal. Creation of thicker vaginal flaps with an attached fibromuscularis may decrease the mesh erosion rate.

Anterior colporrhaphy with bladder neck plication may be effective for treatment of mild stress incontinence associated with urethral hypermobility. However, the cure rate after 1 year is only about 60% and it is less effective than Burch colposuspension and most slings.[32] These findings hold irrespective of the coexistence of pelvic organ prolapse. However, suburethral plication may be satisfactory for some women with mild symptoms of stress incontinence who do not desire a sling or who have significant preoperative voiding dysfunction, or for elderly or medically compromised women in whom surgical risk must be minimized.

For women with potential or occult stress incontinence in association with advanced prolapse, Meschia et al. reported that placement of a TVT results in significantly higher objective continence rates postoperatively compared to suburethral plication (92% versus 56%; $p<0.01$).[16] Thus, placement of a TVT or a transobturator sling is recommended for all women with potential stress incontinence, excepting perhaps for very elderly patients and those with significant voiding dysfunction.

Paravaginal defect repair using the transvaginal approach results in excellent anatomic cure of anterior vaginal prolapse.[17] However, it has been used infrequently as an isolated procedure for treatment of stress urinary incontinence. Evidence suggests that it has less than satisfactory results when used in this capacity. In a report by Mallipeddi et al.,[33] 57% of subjects with anterior vaginal prolapse and stress incontinence treated with a vaginal paravaginal repair and bladder neck plication had persistent urinary incontinence after an average of 1.6 years of follow-up. Thus, while the vaginal paravaginal repair is safe and relatively effective for correction of anterior vaginal prolapse, it has limited applicability in the surgical correction of stress incontinence.

Women with advanced anterior vaginal prolapse, with or without stress incontinence, often have other abnormal bladder symptoms such as urgency, urge incontinence, and voiding difficulty. In a study of surgical repair of large cystoceles by Gardy et al.,[34] stress incontinence resolved in 94%, urge incontinence in 87%, and significant residual urine (>80 ml) in 92% of patients 3 months after needle suspension procedures and anterior colporrhaphy. Approximately 5% of patients developed a recurrent anterior vaginal prolapse, and 8% developed a recurrent enterocele after an average of 2 years of follow-up.

Risk factors for failure of anterior vaginal prolapse repair have not been specifically studied. Vaginal prolapse recurs with increasing age and length of follow-up, but the actual frequency is unknown. Recurrence of anterior prolapse is more likely to occur with more severe initial prolapse[35] and probably with transvaginal, compared to abdominal, repairs.[36] Recurrence may represent a failure to identify and repair all support defects, or weakening, stretching or breaking of patients' tissues, as occurs with advancing age and after menopause. Sacrospinous ligament suspension of the vaginal apex, with exaggerated retrosuspension of the vagina, may predispose patients to recurrence of anterior vaginal prolapse. Other characteristics that may increase chances of recurrence are genetic predisposition, subsequent pregnancy, heavy lifting, chronic pulmonary disease, smoking, and obesity.

COMPLICATIONS

Intraoperative complications are uncommon with anterior vaginal prolapse repair. Excessive blood loss may occur, requiring blood transfusion, or a hematoma may develop in the anterior vagina; this is probably more common after vaginal paravaginal repair than anterior colporrhaphy.[37] The lumen of the bladder or urethra may be entered in the course of dissection. Accidental cystotomy should be repaired in layers at the time of the injury. After repair of cystotomy, the bladder is generally drained for 7–14 days to allow adequate healing. Ureteral damage or obstruction occurs rarely (0–2%),[38] usually with very large cystoceles or with apical prolapse. Other rare complications include intravesical or urethral suture placement (and associated urologic problems) and fistulae, either urethrovaginal or vesicovaginal. If permanent sutures or mesh material are used in the repair, erosion, draining sinuses or chronic areas of vaginal granulation tissue can result. The incidence of these complications is unknown but may be as high as 13%.[24] Urinary tract infections are common (especially with concurrent catheter usage), but other infections such as pelvic or vaginal abscesses are less common.

Voiding difficulty can occur after anterior vaginal prolapse repair. In our hands, the average time to adequate voiding after cystocele repair with suburethral plication is 9 days.[39] This problem may occur more often in women with subclinical preoperative voiding dysfunction. Treatment is bladder drainage or intermittent self-catheterization until spontaneous voiding resumes, usually within 6 weeks.

Sexual function may be positively or negatively affected by vaginal operations for anterior vaginal prolapse. Haase and Skibsted[40] studied 55 sexually active women who underwent a variety of operations for stress incontinence or genital prolapse. Postoperatively, 24% of the patients experienced improvement in their sexual satisfaction, 67% experienced no change, and 9% experienced deterioration. Improvement often resulted from cessation of urinary incontinence. Deterioration was always caused by dyspareunia after posterior colporrhaphy. These authors concluded that the prognosis for an improved sexual life is good after surgery for stress incontinence, but that posterior colpoperineorrhaphy causes dyspareunia in some patients. The current popularity of synthetic or allograft mesh to augment vaginal prolapse repairs could improve sexual function if cure rates improve, or could worsen function if vaginal stiffness, mesh erosions or draining sinuses result. More data with careful follow-up after surgery are needed.

REFERENCES

1. Bump RC, Mattiasson A, Bø K et al. The standardization of terminology of female pelvic organ prolapse and pelvic floor dysfunction. Am J Obstet Gynecol 1996;175:10–17.
2. Weber AM, Walters MD. Anterior vaginal prolapse: review of anatomy and techniques of surgical repair. Obstet Gynecol 1997;89:311–18.
3. DeLancey JOL. Anatomic aspects of vaginal eversion after hysterectomy. Am J Obstet Gynecol 1992;166:1717–28.
4. Nichols DH, Randall CL. Vaginal Surgery, 4th ed. Baltimore: Williams and Wilkins, 1996.
5. White GR. A radical cure by suturing lateral sulci of vagina to white line of pelvic fascia. JAMA 1909;21:1707–10.
6. White GR. An anatomical operation for the cure of cystocele. Am J Obstet Dis Women Child 1912;65:286–90.
7. Richardson AC, Lyon JB, Williams NL. A new look at pelvic relaxation. Am J Obstet Gynecol 1976;126:568–73.
8. Karram MM. Vaginal operations for prolapse. In: Baggish MS, Karram MM (eds) Atlas of Pelvic Anatomy and Gynecologic Surgery. Philadelphia: Saunders, 2001.
9. DeLancey JO. Fascial and muscular abnormalities in women with urethral hypermobility and anterior vaginal wall prolapse. Am J Obstet Gynecol 2002;187:93–8.
10. Aronson MP, Bates SM, Jacoby AF et al. Periurethral and paravaginal anatomy: an endovaginal magnetic resonance imaging study. Am J Obstet Gynecol 1995;173:1702–8.
11. Barber MD, Cundiff GW, Weidner AC et al. Accuracy of clinical assessment of paravaginal defects in women with anterior vaginal wall prolapse. Am J Obstet Gynecol 1999;181:87–90.
12. Whiteside JL, Barber MD, Paraiso MF et al. Clinical evaluation of anterior vaginal wall support defect: interexaminer and intraexaminer reliability. Am J Obstet Gynecol 2004;191:100–4.
13. Tulikangas PK, Lukban JC, Walters MD. Anterior enterocele: a report of three cases. Int Urogynecol J 2004;15:350–2.
14. Beverly CJ, Walters MD, Weber AM et al. Prevalence of hydronephrosis in women undergoing surgery for pelvic organ prolapse. Obstet Gynecol 1997;90:37–41.

15. Bump RC, Fantl JA, Hurt WG. The mechanism of urinary continence in women with severe uterovaginal prolapse: results of barrier studies. Obstet Gynecol 1988;72:291–5.

16. Meschia M, Pifarotti P, Spennacchio M et al. A randomized comparison of tension-free vaginal tape and endopelvic fascia plication in women with genital prolapse and occult stress urinary incontinence. Am J Obstet Gynecol 2004;190:609–13.

17. Shull BL, Benn SJ, Kuehl TJ. Surgical management of prolapse of the anterior vaginal segment: an analysis of support defects, operative morbidity, and anatomic outcome. Am J Obstet Gynecol 1994;171:1429–39.

18. Macer GA. Transabdominal repair of cystocele, a 20-year experience, compared with the traditional vaginal approach. Am J Obstet Gynecol 1978;131:203–6.

19. Weber AM, Walters MD, Piedmonte MA et al. Anterior colporrhaphy: a randomized trial of three surgical techniques. Am J Obstet Gynecol 2001;185:1299–1306.

20. Sand PK, Koduri S, Lobel RW et al. Prospective randomized trial of polyglactin 910 mesh to prevent recurrence of cystoceles and rectoceles. Am J Obstet Gynecol 2001;184:1357–62.

21. Gandhi S, Kwon C, Goldberg RP et al. A randomized controlled trial of fascia lata for the prevention of recurrent anterior vaginal wall prolapse [abstract]. Neurourol Urodyn 2004;23:558.

22. Goldberg RP, Koduri S, Lobel RW et al. Protective effect of suburethral slings on postoperative cystocele recurrence after reconstructive pelvic operation. Am J Obstet Gynecol 2001;185:1307–12.

23. Flood CG, Drutz HP, Waja L. Anterior colporrhaphy reinforced with Marlex mesh for the treatment of cystoceles. Int Urogynecol J 1998;9:200–4.

24. Salvatore S, Soligo M, Meschia M et al. Prosthetic surgery for genital prolapse: functional outcome [abstract]. Neurourol Urodyn 2002;21:296–7.

25. Nicita G. A new operation for genitourinary prolapse. J Urol 1998;160:741–5.

26. Julian TM. The efficacy of Marlex mesh in the repair of severe, recurrent vaginal prolapse of the anterior midvaginal wall. Am J Obstet Gynecol 1996;175:1472–5.

27. Mage P. [Interposition of a synthetic mesh by vaginal approach in the cure of genital prolapse.] Gynecol Obstet Biol Reprod (Paris) 1999;28:825.

28. Migliari R, Usai E. Treatment results using a mixed fiber mesh in patients with grade IV cystocele. J Urol 1999;161:1255–8.

29. Migliari R, De Angelis M, Madeddu G et al. Tension-free vaginal mesh repair for anterior vaginal wall prolapse. Eur Urol 2001;38:151–5.

30. Hardiman P, Oyawoye S, Browning J. Cystocele repair using polypropylene mesh [abstract]. Br J Obstet Gynaecol 2000;107:825.

31. de Tayrac R, Gerviase A, Chauveaud A et al. Tension-free polypropylene mesh for vaginal repair of anterior vaginal wall prolapse. J Reprod Med 2005;50:75–80.

32. Glazener CMA, Cooper K. Anterior vaginal repair for urinary incontinence in women (Cochrane Review). In: The Cochrane Library, Issue 3, 2002. Oxford: Update Software.

33. Mallipeddi PK, Steele AC, Hohli N et al. Anatomic and functional outcome of vaginal paravaginal repair in the correction of anterior vaginal prolapse. Int Urogynecol J 2001;12:83–8.

34. Gardy M, Kozminski M, DeLancey J et al. Stress incontinence and cystoceles. J Urol 1991:145:1211–3.

35. Whiteside JL, Weber AM, Meyn LA et al. Risk factors for prolapse recurrence after vaginal repair. Am J Obstet Gynecol 2004;191:1533–8.

36. Maher CF, Qatawneh AM, Dwyer PL et al. Abdominal sacral colpopexy or vaginal sacrospinous colpopexy vaginal vault prolapse: a prospective randomized study. Am J Obstet Gynecol 2004;190:20–6.

37. Young SB, Daman JJ, Bony LG. Vaginal paravaginal repair: one-year outcomes. Am J Obstet Gynecol 2001;185:1360–6.

38. Kwon CH, Goldberg RP, Koduri S et al. The use of intraoperative cystoscopy in major vaginal and urogynecologic surgeries. Am J Obstet Gynecol 2002;187:1466–72.

39. Kobak WH, Walters MD, Piedmonte MR. Determinants of voiding after three types of incontinence surgery. Obstet Gynecol 2001;97:86–91.

40. Haase P, Skibsted L. Influence of operations for stress incontinence and/or genital descensus on sexual life. Acta Obstet Gynecol Scand 1988;67:659–61.

71

Enterocele

Kaven Baessler, Bernhard Schuessler

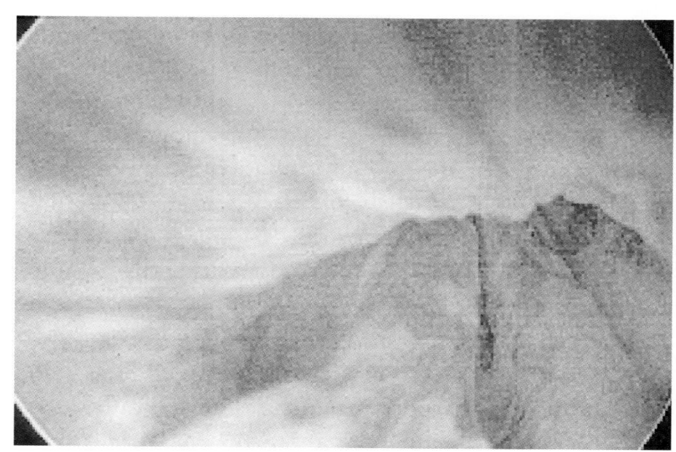

DEFINITION AND SCOPE OF AN ENTEROCELE

The term enterocele is derived form of *enter* (intestine) and *cele* (hernia), i.e. a herniation of the bowel or a hernial tumor containing bowel. In general, a hernia occurs when a rupture in the smooth muscle or connective tissue allows a bodily structure to protrude. An enterocele is usually referred to as a herniation through or into the vagina, typically as a posterior enterocele which develops in the rectovaginal space (pouch of Douglas, or cul-de-sac). The anterior enterocele in the vesicovaginal space is a rare entity.

An enterocele is a form of pelvic organ prolapse: bowel is protruding into the vagina. Why and how this happens are etiologic and pathophysiologic issues which are illustrated in this chapter. Surgical treatment of an enterocele is often concurrent with, or identical to, operations for vaginal vault prolapse. Preventive and therapeutic procedures will be described.

ANATOMY, ETIOLOGY, DEFECTS AND PATHOPHYSIOLOGY

Normal anatomy

The important anatomic structures with regard to enterocele formation are consistent with normal pelvic organ support mechanisms. An enterocele develops in the pouch of Douglas; therefore, the pouch of Douglas is an anatomic structure that plays an imperative and probably predisposing part. The pouch of Douglas is normally closed and does not contain intestine or omentum.

In anatomy textbooks (e.g. *Gray's Anatomy*), the extent of the pouch of Douglas has traditionally been described as 2–3 cm below the uterosacral ligaments. Histologic studies by Uhlenhuth and colleagues have demonstrated that, in the fetus, the pouch of Douglas may extend to the perineal body.[1] The consecutive fusion of the anterior and posterior peritoneum forms the rectovaginal septum and determines the depth of the pouch of Douglas.[1–3] According to Uhlenhuth, the rectovaginal septum is distinguishable from the fascial capsule of the vagina and rectum. In contrast to anatomy textbooks, recent in vivo intra-abdominal measurements of the depth of the pouch of Douglas in young nulliparous women revealed considerable variations, with 25–75% of the posterior vaginal wall covered with peritoneum.[4] The mean depth of the pouch of Douglas was 49% of vaginal length in nulliparas, 46% in parous women and was significantly deeper (72%) in patients with posterior vaginal wall prolapse. The mean vaginal length was 10 cm. Age and parity did not have an influence. It would appear that a deep pouch of Douglas is frequently present in young nulliparous women without pelvic organ prolapse, which implies a congenital variation and predisposition.[4]

A sophisticated concept of normal pelvic organ support accentuates the imperative role of several factors, including integrity of the anterior and posterior endopelvic fasciae with intact attachments as well as normal tone, position, and functionality of the levator ani muscle. Normal pelvic floor muscle and fascial structures are required to hold the perineum in place and ensure normal bladder, bowel, and sexual function. It is apparent that fascial defects in the three levels of vaginal support and the posterior compartment may contribute to pelvic organ prolapse including enteroceles.[5,6] Normal pelvic floor tone and position are essential for the nearly horizontal axis of the vagina which in turn is necessary to allow for a normal pelvic floor protecting intra-abdominal pressure distribution. These elements may well have an important role in keeping the pouch of Douglas closed.

The deep pouch of Douglas as a predisposing factor

Principally, a posterior enterocele develops in the pouch of Douglas which is normally closed. Figure 71.1 illustrates the different characteristics in the development of enteroceles. Intra-abdominal measurements of the depth of the pouch of Douglas have shown that in women with posterior vaginal wall and anterior rectal wall prolapse the pouch of Douglas is significantly deeper and may reach the level of the perineal body.[4] In addition, the anatomy of the pouch of Douglas is considerably different, which is a recognized feature in some studies. In women with severe pelvic organ prolapse, a large or voluminous rectovaginal pouch was a consistent anatomic finding requiring obliteration during pelvic reconstructive surgery.[7–9] Apart from a mobile vaginal axis and a dehiscence of the levator hiatus, French authors reported a 'grande fosse pelvi-périnéale' – a large pelvic pouch – to be a principal lesion in women with enteroceles.[10] Their anatomic observations included a deep and wide rectovaginal pouch and a rectosigmoid colon, which closely follows the sacral curve (Fig. 71.2). Although different positions and courses of the sigmoid colon and its mesentery are known,[11] systematic descriptions in women with pelvic organ prolapse are scarce. Baessler and Schuessler found 64% of women with enteroceles and all women with anterior

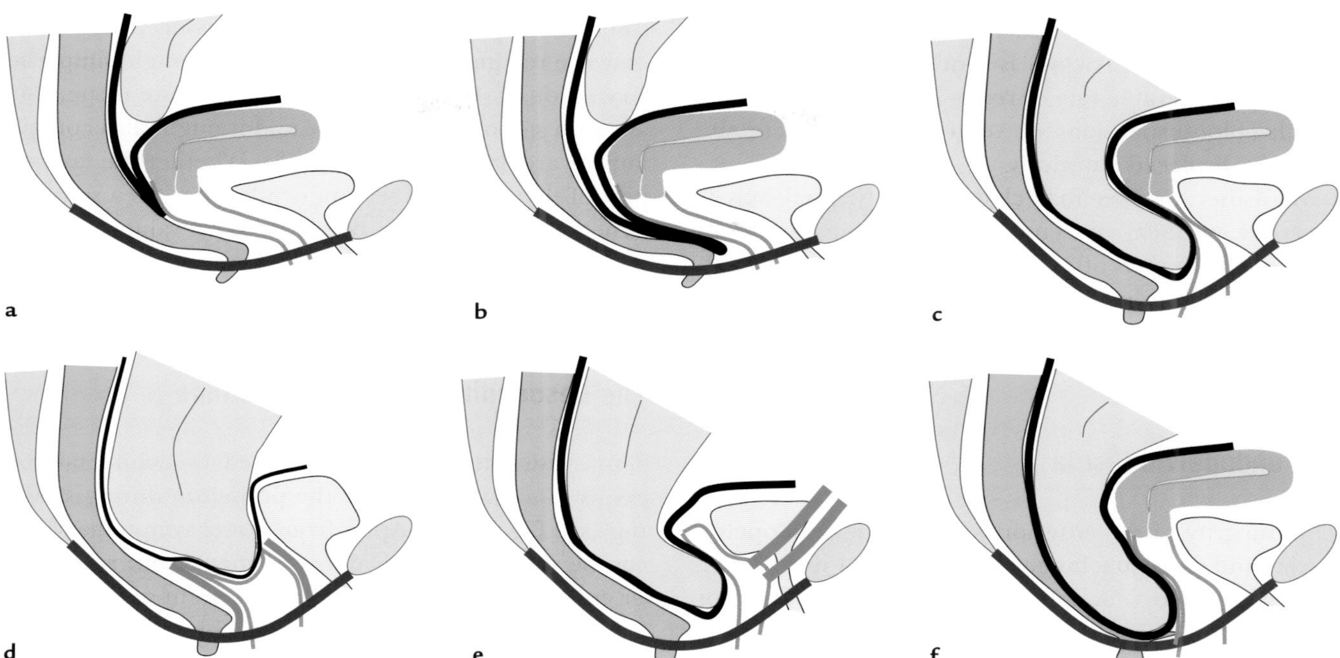

Figure 71.1. *The pouch of Douglas – 'normal' depth, deep, grande fosse pelvienne. (a) The 'normal' pouch of Douglas covers approximately one-third of the posterior vaginal wall and is closed. (b) Deep pouch of Douglas: peritoneum covers the posterior vaginal wall down to the level of the levator ani. Normal pelvic floor support prevents opening and exposure of the pouch of Douglas. (c) An enterocele has developed in the rectovaginal space displacing the posterior vaginal wall. The vaginal and rectal course is more vertical and the pelvic floor position is lower, leaving the pouch of Douglas unprotected. (d) Apical enterocele with separation of the anterior and posterior endopelvic fascia after hysterectomy. (e) Enterocele after Burch colposuspension with ventral displacement of anterior compartment; the pouch of Douglas was not protected. (f) Enterocele bulging primarily into the rectum; anterior rectal wall procidentia; intact posterior endopelvic fascia.*

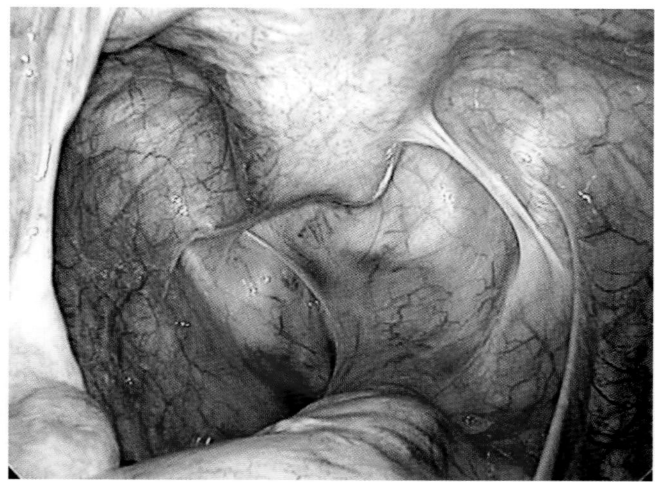

Figure 71.2. *Laparoscopic view of a grande fosse pelvienne: note the deep and wide pouch of Douglas, the lack of prominent uterosacral ligaments and the rectal course close to the sacrum with a short mesentery.*

rectal wall procidentia to have these features, termed a 'grande fosse pelvienne'. A grande fosse pelvienne was also present in six of 43 women (14%) in the control group who did not have pelvic organ prolapse; three were nulliparous.[12] Given these findings, it seems reasonable to regard a deep pouch of Douglas as a risk factor for enterocele formation. However, a deep pouch of Douglas does not necessarily result in an enterocele; an enterocele can only develop when other factors open and expose the (deep) pouch of Douglas.

The vaginal axis

In a woman with normal pelvic organ support, the pouch of Douglas is closed, irrespective of its depth, and lies nearly horizontally between the levator plate and the vagina.[13–15] A recent magnetic resonance imaging (MRI) study measured the mean levator–vaginal angle with a horizontal line at 35–53 degrees in different ethnic nulliparous populations.[16] It is known that operations that change the vaginal axis can lead to increased prolapse in the 'unprotected' area. This is true for the higher incidence of cystoceles after sacrospinous fixations where the position of the vagina is more posterior and also for the considerable rate of recto- and enteroceles after Burch colposuspensions or ventrofixations where the vagina is displaced anteriorly.

A further process that changes the vaginal axis is excessive perineal descent (or descending perineum syndrome) which is often seen clinically in women with significant posterior vaginal wall prolapse (Fig. 71.3). A deep pouch of Douglas is likely to accentuate the process of enterocele development once the vaginal axis is changed.

The endopelvic fascia

The integrity of the anterior and posterior endopelvic fasciae and their attachments is essential for normal pelvic organ support.[6] A defect in the endopelvic fascia or insufficiency is necessary for an enterocele to protrude. However, an intact endopelvic fascia might prevent the enterocele bulging into the vagina, but not into the rectum where it causes anterior rectal wall procidentia.

It is not entirely clear whether the endopelvic fascia is identical to the rectovaginal septum as the latter can be rather short, depending on the depth of the pouch of Douglas. Whole-thickness biopsies of the leading edge of radiologically proven enteroceles showed that in none of the examined 13 women was the vaginal epithelium in direct contact with the perineum and all had a well-defined vaginal wall muscularis.[17] These findings add to the ongoing controversy on whether 'fascia' exists or not. It has been suggested that it is a structure that is artificially created during surgical dissection. This debate is complicated by inconsistent histologic studies, some of which do not substantiate the concept of a fascia between rectum and vagina. However, it might simply be a question of definition: fascia is connective tissue, usually with smooth muscle cells, and it might also contain fatty or areolar tissue[18] (Fig. 71.4). Whether the fascia is part of the vagina or rectum or whether it is a separate structure is of scientific but not clinical value. Fascia in the clinical sense means connective tissue that has tensile strength and is strong enough to hold sutures and support the underlying organs.

The descending perineum syndrome

This syndrome has been described by colorectal surgeons as a 'ballooning' of the perineum during straining (see Fig. 71.3).[19] Apart from bowel symptoms which can be similar to complaints of patients with rectoceles or enteroceles, excessive perineal descent of more than 2 cm (measured in relation to the ischial tuberosities) is seen more frequently in women with posterior vaginal wall prolapse.[20] Solitary rectal ulcer, rectal prolapse, and intussusception are common concomitant findings.[20,21] The etiology is unclear but reduced pelvic floor tone[22] with insufficient perineal and endopelvic fascial attachment, as well as a deep pouch of Douglas and sigmoid colon elongation, have been discussed.

Pulsion, traction, sliding, true and congenital: concepts of enterocele development

There are many different concepts and each one of them might be true in the individual patient. The idea to find a one-fits-all theory is probably in vain. Enteroceles may develop as a *true hernia* with a hernial sac and neck. A

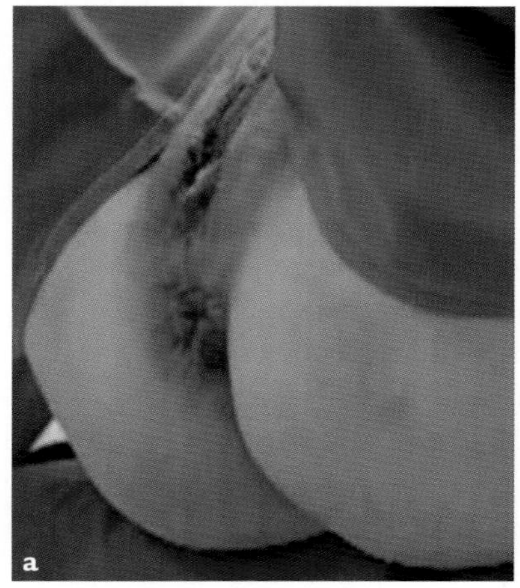

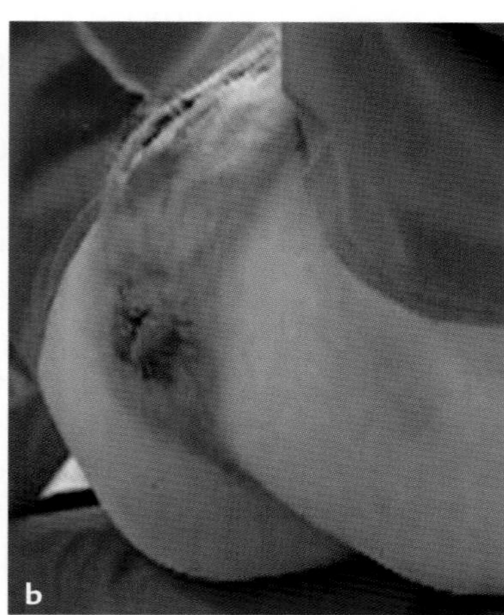

Figure 71.3. *Excessive perineal descent. Nearly normal position of the perineum at rest (a) but a 'ballooning' of the perineum on straining (b). This patient had a large rectoenterocele that did not protrude outside the introitus.*

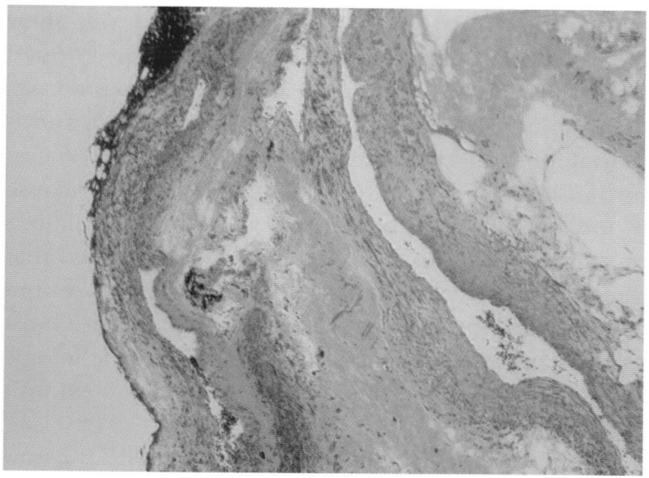

Figure 71.4. *Mallory-trichrome stain of a biopsy taken from the tissue used in posterior vaginal wall repairs. The biopsy site was approximately 2 cm below the ischial spine. This stain is used to differentiate fibrous tissue (green) and smooth muscle (red). Note the amount of smooth muscle, organized connective tissue and areolar tissue. (With permission from Dr Christopher Maher, Auchenflower, Australia.)*

defect in the endopelvic fascia is then a prerequisite. It is argued that a *traction enterocele* is accompanied by loss of pelvic organ support[14] and a greater vault descent with normal anatomic connections between the pouch of Douglas and vagina.[23,24] In contrast, according to Nichols and Genadry,[14] a *pulsion enterocele* is secondary to increased abdominal pressure whereas Zacharin states that a pulsion enterocele occurs as a late complication of pelvic surgery (e.g. hysterectomy) and is associated with a large rectovaginal pouch.[23] However, Zacharin is convinced that the depth of the pouch of Douglas has no bearing on enterocele development. He considers levator incompetence and relaxation of the fascial support to be the primary defects. Nichols and Genadry describe *iatrogenic enteroceles* as a sequela of operations that alter the vaginal axis (e.g. Burch colposuspension) and *congenital enteroceles* which are associated with an 'unusually' deep pouch of Douglas (see Fig. 71.1e).

In theory, an enterocele can only develop when important anatomic factors change: the vagina becomes more vertical and the (deep) pouch of Douglas opens, or the pubocervical and rectovaginal fasciae are separated. Whether a discrete defect in the endopelvic fascia is also required remains a topic for discussion. Therefore, Zacharin's observation of a common deep pouch of Douglas in the Chinese female only corroborates the above: their pelvic floor status including tone and support prevents an exposure of the rectovaginal pouch.

Rectal prolapse

Colorectal surgeons view prolapse with a different attitude but have similar problems defining the etiology of rectal prolapse which might originate from the pouch of Douglas.[25] Altemeier et al. described three types: type 1 is a false prolapse due to mucosal redundancy, type 2 is an intussusception without an association with the pouch of Douglas, and type 3 is a sliding hernia of the rectovaginal pouch.[26] Enteroptosis and elongation of the rectosigmoid colon are considered contributing factors.[27] Similar to vaginal enteroceles, type 3 rectal prolapse develops in the pouch of Douglas and basically is an enterocele bulging into the rectum, sometimes termed anterior rectal wall prolapse (see Fig. 71.1f).

Further factors

Old textbooks often quote other factors that might contribute to enterocele formation. Apart from established confounders for pelvic organ prolapse such as aging, obesity, constipation with excessive defecation straining, connective tissue diseases and parity, malnutrition – particularly in times of war – is mentioned.[28]

EPIDEMIOLOGY

The prevalence of enteroceles is inseparable from the prevalence of other types of pelvic organ prolapse. Isolated enteroceles usually occur after pelvic surgery. The classic example is the development of enteroceles after Burch colposuspension in up to 32% of patients.[29–31] It is also recognized that enteroceles and rectal prolapse frequently coexist with other defects of pelvic floor support.[32–34]

Specific data on enteroceles from women in the community are scarce. In a prevalence study of 639 women aged 45–85 years using the pelvic organ prolapse quantification of the International Continence Society, 22% had no prolapse at all, 37% had stage 1, 29% had stage 2, 9% had stage 3, and 3% had complete eversion.[35]

SYMPTOMS

As with any other type of pelvic organ prolapse, an enterocele can cause prolapse symptoms, including the feeling of a bulge and a dragging sensation, and can interfere with bladder, bowel, and sexual function. Unlike a cystocele or rectocele, an enterocele does not appear to cause any stereotypical and pathognomonic symptoms, and very often symptoms cannot be distinguished from those of any coexisting pelvic organ prolapse. Some women primarily complain of rectal symptoms such as fullness and incomplete or difficult bowel emptying; however, in others the prolapse symptoms are predominant.[36] There might be dyschezia and a frequent, unproductive urge to defecate.

Partial or complete obstruction of the urethra by the enterocele might result in voiding difficulties or retention.[37,37] Dyspareunia, 'slackness at intercourse', vaginal dryness, and coital incontinence are frequently reported by women with pelvic organ prolapse.[38] Mainly a complication of previous pelvic floor surgery and hysterectomy, vaginal rupture and evisceration have been reported in women with enteroceles.[40]

CLINICAL ASSESSMENT AND INVESTIGATIONS

Vaginal and rectal examination with special attention to the endopelvic fascia is probably capable of identifying most enteroceles. Defects in the endopelvic fascia and their location with diminished vaginal rugae are a clue (Fig. 71.5). Simultaneous bimanual examination of the tissues between vagina and rectum under straining or in the standing position usually helps. An enterocele can be located in the anterior vaginal wall where it divides the pubocervical fascia or in the posterior vaginal wall, or it might separate the anterior and posterior endopelvic fasciae at the vaginal vault (apical enterocele). Occasionally peristalsis of the intestine bulging into the vagina establishes the diagnosis. If in doubt, and a diagnosis is necessary before an intraoperative evaluation to ascertain the presence or absence of an enterocele, radiologic assessment is the investigation of choice.

Viscerography or fluoroscopic imaging includes the opacification of bladder, rectum, and vagina with contrast medium. An additional barium meal will show the small bowel. Ideally, the investigation is performed dynamically during straining or coughing and comprises defecography. The bowel evacuation gives room and is crucial for some enteroceles to descend. It will also give further information on bowel emptying, rectal prolapse or intussusception,[41] although there are great variations of 'normal' findings. Shorvon et al. demonstrated that rectoceles and intussusception are frequently present in young and asymptomatic women.[42] It is therefore most valuable when the clinician performs the radiologic investigations and interprets the findings in context with the symptoms.

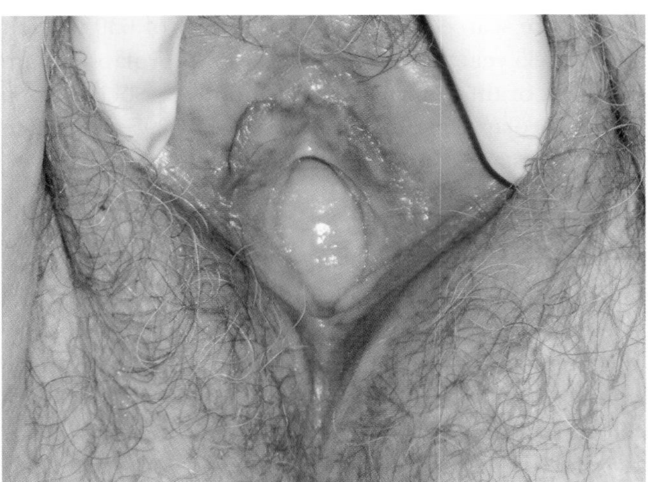

Figure 71.5. *A rectoenterocele with diminished vaginal rugae.*

With the advance of dynamic defecation MRI, we now have an excellent method to evaluate pelvic floor dynamics. However, there are major disadvantages: it is expensive, not widely available and, at present, is performed in the supine position only. Defecation in this situation might be impossible for some patients. However, the images obtained are remarkable and usually provide an accurate diagnosis (Fig. 71.6).[43]

The improving three-dimensional (3D) ultrasound technology can also produce astounding images, especially when acquired as real-time sonography (4D). Although limited in the evaluation of structures located more proximally, it may provide information on fascial defects and also on pelvic floor dynamics. Even with conventional two-dimensional perineal ultrasound, it is still possible to identify an enterocele. Rectal ultrasound can also be helpful; sonographic diagnosis of an enterocele was confirmed intraoperatively in 27 of 29 cases.[44]

PREVENTION OF ENTEROCELES

Theoretically, obliteration of the pouch of Douglas and maintaining a normal vaginal axis should prevent enteroceles from developing. Controlled studies assessing prevention of enteroceles are scarce. Reattachment of the uterosacral ligaments to the vaginal vault during hysterectomy has long been advocated and several techniques are widely used. In a randomized controlled trial undertaken at the time of hysterectomy, Cruikshank and Kovac compared three available methods to prevent an enterocele:[45]

- Obliteration of the pouch of Douglas by suturing the uterosacral ligaments in the midline, called a vaginal Moschcowitz-type operation;
- A McCall-type culdoplasty where the uterosacral ligaments are plicated and attached to the vaginal vault and the sutures externalized;
- Closing of the peritoneum with a purse-string suture.

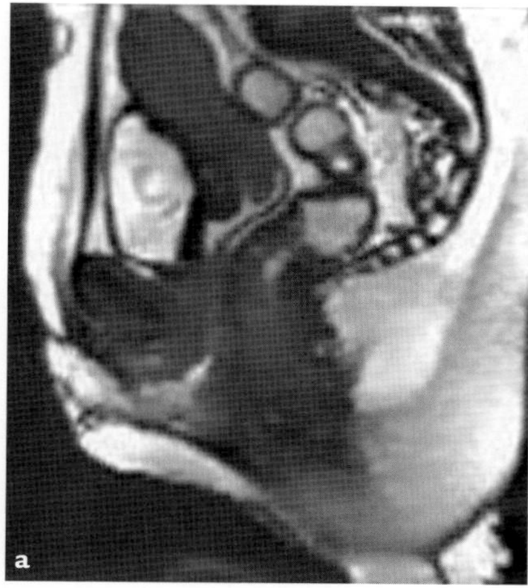

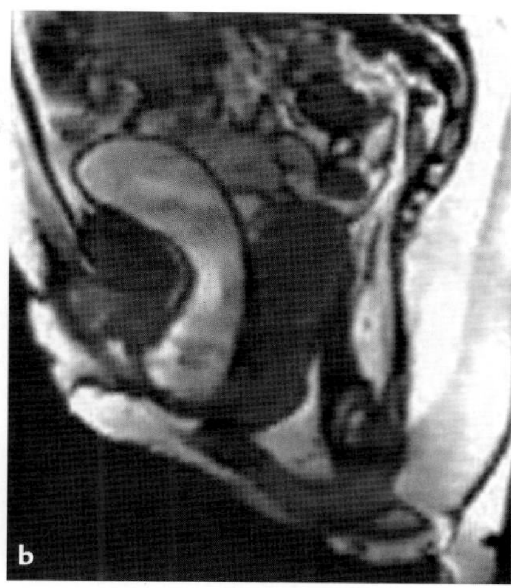

Figure 71.6. *Enterocele, considerable pelvic floor and perineal descent, uterine and bladder prolapse: MRI pictures (a) at rest and (b) during straining.*

Up to 3 months postoperatively all procedures were equally successful (100%). After 3 years, the McCall-type method was found to be superior in terms of enterocele prevention; none of these 32 patients developed a symptomatic enterocele.[45]

The prevention of an enterocele after a Burch colposuspension, with or without additional pouch of Douglas obliteration, by either approximation of the uterosacral ligaments or Moschcowitz-type horizontal purse-string sutures, was reported recently.[29] Without pouch of Douglas obliteration, postoperative enterocele formation after 3–16 years (mean 9 years) occurred in 19%, whereas after the additional Moschcowitz procedure the incidence was 11%, and 2% after uterosacral ligament plication. These differences were significant.[29]

Whether extensive distal preparation of the bladder during abdominal or laparoscopic hysterectomy with exposure of the pubocervical fascia might contribute to the development of anterior enteroceles is unclear. The utilization of intrafascial hysterectomy might be of value but this has not been assessed systematically. During intrafascial hysterectomy, parts of the endopelvic fascia are maintained in their normal position and plicated over the vaginal vault to prevent separation and subsequent enterocele formation.

CONSERVATIVE TREATMENT

Treatment of pelvic organ prolapse depends on associated symptoms, the extent of prolapse, the patient's preferences for management, and whether the patient has completed her family. As subjective and objective success and durability of our current surgical prolapse repairs remain limited, and women's longevity is increasing, more patients might ask for conservative options. Conservative treatment of pelvic organ prolapse in general includes the use of pessaries and pelvic floor training in early prolapse stages. Because of the enterocele etiology, pelvic floor muscle exercises are likely to be ineffective in isolated enteroceles.

Vaginal pessaries might prevent deterioration of the prolapse, as well as alleviating symptoms of prolapse, and are especially useful if there is a long waiting list for surgery. There is an extensive range of mechanical devices available to reduce the prolapse but literature on success and complications is inadequate, especially if isolated enteroceles are considered. Pessaries are a viable option, and a trial of pessary fitting can easily be performed in clinics and be managed by specially trained nurses or continence advisers. In an observational study, 73 of 100 women with at least stage II pelvic organ prolapse had a successful pessary fitting trial. At assessment at 2 months, prolapse-related symptoms had disappeared in most women, in 50% urinary symptoms improved, and 92% were satisfied with their pessary. Dissatisfaction with the pessary treatment was associated with occult stress incontinence.[46]

SURGICAL TREATMENT

There are procedures that obliterate only the pouch of Douglas by plicating the peritoneum (e.g. the Moschcowitz or Halban operation) or the uterosacral ligaments (e.g. the McCall procedure; Fig. 71.7). The failure rates are high if there is insufficient pelvic floor support present or if there has been a previous repair. Peritoneum alone is not a supportive structure. Therefore, best results might only be achieved when the pouch of Douglas obliteration is combined with surgery to support the vaginal vault or uterus. In the Cochrane Review of surgical management of pelvic organ prolapse,

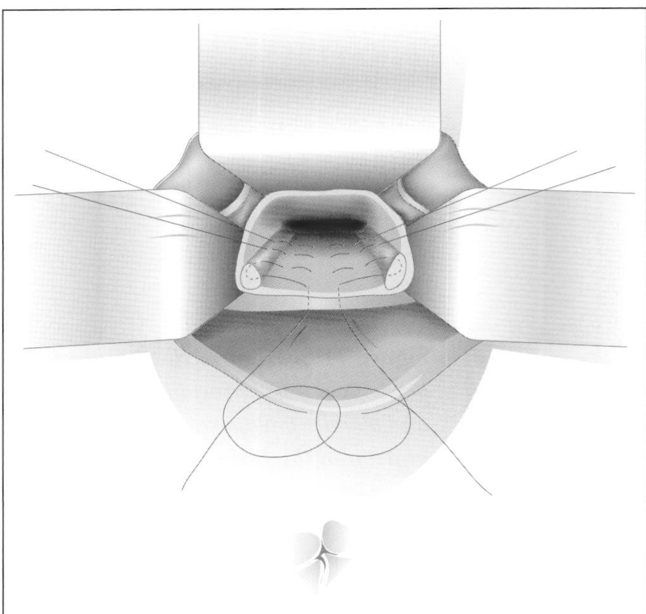

Figure 71.7. *McCall procedure. This is one of several different methods of vaginal suture placement through the uterosacral ligaments.*

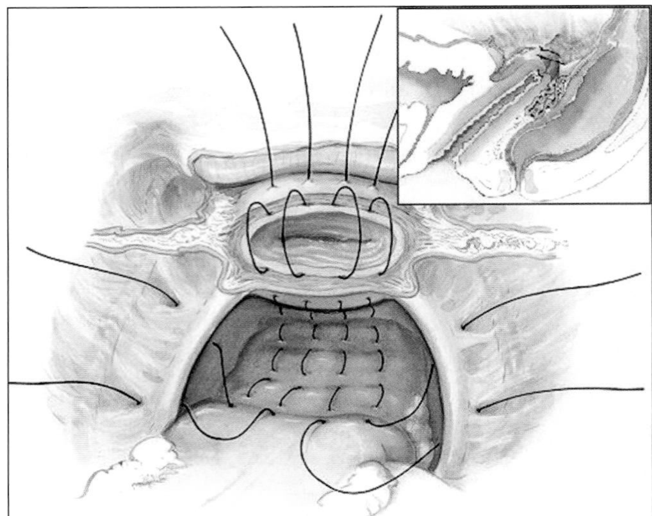

Figure 71.8. *Combination of a Halban-type pouch of Douglas obliteration with sagittal sutures and a McCall part with incorporation of the uterosacral ligaments after concomitant abdominal hysterectomy. Note that the anterior and posterior endopelvic fasciae are joined over the vaginal vault and incorporated in the pouch of Douglas obliteration.*

the lack of randomized controlled trials for enterocele repair was apparent.[47] There are few studies that address enteroceles directly.

Current widely used procedures and their success rates are described below. As with other pelvic floor repairs, the patients' goals should be kept in mind – they might diverge considerably from objective restoration of the anatomy.[48]

Operations to obliterate the pouch of Douglas

Several horizontal circular, purse-string type sutures, beginning at the most distal part of the pouch of Douglas/enterocele form the so-called Moschcowitz procedure which was described by Moschcowitz in 1912 after extensive anatomic studies of rectal prolapse.[25] Although he found it a successful operation in his patients, it has subsequently been associated with a high failure rate and complications such as ureteral kinking and small bowel obstruction[49] although there is a lack of controlled studies. Currently it tends to be used only as an adjunct to major pelvic floor surgery.

Occlusion of the pouch of Douglas, as described by Halban in his 1912 textbook, includes several sagittal sutures positioned along the pouch in a vertical direction (Fig. 71.8).[28] Although there is less risk for ureteral damage, the ureters should be checked carefully. As with the Moschcowitz operation, this approach has not been studied systematically and is currently performed concomitantly with other pelvic floor surgery.

Both the Moschcowitz and Halban operations were initially described as abdominal procedures but can also be achieved transvaginally or laparoscopically.[50,51] The McCall, Halban and Moschcowitz procedures and their extensive variations can be performed prophylactically to obliterate a deep pouch of Douglas or therapeutically to correct an enterocele.

As described above in 'Prevention', there are several methods available to close the rectovaginal pouch, not only vaginally but also abdominally. A popular approach is the simple plication of the uterosacral ligaments in the midline and the McCall culdoplasty with its numerous modifications (see Figs 71.7, 71.8). The principal structure employed is the uterosacral ligaments which are sutured together in the midline with several interrupted stitches or one continuous stitch. Modifications include the incorporation of the vaginal vault or cervix into the sutures. During vaginal hysterectomy after the suture is passed through the uterosacral ligaments on either side, with or without inclusion of the rectosigmoid serosa, it is tied and the ends are passed through the medial aspect of the vaginal vault. Permanent or delayed absorbable sutures should be used although there are no controlled studies to corroborate this. Non-absorbable sutures should not be passed through the vagina to avoid any sinus formation or abscess. Given[52] did not report any enterocele recurrences after an average follow-up of 7 years after McCall culdoplasty and pouch of Douglas obliteration with excision of peritoneum (Torpin wedge culdoplasty).

Vaginal enterocele repair comprises identification, preparation, and opening of the enterocele sac, high closure of the peritoneum with a purse-string suture and excision of the sac if preferred. The failure rate with this repair was reported at 33% in one study, although 72% of women also received a posterior repair and 22% had a Burch colposuspension.[53] A site-specific fascial defect repair with reattachment of the disruption might complete the vaginal repair.

The effect of pelvic organ prolapse operations on enterocele formation

A surgical technique to suspend the vaginal vault and reattach the endopelvic fascia to the uterosacral ligaments has been studied by Shull et al.[54] The concept of prolapse as a hernia is meticulously followed. Using one suture, the anterior and posterior endopelvic fasciae (usually after a concomitant repair) are connected to the uterosacral ligaments, thereby completely covering the vault with fascia. Two or three permanent stitches along the ligament might be passed; the more proximal sutures correspond with more lateral placements in the anterior and posterior fasciae. The success rate for vault prolapse and enteroceles was reported to be 99%. This method was originally described as a vaginal procedure; however, using these principal steps allows it to be performed (at least partly) laparoscopically as illustrated by Miklos et al.[55] and Paraiso et al.[51] Laparoscopically, the sutures are placed through the uterosacral ligaments which are later, during the vaginal part of the operation, passed through the anterior and posterior endopelvic fasciae. Early success rates were 100%; there were no recurrent enteroceles.[55] Similar vaginal procedures that include some form of uterosacral ligament plication and address an enterocele have been described by Karram et al. with a 7% enterocele recurrence rate.[56]

There are two randomized controlled trials that compare the transvaginal and the transanal rectocele repair.[57,58] The authors reported a higher incidence of enteroceles and rectoenteroceles in the transanal repair group. It was suggested that the transvaginal posterior repair with continuous plication of the fascia from the perineal body to the vaginal apex offers protection against enterocele formation.[59] A posterior colporrhaphy augmented with vicryl mesh is not superior to a simple posterior repair in terms of recurrent enterocele according to one randomized controlled trial.[60]

Combined operations for pelvic organ prolapse and concomitant enterocele

There are several vaginal, abdominal and laparoscopic operations that address vaginal vault or uterine prolapse and concomitant enteroceles but there is a paucity of studies that assess long-term objective and subjective outcomes. Open abdominal[61–63] and laparoscopic sacrocolpopexy[51,64,65] may include pouch of Douglas obliteration. Obliteration of the pouch of Douglas with Moschcowitz or Halban sutures or rectovaginal mesh interposition as advocated by Villet et al.[66] has been criticized by several authors because posterior enteroceles have been observed behind the mesh.[62,67] However, on reviewing the available literature, there appears to be no considerably higher incidence of enteroceles in women who did not undergo any form of pouch of Douglas obliteration.[62] There were 12 cases (2.2%) of recurrent vault prolapse or enterocele described out of 549 patients in whom the pouch of Douglas was obliterated. In 548 patients with no obliteration of the pouch of Douglas the failure rate of vault prolapse was 4.0% (22 of 548 cases).[68]

In a meta-analysis of two randomized controlled trials, the abdominal sacrocolpopexy with mesh and vaginal sacrospinous colpopexy were equally effective with regard to occurrence of postoperative enterocele (odds ratio = 0.77; 95% CI: 0.28–2.06).[69,70] Non-randomized comparisons of sacrospinous and iliococcygeus colpopexy did not reveal any difference with respect to postoperative enteroceles.[71] The same applies to fixation of the cervix/uterus or vaginal vault to the sacrospinous ligament.[72]

CONCLUSION

An isolated enterocele is rare and usually occurs after pelvic surgery that displaces the vaginal axis, leads to disruption of the anterior and posterior endopelvic fasciae or exposes the pouch of Douglas. A deep pouch of Douglas might predispose to enterocele formation. Enteroceles are frequently associated with pelvic organ prolapse in other compartments. Symptoms range widely and include prolapse sensation, disturbance of defecation and micturition, and dyspareunia. During careful clinical vaginal and rectal examination, enteroceles can usually be identified but imaging techniques such as viscerography and MRI are helpful.

There are two procedures that close the peritoneum of the pouch of Douglas only: the Moschcowitz operation with horizontal sutures and the Halban method with vertical suture placement. Several other procedures and modifications utilize the uterosacral ligaments. These repairs can be performed vaginally, open abdominally or laparoscopically, and are usually combined with other pelvic floor surgery. Operations that address vaginal vault prolapse might be necessary to accomplish a good anatomic and symptomatic result. To date there are no data available to recommend one particular procedure.

REFERENCES

1. Uhlenhuth E, Wolfe WM, Smith EM et al. The rectogenital septum. Surg Gynecol Obstet 1948;86:148–63.
2. van Ophoven A, Roth S. The anatomy and embryological origins of the fascia of Denonvilliers: a medico-historical debate. J Urol 1997;157(1):3–9.
3. Holley RL. Enterocele: a review. Obstet Gynecol Surv 1994;49:284–93.
4. Baessler K, Schuessler B. The depth of the pouch of Douglas in nulliparous and parous women without genital prolapse and in patients with genital prolapse. Am J Obstet Gynecol 2000;182(3):540–4.
5. DeLancey JO. Structural anatomy of the posterior pelvic compartment as it relates to rectocele. Am J Obstet Gynecol 1999;180:815–23.
6. DeLancey JO. Anatomic aspects of vaginal eversion after hysterectomy. Am J Obstet Gynecol 1992;166 (6 Part 1):1717–24.
7. Lansman HH. Posthysterectomy vault prolapse: sacral colpopexy with dura mater graft. Obstet Gynecol 1984;63:577–82.
8. Maloney JC, Dunton CJ, Smith K. Repair of vaginal vault prolapse with abdominal sacropexy. J Reprod Med 1990;35:6–10.
9. Powell JL, Joseph DB. Abdominal sacral colpopexy in patients with gynecologic cancer and 'Burch' not 'Birch'. Gynecol Oncol 2000;77:483–4.
10. Robert HG, Vayre P. Les élytrocèles. Considérations anatomique et thérapeutiques. A propos de 25 observations. Ann Chir 1964;18:1060–71.
11. Anson BJ. An atlas of human anatomy. Philadelphia: WB Saunders, 1950.
12. Baessler K, Schuessler B. Anatomy of the sigmoid colon, rectum, and the rectovaginal pouch in women with enterocele and anterior rectal wall procidentia. Clin Anat 19, 2006
13. Berglas B, Rubin IC. Study of the supportive structures of the uterus by levator myography. Surg Gynecol Obstet 1953;97:677–92.
14. Nichols DH, Genadry RR. Pelvic relaxation of the posterior compartment. Curr Opin Obstet Gynecol 1993;5:458–64.
15. Singh K, Reid WM, Berger LA. Magnetic resonance imaging of normal levator ani anatomy and function. Obstet Gynecol 2002;99(3):433–8.
16. Rizk DE, Czechowski J, Ekelund L. Dynamic assessment of pelvic floor and bony pelvis morphologic condition with the use of magnetic resonance imaging in a multiethnic, nulliparous, and healthy female population. Am J Obstet Gynecol 2004;191:83–9.
17. Tulikangas PK, Walters MD, Brainard JA et al. Enterocele: is there a histologic defect? Obstet Gynecol 2001;98:634–7.
18. Weber AM, Walters MD. Anterior vaginal prolapse: review of anatomy and techniques of surgical repair. Obstet Gynecol 1997;89(2):311–8.
19. Henry MM, Parks AG, Swash M. The pelvic floor musculature in the descending perineum syndrome. Br J Surg 1982;69:470–2.
20. Fialkow MF, Gardella C, Melville J et al. Posterior vaginal wall defects and their relation to measures of pelvic floor neuromuscular function and posterior compartment symptoms. Am J Obstet Gynecol 2002;187(6):1443–8.
21. Harewood GC, Coulie B, Camilleri M et al. Descending perineum syndrome: audit of clinical and laboratory features and outcome of pelvic floor retraining. Am J Gastroenterol 1999;94:126–30.
22. Baessler K, Stanton SL. Symptomatic pelvic organ prolapse and perineal descent. Int Urogynecol J Pelvic Floor Dysfunct 2001:S24.
23. Zacharin RF. Pulsion enterocele: review of functional anatomy of the pelvic floor. Obstet Gynecol 1980;55(2):135–40.
24. Zacharin RF, Hamilton NT. Pulsion enterocele: long-term results of an abdominoperineal technique. Obstet Gynecol 1980;55:141–8.
25. Moschcowitz AV. The pathogenesis, anatomy, and cure of prolapse of the rectum. Surg Gynecol Obstet 1912;15:7–12.
26. Altemeier WA, Culbertson WR, Schowengerdt CJ, Hunt J. Nineteen years' experience with the one stage perineal repair of rectal prolapse. Ann Surg 1971;173(6):993–1006.
27. Jorge JM, Yang YK, Wexner SD. Incidence and clinical significance of sigmoidoceles as determined by a new classification system. Dis Colon Rectum 1994;37:1112–7.
28. Halban J. Gynäkologische Operationslehre. Berlin: Urban and Schwarzenberg, 1912.
29. Langer R, Lipshitz Y, Halperin R et al. Prevention of genital prolapse following Burch colposuspension: comparison between two surgical procedures. Int Urogynecol J Pelvic Floor Dysfunct 2003;1:13–6.
30. Wiskind AK, Creighton SM, Stanton SL. The incidence of genital prolapse after the Burch colposuspension. Am J Obstet Gynecol 1992;167:399–404.

31. Alcalay M, Monga A, Stanton SL. Burch colposuspension: a 10–20 year follow up. Br J Obstet Gynaecol 1995;102:740–5.

32. Peters WA 3rd, Smith MR, Drescher CW. Rectal prolapse in women with other defects of pelvic floor support. Am J Obstet Gynecol 2001;184(7):1488–94.

33. Thompson JR, Chen AH, Pettit PD et al. Incidence of occult rectal prolapse in patients with clinical rectoceles and defecatory dysfunction. Am J Obstet Gynecol 2002;187:1494–9.

34. Mellgren A, Schultz I, Johansson C et al. Internal rectal intussusception seldom develops into total rectal prolapse. Dis Colon Rectum 1997;40:817–20.

35. Slieker-ten Hover MCP, Vierhout M, Bloembergen H et al. Distribution of pelvic organ prolapse (POP) in the general population: prevalence, severity, etiology and relation with the function of the pelvic floor muscles. Neurourol Urodyn 2004:401–2.

36. Kinzel GE. Enterocele. Am J Obstet Gynecol 1961;81:1166–74.

37. Marinkovic SP, Stanton SL. Incontinence and voiding difficulties associated with prolapse. J Urol 2004;171(3):1021–8.

38. Haylen BT, Law MG, Frazer M et al. Urine flow rates and residual urine volumes in urogynecology patients. Int Urogynecol J Pelvic Floor Dysfunct 1999;10:378–83.

39. Weber AM, Walters MD, Piedmonte MR. Sexual function and vaginal anatomy in women before and after surgery for pelvic organ prolapse and urinary incontinence. Am J Obstet Gynecol 2000;182(6):1610–5.

40. Croak AJ, Gebhart JB, Klingele CJ et al. Characteristics of patients with vaginal rupture and evisceration. Obstet Gynecol 2004;103(3):572–6.

41. Kelvin FM, Maglinte DD, Hornback JA et al. Pelvic prolapse: assessment with evacuation proctography (defecography). Radiology 1992;184:547–51.

42. Shorvon PJ, McHugh S, Diamant NE et al. Defecography in normal volunteers: results and implications. Gut 1989;30:1737–49.

43. Lienemann A, Anthuber C, Baron A et al. Diagnosing enteroceles using dynamic magnetic resonance imaging. Dis Colon Rectum 2000;43:205–12.

44. Vierhout ME, van PD. Diagnosis of posterior enterocele: comparison of rectal ultrasonography with intraoperative diagnosis. J Ultrasound Med 2002;21(4):383–7.

45. Cruikshank SH, Kovac SR. Randomized comparison of three surgical methods used at the time of vaginal hysterectomy to prevent posterior enterocele. Am J Obstet Gynecol 1999;180(4):859–65.

46. Clemons JL, Aguilar VC, Tillinghast TA et al. Patient satisfaction and changes in prolapse and urinary symptoms in women who were fitted successfully with a pessary for pelvic organ prolapse. Am J Obstet Gynecol 2004;190(4):1025–9.

47. Maher CF, Baessler K, Glazener CMA, Adams EJ, Hagen S. Surgical management of pelvic organ prolapse in women (Cochrane Review). Cochrane Database Syst Rev 2004; Issue 4.

48. Hullfish KL, Bovbjerg VE, Steers WD. Patient-centered goals for pelvic floor dysfunction surgery: long-term follow-up. Am J Obstet Gynecol 2004;191:201–5.

49. Dicke JM. Small bowel obstruction secondary to a prior Moschcowitz procedure. Am J Obstet Gynecol 1985;152 (7 Pt 1):887–8.

50. Lyons TL. Minimally invasive treatment of urinary stress incontinence and laparoscopically directed repair of pelvic floor defects. Clin Obstet Gynecol 1995;32(2):380–91.

51. Paraiso MF, Falcone T, Walters MD. Laparoscopic surgery for enterocele, vaginal apex prolapse and rectocele. Int Urogynecol J Pelvic Floor Dysfunct 1999;10:223–9.

52. Given FT Jr. 'Posterior culdeplasty': revisited. Am J Obstet Gynecol 1985;15320:135–9.

53. Tulikangas PK, Piedmonte MR, Weber AM. Functional and anatomic follow-up of enterocele repairs. Obstet Gynecol 2001;98:265–8.

54. Shull BL, Bachofen C, Coates KW et al. A transvaginal approach to repair of apical and other associated sites of pelvic organ prolapse with uterosacral ligaments. Am J Obstet Gynecol 2000;183:1365–73.

55. Miklos JR, Kohli N, Lucente V et al. Site-specific fascial defects in the diagnosis and surgical management of enterocele. Am J Obstet Gynecol 1998;179(6 Pt 1):1418–22; discussion 1822–3.

56. Karram M, Goldwasser S, Kleeman S et al. High uterosacral vaginal vault suspension with fascial reconstruction for vaginal repair of enterocele and vaginal vault prolapse. Am J Obstet Gynecol 2001;185(6):1339–42; discussion 1342–3.

57. Kahn MA, Stanton SL, Kumar D et al. Posterior colporrhaphy is superior to the transanal repair for treatment of posterior vaginal wall prolapse. Neurourol Urodyn 1999;18:70–1.

58. Nieminen K, Hiltunen KM, Laitinen J et al. Transanal or vaginal approach to rectocele repair: a prospective, randomized pilot study. Dis Colon Rectum 2004;47(10):1636–42.

59. Nieminen K, Heinonen PK. Sacrospinous ligament fixation for massive genital prolapse in women aged over 80 years. BJOG 2001;108:817–21.

60. Sand PK, Koduri S, Lobel RW et al. Prospective randomized trial of polyglactin 910 mesh to prevent recurrence of cystoceles and rectoceles. Am J Obstet Gynecol 2001;184(7):1357–62; discussion 1362–4.

61. Baessler K, Schuessler B. Abdominal sacrocolpopexy and

anatomy and function of the posterior compartment. Obstet Gynecol 2001;97:678–84.

62. Timmons MC, Addison WA, Addison SB et al. Abdominal sacral colpopexy in 163 women with posthysterectomy vaginal vault prolapse and enterocele. Evolution of operative techniques. J Reprod Med 1992;37(4):323–7.

63. van Lindert AC, Groenendijk AG, Scholten PC et al. Surgical support and suspension of genital prolapse, including preservation of the uterus, using the Gore-Tex soft tissue patch (a preliminary report). Eur J Obstet Gynecol Reprod Biol 1993;50(2):133–9.

64. Nezhat CH, Nezhat F, Nezhat C. Laparoscopic sacral colpopexy for vaginal vault prolapse. Obstet Gynecol 1994;84(5):885–8.

65. Ross JW. Techniques of laparoscopic repair of total vault eversion after hysterectomy. J Am Assoc Gynecol Laparosc 1997;4(2):173–83.

66. Villet R, Morice P, Bech A et al. Approache abdominale des rectoceles et des elytroceles. Ann Chir 1993:626–30.

67. Addison WA, Timmons MC, Wall LL et al. Failed abdominal sacral colpopexy: observations and recommendations. Obstet Gynecol 1989;74:480–3.

68. Baessler K, Leron E, Stanton SL. Sacrohysteropexy and sacrocolpopexy. In: Stanton SL, Zimmern PE (eds) Female Pelvic Reconstructive Surgery. Berlin: Springer, 2003; 184–91.

69. Maher CF, Qatawneh A, Dwyer PL et al. Abdominal sacral colpopexy or vaginal sacrospinous colpopexy for vaginal vault prolapse: a prospective randomized study. Am J Obstet Gynecol 2004;190(1):20–6.

70. Benson JT, Lucente V, McClellan E. Vaginal versus abdominal reconstructive surgery for the treatment of pelvic support defects: a prospective randomized study with long–term outcome evaluation. Am J Obstet Gynecol 1996;175(6):1418–21; discussion 1421–2.

71. Maher CF, Murray CJ, Carey MP et al. Iliococcygeus or sacrospinous fixation for vaginal vault prolapse. Obstet Gynecol 2001;98:40–4.

72. Maher CF, Cary MP, Slack MC et al. Uterine preservation or hysterectomy at sacrospinous colpopexy for uterovaginal prolapse? Int Urogynecol J Pelvic Floor Dysfunct 2001;12(6):381–4; discussion 384–5.

72

Rectocele – anatomic and functional repair

William A Silva, Mickey M Karram

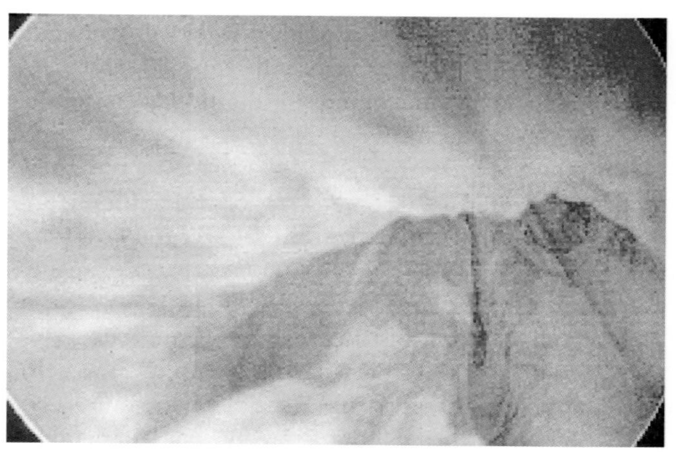

INTRODUCTION

Since the early 19th century, surgeons have performed posterior colporrhaphy to manage complete tears of the perineum. The supports of the genital organs were largely a mystery, and there was little distinction between prolapses of the rectum, bladder, and uterus. As anatomic concepts developed, surgeons ascertained that the main support of the uterus was the vagina, which in turn was supported by the insertion of the levator ani muscles into the perineum. This concept was the basis for the incorporation of plication of the levator ani muscles into posterior colpoperineorrhaphy, with the surgical goals of constriction of the vaginal tube, creation of a perineal shelf, and partial closure of the genital hiatus. Until recently, very little attention has been given to the functional derangements that are commonly associated with rectoceles.

A rectocele is an outpocketing of the anterior rectal and the posterior vaginal wall into the lumen of the vagina.[1] Some rectoceles may be asymptomatic, whereas others may cause such symptoms as incomplete bowel emptying, vaginal mass, pain, and pressure. The prevalence of rectoceles ranges from 20 to 80% in the general population.[2] A rectocele is fundamentally a defect of the rectovaginal septum, not of the rectum. The size of the defect does not necessarily correlate with the amount of functional derangement. This chapter reviews the anatomy, pathophysiology, diagnosis, and management of rectoceles.

ANATOMY

In 1839, Denonvilliers first described a layer of fascia found in males, which he named the 'rectovesical septum'. Nichols and Milley later recorded the existence of this septum in surgical dissections and autopsies of fresh female cadavers.[3] This layer of connective tissue is fused to the undersurface of the posterior vaginal wall.

The rectovaginal fascia extends downwards from the posterior aspect of the cervix and the cardinal–uterosacral ligaments to its attachment on the upper margin of the perineal body and laterally to the fascia over the levator ani muscle. Richardson[3] states that the rectovaginal septum and uterosacral ligaments provide suspensory support of the perineal body from the sacrum. Posterior to the rectovaginal septum lies the rectovaginal space, which provides a plane for dissection. In between the rectovaginal septum and the rectum is the pararectal fascia; inside this fibromuscular layer lie blood vessels, nerves, and lymph nodes, which supply the rectum. The pararectal fascia, originating from the pelvic sidewalls, divides into fibrous anterior and posterior sheaths, which encompass the rectum. These layers provide additional support to the anterior rectal wall.[4]

Further support is provided by the levator ani, which are composed of paired iliococcygeus, puborectalis, and pubococcygeus muscles. These muscles function to maintain a constant basal tone and a closed urogenital hiatus. This constant basal tone prevents the urogenital hiatus from widening and the eventual descent of the pelvic viscera. These muscles also provide a contraction reflex to increased intra-abdominal pressures, preventing incontinence and prolapse. The anterior sacral nerve roots S2–S4, which innervate these muscles, cross the pelvic floor and are stretched and compressed during labor, increasing the risk of injury.[4,5]

ETIOLOGY

Rectocele was once thought to be a condition affecting only multiparous females and resulting from obstetric damage or increased tissue laxity with aging and menopausal atrophy. However, recently, rectoceles and enteroceles have been noted to occur in approximately 40% of asymptomatic parous women.[6] Shorvon et al. performed defecography on healthy, young, nulliparous, asymptomatic volunteers, noting that 17/21 women had small or moderately sized rectoceles.[7] Rectoceles may thus have a wider prevalence than previously thought and may not be a result of parity.

The most common causes of rectoceles are obstetric events. Traumatic obstetric events, which usually occur when the presenting part descends quickly in the second stage of labor, can predispose to rectocele formation. The forces of labor may separate, tear or distend the pelvic floor, altering the functional and anatomic position of the muscles, nerves, and connective tissues. The rectal fascia may separate from the perineal body, causing a transverse defect and low rectocele. Low rectoceles are isolated defects in the suprasphincteric portion of the rectovaginal fascia. They are usually caused by obstetric trauma that disrupts the attachments of the levator ani fascia and bulbocavernosus muscles. An eversion of the introitus will be noted on physical examination. This will aggravate constipation and will result in inefficient bowel movements and the need for stronger Valsalva maneuver.[8–12]

If mid or high rectoceles form, they may alter the vaginal axis.[1,4,8,9] Laxity of the levator ani secondary to the levator detaching from the perineal body along the vaginal axis allows the pelvic organs to slide downwards, following the new altered axis. Women with an android pelvis are at increased risk because labor forces are directed towards the posterior vaginal wall and perineum, leaving the anterior vaginal wall relatively protected.

Mid-vaginal rectoceles are most likely caused by obstetric trauma not involving the levator ani. The rectovaginal fascia is damaged by the stretching and laceration of the tissue, which results in the thinning of the fascia, leading to subsequent adhesion formation. This adhesion of the rectovaginal septum, vagina, and rectal capsule inhibits independent function. Symptoms may include incomplete bowel emptying, rectal pressure, and pain after bowel movements; they may also coexist with a high rectocele.[12]

High rectoceles often occur from pathologic overstretching of the posterior vaginal wall. The cardinal ligaments fuse with the vagina and cervix, causing the cervix to fuse with the anterior vaginal wall. The rectovaginal septum is absent from the posterior vaginal wall, causing loss of the anterior rectal wall support. High rectocele may also coexist with congenital deepness of the pouch of Douglas.[12]

Rectoceles may occur as a result of pathologic stretching of the pudendal nerves during descent of the fetal head, causing atrophy and denervation of the pelvic floor muscles. Sultan reported that most damage to the pelvic support occurs in the first vaginal delivery.[13,14] Electromyographic studies demonstrate an 80% incidence of denervation of the perineal muscles after vaginal delivery.[5,15,16] Denervation will probably recover after the postpartum period; however, it has been demonstrated that injury may be cumulative with increasing parity.[5] Increased labor duration and weight of the baby directly influence the perineal damage and denervation of the pelvic floor. This neuropathy can lead to the weakening of pelvic floor muscles and development of a rectocele. Thus, shortening of the second stage of labor by episiotomy or forceps may decrease the risk of denervation and subsequent pelvic floor damage.[8]

Defecation disorders may account for a subgroup of rectoceles. They may lead to the weakening of the rectovaginal septum by continuous straining against an obstruction. One disorder, the perineal descent syndrome, is clinically diagnosed when the individual strains and the perineal plane descends past the ischial tuberosities;[15] this disorder may be confused with a rectocele. Other conditions, such as paradoxical sphincter reaction (anismus), cause unconscious contraction of the voluntary striated muscles when attempting to defecate. This constant straining with bowel movements has been shown to cause or worsen a pre-existing rectocele and increasingly to weaken the rectovaginal septum by denervation injury.[17] Anismus eventually leads to the accumulation of stool in the rectum, which may complicate pelvic outlet obstruction and cause a progressive cycle, worsening the rectocele.[18]

Congenital absence of the perineum may mimic a rectocele. This pseudorectocele has its posterior vaginal wall exposed because of lack of inferior support; this may be corrected by surgical reconstruction of the perineum. Congenital absence allows for deepening of the cul-de-sac and weakening of the rectovaginal septum, leading to the development of a high rectocele and enterocele.[6,12]

Some studies have found differences in connective tissue strengths between races, which may contribute to rectoceles. Africans have been noted to have a decreased frequency of laceration after normal spontaneous deliveries and a subsequent decrease of uterine prolapse. This may be related to constitutional factors such as pelvis type, connective tissue, and ability to fibrose,[12] whereas Hispanic, Filipino and Chinese women may have an increased risk of laxity of tissue.[19]

CLINICAL PRESENTATION

The symptoms associated with a rectocele are summarized in Table 72.1. Clinical symptoms vary from being non-existent to severe bowel problems. A common complaint is constipation, which may occur in up to 75% of patients with rectoceles.[2] Patients may also complain of incomplete rectal emptying, a sense of rectal pressure or a vaginal bulge.[1,20,21] Patients may describe stool becoming trapped in the rectocele pocket itself. Vaginal digitation or perineal support is sometimes necessary to facilitate defecation.[20] Constipation and straining may worsen the symptoms and lead to left lower quadrant abdominal pain if impaction occurs. Many non-specific symptoms, such as rectal pain, bleeding, fecal or gas incontinence, low back pain worsening throughout the day but relieved

Table 72.1. ***Symptoms associated with a rectocele***

- Sensation of pelvic pressure
- Feeling that something is falling down or falling out from the pelvis
- Symptoms often worsened by standing up and eased by lying down
- Lower abdominal and/or back pain
- Bulging mass felt inside the vagina
- Painful or impossible vaginal intercourse
- Vaginal bleeding
- Constipation
- Problems with passage of stool as it becomes caught in the rectocele
- Sensation of incomplete bowel emptying
- Fecal incontinence
- Asymptomatic

by lying down, and dyspareunia may occur, as well as many other defecatory disorders.[6] The prevalence of fecal incontinence increases to 17% in populations with pelvic organ prolapse and urinary incontinence[22] compared to 2–3% in the general population.[23,24] The most common mechanisms are an incompetent sphincteric mechanism (secondary to a structural defect or pudendal nerve damage) and overflow incontinence. As previously mentioned, the majority of rectoceles are totally asymptomatic.

PHYSICAL EXAMINATION

A rectocele is detected by observing the bulge in the posterior vaginal wall during maximum Valsalva or cough. The patient may be in the dorsal supine position (for the gynecologist) or in the left lateral decubitus position (for the colorectal surgeon). The use of the split blade of a Sims or Graves speculum to support the anterior segment can aid in visualization. A rectocele can be confirmed with a rectal examination during which anterior displacement of the vaginal wall adjacent to the rectum and the perineal body is noted. This can be differentiated from enterocele by noting bowel in the rectovaginal space: with the patient standing, the rectovaginal examination will reveal small bowel herniating into this space when an enterocele is present. Of women with rectoceles, 80% are asymptomatic and can be diagnosed only on physical examination.[7,18]

The current standardized system used for prolapse assessment is termed the pelvic organ prolapse quantification (POPQ) system, and was described by Bump et al. in 1996.[25] The POPQ is a descriptive system that contains a series of site-specific measurements of a patient's anterior, apical, and posterior pelvic organ support. This nomenclature has replaced the respective terms cystocele, enterocele, and rectocele as it is often uncertain which specific structures are contributing to prolapse at each segment. Prolapse is measured in centimeters relative to the hymeneal ring in relation to six defined points. Points proximal to the hymen are denoted as negative and points distal as positive. The other landmarks which complete the examination are the genital hiatus, perineal body, and total vaginal length.

In the POPQ system, the posterior segment includes analogous points ascribed to the anterior segment. Point Ba corresponds to a point 3 cm proximal to the hymen in the midline of the posterior segment. Possible values range from –3 to +3 cm from the hymeneal ring. Point Bp represents the most distal portion of the posterior vaginal wall. The minimum value is –3 in the absence of any posterior wall prolapse. In the presence of complete vaginal eversion, the maximum value equals the value of C.

Richardson described site-specific defects in the rectovaginal septum that occur in various locations including the superior, inferior, right, left, and midline areas.[3] These defects are often noted at the time of surgical intervention.[26] One study has suggested that locating defects during clinical evaluation of the posterior vaginal wall is often inaccurate when compared to surgical assessment at the time of defect-specific repair.[27]

DIAGNOSTIC STUDIES

Imaging studies

Significant strides in the area of prolapse evaluation have occurred in the last decade, largely as a result of advanced technology in the field of radiology. However, the results of imaging studies are only useful when used in combination with other information, especially history, symptomatology, and physical examination, and should not be used alone to make treatment decisions. Potential uses of radiologic investigation include those situations in which: 1) symptomatology and physical findings do not correlate; 2) the pelvic anatomy is unusual or altered due to previous pelvic surgery or a congenital defect; and 3) the patient is unable to exert maximal straining during pelvic examination.

Dynamic proctography or defecography

The use of contrast media in pelvic fluoroscopy allows the various prolapsed organs to be opacified and seen in real time. Traditionally, it has mainly been used in the study of anorectal dysfunction as evacuation proctography, which is also known as defecography. However, the addition of a cystogram (dynamic cystoproctography) to this modality allows further information to be gained during the assessment.[28]

The equipment required includes a thick barium paste, a radiolucent toilet, and video equipment. Images are taken at rest, during straining effort, and during and after evacuation.

Currently, universally accepted radiologic criteria for defining pelvic organ prolapse are lacking.[29] However, prolapse is usually radiologically defined in reference to the pubococcygeal line – a line extending from the inferior pubic ramus to the sacrococcygeal junction.[30] This line is reproducible and includes the attachment sites for the levator muscle.

A rectocele is seen radiologically as an anterior rectal bulge (Fig. 72.1).[31–35] It is usually measured as the depth in relation to a line extended upward through the anterior anal wall. The cut-off value has not been universally agreed, but some authors consider a depth of greater than 3 cm to be abnormal (many asymptomatic women will be found to have a small rectocele 2 cm or less in depth).[7,36] Proctography will also note the finding of postevacuation barium trapping which may help to explain any evacuation dysfunction.[37] During testing, patients can be taught how to apply manual pressure in the vagina to obtain relief from the symptoms associated with incomplete emptying. Proctography may suggest the diagnosis of anismus, which may be the main contributor to a patient's bowel dysfunction rather than a rectocele.[38] This has important implications because anismus is treated with biofeedback therapy rather than with surgery.

An enterocele is noted as a herniation of the small bowel into the cul-de-sac into the vagina, rectovaginal space, or both. The vagina and small bowel in the pelvis need to be opacified to obtain this diagnosis. They are most evident after evacuation as a full rectum may obscure its visualization (Fig. 72.2). Sigmoidoceles are noted in approximately 5% of proctograms.[39] However, there still may be false negatives with proctography due to insufficient filling of contrast media into the sigmoid. This finding is important in that a patient may require sigmoid resection or sigmoidopexy as treatment. Vaginal vault prolapse can also be assessed on postevacuation studies.

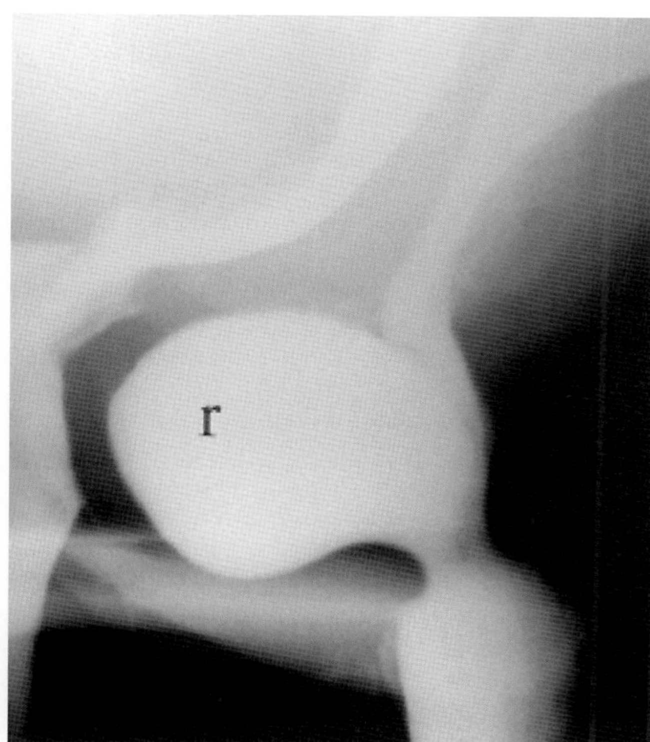

Figure 72.1. *A rectocele (r) with the classic 'hockey puck' appearance is shown to be trapping radiocontrast medium after the evacuation phase. (Reproduced from ref. 35 with permission.)*

Compared with physical examination, evacuation cystoproctography will detect many enteroceles and sigmoidoceles not seen on pelvic examination.[31] Studies have shown that enteroceles are only identified approximately 50% of the time on physical examination, which is less than the rates of identifying rectoceles and cystoceles.[32,39] This has been attributed to the failure of the patient to strain maximally during pelvic examination, an impediment that is removed during the evacuation phase of cystoproctography. One study by Altringer et al. found that patient diagnosis was changed in 75% of cases after dynamic cystoproctography.[32] Another benefit is that fluoroscopy will identify the specific organs involved in the prolapse. However, it is difficult to correlate the degree of prolapse seen on imaging with that seen on physical examination as each has two separate reference points, the pubococcygeal line and hymen, respectively.[29]

Magnetic resonance imaging

Magnetic resonance imaging (MRI) was first introduced as a diagnostic modality for pelvic organ prolapse by Yang et al.[30] It has many advantages over dynamic cystoproctography:

- it is able to contrast soft tissue structures well;
- it provides images in numerous different planes;
- it can examine subtle pelvic floor changes such as superior rectovaginal, paravaginal, and uterine defects;
- it can assess pelvic floor musculature;
- bony landmarks are easier to identify;
- no catheterization is necessary;
- the patient is not exposed to ionizing radiation.

The main limitation is the supine position usually employed by this modality.

As with dynamic proctocystography, the pubococcygeal line is used as the reference point radiographically (Fig. 72.3a). Pelvic organ prolapse is seen as an extension of the pelvic organ below the pubococcygeal line, and can be measured in the same way as with dynamic proctocystography (Fig. 72.3b).[40] It also shares some of

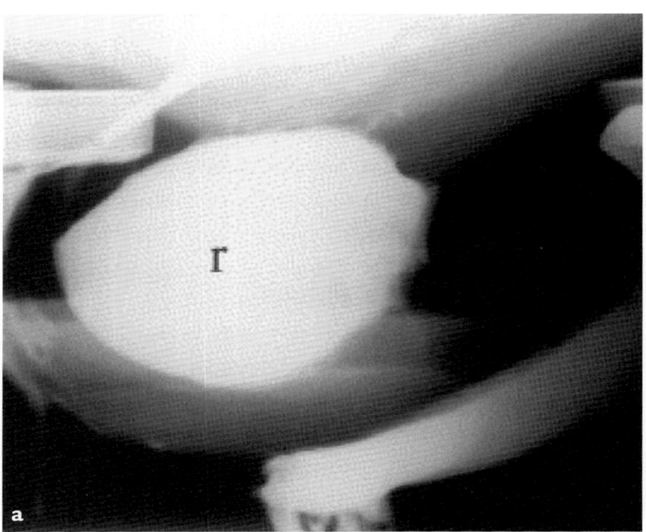

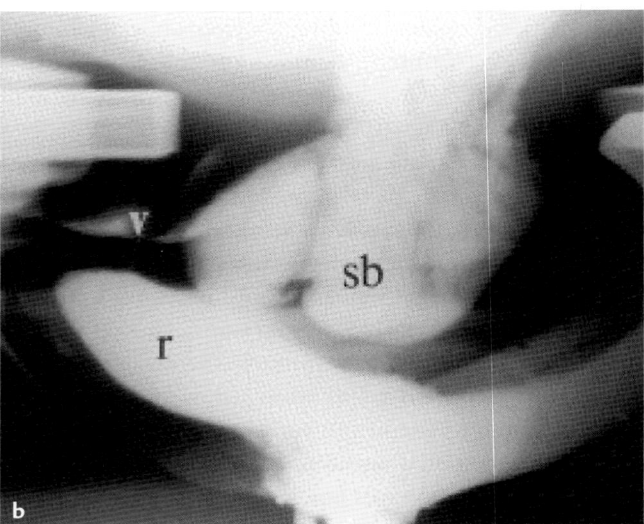

Figure 72.2. *(a, b) A full rectum (r) is partially obscuring complete visualization of the enterocele (sb). The enterocele is then noted to push contrast out of the rectocele, resulting in a better view of the enterocele. v, vagina. (Reproduced from ref. 35 with permission.)*

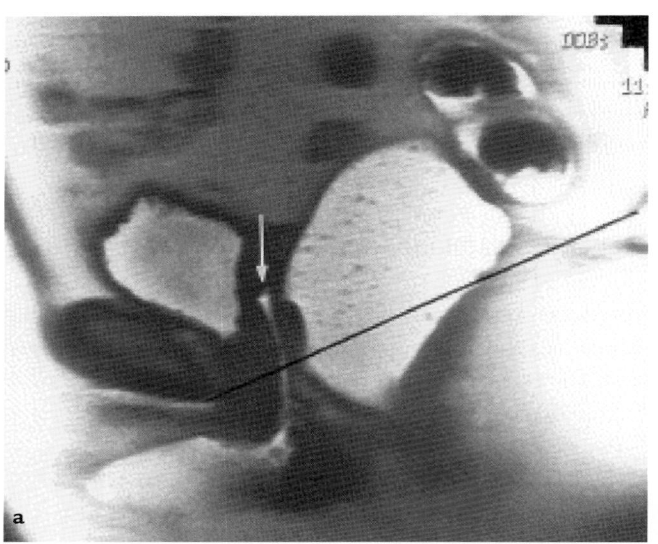

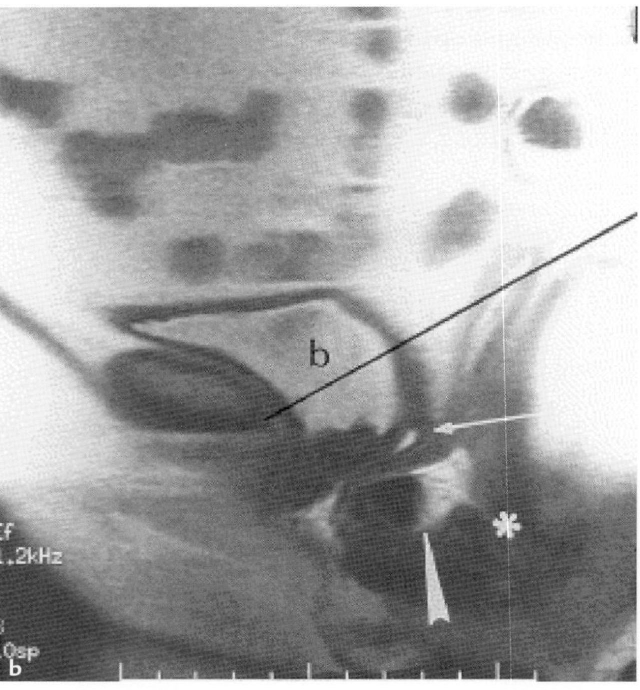

Figure 72.3. *(a) The pubococcygeal line used as a reference point radiographically is drawn from the inferior pubic symphysis to the sacrococcygeal junction (arrow = vaginal vault). (b) Compared to the normal examination in the first image, the second image shows prolapse of the bladder (b) and vaginal vault (long arrow) below the pubococcygeal line, compatible with a cystocele and vaginal vault prolapse. A rectocele is also seen as an anterior bulge (arrowhead) in relation to the anal canal (asterisk). (Reproduced from ref. 40 with permission.)*

the same advantages, including identifying prolapse not noted on physical examination. One study showed that the surgical plan was altered in 41% of cases after MRI and fluoroscopy were employed.[41] Tunn et al. found that rectoceles and enteroceles were easily identifiable with MRI in patients with posthysterectomy vault prolapse.[42]

There is evidence that MRI is equivalent or superior to proctocystography if evacuation studies are performed during the MRI investigation; it also enables an upright assessment to be undertaken.[43,44] In addition, MRI defecography facilitates the diagnosis of anismus and intussusception. Another advantage is that the cervix and vaginal vault are often easier to see on MRI imaging than on fluoroscopy due to leakage of vaginal contrast in the latter. Fluoroscopy may not detect enteroceles in 20% of cases in which small portions of peritoneal fat enter the rectovaginal space.[44] However, due to greater soft tissue contrast with MRI, the various tissue components can be seen with relative clarity.

Disadvantages of MRI include:

- limited access to a vertical configuration magnet;
- increased relative cost to fluoroscopy;
- less physiologic modality than fluoroscopy if performed supine and without evacuation studies;
- lack of available MRI time due to demands from other specialties.

Ultrasonography

Transperineal ultrasound has been described in the assessment of dynamic function of the pelvic floor.[45] Dynamic anorectal endosonography has also been described and may detect the presence of enteroceles.[46] The role of these alternate modalities has not been fully elucidated and needs further study.

Anal manometry

Anal manometry measures rectal pressures by a transducer or balloon. Its measurement of rectal sensation evaluates the first feeling, urge, and discomfort; this information is used to distinguish causes of constipation. When an individual is able to tolerate increased volumes without signs of increased discomfort or the urge to defecate, overflow incontinence may occur. Careful consideration must be given to this evaluation process because individuals able to tolerate only small volumes in the rectum may have an irritable rectum, causing incontinence or urgency. Overflow incontinence and irritable bowel syndrome may mimic rectocele symptoms such as incontinence or incomplete emptying. If misdiagnosis of a rectocele is made, rectocele repair may exacerbate these disorders by causing a worsening of symptoms.[16,17,47]

Electromyography and nerve conduction studies

Electromyography (EMG) and nerve conduction studies also have been used to evaluate defecation disorders. Obstetric trauma denervates and causes atrophy of the pelvic floor muscles and tissue, which may lead to subsequent pelvic floor weakness. This denervation may be detected by EMG studies, and pudendal terminal motor latency can be used as a method to detect the causes of pelvic floor weakness.

Colonic transit studies

For colonic transit studies, the patient ingests radiopaque markers, which are measured and counted in the right colon, left colon, sigmoid colon, and rectum. Clinically slow transit time is defined as less than two bowel movements per week over several years. The utility of this test in individuals with rectoceles is debatable; some have normal transit times whereas others have prolonged times.[48] Patients whose symptoms did not improve after repair were found to have longer transit times preoperatively.[20]

MANAGEMENT

Once the clinical diagnosis has been made and (if necessary) confirmed by ancillary studies, the decision to operate or to treat conservatively must be made. Most non-surgical treatments consist of proper bowel training, following an active lifestyle, and eating an appropriate amount of dietary fibre.[49,50] These steps are most important when the main complaint is constipation.

The only non-surgical therapy available for prolapse symptoms is estrogen replacement therapy in postmenopausal women in the setting of vaginal atrophy, and the use of a vaginal pessary. In our experience, pessaries have not been very effective in women with isolated symptomatic rectoceles.

Indications for surgery should include being symptomatic, having an anatomic defect, or undergoing other pelvic reconstructive surgery with an asymptomatic rectocele.[9] Symptoms that respond well to surgery include pelvic pressure and a vaginal bulge, vaginal digitalization or splinting (which occurs in 20–75% of symptomatic patients) and outlet obstruction constipation. Janssen and van Dijke noted that repair increased rectal sensitivity, causing the urge to defecate earlier as a positive predictor of a good outcome.[47] In the colorectal literature it has been noted that defecography showing a rectocele ≥2 cm with symptoms is also a good indicator for surgery; however, this finding has not been conclusive in all studies.[2] Sullivan et al.[51] reported that anoscopic evidence of the rolling down of the anterior rectal wall will be present before surgical correction;[20] however, this may not be valid for all female patients.[47]

Signs and symptoms that are predictive of a poor surgical outcome include a history of use of potent laxatives, incidence of preoperative pain and (possibly) large rectoceles in women who had previously undergone hysterectomy.[20,21,47,52] A few studies in the colorectal literature have noted that hysterectomy disrupts parasympathetic nerves, causing decreased rectal sensation as well as increased rectal compliance, which may not be improved after anatomic correction.[47,52] The persistence or development of dyspareunia after rectocele repair has been variable and is dependent on the surgical technique: levator plication and overnarrowing of the introitus may lead to increased dyspareunia, whereas defect-specific repair has been associated with disappearance or improvement of dyspareunia.[26]

SURGICAL REPAIR

Indications for use of different approaches

Traditionally, the vaginal and transrectal approaches have been used by gynecologists and colorectal surgeons, respectively, as a result of training and familiarity with each technique. Colorectal surgeons tend to focus on improving symptoms of rectal emptying and constipation and thus advocate transanal surgery in patients with defecation disorders.

The transrectal approach is often used if perianal/rectal pathology such as hemorrhoids, anterior rectal wall prolapse, or rectal mucosal redundancy is surgically treated concurrently with the rectocele. A vaginal approach is advocated when:

- other genital prolapse (i.e. enterocele, perineocele, apical or anterior vaginal wall prolapse) is to be repaired, thus avoiding a second incision;
- compromised anal function exists (a transanal retractor may further compromise function);[53,54]
- an anal sphincteroplasty is also performed;
- a high rectocele exists (as the posterior fornix or vaginal apex is not reached through the transanal approach).[55]

Currently, there are no conclusive data to describe the proper indications for the use of graft material in posterior compartment repairs. Some authors advocate the use of mesh or graft in recurrent rectoceles, in patients with deficient rectovaginal fascia and weak tissue, in the presence of advanced prolapse, or with the coexistence of risk factors such as obesity and chronic constipation.[56]

Defect-specific rectocele repair

According to Richardson, rectoceles are caused by a variety of breaks in the fascia.[3] He described the most common break as being a transverse separation above the attachment to the perineal body, resulting in a low rectocele. Another common fascial break was considered to result from an obstetric tear or episiotomy that was incorrectly repaired. This midline vertical defect may involve the lower vagina and extend to the vaginal apex. Less common separations involving a lateral separation down one side of the fascia were also found to exist (Fig. 72.4). Richardson also stated that a U- or L-shaped tear in the fascia might occur. Since Richardson's observation, there has been an increased movement among gynecologists towards site-specific rectocele repair. Richardson recommended performing the repair with a finger in the rectum, so that defects can be easily identified and fascia can be appropriately approximated with interrupted sutures (Fig. 72.5).

Before starting any rectocele repair, the surgeon should approximate the introitus by using Allis clamps bilaterally to help determine how much perineal and vaginal tissue should be excised to correct a gaping introitus. The repaired opening should accommodate three fingerbreadths, taking into account that the levator ani and perineal muscles are relaxed from general anesthesia and may further constrict postoperatively and with postmenopausal atrophy. The next step is to place Allis clamps on the posterior perineum; a diamond-shaped perineal incision is made and the overlying skin is removed (Fig. 72.6). The length and width of the perineal incision are dependent on the epithelium needed for restoration of the perineal body. Mayo scissors are used to make a plane in the rectovaginal space. As much fascia is left on the rectum as possible. Sharp dissection is usually required over the perineal body because of previous scarring from episiotomies. The surgeon performs blunt and sharp dissection to the apex of the vagina. This is continued laterally to the tendinous arch of the levator ani and extends inferiorly to the perineal body.

If perineal lacerations are present, dissections are continued as follows. For grade 3 perineal lacerations, adequate exposure is needed to reapproximate the divided anal sphincter. In complete or grade 4 perineal lacerations, dissection continues to allow enough tissue exposure for the subsequent edge-to-edge anal mucosal suturing to be tension-free. Hemostasis is ensured and irrigation may be used to attain a clean operative field to allow inspection for defects. The rectovaginal fascia is inspected by the surgeon inserting a finger of the non-dominant hand into the rectum (Fig. 72.7). The rectal

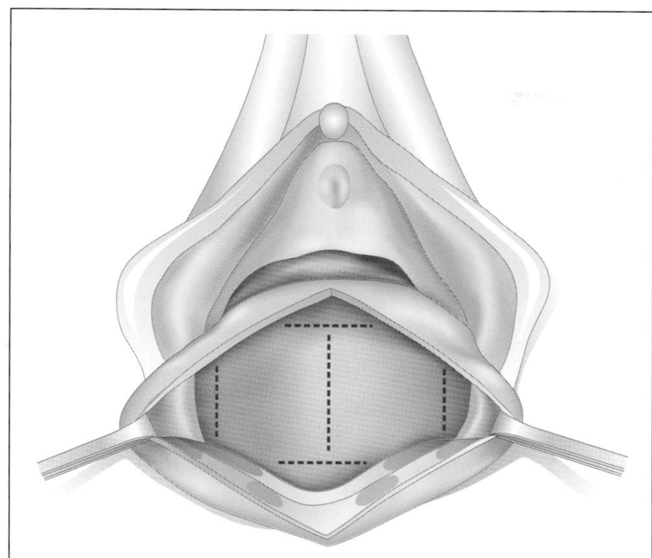

Figure 72.4. *Representation of the various locations where breaks in the rectovaginal septum have been observed in patients with rectocele, as seen through a colporrhaphy incision.*

wall is brought forwards, distinguishing the uncovered muscularis (fascial defect) from the muscularis covered by the smooth semi-transparent rectovaginal septum. According to the plane of dissection and the location of the defect, frequently the rectovaginal fascia must be mobilized off the lateral vaginal epithelium (Fig. 72.8). After the defect has been identified, Allis clamps are used to grasp the connective tissue (perirectal or rectovaginal fascia), which is pulled over the bare area to facilitate repair (Fig. 72.9). The rectal finger is then used to determine if a defect has been corrected. Next, this area is sewn together with interrupted sutures, plicating the fascia over the rectal wall with a No.v 2-0 delayed absorbable suture (Fig. 72.10). The surgeon must continuously examine the vaginal caliber to ensure a smooth contour and a diameter of three fingerbreadths.[3,4,6,57,58]

Whereas rectocele repair is accomplished for identification of the fascial defect and reapproximation of the connective tissue, evaluation of the levator hiatus is an entirely different issue. In women who have an enlarged levator hiatus, it may be appropriate to place another set of interrupted sutures horizontally to narrow the levator hiatus. This portion of the operation is not necessary in all patients and is independent of rectocele repair.

Perineorrhaphy is the next step in posterior segment reconstruction. The perineal body consists of the anal sphincter, the superficial and deep transverse perineal muscles, the bulbocavernosus muscles, and the junction of the rectovaginal fascia with the anal sphincter.

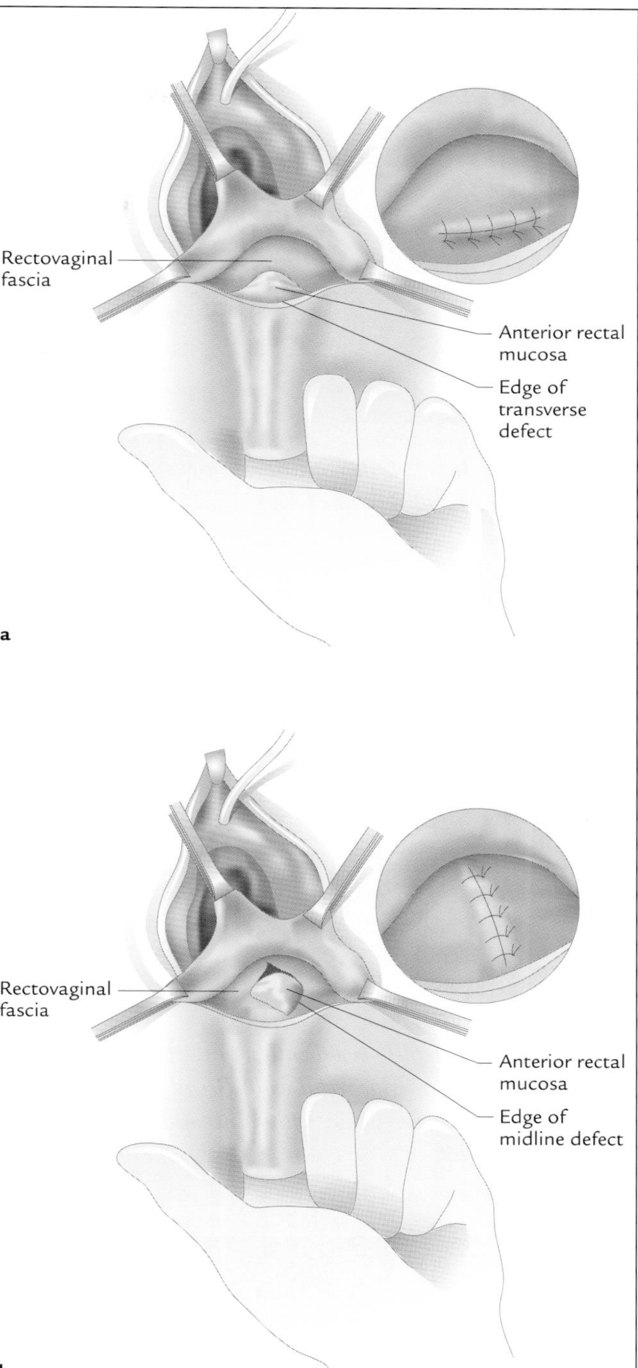

Figure 72.5. *Transverse and midline defects detected on rectal examination. Inset demonstrates a site-specific defect closed with interrupted suture.*

Perineorrhaphy implies identification and reconstruction of these components. The first step in perineorrhaphy is to remove any old scar tissue to the point that fresh viable tissue is revealed. If a grade 4 laceration is present, the rectal mucosa is completely mobilized off

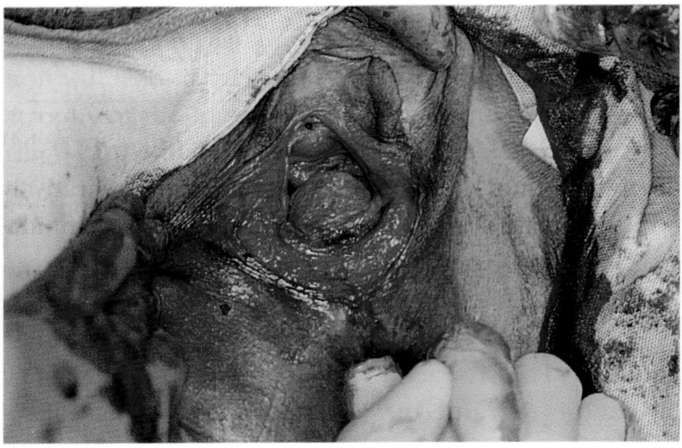

Figure 72.6. *Rectocele demonstrated on rectal examination. Note that the perineal skin has been excised.*

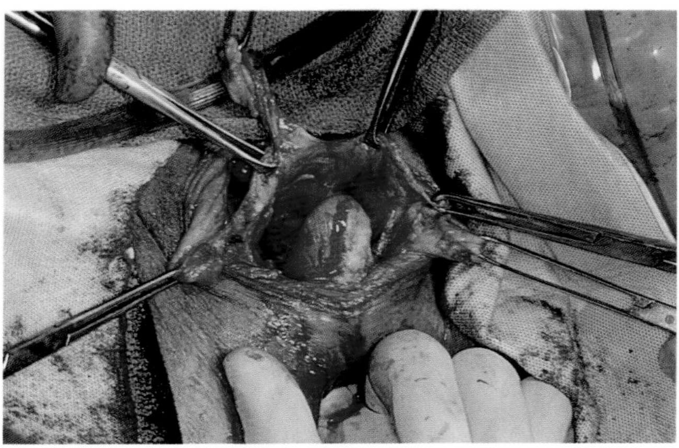

Figure 72.7. *Complete mobilization of the posterior vaginal wall from anterior rectal wall. Rectal examination demonstrates obvious rectocele, with minimal fascia on the anterior rectal wall.*

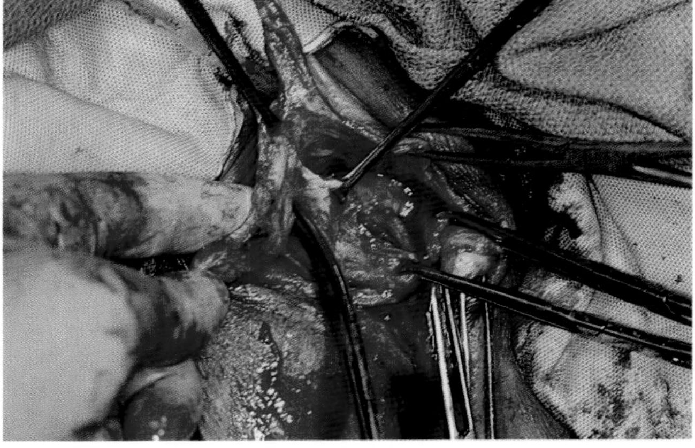

Figure 72.8. *The fascia is being mobilized off the vaginal epithelium.*

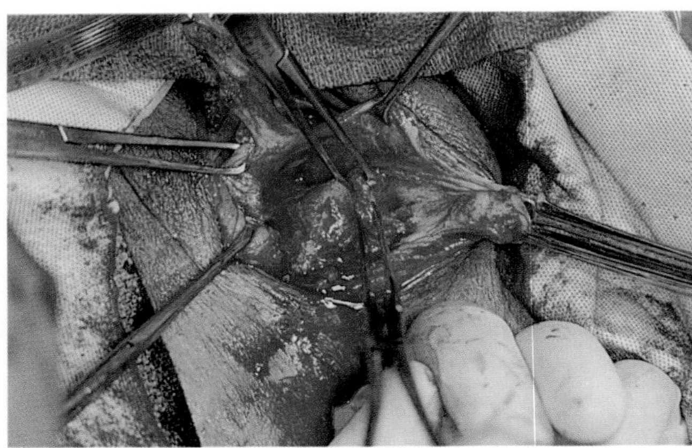

Figure 72.9. *Sufficient fascia has been mobilized to cover the defect.*

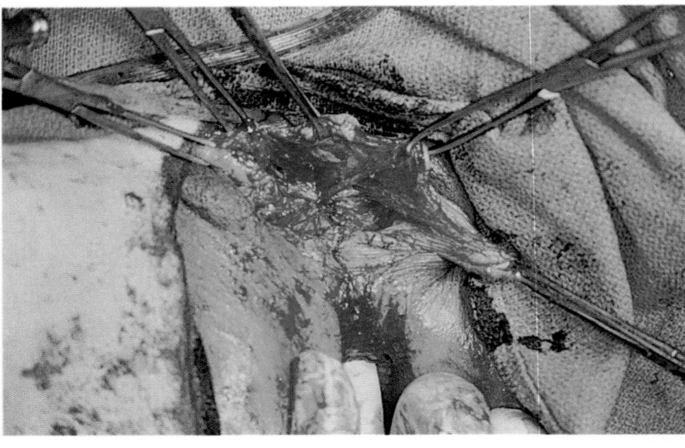

Figure 72.10. *The fascial edges have been sutured together and the defect closed.*

the vaginal wall and reapproximated with interrupted sutures. The external anal sphincter is then reapproximated. After stepwise reapproximation of the transverse perineal muscles, the perineal body is sewn over the sphincter. Finally, the bulbocavernosus muscle ends are attached to the perineal body. This musculofascial complex is covered by suturing the overlying vulvar skin with a No. 3-0 suture in a running fashion. Vaginal packing is removed on postoperative day 1 and diet is advanced as tolerated.[57,58]

Traditional transvaginal repair

The traditional rectocele approach has been described and illustrated by Nichols, Wheeless and others.[59,60] The opening of the vagina is as previously described, via a midline incision or by removal of a triangular wedge of vaginal wall. Some surgeons will place an initial row of No. 2-0 interrupted sutures approximating the rectovaginal fascia. The rectocele is then depressed in the midline with the surgeon's finger to reveal the margin of the puborectalis portion of the levator ani muscle. With the rectocele still depressed, a No. 1-0 absorbable suture is used to suture the margins of the levator ani muscles in an interrupted fashion. After all the sutures have been placed, they are tied.

The posterior vaginal mucosa is appropriately trimmed and closed with either interrupted or continuous 3-0 absorbable suture. The perineal body is repaired as previously described.

Transrectal approach

The transrectal approach was described by Sarles et al.[11] In this method, all patients are treated preoperatively with oral laxatives and are given antibiotics: metronidazole (500 mg twice daily for 2 days prior to surgery) and cefuroxime (250 mg intravenously 1 hour before surgery). The anus and vagina are cleansed with povidone-iodine. A Park retractor is inserted into the anal canal to expose the anterior rectal surface. An incision of the anterior rectal mucosa is made 1 cm above the dentate line. The submucosal plane is sharply dissected 8–10 cm from the anal verge. Bleeding is controlled by diathermy. Dissection is performed anteriorly and laterally; the resulting bare areas are plicated using interrupted polyglycolic acid 2-0 sutures 0.5 cm apart; the suture includes the rectal muscle and the rectovaginal septum. If the vaginal mucosa is perforated, the stitch is removed. A mucosal flap at least 6 cm long is excised. A second layer of polyglycolic acid sutures 3-0 close the mucosal defect. Postoperative care includes delaying food by mouth for 48 hours after surgery and slowly advancing the diet over several days.

Rectocele repair with mesh or graft

Graft materials have been employed in both the traditional posterior colporrhaphy and the defect-specific technique in an attempt to strengthen the repair. In the latter variation, a site-specific repair is first performed (see Figs 72.6–72.10). A dermal allograft is then attached to the rectovaginal and pubocervical fasciae proximally, levator ani muscles laterally, and perineal body distally with a series of interrupted permanent sutures.[56] The repair of a high rectocele can be challenging as there is commonly a deficiency of rectovaginal and pubocervical fasciae proximally. However, this repair can be facilitated by entry into an associated enterocele with attachment of the graft to the distal uterosacral ligaments (Fig. 72.11).

A transperineal approach has been described that starts with a transverse incision over the perineum. A plane of dissection is created between the vaginal epithelium and external anal sphincter and continues apically until the cul-de-sac peritoneum is encountered, but not entered. A strip of mesh or graft is incorporated into the upper region of the dissection over which the levator ani muscles are plicated.[61,62]

During an abdominal approach for vault prolapse and enterocele, the accompanying rectocele may be corrected. For a high posterior defect, the posterior graft of a sacral colpopexy may be extended down the posterior wall.[63,64] In the setting of additional perineal descent, a sacral colpoperineopexy may also be performed through an abdominal or combined abdominal/vaginal approach.[65] In the abdominal approach, the rectovaginal space is entered and a series of sutures are placed along the posterior vaginal wall from the apex to the perineal body which will secure the posterior arm of the colpopexy graft. In the combined approach, the graft is brought into

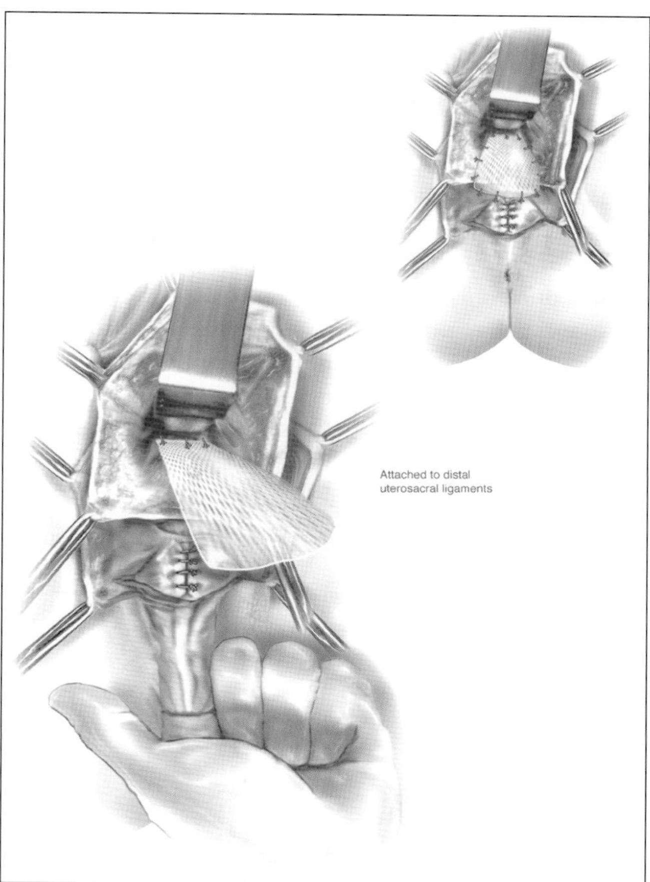

Figure 72.11. *Graft augmentation of rectocele repair.*

the vaginal field from the abdominal field (via the same posterior vaginal wall dissection used for a traditional or defect-specific repair) and sutured to the perineal body.

RESULTS AND COMPLICATIONS

Posterior colporrhaphy without or with levatorplasty

Anatomic cure rates after posterior colporrhaphy without or with levator plication range from 76 to 96% after a mean follow-up period of 12–42 months.[1,48,66–68] One study revealed an 88% cure rate for constipation in 24 patients that were prospectively followed and evaluated pre- and postoperatively with standardized questionnaires, defecography, colon transit studies, anorectal manometry, and electrophysiology.[1]

In comparison, two studies showed a modest improvement (less than 50%)[66] or an increase[50] in constipation rate (from 22 to 33% after a mean follow-up of 52 months). Reasons suggested for these observations include: 1) unselective approach used in offering surgical treatment for persistent constipation;[66] 2) retrospective analysis of the data;[1] and 3) the possibility that patients with a pathologic transit study might have a less favorable outcome with respect to constipation.[1,68] In addition, the study by Kahn and Stanton showed an increase in rates of incomplete bowel emptying and fecal incontinence (4% preoperatively versus 11% postoperatively) after posterior colpoperineorrhaphy.[50]

De novo dyspareunia rates after levatorplasty have been reported to range from 12.5 to 16%. Several studies suggest that this is due to pressure atrophy of the included muscle and the resulting scarring.[50,59] An additional study showed an increased rate of sexual dysfunction (18–27%) after levatorplasty.[50] A study by Weber et al. reported an even higher dyspareunia rate of 26% after posterior repair only (except for one patient who had a levator plication) and 38% after a posterior repair with Burch colposuspension.[67] The postoperative introital calibers in patients with or without dyspareunia were not different. The reasons for the unexpectedly high rate of dyspareunia in that study are unclear.

Defect-specific rectocele repair

The surgical outcomes after defect-specific rectocele repair are summarized in Table 72.2.[26,69–72] Anatomic cure rates range from 82 to 100% after a mean follow-up period of 3–18 months.

Improvements in constipation were seen in 43–84% of patients[26,69,70] with a de novo constipation rate of 3–4%;[26,70] however, Kenton et al. found that the rate of constipation was not statistically significantly different after 1 year of follow-up and attributed this to the predominantly medical etiology for the disorder. In addition, the lack of a standardized definition of constipation contributes to the difference in constipation rates seen in the literature after rectocele repair.[70] Improvements in the symptom of manual evacuation was noted in 36–63%,[26,69,70] with a de novo rate of 7% in one study.[26]

Most studies report some improvement in dyspareunia after site-specific repair (35–92%)[26,69–72] (see Table 72.2). The only study where site-specific rectocele repair was not combined with other prolapse or incontinence surgery followed 42 women for a period of 18 months. Improvement in sexual function was reported in 35% and there were no patients who developed de novo dyspareunia.[72] Other studies report a de novo dyspareunia rate of zero to 8%.[26,69–72]

Table 72.2. *Results of defect-specific rectocele repair*

Study	Cundiff et al.[26]	Porter et al.[69]	Kenton et al.[70]	Glavind & Madsen[71]	Singh et al.[72]
n	67	125	66	67	42
Mean follow-up (months)	12	6	12	3	18
Anatomic cure (%)	82	82	90	100	92
Improvement in vaginal protrusion (%)	–	73	90	–	88
Improvement in difficult defecation (%)	–	55	54	88	81
Improvement in constipation (%)	84	44	43	–	–
Improvement in manual evacuation (%)	63	65	36	–	–
Improvement in dyspareunia (%) de novo dyspareunia (%)	44/3	73/8	92/7	75/4	35/0

Transanal approach

The majority of studies are based on the experience of colorectal surgeons whose primary focus is defecatory dysfunction and anal incontinence. The results are summarized in Table 72.3.[10,20,21,47,51,53,73–76] Anatomic cure rates range from 70 to 98% after a 12- to 52-month follow-up. Reported rates of symptomatic improvement are 58–100% after the transrectal approach. De novo anal incontinence may be a concern, especially in those with occult sphincter lacerations, as a transanal retractor may further compromise function. One study reported a 38% rate of new-onset fecal incontinence after this approach.[66]

In a combined transvaginal/transanal approach, van Dam et al. found an anatomic cure rate of 72% in 89 women after a mean follow-up period of 52 months. Rates of constipation were 63% preoperatively and 33% postoperatively, while difficulty in evacuation decreased from 92% to 27%. However, rates of dyspareunia were found to be 28% preoperatively and 44% postoperatively which the authors attributed to the transvaginal portion of the operation.[54]

Studies comparing the transvaginal and transanal approaches have been mainly retrospective,[49,66,77,78] or prospective and non-randomized.[54] In a recent randomized controlled trial of 30 patients by Nieminen et al.,[79] 15 patients underwent transanal rectocele repair while the other 15 underwent vaginal posterior colporrhaphy. They excluded patients with other symptomatic prolapse or compromised anal sphincter function as evidenced by colon transit study. At 12 months follow-up, 14 (93%) patients in the vaginal group and 11 (73%) in the transanal group reported improvement in symptoms (p=0.08). The need to digitally assist rectal emptying decreased significantly in both groups, from 11 to 1 (73 to 7%) for the vaginal group and from 10 to 4 (66 to 27%) for the trans-

Table 72.3. ***Results of transanal rectocele repair***

Study	*n*	Mean follow-up (months)	Results	Complications
Sullivan et al.[51]	137	18	Anatomic cure 96% Difficult evacuation: 58% pre-op, 2% post-op Fecal incontinence: 39% pre-op, 3% post-op Dyspareunia 0%	1 RV fistula
Schapayak[73]	355		Anatomic cure 98% Constipation: 82% pre-op, 15% post-op	Infection 6% RV fistula 0.3%
Jansen & van Dijke[47]	64	12	Anatomic cure 70% Difficult evacuation: 72% pre-op, 16% post-op Fecal incontinence: 46% pre-op, 9% post-op Vaginal digitation: 26% pre-op, 4% post-op	None
Murthy et al.[21]	32	31	Constipation 84% improvement Vaginal bulge: 58% pre-op, 12% post-op	RV fistula 3%
Karlbom et al.[20]	34	10	Constipation 79% improvement	Bleeding 9%
Khubchandani et al.[10]	123	38	82% improvement Reoperation 10%	Wound dehiscence 2.4% RV fistula 0.8%
Rao et al.[74]	75		Vaginal bulge: 72% pre-op, 14% post-op	None
Ho et al.[53]	21	37	100% improvement ↓ mean resting and maximum squeeze anal pressures	None
Tjandra et al.[75]	59	19	Improved evacuation without anismus 93% Improved evacuation with anismus 38% Vaginal bulge: 88% pre-op, 13% post-op	Bleeding 1.7%
Ayabaca et al.[76]	49	48	Anatomic cure 90% Constipation: 83% pre-op, 32% post-op Fecal incontinence: 71% pre-op, 27% post-op	1 infection 1 pyogenic granuloma 4 dehiscence 1 anal fissure

post-op; postoperatively; pre-op, preoperatively; RV, rectovaginal.

anal group (p=0.17 between groups). Rectocele recurrence rates were 7% and 40%, respectively (p=0.04), and enterocele rates were zero and 27%, respectively (p=0.05). A 27% improvement rate in dyspareunia was noted; none of the patients developed de novo dyspareunia.[79]

Graft-augmented approach

The ideal mesh or graft (allograft or autograft) material used to augment repairs of pelvic fascial defects remains elusive. It should be inexpensive and improve recurrence rates, it should not be rejected, and should cause no detriment to sexual and bowel function.

Currently, there are few long-term data regarding the use of graft materials and mesh in the posterior segment. Results of graft augmentation are summarized in Table 72.4.[56,61,68,80–84] Anatomic cure rates range from 92 to 100% (12–30 month follow-up) with the transvaginal approach, and 89–95% (12–29 month follow-up) with the transperineal approach. De novo dyspareunia rates range from 3 to 20%. Several studies show an improvement in bowel function.[61,80,81]

In a prospective, controlled trial, Sand et al. randomly assigned 160 patients to undergo anterior and posterior colporrhaphy with (80 patients) or without (80 patients) polyglactin 910 mesh reinforcement. Preoperatively, 91 women had a rectocele to the mid-vaginal plane, 31 to the hymeneal ring, and 22 beyond the introitus. In the treatment group, a strip of mesh was incorporated into the imbricating endopelvic fascia during the midline plication. Thirteen recurrent rectoceles were noted at 1 year follow-up, with no differences observed between the two groups (10% versus 8%).[68]

The use of non-synthetic grafts may have a lower erosion rate, although this has yet to be confirmed in

Table 72.4. ***Results of graft augmentation in the posterior segment***

Study	*n*	Graft	Mean follow-up (months)	Results	Complications
Transvaginal					
Osler & Astrup[80]	15	Dermis, autologous	30	Anatomic cure 100% Difficult evacuation: 58% pre-op, 2% post-op Vaginal bulge: 80% pre-op, 0% post-op	1 infection 3 de novo dyspareunia
Sand et al.[68]	73	Polyglactin	12	Anatomic cure 92%	None
Goh & Dwyer[82]	43	Polypropylene	12	Anatomic cure 100%	1 RV fistula 3 erosions
Kohli & Miklos[56]	43	Dermis, cadaveric	12	Anatomic cure 93%	None
Dell & O'Kelley[83]	41	Dermis, porcine	12	Average Ap: 0.3 pre-op, −2.3 post-op Average Bp: 1.2 pre-op, −2.5 post-op 0% dyspareunia	6 vaginal dehiscence
Dwyer & O'Reilly[84]	50	Polypropylene	29	Anatomic cure 100% 0% erosion	1 RV fistula 1 de novo dyspareunia
Transperineal					
Watson et al.[61]	9	Polypropylene	29	Anatomic cure 89% Difficult evacuation: 100% pre-op, 12% post-op Vaginal bulge: 100% pre-op, 0% post-op	1 de novo dyspareunia
Mercer-Jones et al.[81]	22	14 polypropylene 8 polyvinyl	12	Anatomic cure 95% Constipation: 50% pre-op, 14% post-op Difficult evacuation: 95% pre-op, 32% post-op Vaginal bulge: 86% pre-op, 23% post-op	1 de novo dyspareunia

Ap/Bp, two points along the posterior vaginal wall; post-op; postoperatively; pre-op; preoperatively; RV, rectovaginal.

randomized controlled trials. In a recent retrospective review by Dwyer and O'Reilly, polypropylene mesh was used as an overlay for repair of large or recurrent anterior and posterior compartment prolapse. Forty-seven patients had mesh placed under the bladder base with lateral extensions onto the pelvic sidewall, 33 women had a Y-shaped mesh placed from the sacrospinous ligaments to the perineal body, and 17 women had mesh placement in both compartments. Of the erosions that occurred in nine women (9%), six lesions were in the posterior segment. One woman required surgical repair of a rectovaginal fistula.[84] In contrast, at 12 months of follow-up, Kohli and Miklos reported no complications (including erosion or fistula) in 43 women after placement of a cadaveric dermal graft.[56] At 1-year follow-up of 35 women, Dell and O'Reilly noted no erosions after the use of a porcine collagen mesh that contained fenestrations in the graft material. They also described 6/41 patients that experienced wound separation and delayed vaginal healing when they previously employed the non-fenestrated form of the same material. The authors suggested that the fenestrations allowed immediate contact between the vaginal mucosa and underlying host tissues, thus facilitating appropriate tissue ingrowth.[83]

CONCLUSIONS

The prevalence of surgical repair for urinary incontinence or genital prolapse has exceeded more than 10% of all women who reach the eighth decade of life.[85] With society's gradually aging population, there will be a large number of women suffering from rectoceles or defecation disorders.

A thorough pelvic assessment is necessary prior to any planning regarding surgical or non-surgical intervention for pelvic organ prolapse. Patient history will direct the physician to look for appropriate findings on physical examination. The use of pelvic floor imaging may complement the clinical assessment of the pelvic floor, but its use needs to be further studied and defined prior to advocating its routine use. Ultimately, the goal of the evaluation is to fully appreciate the extent of the posterior vaginal wall prolapse and to relate that to any visceral or sexual dysfunction that may coexist.

REFERENCES

1. Mellgren A, Anzen B, Nilsson BY et al. Results of rectocele repair. A prospective study. Dis Colon Rectum 1995;38(1):7–13.
2. Mollen RG, van Larrhoven CM, Kuijpers JC. Pathogenesis and management of rectoceles. Semin Colorectal Surg 1996;7:192–6.
3. Richardson AC. The rectovaginal septum revisited: its relationship to rectocele and its importance in rectocele repair. Clin Obstet Gynecol 1993;36(4):976–83.
4. Babiarz JW, Raz S. Pelvic floor relaxation. In: Raz S (ed) Female Urology, 2nd ed. Philadelphia: WB Saunders, 1996; 445–56.
5. Handa VL, Harris TA, Ostergard DR. Protecting the pelvic floor: obstetric management to prevent incontinence and pelvic organ prolapse. Obstet Gynecol 1996;88(3):470–8.
6. Walters MD. Pelvic floor prolapse: cystocele and rectocele. In: Walters MD, Karram MM (eds) Clinical Urogynecology. St Louis: Mosby-Year Book, 1993; 225–36.
7. Shorvon PJ, McHugh S, Diamant NE, Somers S, Stevenson GW. Defecography in normal volunteers: results and implications. Gut 1989;30(12):1737–49.
8. Nichols DH, Randall CL. Reduction of maternal injuries associated with childbirth. In: Nichols DH, Randall CL (eds) Vaginal Surgery, 4th ed. Baltimore: Lippincott, Williams and Wilkins, 1996; 43–57.
9. Brubaker L. Rectocele. Curr Opin Obstet Gynecol 1996;8(5):876–9.
10. Khubchandani IT, Clancy JP 3rd, Rosen L, Riether RD, Stasik JJ Jr. Endorectal repair of rectocele revisited. Br J Surg 1997;84(1):89–91.
11. Sarles JC, Arnaud A, Selezneff I, Olivier S. Endorectal repair of rectocele. Int J Colorectal Dis 1989;4(3):167–71.
12. Nichols DH, Randall CL. Types of prolapse. In: Nichols DH, Randall CL (eds) Vaginal Surgery, 4th ed. Baltimore: Lippincott Williams and Wilkins, 1996; 101–18.
13. Sultan AH. Anal incontinence after childbirth. Curr Opin Obstet Gynecol 1997;9(5):320–4.
14. Sultan AH, Stanton SL. Preserving the pelvic floor and perineum during childbirth – elective caesarean section? Br J Obstet Gynaecol 1996;103(8):731–4.
15. Benson JT. Vaginal approach to posterior vaginal defects: the perineal site. In: Baden W, Walker T (eds) Surgical Repair of Vaginal Defects. New York: Lippincott, 1992; 219–33.
16. Kahn MA, Stanton SL. Techniques of rectocele repair and their effects on bowel function. Int Urogynecol J Pelvic Floor Dysfunct 1998;9(1):37–47.
17. Johansson C, Nilsson BY, Holmstrom B, Dolk A, Mellgren A. Association between rectocele and paradoxical sphincter response. Dis Colon Rectum 1992;35(5):503–9.
18. Kelvin FM, Maglinte DD, Benson JT. Evacuation proctography (defecography): an aid to the investigation of pelvic floor disorders. Obstet Gynecol 1994;83(2):307–14.
19. Green JR, Soohoo SL. Factors associated with rectal injury

in spontaneous deliveries. Obstet Gynecol 1989;73(5 Pt 1):732–8.

20. Karlbom U, Graf W, Nilsson S, Pahlman L. Does surgical repair of a rectocele improve rectal emptying? Dis Colon Rectum 1996;39(11):1296–302.

21. Murthy VK, Orkin BA, Smith LE, Glassman LM. Excellent outcome using selective criteria for rectocele repair. Dis Colon Rectum 1996;39(4):374–8.

22. Jackson SL, Weber AM, Hull TL et al. Fecal incontinence in women with urinary incontinence and pelvic organ prolapse. Obstet Gynecol 1997;89:423–7.

23. Leigh RJ, Tumberg LA. Fecal incontinence: the unvoiced symptom. Lancet 1982;1:1349–51.

24. Thomas TM, Egan M, Walgrove A et al. The prevalence of fecal and double incontinence. Community Med 1984;6:216–20.

25. Bump RC, Mattiasson A, Bo K et al. The standardization of terminology of female pelvic organ prolapse and pelvic floor dysfunction. Am J Obstet Gynecol 1996;175:10–17.

26. Cundiff GW, Weidner AC, Visco AG et al. An anatomic and functional assessment of the discrete defect rectocele repair. Am J Obstet Gynecol 1998;179:1451–6.

27. Burrows LJ, Sewell C, Leffler KS et al. The accuracy of clinical evaluation of posterior vaginal wall defects. Int Urogynecol J Pelvic Floor Dysfunct 2003;14(3):160–3.

28. Maglinte DD, Kelvin FM, Hale DS et al. Dynamic cystoproctography: a unifying diagnostic approach to pelvic floor and anorectal dysfunction. Am J Roentgenol 1997;169(3):759–67.

29. Kelvin FM, Maglinte DD, Hale DS et al. Female pelvic organ prolapse: a comparison of triphasic dynamic MR imaging and triphasic fluoroscopic cystocolpoproctography. Am J Roentgenol 2000;174(1):81–8.

30. Yang A, Mostwin JL, Rosenshein NB et al. Pelvic floor descent in women: dynamic evaluation with fast MR imaging and cinematic display. Radiology 1991;179(1):25–33.

31. Kelvin FM, Maglinte DD, Hornback JA et al. Pelvic prolapse: assessment with evacuation proctography (defecography). Radiology 1992;184(2):547–51.

32. Altringer WE, Saclarides TJ, Dominguez JM et al. Four-contrast defecography: pelvic 'fluoroscopy'. Dis Colon Rectum 1995;38(7):695–9.

33. Halligan S. Commentary: imaging of anorectal function. Br J Radiol 1996;69(827):985–8.

34. Stoker J, Halligan S, Bartram CI. Pelvic floor imaging. Radiology 2001;218(3):621–41.

35. Kelvin FM, Maglinte DDT. Dynamic evaluation of female pelvic organ prolapse by extended proctography. Radiol Clin North Am 2003;41(2):395–407.

36. Bartram CI, Turnbull GK, Lennard-Jones JE. Evacuation proctography: an investigation of rectal expulsion in 20 subjects without defecatory disturbance. Gastrointest Radiol 1988;13(1):72–80.

37. van Dam JH, Ginai AZ, Gosselink MJ et al. Role of defecography in predicting clinical outcome of rectocele repair. Dis Colon Rectum 1997;40(2):201–7.

38. Halligan S, Bartram CI, Park HJ et al. Proctographic features of anismus. Radiology 1995;197(3):679–82.

39. Kelvin FM, Hale DS, Maglinte DD et al. Female pelvic organ prolapse: diagnostic contribution of dynamic cystoproctography and comparison with physical examination. Am J Roentgenol 1999;173(1):31–7.

40. Pannu HK. Dynamic MR imaging of female organ prolapse. Radiol Clin North Am 2003;41(2):409–23.

41. Kaufman HS, Buller JL, Thompson JR et al. Dynamic pelvic magnetic resonance imaging and cystocolpoproctography alter surgical management of pelvic floor disorders. Dis Colon Rectum 2001;44(11):1575–83.

42. Tunn R, Paris S, Taupitz M et al. MR imaging in posthysterectomy vaginal prolapse. Int Urogynecol J Pelvic Floor Dysfunct 2000;11(2):87–92.

43. Kelvin FM, Maglinte DD. Radiologic investigation of prolapse. J Pelv Surg 2000;6:218–20.

44. Lienemann A, Anthuber C, Baron A et al. Dynamic MR colpocystorectography assessing pelvic-floor descent. Eur Radiol 1997;7(8):1309–17.

45. Beer-Gabel M, Teshler M, Barzilai N et al. Dynamic transperineal ultrasound in the diagnosis of pelvic floor disorders: pilot study. Dis Colon Rectum 2002;45(2):239–45.

46. Karaus M, Neuhaus P, Wiedenmann TB. Diagnosis of enteroceles by dynamic anorectal endosonography. Dis Colon Rectum 2000;43(12):1683–8.

47. Janssen LW, van Dijke CF. Selection criteria for anterior rectal wall repair in symptomatic rectocele and anterior rectal wall prolapse. Dis Colon Rectum 1994;37(11):1100–7.

48. Pucciani F, Rottoli ML, Bologna A et al. Anterior rectocele and anorectal dysfunction. Int J Colorectal Dis 1996;11:1–9.

49. Infantino A, Masin A, Melega E et al. Does surgery resolve outlet obstruction from rectocele? Int J Colorectal Dis 1995;10(2):97–100.

50. Kahn MA, Stanton SL. Posterior colporrhaphy: its effects on bowel and sexual function. Br J Obstet Gynaecol 1997;104(1):82–6.

51. Sullivan ES, Leaverton GH, Hardwick CE. Transrectal perineal repair: an adjunct to improved function after anorectal surgery. Dis Colon Rectum 1968;11(2):106–14.

52. Smith AN, Varma JS, Binnie NR, Papachrysostomou M. Disordered colorectal motility in intractable constipation following hysterectomy. Br J Surg 1990;77(12):1361–5.

53. Ho YH, Ang M, Nyam D et al. Transanal approach to rec-

tocele repair may compromise anal sphincter pressures. Dis Colon Rectum 1998;41(3):354–8.

54. van Dam JH, Huisman WM, Hop WC et al. Fecal continence after rectocele repair: a prospective study. Int J Colorectal Dis 2000;15(1):54–7.
55. Goh JT, Tjandra JJ, Carey MP. How could management of rectoceles be optimized? Aust N Z J Surg 2002;72(12):896–901.
56. Kohli N, Miklos JR. Dermal graft-augmented rectocele repair. Int Urogynecol J Pelvic Floor Dysfunct 2003;14(2):146–9.
57. Baden W, Walker T. Evolution of the defect approach. In: Baden W, Walker T (eds) Surgical Repair of Vaginal Defects. New York: JB Lippincott, 1992; 1–7.
58. Baden W, Walker T. Vaginal approach to posterior vaginal defects: the rectal site. In: Baden W, Walker T (eds) Surgical Repair of Vaginal Defects. New York: JB Lippincott, 1992; 209–18.
59. Nichols DH, Randall CL. Posterior colporrhaphy and perineorrhaphy. In: Nichols DH, Randall CL (eds) Vaginal Surgery, 4th ed. Baltimore: Lippincott Williams and Wilkins, 1996; 257–89.
60. Wheeless CR. Posterior repair. In: Wheeless CR (ed) Atlas of Pelvic Surgery, 3rd ed. Baltimore: Williams and Wilkins, 1997; 46–9.
61. Watson SJ, Loder PB, Halligan S et al. Transperineal repair of symptomatic rectocele with Marlex mesh: a clinical, physiological and radiologic assessment of treatment. J Am Coll Surg 1996;183(3):257–61.
62. Parker MC, Phillips RK. Repair of rectocele using Marlex mesh. Ann R Coll Surg Engl 1993;75(3):193–4.
63. Addison WA, Cundiff GW, Bump RC, Harris RL. Sacral colpopexy is the preferred treatment for vaginal vault prolapse. J Gynecol Tech 1996;2:69–74.
64. Lyons TL, Winer WK. Laparoscopic rectocele repair using polyglactin mesh. J Am Assoc Gynecol Laparosc 1997;4(3):381–4.
65. Cundiff GW, Harris RL, Coates K et al. Abdominal sacral colpoperineopexy: a new approach for correction of posterior compartment defects and perineal descent associated with vaginal vault prolapse. Am J Obstet Gynecol 1997;177(6):1345–53.
66. Arnold MW, Stewart WR, Aguilar PS. Rectocele repair. Four years' experience. Dis Colon Rectum 1990;33(8):684–7.
67. Weber AM, Walters MD, Piedmonte MR. Sexual function and vaginal anatomy in women before and after surgery for pelvic organ prolapse and urinary incontinence. Am J Obstet Gynecol 2000;182(6):1610–15.
68. Sand PK, Koduri S, Lobel RW et al. Prospective randomized trial of polyglactin 910 mesh to prevent recurrence of cystoceles and rectoceles. Am J Obstet Gynecol 2001;184:1357–62.
69. Porter WE, Steele A, Walsh P et al. The anatomic and functional outcomes of defect-specific rectocele repairs. Am J Obstet Gynecol 1999;181(6):1353–8.
70. Kenton K, Shott S, Brubaker L. Outcome after rectovaginal fascia reattachment for rectocele repair. Am J Obstet Gynecol 1999;181(6):1360–3.
71. Glavind K, Madsen H. A prospective study of the discrete fascial defect rectocele repair. Acta Obstet Gynecol Scand 2000;79(2):145–7.
72. Singh K, Cortes E, Reid WM. Evaluation of the fascial technique for surgical repair of isolated posterior vaginal wall prolapse. Obstet Gynecol 2003;101(2):320–4.
73. Schapayak S. Transrectal repair of rectocele: an extended armamentarium of colorectal surgeons. A report of 355 cases. Dis Colon Rectum 1985;28(6):422–33.
74. Rao GN, Carr ND, Beynon J et al. Endorectal repair of rectocoele revisited. Br J Surg 1997;84(7):1034.
75. Tjandra JJ, Ooi BS, Tang CL et al. Transanal repair of rectocele corrects obstructed defecation if it is not associated with anismus. Dis Colon Rectum 1999;42(12):1544–50.
76. Ayabaca SM, Zbar AP, Pescatori M. Anal continence after rectocele repair. Dis Colon Rectum 2002;45(1):63–9.
77. Van Laarhoven CJ, Kamm MA, Bartram CI et al. Relationship between anatomic and symptomatic long-term results after rectocele repair for impaired defecation. Dis Colon Rectum 1999;42(2):204–10.
78. Marti MC, Roche B, Déléaval J. Rectoceles: value of videodefaecography in selection of treatment policy. Colorectal Dis 1999;1:324–9.
79. Nieminen K, Hiltunen KM, Laitinen J et al. Transanal or vaginal approach to rectocele repair: a prospective, randomized pilot study. Dis Colon Rectum 2004;47(10):1636–42.
80. Oster S, Astrup A. A new vaginal operation for recurrent and large rectocele using dermis transplant. Acta Obstet Gynecol Scand 1981;60(5):493–5.
81. Mercer-Jones MA, Sprowson A, Varma JS. Outcome after transperineal mesh repair of rectocele: a case series. Dis Colon Rectum 2004;47(6):864–8.
82. Goh JW, Dwyer PL. Effectiveness and safety of polypropylene mesh in vaginal prolapse surgery. Int Urogynecol J 2001;12:S90.
83. Dell JR, O'Kelley KR. PelviSoft BioMesh augmentation of rectocele repair: the initial clinical experience in 35 patients. Int Urogynecol J Pelvic Floor Dysfunct 2005;16(1):44–7; discussion 47.
84. Dwyer PL, O'Reilly BA. Transvaginal repair of anterior and posterior compartment prolapse with Atrium polypropylene mesh. BJOG 2004;111(8):831–6.
85. Olsen AL, Smith VJ, Bergstrom JO et al. Epidemiology of surgically managed pelvic organ prolapse and urinary incontinence. Obstet Gynecol 1997;89(4):501–6.

73

Vaginal approach to fixation of the vaginal apex

May Alarab, Harold P Drutz

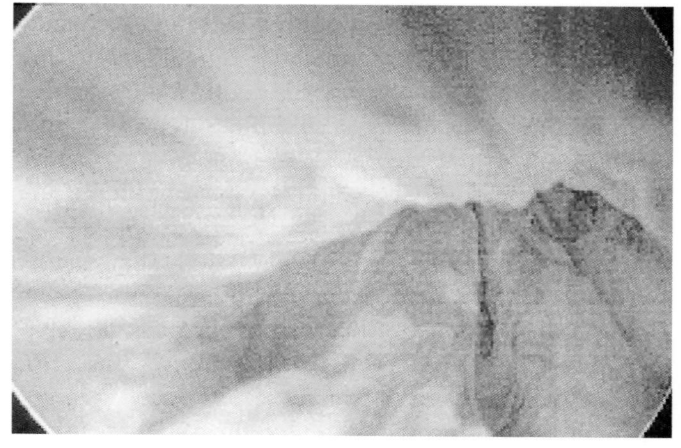

INTRODUCTION

Caring for women with pelvic floor disorders has become an increasingly important component of women's health care. Pelvic organ prolapse is a major health issue for women; it affects almost half of all women over 50 years of age, with a lifetime prevalence of 30–50%.[1] A 1997 study found that women with normal life expectancy will, by the age of 79 years, have an 11–12% chance of undergoing at least one operation for prolapse or incontinence, with a reoperation rate of 29%.[2] With the current generation of women maintaining a more active lifestyle into an older age, it is likely that an increasing number of women will seek treatment for prolapse – a condition requiring increasing expertise on the part of the urogynecologist and pelvic reconstructive surgeon. It has been projected that over the next 30 years, the rate of women seeking care for pelvic floor disorders will double.[3]

Conservative management of pelvic organ prolapse using vaginal pessaries is a known and effective method of treating this problem; however, patients are increasingly inclined towards more permanent solutions to correct their symptoms while maintaining body image and coital function. Numerous surgical operations have been described for the support of the vaginal apex at the time of hysterectomy or for posthysterectomy vault prolapse, and are performed either abdominally or vaginally. In this chapter we will describe the different vaginal approaches for fixation of the vaginal apex.

HISTORY

Genital prolapse in antiquity finds its roots in the Ebers Papyrus (1500 BC).[4]

Soranus of Ephesus (AD 98–138) is commonly considered the foremost gynecologic authority of antiquity. He proposed vaginal hysterectomy for uterine prolapse in AD 120.[5] The vaginal reconstructive approach was first described by Zweifel in 1892[6] and involved suspension of the prolapsed vagina to the sacrotuberous ligament. In 1909, White suspended the vaginal vault to the tendinous arch of the obturator fascia via a transvaginal approach.[7] A transvaginal technique suspending the vaginal vault to the sacrouterine ligaments just below the sacral promontory was reported by Miller in 1927.[8] In 1951, Amreich described a trasgluteal, and later a transvaginal, approach to attach an everted vagina to the sacrotuberous ligament.[9] Sederl first tried the use of the sacrospinous ligament for this purpose in 1958.[10] Richter introduced the sacrotuberous fixation in Europe in 1967, and one year later described the use of the sacrospinous ligament as an improved technique for the suspension of the vaginal vault.[11] This procedure was introduced in the United States by Randall and Nichols in 1971,[12] and has been increasingly popular since then. Cruikshank and Cox have described the use of sacrospinous ligament fixation as an adjuvant to vaginal hysterectomy and colporrhaphy for marked uterovaginal prolapse in the presence of poor integrity of the endopelvic fascia.[13]

ANATOMIC CONSIDERATION

The normal support of the pelvic floor is based on three mechanical principles:

1. the uterus and vagina are attached to the walls of the pelvis by the endopelvic fascia that suspends the organs from the pelvic sidewalls;
2. the levator ani muscle constrict the lumens of these organs until they are closed, forming an occlusive layer on which the pelvic organs may rest;[14]
3. the flap valve, where the vagina is suspended in such a way that it rests against the supporting wall adjacent to it, controls increases in pressure which force the vagina against the wall, pinning it in place.[15]

The part of the pelvic fascia that attaches the uterus to the pelvic walls (i.e. the broad, cardinal, and uterosacral ligaments) is called the parametrium; similar tissue attaching the vagina to the pelvic walls is called the paracolpium. Unlike other ligaments in the body that are made of dense connective tissue, these ligaments contain blood vessels, nerves, and fibrous connective tissue (smooth muscle, collagen, and elastin), a composition that reflects their function as neurovascular and supportive structures. The paracolpium is attached to the upper two-thirds of the vagina, and consists of two portions: Level I (suspension, Fig. 73.1) consist of a relatively long sheet of tissue that converges from its broad origin on the lateral pelvic walls and sacrum to its attachment to the lateral walls of the vagina. Defective suspension at this level presents clinically as uterine or vaginal vault prolapse. At Level II (attachment) the mid-portion of the vagina is attached laterally and more directly to the pelvic walls, and stretches the vagina transversely between the bladder and the rectum. This part includes the pubocervical fascia anteriorly and the rectovaginal fascia posteriorly. At this level the vagina comes closer to the pelvic wall, and failure of level II support presents as cystocele or rectocele, or both. In the distal part of the vaginal wall (Level III: fusion) that extends from the introitus 2–3 cm above the hymeneal ring, the vagina is fused laterally to the levator ani muscle, posteriorly to the perineal body, and anteriorly it blends with the

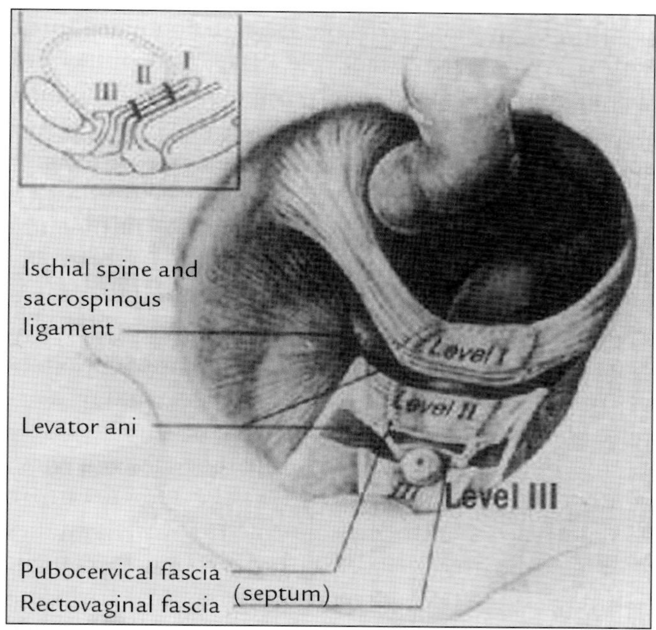

Figure 73.1. *At level I, paracolpium suspends the vagina from the lateral pelvic walls. Fibers of level I extend both vertically and posterior towards the sacrum. At level II, the vagina is attached to the arcus tendineus fasciae pelvis and superior fascia of the levator ani muscles. At level III, the vagina is fused to the medial surface of the levator ani muscles, urethra, and perineal body. (Reproduced from ref. 16 with permission from Elsevier.)*

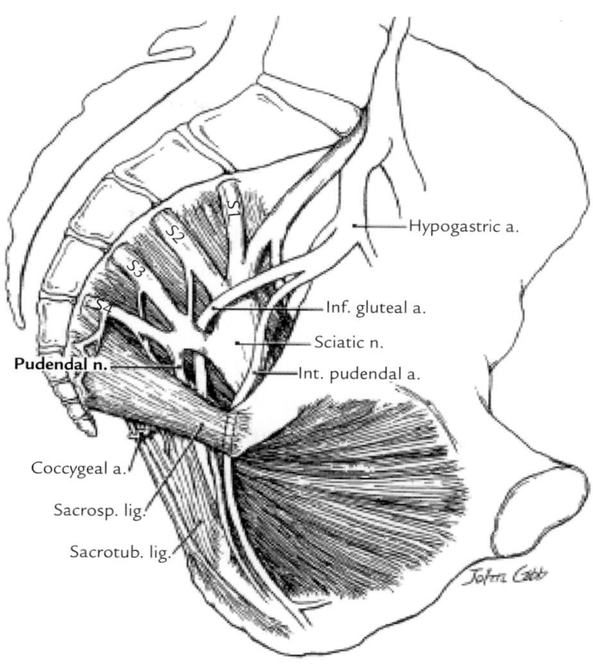

Figure 73.2. *Left hemipelvis. The sacrospinous ligament covered by the coccygeus muscle extends from the ischial spine to the sacrum. The pudendal neurovascular structures pass beneath the sacrospinous ligament at the ischial spine. The inferior gluteal artery passes between the sciatic nerve and the sacrospinous ligament. (Reproduced from ref. 20 with permission.)*

urethra and is embedded in the connective tissue of the perineal membrane, with no intervening paracolpium. The attachments at this level are so dense that the vagina is left with no mobility, and displacement of the levator ani muscle, perineal body or the urethra will carry the vagina along with it.[16]

SURGICAL ANATOMY

Pelvic fascia and ligaments have been used to suspend the prolapsed vagina; however, it should be borne in mind that the nerves and vessels surrounding these anchoring structures are susceptible to injury during surgical repair. In order to reduce hemorrhage and postoperative pain secondary to colpopexy operations, it is essential to understand the anatomic relations of the pelvic organs and their adjacent neurovascular structures.

The pararectal space is filled with fat and loose areolar tissue, and the middle rectal artery and the nerve of the levator ani muscle course through this space.[17] The sacrospinous ligament, located within the substance of the coccygeal muscle,[18] extends from the lateral sacrum to the ischial spine (Fig. 73.2). The average length of the sacrospinous ligament is 43.04±6.58 mm;[19] it divides the sciatic notch into the greater and lesser sciatic foramina. The inferior gluteal artery, after originating from the internal iliac artery, descends inferolaterally, passing through the greater sciatic foramen and leaves the pelvis by crossing the upper border of the sacrospinous ligament 8.54 mm from the ischial spine, accompanied by the inferior gluteal vein. After emerging from the sacral plexus, the inferior gluteal nerve passes close to the vessels and leaves the infrapiriform foramen by crossing the upper border of the sacrospinous ligament 13.82 mm from the ischial spine. Leaving the pelvis, the inferior gluteal complex crosses the sciatic nerve posteriorly, and branches inside the gluteus maximus muscle. The internal pudendal artery, after originating from the internal iliac artery (the anterior branch) and accompanied by the internal pudendal vein, reaches the upper border of the ligament and leaves the infrapiriform foramen accompanied by the pudendal nerve. The pudendal complex lies a maximum of 5.5 mm medial to the spine. The sciatic nerve is the most lateral of the structures emerging from the infrapiriform foramen, situated on average 25.14±3.94 mm lateral to the ischial spine.[19] The coccygeal branch of the inferior gluteal artery passes immediately behind the mid-portion of the sacrospinous ligament and pierces the sacrotuberous ligament at multiple sites.

During the procedure of sacrospinous vault suspension, placing the sutures immediately medial and inferior to the ischial spine may cause injury to the pudendal vessels. However, placing the sutures superior to the mid-portion of the ligament may cause injury to the inferior gluteal artery. The coccygeal branches of the inferior gluteal artery may be injured if any deep suture traverses the full thickness of the ligament. Thompson et al. have shown that, by placing the sutures through the sacrospinous ligament 2.5 cm or more medially from the ischial spine along the superior border of the ligament and not through the full thickness, the risk of complications is minimal.[20]

ETIOLOGY AND PATHOPHYSIOLOGY

The opening in the levator ani muscle, through which the vagina and urethra pass, is called the urogenital hiatus of the levator ani (through which prolapse occurs). Although the rectum also passes through the opening, it is not included in the hiatus because the levator ani muscle attaches directly to the anus and the external anal sphincter. The hiatus is surrounded by the pubic bones anteriorly, the levator ani muscle laterally, and the perineal body and the external anal sphincter posteriorly. The levator ani muscle is always contracting, keeping the urogenital hiatus closed. It closes the vagina, urethra, and rectum by compressing them against the pubic bone, thus preventing any opening in the pelvic floor through which prolapse may occur. As long as the levator ani muscle functions normally, the pelvic floor is closed; the ligaments and fascia are under no tension. When the muscles relax or are damaged, the pelvic floor opens and the pelvic organs lie between the high abdominal pressure and the low atmospheric pressure; here the organs must be held in place by the ligaments, which can sustain the load for only a short period of time and eventually become damaged and fail to hold the vagina in place. This failure is due not only to acute damage, but also from the inability of the ligaments to self-repair. The injury to the connective tissue in the pelvis is due to rupture rather than stretching.[21]

Neuromuscular injuries to the pelvic floor are associated with the development of pelvic organ prolapse (POP).[22] The health and function of the pelvic muscles provide significant protection to the ligaments to avoid POP. The neuromuscular damage to the pelvic floor that occurs during parturition plays a major role in the etiology of prolapse; however, the loads on the pelvic floor resulting from increases in abdominal pressure also play a significant role in the development of this disorder – for example, continuous heavy lifting, chronic obstructive pulmonary disease, obesity, chronic constipation, large fibroids or tumors. Direct damage to the muscle may result from previous pelvic surgery, spinal cord conditions and injury, thinning of the muscle and fascia that occurs with postmenopausal atrophy and attenuation, and finally the collagen status of these groups of patients. It has been shown that women with Marfan or Ehlers–Danlos syndrome have high rates of urinary incontinence and POP. This finding supports the hypothesized etiologic role of connective tissue disorders as a factor in the pathogenesis of these conditions.[23]

These facts have been confirmed by recent studies showing decreased collagen and smooth muscle content in women with POP, with or without stress urinary incontinence (SUI), regardless of age, parity, body mass index or smoking,[24] and increased collagen breakdown in the SUI and POP groups compared to controls.[25]

SYMPTOMS, PRESENTATION AND EVALUATION

Patients with vaginal apical prolapse can vary from being asymptomatic to presenting with various complaints of vaginal pressure, feeling something coming down, coital difficulties, urinary symptoms (urgency, frequency, incontinence or voiding dysfunction), and bowel emptying difficulties due to concomitant anterior and posterior vaginal wall defects. Burrows et al. investigated the correlation of symptoms with the severity of POP, and concluded that the more advanced the prolapse, the less likely the woman would have SUI, and the more likely to manually reduce prolapse to void; however, prolapse severity was not associated with sexual or bowel symptoms.[26] Another study correlating symptoms in women with or without enterocele showed that women with enterocele were more likely to be older, postmenopausal, to have had posthysterectomy or vaginal prolapse repairs, and to have more advanced apical and posterior vaginal prolapse than women without enterocele, but not to differ from them in bowel function.[27]

A patient may present to a gynecologist, a urologist or a colorectal surgeon depending on their major complaint. A detailed history is taken, including a history of the chief complaint, urinary and bowel symptoms, obstetric and medical history, and current medication. A careful speculum and digital examination at rest and with straining is performed to quantify POP and SUI. By placing the Sim's speculum along the posterior vaginal wall and asking the patient to bear down, we look for anterior compartment prolapse; the opposite is done to examine the posterior vaginal wall. A digital rectal–vaginal examination while the patient is straining is performed to differentiate between a high rectocele and an enterocele.

There are numerous grading systems for prolapse.[28–31] The pelvic organ prolapse quantification (POPQ) system[31] produced by the International Continence Society has gained popularity among urogynecologists to describe, measure, and stage prolapse. Careful vaginal examination is vital to identify the site-specific vaginal wall prolapse present, and to identify patients at risk of developing SUI after their reconstructive surgery. SUI has been strongly associated with POP,[32,33] and it has been shown that mild to moderate POP is often associated with SUI; however, women with severe POP rarely complain of urine leakage because of urethral kinking and increased urethral resistance with the urogenital prolapse in an unreduced state.[34–36] In fact, these patients may complain of difficulty in voiding, with an elevated post-void residual volume and recurrent urinary tract infections.[37] Liang et al. showed a 65.8% incidence of trabeculation in preoperative urethrocystoscopic evaluation in patients with marked prolapse; this can be attributed to the obstruction caused by the large prolape.[38]

The leakage problem manifests after correction of the prolapse in what is called occult or latent SUI, one of the common problems seen with complex vault prolapse.[39] The incidence of occult SUI can vary from 22 to 80%, and can be quite distressing.[40,41] Investigating abdominal leak point pressures (ALPPs) in patients with vaginal vault prolapse, Gallentine and Cespedes have shown a 50% incidence of occult SUI, with a mean decrease in ALPP of 59 cmH_2O after prolapse reduction, a drop that is more marked than in patients with cystocele alone.[42]

Traditionally, the prolapse is reduced by inserting a pessary, and a recent study confirmed that continent patients suffering from severe POP, but with a positive pessary test and who did not undergo a concomitant SUI procedure, had a 64.7% risk of urinary leakage after their prolapse surgery.[38] However, Bump et al., in an extensive study, showed that there was a high false-positive rate of incontinence with barrier testing.[43] If occult incontinence is not demonstrated, a concomitant incontinence procedure, with its associated morbidity, may be safely omitted.[35]

Investigations which may be required prior to any prolapse repair include accurate preoperative urodynamic studies (with the prolapse reduced to examine the expected outcome after repair), cystourethroscopy, and abdominal–pelvic ultrasound. In addition, transanal studies may be required if there is a history of fecal incontinence. Other tests include defecography, anorectal motility studies, pudendal motor nerve latency studies, and magnetic resonance imaging of the pelvic floor.

SURGICAL TECHNIQUES IN SUPPORTING THE VAGINAL APEX (VAGINAL APPROACH)

The vaginal approach to prolapse surgery carries significant low postoperative morbidity, and does not require additional skill or the cost of laparoscopy. It provides the option to perform the operation under regional or general anesthesia, and the ability to repair other pelvic defects simultaneously. Various techniques have been described for the treatment of vault prolapse: these include sacrospinous vault suspension, iliococcygeus muscle fixation, uterosacral ligament fixation, McCall culdoplasty, and posterior intravaginal slingoplasty. The different techniques of restoration of the vaginal apical defect are outlined as follows.

Sacrospinous vault suspension

Indications

The main indication for sacrospinous ligament suspension is to correct total procidentia, or posthysterectomy vaginal vault prolapse with an associated weak cardinal uterosacral ligament complex, and in posthysterectomy enterocele.[44,45] Bilateral sacrospinous ligament fixation has been described and recommended in patients with recurrent vault prolapse,[46,47] or a desire to maintain a wide vaginal vault.[48] The procedure has also been described as a prophylactic step at the time of vaginal hysterectomy against subsequent vaginal vault prolapse,[13,49] as well as in patients with marked prolapse who wish to retain their uterus.[50–52]

Contraindications

A short vagina, mainly attributed to previous repeated repairs, is considered the principal contraindication to performing sacrospinous colpopexy; the surgeon needs to ensure that there is an adequate vaginal depth to allow the attachment of the vault to the ligament without any tension. Surgical inexperience is another contraindication, and the procedure should only be performed by experienced reconstructive pelvic surgeons.

Surgical techniques

Postmenopausal patients with vaginal atrophy usually benefit from preoperative local hormone treatment to improve the quality of the tissues, and to help improve the vascularity of the operative site. Preoperative intravenous prophylactic antibiotics as well as measures for prophylaxis against venous thromboembolism (compression stockings and low dose subcutaneous heparin) are recommended. After the patient receives the appropriate anesthesia, bearing in mind the feasibility of regional anaesthesia with the vaginal approach, the surgery is performed with the patient in the dorsal lithotomy position. An intraoperative assessment allows the surgeon to identify the extent of the prolapse, and to confirm that the vault can reach the ligament without tension.

In a marked uterovaginal prolapse, a vaginal hysterectomy is performed initially in the usual fashion; if a cystocele is present, this is dealt with next, usually with standard suburethral buttressing sutures.[16,53] Some authors have suggested the addition of polyglactin mesh as an extra support to the anterior vaginal wall; however, a randomized trial by Weber et al. showed that this technique did not improve the cure rate compared to standard anterior colporrhaphy.[54] Sand et al., in a similar caliber study, found the addition of mesh to be useful in the prevention of recurrent cystocele.[55] Flood et al. have shown that reinforcing anterior colporrhaphy with Marlex mesh is highly effective in preventing recurrence of cystocele with minimal complications.[56]

When an enterocele is identified – usually noted as a distinct loss of the rectovaginal fascia with a sudden protrusion of the enterocele sac – it is demarcated by the pubocervical fascia anteriorly and the rectovaginal septum posteriorly. The sac is dissected free, opened, and a high ligation performed with a 2-0 type permanent purse-string suture.[57]

Sacrospinous ligament suspension is usually performed via the posterior approach. It starts with a longitudinal incision in the posterior vaginal wall after infiltration with a dilute solution of epinephrine (1:200,000). The incision extends from the introitus to the vault, and the epithelium is dissected laterally on both sides, penetrating the right rectal pillar into the pararectal space near the ischial spine. The right ischial spine is palpated and, using a combination of sharp and blunt dissection, a window is created between the ligament and the rectovaginal space. It is important to split the fascia in front of the ligament that is palpated as a cord-like structure to ensure that the suture placement will involve the body of the ligament. The rectum is mobilized medially with the fingers and, with one retractor protecting the rectum medially, the Miya hook ligature carrier[58] (Fig. 73.3a) – loaded with two delayed absorbable sutures and held in the right hand of the surgeon with the tip protected by the surgeon's left index finger – is introduced into the vagina while an assistant retracts the rectum to the left with a Heaney retractor. The sutures are placed into the ligament at two fingerbreadths medial to the spine and just inferior to the superior border of the ligament, thus avoiding injury to the pudendal complex. Care must be taken not to penetrate the full thickness of the ligament to avoid injury to the inferior gluteal vessels and nerve. At the required location at the ligament, the hook is closed and the handle of the hook is lifted upwards, bringing the tip out of the ligament. A notched vaginal speculum is placed just below the tip of the hook (Fig. 73.3b) and the sutures retrieved with a nerve hook. Threading two sutures at the same time avoids the need to repeat the insertion. The two sutures are paired, loaded separately onto a Mayo needle, and passed through the angles of the vaginal epithelium at the level of the vault, 1–2 cm apart, and held for later tying.[59] If bilateral suspension is to be performed, one suture will be placed per site.[60]

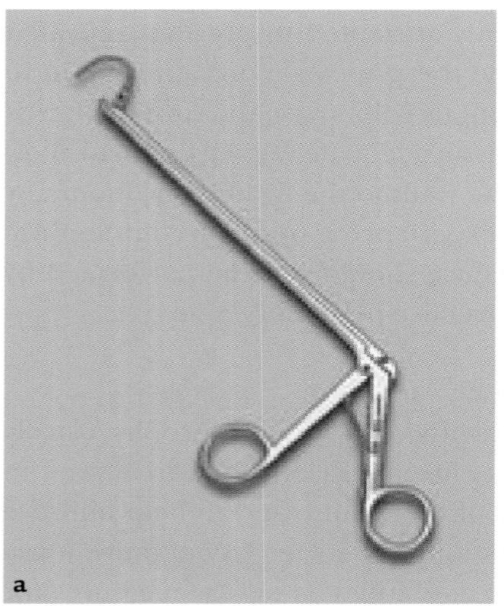

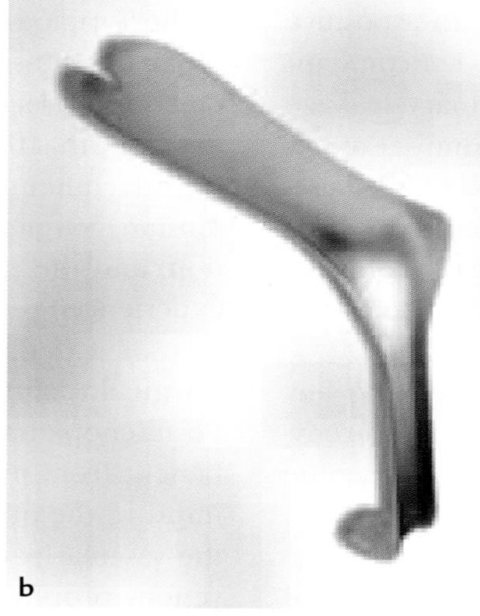

Figure 73.3. *(a) Miya hook; (b) notched speculum.*

The anterior rectocele and the rectovaginal septum are repaired by interrupted absorbable sutures (Vicryl 2-0). The levator muscles are approximated separately with Vicryl No. 1 suture, but left untied at this stage; the ends are held. The bulbocavernosus muscle is approximated and held, and the vaginal skin is closed with a continuous locking suture until the level of the introitus. The sacrospinous sutures are tied, pulling the vault onto the ligament, ensuring a close approximation and avoiding the suture bridge between the vault and the ligament. Finally, the levator and bulbocavernousus muscle sutures are tied, and the vaginal skin is closed. A slight deviation of the vaginal apex to the right may be noted at the end of the procedure; this may be of benefit as the vault will no longer be subjected to intra-abdominal pressure after the operation.[45] At the end of surgery, the bladder is drained transurethrally; a vaginal pack and hemovac drain are inserted if necessary in the reconstructed vagina, both to be removed in 24 hours.

The earlier description of the procedure involves exposure of the ligament and placement of the sutures under direct vision.[45,61] The ligament is grasped with an Allis forceps and a Deschamps ligature carrier is used to place the suture into the ligament; this technique requires more dissection in the pararectal space.[61] Another modification is the Sharp technique, which uses the shut suture punch system.[62] With its automatic suture retrieval, this method proved to be quick and easy, especially in obese patients; the downside, however, is that the sutures need to be of rigid material such as nylon or polypropylene. Watson has described using the Endo Stitch (a laparoscopic suturing instrument) to pass the suture through the sacrospinous ligament; advantages of this tool include a predictable penetration depth, without the need for a retrieval hook.[63] The same advantages have been described with the Raz Anchoring System (RAS).[64] On the other hand, Morley and DeLancey[45] found that, with the help of traditional retractors, a straight or curved needle holder could position the suture with little difficulty. Their other modifications include creating a neovaginal apex via a circumscribing incision at the prolapse proper.[45]

Anterior sacrospinous vault suspension has been described, where the ligament is approached through an anterior vaginal incision. Goldberg et al. have shown that with this technique there will be a slight increase in vaginal length, with a decrease in recurrence of anterior vaginal wall prolapse.[65]

The choice of suture material remains controversial: some advocate the use of absorbable sutures;[11,12,17,45,66] others used delayed absorbable or permanent sutures[13,44–46,58,59,67] to allow adequate time for fibrosis and scarring between the sacrospinous ligament and the vaginal apex. When absorbable sutures are used, they are passed through the full thickness of the vagina and tied over the vaginal mucosa, unlike the permanent sutures which should be passed submucosally in a double helix and tied beneath the vaginal mucosa.[59,60]

Results

Thirty-six studies[13,17,44–47,59–61,64–92] on sacrospinous colpopexy involving more than 2610 patients have been reported; these included women who underwent the procedure for posthysterectomy prolapse and procidentia. The lack of objective outcome measures and the variety of definitions of success made the data difficult to collate. Sze and Karram[93] published a meta-analysis of the available literature, where 86% of patients were followed from 1 month to 11 years. Three investigators[45,72,81] reported subjective or objective cure rates of 77–82%, while other studies did not specify the assessment method of the cure rate.[12,58,61] The cure rate in general ranged between 8[79] and 97%.[61] Based on the vault support alone as a final outcome, success was achieved in 80–90% of cases. The sacrospinous vault suspension distorts the vaginal axis, predisposing to future anterior compartment defects, with an incidence ranging between 20–33%[83,94] and 92%.[79] Goldberg et al. have shown in a retrospective analysis that anterior sacrospinous vault suspension showed a subtle but statistically significant decrease in anterior wall relaxation compared to the traditional posterior approach.[65] Lovatsis and Drutz,[60] in a 5-year case series study with a total of 293 cases, demonstrated a cure rate of 97% with a minimum of 1-year follow-up. The incidence of de novo SUI was 3.1% and anal incontinence 6%. However, 38 out of 43 patients who had preoperative anal incontinence denied any symptoms after surgery, giving a cure rate of 88.4%. The incidence of postoperative cystocele was 8.5%, and rectocele 3.5%. Nieminen and Heinonem investigated sacrospinous ligament fixation in women aged over 80 years with massive genital prolapse.[68] They showed comparative results with younger women, and concluded that, in the absence of major vascular disease, this operation is as safe as the obliterative procedures; they noted, however, that intraoperative bleeding control is important in high risk patients.

Complications

Hemorrhage

Hemorrhage is the most commonly reported complication, the blood loss ranging from 75 to 839 ml. Sze and

Karram, in their review of 1229 cases of sacrospinous ligament suspension, found that only 27 (2%) cases required transfusion.[93] Barksdale et al., in dissecting 10 female cadaveric pelves, concluded that the location of the inferior gluteal artery (because of its perpendicular course relative to the sacrospinous ligament, approximately mid-way between the ischial spine and the sacrum, and lying in a position immediately posterior to the most common location of suture placement) renders it more susceptible to injury. On the other hand, the pudendal neurovascular bundle was found to be relatively protected by the ischial spine, and therefore injury to the pudendal vessels would be uncommon and would respond to ligation of the internal iliac artery. Massive intraoperative bleeding should be dealt with by packing and vascular clips or packing and arterial embolozation.[96] Other causes of bleeding are injury to the perirectal veins,[13] sacral veins,[44] and severe adhesions,[76] mainly attributed to previous surgery.

Nerve injury
Nerve tissue was found in all parts of the sacrospinous ligament, with the highest concentration at the centre of the ligament.[97] Postoperative sciatic neuralgia is induced by traction of the suture on the ligament, the tension being transmitted to the sciatic nerve. Usually the pain resolves in 2–3 weeks; if persistent, transvaginal infiltration of xylocaine may be helpful.[97]

Gluteal pain has been reported after sacrospinous fixation with an incidence of 3%[93] and 6.1%,[60] usually resolving spontaneously within 6 months. Immediate postoperative gluteal pain radiating to the posterior surface of the leg, accompanied by paresthesia, usually indicates posterior cutaneous, pudendal or sciatic nerve injury.[61] The recommended treatment is immediate reoperation to remove the offending suture and to reposition the new suture in a more medial location on the same or the opposite sacrospinous ligament.[61]

Injury to pelvic organs
Injury to pelvic organs such as the bladder and the rectum has been reported[17,45,61,73,80] as a result of their close proximity to the sacrospinous ligament. These injuries should be immediately repaired using conventional techniques. The surgeon must be vigilant regarding this complication, and intraoperative cystoscopy and careful rectal examination after insertion of the suture into the ligament are mandatory.

Dyspareunia
Sexual function following sacrospinous ligament suspension has been evaluated in numerous studies.[17,71,73,75,79,82] Clinically, the vaginal length is maintained after a sacrospinous suspension procedure. Richter and Albrich[17] reported that eight of their patients were afraid to attempt coitus because of a narrowed vagina, while Given et al.[95] found that the procedure did not interfere with coital function. Holley et al.[79] compared pre- and postoperative sexual activity in 35 patients, and found a higher frequency of sexual intercourse postoperatively, with no associated dyspareunia.

Postoperative SUI
This complication may be a consequence of vesicourethral junction straightening that results from restoration of vaginal length and depth, or a significant reduction of urethral closure pressure when the vaginal vault is replaced intra-abdominally.[61,98] It is recommended that all patients with a large prolapse be evaluated preoperatively to rule out the presence of occult SUI.

Voiding dysfunction
This problem has been highlighted in those cases where sacrospinous ligament fixation has been performed in conjunction with an incontinence procedure. This can be attributed to dislocation of the vesicourethral region from the right-sided vaginal vault, and ventral fixation in combination with colposuspension.[97]

Rare complications
Other reported rare complications are death from postoperative coronary thrombosis (two patients)[61,77] and pulmonary embolism (one patient).[68] Evisceration through the vaginal incision has also been reported.[99]

Failures

Failure to maintain the support of the vault after sacrospinous suspension may be attributed to a variety of reasons. Poor approximation of the vault to ligament may play a major role. The presence of the suture bridge will prevent fibrosis taking place between the ligament and the vault, leaving the support mainly dependent on the suture material (this is the main reason why this procedure is contraindicated in patients with short vagina). There is no supporting evidence in the literature that permanent sutures would reduce the incidence of recurrence. Additionally, although bilateral attachment offers better anatomic results with more surface area of attachment, it does not appear to contribute to a reduction in failure rate of the procedure.[47]

Nieminen et al. have shown that postoperative infection is an independent and most important individual risk factor for recurrence of prolapse, and the lack of intravenous antibiotic prophylaxis, preoperative vaginal ulcerations, and low age at operation were significantly associated with infectious complications.[100] Prophylactic antibiotics are highly recommended and should be routine, and vaginal ulceration should always be treated preoperatively.

If the sacrospinous procedure fails, it can be repeated on the opposite side. Bilateral sacrospinous fixation can also be performed in these circumstances, bearing in mind that fibrosis and scarring may make repeating the procedure on the same side extremely difficult.

Vault prolapse repair: vaginal or abdominal route, and why?

Both sacrospinous ligament vault suspension and abdominal sacrocolpopexy (laparoscopy or laparotomy) have their own indications with their separate advantages and disadvantages. Reconstructive pelvic surgeons require the surgical expertise and proficiency to do both, and to make an informed choice taking into consideration the patient's age, weight, medical condition, coital activity, multiple previous laparotomies, and any history of previous failed surgery.

The sacrospinous ligament vault suspension has the following advantages:

- It significantly reduces postoperative morbidity, and does not require the additional skills or cost of laparoscopy.
- The procedure can be performed under either local or regional anesthesia.
- It allows the simultaneous repair of other pelvic defects.
- It has a shorter operating time.

However, orthopedic deformities, coexisting intra-abdominal pathology, and compromised vaginal length may favor the abdominal route. Furthermore, the abdominal route – whether open or laparoscopic – has its own complications of lumbosacral osteomyelitis[101] and mesh erosion into the vagina,[102] bladder,[103] and rectum.[104]

In a retrospective review comparing vaginal sacrospinous colpopexy and abdominal sacral colpopexy, Hardiman and Drutz found the two procedures to be equally effective.[59] Benson et al., in a prospective randomized study, found abdominal sacral colpopexy to be superior to the vaginal procedure (bilateral sacrospinous suspension) in the treatment of POP.[67] However, in both studies, 50% of the women had uterovaginal prolapse, the results of which may be not relevant to women with posthysterectomy vault prolapse.

A recent prospective randomized study by Maher et al. found both the abdominal and the vaginal procedure to be highly effective in the treatment of vaginal vault prolapse. However, the abdominal route was associated with a longer operating time, a slower return to activities, and more cost. Both significantly improved the patients' quality of life.[105]

There are no randomized trials comparing laparoscopic sacral colpopexy to sacrospinous ligament suspension. We would anticipate that the results with regard to the short hospital stay, intraoperative blood loss, preservation of vaginal length, and coital function will be comparable between the two; however, cost effectiveness and the additional skills of laparoscopy may favor the vaginal approach. There have been a few case series studying the laparoscopic approach,[106,107] and well-designed randomized trials in this field are required.

Different vaginal approaches for fixation of the vaginal apex

Iliococcygeal fixation

The suspension of the vaginal cuff to the iliococcygeal fascia was described by Inmon in 1963,[108] and was popularized by Shull and colleagues,[109] with the proposed advantages of decreasing neurovascular injury or further cystocele.[109,110] Using this procedure, the vaginal vault is fixed to the iliococcygeus fascia on both sides, just anterior to the ischial spine, with the muscle being approached by either an anterior or a posterior vaginal incision. Usually no vaginal epithelium needs to be excised, as the upper vagina is attached bilaterally, resulting in good vaginal length and circumference. Meeks et al., in a case series of 110 patients undergoing iliococcygeal vault suspension, reported one bowel injury and one bladder injury, with eight recurrences of anterior wall relaxation.[110] Maher et al., in a case-controlled study comparing sacrospinous vault suspension to iliococcygeal fixation of the vaginal vault,[111] found the two procedures to be equally effective in treating vaginal vault prolapse, with similar rates of postoperative cystocele, buttock pain, and hemorrhage requiring transfusion. However, fixation of the vault to this more distal location may potentially foreshorten the vagina.

McCall culdoplasty

In 1957, McCall described suspension of the vaginal vault from the origins of the uterosacral ligament along with obliteration of the pouch of Douglas.[112] Elkins et al. described a high McCall culdoplasty technique to repair the prolapsed vault at hysterectomy, where the uterosacral ligaments are plicated close to the pelvic sidewall.[82]

Cruikshank and Kovac, in a randomized comparison of three surgical methods used at the time of vaginal hysterectomy, concluded that McCall culdoplasty is superior to a vaginal Moschcowitz-type procedure and to simple peritoneal closure in preventing recurrence of enterocele.[113] Colombo and Milani, in a retrospective case-control study comparing the functional and anatomic outcome of sacrospinous vault suspension and McCall culdoplasty, found no statistical difference in recurrence of vault prolapse between the two procedures.[114] Previous studies by Shull et al.[115] and Karram et al.[116] found that the uterosacral ligaments are durable structures in patients with advanced POP; however, all available data comparing this procedure to sacrospinous ligament suspension are retrospective reviews, and prospective randomized trials are needed.

Posterior intravaginal slingoplasty (IVS)

Papa Petros was the first to describe posterior intravaginal slingoplasty when he reported 75 patients aged 40–70 years with vault prolapse.[117] Seventy-one patients were followed up for between 1 and 4.5 years. Vault prolapse recurred in 6%, and the main complication was tape erosion (5.3%)

The surgical technique (Fig. 73.4) includes level I repair that aims to insert a tape in the position of the uterosacral ligament; this has a vaginal stage and a perineal stage. The vaginal stage starts with a 4–5 cm transverse incision in the posterior vaginal wall 1.5–2 cm below the hysterectomy scar and is opened anteroposteriorly. A rectal examination is performed to identify what is adherent to the vault. At the perineal stage, a tape as an inverted 'U' is passed around the rectum behind the posterior vaginal wall via the ischiorectal fossa. Level II repair aims to approximate the rectovaginal fascia towards the midline, and level III includes restoring the integrity of the perineal body. The total operating time varied between 30 and 60 minutes. Mean blood loss was 120 ml.

Rectal perforation was reported in two patients with no serious consequences. All patients were discharged within 24 hours and were back to normal activities within 7–10 days. Farnsworth reported a larger series of 93 patients, and had a cure rate of 91%. Median follow-up was 12 months (range 2–24 months). There was one rectal perforation and one rectal erosion.[118]

These two papers showed that the IVS procedure had comparable results to other more established surgical techniques. However, it should not be undertaken without adequate training. It is suitable in patients with a short vagina, where sacrospinous fixation is not appropriate. Larger randomized trials comparing it to other known procedures are essential.

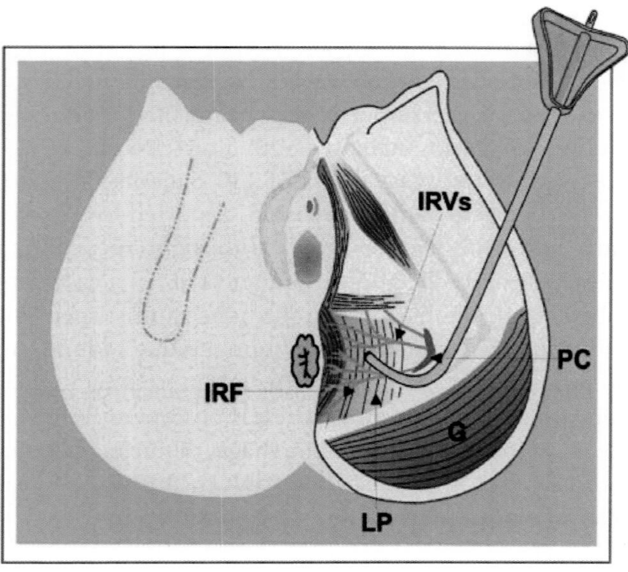

Figure 73.4. *Tunneler insertion. Patient in lithotomy position. The tunneler is seen entering the ischiorectal fossa (IRF) by penetration of levator plate (LP) 2 cm lateral to the external anal sphincter. G, gluteal muscle; IRVs, inferior rectal nerves and veins; PC, pudendal canal. (Reproduced from ref. 117 with permission from Springer-Verlag.)*

CONCLUSION

Appropriate management of vault prolapse is a known problem and, with an increasing aging and yet more active population, there will be an increased need to manage women with complex vaginal prolapse with procedures that restore anatomy, and maintain bladder, bowel, and sexual function.

The reconstructive procedures for vaginal vault prolapse remain controversial, and with the availability of different routes and procedures, it is important to take into consideration the patient's age, medical status, sexual activity, reproductive history, and previous surgery. Bowel and bladder function should also be taken into account in making the decision. It is therefore essential that every clinician dealing with complex vaginal prolapse be well versed in all surgical techniques, and management should be individually tailored for each patient.

Well-designed prospective randomized trials should be undertaken to determine whether or not any of the procedures described truly deserves to be considered the 'gold standard'.

REFERENCES

1. Subak LL, Waetjen LE, Van den Eaden S et al. Cost of pelvic organ prolapse surgery in the United States. Obstet Gynecol 2001;98:646–51.
2. Olsen AL, Smith VJ, Bergstrom JO et al. Epidemiology of surgically managed pelvic organ prolapse and urinary incontinence. Obstet Gynecol 1997;89:501–6.
3. Luber KM, Boero S, Choe JY. The demographics of pelvic floor disorders: current observations and future projections. Am J Obstet Gynecol 2001;184:1496–1501.
4. Emge LA, Durfee RB. Pelvic organ prolapse: four thousands years of treatment. Clin Obstet Gynecol 1996;9:997–1032.
5. van Meekeren J. Heel-en geneeskonstige aenmerkingen. Alphen aan de Rijn: Stafleu, 1728; 313–19.
6. Zweifel P. Vorlesungen über klinische Gynäkologie. Berlin: Hirschwald, 1892; 407–15.
7. White GR. Cystocele a radical cure by suturing lateral sulci of vagina to white line of pelvic fascia. JAMA 1909;53:17–27.
8. Miller NF. A new method of correcting complete inversion of the vagina. Surg Gynecol Obstet 1927;44:550–4.
9. Amreich J. Aetiologie and Operation des Scheidenstumpf prolapses. Wien Klin Wochenschr 1951;63:74–7.
10. Sederl J. Zur Operation des Prolapses der blindendingenden Scheide. Geburtshilfe Frauenheilkd 1958;18:824–8.
11. Richter K. Die chirurgische Anatomie der Vaginaefixation sacrospinalis vaginalis: Ein Beitrag zur operativen Behandlung des Scheiden blindsack prolapses. Geburtshilfe Frauenheilkd 1968;28:321–7.
12. Randall CL, Nichols DH. Surgical treatment of vaginal eversion. Obstet Gynecol 1971;38:72–7.
13. Cruikshank SH, Cox DW. Sacrospinous ligament fixation at the time of transvaginal hysterectomy. Am J Obstet Gynecol 1990;162(6):1611–19.
14. DeLancey JO. The anatomy of the pelvic floor. Curr Opin Obstet Gynecol 1994;6:313–16.
15. DeLancey JO. Anatomy and biomechanics of genital prolapse. Clin Obstet Gynecol 1993;36(4):897–909.
16. DeLancey JO. Anatomic aspects of vaginal eversion after hysterectomy. Am J Obstet Gynecol 1992;166:1717–28.
17. Richter K, Albrich W. Long term results following fixation of the vagina on the sacrospinous ligament by the vaginal route. Am J Obstet Gynecol 1981;141:811–16.
18. Nichols D, Randall C. Pelvic anatomy of the living. In: Nichols D, Randall C (eds) Vaginal surgery, 3rd ed. Baltimore: Williams and Wilkins, 1989; 1–45.
19. Sagsoz N, Erosy M, Kamaci M, Tekdemir I. Anatomical landmarks regarding sacrospinous colpopexy operations performed for vaginal vault prolapse. Eur J Obstet Gynecol Reprod Biol 2002;101(1):74–8.
20. Thompson J, Gibb J, Genadry R et al. Anatomy of pelvic arteries adjacent to the sacrospinous ligament: importance of the coccygeal branch of the inferior gluteal artery. Obstet Gynecol 1999;94:973–7.
21. Richardson AC, Lyons JB, Williams NL. A new look at pelvic relaxation. Am J Obstet Gynecol 1976;126(5):568–73.
22. Smith ARB, Hosker GL, Warrell DW. The role of partial denervation of the pelvic floor in the aetiology of genitourinary prolapse and stress incontinence of urine: a neurophysiological study. Br J Obstet Gynecol 1989;96:24–8.
23. Carley ME, Schaffer J. Urinary incontinence and pelvic organ prolapse in women with Marfan or Ehlers–Danlos syndrome. Am J Obstet Gynecol 2000;182(5):1021–3.
24. Wong MY, Harmanli OH, Agar M et al. Collagen content of non-support tissue in pelvic organ prolapse and stress urinary incontinence. Am J Obstet Gynecol 2003;189:1597–600.
25. Chen BH, Wen Y, Li H, Polan ML. Collagen metabolism and turnover in women with stress urinary incontinence and pelvic prolapse. Int Urogynecol J Pelvic Floor Dysfunct 2002;13(2):80–7.
26. Burrows LJ, Meyn LA, Walters MD, Weber AM. Pelvic symptoms in women with pelvic organ prolapse. Obstet Gynecol 2004;104:982–8.
27. Chou Q, Weber AM, Piedmonte MR. Clinical presentation of enterocele. Obstet Gynecol 2000;96:599–603.
28. Porges RF. A practical system of diagnosis and classification of pelvic relaxation. Surg Gynecol Obstet 1963;117:761–73.
29. Baden WF, Walker TA. Genesis of the vaginal profile: a correlated classification of vaginal relaxation. Clin Obstet Gynecol 1972;15:1048–54.
30. Beecham CT. Classification of vaginal relaxation. Am J Obstet Gynecol 1980;136:957–8.
31. Bump RC, Mattiasson A, Bo K et al. The standardization of terminology of female pelvic floor dysfunction. Am J Obstet Gynecol 1996;175:10–7.
32. Bai SW, Jeon MJ, Kim YJ et al. Relationship between stress urinary incontinence and pelvic organ prolapse. Int Urogynecol J Pelvic Floor Dysfunct 2002;13:256–60.
33. Ng CS, Rackley RR, Appell RA. Incidence of concomitant procedures for pelvic organ prolapse and reconstruction in women who undergo surgery for stress urinary incontinence. Urology 2001;57:911–13.
34. Ellerkmann RM, Cundiff GW, Melick CF et al. Correlation of symptoms with location and severity of pelvic organ prolapse. Am J Obstet Gynecol 2001;185:1332–8.
35. Bergman A, Koonings PP, Ballard CA. Predicting postoperative urinary incontinence in women undergoing operation for genitourinary prolapse. Am J Obstet Gynecol 1988;158:1171–5.

36. Bump R, Fantl A, Hurt G. The mechanism of urinary incontinence in women with severe uterovaginal prolapse: results of barrier studies. Obstet Gynecol 1988;72:291–5.

37. Gardy M, Kozminski M, DeLancey J et al. Stress incontinence and cystoceles. J Urol 1991;145:1211–13.

38. Liang CC, Cang YL, Chang SD et al. Pessary test to predict postoperative urinary incontinence in women undergoing hysterectomy for prolapse. Obstet Gynecol 2004;104:795–800.

39. Cutner AS, Elneil S. The vaginal vault. Br J Obstet Gynecol 2004;111(S1):79–83.

40. Borstad E, Rud T. The risk of developing urinary stress incontinence after vaginal repair in continent women: a clinical and urodynamic follow-up study. Acta Obstet Gynecol Scand 1989;68:545–9.

41. Richardson D, Bent A, Ostergard D. The effect of uterovaginal prolapse on urethrovesical pressure dynamics. Am J Obstet Gynecol 1983;146:901–5.

42. Gallentine ML, Cespedes RD. Occult urinary stress incontinence and the effect of vaginal prolapse on abdominal leak point pressure. Urology 2001;57:40–4.

43. Bump RC, Hurt WG, Theofrastous JP et al. Randomized prospective comparison of needle colposuspension versus endopelvic fascia placation to potential stress incontinence prophylaxis in women undergoing vaginal reconstruction for stage III or IV pelvic organ prolapse. The Continence Program for Women Research Group. Am J Obstet Gynecol 1996;175:326–33.

44. Carey MP, Slack MC. Transvaginal sacrospinous colpopexy for vault and marked uterovaginal prolapse. Br J Obstet Gynecol 1994;101:536–40.

45. Morley GW, DeLancey JO. Sacrospinous ligament fixation for eversion of the vagina. Am J Obstet Gynecol 1988;158:872–81.

46. Imparato E, Aspesi G, Rovetta E, Presti M. Surgical management and prevention of vaginal vault prolapse. Surg Gynecol Obstet 1992;175:233–7.

47. Nichols DH (ed). Massive eversion of the vagina. In: Gynecologic and Obstetric Surgery. St Louis: Mosby, 1993; 431–64.

48. Pohl JF, Frattarelli JL. Bilateral transvaginal sacrospinous colpopexy: preliminary experience. Am J Obstet Gynecol 1997;177:1356–61.

49. Cruikshank SH. Sacrospinous fixation. Should this be performed at the time of vaginal hysterectomy? Am J Obstet Gynecol 1991;164:1072–6.

50. Kovac RC, Cruikshank SH. Successful pregnancies and vaginal deliveries after sacrospinous uterosacral fixation in five of nineteen patients. Am J Obstet Gynecol 1993;168:1778–90.

51. Richardson DA, Scotti RJ, Ostergard DR. Surgical management of uterine prolapse in young women. J Reprod Med. 1989;34:388–92.

52. Hefni M, El-Toukhy T, Bhaumik J, Katsimanis E. Sacrospinous cervicocolpopexy with uterine conservation for uterovaginal prolapse in elderly women: An evolving concept. Am J Obstet Gynecol 2003;188:645–50.

53. Verdeja AM, Elkins TE, Odoi A et al. Transvaginal sacrospinous colpopexy: anatomic landmarks to be aware of to minimise complications. Am J Obstet Gynecol 1995;173:1468–9.

54. Weber AM, Walters MD, Piedmonte MR, Ballard LA. Anterior colporrhaphy: a randomized trial of three surgical techniques. Am J Obstet Gynecol 2001;185:1299–306.

55. Sand PK, Koduri S, Lobel R et al. Prospective randomized trial of polyglactin 010 mesh to prevent recurrence of cystoceles and rectoceles. Am J Obstet Gynecol 2001;184:1357–64.

56. Flood CG, Drutz HO, Waja L. Anterior colporrhaphy reinforced with Marlex mesh for the treatment of cystoceles. Int Urogynecol J 1998;9:200–4.

57. Miklos JR, Kholi N, Lucente V, Saye W. Site-specific fascial defects in the diagnosis and surgical management of enterocele. Am J Obstet Gynecol 1998;179:1418–23.

58. Miyazaki FS. Miya hook ligature for sacrospinous ligament suspension. Obstet Gynecol 1987;70:286–8.

59. Hardiman PJ, Drutz HP. Sacrospinous vault suspension and abdominal colposacropexy: success rates and complications. Am J Obstet Gynecol 1996;175:612–16.

60. Lovatsis D, Drutz HP. Safety and efficacy of sacrospinous vault suspension. Int Urogynecol J 2002;13:308–13.

61. Nichols DH. Sacrospinous fixation for massive eversion of the vagina. Am J Obstet Gynecol 1982;142:901–4.

62. Sharp TR. Sacrospinous suspension made easy. Obstet Gynecol 1993;82:873–5.

63. Watson JD. Sacrospinous ligament colpopexy: new instrumentation applied to a standard gynecologic procedure. Obstet Gynecol 1996;88:883–5.

64. Giberti C. Transvaginal sacrospinous colpopexy by palpation – a new minimally invasive procedure using an anchoring system. Urology 2001;57:666–9.

65. Goldberg RP, Tomezsko JE, Winkler HA, Koduri S, Culligan PL, Sand PK. Anterior or posterior sacrospinous vaginal vault suspension: long-term anatomic and functional evaluation. Obstet Gynecol 2001;98:199–204.

66. Richter K. Massive eversion of true vagina: pathogenesis, diagnosis, and therapy of the 'true' prolapse of the vaginal stump. Clin Obstet Gynecol 1982;25:897–912.

67. Benson JT, Lucente V, McClellan E. Vaginal versus abdominal reconstructive surgery for the treatment of pelvic support defects: a prospective randomized study

with long-term outcome evaluation. Am J Obstet Gynecol 1996;175:1418–21.

68. Nieminen K, Heinonem PK. Sacrospinous ligament fixation for massive genital prolapse in women aged 80 years. Br J Obstet Gynaecol 2001;108:817–21.

69. Lantzch T, Goepel C, Wolters M, Koelbl H. Sacrospinous ligament fixation for vaginal vault prolapse. Arch Gynecol Obstet 2001;265:21–5.

70. Guner H, Noyan V, Tiras MB et al. Transvaginal sacrospinous colpopexy for marked uterovaginal and vault prolapse. Int J Gynecol Obstet 2001;74(2):165–70.

71. Brown WE, Hoffman MS, Bouis PJ et al. Management of vaginal vault prolapse: retrospective comparison of abdominal versus vaginal approach. J Fla Med Assoc 1989;76:249–52.

72. Kettel ML, Herbertson RM. An anatomic evaluation of the sacrospinous ligament colpopexy. Surg Gynecol Obstet 1989;168:318–22.

73. Monk BJ, Ramp JF, Montz FJ, Febherz TB. Sacrospinous fixation for vaginal vault prolapse. Complications and results. J Gynecol Surg 1991;7:87–92.

74. Baker MH. Success with sacrospinous suspension of the prolapsed vaginal vault. J Gynecol Surg 1992;175:419–20.

75. Heinonen PK. Transvaginal sacrospinous colpopexy for vaginal vault and complete genital prolapse in aged women. Acta Obstet Gynecol Scand 1992;71:377–81.

76. Shull BT, Capen CV, Riggs MW, Kuch TJ. Preoperative and postoperative analysis of site-specific pelvic support defects in 81 women treated with sacrospinous ligament suspension and pelvic reconstruction. Am J Obstet Gynecol 1992;166:1764–71.

77. Kaminski PF, Sorosky JI, Pees RC, Rodczkski ES. Correction of massive vaginal prolapse in aged women. J Am Geriatr Soc 1993;41:42–4.

78. Porges RF, Smilen SW. Long-term analysis of the surgical management of pelvic support defects. Am J Obstet Gynecol 1994;171:1518–28.

79. Holley RJ, Varner RE, Gleason BP et al. Recurrent pelvic support defects after sacrospinous ligament fixation for vaginal vault prolapse. J Am Coll Surg 1995;180:444–8.

80. Sauer HA, Klutke CG. Transvaginal sacrospinous ligament fixation for treatment of vaginal prolapse. J Urol 1995;154:1008–12.

81. Peters WA, Christenson ML. Fixation of the vaginal apex to the coccygeal fascia during repair of vaginal vault eversion with enterocele. Am J Obstet Gynecol 1995;172:1894–1902.

82. Elkins TE, Hooper JB, Goodfellow K et al. Initial report of anatomic and clinical comparison of the sacrospinous ligament fixation to the high McCall culdoplasty for vaginal cuff fixation at hysterectomy for uterine prolapse. J Pelvic Surg 1995;1:12–7.

83. Paraiso MF, Ballard LA, Walters MD et al. Pelvic support defects and visceral and sexual function in women treated with sacrospinous ligament suspension and pelvic reconstruction. Am J Obstet Gynecol 1996;175:1423–31.

84. Chapin DS. Teaching sacrospinous colpopexy. Am J Obstet Gynecol 1997;177:1330–6.

85. Schlesinger RE. Vaginal sacrospinous ligament fixation with the Autosuture Endostitch device. Am J Obstet Gynecol 1997;167:1358–62.

86. Penalver M, Mekki Y, Laferty H et al. Should sacrospinous ligament fixation for the management of pelvic support defects be part of a residency program procedure? Am J Obstet Gynecol 1998;178:326–30.

87. Ozcan U, Gungor T, Ekin M, Eken S. Sacrospinous fixation for the prolapsed vaginal vault. Gynecol Obstet Invest 1999;47:65–8.

88. Meschia M, Bruschi F, Amicarelli F et al. The sacrospinous vaginal vault suspension: critical analysis of outcomes. Int Urogynecol J 1990;10:155–9.

89. Vigano R, Ferrari A, Quellari P, Frigerio L. Sacrospinous ligament fixation: long term follow up. Int Urogynecol J 2000;11:i–ii.

90. Febbraro W, Beucher G, Von Theobold P et al. Feasibility of bilateral sacrospinous ligament vaginal suspension with a stapler. Prospective study with the first 34 cases. J Gynecol Obstet Biol Reprod 1997;26:815–21.

91. Brieger GM, MacGibbon AL, Atkinson KH. Sacrospinous colpopexy. Aust N Z J Obstet Gynecol 1995;35:86–7.

92. Hoffman MS, Harris MS, Bouis PJ. Sacrospinous colpopexy in the management of uterovaginal prolapse. J Reprod Med 1996;41:299–303.

93. Sze EH, Karram MM. Transvaginal repair of vault prolapse: a review. Obstet Gynecol 1997;89:466–75.

94. Karram MM, Sze EH, Walters MD. Surgical treatment of vaginal vault prolapse. In: Walters MD, Karram MM (eds) Urogynecology and Reconstructive Pelvic Surgery, 2nd ed. St Louis: Mosby, 1999; 235–56.

95. Given FY, Muhlendorf TK, Browning GM. Vaginal length and sexual function after colpopexy for complete uterovaginal eversion. Am J Obstet Gynecol 1993;169:284–8.

96. Barksdale PA, Elkins TE, Sanders CK et al. An anatomic approach to pelvic hemorrhage during sacrospinous ligament fixation of the vaginal vault. Obstet Gynecol 1998;91:715–18.

97. Barksdale PA, Gasser RF, Gauthier CM, Elkins TE, Wall LL. Intraligamentous nerves as a potential source of pain after sacrospinous ligament fixation of the vaginal apex. Int Urogynecol J Pelvic Floor Dysfunct 1997;8:121–5.

98. Scotti RJ. Repair of genitourinary prolapse in women. Curr Opin Obstet Gynecol 1991;3:404–12.

99. Farrell SA, Scotti RA, Osterrgard DR et al. Massive evisceration: a complication following sacrospinous vaginal vault fixation. Obstet Gynecol 1991;78:560–2.

100. Nieminen K, Huhtala H, Heinonen PK. Anatomic and functional assessment and risk factors of recurrent prolapse after vaginal sacrospinous fixation. Acta Obstet Gynecol Scand 2003;82:471–8.

101. Weidner AC, Cundiff GW, Harris RL et al. Sacral osteomyelitis: an unusual complication of abdominal sacral colpopexy. Obstet Gynecol 1997;90:689–91.

102. Kholi N, Walsh PM, Roat TW, Karram MM. Mesh erosion after abdominal sacrocolpopexy. Obstet Gynecol 1998;92:999–1004.

103. Patsner B. Mesh erosion into the bladder after abdominal sacral colpopexy. Obstet Gynecol 2000;95:1029.

104. Kenton KS, Woods MP, Brubaker L. Uncomplicated erosion of polytetrafluoroethylene grafts into the rectum. Am J Obstet Gynecol 2002;187:233–4.

105. Maher CF, Qatawneh AM, Dwyer PL et al. Abdominal sacral colpopexy or vaginal sacrospinous colpopexy for vaginal vault prolapse: a prospective randomized study. Am J Obstet Gynecol 2004;190:20–6.

106. Mahendran D, Prashar S, Smith ARB et al. Laparoscopic sacrocolpopexy in the management of vaginal vault prolapse. Gynecol Endosc 1996;5:217–22.

107. Cusson M, Bogaert E, Narducci F et al. Laparoscopic sacral colpopexy: short-term results and complications in 83 patients. J Gynecol Obstet Biol Reprod 2000;29:746–50.

108. Inmon WB. Pelvic relaxation and repair including prolapse of the vagina following vaginal hysterectomy. South Med J 1963:56:577–82.

109. Shull BL, Capen MD, Riggs MW et al. Bilateral attachment of the vaginal cuff to iliococcygeus fascia: an effective method of cuff suspension. Am J Obstet Gynecol 1993;168:1669–74.

110. Meeks GR, Wasshburne JF, McGehee RP, Wiser WL. Repair of vaginal vault prolapse by suspension of the vagina to iliococcygeus (prespinous) fascia. Am J Obstet Gynecol 1994;171(6):1444–52.

111. Maher CF, Murray CJ, Carey MP et al. Iliococcygeus or sacrospinous fixation for vaginal vault prolapse. Obstet Gynecol 2001;98:40–4.

112. McCall ML. Posterior culdoplasty: surgical correction of enterocele during vaginal hysterectomy: a preliminary report. Am J Obstet Gynecol 1957;10:595–602.

113. Cruikshank SH, Kovac SR. Randomized comparison of three surgical methods at the time of vaginal hysterectomy to prevent posterior enterocele. Am J Obstet Gynecol 1999;180:859–65.

114. Colombo M, Milani R. Sacrospinous ligament fixation and modified McCall culdoplasty during vaginal hysterectomy for advanced uterovaginal prolapse. Am J Obstet Gynecol 1998;179:13–20.

115. Shull BL, Bachofen C, Coates K et al. A transvaginal approach to repair of apical and other associated sites of pelvic organ prolapse with uterosacral ligaments. Am J Obstet Gynecol 2000;183:1365–74.

116. Karram M, Goldwasser S, Kleeman S et al. High uterosacral vaginal vault suspension with fascial reconstruction for vaginal repair of enterocele and vaginal vault prolapse. Am J Obstet Gynecol 2001;185:1339–43.

117. Papa Petros PE. Vault prolapse II. Restoration of dynamic vaginal supports by infracoccygeal sacropexy, an axial day-case vaginal procedure. Int Urogynecol J 2001;12:296–303.

118. Farnsworth BN. Posterior intravaginal slingoplasty (infracoccygeal sacropexy) for severe posthysterectomy vaginal vault prolapse – a preliminary report on efficacy and safety. Int Urogynecol J 2002;13:4–8.

74

Abdominal approach to fixation of the vaginal apex

Wesley Hilger, Jeffrey Cornella

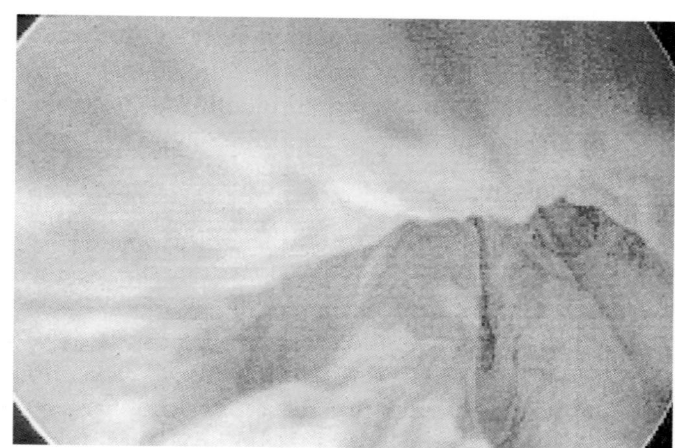

INTRODUCTION

Pelvic organ prolapse is a common condition that can adversely affect a woman's quality of life. A recent study found that in older women with an intact uterus, 25% had prolapse with the leading edge below the hymeneal ring.[1] Up to 14% of all hysterectomies are performed for prolapse and the risk of requiring surgery for prolapse after a hysterectomy has been reported to be up to 5%.[2,3] Each year in the United States approximately 200,000 women undergo surgery for pelvic prolapse or urinary incontinence.[4] One-third of these women will experience recurrent prolapse and require additional surgery within 4 years.[5] As the population in developed countries ages, pelvic organ prolapse will be a condition that all physicians caring for women will encounter with increasing frequency.[6] A full understanding of the pathophysiology, evaluation, and treatment of prolapse will become increasingly important.

There are many surgical approaches to vaginal prolapse. Lane first proposed the abdominal sacrocolpopexy in 1962.[7] Since that time it has undergone several modifications but the basic concept of the procedure has remained the same: support of the vagina with a suspensory bridge connected to the anterior longitudinal ligament of the sacrum.[8] Abdominal sacrocolpopexy has been studied extensively and has been shown to be reliable and durable.[9] This chapter will discuss the pathophysiology of prolapse, the evaluation of the patient with prolapse, the surgical techniques of abdominal sacrocolpopexy, and possible complications of the procedure.

PATHOPHYSIOLOGY

The pathophysiology of vaginal vault prolapse is not fully understood. Support of the female pelvic viscera involves the complex interaction among pelvic floor muscles, nerves, and connective tissue. It is believed that abnormal anatomy and abnormal function of the pelvic viscera result from congenital or acquired weakness of one or more of the components that interact to support them. Risk factors thought to contribute to vaginal prolapse include obesity, chronic bronchitis, vaginal delivery, multiparity, age, and diseases of collagen metabolism.[10]

The levator ani muscles are the primary muscles of support in the pelvis. They are typically the main active source of support for the pelvic viscera. When the muscles relax during micturition or defecation, the connective tissue attachments of the pelvis bear the load of the intra-abdominal pressure. Norton[11] used a 'boat in a dry dock' analogy to describe this relationship between muscle and connective tissue. The muscles act like the water holding up the boat while the moorings are the connective tissue. If the muscles do not function (or the water level is lowered in the dock) due to nerve damage or direct damage then more stress is placed on the connective tissue (moorings). Eventually, this stress can lead to connective tissue damage and prolapse.

The connective tissue supporting the pelvic viscera includes the endopelvic fascia, the arcus tendineus fascia pelvis and the uterosacral and cardinal ligaments. DeLancey[12] divided the connective tissue support in the pelvis into three interconnected levels (Fig. 74.1). Level I support occurs at the cervix or vaginal cuff and consists of the uterosacral and cardinal ligament complexes. These ligaments attach the uterus, cervix, and upper vagina to the pelvic walls. Level II support occurs at the mid-portion of the vagina. These supporting connective tissue layers aid in supporting and separating the bladder anteriorly and rectum posteriorly from the vagina. At level III the vagina fuses directly with the urethra anteriorly, perineal body posteriorly, and levator ani muscles laterally. Damage to or weakness of the support structures at each level will

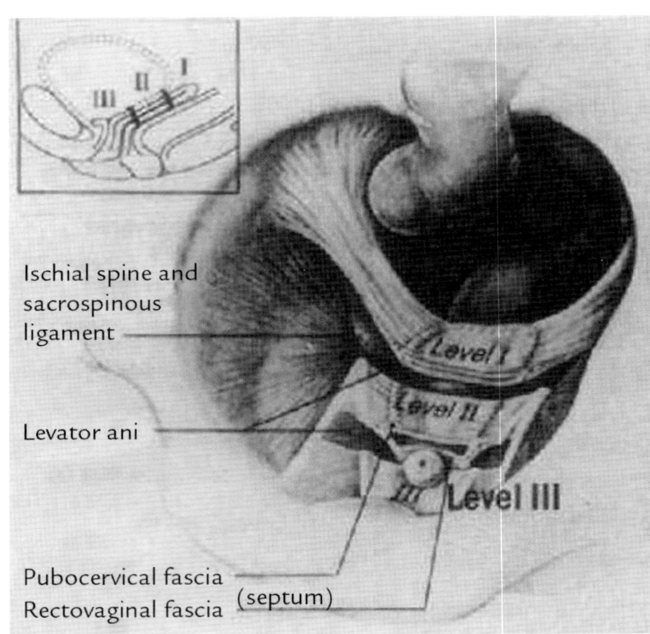

Figure 74.1. *At level I, paracolpium suspends the vagina from the lateral pelvic walls. Fibers of level I extend both vertically and posterior towards the sacrum. At level II, the vagina is attached to the arcus tendineus fasciae pelvis and superior fascia of the levator ani muscles. At level III, the vagina is fused to the medial surface of the levator ani muscles, urethra, and perineal body. (Reproduced from ref. 12 with permission from Elsevier.)*

lead to prolapse of the corresponding pelvic viscera: loss of anterior support can lead to cystocele or urethral hypermobility; deficiencies in the cardinal–uterosacral complex will lead to prolapse of the vaginal apex or uterus; and loss of posterior support can lead to enterocele or rectocele.

PATIENT SELECTION AND PREOPERATIVE EVALUATION

Patients with vaginal apical prolapse are likely to have support defects in other compartments of the vagina (Fig. 74.2). Each patient should be assessed for symptoms related to the anterior, apical, and posterior compartments to help guide the physical examination and plan corrective surgery. Symptoms commonly associated with pelvic organ prolapse include vaginal bulge, low back pain, sense of pelvic pressure and fullness, constipation, urinary and/or fecal incontinence, and the inability to empty the bladder and/or rectum.[13] Studies have shown that there are no symptoms typical of vaginal prolapse and that symptoms do not correlate with the severity of prolapse.[14,15] As an example, as the prolapse increases in severity, symptoms of urinary incontinence may be masked if kinking of the urethra occurs.[14] Patients with prolapse in general, and especially those who describe resolution of stress urinary incontinence symptoms, should be suspected of having occult incontinence. A thorough understanding of the patient's symptoms should precede the physical examination but only

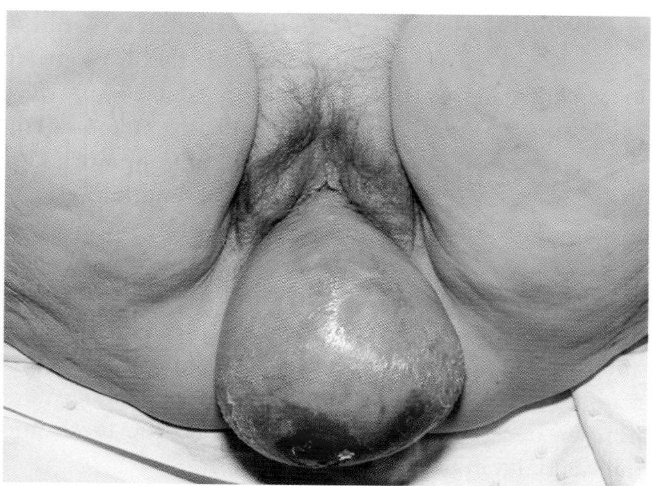

Figure 74.2. *A patient with a massive vaginal vault prolapse and multicompartment defects. (Reproduced with permission from the Mayo Foundation for Medical Education and Research.)*

a thorough physical examination will reveal the degree and site of vaginal support defects.

The physical examination should be performed in a systematic fashion to evaluate all compartments. Standardized staging for pelvic organ prolapse has been described, and currently the International Continence Society advocates use of the pelvic organ prolapse quantification (POPQ) system.[16] Evaluating subjects in the standing as well as the supine position may make a difference in the degree of prolapse noted and it is recommended that both examinations be performed.[17] The anterior compartment should be assessed for paravaginal versus midline defects and urethral hypermobility. Specific findings on examination may indicate a paravaginal defect: persistent rugae in the prolapsed anterior wall or, if the prolapse does not occur with lateral support of the anterior vaginal wall, with ring forceps on examination. Apical or cervical descent should be assessed as should posterior wall and perineal descent. Levator ani tone, anal tone, and perineal reflexes should be tested for neurologic integrity of the pelvic floor.

Stress incontinence can be unmasked after prolapse surgery in 8–60% of patients.[18,19] Provocative maneuvers (i.e. straining or cough) with a full bladder should be performed with the prolapse evident and the prolapse reduced to try to detect occult stress incontinence. A large cotton swab or sponge stick elevating the prolapsed apex to its normal anatomic position is useful for this portion of the examination. Finally, a simple office bladder fill including a post-void residual volume can assess the sensation, capacity, and function of the bladder.

Further evaluation and testing with urodynamics, magnetic resonance imaging (MRI) or defecography should be performed as indicated by the history, symptoms, and physical examination. Currently, urodynamic measures have not been validated in women with prolapse. MRI also lacks standardized protocols and its impact on identifying fascial defects and improving surgical outcomes is not known. At our institution we have found that, in most patients, these modalities add little to our assessment and treatment plan.

The surgery for pelvic prolapse must be individualized for each patient. The patient's medical history, symptoms, examination findings and expectations help to guide the surgeon's decision-making process. In our practice, an abdominal sacrocolpopexy is performed in subjects who are medically stable, have failed prior vaginal suspension procedures, have a short vagina, or need further abdominal surgery. Currently, studies do not indicate who would benefit most from an abdominal sacrocolpopexy. In our practice, additional procedures such as bilateral salpingo-oophorectomy, paravaginal defect repair, Burch procedure, or perineorrhaphy are added as needed.

It is controversial whether a hysterectomy should be performed at the time of abdominal sacrocolpopexy. There is concern for increased risk of mesh erosion due to exposure to the vagina. Studies have noted a range of erosion rates from zero to 27% when the uterus is completely removed but there are no randomized trials.[9] If a hysterectomy is to be carried out, any one of three procedures can be performed to decrease the risk of erosion: a supracervical hysterectomy can be undertaken; the cuff can be closed in two layers; or an intervening portion of biologic graft can be placed between the cuff and the mesh.

Preoperative instructions for our patients include clear liquids the day before surgery, with bowel preparation the evening before surgery. Each patient also has a preoperative visit to discuss the proposed procedure, the risks and the benefits, and to answer any remaining questions.

ABDOMINAL SACROCOLPOPEXY TECHNIQUE

All surgeons should have a standard technique for patient positioning, preparation, and procedure. To form this technique, a thorough understanding of the anatomy, surgical principles, and possible complications of the procedure is required. This knowledge will allow the surgeon to perform an abdominal sacrocolpopexy efficiently, make adjustments in technique as dictated by intraoperative findings, and minimize postoperative complications.

Patients are given thromboembolic stockings and sequential compression devices as deep venous thrombus (DVT) prophylaxis. The patient is placed in a dorsal lithotomy position in Allen-type stirrups. This position allows for access to the vagina, perineum, and rectum during the procedure. The Allen stirrups also allow for elevation of the legs should an additional vaginal procedure need be performed. The abdomen and vagina are prepped with betadine and a single dose of preoperative antibiotics is given.

The choice of entry incision depends on the patient. We have found that a Pfannenstiel incision gives adequate exposure in most patients. A midline incision may be used to gain greater exposure in an obese patient or it may be used if the patient has a prior midline scar. If there is a paravaginal defect that is to be repaired with an abdominal paravaginal repair, or if the patient has stress incontinence that will be repaired with a Burch procedure, we will enter the space of Retzius and perform the retropubic procedures prior to entering the peritoneal cavity.

Once procedures in the space of Retzius are completed, the peritoneal cavity is entered. If there are adhesions of the bowel to the pelvis, these are lyzed and the small bowel is packed above the level of the sacral promontory. We use a Bookwalter retractor with a bladder blade, two side blades, and a malleable blade that retracts the packing.

A device should be placed in the vagina to aid in identification and manipulation of the vagina. Such a device can be a Lucite rod, EEA sizer or sponge stick. We prefer to use the Lucite rod because it manipulates the vagina well, fills the entire cavity, and allows sutures to be easily placed through the entire thickness of the vagina.

Once the vagina is identified, its overlying peritoneum is dissected away. Initially, stay sutures are placed at the apical corners to aid in orientation. Metzenbaum scissors are used to incise the peritoneum transversely. The posterior peritoneum is then dissected down to the rectovaginal septum of the pelvis. Care is taken to avoid the rectum. Another Lucite rod can be placed into the rectum for visualization if it is difficult to identify. Finally, the anterior peritoneum and bladder are dissected off the anterior vagina.

Dissecting the peritoneum widely off the vagina provides a large surface area for attaching the mesh. If there are fascial defects noted at the apex of the vagina these are repaired with 2-0 Vicryl suture but no effort is made to excise the underlying vaginal mucosa. We feel that efforts to maintain the integrity of the vaginal mucosa will reduce the chance of mesh erosion.

Once the vagina is dissected and exposed, the mesh is attached. Typically, a 4×18 cm strip of mesh is required. The mesh is cut in a Y-formation and the appropriate length for each patient is determined intraoperatively. The mesh is folded in half longitudinally and cut along this line to create the arms of the Y. Length required for the arms of the Y is determined by the length of attachment required for the anterior and posterior aspects of the vagina. The folded mesh is then sutured in place at the corners to maintain the fold for easier handling. Other options include using two strips of mesh for the anterior and posterior aspects of the vagina. If the vagina is noted to have significant thinning then an allograft of porcine dermis may be placed between the mesh and the vaginal wall to prevent mesh erosion.

Suture placement is crucial for mesh security. Initially, the sutures are attached to the posterior vagina. We have found that this portion of the vagina can be difficult to visualize if an attempt is made to attach the mesh directly. We recommend a monofilament suture and use a No. 0 Prolene suture on a CT-1 needle. The first two sutures are placed bilaterally as caudad as possible on the posterior vaginal wall. Essentially, full thickness bites are taken with the suture and this can easily be felt as the needle encounters the vaginal rod. The sutures are tagged with curved Kelly clamps for orientation. A second row of bilateral sutures approximately 1–2 cm cephalad is placed in the posterior vagina. (Concerns have been raised regarding mesh erosion with full thickness bites; however, this has not been assessed in controlled studies and we feel our technique is sound based on our clinical outcomes.)

If the position and orientation of the suture appears appropriate, the mesh is attached to the vagina. Sutures are placed through the mesh with the aid of a Mayo needle, the mesh is pushed down over the posterior vagina, and the sutures tied. After the posterior flap of mesh is fixed to the vagina the corresponding apical and anterior portions can easily be fixed. At this point sutures can be placed directly through the mesh and vagina using the Lucite rod as a backstop. The sutures are placed in a bilateral and midline fashion in 1–2 cm increments. The mesh is usually placed 4–5 cm along the anterior vaginal wall. The number of sutures required is typically 8–10 sutures for the posterior, apex, and anterior segments of the vagina. Once the two arms of the Y-segment of the mesh are applied to the vagina, attention is then turned to the sacral promontory.

Important landmarks for the sacral promontory of the pelvis include bifurcation of the aorta at the level of L4–L5, the right ureter, right iliac vessels, the middle sacral vein, the sigmoid colon, and the left common iliac vein that crosses the midline over the sacral promontory.

The peritoneum over the promontory is incised sharply and delicate blunt and sharp dissection is used to expose the anterior longitudinal ligament overlying the sacrum (Fig. 74.3). Care should be taken during this dissection to avoid damaging middle sacral vessels and presacral veins because life-threatening hemorrhage can occur.[20] The peritoneal incision is extended to the posterior cul-de-sac with care taken to avoid the rectum to the left and the ureter to the right of the dissection. Two No. 0 Prolene sutures on a CT-2 needle are placed just below the level of the sacral promontory, approximately 1–2 cm apart (Fig. 74.4). Attachment at the upper third of the sacrum reduces the risk of bleeding from presacral vessels lower in the sacrum without compromising the angle of the vagina.[21] The appropriate length of the graft is determined as one that avoids any tension on the graft and vagina (Fig. 74.5). The excess graft is cut and removed and the promontory sutures are then brought through the remaining graft and tied down.

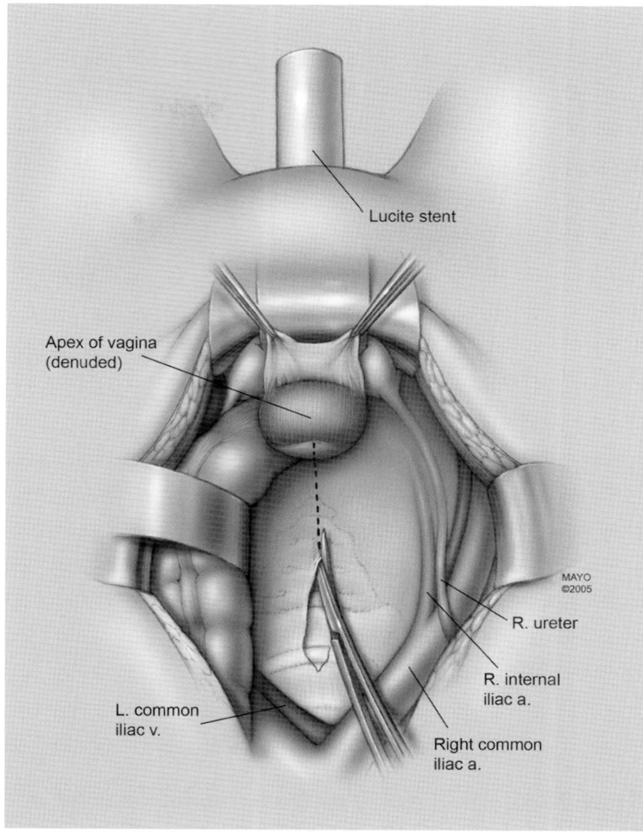

Figure 74.3. *Arial view of the pelvis showing a Lucite rod in the vagina. The peritoneum has been dissected off the apex of the vagina but the mesh has yet to be applied. The peritoneum at the sacral promontory has been incised and anatomic structures can be appreciated: right internal iliac artery, right ureter, right common iliac artery, left common iliac vein, sigmoid colon (retracted). (Reproduced with permission from the Mayo Foundation for Medical Education and Research.)*

Reperitonealization of the graft is performed with a running 2-0 delayed absorbable suture. Care should be taken to ensure that all areas of the graft material are covered with peritoneum. The packs are removed and the abdomen is closed in the usual fashion.

Attention should then be turned to the vagina if needed. Cystoscopy is not routinely performed after abdominal sacrocolpopexy but is performed if indicated by another procedure (e.g. Burch procedure, paravaginal repair, etc.). Posterior colpoperineorrhaphy is performed at this time if a posterior vaginal defect not addressed by the mesh is suspected, or if the perineal body needs to be reconstructed.

The hospital postoperative course is usually uneventful. Pain is controlled with intravenous medication until clear liquids are tolerated. Clear liquids are started as

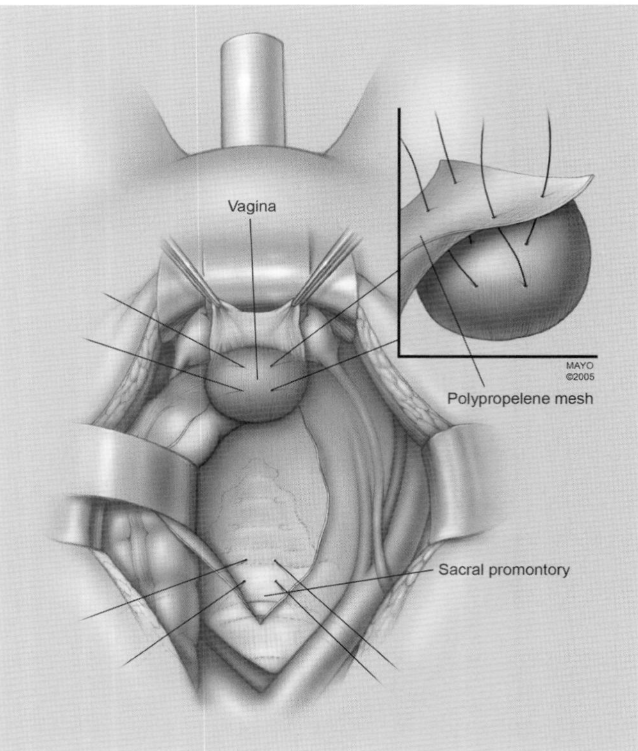

Figure 74.4. *Arial view of the pelvis with sutures noted at the vaginal apex and 1–2 cm below the sacral promontory (mesh not attached). Inset: sutures are placed through the mesh with a Mayo needle. (Reproduced with permission from the Mayo Foundation for Medical Education and Research.)*

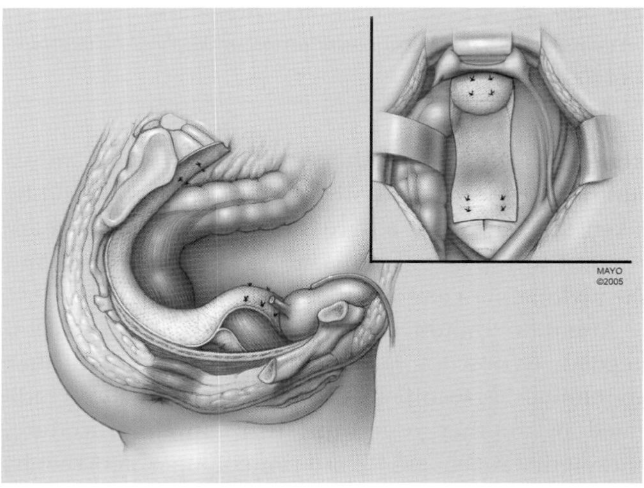

Figure 74.5. *Sagittal view of the pelvis showing attached Y-shaped mesh extending posteriorly and anteriorly along the vagina and attached to the sacrum. The lack of tension on the mesh is noted. (Reproduced with permission from the Mayo Foundation for Medical Education and Research.)*

soon as the patient desires and the diet is advanced as soon as liquids are tolerated. The patient has their Foley catheter removed the next day unless dictated otherwise by another procedure. The typical hospital stay is 2–3 days.

Patients are discharged home with instructions to avoid excessively increasing intra-abdominal pressure (due to heavy lifting or straining) or having anything in the vagina for 6 weeks. Estrogen is not prescribed regularly but is used for symptoms like hot flashes or vaginal dryness. All patients are re-examined 6 weeks after surgery and treated as needed.

RESULTS AND COMPLICATIONS

Many studies have evaluated the success of abdominal sacrocolpopexy. These studies vary in their surgical technique, patient population, definition of success, and length of follow-up. When looking at anatomic success in terms of apical support, success ranges from 78 to 100%; those looking at satisfaction or complete relief of symptoms reported 85–100% success.[9] Studies looking at the durability of the procedure found success rates of 74–91% an average 10–14 years after the procedure.[22,23]

Failures after abdominal sacrocolpopexy typically occur in other compartments. The failure rate in the posterior compartment has been noted in up to 57% of subjects in one study, even when attempts were made to extend the mesh along the posterior vagina.[24] The anterior compartment can be equally problematic with one study noting anatomic failures in 29% of subjects.[25] The surgeon should be aware that sacrocolpopexy is effective and durable for apical support but other compartments may require additional surgeries due to subsequent failure. Further studies are needed to address how to repair all compartment defects optimally at one time.

Abdominal sacrocolpopexy appears to be more effective for vault prolapse when compared to vaginal sacrospinous suspension. Benson et al.[26] were the first to compare sacrocolpopexy to bilateral sacrospinous vault suspension in a randomized trial consisting of 88 subjects. In this trial, with a mean 2.5-year follow-up, the vaginal group had a higher number of unsatisfactory outcomes than the abdominal group (33% versus 16%) and surgical failures were noted 11 months sooner in the vaginal group than the abdominal group (mean 11.2 versus 22.1 months). Lo and Wang[27] randomized 138 women to unilateral sacrospinous ligament suspension or abdominal sacrocolpopexy. Patients were followed for 2.1 years after surgery and there were more optimal surgical results in the abdominal group (94.2%) than in the vaginal group (80.3%). Finally, Maher et al.[28]

randomized 95 subjects to abdominal sacrocolpopexy versus sacrospinous ligament suspension. At the end of the 2-year follow-up period, patients' symptoms and anatomic success were equivalent. However, the vaginal group had a higher percentage of failures extending to the introitus (17% versus 4%) and postoperative cystoceles (14% versus 7%).

In addition to success and failure, it is important to discuss with patients the possible immediate and long-term postoperative complications associated with abdominal sacrocolpopexy. The intra- and postoperative complications as presented by Nygaard et al.[9] in their thorough review of the literature on abdominal sacrocolpopexy are presented in Table 74.1.

The incidence of mesh erosion varies depending on which mesh is used in the procedure and how it is placed. The overall rate of 3.4% has been reported in the literature.[9] Typically, erosion occurs within the first 2 years after surgery but may occur many years later.[29] The lowest rate of erosion is noted in autologous or cadaveric fascia (0%) and the highest rates are noted in Teflon and polyethylene mesh (5%).[9] Placement of mesh via a combined vaginal–abdominal sacral colpoperineopexy has a prohibitively high rate (40%) of erosion.[29]

The ideal mesh should be biocompatible, inert, hypoallergenic, sterile, resistant to mechanical stress or shrinkage, convenient, and affordable[30] – the ideal mesh is currently not available! Autologous fascia has no risk of erosion but takes longer to harvest and has associated morbidities with harvesting that make it unattractive. Freeze-dried cadaveric fascia has been found to have a high rate of failure (83%) due to autolysis.[31] Of the synthetic mesh types available, we feel that a macroporous polypropylene mesh is currently the best option. Studies have found that it has the lowest rate of erosion (0.5%) next to autologous fascia.[9]

Table 74.1. *Complication rates*

Complication	Percentage
Intraoperative	
Cystotomy	3.1
Enterotomy or proctotomy	1.6
Ureteral injury	1.0
Hemorrhage or transfusion or both	4.4
Postoperative	
Urinary tract infection	10.9
Wound problems	4.6
Postoperative ileus	3.6
Deep venous thrombus or pulmonary embolus	3.3
Small bowel obstruction	1.1

Data from ref. 9.

The ability to reduce the risk of mesh erosion depends on preoperative planning and intraoperative technique.[32] Vaginal health should be optimized as indicated by the vaginal skin prior to the procedure. Thin vaginal mucosa may require a period of estrogen cream to help increase tissue strength. Erosive lesions of vaginal epithelium secondary to pessary use should be allowed to heal prior to surgery. Proper technique of placement of the mesh includes using one that has a good track record of minimal mesh erosion. The mesh should be attached to a healthy fibromuscular layer of vaginal tissue; if this is not available then an intervening layer of dermal allograft should be considered to add strength to the tissue. Minimal tension should be placed on the mesh and reperitonealization should be performed.

If mesh erosion occurs after abdominal sacrocolpopexy it can typically be dealt with conservatively. This includes trimming the visible mesh, cauterizing granulation tissue and applying estrogen cream. If resolution of the erosion does not occur, then surgical removal of the mesh can be accomplished via a vaginal, laparoscopic or abdominal route. Typically, the prolapse will not fail after the mesh has been removed. After mesh removal, allowing the sinus tract to drain into the vagina and heal by secondary intention may facilitate a better recovery.[32]

CONCLUSION

Abdominal sacrocolpopexy is a procedure that has continued to evolve since Lane first proposed using a suspensory bridge to support the vaginal apex by attaching it to the sacrum. Surgeons have taken minimally invasive technologies and applied them to the technique of sacrocolpopexy. Nezhat et al.[33] reported the first case series in 1994 and since that time several small case series have followed. The largest series of 83 patients noted that six subjects required a conversion to laparotomy, and at 12 months 62/63 (94%) noted no evidence of recurrent prolapse.[34] The laparoscopic approach is reported to shorten hospitalization, decrease pain, and decrease time to return to normal activities. However, this approach requires advanced laparoscopic training, a skilled laparoscopic assistant, and increased operating room time. Recently, robotic laparoscopic surgery has been used in an effort to overcome the technical skill required for regular laparoscopic surgery.[35] Although promising, the minimally invasive approach to sacrocolpopexy needs further exploration and study to compare its success and complication rate to the open approach.

Abdominal sacrocolpopexy is an effective and durable surgery for the treatment of vaginal vault prolapse. To perform this procedure safely and effectively, knowledge of pelvic anatomy and surgical technique are required. Possible complications after the procedure must be recognized and addressed to minimize the morbidity to the patient. As our understanding of the pathophysiology of prolapse increases and new surgical technologies arise, the technique of abdominal sacrocolpopexy will continue to evolve.

REFERENCES

1. Nygaard I, Bradley C, Brandt D. Pelvic organ prolapse in older women: prevalence and risk factors. Obstet Gynecol 2004;104:489–97.
2. Farquhar CM, Steinar CA. Hysterectomy rates in the United States 1990–1997. Obstet Gynecol 2002;99:229–34.
3. Mant J, Painter R, Vessey M. Epidemiology of genital prolapse: observations from the Oxford Family Planning Association study. Br J Obstet Gynaecol 1997;104:579–85.
4. Boyles SH, Weber AM, Meyn L. Procedures for pelvic organ prolapse in the United States, 1979–1997. Am J Obstet Gynecol 2003;188:108–15.
5. Olsen AL, Smith VJ, Bergstrom JO et al. Epidemiology of surgically managed pelvic organ prolapse and urinary incontinence. Obstet Gynecol 1997;89:501–6.
6. Luber KM, Boero S, Choe JY. The demographics of pelvic floor disorders: current observations and future projections. Am J Obstet Gynecol 2001;184:1496–501; discussion 1501–3.
7. Lane FE. Repair of posthysterectomy vaginal-vault prolapse. Obstet Gynecol 1962;20:72–7.
8. Timmons MC, Addison WA, Addison SB et al. Abdominal sacral colpopexy in 163 women with posthysterectomy vaginal vault prolapse and enterocele: evolution of operative techniques. J Reprod Med 1992;37:323–7.
9. Nygaard IE, McCreery R, Burbaker L et al. Abdominal sacrocolpopexy: a comprehensive review. Obstet Gynecol 2004;104:805–23.
10. Fornell EU, Wingren G, Kjolhede P. Factors associated with pelvic floor dysfunction with emphasis on urinary and fecal incontinence and genital prolapse: an epidemiological study. Acta Obstet Gynecol Scand 2004;83:383–9.
11. Norton PA. Pelvic floor disorders: the role of fascia and ligaments. Clin Obstet Gynecol 1993;36:926–38.
12. DeLancey JO. Anatomic aspects of vaginal eversion after hysterectomy. Am J Obstet Gynecol 166:1992;1717–28.
13. American College of Obstetricians and Gynecologists. Pelvic organ prolapse. ACOG Technical Bulletin 214. Washington, DC: ACOG, 1995.
14. Ellerkamann RM, Cundiff GW, Melick CF et al. Correlation of symptoms with location and severity of pelvic organ prolapse. Am J Obstet Gynecol 2001;185:1332–8.
15. Burrows LJ, Meyn LA, Walters MD et al. Pelvic symptoms in women with pelvic organ prolapse. Obstet Gynecol 2004;104:982–8.
16. Bump RC, Mattiasson A, Bo K et al. The standardization of terminology of female pelvic organ prolapse and pelvic organ dysfunction. Am J Obstet Gynecol 1996;175:10–7.
17. Silva WA, Kleeman S, Segal J et al. Effects of a full bladder and patient positioning on pelvic organ prolapse assessment. Obstet Gynecol 2004;104:37–41.
18. Gallentine ML, Cespedes RD. Occult stress urinary incontinence and the effect of vaginal vault prolapse on abdominal leak point pressures. Urology 2001;57:40–4.
19. Bergman A, Koonings PP, Baddard CA. Predicting postoperative urinary incontinence development in women undergoing operation for genitourinary prolapse. Am J Obstet Gynecol 1988;158:1171–5.
20. Sutton GP, Addison WA, Livengood CH III et al. Life-threatening hemorrhage complicating sacral colpopexy. Am J Obstet Gynecol 1981;140:836–7.
21. Addison WA, Livengood CH, Sutton GP et al. Abdominal sacral colpopexy with mersilene mesh in the retroperitoneal position in the management of posthysterectomy vaginal vault prolapse and enterocele. Am J Obstet Gynecol 1985;153:140–6.
22. Hilger WS, Poulson M, Norton PA. Long-term results of abdominal sacrocolpopexy. Am J Obstet Gynecol 2003;189:1606–10.
23. Lefranc JP, Atallah D, Camatte S et al. Long-term follow-up of posthysterectomy vaginal vault prolapse abdominal repair: a report of 85 cases. J Am Coll Surg 2002;195:352–8.
24. Baessler K, Schuessler B. Abdominal sacrocolpopexy and anatomy and function of the posterior compartment. Obstet Gynecol 2001;97:678–84.
25. Brubaker L. Sacrocolpopexy and the anterior compartment: support and function. Am J Obstet Gynecol 1995;173:1690–6.
26. Benson JT, Lucente V, McClellan E. Vaginal versus abdominal reconstructive surgery for the treatment of pelvic support defects: a prospective randomized study with long-term outcome evaluation. Am J Obstet Gynecol 1996;175:1418–22.
27. Lo T-S, Wang AC. Abdominal colposacropexy and sacrospinous ligament suspension for severe uterovaginal prolapse: a comparison. J Gynecol Surg 1998;14:59–64.
28. Maher CF, Qatawneh AM, Dwyer PL et al. Abdominal sacrocolpopexy or vaginal sacrospinous colpopexy for vaginal vault prolapse: a prospective randomized study. Am J Obstet Gynecol 2004;190:20–6.

29. Visco AG, Weidner AC, Barber MD et al. Vaginal mesh erosion after abdominal sacral colpopexy. Am J Obstet Gynecol 2001;184:297–302.

30. Birch C, Fynes MM. The role of synthetic and biological prostheses in reconstructive pelvic floor surgery. Curr Opin Obstet Gynecol 2002;14:527–35.

31. Fitzgerald MP, Edwards SR, Fenner D. Medium-term follow-up on use of freeze-dried, irradiated donor fascia for sacrocolpopexy and sling procedures. Int Urogynecol J Pelvic Floor Dysfunct 2004;15(4):238–42.

32. Hurt WG. Abdominal sacral colpopexies complicated by vaginal graft extrusion. Obstet Gynecol 2004;103:1033–4.

33. Nezhat CH, Nezhat F, Nezhat C. Laparoscopic sacral colpopexy for vaginal vault prolapse. Obstet Gynecol 1994;84:885–8.

34. Cosson M, Bogaert E, Narducci F et al. Laparoscopic sacral colpopexy: short-term results and complications in 83 patients. J Gynecol Obstet Biol Reprod 2000;29:746–50.

35. Elliott DS, Frank I, DiMarco DS et al. Gynecologic use of robotically assisted laparoscopy: sacrocolpopexy for the treatment of high-grade vaginal vault prolapse. Am J Surg 2004;188:52S–56S.

75

Preservation of the prolapsed uterus

Vasiliki Varela, Adam Magos

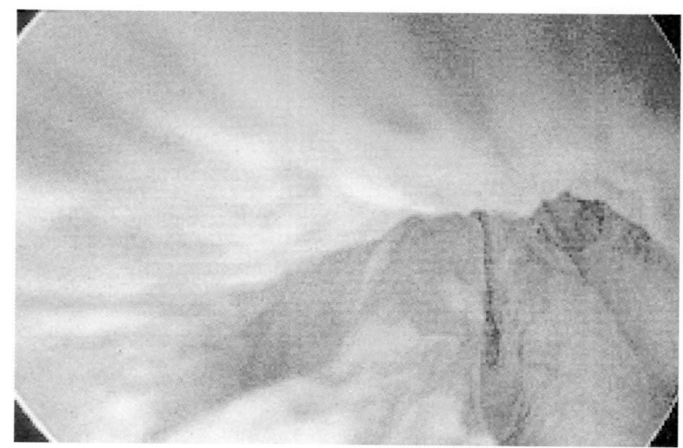

INTRODUCTION

Pelvic organ prolapse is a common condition and a major cause of gynecologic surgery. Women who reach 80 years of age have an 11% risk of undergoing at least one operation for this indication during their lifetime.[1] It is projected that the rate of women seeking treatment for pelvic floor disorders will double over the next 30 years.[2]

The pathogenesis of uterine prolapse is thought to be related to weakness of the supporting connective tissues of the pelvic structures, but is not fully understood. Pelvic floor dysfunction is a possible result of many contributing factors such as pregnancy, multiparity, labor, vaginal birth, obstetric trauma, chronic increased abdominal pressure, and the aging process.

Uterine prolapse can be managed in a number of different ways – some conservative, some radical. The choice of treatment is influenced by the age of the patient, the severity of the symptoms, the degree of prolapse, desire for maintenance (or not) of reproductive and sexual function, and general health. Therapeutic options range from observation, physiotherapy, and the use of vaginal pessaries to surgery, which often involves hysterectomy as part of the pelvic reconstructive process (Table 75.1).

There is an increasing recognition that uterine-preserving procedures have an important role in management. Uterine prolapse does not just affect elderly, postmenopausal women who have completed their family and who are therefore prepared to undergo hysterectomy as part of their treatment. For instance, a recent Swedish study found the prevalence of uterine prolapse to be 5% in women aged 20–59 years.[3] The successful surgical treatment of uterine prolapse when the uterus needs to be preserved is a challenging problem for the pelvic surgeon.

This chapter describes the indications for, and techniques and results of, surgery of prolapse if the uterus is to be maintained.

HISTORY

Uterine prolapse was first recorded on the Kahuun papyri in 2000 BC. Hippocrates described numerous non-surgical treatments for this condition. In AD 98, Soranus of Rome first described the removal of the prolapsed uterus when it became black. The first successful vaginal hysterectomy for the cure of uterine prolapse was self-performed by a peasant woman named Faith Raworth, as described by Willouby in 1670. In 1861, Sammuel Choppin of New Orleans performed the first vaginal hysterectomy under anesthesia and antiseptic conditions. From the early 1800s, other successful surgical procedures were introduced for the treatment of this condition. By the beginning of the 20th century, European and American reports of hysterectomy, colporrhaphy, cervical amputation, transposition/interposition operations, cervical ligament plications, colpocleisis, ventral fixation of the uterus to the abdominal wall, and trachelorrhaphy for procidentia were being published.

In the early 1900s, Bonney emphasized the passive role of the uterus in uterovaginal prolapse, and suggested uterine-preserving surgery.[4] Ross later described the pericervical fascia as the cornerstone of pelvic reconstruction, which is not always addressed during vaginal hysterectomy with anterior–posterior colporrhaphy.[5] Since then, many authors have reported their experiences with uterus-sparing pelvic reconstructive surgery.

INDICATION

The traditional procedure for uterovaginal prolapse has been vaginal hysterectomy together with an anterior and posterior colporrhaphy. Rationales for performing hysterectomy include the removal of a non-functional organ in postmenopausal women, the removal of any concomitant uterine or cervical pathology, as well as

Table 75.1. *Routes of surgery and procedures for uterine prolapse**

Route of surgery	Uterine sparing	Uterine non-sparing
Vaginal	Manchester procedure Uterosacral suspension/plication Sacrospinous fixation Le Fort and other colpocleisis	Vaginal hysterectomy ± culdoplasty ± sacrospinous fixation
Abdominal	Sacrohysteropexy/sacrocervicopexy Pectineal ligament suspension	Abdominal hysterectomy with sacrocolpopexy
Joint vaginal/abdominal	Retropubic suspension	–
Laparoscopic	Ventrosuspension Uterosacral ligament plication Hysteropexy with culdoplasty	Laparoscopic hysterectomy with sacrocolpopexy

* Can be combined with surgery for vaginal prolapse if indicated.

the long-term success of the surgery which can theoretically be compromised by leaving the uterus in situ. However, there is no evidence that hysterectomy affects the efficacy of incontinence surgery with complete pelvic floor reconstruction, or the durability of the repair.[6] In fact, it may increase the risk of pelvic neuropathy and disrupt natural support structures such as the uterosacral–cardinal ligament complex.[7] Some studies suggest that women who undergo hysterectomy may be at increased risk for de novo urinary incontinence, bladder dysfunction and prolapse, as well as increased blood loss, morbidity, and operative and postoperative recovery times.[8,9]

Recent randomized trials comparing subtotal (supracervical) with total hysterectomy came to the same conclusions. For instance, Thakar et al. reported no difference in urinary function or in any measures of bowel function between the two types of hysterectomy.[10] According to the authors, subtotal abdominal hysterectomy results in more rapid recovery and fewer short-term complications but neither subtotal nor total abdominal hysterectomy adversely affects pelvic organ function at 12 months postoperatively; however, it should be noted that patients with symptomatic uterine prolapse were not included in this study.

Another area of debate relates to the effect of hysterectomy on sexual well-being. The traditional view according to Masters and Johnson states that removal of the uterus may affect the patient's sexual and personal life as the uterus and cervix can have a significant role in orgasm and sexual function.[11] Again, data from prospective randomized trials have refuted this. The UK study quoted above also looked at measures of sexual function, including frequency of intercourse and orgasm, and found no significant change in either group after surgery.[10] Similarly, a recent randomized clinical trial conducted in Denmark, comparing total to subtotal abdominal hysterectomy regarding effects on sexuality, also showed that there were no statistically significant differences between the two operation methods.[12]

Considering all of the above, the aims of the surgical procedure should be to correct prolapse with the greatest efficacy, in both the short and long term, but with the least morbidity. Any intervention should have no adverse effect on sexual function and, especially in young women, preserve fertility. According to these criteria, uterine preservation warrants serious evaluation.

A variety of surgical techniques have been described in an attempt to satisfactorily correct uterine prolapse while preserving the uterus, including vaginal, abdominal, laparoscopic, and combined procedures.

SURGERY

Vaginal procedures

The traditional approach to the surgical management of uterovaginal prolapse is via the vagina. This route is considered less invasive than the other routes, with lower morbidity and faster recovery.

Manchester procedure

The Manchester procedure was originally described in 1888 by Archibald Donald of Manchester, England, and subsequently modified by Fothergill as an alternative to vaginal hysterectomy for the management of uterovaginal prolapse in patients with cervical elongation and intact, non-attenuated uterosacral–cardinal ligaments.

The procedure consists of:

1. amputation of the elongated and descended cervix;
2. plication and fixation of the cardinal ligaments in front of the residual cervix;
3. anterior colporrhaphy (posterior colporrhaphy can also be performed if necessary).

The operation begins with an anterior circumcision of the cervix at the level of the bladder sulcus. The anterior wall is divided and dissected off the bladder laterally, the supravaginal septum and the vesicouterine ligaments are divided, and the bladder is displaced upward. The cervix is then circumcised laterally and posteriorly, and the vagina is separated from the cervix. The entire bundle of tissue entering the cervix laterally, which includes the cardinal ligament and cervical branch of the uterine artery, is clamped, divided and suture ligated, and the cervix is amputated with a scalpel. The posterior cervix is covered with the vaginal wall with a Sturmdorf suture, and the cardinal ligaments are sewn to the anterior cervical stump using two Fothergill stitches (Fig. 75.1).[13] Finally, the bladder fascia is plicated as at anterior colporrhaphy, and the vagina is closed.

Many experts claim that the anatomic and functional results of the Manchester operation in suitable cases are good and comparable with those of hysterectomy, but with decreased morbidity and mortality. Studies in this area tend to be retrospective with all their inherent limitations. For instance, a report by Thomas et al. published in 1995 compared data from 88 consecutive Manchester procedures with 105 randomly selected vaginal hysterectomy patients;[14] anterior and/or posterior repairs were performed as indicated. All patients undergoing Manchester procedure or vaginal hysterectomy had uterine prolapse as the pri-

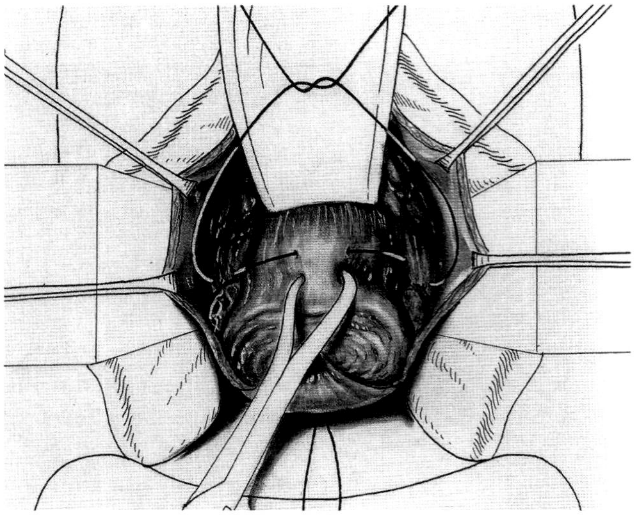

Figure 75.1. *Approximation of cardinal ligaments and posterior Sturmdorf suture at Manchester repair. (Reproduced from ref. 13 with permission.)*

mary indication for surgery. The Manchester patients were older (66 versus 52 years), and more likely to be menopausal (median 14.5 years versus 4 years from last period) and to have advanced prolapse. The median operating time was 100 minutes for the Manchester procedure compared with 130 minutes for vaginal hysterectomy, and the estimated blood loss was lower with the former (200 versus 300 ml). Postoperative cuff abscess or cellulitis occurred in 5% of hysterectomy patients but was not seen after the Manchester procedure. No other differences in postoperative complications were noted. Questionnaire follow-up of 67 patients an average of 2.5 years after Manchester repair revealed that four (6%) experienced recurrent prolapse, the time to recurrence ranging from 8 weeks to 5.5 years. Similar follow-up data for vaginal hysterectomy patients were not recorded.

A prior revue by Conger and Kettel in 1958 involving 960 Manchester procedures reported a prolapse recurrence rate of 4.3%;[15] however, this study was based on a questionnaire sent to patients with a response rate of only 52%.

The ability to conceive is preserved but reduced after the Manchester operation. Approximately one-third of women who desire children become pregnant after this procedure,[16] but the risks of spontaneous abortion and premature delivery are significantly increased as a consequence of cervical incompetence. The rate of cesarean section after the Manchester procedure is 20–50%. The rate of recurrent prolapse after delivery, even after prophylactic cesarean section, is high.

Uterosacral suspension/plication

In 1966, Williams described transvaginal uterosacral–cardinal ligament plication in 20 women ranging from 21 to 37 years of age with uterovaginal prolapse.[17] Eleven patients had uterovaginal prolapse up to 3 cm beyond the introitus, and nine had prolapse beyond this point. The mean parity of the patients was 2.9. The peritoneal cavity was entered via a posterior colpotomy. The uterosacral ligaments were identified and divided from the cervix, plicated across the midline and reinserted into the cervix. A transverse incision was made through the peritoneum between the cervix and the bladder and the cardinal ligaments were plicated across the midline. The plicating sutures were tied tightly and the cervix was drawn upward. In four cases additional procedures for the correction of cystocele, rectocele, and enterocele were concurrently performed. Postoperative complications occurred in five patients and included genitourinary tract infection in one, pelvic cellulites in two, atonic bladder in one, and vaginal bleeding in one patient who subsequently underwent a subtotal vaginal hysterectomy. Three patients (15.5%) experienced a recurrence of uterine prolapse within 6 months of surgery and were all treated with vaginal hysterectomy. Six patients subsequently had full-term pregnancies with no recurrence of prolapse. Williams found this procedure to have low morbidity and high success in women without marked vaginal relaxation. However, the undefined duration of follow-up, the small sample size, and the lack of a control group limit this study. As far as we are aware, no further data are available about this procedure.

Sacrospinous uterosacral fixation (sacrospinous hysteropexy)

Transvaginal sacrospinous ligament fixation is an established treatment for vaginal and uterovaginal prolapse, and is usually undertaken after or with vaginal hysterectomy.[18,19] As a result, data concerning this procedure combined with uterine conservation are relatively scant.

Richardson et al. described the use of this procedure in five women aged 24–31 years with uterine prolapse.[20] The rectovaginal space was entered via a posterior colpotomy and the uterosacral ligaments were identified. The right sacrospinous ligament was then exposed and attached to the uterosacral ligaments and posterior colporrhaphy completed. A Stamey or Pereyra procedure was performed concurrently for stress incontinence in four of the five patients. The follow-up period was 6–24 months, during which there were no recurrences of prolapse and no pregnancies reported. There are no data on preoperative evaluation of degree of uterine prolapse and no comment regarding patient comfort or the development of postoperative dyspareunia. Although this case series supports the concept of uterine preservation in the management of uterine prolapse, it is limited by its very small sample size and its lack of a control group.

Kovac and Cruikshank reported the results of transvaginal sacrospinous uterosacral ligament fixation in 19 women aged 17–37 years with uterovaginal prolapse.[21] Mean patient parity was 1.31 vaginal births (0–4). Eight patients (four parous and four nulliparous) had symptomatic moderate uterovaginal prolapse, and 11 (nine parous and two nulliparous) had severe uterovaginal prolapse. All patients had markedly attenuated but identifiable uterosacral ligaments on pelvic examination and all desired fertility. Four of these procedures were performed unilaterally to the right sacrospinous–coccygeal complex and 15 were performed bilaterally.

Ligament fixation was performed as follows:

1. The posterior vaginal wall was opened to the level of the cervix and the rectovaginal space entered.
2. The rectovaginal space was dissected bluntly to the level of the ischial spines.
3. The descending rectal septum was perforated, opening the pararectal space.
4. Further dissection exposed the uterosacral ligaments; these were grasped for identification, traction, and suture placement.
5. The right sacrospinous–coccygeus complex (for unilateral procedure) or both sacrospinous–coccygeal complexes (for bilateral procedures) were identified; sutures were placed to one side or to each sacrospinous ligament respectively, and then sewn to each uterosacral ligament to be tied (Figs 75.2, 75.3). The uterosacral sutures were tied within 1–2 cm of the cervical attachment of the uterosacral ligament.
6. Traction on the other end of the suture drew the uterosacral ligaments and cervix lateral and cephalad above the levator plate. A McCall culdoplasty was performed concurrently (Fig. 75.4). All sutures were left untied until additional adjunct procedures were completed; the sacrospinous uterosacral sutures were then tied.

In this series, there were no injuries to the bladder or nerves. In one case an accidental rectal perforation occurred which was repaired without sequelae. The average time for sacrospinous uterosacral fixation was 15 minutes, with an average blood loss of 75 ml (200 ml with adjunct procedures). The average hospital stay was 2.4 days and mean follow-up for all 19 patients was 3.1 years with two patients lost to follow-up. Eleven of the 12 patients who failed to conceive had good objective results and have retained excellent uterovaginal support, vaginal depth, and displayed no defect recurrence during follow-up. One patient returned for her 6 weeks

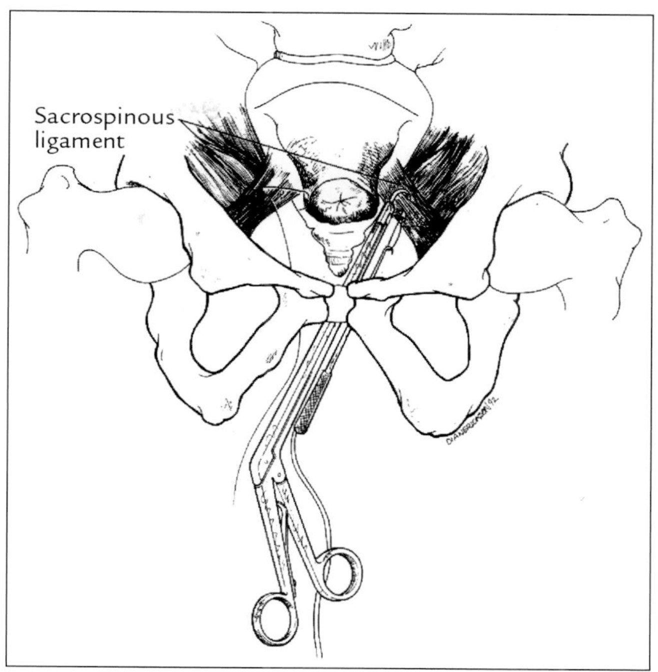

Figure 75.2. *Miya hook with sutures is placed through the sacrospinous ligament. (Reproduced from ref. 21 with permission.)*

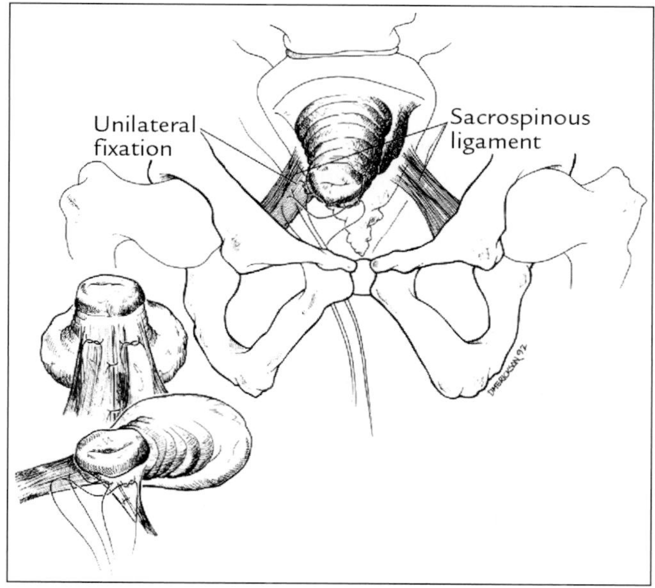

Figure 75.3. *Unilateral sacrospinous uterosacral fixation illustrating closure of the cul-de-sac. (Reproduced from ref. 21 with permission.)*

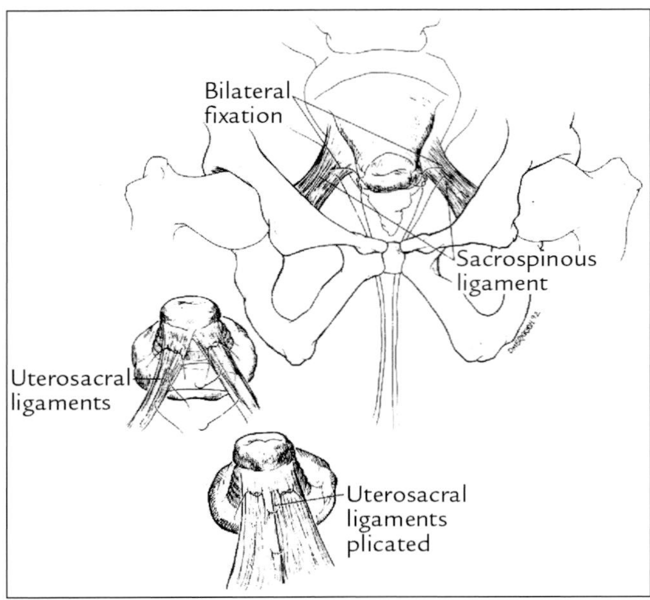

Figure 75.4. *Bilateral sacrospinous uterosacral fixation; uterosacral plication is also shown. (Reproduced from ref. 21 with permission.)*

postoperative visit with moderate uterovaginal prolapse and was cured after a second bilateral operation.

Five patients became pregnant, and all were delivered vaginally without incident; one patient has been delivered twice since the operation. This patient had moderate uterovaginal prolapse after her first delivery, and subsequent to her second vaginal delivery she had a vaginal hysterectomy. Since the original report, eight additional sacrospinous uterosacral fixations with three resultant vaginal deliveries have been reported. The authors feel that this procedure may be used to treat uterovaginal prolapse in parous and nulliparous women desiring uterine preservation or further childbearing. The procedure is less time consuming and has less morbidity than major abdominal surgery, is associated with minimal intra-abdominal manipulation, and avoids the longer recovery needed after a laparotomy. By performing uterosacral plication, enterocele formation is avoided, and vaginal depth, axis, and function are restored. However, pre- and postoperative assessments were not blinded, and subjective data were not routinely collected. In addition, this study is limited by its lack of a control group.

In 2001, Maher et al. reported the results of a retrospective study comparing sacrospinous hysteropexy and vaginal hysterectomy with sacrospinous fixation for symptomatic uterine prolapse.[22] Seventy women aged 23–87 years with symptomatic second or third degree uterovaginal prolapse were included in the study; 34 had a sacrospinous hysteropexy and 36 had a vaginal hysterectomy with sacrospinous vault fixation. All women underwent independent review and examination. The groups were similar in age, parity, body mass index, menopausal status, prior pelvic reconstructive surgical history, presence of stress incontinence, and degree of cervical prolapse. Mean follow-up was 26 months in the hysteropexy group and 33 months in the hysterectomy group, with seven patients in each group being lost to follow up.

The groups were assessed retrospectively for subjective outcomes via site-specific vaginal examinations. Women were independently evaluated by a non-surgical author blinded to the surgery performed. Data regarding operating time, intraoperative blood loss, transfusion requirement, thromboembolic events and full recovery time were also collected. The operating time in the hysteropexy group was 59 minutes compared to 91 minutes in the hysterectomy group ($p<0.01$). The mean intraoperative blood loss in the hysteropexy group was 198 ml compared to 402 ml in the hysterectomy group ($p<0.01$). No patients required blood transfusion or experienced thromboembolic events. The duration of hospitalization was also similar.

In terms of the correction of prolapse, there was no statistically significant difference in either the subjective or the objective success of the surgery. For instance, the subjective success rates were 78% in hysteropexy group and 86% in the hysterectomy group ($p=0.7$). The objective success rates were 74% and 72%, respectively ($p=1.0$). The patient-determined satisfaction rates were 85% and 86%, respectively ($p=1.0$). The authors concluded that vaginal hysterectomy may not be necessary in the surgical treatment of uterine prolapse, and that sacrospinous hysteropexy is an effective alternative in treating uterovaginal prolapse, with a decrease in both mean operating time and intraoperative blood loss.

Neugebauer–Le Fort procedure

For some patients, particularly elderly women who are not sexually active and/or suffer from severe medical illnesses, pelvic organ prolapse can be managed by surgically closing off the vagina, commonly referred to as the 'Le Fort' or 'Neugebauer–Le Fort' colpocleisis.[23,24]

The procedure is performed as follows:

1. A rectangular incision is made in the anterior vaginal wall, extending from 2 cm proximal to the tip of the cervix to 4–5 cm below the external urethral meatus.
2. The vaginal mucosa is undermined and freed with scissors in the area of the vesicovaginal tissue plane.
3. Plication of the bladder neck should be routinely performed because of the high incidence of postoperative stress incontinence.

4. An analogous area of vaginal tissue is excised from the posterior vaginal wall.
5. With the cervix pushed back with a sponge stick, the congruent edges of the incisions at the anterior and posterior vaginal walls are approximated with interrupted absorbable sutures.
6. The vesicovaginal and rectovaginal fasciae are approximated in a second layer and the uterus and vaginal apex are gradually turned inward (Fig. 75.5).
7. After the vagina has been inverted, the superior and inferior margins of the original vaginal incisions are sutured.
8. An aggressive perineorrhaphy should be performed to narrow the introitus.

The classic technique has been modified over the years:

- wider vaginal excision described by Wyatt in 1912;[25]
- pubocervical fascial plication before colpocleisis of Adair and DaSef in 1936;[26]
- excision of a triangular vaginal mucosa, creating a canal permitting sexual intercourse and decreasing the incidence of iatrogenic stress urinary incontinence described by Goodall and Power in 1937 (Fig. 75.6);[27]
- the conceptually similar Labhardt partial colpocleisis;[28]
- circular amputation of the cervix preceding the Le Fort suggested by Mazer and Israel in 1948;[29]
- the Doderlein crossbar colporrhaphy.[28]

In selected patients, total colpocleisis is an alternative to the other procedures which result in partial vaginal obliteration. The surgical procedure consists of stripping the vaginal mucosa from the underlying fascia, everting the uterovaginal prolapse up into the pelvis and suturing the vaginal cavity closed using either purse-string or interrupted anterior/posterior sutures in a stepwise fashion. This operation differs considerably from the Le Fort procedure, because complete vaginal obliteration is achieved.[30–32]

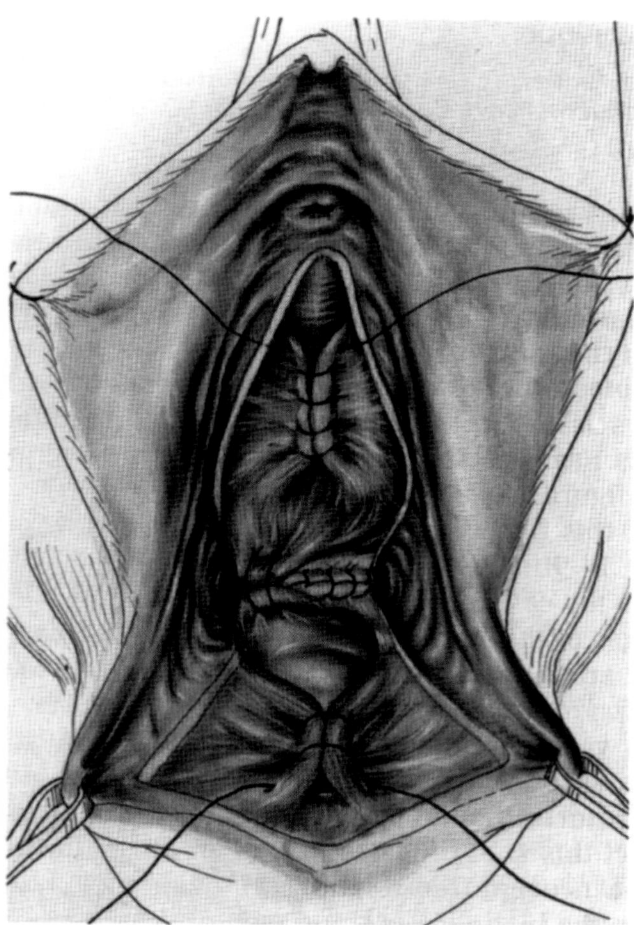

Figure 75.5. *Approximation of vesicovaginal and rectovaginal fascia during Le Fort operation. (Reproduced from ref. 13 with permission.)*

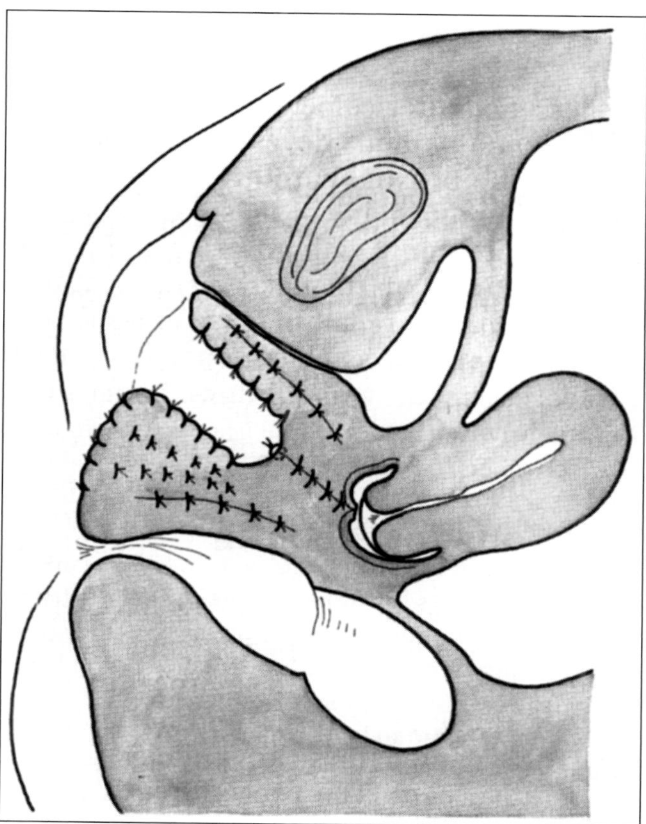

Figure 75.6. *Completed Le Fort operation showing position of sutures. (Reproduced from ref. 13 with permission.)*

Several recent studies have shown that the Le Fort colpocleisis and its modifications offer significant advantages in a select population of elderly, not sexually active or medically compromised patients, and represent a good treatment option when conservative management is not feasible.[33,34] However, colpocleisis is an obliterative procedure which in the main does not allow maintenance of sexual function and leaves little if any access to the uterus should disease of the uterus develop after the operation. With the advances in anesthesia, surgical techniques and perioperative care, these operations are now only rarely performed.

Abdominal procedures

Although the vaginal route for the surgical treatment of prolapsed uterus is considered less invasive, the abdominal approach offers a better and easier access to the peritoneal cavity, the pelvic structures and, especially, the sacrum and sacrospinous ligaments.

Sacrohysteropexy/sacrocervicopexy

The originators of this technique to support the vaginal vault and uterus include Stoesser[35] and Arthure and Savage.[36]

Stoesser described the results of transabdominal sacrocervicopexy in 22 women aged 18–44 years with uterovaginal prolapse and attenuated uterine support ligaments. His technique included the following steps:

1. Through an abdominal incision, a strip of external oblique fascia was excised; Stoesser initially used rectus sheath or abdominal scar derivatives to create sacrocervical ligaments, but found that the external abdominal oblique aponeurosis was superior.
2. The retroperitoneal space was entered via the posterior cul-de-sac. The strip of fascia was then used as a de novo sacrocervical ligament to join the posterior cervix to the sacral periosteum, providing support to the uterus.

Twenty-one of the 22 patients underwent concurrent surgical procedures, including myomectomy, resection of endometriosis, colporrhaphy, presacral neurotomy, and round ligament plication. Simultaneous round ligament plication was abandoned after the first 17 procedures as it was found to be insufficient.

Stoesser reported 'good' operative outcomes with no postoperative failures. There are no data on the baseline degree of uterine prolapse or any details on the pre- and postoperative assessment of the patients. Stoesser's case series supports the concept of uterine preservation in the treatment of uterovaginal prolapse but it is limited by its undefined duration of follow-up and its small sample size.

Practice has changed through the years to the use of synthetic materials to support the vaginal vault with or without the uterus. Various meshes (Gore-Tex, Teflon, polypropylene) and Mersilene suture have all been tried.

In 1997, Banu reported the results of sacrohysteropexy in 19 young women aged 17–27 years with uterine prolapse.[37] Through an abdominal approach, a Mersilene tape was fixed on the posterior surface of the uterus and anchored to the anterior longitudinal ligament over the sacral promontory. There were no significant intra- or postoperative complications and no recurrence was reported during the 3–5 year follow-up period.

Constantini et al. reported satisfactory results in seven patients with uterovaginal prolapse who underwent sacrohysteropexy with Gore-Tex mesh, although first degree cystocele recurred in three women during the 12–68 month follow-up period.[38]

In 2001, Leron and Stanton reported the results of sacrohysteropexy with Teflon mesh for the treatment of uterovaginal prolapse in 13 patients (mean age 38 years) who desired uterine preservation (Fig. 75.7).[39] Twelve women had second degree uterine prolapse and one woman had third degree prolapse. Mean follow-up time was 16 months (range 4–49 months) and only one woman had a recurrence of first degree uterine prolapse during that period.

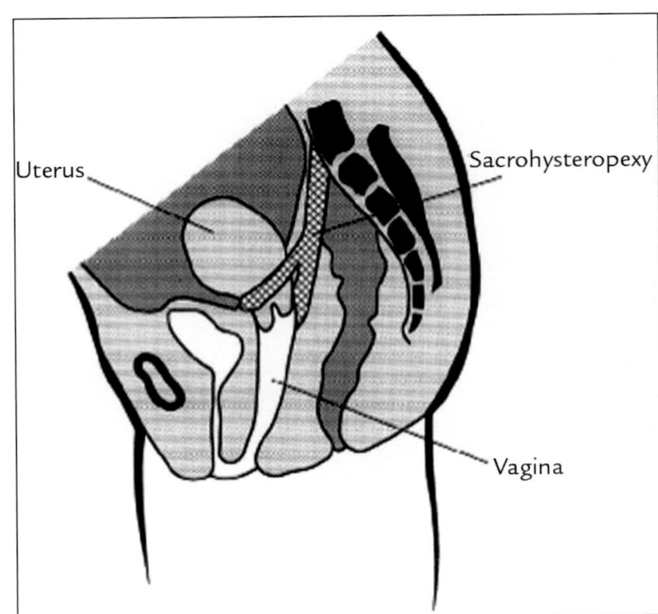

Figure 75.7. *Sacrohysteropexy using a synthetic mesh. (Reproduced from ref. 39 with permission.)*

Most recently, in 2003, Barranger et al. reported the results of abdominal hysteropexy carried out between 1987 and 1999 in 30 women of childbearing age with uterovaginal prolapse, who wanted uterine preservation.[40] Mean age was 35.7 years (range 29–33 years) and mean parity was 2.3 (1–5). Thirteen women had grade 2 uterovaginal prolapse and 17 had grade 3 prolapse. All patients were healthy and active and all of them wished to conserve their uterus and preserve their fertility. Three patients had undergone previous surgery that included Burch colposuspension and periurethral Teflon injection, posterior colporrhaphy and salpingectomy for ectopic pregnancy. Eleven patients (36.6%) were urinary continent but the remainder had some type of urinary incontinence.

Abdominal sacrohysteropexy was performed under general anesthesia. The peritoneal cavity was entered through a Pfannenstiel or midline infraumbilical incision. Thereafter, the technique was as follows:

1. A transverse incision was made through the peritoneum between the uterus and the bladder.
2. The bladder was mobilized and a polyester fiber mesh was attached to the anterior vaginal wall and passed through the right and the left broad ligaments next to the uterus.
3. After the rectum was mobilized from the vaginal wall, another polyester mesh was attached to the posterior vaginal wall.
4. An incision was made in the posterior peritoneum over the sacral promontory, which extended inferiorly along the right lateral aspect of the rectum. The anterior and posterior meshes were then attached to the ligaments with two non-absorbable sutures in such a way that the vagina and the uterus were elevated without tension.
5. The peritoneal incision over the anterior vaginal wall was closed transversally.

A Burch procedure and posterior colporrhaphy were performed in all cases of sacrohysteropexy. Intraoperative and early postoperative complications occurred in two (6.6%) and four patients (13.3%), respectively. The average hospital stay was 7 days (range 6–9 days). The mean objective and subjective follow-up periods were 44.5 months (range 2–156 months) and 94.6 months (range 8–160 months), respectively. Follow-up consisted of a history, physical examination, and urodynamic study. The same questions were asked before and after the operation to assess symptoms. To assess subjective results an independent party asked the patients by phone to answer a questionnaire about symptoms of recurrent uterovaginal prolapse, constipation, dyspareunia, symptoms of urinary incontinence, and reproductive performance. With regard to pregnancy, an assessment was made concerning their number and their outcome. The pelvic floor support was evaluated and categorized as cured (grade 0 or 1 uterovaginal prolapse, asymptomatic) or failed (grade 2–4 uterovaginal prolapse, symptoms of recurrent uterovaginal prolapse or recurrent prolapse surgery).

At the time of the last physical examination, there were two cases of recurrent uterovaginal prolapse (6.6%) of which one was symptomatic and required repeat surgical treatment. At the time of the last questionnaire, apart from the patient who underwent repeat surgery, no patients had any uterovaginal prolapse symptoms. Three women had pregnancies that were conceived spontaneously, which led to three early legal abortions. The authors concluded that, although abdominal sacrohysteropexy is a more invasive procedure than the vaginal approach, it is safe and effective in the treatment of uterovaginal prolapse in women of childbearing age. The long-term results were excellent in the correction of prolapse without a time-dependent decrease in efficiency. It was, however, difficult to draw a conclusion about reproductive performance as well as continued uterovaginal support after pregnancy and delivery in this study.

Pectineal ligament suspension

In 1993, Joshi described a new technique of uterine suspension to the pectineal ligaments as an alternative to traditional procedures in 20 women who averaged 27.5 years of age (range 17–32 years).[41] Utilizing a wide Cherney incision, the procedure involved the following steps:

1. The abdomen and subsequently the retropubic space are entered.
2. The uterus is pulled up and the peritoneum incised transversely at the level of the internal cervical os.
3. A Mersilene tape measuring 30×0.5 cm is anchored at its midpoint to the anterior wall of the uterus, just above the level of the internal os.
4. The retropubic space is developed and the pectineal ligaments on either side are cleared of loose areolar tissue as laterally as possible.
5. A long artery forceps is passed subperitoneally from the retropubic space, just below the lateral end of the round ligament toward the lateral edge of the peritoneal incision over the uterus to grasp the lateral end of the Mersilene tape; the lateral end of the tape is drawn to the retropubic space and the procedure is repeated on the other side.

6. The visceral peritoneum is closed, keeping the tape outside the peritoneum.
7. The lateral end of the Mersilene tape is passed through an adequate thickness of the pectineal ligament on each side as laterally as possible. The two ends of the tape are drawn to elevate the uterus and are anchored to the pectineal ligaments using three to four firm knots of the tape.
8. The knots are fixed with sutures to prevent loosening, and the excess portion of the tape is cut off.

A simultaneous Burch colposuspension was performed in five patients, posterior colporrhaphy in three, anterior colporrhaphy in one, and Moschcowitz culdoplasty in one case. There were no intra- or postoperative complications reported and no early or late morbidity during the follow-up period of 6–30 months. Of nine women desiring further childbearing, seven conceived within 6 months of surgery; at the time this case series was initially reported, five had an uneventful vaginal delivery at term and the other two had continuing normal gestations. There was no recurrence of prolapse at 6 weeks postpartum in any of the women.

According to the author, suspension of the uterus from strong ligaments such as the pectineal ligaments minimizes the chance of prolapse recurrence and the procedure requires only minimal dissection in an area distant from important structures; therefore it may be considered a simple, safe and effective treatment for uterine prolapse in young women. However, it is acknowledged that the sample size of the study was small with limited duration of follow-up and, even now, further evaluation is awaited.

Combined procedures

Uterovaginal prolapse is often associated with stress urinary incontinence. A combined vaginoabdominal procedure may restore both the pelvic anatomy and urinary continence without the need for hysterectomy and extensive dissection and plications of the anterior vaginal wall.

Retropubic suspension

In 1989, Nesbitt described a new operative approach designed to correct uterovaginal prolapse as well as stress urinary incontinence while preserving the uterus.[42] It consisted of a combined vaginoabdominal retropubic ventral suspension of both the uterine isthmus and the vesical neck:

1. First, the vesical neck, paraurethral tissues, uterine isthmus and uterosacral–cardinal ligament complex are mobilized transvaginally.
2. Sutures are placed at the uterosacral–cardinal ligaments bilaterally and the suture ends are left long and tagged.
3. The retropubic spaces are entered with gentle digital dissections.
4. Suspensory sutures are placed in the endopelvic fascia and vaginal wall lateral to the bladder neck, three on each side.
5. A Moschcowitz-type culdoplasty is performed.
6. The suspensory sutures are retrieved through a transverse suprapubic incision, and the paraurethral endopelvic fascia and the uterosacral–cardinal ligaments are suspended from Cooper's ligaments.

The operation was performed on 16 patients aged 30–80 years, seven of whom had previously undergone up to three anti-incontinence procedures. The follow-up period was 5 years or longer, during which time no significant postoperative complications or recurrences of symptomatic uterine prolapse or stress incontinence were reported. Although the results of the study are limited by the small sample size and the lack of controls, the author felt that this procedure was simple, conservative, and effective, and could safely be performed as an alternative to the traditional vaginal hysterectomy with anterior/posterior colporrhaphy.

Laparoscopic procedures

With modern innovations in minimally invasive surgery, several laparoscopic procedures have been described for the treatment of uterine prolapse with uterine preservation and these are addressed later in the book. Suffice to say, that some very simple laparoscopic techniques have been tried as well as those that try to reproduce complex abdominal procedures. However successful some of these operations prove to be in the short term, even the keenest laparoscopic surgeon has to admit that long-term data are currently not available.

CONCLUSION

The traditional surgical treatment for uterovaginal prolapse has long been vaginal hysterectomy with an anterior/posterior colporrhaphy. However, women who wish to preserve their fertility may desire uterine preservation. Furthermore, hysterectomy may not be necessary in the surgical correction of uterovaginal prolapse and may serve to increase the morbidity of the surgical procedure and cause psychological misgivings.

The idea of uterine preservation at prolapse surgery is not new. The Manchester procedure, one of the earlier surgical options for the treatment of uterovaginal prolapse, is an attractive option but is limited by the postoperative decrease in fertility and the high rates of pregnancy wastage and recurrence of prolapse. As a result, the search has continued for alternative uterine-preserving procedures and now the gynecologist has a choice of several vaginal, abdominal, combined vagino-abdominal, and laparoscopic techniques. These reconstructive operations aim to correct prolapse, maintain urinary and fecal continence, and preserve coital and childbearing function. As a result of our better understanding of the anatomy of the pelvis, its supports and attachments, modern surgical techniques have evolved to be site specific.

The question remains as to which patients are suitable candidates for uterine preservation and which procedure is the ideal for a given patient. There is a paucity of information available on the efficacy of the uterus-sparing procedures and there are few if any comparative studies of pelvic floor reconstruction with and without hysterectomy. In order to routinely recommend uterine preservation at the time of uterovaginal prolapse surgery, studies with more patients, objective evaluation techniques, control subjects and longer follow-up are necessary. However, the current literature suggests that pelvic floor reconstruction with uterine preservation is feasible and safe and may be considered by the pelvic surgeon for selected women who desire it.

REFERENCES

1. Olsen AL, Smith VJ, Bergstrom JO et al. Epidemiology of surgically managed pelvic organ prolapse and urinary incontinence. Obstet Gynecol 1997;89:501–6.
2. Luber KM, Boero S, Choe JY. The demographics of pelvic floor disorders: current observations and future projections. Am J Obstet Gynecol 2001;184:1496–1501.
3. Samuelsson EC, Victor FTA, Tibblin G et al. Five-year incidence and remission rates of female urinary incontinence in a Swedish population less than 65 years old. Am J Obstet Gynecol 2000;183:568–74.
4. Bonney V. The principles that should underline all operations for prolapse. J Obstet Gynaecol Br Emp 1934;41:669–83.
5. Ross JW. Apical vault repair, the cornerstone of pelvic vault reconstruction. Int Urogynecol J 1997;8:146–52.
6. Langer R, Ron-El R, Neuman M et al. The value of simultaneous hysterectomy during Burch colposuspension for urinary stress incontinence. Obstet Gynecol 1988;72:866–9.
7. Nesbitt RE Jr. Uterine preservation in the surgical management of genuine stress urinary incontinence associated with uterovaginal prolapse. Surg Gynecol Obstet 1989;168:143–7.
8. Kjerluff KH, Langenberg PW, Greenaway L et al. Urinary incontinence and hysterectomy in a large prospective cohort study in American women. J Urol 2002;167:2088–92.
9. Petros PE. Influence of hysterectomy on pelvic-floor dysfunction. Lancet 2000;356:1275.
10. Thakar R, Ayers S, Clarkson P et al. Outcomes after total versus subtotal abdominal hysterectomy. N Engl J Med 2002;347:1318–25.
11. Masters WH, Johnson VE. Human Sexual Response. Boston: Little, Brown, 1966.
12. Zobbe V, Gimbel H, Andersen MA et al. Sexuality after total vs. subtotal hysterectomy. Acta Obstet Gynecol Scand 2004;83:191–6.
13. Hirsch HA, Kaser O, Ikle FA. Atlas of Gynecologic Surgery, 3rd ed. Stuttgart: Thieme, 1997.
14. Thomas AG, Brodman ML, Dottino PR et al. Manchester procedure vs. vaginal hysterectomy for uterine prolapse. J Reprod Med 1995;40:299–304.
15. Conger GT, Kettel WC. The Manchester–Fothergill operation: its place in gynecology. Am J Obstet Gynecol 1958;76:634–40.
16. Taylor RW. Pregnancy after pelvic floor repair. Am J Obstet Gynecol 1966;94:35–9.
17. Williams BF. Surgical treatment for uterine prolapse in young women. Am J Obstet Gynecol 1966;95:967–71.
18. Randall CL, Nichols DH. Surgical treatment of vaginal inversion. Obstet Gynecol 1971;38:327–32.
19. Cruikshank SH, Cox DW. Sacrospinous fixation at the time of transvaginal hysterectomy. Am J Obstet Gynecol 1990;162:1611–19.
20. Richardson DA, Scotti RJ, Ostergard DR. Surgical management of uterine prolapse in young women. J Reprod Med 1989;34:388–92.
21. Kovac RS, Cruikshank SH. Successful pregnancies and vaginal deliveries after sacrospinous uterosacral fixation in five of nineteen patients. Am J Obstet Gynecol 1993;168:1778–86.
22. Maher CF, Cary MP, Slack MC et al. Uterine preservation or hysterectomy at sacrospinous colpopexy for uterovaginal prolapse? Int Urogynecol J 2001;12:381–5.
23. Le Fort L. Nouveau procede pour la guerison du prolapsus uterin. Bull Gen Ther 1887;92:337.
24. Neugebauer LA. Einige Worte uber die mediane Vaginal-

naht als Mittel zur Beseitigung des Gebarmuttervorfalls. Zbl Gynakol 1881;5:25.

25. Wyatt J. Le Fort's operation for prolapse with an account of eight cases. J Obstet Gynaecol Br Emp 1912;22:266.
26. Adair F, DaSef L. The Le Fort colpocleisis. Am J Obstet Gynecol 1936;32:218–26.
27. Goodall J, Power R. A modification of the Le Fort operation for increasing its scope. Am J Obstet Gynecol 1937;34:968–76.
28. Reiffenstuhl G, Platzer W, Knapstein PG. Vaginal Operations. Surgical Anatomy and Technique, 2nd ed. Baltimore: Williams and Wilkins, 1996; 161–75.
29. Mazer C, Israel S. The Le Fort colpocleisis: an analysis of 43 operations. Am J Obstet Gynecol 1948;56:944–9.
30. Nichols DH, Randall CL. Vaginal Surgery, 4th ed. Baltimore: Williams and Wilkins, 1996.
31. Adams HD. Total colpocleisis for pelvic eventeration. Surg Gynecol Obstet 1951;92:321–4.
32. Morley GW. Treatment of uterine and vaginal prolapse. Clin Obstet Gynecol 1996;39:959–69.
33. Neimark M, Davila GW, Kopka SL. Le Fort colpocleisis: a feasible treatment option for pelvic organ prolapse in the elderly woman. J Pelvic Med Surg 2003;9:83–9.
34. Denehy TR, Choe JY, Gregori CA et al. Modified Le Fort colpocleisis with Kelly urethral plication and posterior colpoperineoplasty in the medically compromised elderly: a comparison with vaginal hysterectomy, anterior colporrhaphy, and posterior colpoperineoplasty. Am J Obstet Gynecol 1995;173:1697–1702.
35. Stoesser FG. Construction of a sacrocervical ligament for uterine suspension. Surg Gynecol Obstet 1955;101:638–41.
36. Arthure HGE, Savage D. Uterine prolapse and prolapse of the vaginal vault treated by sacral hysteropexy. J Obstet Gynaecol Br Emp 1957;64:355–60.
37. Banu LF. Synthetic sling for genital prolapse in young women. Int J Gynecol Obstet 1997;57:57–64.
38. Constantini E, Lombi R, Micheli C et al. Colposacropexy with Gore-tex mesh in marked vaginal and uterovaginal prolapse. Eur Urol 1998;34:111–17.
39. Leron E, Stanton SL. Sacrohysteropexy with synthetic mesh for the management of uterovaginal prolapse. Br J Obstet Gynaecol 2001;108:629–33.
40. Barranger E, Fritel X, Pigne A. Abdominal sacrohysteropexy in young women with uterovaginal prolapse: long-term follow-up. Am J Obstet Gynecol 2003;189:1245–50.
41. Joshi VM. A new technique of uterine suspension to pectineal ligaments in the management of uterovaginal prolapse. Obstet Gynecol 1993;81:790–3.
42. Nesbitt RE. Uterine preservation in the surgical management of genuine stress urinary incontinence associated with uterine prolapse. Surg Gynecol Obstet 1989;168:143–7.

76

Urinary incontinence following prolapse surgery

Brigitte Fatton, Bernard Jacquetin, Rufus Cartwright

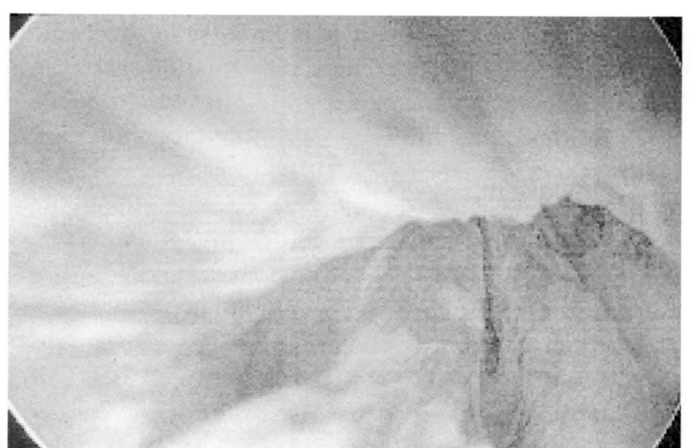

INTRODUCTION

The development or persistence of urinary incontinence following surgery for urogenital prolapse remains a problem for all urogynecologists and female urologists. Although the quoted risk varies widely between different authors and different case series,[1–7] recent publications have estimated rates of between 11%[8] and 28%.[3]

A recent prospective epidemiologic study[9] reported a 7.5% rate of surgery for stress urinary incontinence following 'successful' prolapse surgery at 5-year follow up. This is clearly an underestimate as few patients actually present for repeat surgery in these circumstances. Minimally invasive techniques such as midurethral tension-free slings may present a simple solution for postoperative stress urinary incontinence following prolapse surgery. However, even an appropriately counseled patient following skilled surgery will regard the original operation as being unsuccessful if they subsequently develop urinary incontinence which was not a pre-existing problem for them. It is therefore important to try to identify those patients who are at risk of stress urinary incontinence following surgery for urogenital prolapse and to evaluate any possible preventive measures. This type of screening is difficult and it is inappropriate to develop a wholesale preventive approach as this can cause unacceptable morbidity for uncertain benefit. Based on a review of the literature, the authors wish to propose a rational management pathway.

DEFINITIONS

The concepts of 'masked' and 'potential' in urinary incontinence are frequently confused. This explains the discrepancies between some studies. In the English literature the terms 'potential', 'occult', 'masked', 'latent', and 'iatrogenic' appear to be used interchangeably to describe stress urinary incontinence that develops following prolapse surgery in a previously continent patient. Classic 'masked' incontinence is labeled as 'potential' incontinence, even though it is impossible to predict the latter preoperatively. These two situations are completely different, with separate pathophysiologic mechanisms, and require different diagnostic techniques and management.

Stress urinary incontinence can present in conjunction with urogenital prolapse. Even if the patient fails to mention it, it should become obvious by taking a thorough history. In such cases, a combined procedure to deal with both the prolapse and the stress incontinence should be undertaken.

Masked stress urinary incontinence will not be revealed from the history alone but should be identified following clinical examination. It represents true incontinence which has not been apparent because of the protective role of the prolapse maintaining continence because of outflow obstruction of the lower urinary tract.

Potential stress urinary incontinence is identified in a woman who does not have preoperative urinary incontinence, either on history or on clinical examination, but who is predisposed to develop incontinence secondary to a procedure to correct her urogenital prolapse. This may occur because of inappropriate transmission of intra-abdominal pressure during stress or because of intrinsic urethral sphincter incompetence.

PATHOPHYSIOLOGIC PRINCIPLES

Masked stress urinary incontinence can be explained by the mechanical prevention of urinary incontinence due to the position of the prolapse.[4] The 'ball effect' can be caused by uterine prolapse or a large cystocele, kinking of the urethra or even a rectocele. All of these may prevent urinary leakage.[4,10–12] However, it is important to distinguish between the two main mechanisms underlying masked incontinence: urethral compression and kinking of the urethra.

- *Intrinsic urethral compression* is due to significant uterine descent or a large posterior vaginal prolapse. This can be corrected by a speculum preventing the protrusion of the posterior vaginal wall or the uterine descent. Many consider the use of reduction techniques to be fairly reliable and reproducible and therefore find them useful in screening for masked incontinence.[10]
- *Kinking of the urethra* due to herniation of the anterior vaginal wall can be more difficult to correct. Reduction of the prolapse with excessive traction on the posterior vaginal wall may, in fact, open the bladder neck. This will lead to an overdiagnosis of 'masked stress incontinence'.

The practical methods for reducing prolapse are variable. Some people prefer the pessary test, while others prefer an intravaginal tampon[13,14] and/or a speculum blade.[4]

The pathophysiology of '**potential urinary incontinence**' remains unknown, which partially explains the difficulty in preventing it, and several hypotheses have been suggested. In considering these theories, it is important to employ precise terminology. 'Potential urinary incontinence' should not be used to describe all types of postoperative incontinence occurring in previously dry women. In the authors' opinion, potential urinary incontinence should only refer to stress urinary incontinence excluding de novo cases of overactive bladder. Detrusor overactivity has very different causes, notably surgical overcorrection. Overactive bladder is frequently found to coexist with severe urogenital prolapse, which may be exacerbated or alleviated by surgery.[15]

DIAGNOSIS

Masked urinary incontinence is not identified in the *history*. It can be suspected if the patient gives a history of stress urinary incontinence which improves with the onset or exacerbation of a prolapse. This transitory stress urinary incontinence deserves attention.

The diagnosis of masked stress urinary incontinence should only be made at clinical examination. Urinary leakage may be observed following reduction of the prolapse during a thorough clinical examination. It is important to know whether or not the woman's bladder is full prior to the examination as clinical examination with an empty bladder is unhelpful, whereas examination with an overfull bladder may lead to overdiagnosis. Reduction of the prolapse is important. A forceps can be placed on the cervix to realign the cervix in its anatomic position and the anterior and posterior blades of a vaginal speculum can be used to correct a cystocele and a rectocele, respectively. The patient can then be asked to cough or strain.

It is important to position the patient appropriately for the examination. Although it is usually most convenient to start the examination on a gynecologic couch, if this does not give conclusive results it may be necessary to examine the patient in the sitting or standing position. It is important to recognize that even these examination techniques cannot always replicate the anatomic correction produced by surgery.

Some surgeons have suggested further intraoperative tests to improve the reliability of screening. These tests require the cooperation of the patient and can only be attempted under regional or local anesthesia. At the end of the procedure, the bladder is filled with 250–300 ml of fluid and the patient is asked to cough. If there is an objective leak under these circumstances, a preventive continence procedure is indicated. Other authors have suggested that this is not a physiologic stress test as anesthesia alters the angle of the urethrovesical junction and this serves local sanitation.

Another alternative to a well-conducted clinical examination is the pessary test conducted over several days. It corrects prolapse and allows screening of masked incontinence during the patient's normal daily life. There are, however, limitations to this procedure: either unwillingness on the part of the patient or anatomic difficulties such as previous hysterectomy, discomfort from a ring, or local atrophy. A recent study evaluating patient satisfaction at 2 months following placement of a pessary reported a 21% rate of unmasked incontinence.[16]

It is not possible to establish a diagnosis of **potential urinary incontinence** although certain risk factors may be identified in the assessment of a woman with urogenital prolapse.

- *history:* Mild stress urinary incontinence, which affects 30–50% of women, is usually reasonably well tolerated and may not be mentioned during the course of a consultation. Severe constipation, chronic bronchitis or asthma may be causes of raised intra-abdominal pressure with consequent deleterious effects on the pelvic floor. Some professional, sporting or domestic activities may also involve regular increases in intra-abdominal pressure. Although these factors may predispose to pelvic floor laxity, they do not in themselves predict postoperative stress urinary incontinence.
- *clinical examination:* Hypermobility of the urethrovesical junction may be demonstrated with the Q-tip test or observed with the naked eye. Obesity is known to have a negative impact on the pelvic floor. Abdominoperineal asynchronicity should be sought and, if present, may be treated with pelvic floor re-education; however, this has not been shown to be of any particular value.
- *investigations:* It is contentious whether or not urodynamic studies should be carried out on all women prior to prolapse surgery. However, the authors feel that such investigations are important and may reveal preoperative risk or provide objective evidence of postoperative complications. Despite this, the majority of authors consider that urodynamic studies have a low predictive value for potential urinary incontinence. However, urodynamics may reveal additional information such as urethral sphincter weakness or a low baseline Valsalva leak point pressure.[13,17]

Thus, the quality of the clinical assessment including a pessary test or other maneuvers to reduce the prolapse, together with controlled bladder filling, are most important. For women with prolapse who are to undergo surgery, conventional radiology[18] such as cystourethrography does not distinguish between continent and incontinent women. Therefore, radiology does not help to screen for patients at risk of postoperative incontinence.[3] Ultrasound may prove more useful[19] as it can help in the evaluation of urethral/bladder neck support preoperatively. In the future it may help to select those women who need to undergo a concomitant continence procedure; however, this has proved difficult to date.

Even when the possible risk factors have been established it is not possible to give a precise estimation of the risk of developing urinary incontinence following surgery for urogenital prolapse. However, some operations for prolapse are more likely to cause problems than others. Richter's sacrospinous fixation causes backward angulation of the vagina, so when there is overcorrection of the vaginal vault prolapse it tends to open the bladder neck, increasing the risk of incontinence. It is also important to consider the type of pelvic floor repair as a residual prolapse may be protective against the development of urinary incontinence.[3]

MANAGEMENT

Although it is difficult to reach a consensus, there are certain important questions that should be considered.

When should a combined prolapse and urinary incontinence procedure be carried out?

If stress incontinence and prolapse are both known to be present, then it is important to treat both at the same time. A recent study by Liang et al.[20] revealed that 64.7% of patients with a positive preoperative pessary test who were not offered a primary continence procedure developed incontinence after prolapse surgery. Some surgeons will always perform a continence procedure; however, this may be unnecessary for 35% of patients, thus justifying a delayed approach.

Some pelvic floor surgeons who operate with patients under regional anesthesia employ a cough test at the end of the prolapse procedure.[21,22] In a prospective study (personal communication), Pigné observed that of 70 patients with stress incontinence prior to prolapse surgery, only 60 had a positive cough test following the prolapse procedure, and of the remaining 10 only one developed postoperative stress incontinence requiring a later insertion of a tension-free vaginal tape (TVT). In the same study, of the 76 patients without stress incontinence prior to surgery, the cough test was positive in 18 (24%) which, in the author's opinion, justified a combined continence procedure. Of the remaining 58 patients, six developed postoperative incontinence and four required further surgery. For patients with prolapse and stress incontinence an intraoperative cough test will avoid a continence procedure in 14% (10 out of 70), with an expected risk of requiring a secondary procedure for incontinence (1 out of 10). For patients with prolapse but no stress incontinence carrying out a cough test, this still leaves a 10% rate of postoperative incontinence and necessitates a continence procedure in 24%. Some authorities would consider that, if there is no urinary leakage demonstrated preoperatively (after reduction of the prolapse), there is no reason to carry out a continence procedure. In such circumstances, several studies have shown that the risk of urinary incontinence after prolapse surgery is very small.

In the case of mild stress incontinence, and depending on the preference of both the surgeon and the patient, the management choices are shown in Figure 76.1. In all other cases, a prophylactic continence procedure would appear unnecessary except for those surgeons who undertake an intraoperative cough test at the end of the prolapse procedure (Fig. 76.2).

The reliability of the cough test during pelvic floor surgery is controversial. Some consider that it has only weak discriminative power. However, systematic use of the cough test under controlled intraoperative conditions (position on the operating table, method of anesthesia, disturbance of neuromuscular tone) can identify some false negatives and avoid overtreatment of other patients. This will only affect a small proportion of women. Those who support this method emphasize its advantages. It is the only useful intraoperative test carried out in an anatomic position. Preoperative tests cannot be undertaken in this position, and under- or overcorrection will distort the final outcome. It appears likely that, taking into account the views of different published case series, preoperative maneuvers to reduce prolapse tend to produce more false positives than false negatives.

Which continence procedure?

This is based on the views and preferences of the surgeon but the reliability and low morbidity of suburethral slings (either retropubic or transobturator) are good choices.[23] It is important to avoid procedures with unknown long-term reliability[24] and to opt for the procedure which would be best for stress incontinence alone. Needle suspensions and Kelly bladder neck plication have been abandoned because of their poor results.[24,25] Burch colposuspension[26] is also being superseded by procedures which are as effective but with lower morbidity.

How can we prevent 'potential urinary incontinence'?

As our understanding of the pathophysiologic mechanism underlying potential stress incontinence is so poor, prevention therefore relies on good practice in urogynecologic surgery. Preventive efforts on their own may be

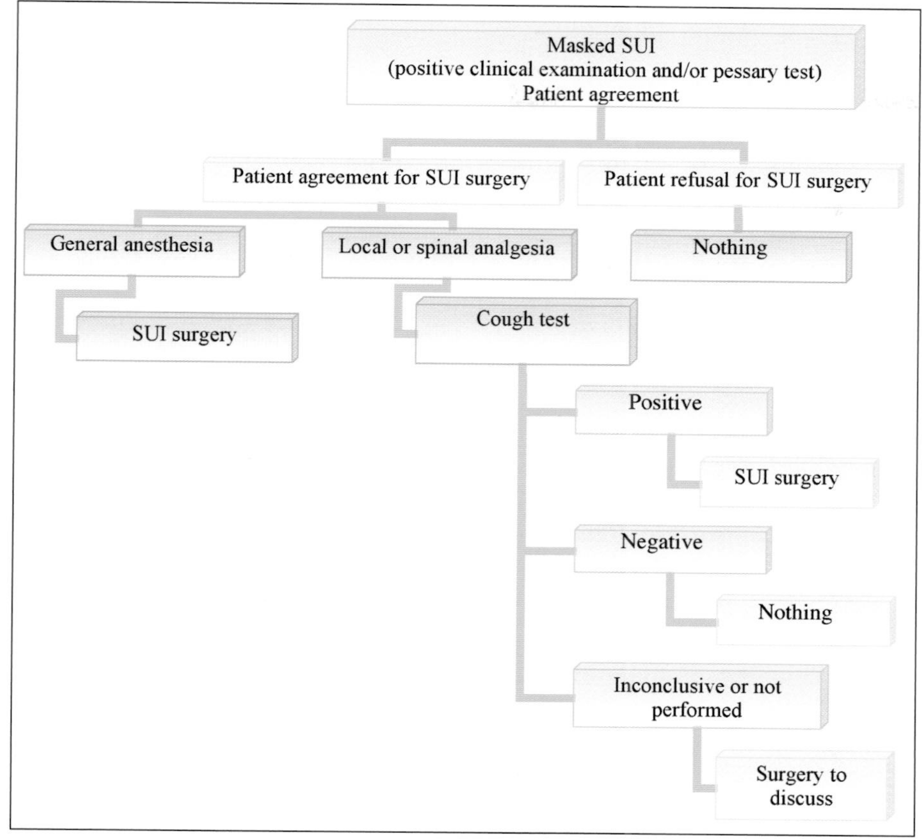

Figure 76.1. *Management of women with masked stress urinary incontinence (SUI).*

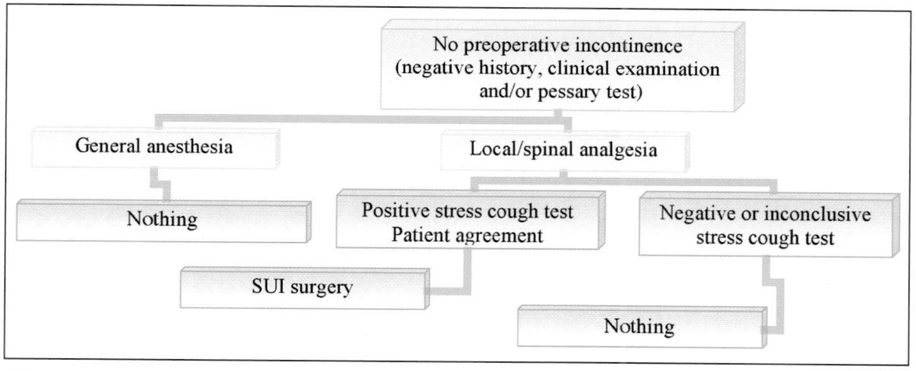

Figure 76.2. *Management of women with no preoperative urinary incontinence. SUI, stress urinary incontinence.*

insufficient but by neglecting them there is an increased risk of postoperative complications. Excessive tension in a repair should be avoided, particularly at the level of the anterior vaginal wall and the vaginal vault.

Many authors have emphasized the increased risk and additional problems associated with procedures such as sacrospinous fixation. In a retrospective study of 62 women,[27] the results in terms of postoperative incontinence were significantly better for the group having a Pereyra suspension alone (34 patients, median follow-up 23 months, subjective cure of stress incontinence 91%, objective cure of stress incontinence 88%) compared to the group having a Pereyra suspension in addition to a sacrospinous ligament fixation (28 patients, median follow-up 26 months, subjective cure of stress incontinence 68%, objective cure of stress incontinence 61%). The posterior angulation of the vaginal axis as a result of the sacrospinous fixation predisposes to opening of the bladder neck by a fraction on the posterior wall. This has been confirmed by Sze et al.[28] in a retrospective comparison of abdominal sacrocolpopexy with Burch colposuspension versus sacrospinous fixation with needle suspension. The rate of recurrent incontinence in the former group was 4% but in the latter was 9%. The choice of continence procedure may have biased this study.

Table 76.1. *Urinary results according to incontinence type and surgical procedure*

Author/year/trial	Incontinence type	Surgery	Follow-up	Results	Comments
Bump et al. (1996)[29] Prospective randomized	Potential or masked, n=20 Transmission <90% or positive pessary test	Transcutaneous needle colposuspension (Muzsnaï), n=10	6 w. and 6 m.	Colposuspension: SUI=7% at 6 w., 14% at 6 m.	Colposuspension – detrusor instability: 36%
		Colporrhaphy, n=10		Suburethral plication: SUI=21% at 6 w., 7% at 6 m.	Plication – detrusor instability: 7%
	Without UI, n=9 (hypermobility only)	Colposuspension, n=4			
		Plication, n=5			
Colombo et al. (1996)[30] Randomized	Potential UI	Cystopexy, n=52	2.6±1.7 y.	SUI: 8% (n=4)	1 reoperation Long-term micturition difficulties: 0% Symptomatic detrusor instability: 2%
		Cystopexy + pubourethral ligaments plication, n=50	2.9±1.8 y.	SUI: 8% (n=4)	1 reoperation Long-term micturition difficulties: 10% Symptomatic detrusor instability: 2%
Colombo et al. (1997)[31] Randomized	Patent SUI	15 Kelly Nichols	>5 y.	SUI: 40%	Detrusor instability after Kelly Nichols: 4%
		21 Pereyra	>5 y.	SUI: 29%	
	Masked SUI	40 Kelly Nichols	>5 y.	SUI: 15%	Detrusor instability after Pereyra: 2%
		33 Pereyra	>5 y.	SUI: 0%	
Gordon et al. (1999)[24] Prospective	Masked SUI, n=30	Kelly plication	25.5 m.	Subjective and objective SUI: 50% Objective SUI: 37%	–
Chaikin et al. (2000)[32] Prospective	Masked SUI, n=14	Pubovaginal sling	47 m. (range 12–108)	SUI: 14%	1 de novo urge incontinence
	Without SUI, n=10	No surgery	44 m. (range 12–96)	SUI: 0%	De novo urge incontinence: 0%
Klutke & Ramos (2000)[26] Retrospective	Masked SUI, n=55	Burch, n=52	3.5 y.	SUI: 4%	De novo detrusor instability: 30%
		Needle colposuspension, n=3	3.5 y.	SUI: 4%	–
	Without SUI, n=70	No surgery	3.5 y.	SUI: 0%	De novo detrusor instability: 5%
Groutz et al. (2000)[25] Prospective	Masked SUI, n=30	Stamey	8 m. (range 3–9)	Subjective and objective SUI: 23.3%	–

Table 76.1. *Urinary results according to incontinence type and surgical procedure (cont.)*

Author/year/trial	Incontinence type	Surgery	Follow-up	Results	Comments
Gordon et al. (2001)[33] Prospective	Masked SUI	TVT	14.25 m. (range 12–24)	Subjective SUI: 0% Objective SUI: 10%	De novo detrusor instability (without obstruction): 13.33%
Barnes et al. (2002)[34] Retrospective	Masked SUI, n=38	Pubovaginal sling	15 m. (range 6–39)	SUI: 5%	De novo urge incontinence: 9.5% Permanent retention: 0%
Groutz et al. (2004)[35] Prospective	Masked SUI, n=100	TVT	27 m. (range 12–52)	Subjective and objective SUI at 1 year follow-up: 2%	De novo urge incontinence: 8%
Meschia et al. (2004)[23] Prospective randomized	Masked SUI	TVT	26 m.	Subjective SUI: 4% Objective SUI: 8%	De novo urge incontinence: 12%
		Plication	24 m.	Subjective SUI: 36% Objective SUI: 44%	De novo urge incontinence: 4%
Liang et al. (2004)[20] Prospective	Masked SUI (positive pessary test), n=49	TVT, n=32	Unknown	Subjective SUI : 9.4% Objective SUI: 0%	Idiopathic detrusor overactivity: 16%
		No TVT, n=17	Unknown	Subjective SUI: 64.7% Objective SUI: 52.9%	Idiopathic detrusor overactivity: 5.9%
	No masked SUI (negative pessary test), n=30	No TVT, n=30	Unknown	No postoperative SUI	Idiopathic de novo overactivity: 0%

SUI, stress urinary incontinence; TVT, tension-free vaginal tape; UI, urinary incontinence; w, week; m, month; y, year.

What information should we give to patients before surgery?

It is important that patients understand the possibilities. They need to know that there is a de novo incidence of stress incontinence following correction of a prolapse. This varies with the type of prolapse and the surgical procedure chosen to repair the pelvic floor as well as the quality of repair. This can change over time; the literature suggests a rate of between 10 and 30%. The specific possible complications must be clearly explained as people often regard minimally invasive procedures as routine and complication-free. The most common urinary problems are dysuria and overactive bladder (Table 76.1). The complications and their management have been the subject of a recent literature review.[36] Estimates of the rate of postoperative dysuria vary from 2 to 22% depending upon the operative technique employed[36] (needle suspensions 5–7%,[37] suburethral sling 4–10%,[38] TVT 2–4%,[22] Marshall–Marchetti–Kranz procedure 5–20%,[39,40] Burch colposuspension 4–22%[41,42]). Symptoms of overactive bladder are even more frequently encountered, varying from 6 to 25% depending upon the choice of technique[36] (sling 8–25%,[43] TVT 6–12%,[44–46] retropubic urethropexies 6–16%[41,47]). Failure of the procedure is possible regardless of the choice of operation and the patient must be forewarned. For suburethral support techniques it is reasonable to suggest a figure of 10% when treating masked stress incontinence.[20,23,33,35]

The major risks of a preventive procedure are the morbidity associated with an initial operation that is poorly tolerated by patients who may regard a preventive procedure as pointless. They must also be informed about the possible treatment that would be available should stress incontinence occur following pelvic floor surgery. It is important to reassure patients that if postoperative complications do recur they will benefit from having had appropriate preoperative counseling.

REFERENCES

1. Bergman A, Koonings PP, Ballard CA. Predicting postoperative urinary incontinence development in women undergoing operation for genitourinary prolapse. Am J Obstet Gynecol 1988;158:1171–5.
2. Borstad E, Rud T. The risk of developing urinary stress-incontinence after vaginal repair in continent women: a clinical and urodynamic follow-up study. Acta Obstet Gynecol Scand 1989;68:545–9.
3. Borstad E, Skrede M, Rud T. Failure to predict and attempts to explain urinary stress incontinence following vaginal repair in continent women by using a modified lateral urethrocystography. Acta Obstet Gynecol Scand 1991;70:501–6.
4. Bump RC, Fantl JA, Hurt WG. The mechanism of urinary continence in women with severe uterovaginal prolapse: results of barrier studies. Obstet Gynecol 1988;72:291–5.
5. Richardson DA, Bent AE, Ostergard DR. The effect of uterovaginal prolapse on urethrovesical pressure dynamics. Am J Obstet Gynecol 1983;15:901–5.
6. Rosenzweig BA, Pushkin S, Blumenfeld D, Bhatia NN. Prevalence of abnormal urodynamic test results in continent women with severe genitourinary prolapse. Obstet Gynecol 1992;79:539–42.
7. Scheepers HC, Wolterbeek JH, Gerretsen G, Venema P. [Inventory and follow-up of patients with surgery for (uterine) vaginal prolapse, combined with or without (masked) stress incontinence.] Ned Tijdschr Geneeskd 1998;142:79–83.
8. Beck RP, McCormick S, Nordstrom L. A 25-year experience with 519 anterior colporrhaphy procedures. Obstet Gynecol 1991;78:1011–18.
9. Clark AL, Gregory T, Smith VJ, Edwards R. Epidemiologic evaluation of reoperation for surgically treated pelvic organ prolapse and urinary incontinence. Am J Obstet Gynecol 2003;189:1261–7.
10. Karram MM. What is the optimal anti-incontinence procedure in women with advanced prolapse and 'potential' stress incontinence? Int Urogynecol J Pelvic Floor Dysfunct 1999;10:1–2.
11. Long CY, Hsu SC, Wu TP, Sun DJ, Su JH, Tsai EM. Urodynamic comparison of continent and incontinent women with severe uterovaginal prolapse. J Reprod Med 2004;49:33–7.
12. Romanzi LJ. Management of the urethral outlet in patients with severe prolapse. Curr Opin Urol 2002;12:339–44.
13. Gallentine M, Cespedes D. Occult stress urinary incontinence and the effect of vaginal vault prolapse on abdominal leak point pressures. Urology 2001;57:40–4.
14. Ghoneim GM, Walters F, Lewis V. The value of the vaginal pack test in large cystoceles. J Urol 1994;152:931–4.
15. Cardozo LD, Stanton SL, Williams JE. Detrusor instability following surgery for genuine stress incontinence. Br J Urol 1979;51:204–7.
16. Clemons JL, Aguilar VC, Tillinghast TA, Jackson ND, Myers DL. Patient satisfaction and changes in prolapse and urinary symptoms in women who were fitted successfully with a pessary for pelvic organ prolapse. Am J Obstet Gynecol 2004;190:1025–9.
17. Veronikis DK, Nichols DH, Wakamatsu MM. The incidence of low-pressure urethra as a function of prolapse-reducing technique in patients with massive pelvic organ prolapse (maximum descent at all vaginal sites). Am J Obstet Gynecol 1997;177:1305–13.

18. Bergman A, McKensie C, Ballard CA, Richmond J. Role of cystourethrography in the preoperative evaluation of stress urinary incontinence in women. J Reprod Med 1988;33:372–6.

19. Bergman A, Koonings PP, Ballard CA, Platt LD. Ultrasonic prediction of stress urinary incontinence development in surgery for severe pelvic relaxation. Gynecol Obstet Invest 1988;26:66–72.

20. Liang CC, Chang YL, Chang SD, Lo TS, Soong YK. Pessary test to predict postoperative urinary incontinence in women undergoing hysterectomy for prolapse. Obstet Gynecol 2004;104:795–800.

21. Bombieri L, Freeman RM. Recurrence of stress incontinence after vault suspension: can it be prevented? Int Urogynecol J Pelvic Dysfunct 1998;9:58–60.

22. Pigné A. Peut-on améliorer la continence des patients lors de la chirurgie du prolapsus. XXVII ème congrès de la Société Francophone d'UroDynamique, Bucarest; 3–5 Juin 2004 (unpublished data).

23. Meschia M, Pifarotti P, Spennacchio M, Buonaguidi A, Gattei U, Somigliana E. A randomized comparison of tension-free vaginal tape and endopelvic fascia plication in women with genital prolapse and occult stress urinary incontinence. Am J Obstet Gynecol 2004;190:609–13.

24. Gordon D, Groutz A, Wolman I, Lessing JB, David MP. Development of postoperative urinary stress incontinence in clinically continent patients undergoing prophylactic Kelly placation during genitourinary prolapse repair. Neurourol Urodyn 1999;18:193–7.

25. Groutz A, Gordon D, Wolman I, Jaffa AJ, Kupferminc MJ, David MP, Lessing JB. The use of prophylactic Stamey bladder neck suspension to prevent post-operative stress urinary incontinence in clinically continent women undergoing genitourinary prolapse repair. Neurourol Urodyn 2000;19:671–6.

26. Klutke JJ, Ramos S. Urodynamic outcome after surgery for severe prolapse and potential stress incontinence. Am J Obstet Gynecol 2000;182:1378–81.

27. Nguyen JK, Bhatia NN. Risk of recurrent stress incontinence in women undergoing the combined modified Pereyra procedure and transvaginal sacrospinous ligament vault suspension. Urology 2001;58:947–52.

28. Sze EHM, Kohli N, Miklos R, Roat T, Karram MM. A retrospective comparison of abdominal sacrocolpopexy with Burch colposuspension versus sacrospinous fixation with transvaginal needle suspension for the management of vaginal vault prolapse and coexisting stress incontinence. Int Urogynecol J 1999;10:390–3.

29. Bump RC, Hurt WG, Theofrastous JP et al. Randomized prospective comparison of needle colposuspension versus endopelvic fascia plication for potential stress incontinence prophylaxis in women undergoing vaginal reconstruction for stage III or IV pelvic organ prolapse. Am J Obstet Gynecol 1996;175:326–33.

30. Colombo M, Maggioni A, Scalambrino S, Zanetta G, Vignali M, Milani R. Prevention of postoperative urinary stress incontinence after surgery for genitourinary prolapse. Obstet Gynecol 1996;87:266–71.

31. Colombo M, Maggioni A, Scalambrino S, Vitobello D, Milani R. Surgery for genitourinary prolapse and stress incontinence: a randomized trial of posterior pubourethral ligament plication and Pereyra suspension. Am J Obstet Gynecol 1997;176:337–43.

32. Chaikin DC, Groutz A, Blaivas JG. Predicting the need for anti-incontinence surgery in continent women undergoing repair of severe urogenital prolapse. J Urol 2000;163:531–4.

33. Gordon D, Gold RS, Pauzner D, Lessing JB, Groutz A. Combined genitourinary prolapse repair and prophylactic tension-free vaginal tape in women with severe prolapse and occult stress urinary incontinence: preliminary results. Urology 2001;58:547–50.

34. Barnes NM, Dmochowski RR, Park R, Nitti VW. Pubovaginal sling and pelvic prolapse repair in women with occult stress urinary incontinence: effect on post-operative emptying and voiding symptoms. Urology 2002;59:856–60.

35. Groutz A, Gold R, Pauzner D, Lessing JB, Gordon D. Tension-free vaginal tape (TVT) for the treatment of occult stress urinary incontinence in women undergoing prolapse repair: a prospective study of 100 consecutive cases. Neurourol Urodyn 2004;23:632–5.

36. Dunn JS, Bent AE, Ellerkman RM, Nihira MA, Melick CF. Voiding dysfunction after surgery for stress incontinence: literature review and survey results. Int Urogynecol J 2004;15:25–31.

37. Spencer JR, O'Connor VJ Jr, Schaeffer AJ. A comparison of endoscopic suspension of the vesical neck with suprapubic vesicourethropexy for treatment of stress urinary incontinence. J Urol 1987;137:411–15.

38. Horbach NS. Suburethral sling procedures. In: Ostergard DR, Bent AE (eds) Urogynecology and Urodynamics: Theory and Practice, 4th ed. Baltimore: Williams and Wilkins, 1996; 569–79.

39. McDuffie RW Jr, Litin RB, Blundon KE. Urethrovesical suspension (Marshall–Marchetti–Krantz). Experience with 204 cases. Am J Surg 1981;141:297–8.

40. Zimmern PE, Hadley HR, Leach GE, Raz S. Female urethral obstruction after Marshall–Marchetti–Krantz operation. J Urol 1987;138:517–20.

41. Alcalay M, Monga A, Stanton SL. Burch colposuspension: a 10–20 year follow-up. Br J Obstet Gynecol 1995;102:740–5.

42. Maher C, Dwyer P, Carey M, Gilmour D. The Burch colposuspension for recurrent urinary stress incontinence following retropubic continence surgery. Br J Obstet Gynecol 1999;106:719–24.

43. Weinberger MW, Ostergard DR. Long term clinical and

urodynamic evaluation of polytetrafluoroethylene suburethral sling for treatment of genuine stress incontinence. Obstet Gynecol 1995;86:92–6.

44. Karram MM, Segal JL, Vassallo BJ, Kleeman SD. Complications and untoward effects of the tension-free vaginal tape procedure. Obstet Gynecol 2003;101:929–32.

45. Kuuva N, Nilsson CG. A nationwide analysis of complications associated with the tension-free vaginal tape (TVT) procedure. Acta Obstet Gynecol Scand 2002;81:72–7.

46. Rackley RR, Abdelmalak JB, Tchetgen MB, Madjar S, Jones S, Noble M. Tension-free vaginal tape and percutaneous vaginal tape sling procedures. Tech Urol 2001;7:90–100.

47. Langer R, Lipshitz Y, Halperin R, Pansky M, Bukovsky I, Sherman D. Long-term (10–15 years) follow-up after Burch colposuspensions for urinary stress incontinence. Int Urogynecol J 2001;12:323–6.

77

Episiotomy and perineal repair

Ranee Thakar, Christine Kettle

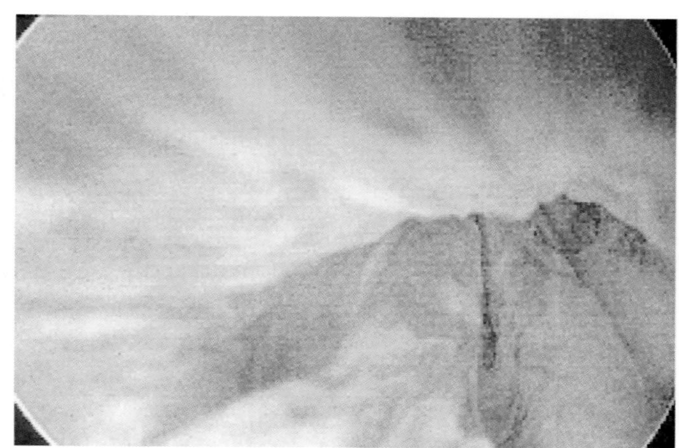

INTRODUCTION

Perineal injury is inherent in childbirth and various methods and materials were used by accoucheurs in an attempt to restore perineal integrity. Surgical treatment in the form of a crossed or bootlace suture is first mentioned in Avicenna's famous Arabic book. However, the first recorded perineal suture was that of Guillemeau in 1610.[1]

Perineal trauma resulting from childbirth remains a common problem[2] that causes a significant increase in maternal morbidity and may also have devastating effects on family life and sexual relationships.[3] More than 85% of women sustain perineal trauma after childbirth,[4] and up to two-thirds need suturing.[2] Perineal pain and discomfort affect up to 42% of women at 10 days postpartum and in 10% of women these problems persist at 18 months following childbirth.[5] Moreover, up to 58% of women experience superficial dyspareunia at 3 months postpartum.[6]

This chapter covers management and repair of episiotomy and first and second degree tears. Preventive measures are also discussed.

APPLIED ANATOMY

Anatomy of the perineum

The perineum corresponds to the outlet of the pelvis and is somewhat lozenge- shaped. The perineum can be divided into two triangular parts by drawing a line transversely between the ischial tuberosities. The anterior triangle, which contains the external urogenital organs, is known as the *urogenital triangle* and the posterior triangle, which contains the termination of the anal canal, is known as the *anal triangle*.

Urogenital triangle

The muscles are classified into a superficial and a deep group relative to the perineal membrane (urogenital diaphragm). The bulbospongiosus, superficial transverse perineal, and the ischiocavernosus muscles lie in the superficial compartment (Fig. 77.1). The bulbospongiosus muscle encircles the vagina and inserts anteriorly into the corpora cavernosa clitoridis. Posteriorly, some of its fibers may merge with those of the superficial transverse perineal muscle and also with the external anal sphincter. Beneath the bulbospongiosus muscles lie the vestibular bulbs anteriorly and the Bartholin's glands posteriorly. The Bartholin's gland is a pea-shaped structure and its duct opens at the introitus just superficial to the hymen at the junction of the upper two-thirds and the lower third of the labia minora. The deep transverse perineal muscle lies below the perineal membrane. It is thin and difficult to delineate and hence some authors deny the existence of this muscle.[7]

Anal triangle

This area includes the anal sphincters and ischiorectal fossae. The external anal sphincter is subdivided into three parts – subcutaneous, superficial, and deep – and

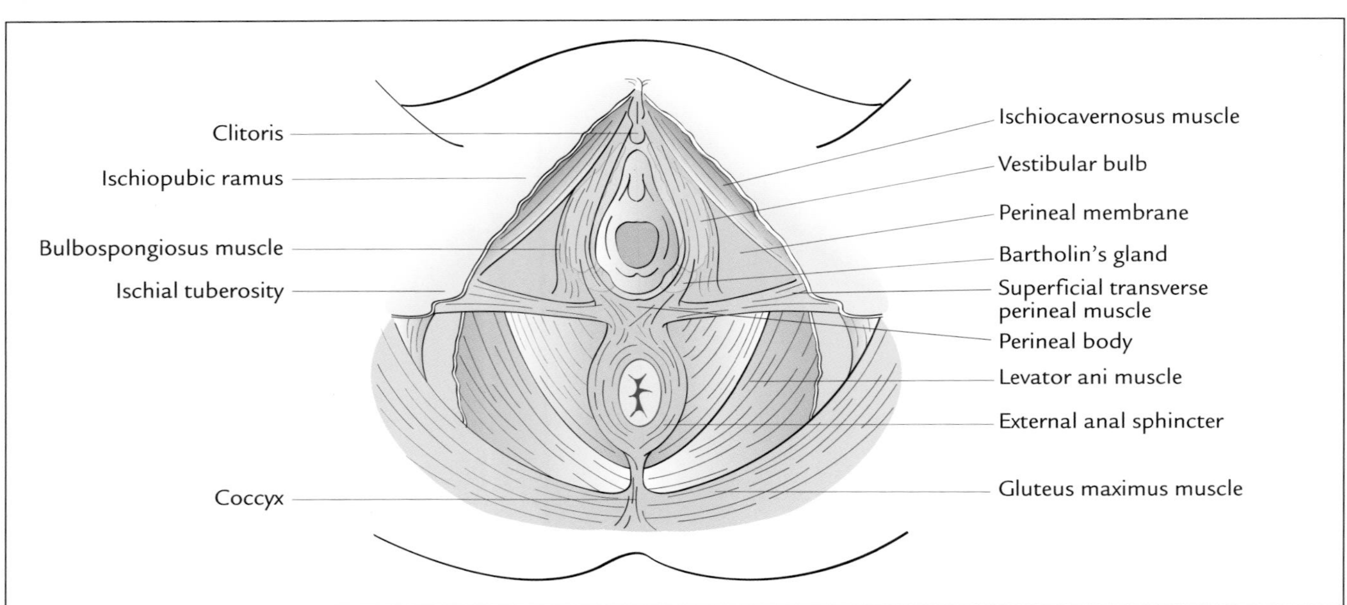

Figure 77.1. *The superficial muscles of the perineum.*

is inseparable from the puborectalis muscle posteriorly (Fig. 77.2). The internal anal sphincter is a thickened continuation of the circular smooth muscle of the bowel. It is separated from the external anal sphincter (striated muscle) by the conjoint longitudinal muscle which is a continuation of the longitudinal smooth muscle of the bowel but may receive contributions from the puborectalis muscle and the deep external sphincter[8] (see Chapter 78).

Perineal body

The perineal body is the central point between the urogenital and the anal triangles of the perineum. Its three-dimensional form has been likened to that of the cone of the red pine, with each 'petal' representing an interlocking structure, such as an insertion site of fascia or a muscle of the perineum.[9] Within the perineal body there is interlacing of muscle fibers from the bulbospongiosus, superficial transverse perineal, and external anal sphincter muscles. Above this level there is a contribution from the longitudinal rectal muscle and the medial fibers of the puborectalis muscle.

DEFINITION OF PERINEAL TRAUMA

Perineal trauma may occur spontaneously during vaginal birth or when a surgical incision (episiotomy) is intentionally made to facilitate delivery. It is possible to have an episiotomy and a spontaneous tear (e.g. extension of an episiotomy). Anterior perineal trauma is defined as injury to the labia, anterior vagina, urethra or clitoris; posterior perineal trauma is defined as any injury to the posterior vaginal wall or perineal muscles and may include disruption of the anal sphincters.

Structures involved

First degree perineal trauma is very superficial and may involve the skin and subcutaneous tissue of the anterior and posterior perineum, the vaginal mucosa, or a combination of these. Second degree tears or mediolateral episiotomy involves the superficial perineal muscles (bulbocavernosus, transverse perineal) or the perineal body if a midline episiotomy incision is made. If the trauma is very deep the pubococcygeus muscle may be disrupted. Rarely, more complex trauma can occur, whereby the tear extends in a circular direction, behind the hymeneal remnants, bilaterally upwards towards the clitoris, causing the lower third of the vagina to detach from the underlying structures.[7]

EPISIOTOMY

Episiotomy is a surgical incision made with scissors or a scalpel into the perineum in order to increase the diameter of the vulval outlet and facilitate delivery.[10] The two main types of episiotomy incision are midline and mediolateral.[11] When a midline episiotomy is undertaken, the incision is made from the midpoint of the introitus and is directed vertically towards the anus; with a mediolateral episiotomy, the incision begins in the midline but is directed directly away from the anal sphincter and rectum. Hudson et al.[12] have suggested that the term 'mediolateral' is a misnomer and they call this type of incision a 'posterolateral episiotomy' as it commences in the midline and is aimed to one side of

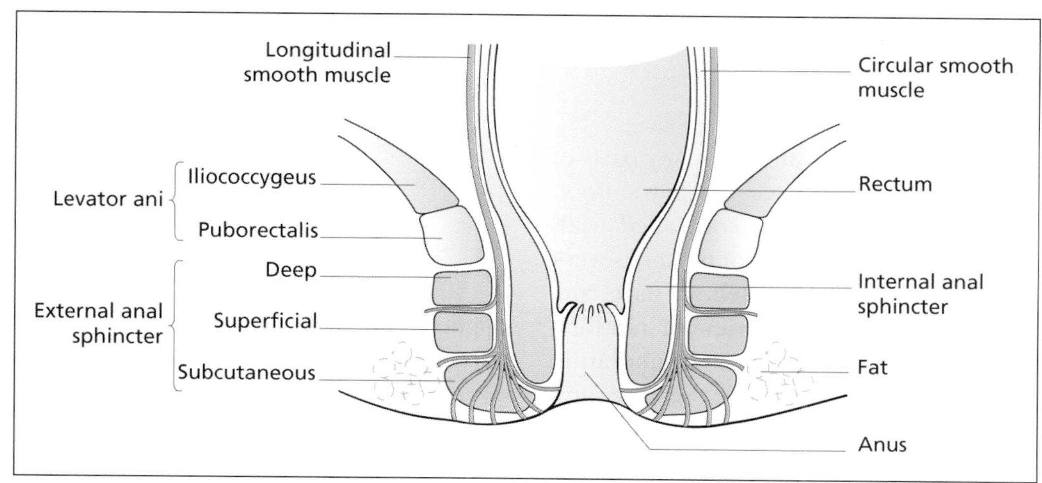

Figure 77.2. *The anal sphincter.*

the perineum in order to avoid the anal sphincter. It is claimed that the midline incision is easier to repair and that it is associated with less blood loss, better healing, less pain, and earlier resumption of sexual intercourse. However, there is no reliable evidence to support these claims.[5] Limited evidence from one quasi-randomized trial suggested that the midline incision may increase the risk of third and fourth degree tears compared with the mediolateral incision.[13] However, these data should be interpreted with caution as there may be an increased risk of selection bias due to quasi-random treatment allocation; in addition, analysis was not by intention to treat.

Incidence

There is a wide variation in the incidence of episiotomies performed in different countries. Clinicians' experiences, practices, and preferences in terms of intrapartum interventions may influence the rate and severity of perineal trauma. Moreover, episiotomy rates may vary considerably according to individual practices and policies of staff and institutions.[3] In the United Kingdom, it is estimated that over 85% of women who give birth will sustain some degree of perineal trauma and, of these, 60–70% will require suturing.[14] However, episiotomy rates have reduced in English-speaking countries and Europe over the last 20 years, probably due to the accumulation of evidence supporting restrictive use of the procedure.

Episiotomy is a common obstetrical procedure, yet statistics relating to prevalence are not always easily located. Figure 77.3 presents data graphically to illustrate the considerable variation in the use of episiotomy.[15] Episiotomy rates that include both primiparous and multiparous women range from as low as 9.7% (Sweden) to 100% (Taiwan); rates for primiparous women range from 63.3% (South Africa) to 100% (Guatemala).[15]

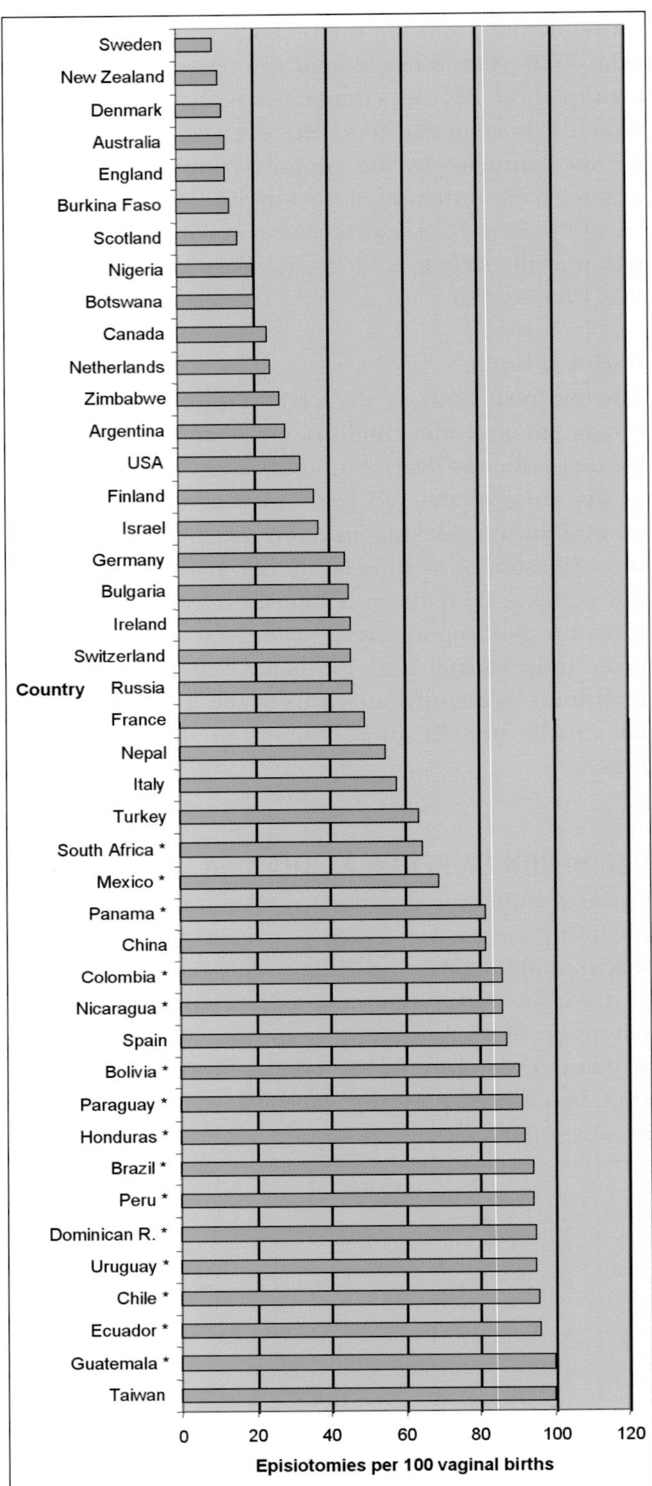

Figure 77.3. *Graphical presentation of the considerable variation in the use of episiotomy: rates by country, 1995–2003.* * *indicates primiparous data only. (Reproduced from ref. 15 with permission.)*

Indications for episiotomy

Episiotomy is still performed routinely in many parts of the world in the belief that it protects the pelvic floor. However, evidence from randomized controlled trials suggests that routine episiotomy does not prevent severe posterior perineal tears. Carroli and Belizan have conducted the most recent systematic review of randomized clinical trials using the Cochrane Collaboration methodology to determine the possible benefits and risks of restrictive episiotomy versus routine episiotomy. Mediolateral episiotomy was the method of incision for all six trials included in the review except for a North American trial where midline episiotomy was performed.

The review revealed that there is a lower risk of posterior perineal trauma, need for suturing and healing complications associated with the restrictive use of episiotomy at 7 days postpartum. However, there is no difference in the incidence of major outcomes such as severe vaginal or perineal trauma, pain, dyspareunia or urinary incontinence between the restrictive and routine/liberal use of episiotomy. The only disadvantage shown in restrictive use of episiotomy is an increased risk of anterior perineal trauma. This systematic review concluded that there is evidence to support the restrictive use of episiotomy compared to routine episiotomy (irrespective of the type of episiotomy performed). This finding applied to both primiparous and multiparous women.[5]

There is currently an absence of clear, evidence-based clinical indications for the use of episiotomy. However, it is reasonable to suggest that an episiotomy should be performed to accelerate vaginal delivery in cases of fetal distress, to facilitate safe delivery if shoulder dystocia occurs, to prevent severe perineal trauma during an instrumental delivery (forceps or ventouse), to aid vaginal delivery in cases where the perineal tissue is thick or rigid causing serious delay, and in cases in which prolonged 'bearing down' maybe harmful for the mother (e.g. severe hypertensive or cardiac disease). However, these indications are not absolute and clinical discretion should always be used.

Episiotomy rate

Although there is clear evidence to recommend restrictive use of episiotomy, there appears to be no consensus regarding the ideal episiotomy rate. Henriksen et al.[16] performed an observational study involving 2188 pregnant women and found that those allocated to the group of midwives with the lowest rate of episiotomies were more likely to have an intact perineum, more spontaneous perineal tears, but no increased risk of having an anal sphincter tear. In a further publication[17] the authors reported a relative decrease of 18% in episiotomy rates after distributing awareness profiles to the midwives, but the rate of anal sphincter tears did not change. There was a tendency towards an increased risk of tears if the midwives tried to reduce episiotomy rates below 20%. This supports the view that the overall ideal episiotomy rate should be between 20 and 30% but fails to indicate the ideal rate for nulliparae versus multiparae. The World Health Organization recommended that an episiotomy rate of 10% for spontaneous vaginal deliveries would be the ideal.[18] Moreover, the figures on what is the appropriate episiotomy rate are not based on robust evidence.

MANAGEMENT OF PERINEAL TRAUMA

For many centuries, there has been longstanding debate relating to suturing of perineal trauma following childbirth. Some accoucheurs believe that it is much better to leave perineal trauma unsutured to facilitate 'ensuing' deliveries, while others argue that the outcome for women and their partners is considerably improved if the trauma is sutured.

Non-suturing of perineal trauma

Non-suturing of perineal skin

Results from two large randomized controlled trials carried out in Ipswich, UK (single center) and the other in Nigeria (multicenter)[19,20] show that there are no major adverse effects associated with leaving the perineal skin unsutured. The trials compared leaving the skin unsutured but apposed (the vagina and perineal muscles were sutured) to the traditional repair whereby all three layers (vagina, perineal muscles and skin) were sutured. The trials showed conflicting results for perineal pain, with the UK trial showing no difference in short- and long-term perineal pain but the Nigerian trial showing that leaving the skin unsutured was associated with a reduction in perineal pain up to 3 months postpartum. Both trials reported lower rates of dyspareunia at 3 months and a significant increase in wound gaping at 2 days in the groups that had perineal skin unsutured. Wound gaping persisted up to 10 days in the UK trial but there was only a non-significant increase at 14 days postpartum in the Nigerian trial.

Non-suturing of perineal trauma

There have been two small randomized controlled trials[21,22] and two small retrospective studies[23,24] carried out to compare the effects of non-suturing versus suturing of first and second degree tears. One of these trials (n=74 primiparous women) carried out in Scotland by Fleming and colleagues[21] found no significant difference between non-suturing and suturing in terms of perineal pain but reported significantly more women in the sutured group had good wound approximation at 6 weeks postpartum. Perineal pain and healing were assessed using standardized measures at 1 day, 10 days and 6 weeks following birth. In the other small Swedish trial (n=78 primiparous women) carried out by Lundquist and colleagues[22] that compared non-suturing to suturing of spontaneous tears which involved the labia, vagina, and perineum found a non-significant increase in short-term discomfort with non-suturing but no difference in wound healing between the groups. Data from this trial must be interpreted with caution, as the sample size was small, it was unclear how healing was defined and measured, and most results did not reach statistical significance. The two small retrospective studies found no difference in short-term morbidity or wound healing rates.[23,24] The practice of leaving first and second degree tears unsutured is associated with poorer wound healing and nonsignificant differences in short-term discomfort.[3]

Suture material

A Cochrane systematic review of eight randomized controlled trials[25] involving 3642 primiparous and multiparous women found that absorbable synthetic material (polyglycolic acid and polyglactin 910) when compared with catgut suture material was associated with less short-term morbidity. Although all the trials showed consistently lower rates of perineal pain, analgesia use, suture dehiscence, and resuturing in the polyglycolic acid and polyglactin 910 groups, two trials found that polyglycolic acid and polyglactin 910 were associated with an increased risk of suture removal up to 3 months postpartum. Standard polyglactin 910 is not totally absorbed from the wound until 60–90 days. However, a more rapidly absorbable form of material is now available. This material has the same chemical composition as polyglactin 910 but is sterilized by gamma irradiation, which causes loss in tensile strength at 10–14 days and complete absorption from the tissue by 42 days.[26]

Three randomized controlled trials[2,27,28] comparing rapid-absorption polyglactin 910 to standard polyglactin 910 found no clear difference in short-term pain between the groups. However, two of the trials[2,27] found a significant reduction in 'pain when walking' at 10–14 days postpartum.[28] Only one of the trials reported a reduction in superficial dyspareunia at 3 months postpartum. All three trials found that rapid-absorption polyglactin 910 was associated with a significant reduction in the need for suture removal up to 3 months following childbirth. In light of current evidence, rapid-absorption polyglactin 910 is the most appropriate suture material for perineal repair.[3]

Method of repair

Skin closure

A Cochrane systematic review of four randomized controlled trials involving 1864 primiparous and multiparous women compared the continuous subcuticular suture technique of perineal skin closure to interrupted sutures. The subcuticular technique was associated with less pain for up to 10 days postpartum compared with interrupted sutures. No differences were seen in the need for analgesia, resuturing of the wound or in dyspareunia. Based on one trial only, there was no difference in long-term pain and failure to resume pain-free intercourse within 3 months of the birth. The continuous technique was associated with less need for the removal of sutures. These results suggest that the continuous subcuticular technique for skin closure is associated with less short-term pain than techniques employing interrupted sutures.[29]

Continuous non-locking method

Based on an observational study by Fleming,[30] Kettle et al.[2] conducted a large factorial randomized controlled trial (n=1542) comparing the loose non-locking continuous suture for all layers to the traditional interrupted method. The trial found a significant reduction in perineal pain at 10 days, which persisted up to 12 months after childbirth but did not reach statistical significance. There was no statistical difference in the rates of superficial dyspareunia between the groups at 3 months postpartum. Suture removal was significantly less in the continuous suturing group.

The reason for the reduction in pain is probably due to the fact that the skin sutures are placed in the subcutaneous tissue, thus avoiding the profusion of nerve endings in the superficial skin surface. The rationale behind using the continuous technique is that stitch tension due to reactionary edema is transferred throughout the whole length of the single knotless suture in comparison to interrupted sutures which are placed transversely across the wound.

Another advantage of the continuous suturing technique is that only one piece of suture material is required to complete the perineal repair as compared to two to three pieces for the interrupted method, thus reducing the overall expenditure.

Based on the above evidence it can be concluded that perineal trauma should be repaired using the continuous non-locking technique to reapproximate all layers (vagina, perineal muscles, and skin) with rapid-absorption polyglactin 910.

Procedure for perineal repair

Assessment of perineal trauma

The person responsible for the woman's care must inspect the perineum thoroughly as soon as possible following the birth, using good lighting. Prior to commencing suturing it is important that the health professional explains the procedure to the woman and her partner and obtains consent. The woman is placed in a comfortable position so that the trauma is easily visualized. It is not necessary to use lithotomy poles to support the woman's legs during the procedure unless she has a working epidural or spinal anesthesia. Rectal examination should be carried out prior to commencement of repair. This helps in the identification of anal sphincter trauma. If the woman does not have an epidural, the woman should be asked to squeeze the anal sphincter. If the external anal sphincter is torn, the separated ends will retract towards the ischiorectal fossa.

The continuous suturing technique[31] (Fig. 77.4)

The first stitch is inserted above the apex of the vaginal trauma to secure any bleeding points that may not be visible. Vaginal trauma, perineal muscles, and skin are approximated with a loose, continuous non-locking technique. The skin sutures are placed loosely and fairly deeply in the subcutaneous tissue, reversing back and finishing with a terminal knot placed in the vagina beyond the hymeneal remnants.

The interrupted suturing method (Fig. 77.5)

The first stitch is inserted above the apex of the vaginal trauma to secure any bleeding points. Vaginal trauma is repaired with a continuous locking (blanket) stitch and the suture is tied at the fourchette with a loop knot. Interrupted sutures are inserted to close the perineal muscle (deep and superficial) and interrupted transcutaneous stitches are inserted to reapproximate the skin edges.

A rectal examination should be performed after completing the repair to ensure that suture material has not been accidentally inserted through the rectal mucosa. Following completion of the repair, the extent of the injury sustained, the suture technique, and the materials used must be documented in the case notes in black

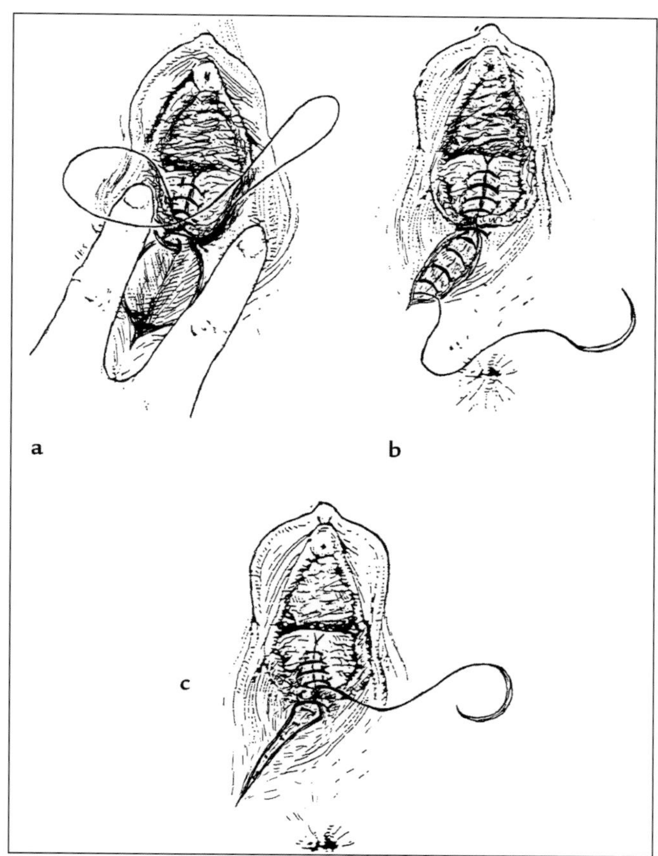

Figure 77.4. *The continuous suturing technique. (a) Vaginal trauma is repaired using a loose, continuous non-locking stitch to the vagina; (b) perineal muscle is repaired using a loose, continuous non-locking stitch; (c) skin is closed using a loose subcutaneous stitch. (Reproduced from ref. 31 with permission.)*

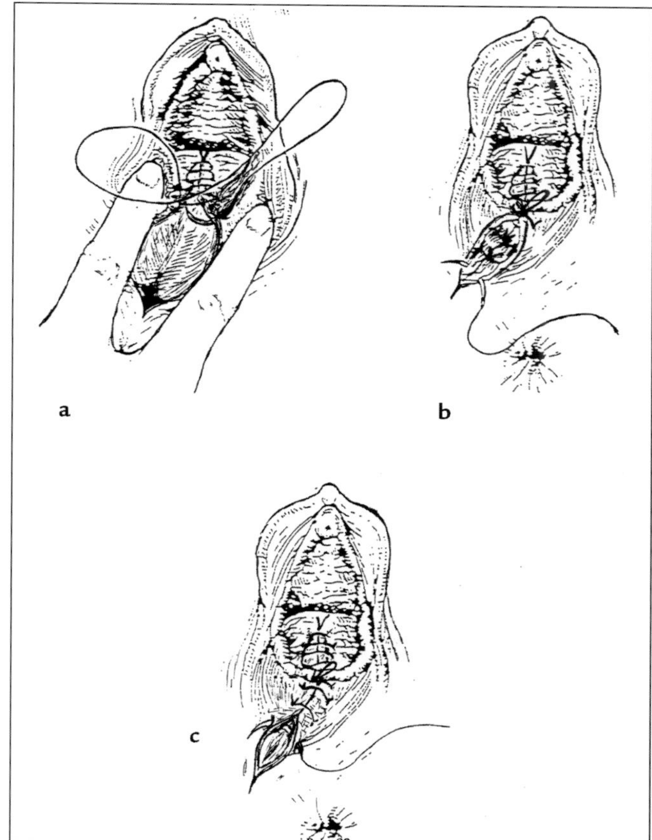

Figure 77.5. *Suturing the vagina using the interrupted suturing method. (a) Vaginal trauma is repaired with a continuous locking (blanket) stitch to the vaginal wall; (b) interrupted sutures are inserted to close the perineal muscles (deep and superficial); (c) interrupted transcutaneous stitches are inserted to reapproximate the skin edges.*

ink. It is also useful to include a diagram to illustrate the extent of the trauma.

Prevention of perineal trauma

Although the case for prevention of perineal trauma is compelling, how to accomplish this is less clear. Certain antenatal risk factors such as maternal nutritional status, body mass index, ethnicity, infant birth weight,[32] race, and age[33] cannot be altered at the time of delivery but awareness of them might prompt modifications in the care pathway.

Cesarean section

Elective cesarean section is the only form of delivery that can totally ensure absence of perineal trauma. However, compared to vaginal delivery, cesarean section is associated with an increase in mortality and morbidity.[34–36] Furthermore, the case for elective cesarean section to prevent perineal trauma cannot be substantiated.

Ventouse versus forceps delivery

A recent Cochrane Review found that the use of the vacuum extractor for assisted vaginal delivery when compared to forceps is associated with significantly less maternal trauma and with less general and regional anesthesia. Overall there were more deliveries with vacuum extraction and fewer cesarean sections were carried out in the vacuum extractor group. However, the vacuum extractor was associated with an increase in neonatal cephalhematomata and retinal hemorrhages. Serious neonatal injury was uncommon with either instrument.[37]

Delivery positions

It has been postulated that position at delivery (upright or lying down) may influence the risk of perineal trauma. One systematic review found that any upright position marginally reduced episiotomies compared with the supine or lithotomy positions for delivery but this was offset by an increase in second degree tears. Rates of assisted deliveries were slightly reduced in the upright group. The findings of this systematic review should be interpreted with caution because of the variable qualities of the trials and the diversity of the treatment interventions (squatting, kneeling, Gardosi cushion, birthing chair).[38]

Delivery techniques

Traditionally, manual support of the perineum has been regarded as mandatory for protecting maternal tissue during delivery. It is widely believed that guarding the perineum during delivery of the fetal head prevents or reduces perineal trauma. The National Perinatal Epidemiological Unit at Oxford conducted a randomized controlled trial of the hands-on or poised (HOOP) method of delivery.[14] At the end of second stage of labor women were allocated to either 'hands on' (the midwife's hands applied pressure on the baby's head and supported the perineum; lateral flexion was then used to facilitate the delivery of the shoulders) or the 'hands poised' (the midwife kept her hands poised, not touching the head or perineum and allowing spontaneous delivery of the shoulders). The trialists found that a reduction in pain at 10 days was noted in the hands-on group (31.1% versus 34.1%, p=0.02), but the rate of episiotomy was significantly lower in the hands-poised group. However, analysis was based on intention to treat and it must be noted that following randomisation 30% of the hands-poised group converted to the hands-on method. Mayerhofer et al.,[39] in a similar randomized study using perineal trauma as a primary outcome measure, found that women receiving hands-on care had a significantly higher rate of third degree perineal tears (2.7% versus 0.9%). Likewise, the episiotomy rate was significantly higher in the hands-on group (17.9% versus 10.1%), but there was no statistically significant difference in overall perineal trauma between the two groups.

Epidural analgesia

There are conflicting data on the effect of epidural analgesia on perineal trauma. Robinson et al.[40] showed that women who had epidural analgesia were more likely to have perineal trauma, but this was due to the increased risk of operative vaginal deliveries and episiotomies with epidurals. Poen et al.[41] found an increased risk of anal sphincter injury due to epidurals and suggested that this could be due to blocking the pain, which normally functions as an alarm for perineal stretching. In contrast, others have found a significant increase in episiotomy rate during vaginal delivery associated with epidurals but without an increase in perineal tears.[42] Overall it appears that the increased perineal trauma is related to the associated increase in instrumental delivery.[43]

Perineal massage

Stretching and massaging of the perineum in the antenatal period and during the second stage of labor has been promoted as a means of increasing the elasticity of the perineum and reducing the need for episiotomy. The protective value of perineal massage during the antenatal period has been evaluated in two randomized studies. It involves digital perineal stretching with oil lubrication from 35 weeks' gestation for about 10 minutes every day. In the United Kingdom, Shipman et al.[44] randomized 861 nulliparous women and found a non-significant benefit of 6% in the prevalence of perineal trauma (75% versus 69%, $p<0.07$), but a secondary analysis by maternal age showed a much larger benefit (12.1%) with massage among those aged 30 years and over.

In a larger randomized study, Labrecque et al.[45] found that among participants without a previous vaginal birth, a significantly greater number of women in the experimental group (24%) delivered with an intact perineum compared to the control group (15%). A dose–response effect was observed. However, for women who had a previous vaginal delivery, there were no differences in intact perineum rates between the experimental and control groups. This effect means that for every 10 women doing perineal massage there will be one additional woman whose perineum remains intact after delivery. More importantly, pregnant women find perineal massage acceptable. This study is encouraging in demonstrating the effectiveness of a simple, woman-controlled intervention to maintain perineal integrity. At 3 months postpartum there was no difference in perineal function between women who had and those that had not received perineal massage.[46]

Perineal massage has also been advocated in the second stage of labor, which is provided by the midwife by inserting two fingers in the vagina, and using a sweeping motion to stretch the perineum with lubricating gel during each uterine contraction. In a randomized study, Stamp et al.[47] found no benefit from massage in terms of an intact perineum or pain.

Available evidence suggests that perineal massage may be beneficial to mothers if performed during the antenatal period, especially if they have not had a previous vaginal delivery. Although perineal massage in labor does not increase the likelihood of an intact perineum, it is a harmless practice and midwives can follow their usual practice while taking into account the preferences of the woman.

Water births

Anecdotal reports suggest that the perineum is more pliable in water and can stretch more easily, resulting in less trauma. However, a recent Cochrane Review[48] showed no difference in episiotomy or perineal tears after immersion in water during the first and second stages of labor. However, there is evidence that water immersion during the first stage of labor reduces maternal pain and the use of analgesia, without adverse outcomes on labor duration, operative delivery or neonatal outcomes.

Home delivery

In a prospective observational study of 1068 women, Murphy and Feinland[49] investigated perineal outcomes in a home birth setting. In this sample, 69.6% had an intact perineum, 1.4% had an episiotomy, 29% had a first or second degree tear, and 0.7% had obstetric anal sphincter injury. Logistic regression analysis showed that in multiparae, low socioeconomic status and higher parity were associated with an intact perineum, whereas increased age (≥40 years), previous episiotomy, weight gain over 40 pounds, prolonged second stage, and the use of oils and lubricants were associated with perineal trauma. Among nulliparas, low socioeconomic status, kneeling or hands-and-knees position at delivery, and manual support of the perineum at delivery were associated with an intact perineum, whereas perineal massage during delivery was associated with perineal trauma. The results of this study suggest that it is possible for midwives to achieve a high rate of intact perineums and a low rate of episiotomy in a selected setting and population group.

TRAINING

Throughout the centuries, midwives have received very little formal training in the art of perineal suturing. In June 1967, midwives working in the United Kingdom were permitted by the Central Midwives Board (CMB) to perform episiotomies, but they were not allowed to suture perineal trauma.[50,51] In June 1970 the Chairman of the CMB issued a statement that midwives who were working in 'remote areas overseas' may be authorized by the doctor concerned to repair episiotomies, provided they have been taught the technique and were judged to be competent, but the final responsibility lay with the doctor. However, it was not until 1983 that perineal repair was included in the midwifery curriculum in the UK when European Community Midwives Directives came into force and the CMB issued the following statement: 'Midwives may undertake repair of the perineum provided they have received instruction and are competent in this procedure'.

However, there has not been enough emphasis on training. In 1995, Sultan et al.[52] carried out a survey in London to assess junior doctors' and qualified midwives' knowledge relating to perineal trauma and anatomy and to establish if they were satisfied with their training. Only 20% of junior doctors and 48% of midwives considered their training to be of a good standard when allowed to perform their first unsupervised perineal repair. Furthermore, many of the answers relating to anatomy and classification of tears were incorrect. To improve training we have recently introduced a course using video presentations and specially designed models to demonstrate anatomy and techniques of repair (www.perineum.net) (Thakar, Kettle and Sultan, personal communication).

In a questionnaire survey of 208 health professionals attending this course, 64% were dissatisfied with their training prior to performing their first unsupervised perineal repair. Evaluation of the course carried out by administration of questionnaires 8 weeks following the course showed a significant increase in the participant's ability to classify degree of perineal trauma accurately. Participants changed their practice to evidence-based care after the course with significantly more performing the continuous suturing technique for repair of second degree tears and episiotomy.

It has also been demonstrated that practitioners require more focused training relating to performing mediolateral episiotomies. Andrews et al.[53] carried out a prospective study over a 12-month period of women having their first vaginal delivery to assess positioning of mediolateral episiotomies. The depth, length, distance from the midline, the shortest distance from the midpoint of the anal canal, and the angle subtended from the sagittal or parasagittal plane were measured following suturing of the episiotomy. Results of the study demonstrated that no midwives and only 13 (22%) doctors performed a truly mediolateral episiotomy and that the majority of the incisions were in fact directed closer to the midline.[52]

CONCLUSION

Obstetric perineal trauma can have a devastating effect on a woman's social life with associated psychological sequelae. Consequently, every attempt should be made to prevent such trauma, which may lead to short-term problems such as pain and dyspareunia or more long-term effects such as prolapse and incontinence. Practitioners must base their care on current research evidence and be aware of the potential maternal morbidity that may occur as a result of perineal injury following childbirth. Furthermore, there is a need for more structured training programs and national guidelines to ensure practitioners are appropriately skilled to identify, correctly classify, and repair perineal trauma in order to minimize morbidity and associated problems. Reducing the adverse sequelae of perineal trauma may make vaginal birth more desirable and could possibly decrease the escalating interest in cesarean section.

REFERENCES

1. Magdi I. Obstetric injuries of the perineum. J Obstet Gynaecol Br Commw 1949;49:687–700.
2. Kettle C, Hills RK, Jones P et al. Continuous versus interrupted perineal repair with standard or rapidly absorbed sutures after spontaneous vaginal birth: a randomised controlled trial. Lancet 2002;359:2217–23.
3. Royal College of Obstetricians and Gynaecologists. Methods and materials used in perineal repair. RCOG Guideline No. 23. London: RCOG, 2004.
4. Sleep J, Grant A. Pelvic floor exercises in postnatal care. Br J Midwifery 1987;3:158–64.
5. Carroli G, Belizan J. Episiotomy for vaginal birth. Cochrane Database Syst Rev 2004;(1):CD000081.
6. Barrett G, Pendry E, Peacock J et al. Women's sexuality after childbirth: a pilot study. Arch Sex Behav 1999;28:179–91.
7. Sultan AH, Kamm MA, Bartram CI. Perineal damage at delivery. Contemp Rev Obstet Gynaecol 1994;6:18–24.
8. Thakar R, Sultan AH. Management of obstetric anal sphincter injuries. Obstetrician Gynaecologist 2003;5:72–8.
9. Woodman P, Graney AO. Anatomy and physiology of the female perineal body with relevance to obstetrical injury and repair. Clin Anat 2002;15:321–34.
10. Thacker SB, Banta HD. Benefits and risks of episiotomy: an interpretative review of the English language literature, 1860–1980. Obstet Gynecol Surv 1983;38(6):322–38.
11. Cunningham F, Gant N, Leveno K, Gilstrap L, Hauth J, Wenstrom K (eds) Williams Obstetrics, 21st ed. New York: McGraw-Hill, 2001.
12. Hudson C, Sohaib S, Shulver HM et al. The anatomy of the perineal membrane: its relationship to injury in childbirth and episiotomy. Aust N Z J Obstet Gynaecol 2004;42:193–6.
13. Coats PM, Chan KK, Wilkins M, Beard RJ. A comparison between midline and mediolateral episiotomies. Br J Obstet Gynaecol 1980;87:408–12.
14. McCandlish R, Bowler U, Van Asten H et al. A randomised controlled trial of care of the perineum during second stage of normal labour. Br J Obstet Gynaecol 1998;105:1262–72.
15. Graham ID, Davies C. Episiotomy: the unkindest cut that persists. In: Henderson C, Bick D (eds) Perineal Care: An International Issue. Salisbury: Quay Books, 2004; 58–86.
16. Henriksen TB, Bek KM, Hedegaard M, Secher NJ. Episiotomy and perineal lesions in spontaneous vaginal deliveries. Br J Obstet Gynaecol 1992;99:950–4.
17. Henriksen TB, Bek KM, Hedegaard M, Secher NJ. Methods and consequences of changes in use of episiotomy. BMJ 1994;309:1255–8.

18. World Health Organization Maternal and Newborn Health/Safe Motherhood Unit. Care in normal birth: a practical guide. Report of a Technical Working Group. Doc. No. WHO/FRH/MSM/96.24. Geneva: WHO, 1996; 29.

19. Gordon B, Mackrodt C, Fern E et al. The Ipswich Childbirth study: a randomised evaluation of two stage after birth perineal repair leaving the skin unsutured. Br J Obstet Gynaecol 1998;105:435–49.

20. Oboro VO, Tabowei TO, Loto OM et al. A multicentre evaluation of the two layer repair of after birth perineal trauma. J Obstet Gynaecol 2003;1:5–8.

21. Fleming EM, Hagen S, Niven C. Does perineal suturing make a difference? The SUNS Trial. Br J Obstet Gynaecol 2003;110:684–9.

22. Lundquist M, Olsson A, Nissen E et al. Is it necessary to suture all lacerations after vaginal birth? Birth 2000;27:79–85.

23. Head M. Dropping stitches. Nursing Times 1993;89:64–5.

24. Clement S, Reed B. To stitch or not to stitch? A long term follow-up study of women with unsutured perineal tears. Practicing Midwife 1999;2:20–8.

25. Kettle C, Johanson RB. Absorbable synthetic versus catgut suture material for perineal repair (Cochrane Review). In: Cochrane Library, Issue 1. Chichester: Wiley, 2004.

26. Ethicon. A unique product completes the family: Ethicon Vicryl Rapide. Edinburgh: Ethicon, 1991.

27. Gemymthe A, Langhoff-Roos J, Sahl S et al. New Vicryl formulation: an improved method of perineal repair? Br J Midwifery 1996;4:230–4.

28. McElhinney BR, Glen DRJ, Harper MA. Episiotomy repair: Vicryl versus Vicryl Rapide. Ulster Med J 2000;69:27–9.

29. Kettle C, Johanson RB. Continuous versus interrupted sutures for perineal repair (Cochrane Review). In: The Cochrane Library, Issue 1. Chichester: Wiley, 2004.

30. Fleming N. Can the suturing method make a difference in postpartum perineal pain. J Nurse-Midwifery 1990;35:19–25.

31. Kettle C. The management of perineal trauma. In: Henderson C, Bick D (eds) Perineal Care: An International Issue. Salisbury: Quay Books, 2004; 58–86.

32. Renfrew MJ, Hannah W, Albers L, Floyd E. Practices that minimize trauma to the genital tract in childbirth: a systematic review of the literature. Birth 1998;25:143–60.

33. Howard D, Davies PS, DeLancey JOL, Small Y. Differences in perineal lacerations in black and white primiparas. Obstet Gynecol 2000;96:622–4.

34. Hall MH, Bewley S. Maternal mortality and mode of delivery. Lancet 1999;354:776.

35. Sultan AH, Stanton SL. Preserving the pelvic floor and perineum during childbirth – elective caesarean section? Br J Obstet Gynaecol 1996;103:731–4.

36. Clarke SL, Koonings PP, Phelan JP. Placenta praevia, baccreta and prior cesarean section. Obstet Gynecol 1985;89:89–92.

37. Johanson RB, Menon V. Vacuum extraction versus forceps for assisted vaginal delivery. Cochrane Pregnancy and Childbirth Group. Cochrane Database Syst Rev 2004;(4): CD000224.

38. Gupta JK, Nikodem VC. Woman's position during second stage of labour (Cochrane Review). In: The Cochrane Library, Issue 2. Chichester: Wiley, 2004.

39. Mayerhofer K, Bodner-Adler B, Bodner K et al. Traditional care of the perineum during birth: a prospective, randomized study of 1,076 women. J Reprod Med 2002;47:477–82.

40. Robinson JN, Norwitz ER, Cohen AP et al. Epidural analgesia and third- or fourth-degree lacerations in nulliparas. Obstet Gynecol 1999;94:259–62.

41. Poen AC, Felt-Bersma RJF, Dekker GA et al. Third-degree obstetric perineal tear: risk factors and the preventative role of mediolateral episiotomy. Br J Obstet Gynaecol 1997;104:563–6.

42. Bodner-Adler B, Bodner K, Kimberger O et al. The effect of epidural analgesia on the occurrence of obstetric lacerations and on the neonatal outcome during spontaneous vaginal delivery. Arch Gynecol Obstet 2002;267:81–4.

43. Lieberman E, O'Donoghue C. Unintended effects of epidural analgesia during labor: a systematic review. Am J Obstet Gynecol 2002;186:S31–68.

44. Shipman MK, Boniface DR, Tefft ME, McGlohry FM. Antenatal perineal massage and subsequent perineal outcomes: a randomised controlled trial. Br J Obstet Gynaecol 1997;104:787–91.

45. Labrecque M, Eason E, Marcoux S et al. Randomised controlled trial of prevention of perineal trauma by perineal massage during pregnancy. Am J Obstet Gynecol 1999;180:593–600.

46. Labrecque M, Eason E, Marcoux S. Randomized controlled trial of prevention of perineal trauma by perineal massage during pregnancy. Am J Obstet Gynecol 2000;182:76–80.

47. Stamp G, Kruzins G, Crowther C. Perineal massage in labour and prevention of perineal trauma: randomised controlled trial. BMJ 2001;322:1277–80.

48. Cluett ER, Nikodem VC, McCandlish RE, Burns EE. Immersion in water in pregnancy, labour and birth. Cochrane Database Syst Rev 2004;(2):CD000111.

49. Murphy PA, Feinland JB. Perineal outcomes in a home birth setting. Birth 1998;25:226–33.

50. Myles MF. Textbook for Midwives, 7th ed. London: Churchill Livingstone, 1971.

51. Silverton L. The Art and Science of Midwifery, 1st ed. London: Prentice Hall, 1993.

52. Sultan AH, Kamm MA, Hudson CN. Obstetric perineal trauma: an audit of training. J Obstet Gynaecol 1995;15:19–23.

53. Andrews V, Thakar R, Sultan AH, Jones PW. Are mediolateral episiotomies actually mediolateral? BJOG 2005;112(8):1156–8.

78

Primary repair of obstetric anal sphincter injury

Abdul H Sultan

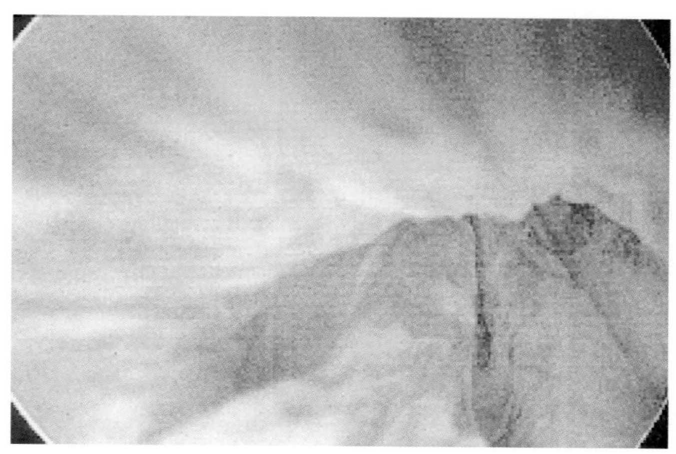

INTRODUCTION

Obstetric anal sphincter injuries (OASIS) are the major cause of anal incontinence and can have a devastating effect on a woman's quality of life. Until the advent of anal endosonography the cause was attributed largely to pelvic neuropathy. However, despite identification and immediate repair of OASIS, the outcome is suboptimal as more than a third of women suffer from impaired continence. This chapter deals with acute OASIS and a description of the various repair techniques is given.

DEFINITION

To avoid confusion, the terms 'primary' and 'secondary' when referring to anal sphincter repair need to be clarified. Following OASIS, repair of the anal sphincter in the immediate postpartum period is usually performed by an obstetrician as a primary procedure. When a repair of the anal sphincter is performed to treat fecal incontinence (usually years after childbirth), it is regarded as a secondary sphincter repair even though a direct primary repair may or may not have been attempted in the postpartum period. Indeed, there is now considerable evidence to suggest that occult[1,2] or missed[3] mechanical trauma to the anal sphincter during childbirth is a major etiologic factor in the development of fecal incontinence.[4] In the UK, primary repair is conducted by obstetricians while secondary repairs are predominantly performed by colorectal surgeons.

CLASSIFICATION OF PERINEAL TEARS

There is considerable inconsistency in the literature regarding the classification of perineal tears, especially relating to third and fourth degree tears.[5] In order to standardize description of anal sphincter injury. Sultan[6] modified the existing classification of perineal tears and the new classification has been accepted by the Royal College of Obstetricians and Gynaecologists[7] as well as the International Consultation on Incontinence:[8]

1. *First degree:* laceration of the vaginal or perineal skin only.
2. *Second degree:* involvement of the vaginal/perineal skin, perineal muscles and fascia but not the anal sphincter.
3. *Third degree:* disruption of the vaginal/perineal skin, perineal body and anal sphincter muscles. This should be subdivided into (Fig. 78.1):
   - 3a: partial tear of the external sphincter involving less than 50% thickness.
   - 3b: more than 50% of external sphincter thickness torn.
   - 3c: internal sphincter also torn.
4. *Fourth degree:* a third degree tear with disruption of the anal epithelium

Isolated tears of the rectal mucosa without involvement of the anal sphincter (Fig. 78.2) are a rare event and should not be included in the above classification.

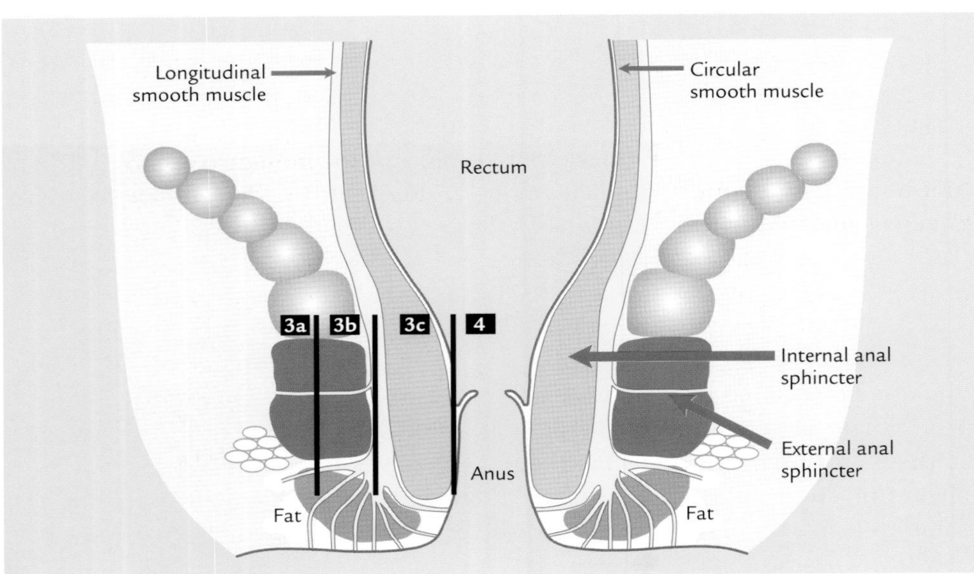

Figure 78.1. *The anal sphincter demonstrating the new classification of anal sphincter injury (see text for full explanation).*

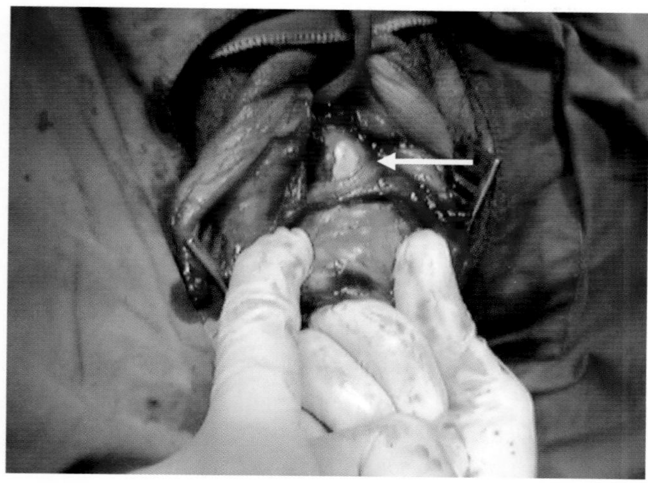

Figure 78.2. *An isolated 'button hole' tear of the rectal mucosa (arrow) inferior to which can be seen an intact anal sphincter.*

INCIDENCE OF OASIS AND OUTCOME OF REPAIR

The reported incidence of OASIS varies from one unit to the next according to obstetric practice but appears to be more specifically related to the type of episiotomy practiced. OASIS is reported to occur between 0.5 and 2.5% of deliveries in centers where mediolateral episiotomy is practiced[9–11] and 11%[12] (19% in primiparae[13]) in centers where midline episiotomy is practiced. Midline episiotomies are favored in North American practice while mediolateral episiotomies are favoured in Europe. To date, 28 studies have evaluated outcome following anal sphincter rupture (Table 78.1). Apart from two studies[22,23] all were performed in centers practicing mainly mediolateral episiotomy. On average, approximately 37% of women continue to suffer from anal incontinence despite primary sphincter repair (Table 78.1). The morbidity would be much higher if other symptoms such as fecal urgency,[9] anal discomfort and dyspareunia[35] are evaluated. The embarrassing symptom of anal incontinence during sexual intercourse is encountered in 72% of symptomatic women.[35]

Anal resting and squeeze pressures are consistently lower in women who previously sustained anal sphincter rupture.[9,16,25,27,30,32,35] The anal canal is shorter after repair.[9,19] The development of incontinence does not appear to be directly related to a pelvic neuropathy as demonstrated by EMG[10,21] and pudendal nerve motor latency conduction studies.[4,9,25] Tetzschner et al.[10] reported that 3-month pudendal latency measurements are longer in women at risk for incontinence. However, these measurements were still within the normal range and no relationship was demonstrated between abnormal latency and incontinence. Although anal sphincter disruption and repair are invariably associated with some degree of denervation and atrophy, current neurophysiologic tests available are not sensitive or specific enough to quantify pudendal neuropathy. There is, however, evidence to show that poor outcome following primary[9,21,25] and secondary[4] repair may be related more to persistent mechanical disruption as demonstrated by anal endosonography rather than 'pudendal neuropathy'.

Unsatisfactory outcome following primary sphincter repair may be attributed either to operator inexperience or to repair technique and subsequent management. Training and experience of clinicians performing perineal repair have been questioned,[38,39] and hands-on training workshops have been shown to influence a change in clinical practice.[40]

TECHNIQUE OF PRIMARY REPAIR

In 1930, Royston[41] described a commonly practiced technique of repair following OASIS: the ends of the torn sphincter were approximated by inserting a deep catgut suture through the inner third of the sphincter muscle and a second set (mattress or interrupted) through the outer third of the sphincter. Subsequently, Ingraham et al.[42] described a modification of the Royston technique[41] such that the sutures were only inserted in the fascial sheath or capsule of the sphincter ani. Fulsher and Fearl[43] also described this technique but emphasized that no sutures should pass through the sphincter muscle. More specifically, Cunningham and Pilkington[44] inserted four interrupted sutures in the capsule of the external sphincter at the anterior, posterior, superior, and inferior points. In 1948, Kaltreider and Dixon[45] described the end-to-end repair technique that had been used since 1935 in which one mattress or figure-of-eight suture was inserted to approximate the sphincter ends.

Obstetricians have used the end-to-end repair technique for decades, using either interrupted or figure-of-eight sutures (Fig. 78.3).[9,46] However, as shown in Table 78.1, despite repair, anal incontinence occurs in 37% of women (range 15 to 61%). In addition, fecal urgency can affect a further 6[9,36] to 28%.[35] Frank fecal incontinence affected 9% (range 2[26] to 23%[35]). Persistent anal sphincter defects following repair have been reported in 34[20] to 91%[36] of women (Fig. 78.4).

By contrast, when fecal incontinence is due to sphincter disruption, colorectal surgeons favor the 'overlap technique' of sphincter repair (secondary) as described by Parks and McPartlin.[47] Jorge and Wexner[48] reviewed the literature and reported on 21 studies using the overlap repair with good results ranging from 74 to 100%. Engel et al.[4] prospectively studied 55 patients with fecal

Table 78.1. *Prevalence of anal incontinence following primary repair of obstetric anal sphincter rupture*

Authors	Year	Country	*n*	Follow-up (months)	Anal incontinence (%)
Sangalli et al.[14]	2000	Switzerland	177	13 years	15
Wood et al.[15]	1998	Australia	84	31	17*
Walsh et al.[16]	1996	UK	81	3	20
Sander et al.[17]	1999	Denmark	48	1	21
Crawford et al.[18]	1993	USA	35	12	23
Sorensen et al.[19]	1993	Denmark	38	3	24
Mackenzie M[20]	2004	England	53	3	25
Nielsen et al.[21]	1992	Denmark	24	12	29
Go & Dunselman[22]	1988	Netherlands	20	6	30
Fenner et al.[13]	2003	USA	165	6	30
DeLeeuw et al.[23]	2001	Netherlands	125	14 years	31
Wagenius & Laurin[24]	2003	Sweden	186	4 years	33
Uustal Fornell et al.[11]	1996	Sweden	51	6	40
Poen et al.[25]	1998	Netherlands	117	56	40
Sultan et al.[9]	1994	UK	34	2	41
Zetterstrom et al.[26]	1999	Sweden	46	9	41
Sorensen et al.[27]	1988	Denmark	25	78	42
Tetzschner et al.[10]	1996	Denmark	72	24–48	42
Williams et al.[28]	2003	UK	124	?	42
Kammerer-Doak et al.[29]	1999	New Mexico	15	4	43
Haadem et al.[30]	1988	Sweden	62	3	44
Bek & Laurberg[31]	1992	Denmark	121	?	50
Davis et al.[32]	2003	UK	52	3.6	50
Fitzpatrick et al.[33]	2000	Ireland	154	3	53
Nazir et al.[34]	2003	Norway	100	18	54
Gjessing et al.[35]	1998	Norway	38	12–60	57
Goffeng et al.[36]	1998	Sweden	27	12	59
Pinta et al.[37]	2004	Finland	52	15	61
Mean					37

* Includes two with secondary sphincter repair.

incontinence undergoing overlap anterior anal sphincter repair and reported a good clinical outcome in 80%. A poor result was found to be associated with an external anal sphincter (EAS) defect, while demonstration of an overlap by anal endosonography (Fig. 78.5) correlated with a favorable outcome.

It is now known that – like other incontinence procedures – outcome can deteriorate with time, and one study has reported 50% continence at 5-year follow-up.[49] However, a number of women in this study had more than one attempt at sphincter repair.[49] Sultan et al.[50] were the first to describe the EAS overlap technique for acute OASIS and, in addition, advocated separate identification and repair (Fig. 78.6) of the internal anal sphincter (IAS). Despite scepticism from surgeons that overlapping friable torn muscle as a primary procedure is not possible, Sultan et al.[50] evaluated the feasibility of this technique in 27 women and demonstrated that EAS overlap repair as well as identification and end-to-end repair of the IAS was possible following acute OASIS. They observed that, compared to matched historical controls[51] who had an end-to-end repair, anal incontinence could be reduced from 41 to 8% using the overlap technique and separate repair of the internal

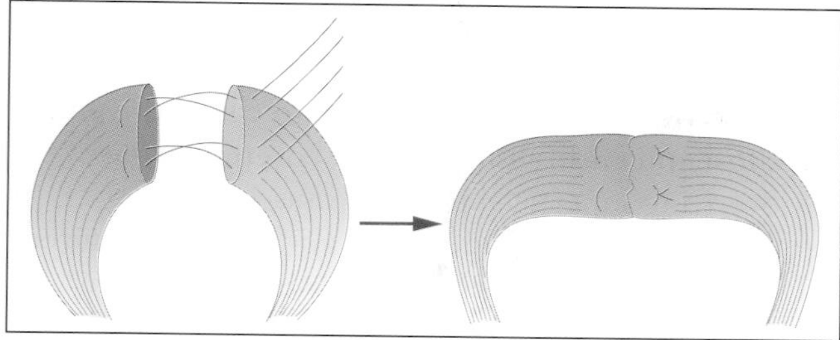

Figure 78.3. *Conventional end-to-end approximation of the disrupted anal sphincter with two figure-of-eight sutures.*

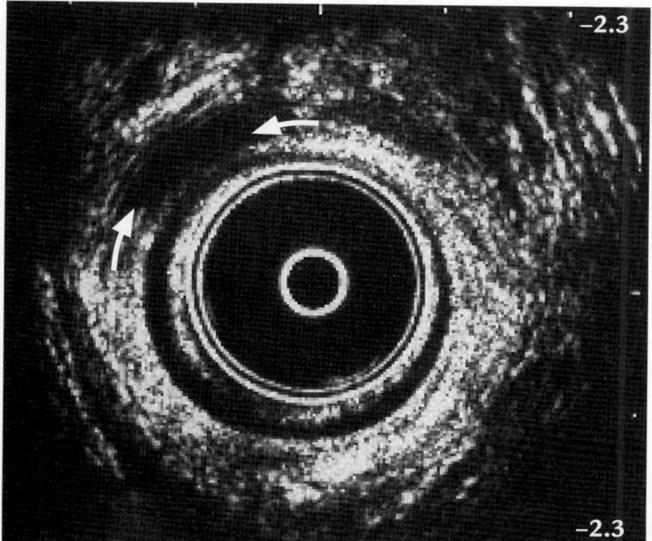

Figure 78.4. *Anal endosonographic image demonstrating an external sphincter defect (between arrows) in a woman complaining of fecal incontinence following an end-to-end repair. The arrows overlie the two retracted ends of the muscle. (Reproduced from ref. 50 with permission.)*

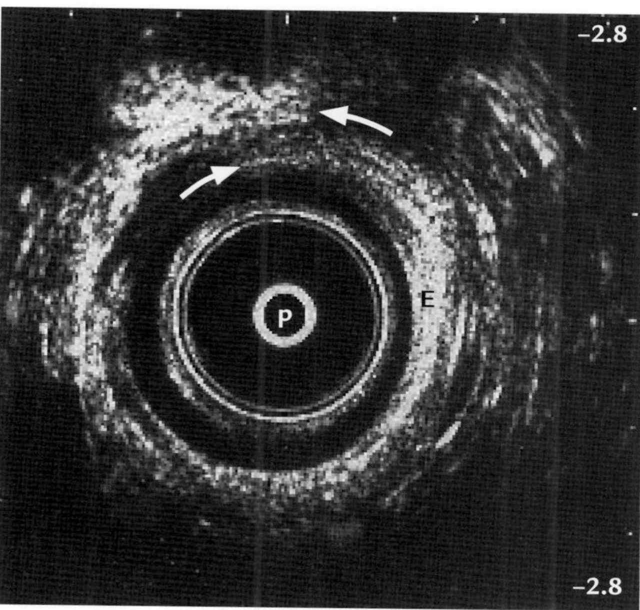

Figure 78.5. *Anal endosonographic image demonstrating overlap of the two ends of the external sphincter. P, probe in anal canal with arrow showing its outer limit. Immediately adjacent to this is the anal epithelium. E, external sphincter; I, internal sphincter. The overlap can be seen between the open arrows. (Reproduced from ref. 50 with permission.)*

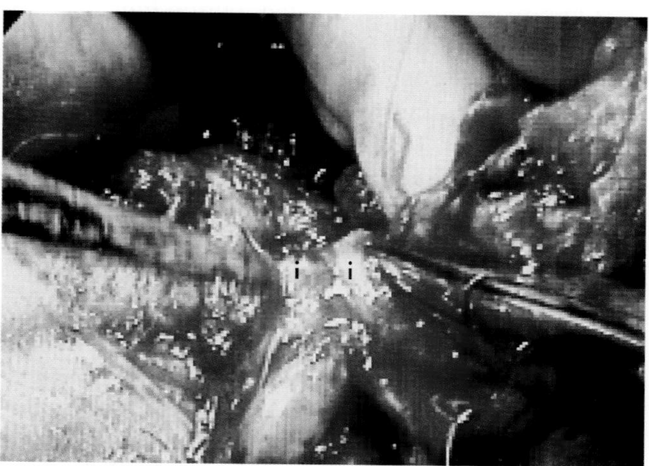

Figure 78.6. *End-to-end approximation of the torn ends of the internal anal sphincter (i). (Reproduced from ref. 50 with permission.)*

sphincter.[50] Based on this they recommended a randomized trial between end-to-end and overlap repair.

The only published randomized trial published to date is by Fitzpatrick et al. in Dublin[33] who found no significant difference between the two methods of repair although there appeared to be a trend towards more symptoms in the end-to-end group. There were methodologic differences in that the torn IAS was not identified and repaired separately and they used a constipating agent for 3 days after the repair. Unfortunately, they included partial EAS tears in their randomized study. A true overlap is not possible if the sphincter ends are not completely divided. Nevertheless, as the authors concur, a better outcome would be expected with both techniques as a consequence of focused education and training in anal sphincter repair.

Fernando et al.[52] performed a multicenter randomized trial of end-to-end versus overlap using the technique described by Sultan et al.[50] At 1-year follow-up they found significantly more urge fecal incontinence in the end-to-end group (24% versus 0; p=0.006).[52]

PRINCIPLES AND TECHNIQUE OF REPAIR

1. OASIS should only be repaired by a doctor experienced in anal sphincter repair or by a trainee under supervision.
2. Repair should be conducted in the operating theater where there is access to good lighting, appropriate equipment, and aseptic conditions. In our unit we have a specially prepared instrument tray containing a Weislander self-retaining retractor, four Allis tissue forceps, McIndoe scissors, tooth forceps, four artery forceps, stitch scissors, and a needle holder (www.perineum.net).
3. General or regional (spinal, epidural, caudal) anesthesia is an important prerequisite, particularly for overlap repair as the inherent tone of the EAS can result in retraction of the torn muscle ends within its sheath. Muscle relaxation is necessary to retrieve the ends, especially if the intention is to overlap the muscles without tension.
4. The full extent of the injury should be evaluated by a careful vaginal and rectal examination in lithotomy and graded according to the classification above (see Fig. 78.1). If there is any uncertainty about the grading it should always be given the higher grade.
5. On rare occasions an isolated 'button hole' type tear (see Fig. 78.2) can occur in the rectum without disrupting the anal sphincter. This is best repaired transvaginally using interrupted Vicryl sutures. To minimize the risk of a persistent rectovaginal fistula, a second layer of tissue should be interposed between the rectum and vagina by approximating the rectovaginal fascia. A colostomy is rarely indicated unless there is a large tear extending above the pelvic floor or there is gross fecal contamination of the wound.
6. In the presence of a fourth degree tear, the torn anal epithelium is repaired with interrupted polyglactin (Vicryl) 3-0 sutures with the knots tied in the anal lumen. A subcuticular repair of the anal epithelium via the transvaginal approach has also been described.[5]
7. The sphincter muscles are repaired with polydioxanone (PDS) 3-0 dyed sutures (see Fig. 78.3). Compared to a braided suture these monofilamentous sutures are less likely to precipitate infection. Non-absorbable monofilament sutures such as nylon or polypropylene (Prolene) are preferred by some colorectal surgeons and can be equally effective. However, they can cause stitch abscesses and the sharp ends of the suture can cause discomfort, necessitating removal. As complete absorption of PDS takes longer than Vicryl, to avoid suture migration care should be taken to cut suture ends short and ensure that they are covered by the overlying superficial perineal muscles.
8. The IAS should be identified and, if torn, repaired separately from the EAS. The IAS lies between the EAS and the anal epithelium. It is thinner and paler than the striated EAS. The appearance of the IAS can be described as being analogous to the flesh of raw fish as opposed to the red meat appearance of the EAS. The ends of the torn muscle are grasped with Allis forceps and an end-to-end repair is performed with interrupted or mattress PDS 3-0 sutures. A torn IAS should be approximated with interrupted sutures as overlapping can be technically difficult. There is some evidence that repair of isolated IAS defects is beneficial in patients with established anal incontinence.[53]
9. The torn ends of the EAS are identified and grasped with Allis tissue forceps (Fig. 78.7). In order to perform an overlap, the muscle may need mobilization by dissection with a pair of McIndoe scissors separating it from the ischioanal fat laterally. When performing an overlap repair, the EAS should be grasped with Allis forceps (Fig. 78.8) and pulled across to overlap in a 'double-breast' fashion. The torn ends of the EAS can then be overlapped (Fig. 78.9) using PDS 3-0 sutures. A proper overlap is only possible when the full length of the torn ends of the EAS are identified; overlapping allows for a greater surface area of contact between muscles (see Fig. 78.9). By contrast, an end-to-end repair can be performed without identifying the full length of the EAS, giving rise to incomplete apposition (Fig. 78.10). Consequently, the woman may remain continent but would be at an increased risk of developing incontinence later in life.

A shorter anal length has been reported following end-to-end primary repair of the external anal sphincter.[9] It has also been shown that a shorter anal length is the best predictor of fecal incontinence following secondary sphincter surgery.[54] Unlike end-to-end repair, if further retraction of the overlapped muscle ends were to occur, it is highly probable that muscle continuity would be maintained. However, if the operator is not familiar with the overlap technique or if the EAS is only partially torn (Grade 3b) then an end-to-end repair should be performed. Instead

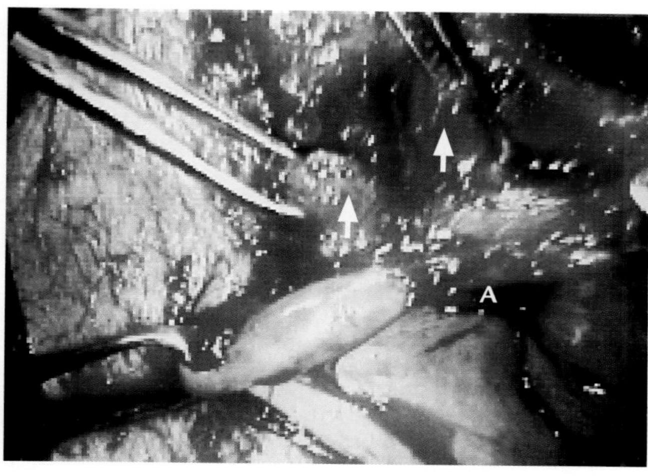

Figure 78.7. *The torn ends of the external anal sphincter (arrows) being elevated by two pairs of Allis forceps. A, anal epithelium. (Reproduced from ref. 50 with permission.)*

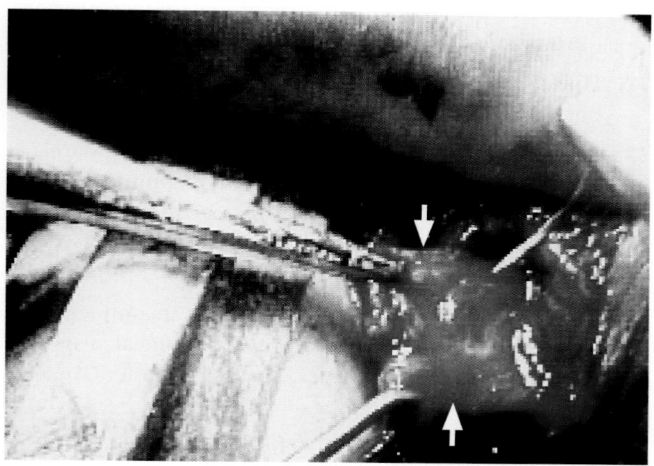

Figure 78.8. *The full width of the external sphincter (arrows) after mobilization. (Reproduced from ref. 50 with permission.)*

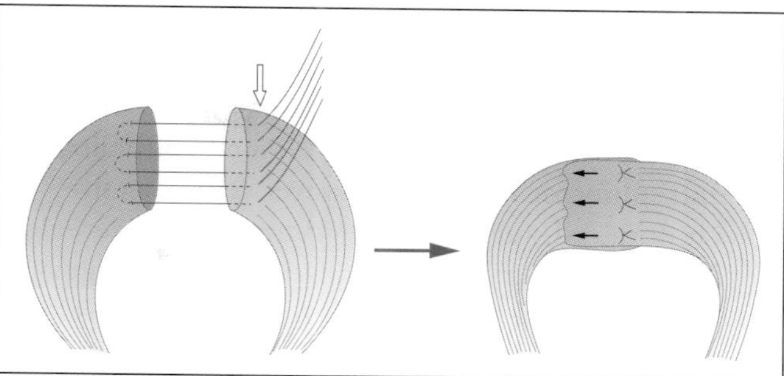

Figure 78.9. *The technique of overlap repair of the external anal sphincter. The first suture is inserted approximately 1.5 cm from the torn edge of the muscle (open arrow) and carried through to within 0.5 cm of the edge of the other arm of the external sphincter. A second row of sutures (small arrows) is inserted to attach the loose end of the overlapped muscle.*

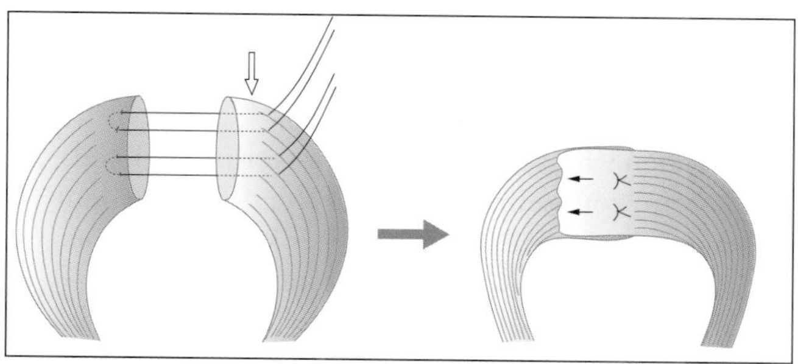

Figure 78.10. *Diagram showing how incomplete apposition can occur with the end-to-end repair of the external sphincter.*

of using hemostatic figure-of-eight sutures, two or three mattress sutures should be used (similar to IAS repair).

10. After repair of the sphincter, the perineal muscles should be sutured to reconstruct the perineal body. A short deficient perineum would make the anal sphincter more vulnerable to trauma during a subsequent vaginal delivery. Finally, the vaginal skin is sutured and the perineal skin is approximated with a Vicryl 3-0 subcuticular suture.
11. A rectovaginal examination should be performed to confirm complete repair and ensure that all tampons or swabs have been removed.
12. Intravenous broad spectrum antibiotics such as cefuroxime 1.5 g and metronidazole 500 mg should be commenced intraoperatively and we prefer to continue this orally for 5–7 days. Although there are no randomized trials to substantiate benefit of this practice, the development of infection could jeopardize repair and lead to incontinence or fistula formation.
13. Severe perineal discomfort, particularly following instrumental delivery, is a known cause of urinary retention and following regional anesthesia it can take up to 12 hours before bladder sensation returns. A Foley catheter should be inserted for about 24 hours unless midwifery staff can ensure that spontaneous voiding occurs at least every 3 hours.
14. Detailed notes should be made of the findings and repair. A pictorial representation of the tears can prove very useful when notes are being reviewed following complications, audit or litigation.
15. As passage of a large bolus of hard stool may disrupt the repair, a stool softener (lactulose 15 ml bd) and a bulking agent such as Fybogel (ispaghula husk, 1 sachet bd) is prescribed

for at least 10–14 days postoperatively. Bowel confinement was practiced by some clinicians who were concerned that the passage of formed stool might disrupt a freshly repaired anal epithelium and sphincter muscle.[52] However, a prospective, randomized, surgeon-blinded trial (*n*=54) revealed that outcome of reconstructive anorectal surgery was not adversely affected by omission of bowel confinement and was associated with fewer episodes of fecal impaction.[55]

16. It is important that the woman understands the implications of sustaining OASIS and should be told how to seek help if symptoms of infection or incontinence develop.
17. Ideally, these women should be followed up in a dedicated perineal clinic by a team with a special interest in OASIS. All women should be given advice on pelvic floor exercises while others with minimal sphincter contractility may need electrical stimulation.[56]
18. Women who sustain anal sphincter injury need careful counseling regarding their management in a subsequent pregnancy. It is known that the risk of recurrence of anal sphincter injury in centers that practice mediolateral episiotomy is only 4.4%.[57] Therefore, asymptomatic women who have no evidence of compromised anal sphincter function (ideally confirmed by anal ultrasound and manometry) should be encouraged to have a vaginal delivery.[5] As cesarean section is associated with increased morbidity and mortality,[58] it should be reserved for those who are symptomatic and women who had undergone a secondary anal sphincter repair for fecal incontinence.

REFERENCES

1. Sultan AH, Kamm MA, Hudson CN. Anal sphincter disruption during vaginal delivery. N Engl J Med 1993:329;1905–11.
2. Donnelly V, Fynes M, Campbell D, Johnson H, O'Connell R, O'Herlihy C. Obstetric events leading to anal sphincter damage. Obstet Gynecol 1998;92:955–61.
3. Andrews V, Thakar R, Sultan AH. Occult anal sphincter injuries – myth or reality? Neurourol Urodyn 2004;23(5/6):442–4.
4. Engel AF, Kamm MA, Sultan AH, Bartram CI, Nicholls RJ. Anterior anal sphincter repair in patients with obstetric trauma. Br J Surg 1994:81:1231–4.
5. Sultan AH, Thakar R. Lower genital tract and anal sphincter trauma. Best Pract Res Clin Obstet Gynaecol 2002;16(1):99–116.
6. Sultan AH. Editorial: Obstetric perineal injury and anal incontinence. Clin Risk 1999;5(5):193–6.
7. Royal College of Obstetricians and Gynaecologists. Management of third and fourth degree perineal tears following vaginal delivery. RCOG Guideline No. 29. London: RCOG Press, 2001.
8. Norton C, Christiansen J, Butler U et al. Anal incontinence. In: Abrams P, Cardozo L, Khoury S, Wein A (eds) Incontinence, 2nd ed. Plymouth: Health Publication, 2002; 985–1044.
9. Sultan AH, Kamm MA, Hudson CN, Bartram CI. Third degree obstetric anal sphincter tears: risk factors and outcome of primary repair. BMJ 1994;308:887–91.
10. Tetzschner T, Sorensen M, Lose G, Christiansen J. Anal and urinary incontinence in women with obstetric anal sphincter rupture. Br J Obstet Gynaecol 1996;103:1034–40.
11. Uustal Fornell EK, Berg G, Hallbook O, Matthiesen LS, Sjodahl R. Clinical consequences of anal sphincter rupture during vaginal delivery. J Am Coll Surg 1996;183:553–8.
12. Hueston WJ. Factors associated with the use of episiotomy during vaginal delivery. Obstet Gynecol 1996;87:1001–5.
13. Fenner DE, Becky-Genberg MPH, Brahma P, Marek L, DeLancey JOL. Fecal and urinary incontinence after vaginal delivery with anal sphincter disruption in an obstetrics unit in the United States. Am J Obstet Gynecol 2003;189:1543–50.
14. Sangalli MR, Floris L, Weil A. Anal incontinence in women with third or fourth degree perineal tears and subsequent vaginal deliveries. Aust N Z J Obstet Gynaecol 2000;40:244–8.
15. Wood J, Amos L, Rieger N. Third degree anal sphincter tears: risk factors and outcome. Aust N Z J Obstet Gynaecol 1998;38:414–17.
16. Walsh CJ, Mooney EF, Upton GJ, Motson RW. Incidence of third-degree perineal tears in labour and outcome after primary repair. Br J Surg 1996;83:218–21.
17. Sander P, Bjarnesen L, Mouritsen A, Fuglsang-Frederiksen A. Anal incontinence after third/fourth degree laceration. One-year follow-up after pelvic floor exercises. Int J Urogynecol 1999;10:177–81.
18. Crawford LA, Quint EH, Pearl ML, DeLancey JOL. Incontinence following rupture of the anal sphincter during delivery. Obstet Gynecol 1993;82:527–31.
19. Sorensen M, Tetzschner T, Rasmussen OO, Bjarnessen J, Christiansen J. Sphincter rupture in childbirth. Br J Surg 1993;80:392–4.
20. Mackenzie N, Parry L, Tasker M, Gowland MR, Michie MR, Hobbiss JH. Anal function following third degree tears. Colorect Dis 2004;6:92–6.
21. Nielsen MB, Hauge C, Rasmussen OO, Pedersen JF, Christiansen J. Anal endosonographic findings in the follow-

up of primarily sutured sphincteric ruptures. Br J Surg 1992;79:104–6.

22. Go PMNYH, Dunselman GAJ. Anatomic and functional results of surgical repair after total perineal rupture at delivery. Surg Gynecol Obstet 1988;166:121–4.

23. DeLeeuw JW, Vierhout ME, Struuk PC, Hop WCJ, Wallenberg HCS. Anal sphincter damage after vaginal delivery: functional outcome and risk factors for fecal incontinence. Acta Obstet Gynecol Scand 2001;80:830–4.

24. Wagenius J, Laurin J. Clinical symptoms after anal sphincter rupture: a retrospective study. Acta Obstet Gynecol Scand 2003;82:246–50.

25. Poen AC, Felt-Bersma RJF, Strijers RLM, Dekkers GA, Cuesta MA, Meuwissen SGM. Third-degree obstetric perineal tear: long-term clinical and functional results after primary repair. Br J Surg 1998;85:1433–8.

26. Zetterstrom J, Lopez A, Anzen B, Norman M, Holmstrom B, Mellgren A. Anal sphincter tears at vaginal delivery: Risk factors and clinical outcome of primary repair. Obstet Gynecol 1999;24:21–8.

27. Sorensen SM, Bondesen H, Istre O, Vilmann P. Perineal rupture following vaginal delivery. Acta Obstet Gynecol Scand 1988;67:315–18.

28. Williams A, Adams EJ, Bolderson J, Tincello DG, Richmond D. Effect of new guideline on outcome following third degree perineal tears: results of a three-year audit. Int Urogynecol J 2003;14:385–9.

29. Kammerer-Doak DN, Wesol AB, Rogers RG, Dominguez CE, Dorin MH. A prospective cohort study of women after primary repair of obstetric anal sphincter laceration. Am J Obstet Gynecol 1999;181(6):1317–23.

30. Haadem K, Ohrlander S, Lingman G. Long-term ailments due to anal sphincter rupture caused by delivery – a hidden problem. Eur J Obstet Gynecol Reprod Biol 1988;27:27–32.

31. Bek KM, Laurberg S. Risks of anal incontinence from subsequent vaginal delivery after a complete obstetric anal sphincter tear. Br J Obstet Gynaecol 1992;99:724–7.

32. Davis I, Kumar D, Stanton SL, Thakar R, Fynes M, Bland J. Symptoms and anal sphincter morphology following primary repair of third degree tears. Br J Surg 2003;90:1573–9.

33. Fitzpatrick M, Behan M, O'Connell R, O'Herlihy C. A randomized clinical trial comparing primary overlap with approximation repair of third degree obstetric tears. Am J Obstet Gynecol 2000;183:1220–4.

34. Nazir M, Stien R, Carlsen E, Jacobsen AF, Nesheim B. Early evaluation of bowel symptoms after primary repair of obstetric perineal rupture. Dis Colon Rectum 2003;46:1245–50.

35. Gjessing H, Backe B, Sahlin Y. Third degree obstetric tears: outcome after primary repair. Acta Obstet Gynecol Scand 1998;77:736–40.

36. Goffeng AR, Andersch B, Berndtsson I, Hulten L, Oresland T. Objective methods cannot predict anal incontinence after primary repair of extensive anal tears. Acta Obstet Gynecol Scand 1988;77:439–43.

37. Pinta TM, Kylanpaa M, Salmi TK. Primary sphincter repair: are the results of the operation good enough? Dis Colon Rectum 2004;47:18–23.

38. Sultan AH, Kamm MA, Hudson CN. Obstetric perineal tears: an audit of training. J Obstet Gynaecol 1995;15:19–23.

39. Fernando RJ, Sultan AH, Radley S, Jones PW, Johanson RB. Management of obstetric anal sphincter injury: a systematic review and national practice survey. BMC Health Services Research 2002;2:9.

40. Thakar R, Sultan AH, Fernando R, Monga A, Stanton S. Can workshops on obstetric anal sphincter rupture change practice? Int Urogynecol J 2001;12(3):S5.

41. Royston GD. Repair of complete perineal laceration. Am J Obstet Gynecol 1930;19:185–95.

42. Ingraham HA, Gardner MM, Heus GE. A report on 159 third degree tears. Am J Obstet Gynecol 1949;57:730–5.

43. Fulsher RW, Fearl CL. The third-degree laceration in modern obstetrics. Am J Obstet Gynecol 1955;69:786–93.

44. Cunningham CB, Pilkington JW. Complete perineotomy. Am J Obstet Gynecol 1955;70:1225–31.

45. Kaltreider DF, Dixon McC. A study of 710 complete lacerations following central episiotomy. Southern Med J 1948;41:814–20.

46. Hauth JC, Gilstrap LC III, Ward SC, Hankins CD. Early repair of an external sphincter ani muscle and rectal mucosal dehiscence. Obstet Gynecol 1986;67(6):806–9.

47. Parks AG, McPartlin JF. Late repairs of injuries of the anal sphincter. Proc R Soc Med 1971;64:1187–9.

48. Jorge JMN, Wexner SD. Etiology and management of fecal incontinence. Dis Colon Rectum 1993;36:77–97.

49. Malouf AJ, Norton CS, Engel AF, Nicholls RJ, Kamm MA. Long term results of overlapping anterior anal-sphincter repair for obstetric trauma. Lancet 2000;355:260–5.

50. Sultan AH, Monga AK, Kumar D, Stanton SL. Primary repair of obstetric anal sphincter rupture using the overlap technique. Br J Obstet Gynaecol 1999;106:318–23.

51. Sultan AH. Third degree tear repair. In: MacClean AB, Cardozo L (eds) Incontinence in Women. London: RCOG Press, 2002; 379–90.

52. Fernando RJ, Sultan AH, Kettle C, Jones P, O'Brien PMS. A randomised trial of overlap vs end-to-end primary repair of the anal sphincter. Neurourol Urodyn 2004;23:411–12.

53. Meyenberger C, Bertschinger P, Zala GF, Buchmann P. Anal sphincter defects in fecal incontinence: correla-

tion between endosonography and surgery. Endoscopy 1996;28:217–24.

54. Hool GR, Lieber ML, Church JM. Postoperative anal canal length predicts outcome in patients having sphincter repair for fecal incontinence. Dis Colon Rectum 1999;42:313–18.

55. Nessim A, Wexner SD, Agachan F et al. Is bowel confinement necessary after anorectal reconstructive surgery? A prospective, randomized, surgeon-blinded trial. Dis Colon Rectum 1999;42:16–23.

56. Sultan AH, Nugent K. Pathophysiology and non-surgical treatment of anal incontinence. Br J Obstet Gynaecol 2004;111(Suppl 1):84–90.

57. Harkin R, Fitzpatrick M, O'Connell PR, O'Herlihy C. Anal sphincter disruption at vaginal delivery: is recurrence predictable? Eur J Obstet Gynecol Reprod Biol 2003;109:149–52.

58. Sultan AH, Stanton SL. Preserving the pelvic floor and perineum during childbirth – elective caesarean section? Br J Obstet Gynaecol 1996;103:731–4.

79

Surgery for fecal incontinence

Klaus E Matzel, Manuel Besendörfer

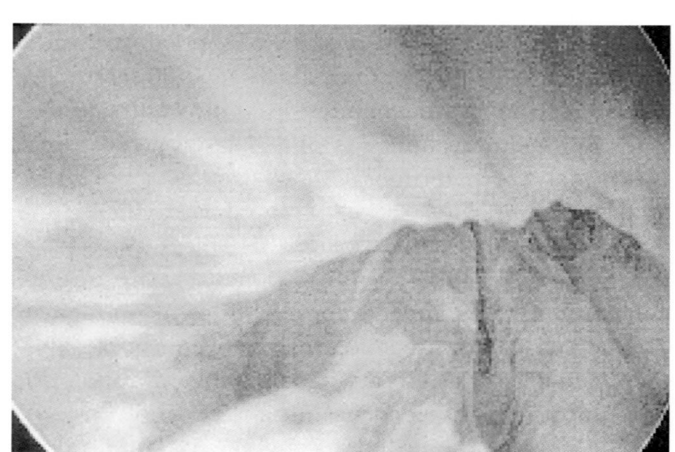

INTRODUCTION

The true prevalence of fecal incontinence is unknown. Approximately 2% of the general population suffers from the inability to control bowel emptying,[1] but this rate rises with age, affecting up to 11% of men and 26% of women over the age of 50,[2] and, in combination with urinary incontinence, up to 40% of nursing home patients.[3]

Recent advances in diagnostic methods have led to a better understanding of the physiology of the various components of the continence organ. Today, fecal continence is understood to be maintained by coordinated, synergistic, and organic functions of three organs: the reservoir system of the rectum, the outlet resistance of the sphincteric complex, and the sensory lining of the anal canal. Their functional interaction is attained by a convergence of somatomotor, somatosensory, and autonomic innervation.

Rectal reservoir function can be addressed therapeutically with surgical resection, but most surgical procedures for fecal incontinence aim to improve, augment, or substitute sphincteric function.

DIAGNOSTIC TECHNIQUES AND TREATMENT CONSIDERATIONS

Causes of fecal incontinence are multiple. To establish a meaningful therapeutic concept, it is important to identify morphologic and functional deficits of the various anatomic components contributing to anal continence. Endoanal ultrasound and magnetic resonance imaging (MRI) enable us to detect morphologic defects of the rectum and sphincteric complex. With anorectal manometry we can test and quantify the muscular function of the smooth muscle internal anal sphincter and the striated muscular external anal sphincter, the perception of rectal filling and distension, the compliance of the rectal reservoir, and the reflexive interaction of the rectum and anal sphincter. Electromyographic recording of the striated muscles of the external anal sphincter and the pelvic floor allows us to differentiate muscular from neurogenic defects and to estimate the extent of reinnervation. Peripheral latency recording (pudendal nerve terminal motor latency [PNTML]) helps to identify the location of neural damage.

To a certain extent, isolated deficits within each functional component of the continence organ can be compensated for – indeed, most cases of incontinence can be sufficiently treated with relatively simple and pragmatic measures. Because comparable morphologic and functional lesions may result in clinical pictures of varying severity, the use of advanced diagnostic procedures should be determined by the desired therapeutic consequence.

The diagnosis of fecal incontinence is based on a standard anorectal examination (to exclude pathologic conditions that may result in secondary incontinence) and a focused history. Standardized questionnaires and general and disease-specific quality-of-life scores[4,5] have become widely used in recent years to quantify the extent and severity of fecal incontinence and its impact on quality of life and to monitor therapeutic effects. If a muscular defect is suspected, endoanal ultrasound should be added.

If sphincteric lesions amenable to direct repair are excluded, conservative treatment such as diet, medication and retrograde irrigation can – without further diagnostic steps – be initiated to improve stool consistency, delay colonic transit, and establish a normal periodicity to bowel emptying. If these fail or do not produce adequate results, further diagnostic procedures are indicated to differentiate muscular from neurogenic and combined lesions. Based on the diagnostic findings, two concepts of treatment can be discussed: functional rehabilitation and morphologic reconstruction. The former is indicated in patients with no morphologic defects, and aims to recruit residual function of the continence organ; the latter is indicated in patients with morphologic defects of functional relevance, and aims to re-establish morphologic integrity.

FUNCTIONAL REHABILITATION

Biofeedback is the first choice for functional rehabilitation. Based on the principle of operant conditioning, visual or acoustic signals are used to teach the patient awareness and use of specific physiologic functions and thus to recruit residual function. Success ranges widely, from 38 to 100%.[6] Retrograde irrigation is intended to improve rectal reservoir function (by distension and improved perception through a defined stimulus) and to establish a rhythm for sufficient bowel emptying (to ensure time intervals free of fecal loss). If these conservative therapies fail to improve symptoms, surgical intervention should be considered.

Sacral nerve stimulation

Sacral nerve stimulation (SNS) is based on the concept of recruiting residual function of the continence organ by stimulation of its peripheral nerve supply. The sacral spinal nerves are the most distal common location of a dual peripheral nerve supply of the striated pelvic floor and anal sphincter muscles.[7] Various physiologic functions contributing to continence are activated by low frequency electrostimulation of one or more sacral spinal nerves by a fully implantable neurostimulation device.[8] The indication for the implantation of a permanent neuroprosthesis is based on the results of the following two-step test stimulation.[9]

Acute percutaneous/peripheral nerve evaluation (PNE)

PNE[10] determines whether, in the prospective patient, contraction of the striated pelvic floor muscles can be elicited by SNS (thus establishing the integrity of the sacral spinal nerves), and tests the individual relevance of each sacral spinal nerve to anal sphincteric contraction and anal canal closure (thus identifying the optimal site of stimulation).[10] The procedure can be performed under general or local anesthesia.

For acute PNE, needle electrodes are inserted into the dorsal sacral foramina of S2, S3, and S4. This positioning aims for placement close to the site where the sacral spinal nerves enter the pelvic cavity through the ventral opening of the sacral foramen and proximal to the sacral plexus.

Stimulation can provoke contraction of the external anal sphincter, pelvic floor, and lower extremities.[11] The concomitant reactions of the leg and foot are helpful to ensure adequate placement of the needle electrode. With different parameters applied during testing, these side effects will be eliminated during therapeutic stimulation. If this acute stimulation successfully elicits contraction of the pelvic floor, subchronic percutaneous stimulation is initiated.

Subchronic percutaneous/peripheral nerve evaluation

The sacral spinal nerve(s) found in acute testing to be most effective with regard to muscular contraction (most commonly, but not consistently, S3) is/are stimulated continuously for a period of time sufficient to demonstrate a potential beneficial effect. The length of the observation period depends on the frequency and severity of the incontinence.

Two technical options can be used for subchronic PNE: a temporary, percutaneously placed, test stimulation lead (or multiple leads) that will be removed at the end of this phase,[10] or a surgically placed quadripolar lead, the so-called 'foramen electrode'. Both types of lead are connected to an external pulse generator for screening. The latter electrode can be connected to an implanted pulse generator (so-called 'two-stage implant') if the test stimulation is effective. With both techniques the selected sacral spinal nerve is continuously stimulated (pulse width 210 μsec; frequency 15 Hz), except during voiding and defecation.

The results of the test stimulation are highly predictive: most commonly a >50% reduction in incontinent episodes or in days with incontinence is generally accepted as the indication for the implantation of a permanent neurostimulation device.

Chronic stimulation with a permanent implant

Permanent stimulation with a fully implantable device aims to make use of the therapeutic effect achieved by subchronic PNE. The permanent system consists of the quadripolar foramen lead and the pulse generator: the electrode is placed close to the sacral spinal nerve successfully tested during subchronic stimulation,[10] and the generator is positioned subcutaneously in the abdomen or gluteal area (Fig. 79.1). Placement is performed under general anesthesia.

Recently, a less invasive technique that uses a foramen electrode with a modified anchoring device placed through a trocar has been proposed[12] (Fig. 79.2). This technique can be used either for stage one of the two-stage implant or for electrode placement after successful screening with wire electrodes. It can be performed under local anesthesia.

The foramen electrode contains four contact electrodes. The combination most effective with regard to required voltage and the patient's perception of muscle contraction of the perineum and anal sphincter is chosen for permanent low frequency stimulation (pulse width

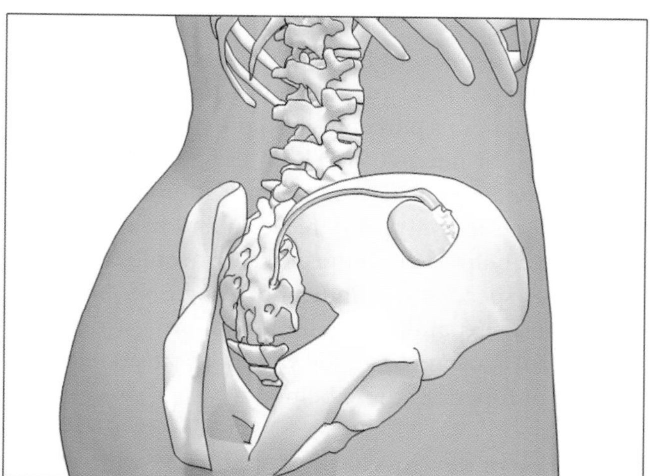

Figure 79.1. *Sacral nerve stimulation: foramen electrode with impulse generator.*

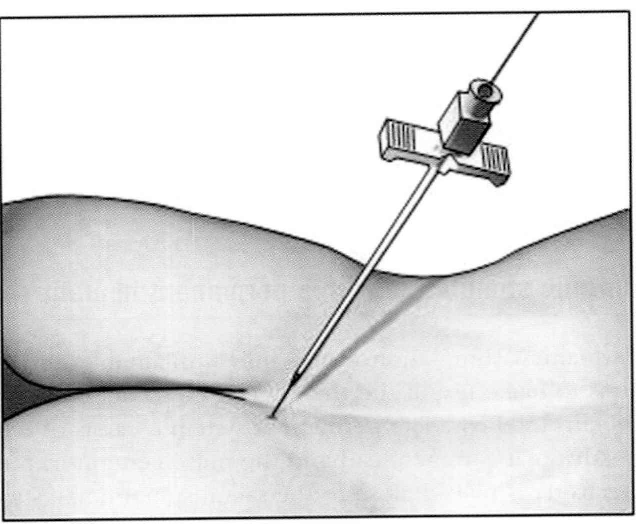

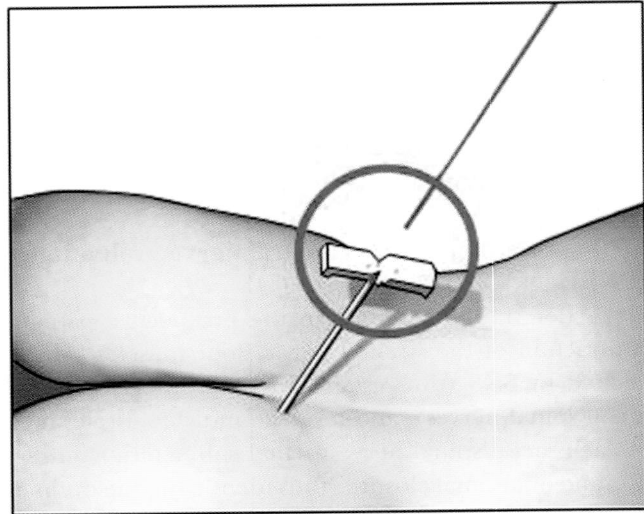

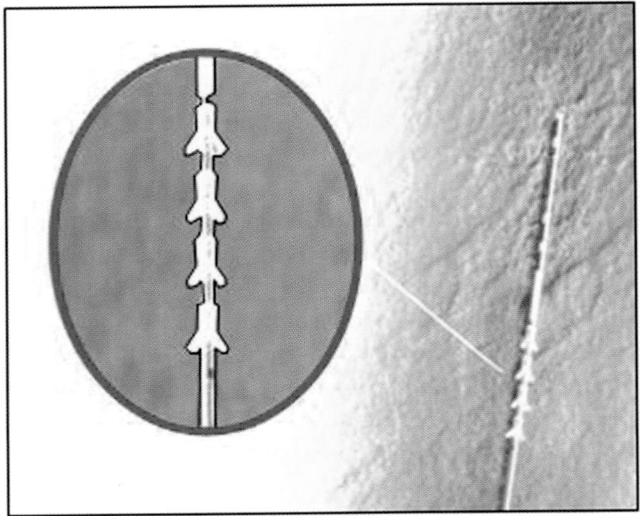

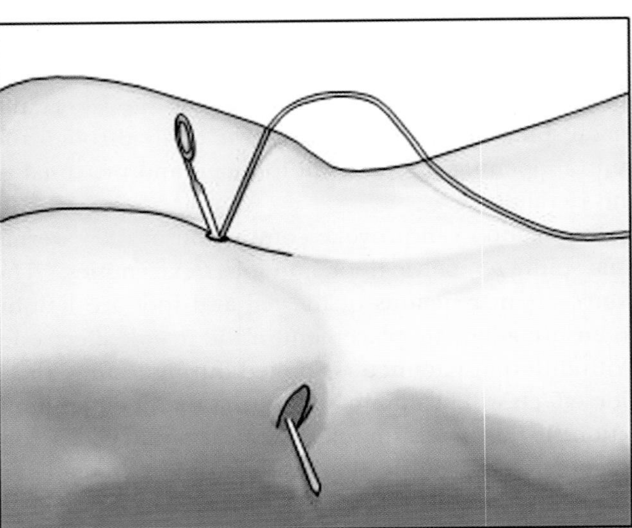

Figure 79.2. *Sacral nerve stimulation: placement of a so-called 'tined lead' electrode through a trocar.*

210 µsec; frequency 15 Hz; on/off: 5 s/1 s or continuous stimulation; level of stimulation usually above the individual patient's perception of muscular contraction, and adjusted if necessary). The pulse generator is activated by telemetry. Patients interrupt stimulation with a hand-held device only for defecation and urination.

With the help of the acute and subchronic test stimulation, the spectrum of indications for SNS has been continuously expanded to patients suffering from fecal incontinence, owing to a wide variety of causes resulting in a lack of function, these being:

- weakness of the external anal sphincter[13] with concomitant urinary incontinence[14] or a defect and/or deficit of the smooth muscle internal anal sphincter;[15]
- status following rectal resection;[16]
- limited structural defects of the external anal sphincter combined with limited defect of the internal anal sphincter;[15]
- neurogenic incontinence.[17]

During the evolution of SNS as a treatment for fecal incontinence, a standard evaluation of outcome became broadly accepted. Not only is the effect on bowel control measured, but also the effect on quality of life.

The short- and long-term effects of SNS have been demonstrated in multiple single and multicenter trials (Table 79.1). With chronic SNS the frequency of involuntary loss of bowel content is reduced, the ability to postpone defecation is improved,[24] and a substantial percentage of patients gain full continence.[10] Quality of

Table 79.1. ***Results of sacral nerve stimulation***

Reference	Year	Study	*n*	Pretreatment	PNE	Treatment*	Follow-up (months)
Incontinent episodes: liquid or solid/1 week							
Altomare et al.[18]	2004	SC	14	14 (11–14)†	–	0.5 (0–2)	14 (6–48)
Ganio et al.[19]	2001	SC	5	3 (2–14)	0	0	14 (5–37)
Ganio et al.[20]	2001	MC	16	5.5 (1–19)	–	0 (0–1)	10.5 (3–45)
Jarrett et al.[21]	2004	MC	46	7.5 (1–78)	–	1 (0–39)	12 (1–72)
Kenefick et al.[22]	2002	SC	15	11 (2–30)	0 (0–7)	0 (0–4)	24 (3–80)
Leroi et al.[14]	2001	SC	6	2 (1–7)	0 (0–4)	0.5 (0–2)	6 (3–6)
Matzel et al.[23]	2001	SC	6	9 (2–19)	1.5 (1–5)	0 (0–1)	59 (5–70)
Matzel et al.[24]	2004	MC	34	8.3 (1.7–78.7)	–	0.75 (0–25)	23.9 (1–36)
Ripetti et al.[25]	2002	SC	4	12‡	–	2‡, §	24
Rosen et al.[17]	2001	SC	16	2 (1–5)	–	0.7 (0–5)	15 (3–26)
Uludag et al.[26]	2002	SC	27	8.7 (2–38)	0.7 (0–10)	0.5 (0.5–0.7)§	6.0‡
Cleveland Clinic Score**							
Altomare et al.[18]	2004	SC	14	15 (12.5–17.5)	–	5.7 (2–6)§	14 (6–48)
Jarrett et al.[21]	2004	MC	27	14 (5–20)	–	6 (1–20)	–
Malouf et al.[15]	2000	SC	5	16 (13–20)	–	2 (0–13)	16
Matzel et al.[13]	2003	SC	16	16 (12–19)	–	2 (0–7)	32.5 (3–99)
Rasmussen & Christiansen[27]	2002	SC	10	19.5 (14–20)	–	5.5 (0–20)	4.5 (1–12)
Rasmussen et al.[28]	2004	MC	37	16 (9–20)	–	6 (0–20)	6 (0–36)

Data: median (range), if not noted otherwise.
*Data at last follow-up; † Median value over 2 weeks; ‡ Mean (SD and range not available); § Follow-up value (median of values at published follow-up intervals); ** Cleveland Clinic Score: 0 continent, 20 incontinent.
MC, multicenter; SC, single center; PNE, peripheral nerve evaluation.

life is improved postoperatively, both in subscales of general quality-of-life instruments[15,22,24] and, significantly, in all categories of the disease-specific Fecal Incontinence Quality of Life Index.[4,17,18,24]

Complications are rare. In less than 5% of patients has device removal become necessary,[10,29] mostly because of pain or infection. After removal because of infection, reimplanation can be performed successfully at a later date.[8]

The physiologic mode of action of SNS is not yet clearly understood. Its effect is complex and multifactorial, involving somatomotor, somatosensory, and autonomic functions of the anorectal continence organ.[10,29]

RECONSTRUCTIVE TECHNIQUES

Morphologic reconstruction is indicated if a defined, functionally relevant, sphincteric defect is diagnosed. Several techniques, such as direct overlapping sphincter repair, postanal repair, and total pelvic floor repair, have been advocated in the past, and sphincter repair is now generally accepted as first line treatment for incontinence owing to sphincteric defects. Electromyography of the external sphincter may be helpful to estimate the functional outcome and to counsel the patient properly, as some studies suggest that the presence of pudendal neuropathy adversely affects results.[6]

Sphincter repair aims to re-establish function by reconstructing the morphologic defect; a muscular gap is closed by adaption of the dehiscent muscle. With a curved incision over the perineal body, the scar tissue is dissected until healthy muscle on either side can be identified. The scar can be used in the readaption of the muscular anal ring (Figs 79.3, 79.4). The muscle can be sutured either in an overlapping fashion or by adaption.[30] Anterior plication of the levator muscles can be added.

The results of sphincter repair are not reported uniformly and thus it is difficult to evaluate series and to compare the outcome of this technique with that of other procedures. Moreover, prospective outcome recording is rare; most reported results are based on patients' recall

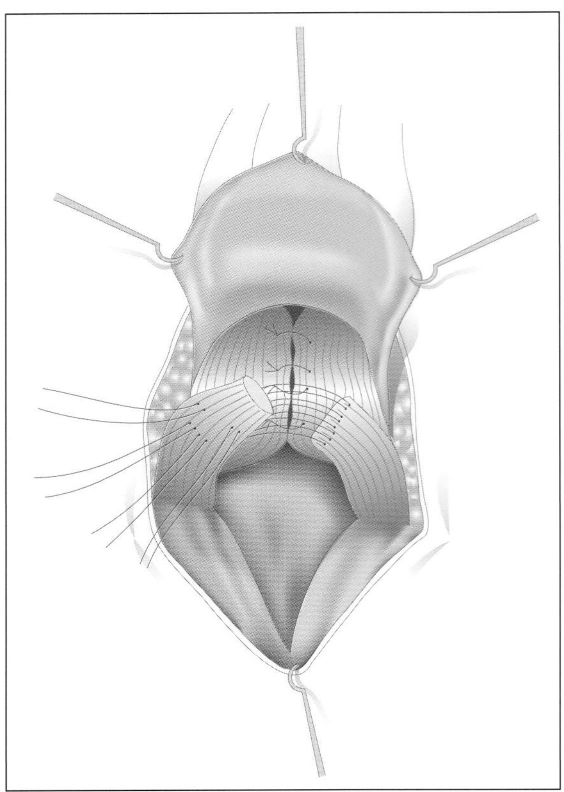

Figure 79.3. *Mattress sutures placed through the mobilized external anal sphincter muscle to achieve an overlap sphincter repair.*

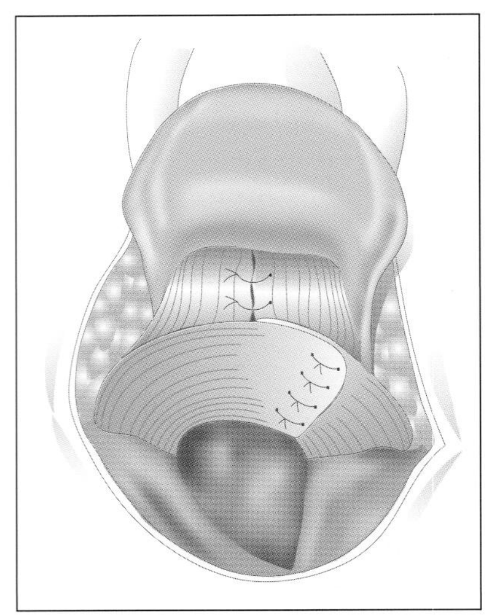

Figure 79.4. *Firm (but not tight) tied sutures with overlapping muscle ends.*

and are limited to functional issues without addressing the quality of life of the patient. Approximately two-thirds of patients report a significant improvement in continence (Table 79.2). However, the long-term therapeutic effect of sphincter repair has recently been questioned as several studies have reported a deterioration in function over time.[41–43]

If sphincter repair – despite re-establishment of morphologic integrity – fails to achieve success, or if function deteriorates over time, patients can be considered for functional rehabilitation, such as biofeedback, irrigation, and sacral nerve stimulation.

Table 79.2. *Results of anterior overlapping sphincter repair**

Reference	Year	Study	*n*	Excellent/ good (%)	Fair (%)	Poor (%)	Follow-up (months)
Buie et al.[31]	2001	SC	158	62	26	12	43 (6–120)
Engel et al.[32]	1994	SC	55	79	17	4	15 (6–36)
Fleshman et al.[33]	1991	SC	55	71	22	6	– (12–24)
Gibbs & Hook[34]	1993	SC	16	73	15	12	na
Gilliland et al.[35]	1998	SC	100	60	19	21	24 (2–96)†
Jacobs et al.[36]	1990	SC	30	83	17	0	– (7–60)
Londono-Schimmer et al.[37]	1994	SC	60	60	18	22	na
Nikiteas et al.[38]	1996	SC	42	67	14	19	38 (12–66)†
Oliveira et al.[39]	1996	SC	55	71	9	20	29
Rasmussen et al.[40]	1999	SC	38	68	13	18	3

Data: mean (range), if not noted otherwise.
*Adapted from ref. 6; † Median (range).
na, not applicable.

Sphincter replacement

Sphincter replacement procedures are indicated if functional rehabilitation is not successful, if incontinence is the result of a substantial muscular defect that is not suitable for sphincter repair, or if a neurologic defect is present. Two techniques have gained broad acceptance: dynamic graciloplasty (DGP)[44] and the artificial bowel sphincter (ABS).[45]

Dynamic graciloplasty

DGP is a modification of the transposition of the gracilis muscle around the anus to function as a neosphincter, described in the early 1950s.[46] The gracilis muscle is mobilized through an incision on the inner thigh and detached at its proximal attachment at the tuberositas tibiae. Only the proximal vascular pedicle and its neural supply are preserved (Fig. 79.5). With two perianal incisions the mobilized gracilis muscle is placed around the anus. The aim of this transposition is to encircle the anal canal completely with muscle tissue. Thus, the configuration of the muscle sling – the alpha, gamma, epsilon configuration – is determined by the length of the muscle and its tendon. This passive muscle wrap is rendered dynamic by the implantation of a neurostimulation device (Fig. 79.6). The system consists of two electrodes, placed intramuscularly, close to the nerve, connected to a pulse generator and positioned subcutaneously or beneath the fascia in the lower abdominal wall.[44] The implantation can be performed either during the muscle transposition or with a timely delay.[47]

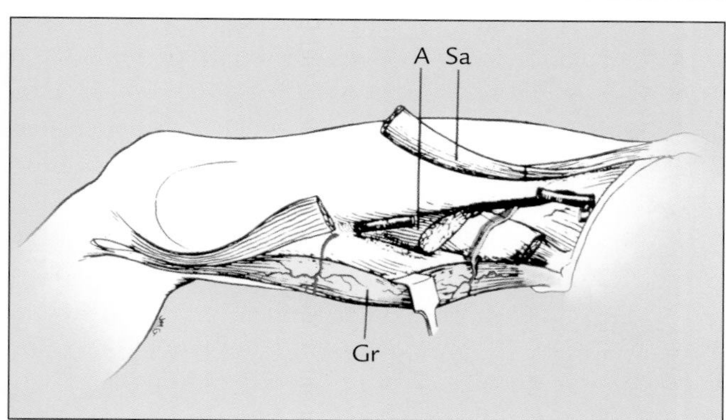

Figure 79.5 *Gracilis (Gr) muscle with proximal neuromuscular pedicle and distal vascular pedicle. A: artery; Sa: sartorius muscle.*

To adapt the muscle to prolonged contraction, the periods of stimulation are increased in a stepwise fashion. Chronic low frequency stimulation causes muscle fiber transformation. The gracilis muscle is predominately composed of fast-twitch, fatigue-prone, type II muscle fibers, which low frequency stimulation will convert to slow-twitch, fatigue-resistant type I fibers. The increase of type I fibers ensures an adequate physiologic condition for continuous contraction of the transposed muscle (induced by permanent stimulation without continuous conscious patient effort) with subsequent closure of the anal canal.[48] The stimulator is deactivated by an external magnet. Thus, bowel emptying becomes a voluntary act.

The short- and long-term efficacy of dynamic graciloplasty is reported in several single and multicenter trials (Table 79.3), but not uniformly. Data collection, outcome measurement, and criteria for success vary. Nevertheless, the therapeutic effect is not limited to an improvement in bowel emptying, but also to quality of life.[44,57]

Artificial bowel sphincter

The artificial bowel sphincter (ABS) consists of three components (Fig. 79.7): an inflatable Silastic cuff placed

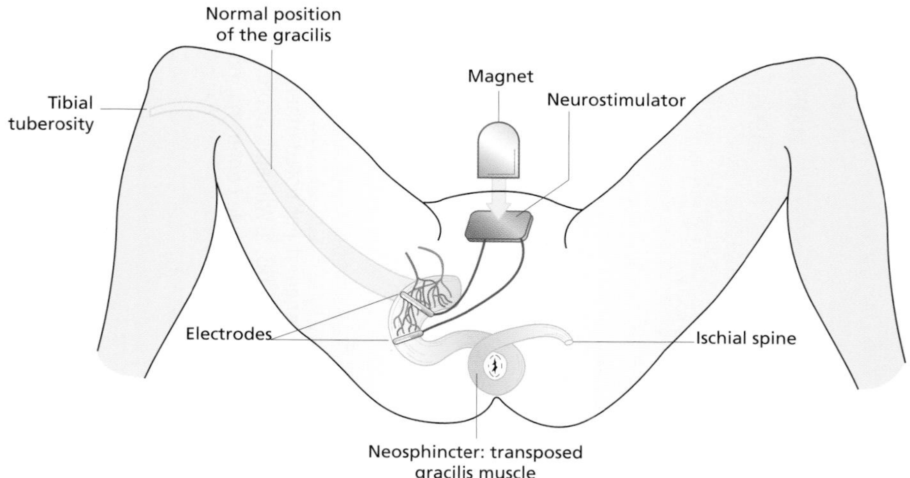

Figure 79.6. *Dynamic graciloplasty (DGP): transposed gracilis muscle configured as a gamma loop with implanted neurostimulation device.*

Table 79.3. ***Results of dynamic graciloplasty****

Reference	Year	Study	*n*	Continent (%)	Pretreatment	Treatment		Follow-up (months)
				Level 1/2	Level 4/5	Level 3,	Level 4/5	
Williams Score†								
Baeten et al.[49]	1995	SC	52	73	100%	4%	23%	25 (3–89)
Baeten et al.[44]	2000	MC	72	63	100%	11%	26%	23 (1–52)‡
Baeten et al.[50]	2001	SC	200	76	100%		24%	na
Cavina et al.[51]	1998	SC	26	85	100%	15%		37.8 (4–68)‡
Rosen et al.[52]	1998	SC	28	64	100%	7%	29%	19.2 (3–53)
Cleveland Clinic Score§								
Altomare et al.[53]	1997	SC	5	–	16.4	5.4		24 (6–58)
Mander et al.[54]	1999	MC	64	69	19	6		16 (15–67)
Ortiz et al.[55]	2002	SC	8	–	18±4	18±12		Median 39
Penninckx[56]	2004	MC	47	–	18.4±9	5.5±4.6		48 (13–117)
Percentage improvement in incontinence during therapy								
Baeten et al.[44]	2000	MC	72	–		>50%: 63%, <50%: 11%, ø: 26%		12
			61	–		>50%: 57%, <50%: 13%, ø: 30%		18
Wexner et al.[57]	2004	MC	76	15		>50%: 57%, <50%: 10%, ø: 33%		24

Data: median (range) if not noted otherwise.
*Adapted from ref. 58; † Williams Score: 1 continent, 5 incontinent; ‡ Mean (range); § Cleveland Clinic Score: 0 continent, 20 incontinent.
MC, multicenter; SC, single center; na, not applicable.

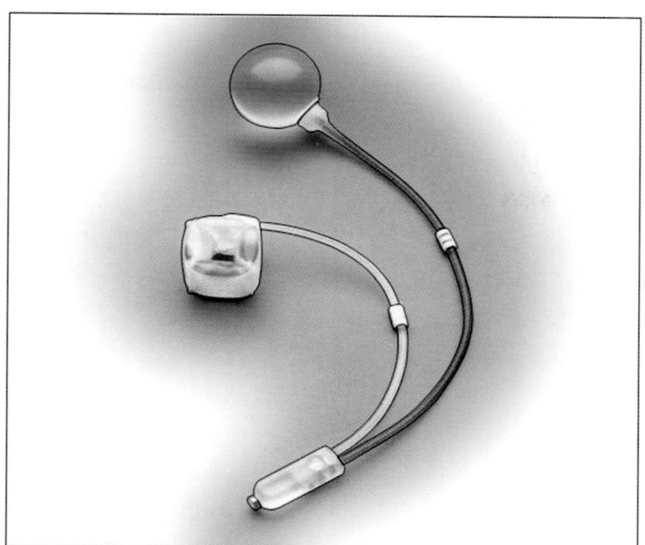

Figure 79.7. *The artificial bowel sphincter consists of a cuff, a pump and a reservoir.*

around the anus via perianal tunnels; a liquid-filled, pressure-regulating balloon positioned in the preperitoneal fat; and a manual pump connecting these components, which is placed in either the right or left labium majus or the scrotum[45] (Fig. 79.8). The anal canal is closed as the cuff fills with liquid. At the time for defecation the device is deactivated via the manual pump, the cuff empties, and the anus opens to pass stool. The cuff is refilled and the anus is closed after a few minutes.[59]

As with dynamic graciloplasty, opening of the ABS becomes a voluntary act and closure of the anal canal is maintained without conscious effort – mimicking the initiation of defecation in the healthy.

Short- and long-term effects on the function and quality of life have been published in several studies (Table 79.4), both single and multicenter.[58,62] Again, outcome measurement is inconsistent and data must be interpreted cautiously.

The indications for both procedures are similar: end-stage incontinence in patients with a substantial muscular and/or neural defect of the anal sphincter complex. Both procedures represent an alternative to the creation of a stoma. Each has advantages and disadvantages in certain anatomic and morphologic conditions. The innervation of the gracilis muscle must be intact for DGP to be successful. If the Silastic cuff of the ABS cannot provide sufficient coverage, the risk of infection with this implanted artificial material is higher.

Both sphincter replacement procedures are associated with substantial morbidity[58,70] in virtually all reports. In larger multicenter trials the need for operative revision reached 42% for DGP[71] and 46% for ABS;[64] treatment had to be discontinued in 8% and 30% of cases, respectively. The most severe complications were infections,[58,70] not surprising when the operation is performed in a naturally contaminated area.[71,72] In most cases device removal is unavoidable. The functional complication most relevant clinically is outlet obstruction,[70,71] caused either by a pre-existing obstruction not identifiable because of incontinence or by 'hypercontinence' subsequent to neosphincter creation. In most cases, this functional problem can be treated with regular enemas.[70,73]

Stoma creation

The creation of a diverting stoma should be considered as an alternative to surgery for end-stage incontinence, despite not addressing incontinence per se, if co-morbidity or intellectual or physical inability precludes the above-described sphincter replacements. Stoma creation carries its own risks, however, and patient counseling and performance of the procedure and postoperative management should be undertaken with great care.

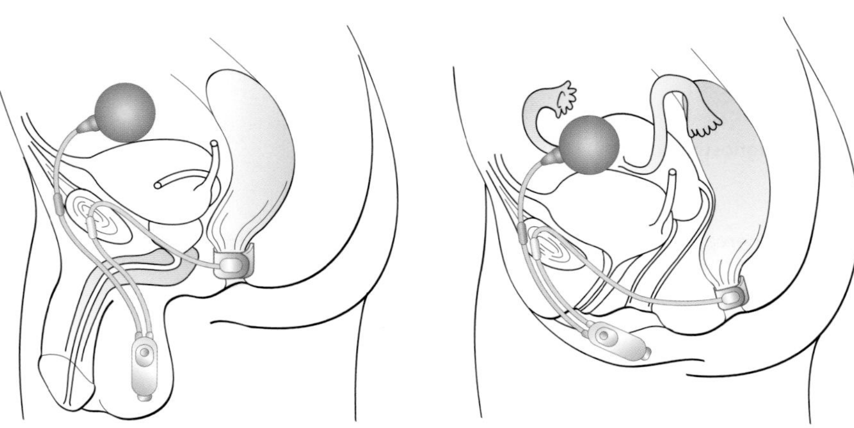

Figure 79.8. *Artificial bowel sphincter implanted; pump easily accessible.*

Table 79.4. ***Results of artificial bowel sphincter****

Reference	Year	Study	*n*	Pretreatment	Treatment	Follow-up (months)
AMS Scale†						
Altomare et al.[60]	2001	MC	24	98.5 (75–120)‡	5.5 (0–49)‡	19 (7–41)
Dodi et al.[61]	2000	SC	8	95.0 (±120)	19.4 (±19.3)	10.5 (4–23)
Lehur et al.[45]	2000	MC	24	106 (±13)	25 (±25)	20 (6–35)
Lehur et al.[62]	2002	SC	16	105 (±14)	23 (±22)	25 (7–49)
Parker et al.[63]	2004	SC	28	103 (74–120)‡	59 (0–108)‡	12
Wong et al.[64]	2002	MC	101	106 (71–120)‡	48 (0–108)‡	12
Cleveland Clinic Score§						
Altomare et al.[60]	2001	MC	24	14.9 (11–20)‡	2.6 (0–6)‡	19 (7–41)
Devesa et al.[65]	2002	SC	53	17 (±3)	4 (±3)	26.5 (7–55)
Lehur et al.[59]	1998	SC	13	17 (±1.8)	4.5 (±3.4)	30 (5–76)
O'Brien & Skinner[66]	2000	SC	13	18.7 (±1.6)	2.1 (±2.6)	–
Ortiz et al.[67]	2002	SC	22	18 (14–20)‡	4 (0–14)‡	28 (6–48)
Vaizey et al.[68]	1998	SC	6	19.5 (0.8)	4.5 (4.9)	10 (5–13)
Williams Score**						
Christiansen et al.[69]	1999	SC	17	5.0 (0.0)	2.5 (0.9)	60 (60–120)

Data: mean (SD) if not noted otherwise.
*Adapted from ref. 70; † AMS: 0 continent, 120 incontinent; ‡ Median (range); § Cleveland Clinic Score: 0 continent, 20 incontinent; **Williams Score: 1 continent, 5 incontinent. MC, multicenter; SC, single center.

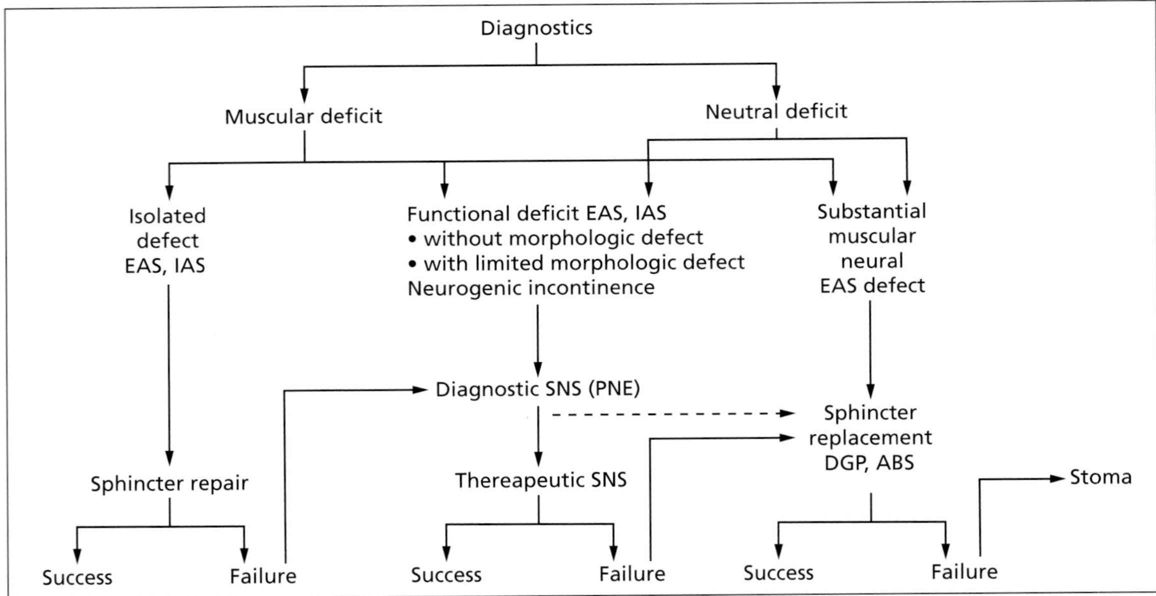

Figure 79.9. *Surgery for fecal incontinence. ABS, artificial bowel sphincter; DGP, dynamic graciloplasty; EAS, external anal sphincter; IAS, internal anal sphincter; PNE, peripheral nerve evaluation; SNS, sacral nerve stimulation.*

SUMMARY

The surgical options for fecal incontinence have increased during recent years, and a new treatment algorithm has evolved (Fig. 79.9). Symptoms and quality of life can be improved if patient selection is appropriate. Although these procedures carry some morbidity, they may offer an alternative to the creation of a diverting stoma.

REFERENCES

1. Nelson R, Norton N, Cautley E, Furner S. Community based prevalence of anal incontinence. JAMA 1995;274:559–61.
2. Roberts RO, Jacobsen SJ, Reilly WT, Pemberton JH, Lieber MM, Talley NJ. Prevalence of combined fecal and urinary incontinence: a community-based study. J Am Geriatr Soc 1999;47:837–41.
3. Chiang L, Ouslander J, Schnelle J, Reuben DB. Dually incontinent nursing home residents: clinical characteristics and treatment differences. J Am Geriatr Soc 2000;48:673–6.
4. Rockwood TH, Church JM, Fleshman JW et al. Fecal Incontinence Quality of Life Scale: quality of life instrument for patients with fecal incontinence. Dis Colon Rectum 2000;43:9–16.
5. Brazier JE, Harper R, Jones NM et al. Validating the SF-36 health survey questionnaire: a new outcome measure for primary care. BMJ 1992;305:160–4.
6. Madoff RD, Parker SC, Varma MV, Lowry AC. Fecal incontinence in adults. Lancet 2004;364:621–32.
7. Matzel KE, Schmidt RA, Tanagho EA. Neuroanatomy of the striated muscular anal continence mechanism: implications for the use of neurostimulation. Dis Colon Rectum 1990;33:666–73.
8. Matzel KE, Stadelmaier U, Hohenberger W. Innovations in fecal incontinence: sacral nerve stimulation. Dis Colon Rectum 2004;47:1720–8.
9. Matzel KE, Stadelmaier U, Hohenfellner M, Gall FP. Electrical stimulation for the treatment of faecal incontinence. Lancet 1995;346:1124–7.
10. Hohenfellner M, Matzel KE, Schultz-Lampel D et al. Sacral neuromodulation for treatment of micturition disorders and fecal incontinence. In: Hohenfellner R, Fichtner J, Novick A (eds) Innovations in Urologic Surgery. Oxford: ISIS Medical Media, 1997; 129.
11. Matzel KE, Stadelmaier U, Gall FP. Direkte Elektrostimulation der sakralen Spinalnerven im Rahmen der anorektalen Funktionsdiagnostik. Langenbecks Arch Chir 1990;380:184–8.
12. Spinelli M, Giardiello G, Arduini A, van den Hombergh U. New percutaneous technique of sacral nerve stimulation has high initial success rate: preliminary results. Eur Urol 2002;208:1–5.
13. Matzel KE, Bittorf B, Stadelmaier U, Hohenberger W. Sakralnervstimulation in der Behandlung der Stuhlinkontinenz. Chirurg 2003;74:26–32.
14. Leroi AM, Michot F, Grise P, Denis P. Effect of sacral nerve stimulation in patients with fecal and urinary incontinence. Dis Colon Rectum 2001;44:779–89.
15. Malouf AJ, Vaizey CJ, Nicholls RJ, Kamm M. Permanent sacral nerve stimulation for fecal incontinence. Ann Surg 2000;232:143–8.
16. Matzel KE, Stadelmaier U, Bittorf B, Hohenfellner M, Hohenberger W. Bilateral sacral spinal nerve stimulation for fecal incontinence after low anterior resection. Int J Colorect Dis 2002;17:430–4.
17. Rosen HR, Urbarz C, Holzer B, Novi G, Schiessel R. Sacral nerve stimulation as a treatment for fecal incontinence. Gastroenterology 2001;121:536–41.
18. Altomare DF, Rinaldi M, Petrolino M et al. Permanent sacral nerve modulation for fecal incontinence and associated urinary disturbances. Int J Colorect Dis 2004;19:203–9.
19. Ganio E, Luc AR, Clerico G, Trompetto M. Sacral nerve stimulation for treatment of fecal incontinence. Dis Colon Rectum 2001;44:619–31.
20. Ganio E, Ratto C, Masin A et al. Neuromodulation for fecal incontinence: outcome in 16 patients with definitive implant. The Initial Italian Sacral Neuromodulation Group (GINS) experience. Dis Colon Rectum 2001;44:965–70.
21. Jarrett MED, Varma JS, Duthie GS, Nicholls RJ, Kamm MA. Sacral nerve stimulation for faecal incontinence in the UK. Br J Surg 2004;91:755–61.
22. Kenefick NJ, Vaizey CJ, Cohen CG, Nicolls RJ, Kamm MA. Medium-term results of permanent sacral nerve stimulation for faecal incontinence. Br J Surg 2002;89:896–901.
23. Matzel KE. Sacral spinal nerve stimulation in treatment of fecal incontinence. Semin Colon Rectal Surg 2001;12:121–30.
24. Matzel KE, Kamm MA, Stösser M et al. Sacral nerve stimulation for fecal incontinence: a multicenter study. Lancet 2004;363:1270–6.
25. Ripetti V, Caputo D, Ausania F, Esposito E, Bruni R, Arullani A. Sacral nerve neuromodulation improves physical, psychological and social quality of life in patients with fecal incontinence. Tech Coloproctol 2002;6:147–52.
26. Uludag Ö, Darby M, Dejong CHC, Schouten WR, Baeten CGM. Sacrale neuromodulatie effectif bij fecale incontinentie en intacte kringsspieren; een perspectieve studie. Ned Tijdschr Geneeskd 2002;146:989–93.
27. Rasmussen O, Christiansen J. Sakralnervestimulation ved analinkontinens. Ugeskr Laeger 2002;164:3866–8.
28. Rasmussen OO, Buntzen S, Sorensen M, Laurberg S,

Christiansen J. Sacral nerve stimulation in fecal incontinence. Dis Colon Rectum 2004;47:1158–62.

29. Tjandra JJ, Lim JF, Matzel KE. Sacral nerve stimulation – an emerging treatment for faecal incontinence. Aust N Z J Surg 2004;74:1098–106.

30. Tjandra JJ, Han WR, Goh J, Carey M, Dwyer P. Direct repair versus overlapping sphincter repair: a randomized controlled trial. Dis Colon Rectum 2003;46:937–43.

31. Buie WD, Lowry AC, Rothenberger DA, Madoff RD. Clinical rather than laboratory assessment predicts continence after anterior sphincteroplasty. Dis Colon Rectum 2001;44:1255–60.

32. Engel AF, Kamm MA, Sultan AH, Bartram CI, Nicholls RJ. Anterior anal sphincter repair in patients with obstetric trauma. Br J Surg 1994;81:1231–4.

33. Fleshman JW, Dreznik Z, Fry RD, Kodner IJ. Anal sphincter repair for obstetric injury: manometric evaluation of functional results. Dis Colon Rectum 1991;34:1061–7.

34. Gibbs DH, Hooks VH 3rd. Overlapping sphincteroplasty for acquired anal incontinence. South Med J 1993;86:1376–80.

35. Gilliland R, Altomare DF, Moreira H Jr, Oliveira L, Gilliland JE, Wexner SD. Pudendal neuropathy is predictive of failure following anterior overlapping sphincteroplasty. Dis Colon Rectum 1998;41:1516–22.

36. Jacobs PP, Scheuer M, Kuijpers JH, Vingerhoets MH. Obstetric fecal incontinence. Role of pelvic floor denervation and results of delayed sphincter repair. Dis Colon Rectum 1990;33:494–7.

37. Londono-Schimmer EE, Garcia-Duperly R, Nicholls RJ, Ritchie JK, Hawley PR, Thomson JP. Overlapping anal sphincter repair for faecal incontinence due to sphincter trauma: five year follow-up functional results. Int J Colorectal Dis 1994;9:110–3.

38. Nikiteas N, Korsgen S, Kumar D, Keighley MR. Audit of sphincter repair. Factors associated with poor outcome. Dis Colon Rectum 1996;39:1164–70.

39. Oliveira L, Pfeifer J, Wexner SD. Physiological and clinical outcome of anterior sphincteroplasty. Br J Surg 1996;83:502–5.

40. Rasmussen OO, Puggard L, Christiansen J. Anal sphincter repair in patients with obstetric trauma. Age affects outcome. Dis Colon Rectum 1999;42:193–5.

41. Malouf AF, Norton CS, Engel AF, Nicholls RJ, Kamm MA. Long-term results of overlapping anterior anal sphincter repair for obstetric trauma. Lancet 2000;366:260–5.

42. Karoui S, Leroi AM, Koning E, Menard JF, Michot F, Denis P. Results of sphincteroplasty in 86 patients with anal incontinence. Dis Col Rectum 2000;43:813–20.

43. Halverson AL, Hull TL. Long-term outcome of overlapping anal sphincter repair. Dis Colon Rectum 2002;45:345–8.

44. Baeten C, Bailey RA, Bakka A et al. Safety and efficacy of dynamic graciloplasty for fecal incontinence: report of a prospective multicenter trial. Dis Colon Rectum 2000;43:743–51.

45. Lehur PA, Roig J, Duinslaeger M. Artificial anal sphincter: prospective clinical and manometric evaluation. Dis Colon Rectum 2000;43:1213–16.

46. Pickrell KL, Broadbent TR, Masters FW, Metzger JT. Construction of a rectal sphincter and restoration of anal continence by transplanting the gracilis muscle; a report of four cases in children. Ann Surg 1952;135:853–62.

47. Rongen MJ, Adang EM, van der Hoop AG, Baeten CGMI. One-step vs. two-step procedure in dynamic graciloplasty. Colorectal Dis 2001;3:51–7.

48. Baeten CG, Konsten J, Spaans F et al. Dynamic graciloplasty for treatment of fecal incontinence. Lancet 1991;338:1163–5.

49. Baeten CG, Geerdes BP, Adang EM et al. Anal dynamic graciloplasty in the treatment of intractable fecal incontinence. N Engl J Med 1995;332:1600–5.

50. Baeten CG, Uludag OO, Rongen MJ. Dynamic graciloplasty for fecal incontinence. Microsurgery 2001;21:230–14.

51. Cavina E, Seccia M, Banti P, Zocco G. Anorectal reconstruction after abdominoperineal resection. Experience with double-wrap graciloplasty supported by low-frequency electrostimulation. Dis Colon Rectum 1998;41:1010–16.

52. Rosen HR, Novi G, Zoech G, Feil W, Urbarz C, Schiessel R. Restoration of anal sphincter function by single-stage dynamic graciloplasty with a modified (split sling) technique. Am J Surg 1998;175:187–93.

53. Altomare DF, Rinaldi M, Pannarale OC, Memeo V. Electrostimulated gracilis neosphincter for faecal incontinence and in total anorectal reconstruction: still an experimental procedure? Int J Colorectal Dis 1997;12:308–12.

54. Mander BJ, Wexner SD, Williams NS et al. Preliminary results of a multicentre trial of the electrically stimulated gracilis neoanal sphincter. Br J Surg 1999;86:1543–8.

55. Ortiz H, Armendariz P, DeMiguel M, Solana A, Alos R, Roig JV. Prospective study of artificial anal sphincter and dynamic graciloplasty for severe anal incontinence. Int J Colorectal Dis 2003;18:349–54.

56. Penninckx F. Belgian Section of Colorectal Surgery. Belgian experience with dynamic graciloplasty for faecal incontinence. Br J Surg 2004;91:872–8.

57. Wexner S, Baeten C, Bailey R et al. Long term efficacy of dynamic graciloplasty for fecal incontinence. Dis Colon Rectum 2002;45:809–18.

58. Chapmann AE, Geerdes B, Hewett P, Young J, Eyers T, Kiroff G, Maddern GJ. Systematic review of dynamic graciloplasty in the treatment of faecal incontinence. Br J Surg 2002;89:138–53.

59. Lehur PA, Glemain P, Bruley des Varannes S, Buzelin JM, Leborgne J. Outcome of patients with an implanted artificial anal sphincter for severe faecal incontinence. A single institution report. Int J Colorectal Dis 1998;13:88–92.

60. Altomare DF, Dodi G, La Torre F, Romano G, Melega E, Rinaldi M. Multicentre retrospective analysis of outcome of artificial anal sphincter implantation for severe fecal incontinence. Br J Surg 2001;88:1481–6.

61. Dodi G, Melega E, Masin A, Infantion A, Cavallari F, Lise M. Artificial bowel sphincter (ABS) for severe fecal incontinence: a clinical and manometric study. Colorectal Dis 2000;2:207–11.

62. Lehur PA, Zerbib F, Neunlist M, Gemain P, Bruley des Varannes S. Comparison of quality of life and anorectal function after artificial bowel sphincter implantation. Dis Colon Rectum 2002;45:508–13.

63. Parker SC, Spencer MP, Madoff RD, Jensen LL, Wong WD, Rothenberger DA. Artificial bowel sphincter. Long-term experience at a single institution. Dis Colon Rectum 2003;46:722–9.

64. Wong WD, Congliosi SM, Spencer MP et al. The safety and efficacy of the artificial bowel sphincter for fecal incontinence: results from a multicenter cohort study. Dis Colon Rectum 2002;45:1139–53.

65. Devesa JM, Rey A, Hervas PL, Halawa KS, Larranaga I, Svidler L, Abraira V, Muriel A. Artificial anal sphincter: complications and functional results of a large personal series. Dis Colon Rectum 2002;45:1154–63.

66. O'Brien PE, Skinner S. Restoring control: the Acticon Neosphincter artificial bowel sphincter in the treatment of anal incontinence. Dis Colon Rectum 2000;43:1213–16.

67. Ortiz H, Armendariz P, DeMiguel M, Ruiz MD, Alos R, Roig JV. Complications and functional outcome following artificial anal sphincter implantation. Br J Surg 2002;89:877–81.

68. Vaizey CJ, Kamm MA, Gold DM, Bartram CI, Halligan S, Nicholls RJ. Clinical, physiological and radiological study of a new purpose-designed artificial bowel sphincter. Lancet 1998;352:105–9.

69. Christiansen J, Rasmussen OO, Lindorff-Larsen K. Long-term results of artificial anal sphincter implantation for severe anal incontinence. Ann Surg 1999;230:45–8.

70. Mundy L, Merlin TL, Maddern GJ, Hiller JE. Systematic review of safety and effectiveness of an artificial bowel sphincter for faecal incontinence. Br J Surg 2004;91:665–72.

71. Matzel KE, Madoff R, LaFontaine LJ, Baeten CGMI, Buie WD, Christiansen J, Wexner S and the Dynamic Graciloplasty Therapy Study Group. Complications of dynamic graciloplasty: incidence, management and impact on outcome. Dis Colon Rectum 2001;44:1427–35.

72. Christiansen J. The artificial anal sphincter. Can J Gastroenterol 2000;14:152–4.

73. Rongen MJGM, Uludang Ö, El Naggar K, Geerdes BP, Konsten J, Baeten CGMI. Long-term follow-up of dynamic graciloplasty for fecal incontinence. Dis Colon Rectum 2003;46:716–21.

80

Combined genital and rectal prolapse

Vanessa Banz, Jürg Metzger, Bernhard Schuessler

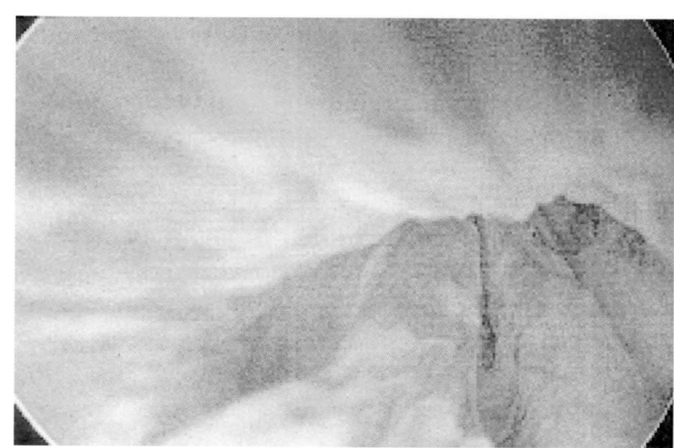

INTRODUCTION

Pelvic floor dysfunction comprises a multitude of diagnoses and symptoms ranging from urinary and fecal incontinence to different forms of prolapse, chronic constipation, sexual dysfunction or pelvic heaviness and backache. The etiology of pelvic organ prolapse is complex and multifactorial with possible risk factors being pregnancy, childbirth, congenital or acquired connective tissue abnormalities, denervation or weakness of the pelvic floor. Additional causes may include aging, previous hysterectomy, menopause, and pathologies such as asthma and bronchitis which lead to chronically increased intra-abdominal pressure. As far as rectal prolapse and rectocele are concerned, chronic constipation is identified as a major contributor.[1–3] This mixed bouquet of causes and effects requires well-differentiated diagnostic tools and an interdisciplinary approach.

Today, prolapse of the anterior and middle compartment, i.e. bladder and uterus, as well as the anterior and posterior vaginal wall, is best managed by a urogynecologic pelvic surgeon. It is equally clear that prolapse of the rectum is the domain of the colorectal surgeon.

Rectal prolapse disease is predominant in females; up to 85% of these patients are women.[4] As its etiology is shared at least partly with the pathology of genital prolapse, incontinence, etc., it is to be expected that in many patients the problems are not confined to one anatomic compartment. This is supported by Peters et al. who found 52 out of 55 patients with rectal prolapse to suffer from other defects of pelvic floor support.[5] If genital prolapse alone is addressed, more than one-third (34.3%) of patients with rectal prolapse also show signs of genital prolapse.[6]

In order to serve patients' needs best, it is essential that there is cooperation between all disciplines involved (i.e. urogynecologist, colorectal surgeon, gastroenterologist and sometimes a neurologist), not only for optimizing surgical treatment but also for diagnosis and indication.

As well as being an introduction to the understanding of rectal prolapse and the different types of surgical management available, this chapter aims to improve shared management of combined genital and rectal prolapse in the individual patient. As the evidence of knowledge in this field to date is poor, personal views and preferences could not be neglected in this chapter.

PATHOPHYSIOLOGY AND ETIOLOGY

Enterocele/sigmoidocele

The descent of the peritoneum between the anterior rectal wall and the vagina into the pouch of Douglas is defined as an enterocele. In the enterocele sac ('cul-de-sac syndrome') one may find small intestine – the actual enterocele – or the sigmoid colon, the 'sigmoidocele'. An elongated sigmoid colon may lead to an obstruction of the rectum upon defecation. Often the enterocele or sigmoidocele will be combined with other pathologic changes such as a rectocele or perineal descent (Fig. 80.1).

Classification of a sigmoidocele according to Jorge et al.[7] is based on the images obtained at defecography. This classification takes into account the lowest part of the sigmoidocele. Grade I sigmoidoceles have their deepest end above the pubococcygeal line. Grade II are below this line but above the ischiococcygeal line, and Grade III sigmoidoceles descend beyond.

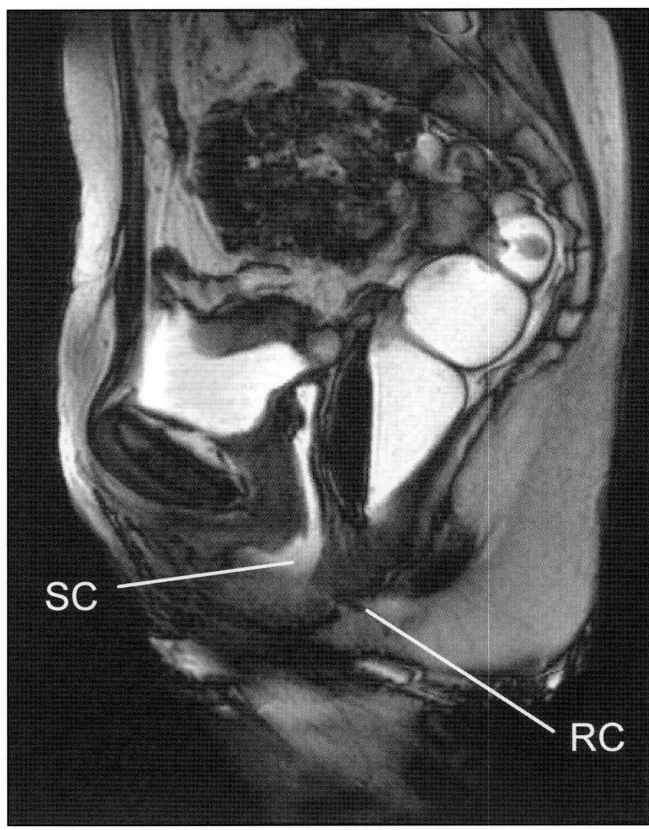

Figure 80.1. *MRI defecography during straining. A large sigmoidocele is present (SC) in combination with a rectocele (RC).*

Enteroceles can bulge into the vagina or the rectum, a condition known as intussusception, or into both.

Rectal prolapse

Complete rectal prolapse (procidentia) is defined as the circumferential protrusion of all layers of the rectal wall through the anal sphincter (Fig. 80.2). Compared to this is the rectal intussusception, which may be seen as a telescope-like invagination of the rectal wall (commonly anterior rectal wall). Synonymously used to describe this condition are the terms 'interior', 'incomplete' or 'occult' rectal prolapse. It is sometimes regarded as an early manifestation of a complete prolapse. Although distinctly different from a complete rectal wall prolapse, anterior rectal wall intussusception can also protrude into and even through the anal canal (Fig. 80.3a). These two conditions are distinctly different from mucosal prolapse, which, as the name implies, is a prolapse solely of the rectal mucosa.

Grade I prolapses are usually only diagnosed using a proctorectoscope or on contrast enema studies. Grade II prolapses can be seen upon pressing, and manifest themselves clinically as soiling of stool. A grade III prolapse is, in its maximal form, a permanent prolapse of

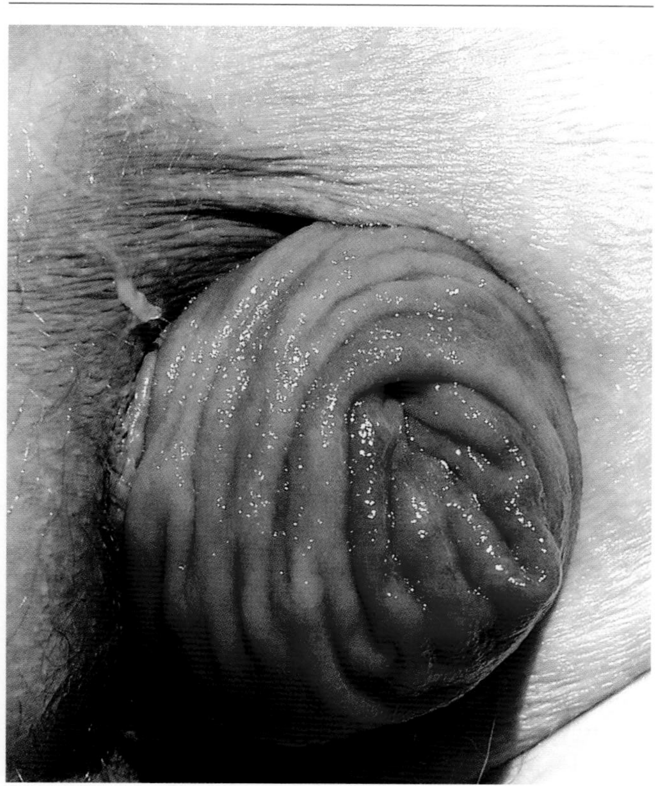

Figure 80.2. *Full thickness, circumferential rectal prolapse – 'rectal procidentia'.*

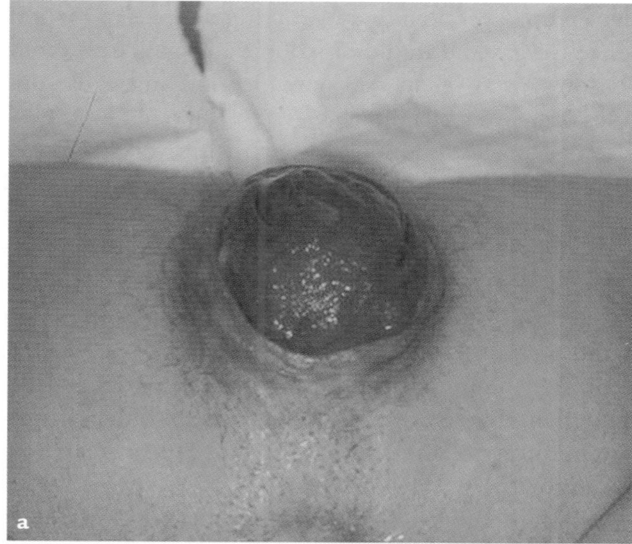

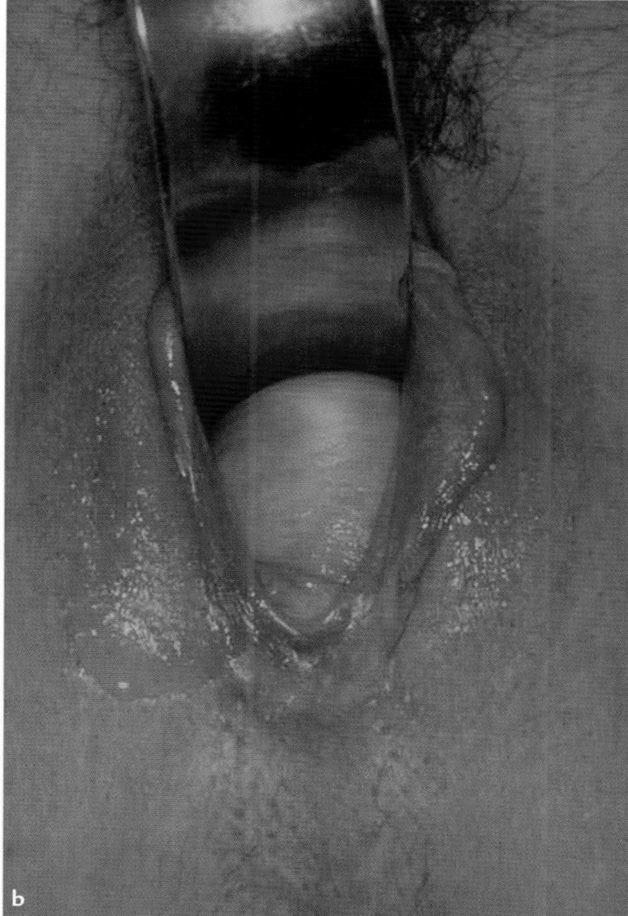

Figure 80.3. *A 38-year-old patient with four uncomplicated and fast vaginal deliveries complained about increasing obstructed defecation. (a) During forced Valsalva maneuver an anterior rectal wall prolapse was found to be the major source of the defecatory symptoms. (b) Vaginal inspection with Preisky speculum. Transanal digital examination revealed a rectocele.*

the rectum, accompanied by varying degrees of incontinence for gas and liquid or stool of normal consistency. The prolapsed rectal wall may ulcerate and cause episodes of heavier bleeding.

Rectal prolapse is seen either in the very young or in the elderly. In infants the as yet undeveloped sacral curve and the reduced resting tone predispose to rectal prolapse. In children it usually commences after episodes of violent diarrhea or after rapid and excessive weight loss. It is also associated with maldevelopment of the pelvis, neurologic defects or fibrocystic disease. A torn perineum predisposes in women, as does straining in men due to urethral obstruction. In older people, general atony of the sphincteric mechanism may be a risk factor.

Although the etiology remains unclear, a series of accompanying or casual anatomic peculiarities appear to play a role. Prolapse patients often have a deep rectovaginal or rectovesical cul-de-sac, a loose attachment of the rectum to the presacral fascia or a general loosening of the mesorectal structures.[8] Nearly all patients with complete rectal prolapse show signs of a weak sphincter, most certainly originating from constant constipation.

Pelvic floor dysfunction

Although from an etiologic point of view the morphologic and functional pathologies may be quite different, the clinical symptoms may be very similar.

Normally, the internal and external sphincters and the puborectal sling relax simultaneously. Together with the propulsive force of the rectum a coordinated defecation takes place. Patients with functional problems show a paradox reaction of the pelvic floor and external sphincter muscles, or failure to relax the internal sphincter, leading to obstruction upon defecation. Patients with pelvic floor dyssynergia with its involuntary, unconscious contraction of the pelvic floor muscles (anismus), with an involuntary contraction of the puborectal muscles – the so-called 'paradoxical puborectalis syndrome' – may thus present with symptoms identical to those seen in patients with pelvic organ prolapse.

Differentiating between functional disorders (which in turn may also be combined with other anatomic pathologies) and purely mechanical–anatomic problems is often very challenging and is usually preceded by years of previous diagnostic steps and fruitless therapies. The distinction between the two entities is also of great importance as far as therapy strategies are concerned, as these will vary enormously – for example, biofeedback for pelvic floor dyssynergia rather than operative treatment options.[9]

DIAGNOSTIC TOOLS

Even nowadays, with our extraordinarily high-tech, specific and exact diagnostic tools, a detailed history of the patient's problems and symptoms is of enormous value. The complexity of pelvic floor dysfunction may become simpler as the patient unknowingly gives valuable hints, resulting in a narrowing down of the working hypothesis to a few probable causes. Irrespective of the specialism of the primarily consulted physician, it is important to obtain the best possible overview of the patient's coloproctologic and urogynecologic problems. The subjective problems may then be transformed into objective, measurable data – for example, when using various scores such as the Rome criteria for constipation or the Faecal Incontinence Severity Index (FISI score) for fecal incontinence. An advantage of such scores is of course the opportunity to compare the results before and after the implemented therapy, thus indicating a certain measure of success, or failure.

Proctologic examination

Every clinical examination should commence with a thorough proctologic check-up including inspection, palpation, and proctorectoscopy, The experienced examiner will often be able to make an accurate diagnosis solely on initial examination. However, considering the complexity of pelvic floor dysfunction, a clinical examination frequently does not suffice and further diagnostic imaging is required.

Endoanal sonography and anorectal manometry

As stool incontinence/soiling is, along with obstructive defecation, the leading symptom in patients suffering from rectal prolapse, it is mandatory to rule out additional sphincter defects. Thus endoanal sonography and anorectal manometry serve best to identify whether incontinence may persist after rectal prolapse surgery.

Anal manometry is a helpful diagnostic tool that allows accurate measurement of the sphincter complex. It can be used for measurement of the resting tone (as given by the function of the internal anal sphincter), the maximal contraction (as dominated by the external sphincter), and general functional coordination, as well as allowing estimation of the length of the anal canal.

Endoanal sonography is the method of choice to identify muscular sphincter defects as well as providing a means of visualizing dynamic changes of accompanying pathologies such as entero- or rectoceles.[10,11]

Colonic transit time measurement

In order to allow for differentiation between obstructed defecation and slow transit constipation one elegant and patient friendly method involves the swallowing of 10 markers per day over a time span of 6 or more days. A plain abdominal radiograph is taken the day after the last marker has been swallowed. Depending on the number of markers still seen, the transit time can be estimated, with a passage time of more than 72 hours being clearly pathologic.

Conventional defecography versus dynamic pelvic floor MRI

If the main problem of a patient with pelvic floor dysfunction is 'obstructed defecation', defecography is a highly sensitive and specific method for the detection of functional rectoceles, sigmoidoceles, and rectal prolapse, and also important for the detection of an intussusception.[12,13] The addition of enteral and rectal contrast agent enhances the outcome of defecography.[12,14]

The main problem with defecography is its failure to optimally visualize the anterior and middle compartments. With many patients showing clinical involvement of more than one compartment, defecography is insufficient for understanding pathology within all three compartments. This is where dynamic pelvic floor magnetic resonance imaging (MRI) plays an important role. It allows complete visualization of the pelvic floor, inclusive of all organs, not only as a summary of images which conventional radiologic imaging provides but also in multiple slices and in different planes without the side effects of irradiation. As of yet, no true agreement exists regarding the exact indication for MRI defecography, whether or not rectal contrast should be applied, where the exact reference lines lie, and in what position the patient should be examined (lying or sitting; the latter technique with an important loss of image resolution).

As the formation of prolapse – whether of rectal or urogenital origin – is often the result of dynamic changes, the sequence of images taken during a Valsalva maneuver gives further insight into the interaction of organs leading to the pathology responsible for the patient's complaints.

The additional information obtained by dynamic MRI as compared to defecography alone may influence and even change therapeutic strategies. Kaufmann et al. showed that, of 22 patients who underwent dynamic pelvic MRI, 41% had a modification of their planned operative procedure, which had been based on previous clinical and conventional radiologic data.[15] Diagnosis of levator hernias was only possible using pelvic MRI.

In summary, one should – as with all potentially complex pathologies – start with a basic diagnosis. It cannot be overemphasized that detailed history taking and clinical examination are of primary importance for all further examinations. Whenever combined prolapse entities are suspected the patient should be examined in an interdisciplinary clinic combining colorectal, urogynecologic and, if necessary, gastroenterologic knowledge.

CONCOMITANT RECTAL PROLAPSE IN GENITAL PROLAPSE PATIENTS

Patients with genital prolapse of any type warrant careful history taking as well as clinical examination in order not to miss concomitant or combined rectoanal pathology. In particular, if a posterior enterocele is suspected, or if symptoms of bowel dysfunction are found which cannot otherwise be explained, colorectal investigation is mandatory.

Not only is careful inspection of the vaginal and introital areas during rest and at maximal Valsalva necessary, but an overview of the complete posterior compartment including the anal region is also essential. If this is neglected – for example, in a patient complaining of stool outlet obstruction as shown in Figure 80.3 – anterior rectal prolapse could well be overlooked in favor of a simple rectocele. Also important is the fact that different entities often share many of the bowel symptoms (Fig. 80.4). Whenever a patient complains about obstructed defecation, stool incontinence or soiling, prolonged defecation time, rectal lump or fragmented defecation, it is mandatory that – as well as a careful digital transanal examination – proctoscopy, defecography (preferably by fast image MRI), and radiologic investigation of the colonic transit time be performed.

RECTAL PROLAPSE

Conservative methods of treatment rarely achieve the hoped-for success for adults with complex rectal prolapse in which the prolapse comprises the entire rectal wall. To date, there have been no randomized studies in which conservative treatment options were compared to operative management.[16]

Many different surgical techniques have already been proposed for the repair of rectal prolapse. The main difference lies with the surgical approach, for which there are two options: perianal and transabdominal (Fig. 80.5).

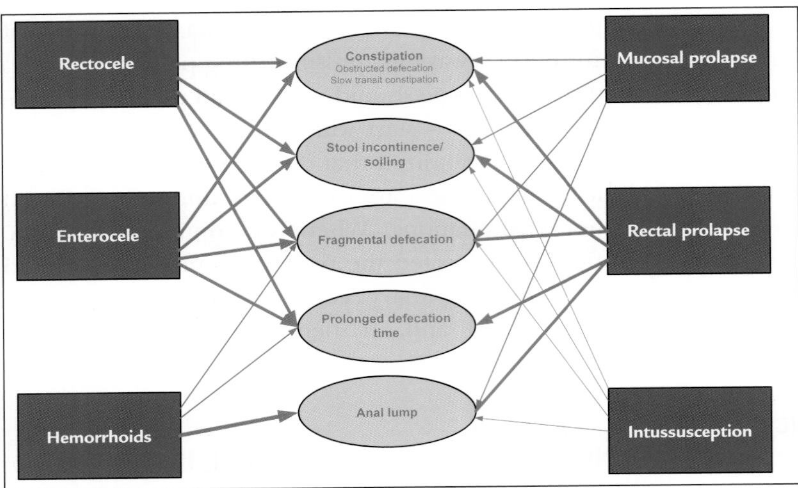

Figure 80.4. *Rectal pathologies in comparison to the spectrum of symptoms. Note that completely different diagnoses nearly always share the same symptoms.*

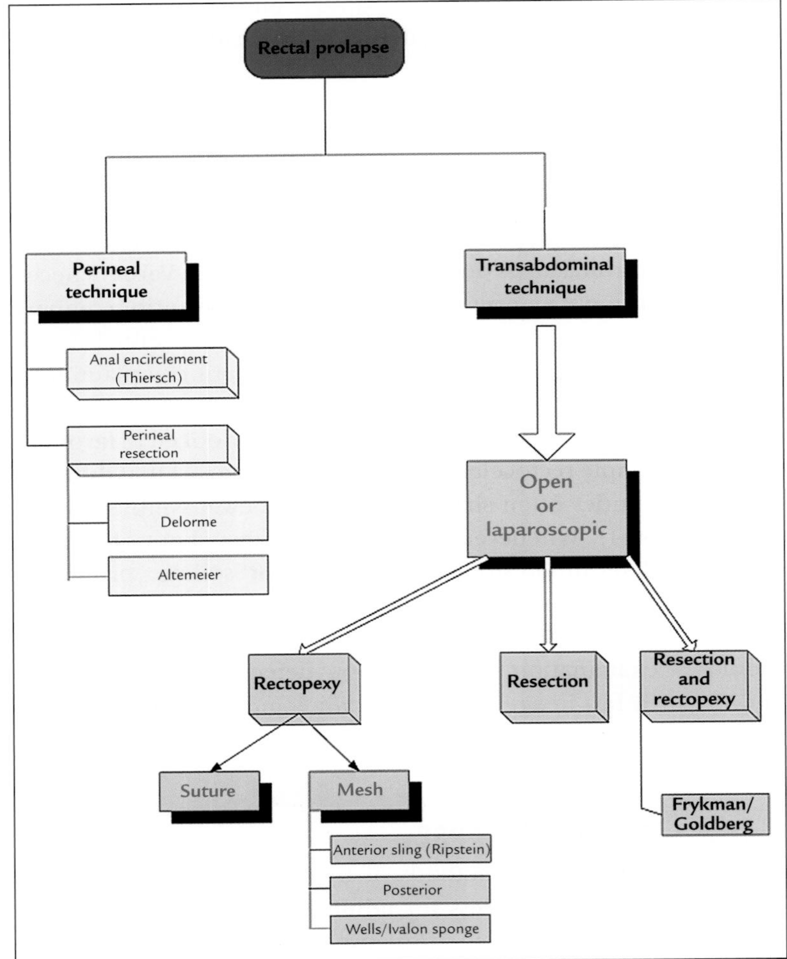

Figure 80.5. *Operative techniques for repair of rectal prolapse.*

Perianal resection – for example, the operations according to Delorme and Altemeier – are nowadays usually only performed for the old and frail.[16,17] One advantage of the perianal techniques is that they may be performed under regional or even local anesthesia. The transabdominal technique is usually used for the younger, otherwise healthy patient. Transabdominal surgical techniques vary in the choice of approach (e.g. laparoscopy versus laparotomy), the extent to which the rectum is mobilized, the method of pexation of the rectum, and the option of combining rectopexy with resection.[17] The primary goal of every surgical technique is to eliminate functional problems such as incontinence and constipation while aiming for the lowest recurrence rate and minimal morbidity and mortality. A Cochrane meta-analysis first published in 1999 included 10 studies with a total of 324 patients.[16] The aim of this specific review was to answer the following four principal questions:

1. Is the abdominal approach more advantageous than the perianal approach?
2. Is one method of rectopexy superior to another?
3. Is laparoscopy better than laparotomy?
4. Should every rectopexy be combined with a resection?

The authors of this particular study came to the conclusion that the small sample sizes of the included studies, some of which were methodically incorrect, make it difficult to publish practical guidelines. Overall, there does not appear to be a significant tendency towards an increased recurrence rate for either of the techniques. Postoperative fecal incontinence, however, was seen less frequently after an abdominal approach as compared to a perianal approach. No difference was seen between the various methods of fixation for rectopexy (mesh versus suture technique). The rate of postoperative constipation was lower for rectopexy, which had been combined with a resection as compared to rectopexy alone. An interesting study currently being conducted in England and Ireland was started in April 2000. The Association of Coloproctology launched a national study in which patients with full-thickness rectal prolapse were included. The aim is to collect data from 950 patients and to compare the abdominal approach with the perianal approach. The Delorme operation will be compared to the Altemeier, which in turn will be compared to suture rectopexy and resection rectopexy. Prolapse recurrence, defecography performance, and quality of life will be the measured outcomes. The study is likely to terminate in December 2005.[16]

Perianal operative techniques

There is a wide spectrum of perianal operative techniques ranging from anal encirclement (according to Thiersch), rectal mucosectomy and muscle plicature according to Delorme, and transsphincteric and parasacral resection of the rectum.

The operation of Delorme is widespread in England and is especially suitable for high-risk patients as it can be carried out under local anesthesia with slight sedation. First described in 1900, it combines the circular mucosectomy of the prolapsed rectum, followed by a plicature of the underlying muscles (Fig. 80.6). Of utmost importance is that at least 10–12 cm of rectal mucosa is completely excised. Together with the plicature of the muscles by means of individual sutures, the prolapse is shortened and reduced back into the anal canal. The newly formed, circular muscle ring acts as a pessary. Recurrence rates of the Delorme technique are summarized in Table 80.1 and range from 14 to 30%.

Another relatively frequently applied perianal operative technique is the rectum resection according to Altemeier.[18] It involves the full thickness excision of the rectum and, if possible, the distal part of the sigma. Recurrence rates in the literature lie between 3 and 16% (Table 80.1). Postoperative convalescence is usually without any complications. However, potentially life-threatening complications such as pelvic sepsis have been described in the literature.[19]

Postoperative complications for both techniques are relatively common, those most frequently seen being constipation and incontinence. The Delorme technique reduces rectal capacity, compliance, and sensitivity[20] whereas the Altemeier operation, with its coloanal anastomosis, often compromises the usually already existing sphincter defect. A levatorplasty is recommended to increase postoperative continence.[21]

A small trial, which included 10 patients per group, compared the abdominal with the perianal approach.[22] Postoperative measurements of resting anal pressure, maximum squeeze pressure, and rectal compliance showed significantly better results for the abdominal group as compared to the perianal group.

Abdominal operative techniques

Many different abdominal techniques have been described in the literature comparing the extent of rectum mobilization, method of rectal fixation, and additional resection of the rectum or sigma. The simple suture rectopexy finds its roots back in the 1950s with complete mobilization of the rectum and proximal fixation. Postoperative fibrosis leads to a permanent fixation of the elevated rectum onto the presacral fascia.[39] Various other materials such as non-resorbable mesh, polyvinyl alcohol (Ivalon) and Teflon have been used to increase the presence of scar tissue formation.[17]

Until the beginning of the 1990s the Ivalon sponge rectopexy, first described by Wells, was the method of choice. A rectangular piece of Ivalon sponge is fixed with a couple of sutures to the sacrum; the elongated rectum is then enclosed posteriorly in a semi-circular fashion and is fixed to the sponge. Some studies show that the implantation of Ivalon sponge has been associated with an increase in postoperative infection rates.[40,41] Nowadays Ivalon sponge has been replaced by synthetic meshes, with the resorbable and the non-resorbable meshes achieving similar results.[31,42,43]

Anterior sling rectopexy was first described in 1952 by Ribstein.[44] Here an anteriorly placed sling consisting of synthetic material is placed in front of the rectum, after having fully mobilized the latter, and is fixed to the sacral promontory. The concept behind this technique lies in the reconstruction of the posterior curvature of the rectum. Despite low mortality rates, frequent strictures at the point of fixation and a high recurrence rate led to this technique being abandoned very quickly.

Results after posterior mesh rectopexy show that recurrence rates range between zero and 6%, although postoperative fecal incontinence or constipation is present in up to 60% of all patients, which is far too high a rate[17] (see Table 80.1).

A comparative study from Novell et al.[32] showed that patients who had undergone Ivalon sponge rectopexy had more problems related to constipation than those operated on according to the suture rectopexy technique. As of yet, there have been no large, randomized trials comparing suture rectopexy and mesh rectopexy. However, there does appear reason to believe that the rate of infection and pelvic abscess formation, as well as postoperative constipation, is higher for the mesh group. Overall, there appears to be a slight advantage for the suture technique compared to mesh rectopexy.[32,45,46]

One important point to bear in mind is whether or not the lateral ligaments should be preserved when performing a rectopexy. Two trials[47,48] with a total of 46 patients tried to answer this specific question. Postoperative constipation was significantly less common in those patients in whom the ligaments had been conserved (one patient versus seven), and postoperative continence and resting as well as squeeze pressure appeared to be positively influenced if the ligaments were preserved.

Resection rectopexy

Opposed to the simple suture and mesh rectopexies are the resection rectopexies. The currently preferred surgical technique was first described in 1969 by Frykman and Goldberg.[36] While taking great care to spare the hypogastric nerves, the rectum is mobilized

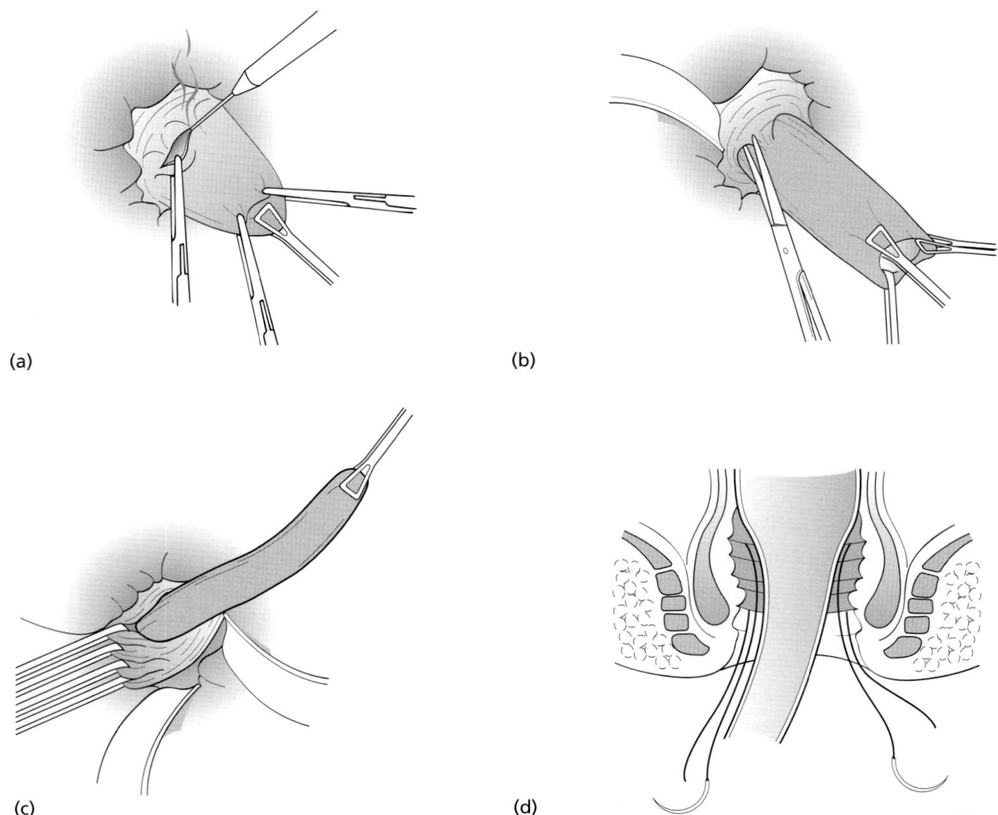

Figure 80.6. *Delorme procedure.*

Table 80.1. ***Recurrence rates after surgical treatment of full-thickness rectal prolapse***

Author	Year	Technique	Patients (*n*)	Recurrence (%)	Follow-up (months)
Oliver et al.[23]	1994	Delorme	41	22	47
Tobin & Scott[24]	1994	Delorme	43	26	20
Lechaux et al.[25]	1995	Delorme	85	14	33
Watts & Thompson[26]	2000	Delorme	101	30	36
Altemeier et al.[18]	1971	Altemeier	106	3	228
Agachan et al.[27]	1997	Altemeier	21	5	30
Kim et al.[28]	1999	Altemeier	183	16	47
Keighley et al.[29]	1983	Posterior mesh rectopexy	100	0	24
Aitola et al.[30]	1999	Posterior mesh rectopexy	96	6	78
Galili & Rabau[31]	1997	Posterior mesh rectopexy	37	3	44
Novell et al.[32]	1994	Suture rectopexy	32	3	47
Khanna et al.[33]	1996	Suture rectopexy	65	0	65
Kessler et al.[34]	1999	Laparoscopic suture rectopexy	32	6	48
Bruch et al.[35]	1999	Laparoscopic suture rectopexy	32	0	30
Frykman & Goldberg[36]	1969	Resection/rectopexy	80	0	–
Watts et al.[37]	1985	Resection/rectopexy	138	2	48
Kim et al.[28]	1999	Resection/rectopexy	176	5	98
Stevenson et al.[38]	1998	Laparoscopic resection/rectopexy	34	0	18

along the lines of the presacral fascia down to the pelvic floor. The anterior mobilization, which needs to be undertaken in order to allow optimal elongation of the rectum, is carried out in a similar fashion. After elongation of the rectum, the excessive colon is resected. The resection prevents the siphon effect and with it the problems of constipation. Fixation of the rectum occurs just below the sacral promontory onto the presacral fascia (Fig. 80.7). A new pouch of Douglas is then reconstructed at a higher level by means of peritoneal closure at promontory level. Long-term results demonstrate recurrence rates of 2–5%. This technique is particularly suitable for those patients with an elongated, redundant sigma and a long history of refractory constipation.[49]

Only two trials exist in which rectopexy alone is compared to rectopexy with resection.[43,50] The only truly significant postoperative difference found was the rate of constipation. Whereas two out of 23 patients in the resection rectopexy group suffered from constipation, this problem was evident in 12 out of 23 patients in the simple rectopexy group without additional resection. More of these operations are performed laparoscopically.[51–55] The postoperative results appear to be as good as those obtained from open surgery. Advantages of laparoscopic rectopexy are, of course, as with any laparoscopic operation: less postoperative pain, shorter hospital stay, and shorter time off work. Disadvantages are the sometimes very long operating times with accordingly long anti-Trendelenburg positioning, which can be especially problematic for the older patient.[56]

Laparoscopic methods

Two small, randomized, single-center studies[57,58] have so far compared laparoscopic mesh rectopexy with open mesh rectopexy. Both trials show a shorter hospital stay and fewer postoperative complications for the laparoscopic group with, however, notably longer operating times. Mortality for laparoscopic rectopexy is between zero and 3%, with recurrence rates lying between zero and 10% after a mean follow-up of 8–30 months.[17] These results compare well with similar trials carried out for the open technique only.

Recently, Benoist et al.[46] published results of 14 patients who had undergone laparoscopic posterior mesh rectopexy compared with results from 18 patients with laparoscopic suture rectopexy with sigma resection, and a further 16 patients with suture rectopexy minus the resection. Mortality and morbidity were comparable for all three groups. On the other hand, postoperative

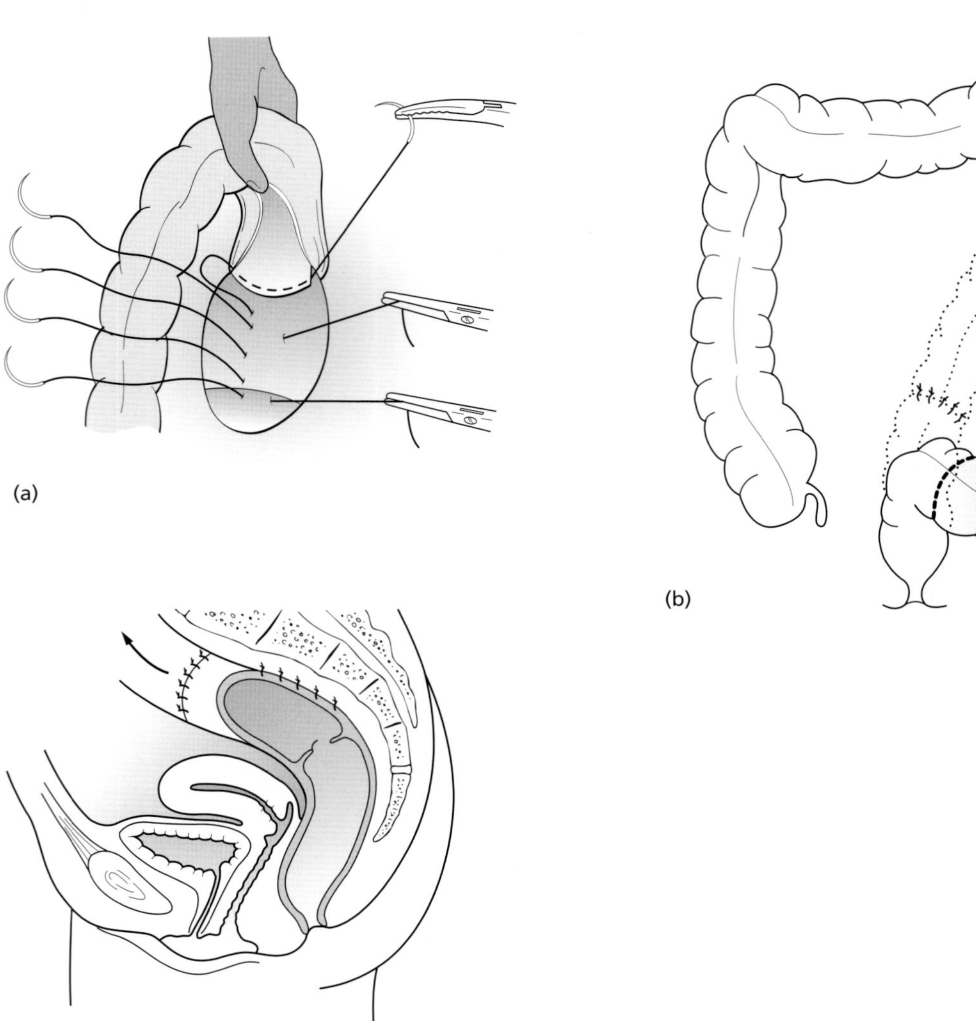

Figure 80.7. *Resection rectopexy according to Frykman and Goldberg.*[36]

constipation was distinctly higher for rectopexy alone (62% with mesh and 64% without mesh) compared to laparoscopic rectopexy with resection (11%).

Salkeld et al.[59] recently published the economic aspects of laparoscopic rectopexy surgery compared to the open technique. A cost-efficiency analysis showed that although operating time is on average 51 minutes longer for laparoscopic surgery and the costs for one-way surgical instruments are £291 more per patient, the shorter hospital stay reduces the actual cost by £357 per patient as compared to the open technique.

Summary/conclusion

From a surgical point of view there is no single ideal operative technique for complete rectal prolapse. Different clinical criteria influence the choice of operation.[60] Older patients with relevant co-morbidities who are unfit for abdominal surgery benefit from the perianal approach, which can be performed under regional or even local anesthesia. For all other patients we opt for the abdominal approach, as functional results regarding constipation and incontinence are better and the recurrence rate definitively lower. In selected patients without any previous major abdominal surgery or relevant anesthesiologic contraindications for the long intraoperative anti-Trendelenburg positioning, we prefer laparoscopic operations. Patients with pre-existing constipation who had been preoperatively diagnosed with MRI defecography (outlet obstruction) or colon transit time (slow transit constipation), or patients with an intraoperatively diagnosed dolichosigma, are ideal candidates for laparoscopic resection rectopexy. We fix the mobilized rectum with sutures to the presacral fascia, as mesh implantation does not show any relevant advantages. As far as the perianal procedures are concerned, the choice of surgical treatment (Delorme versus perianal rectosigmoidectomy) should be chosen according to the experience and preference of the operating surgeon.

Organ prolapse, which affects the middle as well as the posterior compartment, lies on the watershed of two specialties. This occurs if full-thickness rectal prolapse is combined with an entero- or rectocele. Here a combined diagnostic and therapeutic algorithm is important and will be discussed in the following section.

COMBINED SURGERY FOR GENITAL AND RECTAL PROLAPSE

The literature on techniques and results of combined surgery for rectal and genital prolapse is scarce and consists of a few and mostly small case series. No data are yet available in a Medline research with regard to comparison of different methods. Based on logic and reason, however, it is obvious that single-step combined surgery offers the best solution for the patient and should be the primary aim. Even for a transvaginal repair of genital prolapse, together with a perineal approach for rectal prolapse – obviously a combination of two separate operations and two-step surgery – would add only a second anesthesia without beneficial effect. The only issue to debate is whether to perform the genital or the rectal operation first. To start with the correction of the genital prolapse is reasonable, provided a high peritonealization of the pouch of Douglas is planned.

As is the case for rectal prolapse surgery, urogenital prolapse could also be repaired from below (transvaginal route) or above (laparotomy or laparoscopy). Which route is to be chosen for the individual patient is a matter of discussion between the urogynecologic and the colorectal surgeons. Choosing the perineal/transvaginal route is in favor of less invasive surgery against less successful outcome in the posterior compartment, i.e. risk of rectal prolapse recurrence and anal incontinence. As far as the vagina is concerned, cohabitation problems are more likely to be expected. Based on that, it is obvious that these techniques are preferred if the patient is frail and elderly or carries other risk factors for major surgery.

The abdominal (endoscopic) approach necessitates one-step surgery. Two-step surgery, independent of the remaining genital or rectal prolapse, is expected to bear more unnecessary risks for patients. This implies that one-step surgery needs sophisticated preoperative exploration of all compartments.

Depending on the existing genital prolapse situation, concomitant surgery for genital prolapse consists of four steps:

1. Fixation of the vaginal cuff;
2. Obliteration of the pouch of Douglas;
3. Rectocele repair;
4. Cystocele repair.

For the abdominal approach there is universal agreement to fix the vaginal cuff and close the pouch of Douglas from above.[61–64] In one of the largest prospective case series of 89 hysterectomized patients, Collopy et al.[62] preferred to repair the remaining vaginal descent from below following the abdominal procedure, whereas Sullivan et al.[64] used a total mesh repair, extending the mesh lateral to the vagina and the bladder to the symphysis pubis. The high recurrence rate of more than 30% re-operations compared to nil in the series of Collopy, however, does not seem to favor this approach. Fixation of the vaginal cuff to the rectal ligament as used for mesh-free rectopexy has been shown to be successful in the hands of the authors, provided the vagina is long enough to be suspended without tension (Fig. 80.8).

Routine fixation of the vaginal cuff or even the uterus, if still in place, because 'there is genital prolapse present in 25% and if not yet present may occur later in life' does not appear to be a meaningful prevention strategy but strongly supports preoperative interdisciplinary assessment[63,65] (see the discussional remark in ref. 62).

From the authors' point of view, adequate cystocele repair is feasible with an extension of the mesh at the anterior vaginal wall,[62,66] whereas for the effective recto-/perineocele, extension and fixation of the posterior mesh down to the level of the perineum and fixation to the adjacent puborectalis sling appears to be necessary. The feasibility of this technique is simplified by the laparoscopic approach with a 30-degree optic. Techniques that introduce and fix the mesh from an introital incision have been shown to be burdened with a high mesh erosion rate.

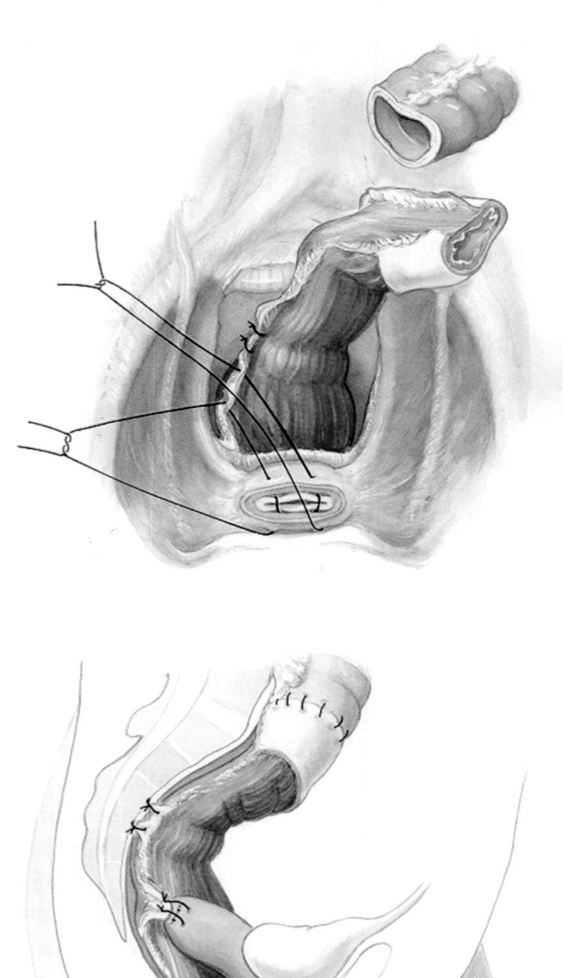

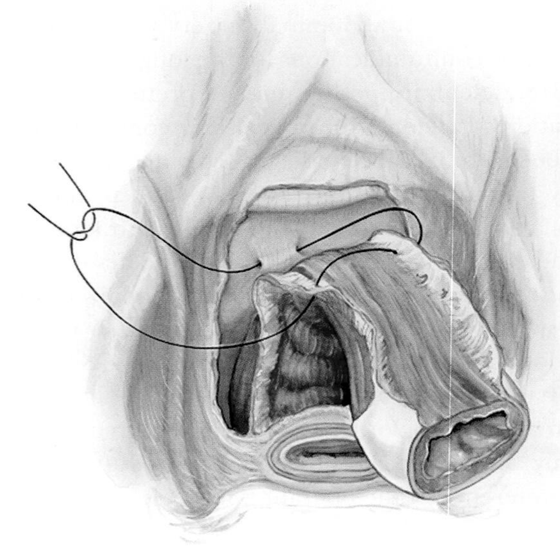

Figure 80.8. *Technique of mesh-free vaginal cuff fixation to the ventral ligament used for sacral rectopexy.*

A large enterocele bulging into the vagina as well as causing the anterior rectal wall to intussuscept into the lumen of the rectum marks the 'gray zone' between the genital prolapse surgeon and the colorectal surgeon. Baessler and Schuessler have shown vaginal double pedicle fixation at the vaginal cuff concomitant with an obliteration of the pouch of Douglas to treat rectal intussusception successfully.[62,66] However, contrary to the good anatomic results, symptoms of a high stool outlet obstruction developed after the surgery. It therefore seems reasonable to discuss concomitant rectal surgery if symptoms of stool outlet obstruction are found in conjunction with anterior rectal wall intussusception without overt rectal prolapse.

REFERENCES

1. Bump RC, Norton PA. Epidemiology and natural history of pelvic floor dysfunction. Obstet Gynecol Clin North Am 1998;25:723–46.
2. Gill EJ, Hurt WG. Pathophysiology of pelvic organ prolapse. Obstet Gynecol Clin North Am 1998;25:757–69.
3. MacLennan AH, Taylor AW, Wilson DH et al. The prevalence of pelvic floor disorders and their relationship to gender, age, parity and mode of delivery. BJOG 2000;107:1460–70.
4. Goligher JC. Prolapse of the rectum. In: Surgery of the Anus, Rectum and Colon. London: Baillière Tindall, 1980; 224–58.
5. Peters WA III, Smith MR, Drescher CW. Rectal prolapse

in women with other defects of pelvic floor support. Am J Obstet Gynecol 2001;184:1488–94.

6. Gonzalez-Argente FX, Jain A, Nogueras JJ et al. Prevalence and severity of urinary incontinence and pelvic genital prolapse in females with anal incontinence or rectal prolapse. Dis Colon Rectum 2001;44:920–6.
7. Jorge JM, Yang YK, Wexner SD. Incidence and clinical significance of sigmoidoceles as determined by a new classification system. Dis Colon Rectum 1994;37:1112–17.
8. Heitland W. [Rectal prolapse in adults.] Chirurg 2004;75:882–9.
9. Battaglia E, Serra AM, Buonafede G et al. Long-term study on the effects of visual biofeedback and muscle training as a therapeutic modality in pelvic floor dyssynergia and slow-transit constipation. Dis Colon Rectum 2004;47:90–5.
10. Barthet M, Portier F, Heyries L et al. Dynamic anal endosonography may challenge defecography for assessing dynamic anorectal disorders: results of a prospective pilot study. Endoscopy 2000;32:300–5.
11. Lohnert M, Doniec JM, Kovacs G et al. New method of radiotherapy for anal cancer with three-dimensional tumor reconstruction based on endoanal ultrasound and ultrasound-guided afterloading therapy. Dis Colon Rectum 1998;41:169–76.
12. Agachan F, Pfeifer J, Wexner SD. Defecography and proctography. Results of 744 patients. Dis Colon Rectum 1996;39:899–905.
13. Pfeifer J, Oliveira L, Park UC et al. Are interpretations of video defecographies reliable and reproducible? Int J Colorectal Dis 1997;12:67–72.
14. Herold A, Muller-Lobeck H, Jost WH et al. [Diagnostic evaluation of the rectum and pelvic floor in chronic constipation.] Zentralbl Chir 1999;124:784–95.
15. Kaufman HS, Buller JL, Thompson JR et al. Dynamic pelvic magnetic resonance imaging and cystocolpoproctography alter surgical management of pelvic floor disorders. Dis Colon Rectum 2001;44:1575–83.
16. Brazzelli M. Surgery for complete rectal prolapse in adults. Cochrane Database Syst Rev 2005; Issue 2.
17. Madiba TE, Baig MK, Wexner SD. Surgical management of rectal prolapse. Arch Surg 2005;140:63–73.
18. Altemeier WA, Culbertson WR, Schowengerdt C et al. Nineteen years' experience with the one-stage perineal repair of rectal prolapse. Ann Surg 1971;173:993–1006.
19. Takesue Y, Yokoyama T, Murakami Y et al. The effectiveness of perineal rectosigmoidectomy for the treatment of rectal prolapse in elderly and high-risk patients. Surg Today 1999;29:290–3.
20. Penninckx F, D'Hoore A, Sohier S et al. Abdominal resection rectopexy versus Delorme's procedure for rectal prolapse: a predictable outcome. Int J Colorectal Dis 1997;12:49–50.
21. Williams JG, Rothenberger DA, Madoff RD et al. Treatment of rectal prolapse in the elderly by perineal rectosigmoidectomy. Dis Colon Rectum 1992;35:830–4.
22. Deen KI, Grant E, Billingham C et al. Abdominal resection rectopexy with pelvic floor repair versus perineal rectosigmoidectomy and pelvic floor repair for full-thickness rectal prolapse. Br J Surg 1994;81:302–4.
23. Oliver GC, Vachon D, Eisenstat TE et al. Delorme's procedure for complete rectal prolapse in severely debilitated patients. An analysis of 41 cases. Dis Colon Rectum 1994;37:461–7.
24. Tobin SA, Scott IH. Delorme operation for rectal prolapse. Br J Surg 1994;81:1681–4.
25. Lechaux JP, Lechaux D, Perez M. Results of Delorme's procedure for rectal prolapse. Advantages of a modified technique. Dis Colon Rectum 1995;38:301–7.
26. Watts AM, Thompson MR. Evaluation of Delorme's procedure as a treatment for full-thickness rectal prolapse. Br J Surg 2000;87:218–22.
27. Agachan F, Reissman P, Pfeifer J et al. Comparison of three perineal procedures for the treatment of rectal prolapse. South Med J 1997;90:925–32.
28. Kim DS, Tsang CB, Wong WD et al. Complete rectal prolapse: evolution of management and results. Dis Colon Rectum 1999;42:460–6.
29. Keighley MR, Fielding JW, Alexander-Williams J. Results of Marlex mesh abdominal rectopexy for rectal prolapse in 100 consecutive patients. Br J Surg 1983;70:229–32.
30. Aitola PT, Hiltunen KM, Matikainen MJ. Functional results of operative treatment of rectal prolapse over an 11-year period: emphasis on transabdominal approach. Dis Colon Rectum 1999;42:655–60.
31. Galili Y, Rabau M. Comparison of polyglycolic acid and polypropylene mesh for rectopexy in the treatment of rectal prolapse. Eur J Surg 1997;163:445–8.
32. Novell JR, Osborne MJ, Winslet MC, Lewis AA. Prospective randomized trial of Ivalon sponge versus sutured rectopexy for full-thickness rectal prolapse. Br J Surg 1994;81:904–6.
33. Khanna AK, Misra MK, Kumar K. Simplified sutured sacral rectopexy for complete rectal prolapse in adults. Eur J Surg 1996;162:143–6.
34. Kessler H, Jerby BL, Milsom JW. Successful treatment of rectal prolapse by laparoscopic suture rectopexy. Surg Endosc 1999;13:858–61.
35. Bruch HP, Herold A, Schiedeck T et al. Laparoscopic surgery for rectal prolapse and outlet obstruction. Dis Colon Rectum 1999;42:1189–94.
36. Frykman HM, Goldberg SM. The surgical treatment of rectal procidentia. Surg Gynecol Obstet 1969;129:1225–30.
37. Watts JD, Rothenberger DA, Buls JG et al. The manage-

ment of procidentia. 30 years' experience. Dis Colon Rectum 1985;28:96–102.

38. Stevenson AR, Stitz RW, Lumley JW. Laparoscopic-assisted resection-rectopexy for rectal prolapse: early and medium follow-up. Dis Colon Rectum 1998;41:46–54.
39. Jacobs LK, Lin YJ, Orkin BA. The best operation for rectal prolapse. Surg Clin North Am 1997;77:49–70.
40. Lake SP, Hancock BD, Lewis AA. Management of pelvic sepsis after Ivalon rectopexy. Dis Colon Rectum 1984;27:589–90.
41. Ross AH, Thomson JP. Management of infection after prosthetic abdominal rectopexy (Wells' procedure). Br J Surg 1989;76:610–2.
42. Winde G. Clinical and functional results of abdominal rectopexy with absorbable mesh-graft for treatment of complete rectal prolapse. Eur J Surg 1993;159:301–5.
43. Luukkonen P. Abdominal rectopexy with sigmoidectomy vs. rectopexy alone for rectal prolapse: a prospective, randomized study. Int J Colorectal Dis 1992;7:219–22.
44. Ribstein C. Treatment of massive rectal prolapse. Am J Surg 1952;83:68–71.
45. Madbouly KM, Senagore AJ, Delaney CP et al. Clinically based management of rectal prolapse. Surg Endosc 2003;17:99–103.
46. Benoist S, Taffinder N, Gould S et al. Functional results two years after laparoscopic rectopexy. Am J Surg 2001;182:168–73.
47. Selvaggi F. Surgical treatment of rectal prolapse: a randomized study. Br J Surg 1993;80:S89.
48. Speakman CT, Madden MV, Nicholls RJ et al. Lateral ligament division during rectopexy causes constipation but prevents recurrence: results of a prospective randomized study. Br J Surg 1991;78:1431–3.
49. Azimuddin K, Khubchandani IT, Rosen L et al. Rectal prolapse: a search for the 'best' operation. Am Surg 2001;67:622–7.
50. McKee RF, Lauder JC, Poon FW et al. A prospective randomized study of abdominal rectopexy with and without sigmoidectomy in rectal prolapse. Surg Gynecol Obstet 1992;174:145–8.
51. Kairaluoma MV, Viljakka MT, Kellokumpu IH. Open vs. laparoscopic surgery for rectal prolapse: a case-controlled study assessing short-term outcome. Dis Colon Rectum 2003;46:353–60.
52. Tsugawa K, Sue K, Koyanagi N et al. Laparoscopic rectopexy for recurrent rectal prolapse: a safe and simple procedure without a mesh prosthesis. Hepatogastroenterology 2002;49:1549–51.
53. Chiu HH, Chen JB, Wang HM et al. Surgical treatment for rectal prolapse. Zhonghua Yi Xue Za Zhi (Taipei) 2001;64:95–100.
54. Zittel TT, Manncke K, Haug S et al. Functional results after laparoscopic rectopexy for rectal prolapse. J Gastrointest Surg 2000;4:632–41.
55. Heah SM, Hartley JE, Hurley J et al. Laparoscopic suture rectopexy without resection is effective treatment for full-thickness rectal prolapse. Dis Colon Rectum 2000;43:638–43.
56. Xynos E, Chrysos E, Tsiaoussis J et al. Resection rectopexy for rectal prolapse. The laparoscopic approach. Surg Endosc 1999;13:862–4.
57. Solomon MJ, Young CJ, Eyers AA, Roberts RA. Randomized clinical trial of laparoscopic versus open abdominal rectopexy for rectal prolapse. Br J Surg 2002;89:35–9.
58. Boccasanta P. Comparison of laparoscopic rectopexy with open technique in the treatment of complete rectal prolapse: clinical and functional results. Surg Laparosc Endosc 1998;8:460–5.
59. Salkeld G, Bagia M, Solomon M. Economic impact of laparoscopic versus open abdominal rectopexy. Br J Surg 2004;91:1188–91.
60. Brown AJ, Anderson JH, McKee RF et al. Strategy for selection of type of operation for rectal prolapse based on clinical criteria. Dis Colon Rectum 2004;47:103–7.
61. Barham K, Collopy BT. Posthysterectomy rectal and vaginal prolapse: a commonly overlooked problem. Aust N Z J Obstet Gynaecol 1993;33:300–3.
62. Collopy BT, Barham KA. Abdominal colporectopexy with pelvic cul-de-sac closure. Dis Colon Rectum 2002;45:522–6.
63. Kuijpers HC. Treatment of complete rectal prolapse: to narrow, to wrap, to suspend, to fix, to encircle, to plicate or to resect? World J Surg 1992;16:826–30.
64. Sullivan ES, Longaker CJ, Lee PY. Total pelvic mesh repair: a ten-year experience. Dis Colon Rectum 2001;44:857–63.
65. Mollen RM, Kuijpers JH, van Hoek F. Effects of rectal mobilization and lateral ligaments division on colonic and anorectal function. Dis Colon Rectum 2000;43:1283–7.
66. Baessler K, Schuessler B. Abdominal sacrocolpopexy and anatomy and function of the posterior compartment. Obstet Gynecol 2001;97:678–84.

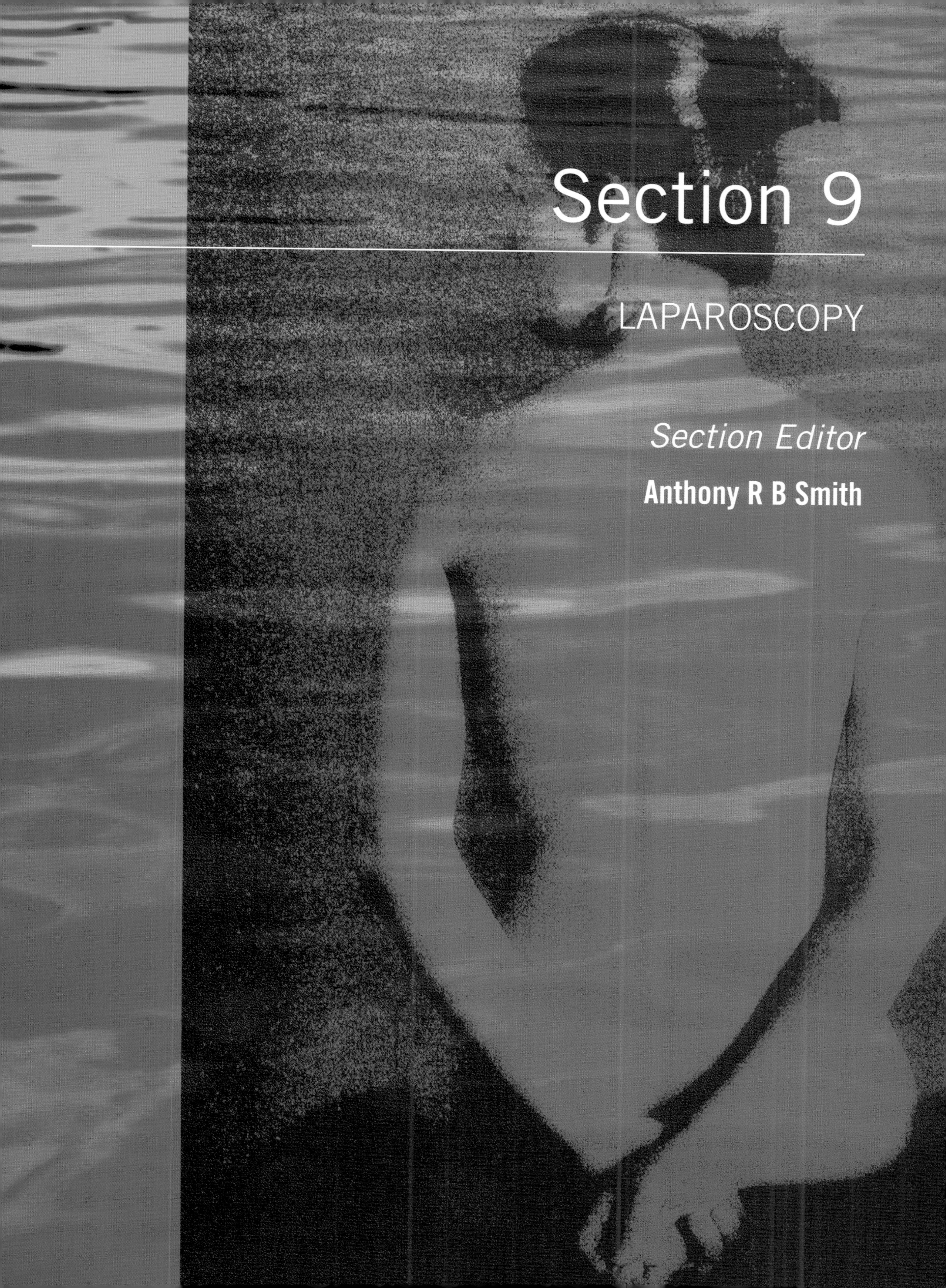

Section 9

LAPAROSCOPY

Section Editor

Anthony R B Smith

81

The role of laparoscopic surgery

Anthony R B Smith

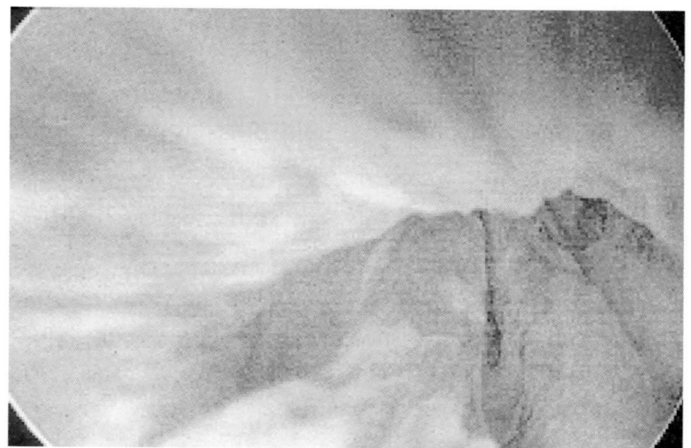

INTRODUCTION

The role of laparoscopic surgery in urogynecology/pelvic reconstructive surgery is not yet clear. This section identifies some of the issues that need to be addressed to clarify whether such surgery is merely a diversion to stimulate the whims of the gynecologic/urologic surgeon or a real advance in an area already clouded by uncertainty with respect to outcome and outcome assessment.

ADVANTAGES

Postoperative pain and recovery

Laparoscopic surgery is frequently heralded as progress on the basis of smaller wounds leading to less postoperative pain and a faster recovery. While there is some evidence that postoperative pain is reduced, there are also randomized studies in which patients are blinded to the type of intervention (laparoscopic or open) and have been unaware, both in pain or speed of recovery, of which operation was performed. It is possible that factors other than wound size may influence postoperative pain in which case reconstructive procedures might be expected to gain more from the laparoscopic approach than ablative procedures such as hysterectomy. Furthermore, the avoidance of digital manipulation by gloved hands and abdominal packs should reduce the risk of ileus which is common following procedures such as open sacrocolpopexy. Small, fine instruments may produce less tissue trauma and reduce postoperative pain. It is also possible that less tissue trauma may induce less fibrosis which may be an important component of a successful repair procedure. These questions can only be answered by well-conducted, randomized trials. There have been very few performed to date.

Visualization

The view of the deep pelvis (including the pelvic floor) is better through the laparoscope than through either a low transverse or a longitudinal incision. Since a fundamental requirement of good surgery is clear visualization of the anatomy, surgery through the laparoscope should have an advantage. In addition, access to new areas with the clearer visualization provides the opportunity to develop pelvic floor reconstructive surgery. This area needs further study.

DISADVANTAGES/PROBLEMS

New skills training

The learning of new laparoscopic surgical skills is a challenge for both the inexperienced and the experienced surgeon. Some surgeons are temperamentally happier with open surgery and should not be pushed into laparoscopic surgery unless there is clear evidence (as with laparoscopic surgery for ectopic pregnancy) that the open alternative is inferior. The surgeon is but one member of the theater team and it is equally important that all members of the theater staff receive training, particularly in the use of the complex range of new equipment that is often required.

As with all surgery, medical staff must be appropriately accredited before they undertake laparoscopic procedures to minimize the influence of the learning curve on the outcome of the procedure. There is some evidence from the published series on laparoscopic colposuspension that surgical inexperience had a significant influence on the stress incontinence cure rate. Furthermore, established procedures should not be modified to accommodate surgical ineptitude while still attributing the same prognosis for the procedure; for example, a colposuspension performed with mesh and staples is not necessarily the same procedure as one performed with sutures.

Anesthetic risks are also important and the use of high CO_2 pressures and the steep Trendelenburg position for prolonged periods may cause additional problems for the patient. While obese patients may gain from laparoscopic surgery by a reduction in wound infections, they also provide additional challenges with ventilation.

Managing complications

The chapter in this section on complications and their management (Chapter 87) highlights the need to appraise patients of the potential hazards of laparoscopic surgery which include the risks peculiar to the laparoscopic approach in addition to the reconstructive procedure itself. Patient expectations of risk and prognosis may be different following 'minimally invasive' surgery and they must be advised that such surgery may result in significant complications including laparotomy and visceral injury. The mindset of patients and staff must be adjusted to recognize problems when they occur and to respond rapidly. The use of day case facilities and rapid discharge from hospital must include the easy provision of telephone advice and access to hospital for immediate review if required.

82

Pelvic anatomy through the laparoscope

Edmund Edi-Osagie

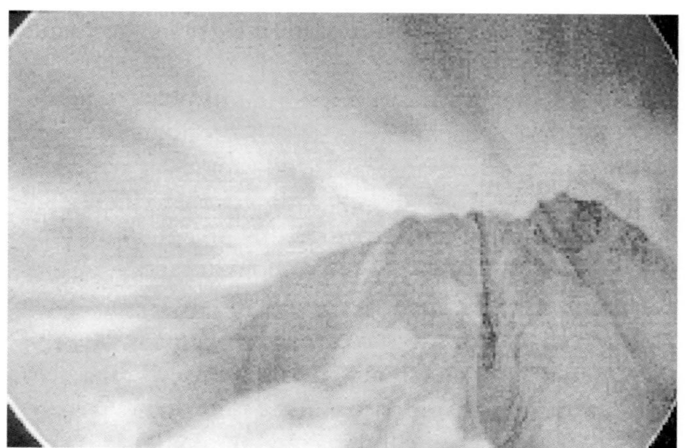

INTRODUCTION

Gynecologic surgeons have advanced the use of the laparoscope as both a diagnostic and a therapeutic tool over the last two decades. The reasons for this include the ease and relative safety with which a laparoscopy can be performed, facilitating diagnosis and treatment of pelvic pathology, and obviating the need for laparotomies with their higher risks and costs to both the patient and healthcare establishment. The modern laparoscope offers access to the pelvis that cannot be obtained by laparotomy, with unequalled and magnified views of the pelvic viscera. These magnified views make it easier to identify and operate on small structures, thereby reducing the overall risks of surgery. This has radically altered the gynecologic approach to pelvic surgery, previously the preserve of abdominal surgeons, allowing the safe laparoscopic accomplishment of sophisticated pelvic surgery such as hysterectomies (total and extended), myomectomies, reversals of tubal sterilization, excision of rectovaginal endometriotic disease, colposuspension, sacrocolpopexy, paravaginal repair, and pelvic lymphadenectomy, as well as resection and re-anastomosis of the ureters, sigmoid colon, and rectum.

The safe performance of any, but especially laparoscopic, pelvic surgery is dependent on a comprehensive and thorough knowledge of pelvic anatomy. The effective placement of laparoscopic instruments such as the Veress needle, laparoscope trocar and ancillary ports depends on this knowledge to facilitate surgery and avoid damage to intra-abdominal and pelvic viscera, as well as to correct any damage that might occur. Gynecologic laparoscopic surgery does not necessarily entail totally new operations but rather the application of a new (minimal access) approach to the accomplishment of known gynecologic procedures. It is, however, peculiar in that the magnification it achieves, the pneumoperitoneum and the positioning of the patient can all affect the visualized image and alter the relationships of pelvic viscera. This knowledge is vital for the training and accreditation process for aspiring gynecologic laparoscopic surgeons.

This chapter hopes to refresh and update readers' knowledge of pelvic anatomy that is especially relevant to the safe performance of gynecologic laparoscopic surgery. It does not attempt a didactic description of all pelvic anatomy, as there are many notable published texts that do this perfectly, but will instead relate various pertinent aspects of pelvic anatomy to gynecologic laparoscopic surgery. It sets out by reviewing the anatomy of the anterior abdominal wall and then reviews the pelvic walls, peritoneum and viscera, relating them to gynecologic laparoscopic surgery and highlighting potential areas of difficulty and pitfalls that might befall the unwary during such surgery.

ANTERIOR ABDOMINAL WALL

The anterior abdominal wall (Fig. 82.1) consists of several layers of tissue including, from outside in:

1. Skin – attaches loosely to the underlying subcutaneous connective tissue except at the umbilicus where it is firmly adherent;
2. Subcutaneous tissue – consists of two distinct layers, the superficial fatty layer (Camper's fascia) and the deep membranous layer (Scarpa's fascia);
3. Fatty layer;
4. Muscle layer – consists of the five muscles of the abdominal wall, i.e. the internal and external oblique, transversus and rectus abdominis, and pyramidalis muscles. The internal and external oblique and transversus abdominis muscles end anteriorly in a strong sheet-like aponeurosis (the rectus sheet) which interlaces with that from the opposite side at the linea alba (white line). All the layers of the linea alba fuse at the umbilicus to create a defect (the umbilical ring) directly underneath, making the umbilical site the thinnest part of the anterior abdominal wall and very amenable to laparoscope ports;
5. Deep fascia – consists essentially of the fascia investing the external oblique muscle as well as the transversalis fascia, a firm membranous sheet that lines most of the abdomen;
6. Endoabdominal fat and fascia – essentially a potential space (of Bogros);
7. Parietal peritoneum.

The umbilicus overlies the fourth lumbar vertebra, the most anterior point of the lumbar lordosis, in 67% of people. However, the level of the umbilicus appears to descend with age and in the overweight, altering its relationship to the internal organs (such as the aorta and rectum) that remain fixed. Knowledge of this should help to ensure safe introduction of the Veress needle and other umbilical ports in these groups of patients.

PELVIC WALL

The pelvic wall consists of bony, ligamentous, and muscular components, and houses the pelvic cavity, which communicates superiorly with the abdominal cavity. The pelvic brim artificially divides the pelvic cavity into superior (the greater or false pelvis) and inferior (the

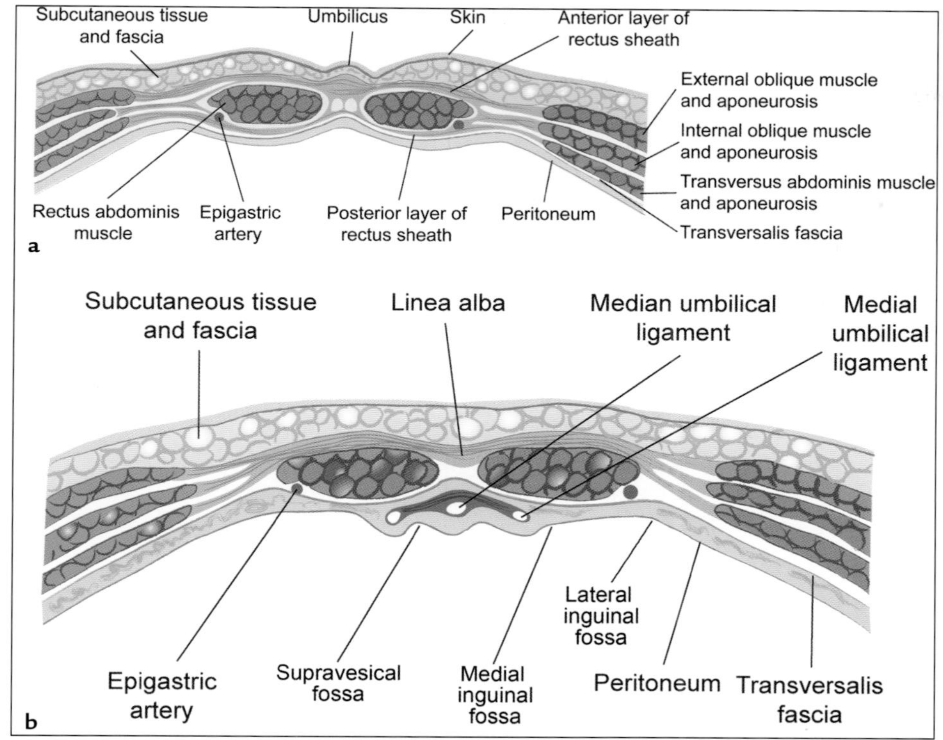

Figure 82.1. *Transverse section of the anterior abdominal wall: (a) at the level of the umbilicus; (b) below the level of the umbilicus.*

lesser or true pelvis) compartments (Fig. 82.2). The pelvic girdle (bony pelvis) forms a protective wall around the pelvis and is made up of the two hipbones (each consisting of the pubis, ilium, and ischium), the sacrum, and the coccyx. The bodies and rami of the pubic bones and the pubic symphysis form the anterior pelvic wall, while the lateral pelvic walls are formed by the hipbones covered by the obturator internus muscle, the obturator nerves and vessels, and branches of the internal iliac vessels (Fig. 82.3). The posterior pelvic wall is formed by the sacrum and coccyx.

The pelvic diaphragm, consisting of the levator ani and coccygeus muscles and their fascia, is stretched between the pubis anteriorly, the coccyx posteriorly and both lateral pelvic walls, and forms the inferior wall of the pelvic cavity. The levator ani muscles consist of the

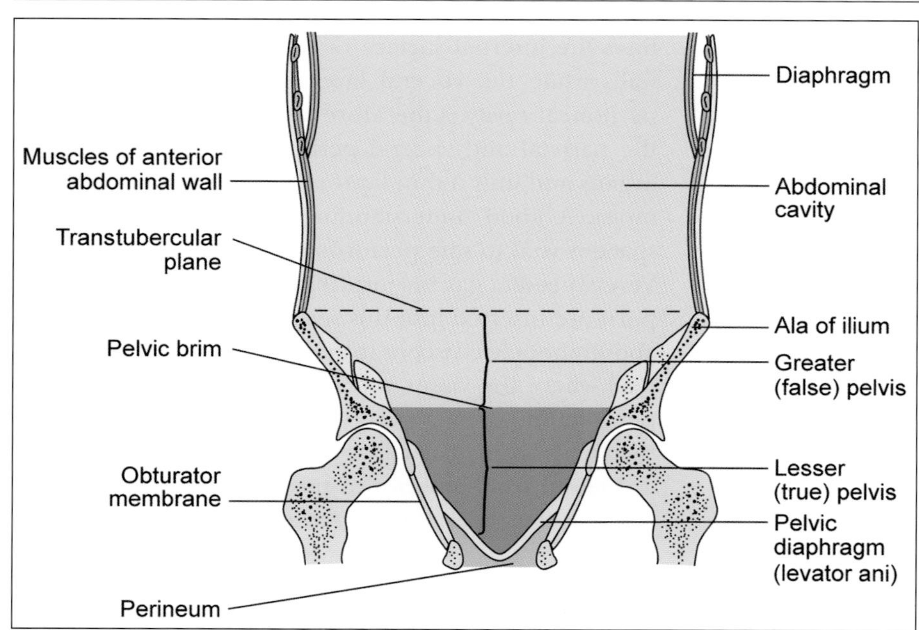

Figure 82.2. *Coronal section of the abdominopelvic cavity showing the greater (false) and lesser (true) pelvis separated by the pelvic brim.*

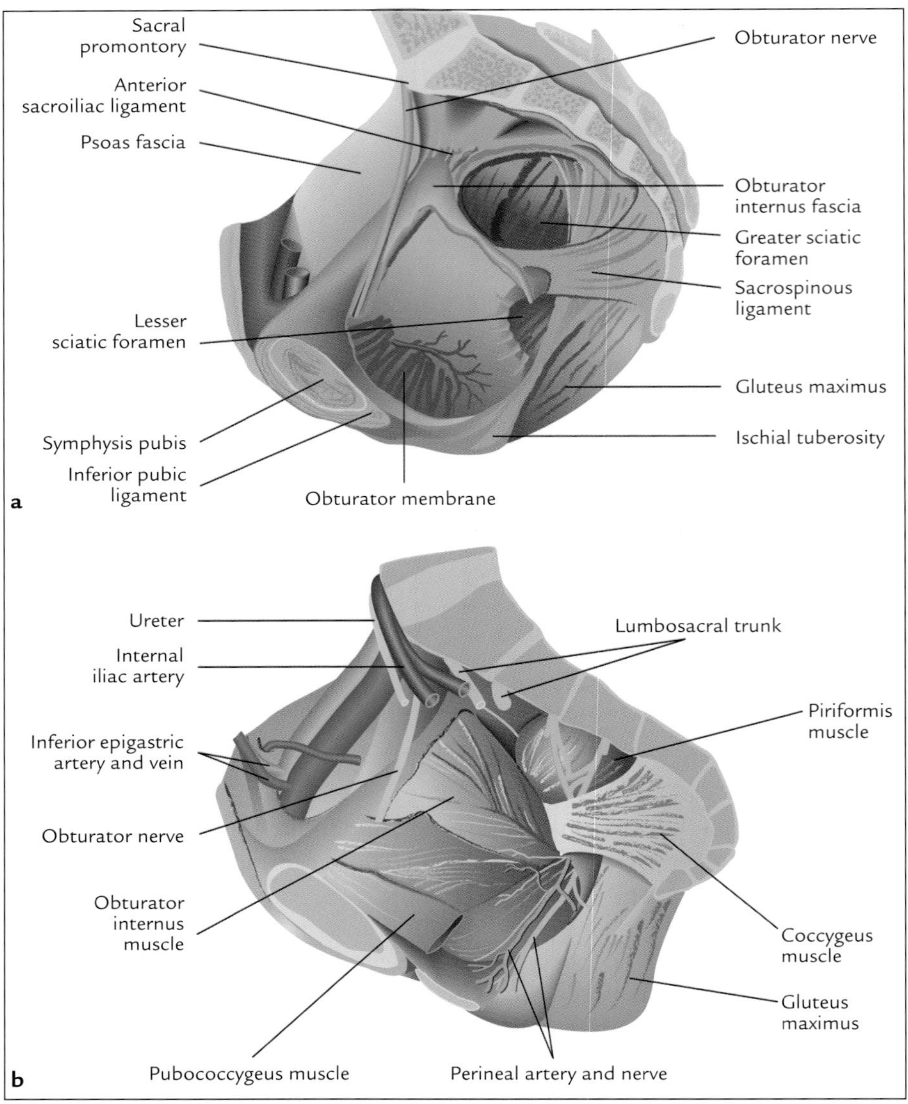

Figure 82.3. *Medial view of the structures which make up the walls and floor of the true pelvis: (a) the bony and ligamentous structures of the pelvic wall; (b) the muscular, nervous and vascular structures of the pelvic wall.*

pubococcygeus (which encircles and supports the urethra, vagina, and anal canal), the puborectalis (which forms a U-shaped muscular sling that passes posterior to the anorectal junction), and the iliococcygeus (the posterior-most part of the levators). The levator ani muscles and pelvic fascia are susceptible to damage by stretching or tearing during childbirth, often leading to an alteration of the position of the bladder neck and urethra and/or anorectal flexure, predisposing to urinary and/or fecal incontinence.

PELVIC PERITONEUM, FASCIA, FOSSAE AND LIGAMENTS

Peritoneum is a continuous, glistening, transparent serous membrane that lines the abdominal and pelvic cavities and invests their viscera. It consists of two layers, both made up of mesothelium: the parietal layer lines the internal surface of the abdominal and pelvic walls while the visceral layer invests the viscera. The peritoneal cavity is therefore a potential space between the parietal and visceral peritoneum that contains no organs and only a thin layer of fluid to keep its surfaces moist. A good understanding of the anatomy of this space is vital to safe performance of laparoscopy as the Veress needle, gas for insufflation, and all laparoscopic ports are inserted into this space. Peritoneum relates to abdominopelvic viscera in one of two ways: intraperitoneal where the viscus is completely covered by visceral peritoneum, or extraperitoneal (retroperitoneal) where the viscus is only partially covered by peritoneum.

Viewed from anterior to posterior through the laparoscope (Fig. 82.4), pelvic peritoneum covers the:

1. retropubic space of Retzius – a potential space that lies behind the pubic symphysis and in front of the

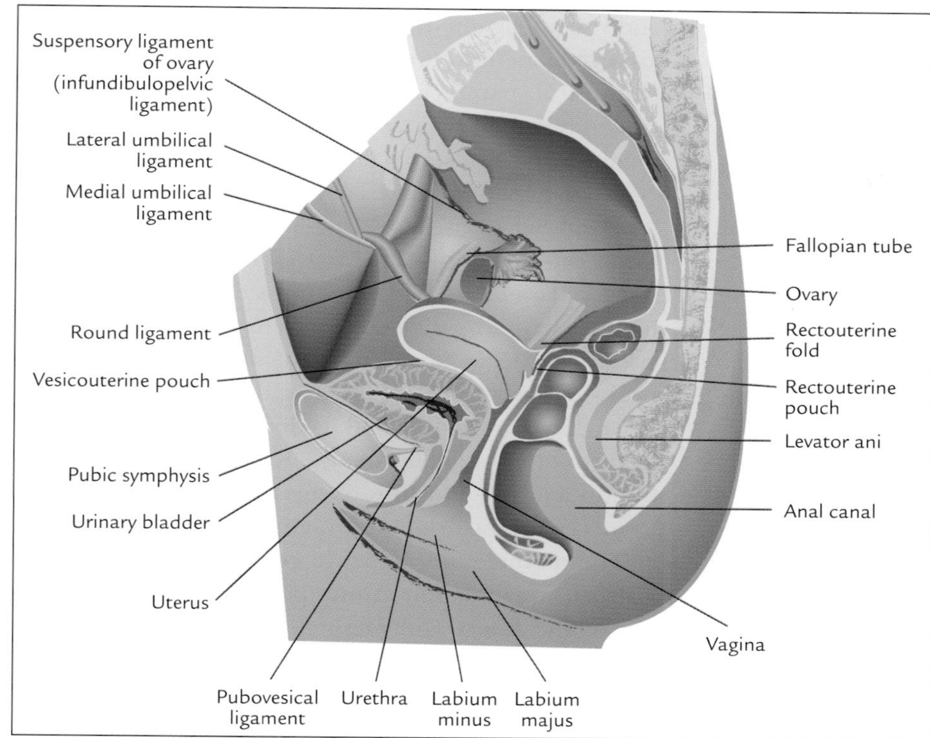

Figure 82.4. *Median section of the pelvis showing the pelvic organs and their peritoneal reflections.*

bladder, and is normally occupied only by venous plexuses;

2. transverse vesical fold on the bladder;
3. vesicouterine pouch between the bladder and the uterine isthmus;
4. opening of the vesicouterine pouch – leading to the vesicouterine septum that ends inferiorly in the fascia between the ureters and vagina;
5. body of the uterus and its appendages;
6. rectouterine pouch (of Douglas) – bordered anteriorly by the vagina and uterus, posteriorly by the rectum and its fascia, and laterally by the rectouterine folds that extend posteriorly towards the pararectal fossae;
7. opening of the rectouterine pouch – leading to the rectovaginal septum that ends at the union of the two uterosacral ligaments behind the cervix;
8. retrorectal space – situated between the rectal and retrorectal fascia.

Laterally, pelvic peritoneum covers the lateral pelvic wall overlying the common iliac vessels and their continuations (the internal and external iliac vessels) and the obturator membrane and fascia.

Peritoneal reflections over the pelvic organs give rise to five umbilical peritoneal folds, which in turn give rise to five peritoneal fossae (see Fig. 82.1):

1. Median umbilical fold – extending from the apex of the bladder to the umbilicus and covering the median umbilical ligament, which is the remnant of the urachus (reduced allantoic stalk) that joined the fetal bladder to the umbilicus;
2. Two medial umbilical folds – lying on either side of the midline lateral to the median folds and covering the medial umbilical ligaments, which contain the remnants of the occluded fetal umbilical arteries;
3. Two lateral umbilical folds – lying on either side of the midline lateral to the medial folds and covering the inferior epigastric vessels.

These umbilical folds give rise to five peritoneal fossae:

1. Supravesical fossa – lying between the medial umbilical folds and bisected by the median umbilical fold;
2. Two medial inguinal fossae – lying on each side between the medial and lateral umbilical folds;
3. Two lateral inguinal fossae –lying on each side lateral to the lateral umbilical folds and containing the inguinal rings.

Peritoneal relationships with the pelvic viscera give rise to specific mesenteries, ligaments, and fossae. The *broad ligament* is a double layer of peritoneum extending from the uterus to the pelvic sidewalls and consisting of three peritoneal mesenteries: funicular (round ligament) meso, mesosalpinx and meso-ovarium (see Fig. 82.4).

1. The funicular meso (mesentery of the round ligament) extends from the uterine horn to the deep inguinal ring. Opening this mesentery provides access to the paravesical fossa which is bounded superiorly by the umbilical artery medially and iliac vascular pedicle laterally, and inferiorly by the levator ani muscles and Cooper's ligament. The paravesical space contains the obturator nerve, the obturator and external iliac lymph nodes, and sometimes an accessory obturator vein.
2. The mesosalpinx (mesentery of the fallopian tube) is triangular when spread out and contains vascular archways (infratubal, infraovarian, and tubal branches of the ovarian vessels) and the infratubal nervous plexus. It is bordered superiorly by the fallopian tube and infundibulopelvic ligaments and laterally by the tubo-ovarian ligament and Richard's fimbrial fringe.
3. The meso-ovarium (mesentery of the ovary) contains the ovarian vessels and nerves.

The pre-ovarian fossa is triangle-shaped and lies between the funicular meso anteriorly, the mesosalpinx posteriorly, the external iliac vessels laterally, and the uterine horns medially. It overlies the obturator fossa and is opposite the appendix on the right and sigmoid colon on the left. The tubo-ovarian recess lies between the mesosalpinx and the meso-ovarium, while the ovarian fossa lies between the meso-ovarium anteriorly, the iliac vessels laterally, and the ureters and uterine vessels posteriorly, and overlies the obturator pedicle which contains the obturator nerves. The infundibulopelvic ligament contains the ovarian vessels and lies lateral to the ovary, crossing the external iliac vessels approximately 2 cm anterior to the ureter, and ending on the tubal extremity of the ovary. The ovarian ligament attaches the medial end of the ovary to the uterine horn below and behind the fallopian tube. The pararectal fossa opens superiorly into the sacroiliac sinus and is bordered anteriorly by the paracervix, medially by the rectum and uterosacral folds, laterally by the piriformis muscle, inferiorly by the levator ani muscle, and posteriorly by the lateral rectal ligament. The ureter runs across the pararectal fossa underneath peritoneum.

There are two distinct types of pelvic cellular tissue: slack tissues (easily dissected) and dense tissues (fascia and visceral ligaments). The slack tissues contain mostly areolar tissue and are predominant in the retropubic, paravesical, pararectal, and retrorectal spaces, and the vesicovaginal and rectovaginal septa. The dense tissues include the pelvic parietal and visceral fasciae. Pelvic fascia is a dense conjunctive lamina covering the pelvic wall (parietal pelvic fascia or urogenital diaphragm); it also forms the adventitia of the pelvic viscera (visceral pelvic fascia). Parietal pelvic fascia forms an effective support for the pelvic organs because of its continuity with the visceral pelvic fascia which invests the visceral subperitoneal surfaces of the organs. The density of the parietal pelvic fascia is variable and its deficiency in the midline leads to uterovaginal prolapse. Knowledge of the distribution and relationships of this fascia is therefore vital to successful repair of uterovaginal prolapse.

The architecture of pelvic cellular tissue resembles a mesh, with traction at one point provoking shortening of the fibers and mesh densification: the greater the traction, the more pronounced the densification near the point of traction. The pelvic fasciae exchange fibers, making anatomic relationships tight and surgical dissection more difficult, thereby increasing the risks of visceral injury, particularly around the points of connection between parietal and visceral fasciae. Pelvic visceral ligaments arise from densifications of pelvic cellular tissue whose visceral insertions intermingle with the perivisceral fascia and are generally of two types:

1. lateral ligaments which relate to the internal iliac arteries and include the vesical, genital, and rectal ligaments;
2. sagittal ligaments which relate to the branches of the inferior hypogastric plexus and include the uterosacral, vesicouterine, and pubovesical ligaments.

The vesical ligament is located around the anterior vesical arteries (branches of the umbilical artery) and attaches to the paracervix anteriorly. The genital ligament is the strongest of the pelvic ligaments, attaches the uterus to the pelvic sidewall, and provides its main support. It has three constituent parts: the parametrium, paracervix, and paravagina. The parametrium lies just above the ureters and contains the uterine vessels and lymphatics, while the paracervix lies beneath the ureters and contains the vaginal arteries and venous plexus and the uterovaginal lymph nodes. The rectal ligament is located around the middle rectal vessels, is thick and disposed almost transversely on each side of the rectum, separating the retrorectal from the pararectal space. The uterosacral ligaments arise from the posterolateral aspects of the cervix and vaginal fornix, the fibers from opposite sides intermingling at the point of origin from the uterus to form the torus uterinus. The ligament runs alongside the lateral aspects of the rectum to fan out into the sacral foramina of S2–S4. It contains few blood vessels but carries the inferior hypogastric nervous plexus of Lee and Frankenhauser. The vesicouterine ligaments extend from the uterine isthmus and cervix to the area around the urethral meatus in front of the parametrium. The pubovesical ligaments extend from the posterior wall of the symphysis pubis to the bladder neck.

REPRODUCTIVE SYSTEM

The *vagina* averages 7–9 cm in length, links the cervix with the vestibule, and is bordered anteriorly by the bladder and urethra, posteriorly by the rectovaginal pouch, rectum and anal canal, and laterally by the ureters, visceral pelvic fascia, and levator ani (Fig. 82.5). It is normally collapsed so its anterior and posterior walls lie together except at its superior end where the cervix holds them apart. Innervation of the upper three-quarters of the vagina is visceral from the uterovaginal plexus while the lower one-quarter is somatic from the pudendal nerve; hence only the lower end of the vagina is sensitive to touch and temperature.

The *uterus* consists of a body (which includes the fundus and isthmus) that forms the upper two-thirds and a cervix that makes up the lower third; its position changes with the degree of fullness of the bladder and rectum (Fig. 82.6). It is covered anteriorly and posteriorly by peritoneum and relates anteriorly to the vesicouterine pouch and bladder, posteriorly to the rectouterine pouch and rectum, and laterally to the broad ligaments, transverse cervical ligaments, and ureters (see Fig. 82.4). The uterus gets its blood supply from the uterine arteries (Fig. 82.7) and nerve supply from the uterovaginal plexus, and has both passive (transverse cervical and uterosacral ligaments) and dynamic (pelvic diaphragm) supports.

The *fallopian tubes* average 10 cm in length and extend laterally from the uterine horns along the free

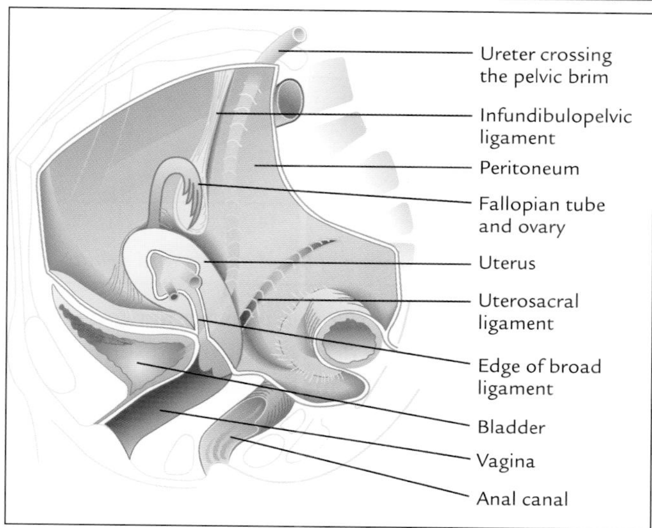

Figure 82.6. *Sagittal section of the pelvis showing the relationships of the pelvic organs and peritoneum.*

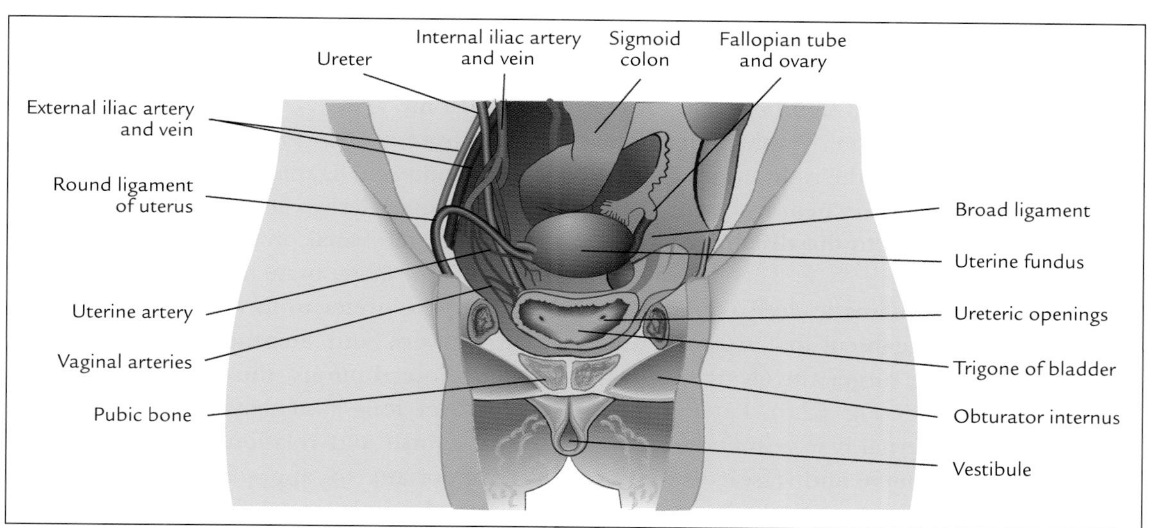

Figure 82.5. *Anterior view of the lower abdominal and pelvic cavities showing coronal sections of the bladder and anterior pelvis. Part of the superior rami and bodies of the pubic bones, anterior aspect of the bladder, right adnexal structures, and peritoneum covering the right lateral pelvic wall are removed for illustration.*

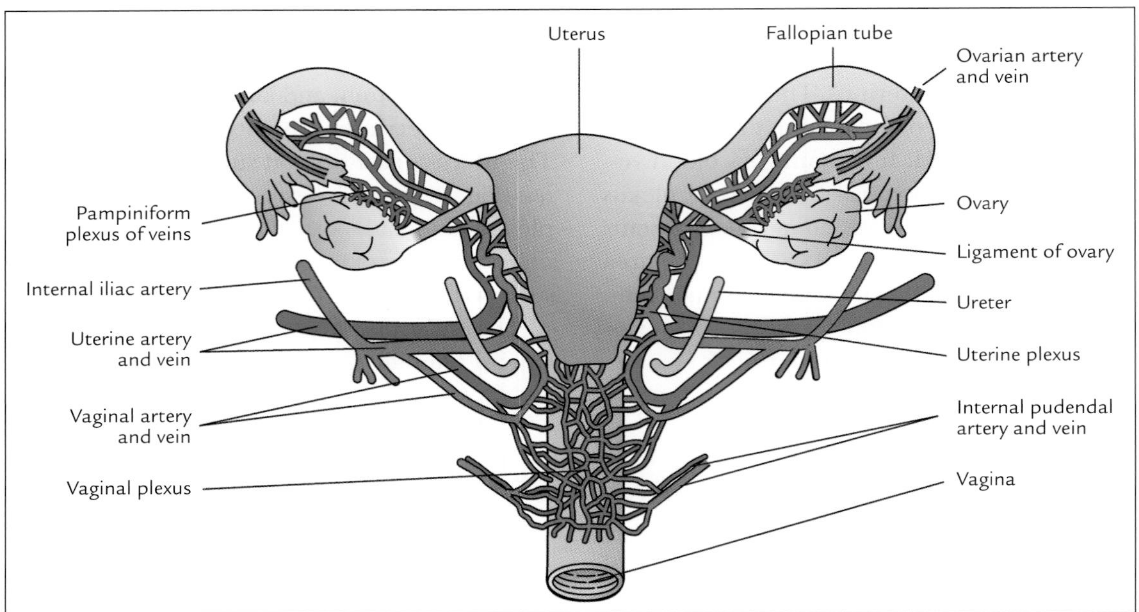

Figure 82.7. *Posterior view of blood supply and venous drainage of the uterus, vagina, fallopian tubes and ovaries.*

edge of the mesosalpinx to open into the peritoneal cavity near the ovaries. They derive their blood supply from the tubal branches of the uterine and ovarian arteries and are innervated jointly by the uterine and ovarian nervous plexuses.

The *ovaries* are located on the pelvic sidewalls suspended by the meso-ovarium and held in position by the ovarian ligaments medially and infundibulopelvic ligaments laterally, through which they receive the ovarian vessels and nervous plexuses.

URINARY SYSTEM

The *lumbar ureter* lies on the psoas muscle on each side of the rachis and is usually only of significance to gynecologic oncologists who perform lymphadenectomy. After descending into the pelvis, the right ureter crosses anterior to the external iliac artery near its origin while the left ureter crosses anterior to the distal end of the common iliac artery.

The *descending ureter* maintains a close relationship with the infundibulopelvic ligament that crosses it and so it is liable to injury during surgery involving this ligament and/or the ovaries (see Fig. 82.6). Laterally, the ureter is adjacent to the internal iliac vein and in close proximity to the obturator nerve and vessels, as well as the umbilical, uterine and vaginal vessels. It is easy to identify in this position in slim patients because of its characteristic peristaltic motion under the peritoneum.

The *retroligamentary ureter* runs forwards and medially along the posteromedial aspect of the uterine artery towards the origin of the uterosacral ligament, where it is normally only 1–3 cm from the ligament. This relationship could be altered by endometriosis, cancer, infection or previous surgery, sometimes bringing the ureter into closer proximity to the uterosacral ligament and/or ovary.

The *intraligamentary ureter* is not visible to the gynecologic surgeon and runs anteriorly across the transverse cervical ligament towards the bladder, crossing beneath the uterine artery at a point approximately 1.5 cm from the uterine isthmus and 1 cm from the lateral vaginal fornix. Diseases such as endometriosis can alter its relationships around this point, significantly increasing the risks of injury during procedures such as laparoscopic hysterectomy.

The *retrovesical ureter* enters the vesical extremity of the vesicouterine ligament to reach the bladder.

The ureter derives its blood supply from contributions from the renal, ovarian, common iliac and uterine arteries: these branches divide into a T-shape on reaching the ureter to form a rich surrounding adventitial network and anastomosis that compensate for vascular interruptions, thus allowing dissection of the ureter over long distances. In addition to knowledge of the course and relationships of both ureters, it is also important to appreciate the subtle differences between the right and left ureters, and to be able to identify, dissect, and protect the ureters from surgical injury (Fig. 82.8). Mobilizing the uterus anteriorly often helps to localize the ascending segment of the uterine artery correctly without altering the posi-

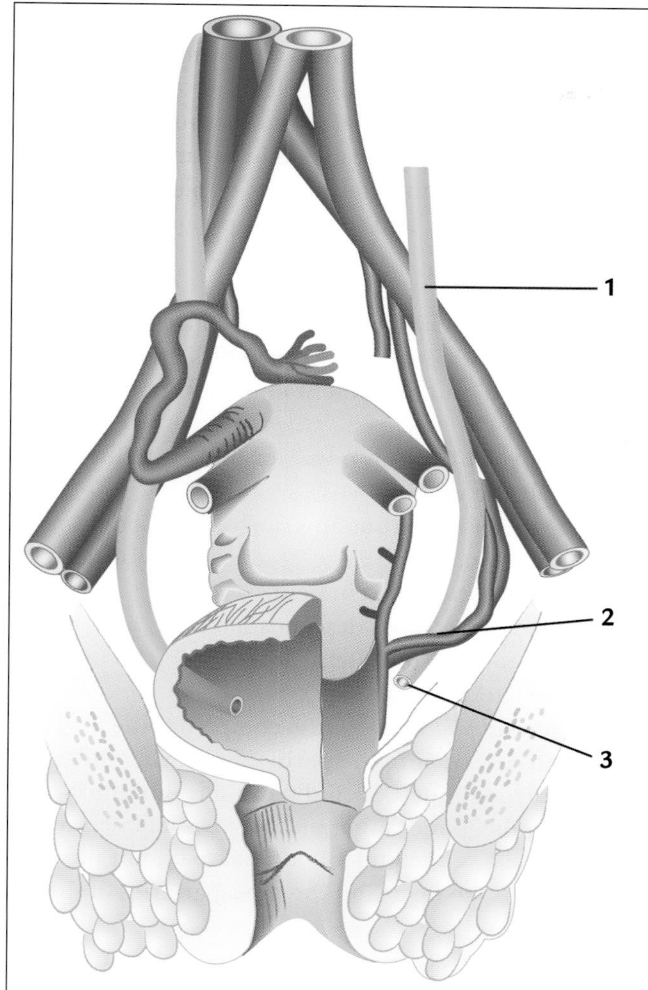

Figure 82.8. *Course of the pelvic ureter showing the three points where it is at most risk of surgical injury: (1) where it crosses the iliac vessels; (2) where it crosses the uterine artery; (3) at the level of the vaginal fornix.*

tion of the ureter. Transecting the correctly localized uterine artery at the level of the uterine isthmus, and pulling its proximal end laterally, helps to mobilize the ureter away from the uterus, further protecting it from injury. Similarly, opening the vesicouterine space to dissect out and mobilize the retrovesical ureter from the vesicouterine ligament can help to protect the ureter.

The retropubic space (of Retzius) is an anterior preperitoneal space containing mostly loose fatty tissue; it is bordered:

- anteriorly by the pubic symphysis, pubovesical ligaments, tendinous arch of the parietal pelvic fascia, and retropubic branches of the obturator and pudendal nerves;
- posteriorly by the inferolateral aspect of the bladder, the urethra, and pelvic vagina;
- laterally by the superior pubic ramus and pectineal ligament (of Cooper);
- inferiorly by the pelvic diaphragm.

The vesical base of the retropubic space includes the trigone and retrotrigonal fossa; it increases in depth with age, a factor in the causation of postmicturition dribbling.

The urethrovesical junction is situated approximately 2.5 cm from the pubic symphysis to which it is secured by the pubovesical ligaments to create an angle of 90–100 degrees between the urethra and bladder base, an angle that is crucial for urinary continence. The urethra descends inferiorly and anteriorly at an angle of 30 degrees from the vertical and is conventionally divided into three segments: supradiaphragmatic, diaphragmatic, and infradiaphragmatic. The pubovesical ligaments support the supradiaphragmatic urethra while the infradiaphragmatic urethra is supported by the pubourethral ligament and suspensory ligament of the clitoris.

Urinary continence and micturition require cooperation and synergy between the bladder, urethra, and abdominopelvic pressure. During bladder filling, abdominopelvic pressure acts as a passive occlusive force on the supradiaphragmatic urethra, apposing the pelvic diaphragm against which the urethra pushes. During the micturition phase, the combined higher intravesical pressure and intraparietal tension caused by detrusor contractions are directed towards the urethrovesical junction, overcoming the urethral closure pressure and leading to opening of the urethra. Weakness or loss of the normal angle of the urethrovesical junction and shortening or increased horizontalization of the urethra predispose to urinary stress incontinence.

INTESTINAL SYSTEM

The common laparoscopic gynecologic operations do not involve the intestinal system but adequate knowledge of the pelvic part of this system is important for safe surgery.

The *rectum* is at considerable risk of injury during certain procedures such as resection of rectovaginal endometriotic disease, surgery for pelvic cancer, and sacrocolpopexy. Placing a patient in the Trendelenburg position normally utilized for gynecologic laparoscopic surgery effectively moves most of the intestines out of the pelvis, leaving only the sigmoid colon and rectum.

The *rectosigmoid junction* overlies the S3 vertebra and is marked by discontinuation of the fatty omental appendices and a spreading out of the teniae of the sigmoid to form a continuous outer longitudinal layer of smooth muscle.

The rectum follows the curve of the sacrum and coccyx (the *sacral flexure*) and ends anteroinferior to the tip of the coccyx by turning sharply posteroinferiorly (the *anorectal flexure*) as it perforates the pelvic diaphragm to become the anal canal. The anorectal flexure is maintained at an angle of approximately 80 degrees by the *puborectalis muscle*, a vital function for fecal continence.

The dilated terminal end of the rectum (*ampulla*) lies directly above and is supported by the pelvic diaphragm and *anococcygeal ligament*, and acts as a reservoir for feces pending defecation.

Peritoneum covers the anterior and lateral surfaces of the superior third of the rectum, only the anterior surface of the middle third, and none of the inferior third (the subperitoneal portion). Medially the visceral peritoneum over the rectum is reflected forward onto the vagina to form the *rectouterine pouch* (beneath which lies the rectovaginal septum) while laterally it is reflected onto the pelvic wall to form the *pararectal fossae*.

PELVIC VASCULAR SYSTEM

The pelvis derives its vascular supply mainly from two paired (internal iliac and ovarian) and two unpaired (median sacral and superior rectal) arteries.

The *internal iliac artery* arises from the bifurcation of the common iliac artery at the point where it is crossed by the ureter anterior to the sacroiliac joint, and descends posteriorly along the pelvic wall to the greater sciatic foramen (GSF). There, it divides into anterior (visceral) and posterior (parietal) branches to provide most of the blood supply to the pelvis. The visceral branch gives off the umbilical, uterine, vaginal, obturator, middle rectal, and internal pudendal arteries while the parietal branch gives off the iliolumbar, lateral sacral, and superior gluteal arteries.

The *umbilical artery* runs along the superior aspect of the inferolateral part of the bladder to end as the *superior vesical artery* and constitutes a surgical landmark denoting the origin of the uterine artery. The *uterine artery* consists of three segments:

- from its origin, the parietal segment descends on the pelvic sidewall down to the ischial spine accompanied by the umbilical and obturator arteries anteriorly and the ureter medially;
- the parametrial segment runs medially beneath the parametrium and anterior to the ureter surrounded by lymph nodes and venous plexuses;
- the tortuous mesometrial segment runs alongside the lateral aspect of the uterus in the mesometrium accompanied by the uterine venous plexus, lymphatic vessels, and sometimes parauterine lymph nodes.

The uterine artery gives off several collateral branches including vesicovaginal, cervicovaginal, sinuous cervical, corporeal, and round ligament branches.

- The *vaginal artery* runs posterior to the uterine artery to supply the vagina.
- The *obturator artery* runs anteriorly towards the obturator foramen in between the obturator nerve above and obturator vein below.
- The *middle rectal artery* descends inferiorly and medially towards the lateral aspect of the rectum and into the lateral rectal fossa.
- The *internal pudendal artery* accompanies the pudendal nerve into the perineum, leaving the pelvis through the GSF and passing round the sciatic spine, penetrating the ischiorectal fascia and running along the pudendal canal to end in two branches – the deep and the dorsal arteries of the clitoris.
- The *ovarian artery* emerges from the abdominal aorta at the level of the L2 vertebra and descends to reach the ovary through the infundibulopelvic ligament.
- The *superior rectal artery* emerges from the *inferior mesenteric artery* to run in the superior rectal ligament to supply the rectum.
- The *median sacral artery* arises from the posterior aspect of the aorta just above its bifurcation and descends on the anterior aspect of the L4 and L5 vertebrae and the sacrum. This artery is exposed to significant risks of injury in this position during the tissue stripping and fixation that is undertaken for laparoscopic sacrocolpopexy or pelvic lymphadenectomy.

In the vast majority (80%) of people the umbilicus is situated at a level that is within 2 cm of the aortic bifurcation, and in slim people it often overlies the bifurcation or left common iliac vessels, placing them at significant risk of injury during umbilical port placement. This risk is further magnified in very slim women in whom the aorta could be less than 3 cm from the anterior abdominal wall. The lumbar lordosis sags on placing a patient in the modified lithotomy position that is normally utilized for gynecologic laparoscopic surgery, effectively moving the aorta further away from the anterior abdominal wall. Manually elevating the anterior abdominal wall and ensuring there is adequate pneumoperitoneum before trocar placement achieves the same objective.

PELVIC LYMPHATIC SYSTEM

The pelvic lymphatic system consists of groups of lymph nodes organized around major pelvic blood vessels to drain the pelvic organs:

1. Lumbar (lateral aortic) nodes – drain the ureters, uterus, fallopian tubes, ovaries, and rectum;
2. Inferior mesenteric nodes – drain the rectum;
3. Common iliac nodes – drain the ureters, bladder, and vagina;
4. External iliac nodes – drain the ureters, bladder, vagina, and uterus;
5. Internal iliac nodes – drain the ureters, bladder, urethra, vagina, uterus, and rectum;
6. Superficial inguinal nodes – drain the urethra, vagina, and uterus;
7. Deep inguinal nodes – drain the urethra;
8. Sacral nodes – drain the bladder, urethra, vagina, and uterus;
9. Pararectal nodes – drain the rectum.

PELVIC NERVOUS SYSTEM

The sacral and coccygeal nerves and the pelvic part of the autonomic nervous system form the main innervations of the pelvis.

Sacral plexus

The sacral nervous plexus is located on the posterior wall of the lesser (true) pelvis, closely applied to the anterior surface of the piriformis muscle, and gives off two main nerves – the sciatic and pudendal.

The sciatic nerve arises from the ventral rami of L4–S3 and leaves the pelvis through the GSF to supply the posterior aspects of the lower limbs. The pudendal nerve arises from the anterior divisions of the ventral rami of S2–S4, accompanies the internal pudendal artery out of the pelvis through the GSF, and hooks round the ischial spine and sacrospinous ligament to enter the perineum through the lesser sciatic foramen. It supplies the skin and muscles of the perineum and terminates as the dorsal nerve of the clitoris. The pudendal nerve also supplies visceral branches to the bladder, the reproductive organs, and the rectum, providing sensory innervation and the nervous control of micturition and defecation.

The superior gluteal nerve arises from the posterior divisions of the ventral rami of L4–S1 and leaves the pelvis through the GSF to supply the gluteal muscles. The inferior gluteal nerve arises from the posterior divisions of the ventral rami of L5–S2 and leaves the pelvis through the GSF to supply the gluteus maximus muscle.

Obturator nerve

The obturator nerve arises from the lumbar nervous plexus (L2–L4) in the greater pelvis and enters the lesser pelvis through the GSF to run in the extraperitoneal fat along the lateral wall to the obturator canal. It divides into anterior and posterior branches that leave the pelvis through this canal to supply the medial thigh muscles.

Coccygeal plexus

The coccygeal plexus is a small network of nerve fibers formed by the ventral rami of S4 and S5, and the coccygeal nerves. It lies on the pelvic surface of the coccygeus muscle and supplies this muscle, part of the levator ani and the sacrococcygeal joint. It gives off the anococcygeal nerves, which pierce the sacrotuberous ligament to supply an area of skin in the coccygeal region.

Pelvic autonomic nerves

The sacral sympathetic trunks are the inferior continuation of the lumbar sympathetic trunks and have the primary function of providing postsynaptic fibers to the sacral plexus for sympathetic (vasomotor, pilomotor, sudomotor) innervation of the lower limbs. They contain four sympathetic ganglia each, and descend on the pelvic surface of the sacrum medial to the sacral foramina to converge into the small ganglion impar (coccygeal ganglion) anterior to the coccyx. These send communicating branches to each of the ventral rami of the sacral and coccygeal nerves and small branches to the median sacral artery and inferior hypogastric plexus.

The hypogastric plexuses consist of two networks of autonomic nerves – superior and inferior. The superior hypogastric plexus lies just inferior to the bifurcation of the aorta at the level of L5 and descends into the pelvis on either side anterior to the sacrum as the right and left hypogastric nerves. These descend within the hypogastric sheaths lateral to the rectum and then spread out in a fan-like fashion to merge with the pelvic splanchnic nerves and form the inferior hypogastric plexus. The inferior hypogastric plexus (Lee and Frankenhauser's ganglion) is a 4 cm long nervous quadrilateral lamina located in the lateral aspect of the uterosacral ligament. Extensions of this plexus (the pelvic plexus) pass to the cervix, lateral vaginal fornices, and the inferolateral surfaces of the bladder. Pelvic splanchnic nerves contain parasympathetic fibers from S2–S4 spinal cord segments, and visceral efferent fibers from cell bodies in the spinal ganglia of the corresponding spinal nerves. The inferior hypogastric and pelvic plexuses thus contain both sympathetic and parasympathetic fibers, which pass along the branches of the internal iliac arteries to form subplexuses (rectal, visceral, uterovaginal) on the pelvic viscera.

The ovarian plexus originates from the aortic plexus to innervate the ovaries and distal half of the fallopian tubes and receives parasympathetic fibers from the pneumogastric nerve, explaining the vagal intestinal response to ovarian manipulation or torsion.

The motor response to pelvic nociceptive stimuli correlates with pelvic innervation. For instance, the parietal pain of acute salpingitis is in fact pain from a viscus transmitted through the closest somatic nerve into the corresponding iliac fossa. The dyspareunia associated with rectovaginal endometriotic disease is accentuated by stimulation of the sympathetic fibers inside the rectovaginal septum causing the sympathetic motor cells to induce a reflex contraction of the pelvic diaphragm.

Laparoscopic surgery, by avoiding large abdominal incisions, avoids transection of the anterior branches of the iliohypogastric and ilioinguinal nerves, which can lead to reversible cutaneous anesthesia of the pubic region, the insides of the upper thighs, and the labia majora, as well as weakness of the muscles of the anterior abdominal wall predisposing to hernia formation. Attention should therefore be paid to correct localization and closure of lateral ports to avoid nerve injury during port placement or nerve entrapment in a stitch during fascial closure of port sites that are placed too close to the anterior superior iliac spines. Such nerve entrapments could give rise to unexplained abdominal pain that only resolves with removal of the stitch. The obturator nerves may become affected by pelvic endometriotic disease or infection at the level of the obturator foramen, leading to obturator neuralgia on the superomedial aspect of the thighs and knees.

ACKNOWLEDGMENTS

I am grateful to Mr Harry Heyes of the Medical Illustration Department of Central Manchester and Manchester Children's University Hospitals Trust for meticulously producing the color images used throughout this chapter.

BIBLIOGRAPHY

1. Abu-Rustum NR. Laparoscopy 2003: oncologic perspective. Clin Obstet Gynecol 2003;46:61–9.
2. Bradley WE. Neural control of urethrovesical function. Clin Obstet Gynecol 1978;21:653–67.
3. Cahill DR, Orland MJ, Miller G. Atlas of Human Cross-sectional Anatomy, 3rd ed. New York: Wiley-Liss, 1996.
4. Dargent D. Laparoscopic surgery in gynaecologic oncology. J Gynecol Obstet Biol Reprod 2000;29:282–4.
5. Donnez J, Chantraine F, Nisolle M. Complications of laparoscopic surgery in gynecology. In: Donnez J, Nisolle M (eds) An Atlas of Operative Laparoscopy and Hysteroscopy, 2nd ed. New York: Parthenon, 2001; 373–87.
6. Ellis H. Clinical Anatomy. A Revision and Applied Anatomy for Clinical Students, 8th ed. Oxford: Blackwell Scientific, 1992.
7. Faucheron JL. Surgical anatomy of pelvic nerves. Ann Chir 1999;53:985–9.
8. Fauconnier A, Delmas V, Lassau JP et al. Ventral tethering of the vagina and its role in the kinetics of urethra and bladder neck straining. Surg Radiol Anat 1996;18:81–7.
9. Healy JE Jr, Hodge J. Surgical Anatomy, 2nd ed. Toronto: BC Decker, 1990.
10. Moore KL, Dalley AF. Clinically Oriented Anatomy, 4th ed. Baltimore: Lippincott, Williams and Wilkins, 1999.
11. Nezhat CH, Nezhat F, Brill AI et al. Normal variations of abdominal and pelvic anatomy evaluated at laparoscopy. Obstet Gynecol 1999;94:238–42.
12. Ploteau S, Donnez J. Anatomy in relation to gynecological endoscopy. In: Donnez J, Nisolle M (eds) An Atlas of Operative Laparoscopy and Hysteroscopy, 2nd ed. New York: Parthenon, 2001; 33–45.
13. Robert R, Brunet C, Faure A et al. Surgery of the pudendal nerve in various types of perineal pain: course and results. Chirurgie 1993–94;119:535–9.
14. Robert R, Prat-Pradal D, Labat JJ et al. Anatomic basis of chronic pelvic pain: role of the pudendal nerve. Surg Radiol Anat 1998;20:93–8.
15. Weber AM. New approaches to surgery for urinary incontinence and pelvic organ prolapse from the laparoscopic perspective. Clin Obstet Gynecol 2003;46:44–60.
16. Williams PL, Bannister LH, Berry MM, Collins P, Dussek JE, Ferguson MWJ (eds) Gray's Anatomy, 38th ed. Edinburgh: Churchill Livingstone, 1995.
17. Woodburne RD, Burkel WE. Essentials of Human Anatomy, 9th ed. New York: Oxford University Press, 1994.

83

Laparoscopic treatment of pelvic pain

Christopher Sutton, Richard Dover

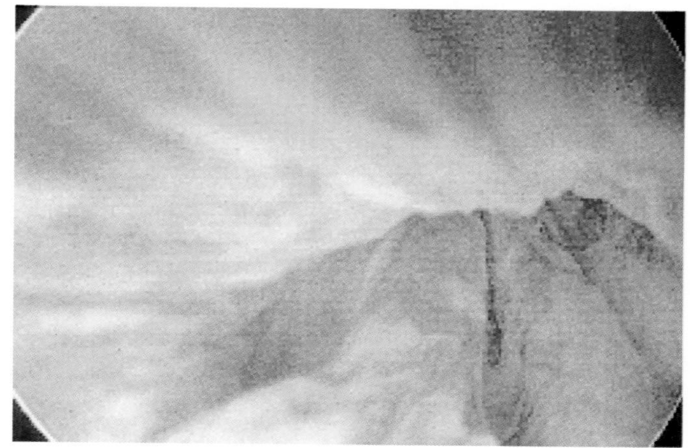

INTRODUCTION

Pelvic pain is a common symptom among women of reproductive age, and its diagnosis and management constitute a considerable part of a gynecologist's workload. Women with acute pain usually present via the Accident and Emergency department. The pain is usually severe and of recent onset, and requires skilled assessment in order to distinguish gynecologic causes from diseases of adjacent organs or structures (Table 83.1).

Pelvic pain of more than 6 months' duration is usually labeled as chronic pelvic pain, and the differential diagnosis is usually more complex and requires careful evaluation of the physical, psychological, and emotional state of the patient[1] (Table 83.2).

Table 83.1. *Causes of acute pelvic pain*

Gynecologic	Non-gynecologic
Uterus	Gastrointestinal
miscarriage	appendicitis
acute degeneration of fibroid	diverticulitis
endometritis	obstruction (adhesions/ volvulus)
perforation (after insertion of IUCD/surgery)	constipation
Fallopian tubes	ischemia
ectopic pregnancy	gastroenteritis
acute salpingitis	Urologic
torsion (e.g. hydrosalpinx)	cystitis/pyelonephritis
Ovary	renal/ureteric colic
cyst accident/ovulation	retention
torsion	Other
tubo-ovarian abscess	musculoskeletal
metabolic	
idiopathic	

IUCD, intrauterine contraceptive device.

Table 83.2. *Causes of chronic pelvic pain*

Gynecologic	Non-gynecologic
Uterus	Gastrointestinal
primary dysmenorrhea	adhesions
adenomyosis	constipation
fibroids	diverticular disease
Fallopian tube	irritable bowel syndrome
chronic salpingitis	Urologica
Ovary	retention
benign and malignant cysts	urethral syndrome
endometriotic cysts	interstitial cystitis
entrapment by adhesions	Other
remnant syndrome	musculoskeletal
General	nerve entrapment
endometriosis	idiopathic
venous congestion	

If one overlooks the difficulties of defining the condition, and focuses on the patients themselves, the magnitude and importance of the problem become obvious. One author comments that chronic pelvic pain is responsible for approximately 5% of new gynecological referrals at his hospital,[2] but unfortunately there is no community-based study from the UK that allows us to estimate the prevalence of chronic pelvic pain within the whole population. Such a study in the United States has been published, quoting a prevalence rate of 15%.[3] This study also made an economic assessment of the problem: in addition to the medical costs associated with hospital attendance and treatments, 15% of the employed women reported time lost from work and 45% reported reduced productivity. Although there is no population-based UK study, a recent paper[4] has reviewed all published work and quotes prevalence rates for dysmenorrhea of 45–97% and for abdominal pain of 23–29%. The authors make the valid point that the definitions used vary widely, and that the selection criteria in some cases may not have been truly representative of the population as a whole.

The next step, once these patients have been identified, is to attempt to reach a diagnosis. The literature is replete with the potential difficulties of assessment in these women, and stresses the importance of the medical history as potentially the most important part of the process.[2,5] The other issue that is constantly highlighted is the possibility of previous sexual abuse, which is more prevalent in women with chronic pelvic pain. This issue in the UK setting has been reviewed by Collett et al.[6] Some clinicians have a special interest in this area and will take the time to explore all aspects of the history. However, it is most likely that the patient will undergo a diagnostic laparoscopy. Because of the number of patients who may suffer from pelvic pain it is not surprising that their investigation may account for more than 40% of all laparoscopic procedures in some units.[7]

The next area of interest is to consider the pathology encountered at the time of the diagnostic laparoscopy. In view of the confusion surrounding the definition of the condition under investigation, it should come as no surprise that the reported findings vary considerably from one unit to the next. It must be remembered, however, that these differences could also be explained in terms of different local referral practices, and the special interest and reputation of the clinician involved. With these reservations in mind, a superficial review of the published literature reveals that, at the time of diagnostic laparoscopy for chronic pelvic pain, the incidence of endometriosis is 16–33.3%, and the incidence of adhesions is 23.1–40%; negative findings may be encountered in 14.8–30% of cases.[8–11] There appears to be considerable variation in these figures, and other papers quoting negative laparoscopy rates of 65%[1] and 10–90%[12] do little to clarify the issue.

It is possible to discern some common themes from these confusing statements. While the exact proportions may vary considerably, it does appear that endometriosis and pelvic adhesions will be diagnosed in a large subgroup; however, the fact that pathology is demonstrable does not imply that the relationship between it and the symptoms is a causal one. There is also the indisputable fact that diagnostic laparoscopy will be negative in a percentage of patients.

One of the reasons for the huge variability in these figures is that, even now, many gynecologists are unable to recognize the protean manifestations of the appearance of endometriosis (Figs 83.1–83.5). The classic appearance of hemosiderin (black powder burns – typical lesions) often represents old burnt-out disease whereas red telangiectases, flame-like lesions, yellow–brown peritoneum, subovarian adhesions, peritoneal defects, and neoangiogenesis (so-called subtle or atypical lesions) are often only recognized by experts in this condition.

The rest of this chapter focuses on the various laparoscopic techniques that are available to treat endometriosis and pelvic adhesions and gives some measure of their success. The treatment of other pathologies such as chronic infection will not be covered, but options for laparoscopic treatment in cases where no pathology has been demonstrated are discussed briefly in the section on denervation.

LAPAROSCOPIC TREATMENT OF ENDOMETRIOSIS

Endometriosis may be present in the pelvis in three main areas: peritoneal deposits, ovarian endometriomas, and rectovaginal septum deposits, and it has been suggested that these are in fact three separate conditions.[13] The treatment of disease in each of these sites will be considered separately.

Peritoneal disease

Endometriosis of the pelvic peritoneum may be superficial or deep. Indeed it has been suggested that deep deposits (3 mm) may be present in up to 60% of patients with this condition.[14] The identification of deep disease

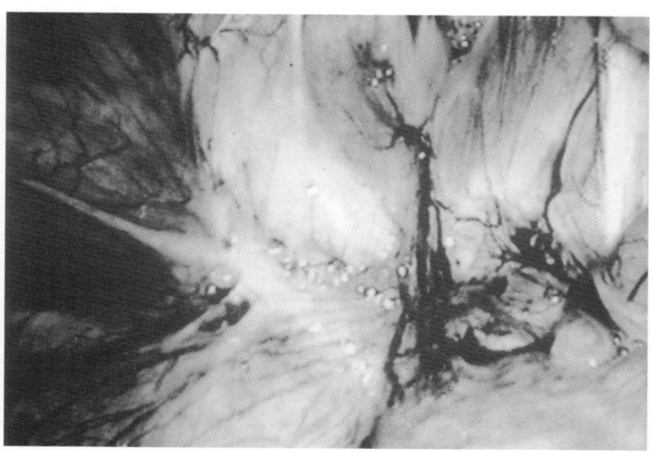

Figure 83.1. *Red flame-like lesions and telangiectases and marked neoangiogenesis.*

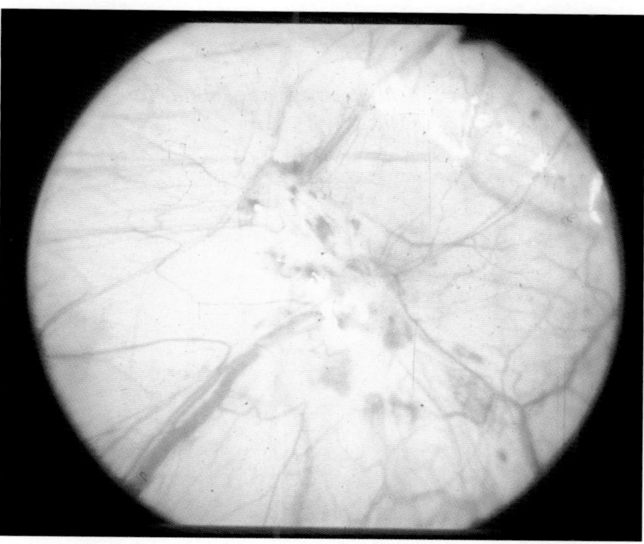

Figure 83.2. *Endometriotic vesicular implant (sago-grain) with telangiectases and neoangiogenesis. Note the straight vessels of varying diameter.*

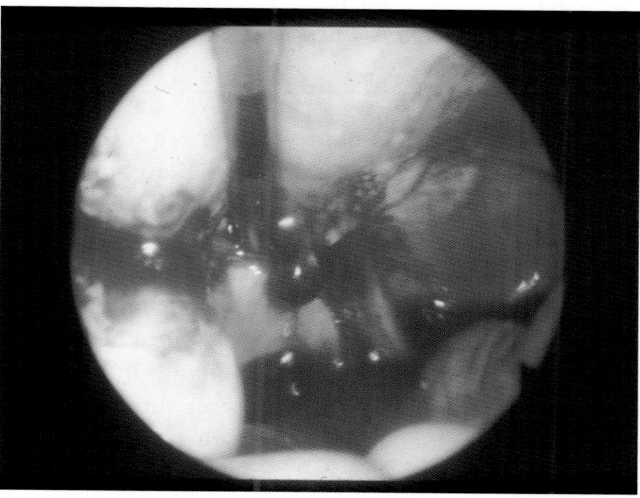

Figure 83.3. *Glandular tissue-like endometrium and hemorrhagic vesicles secreting large amounts of blood and other substances into a pool in the cul-de-sac.*

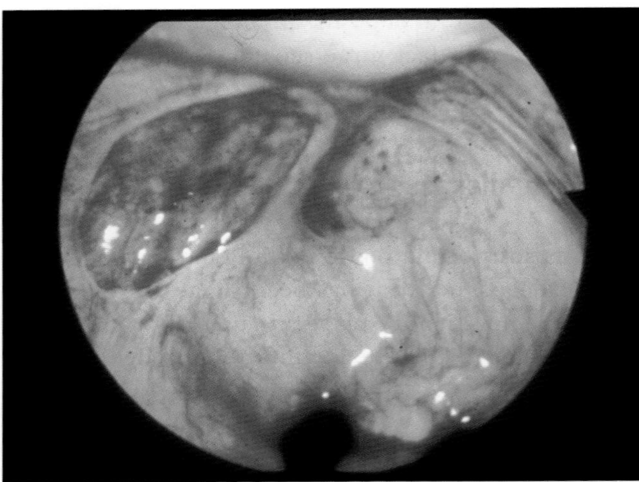

Figure 83.4. *Peritoneal pouches with endometriosis in the base (Allen–Masters syndrome).*

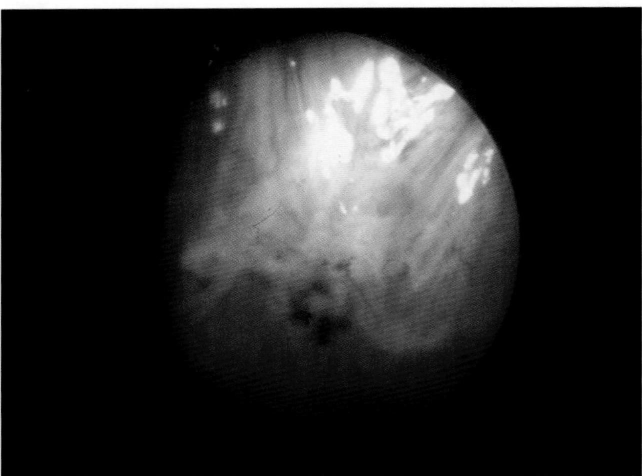

Figure 83.5. *Subovarian adhesion between the interior surface of the ovary and typical deposits of hemosiderin (black lesions).*

is essential, since treatment – either vaporization or excision – needs to extend down to the level of normal tissue. Failure to appreciate the depth of a lesion may therefore lead to inadequate treatment and incomplete relief of symptoms. This is particularly true for deposits infiltrating deeply into the bladder, which may penetrate through the mucosa and give rise to cyclical hematuria. If this is the case, cure can be achieved only by complete excision of the lesion and laparoscopic suturing of the defect in the bladder, followed by catheter drainage for a 'urologic week'.

Most lesions do not penetrate the full thickness of the bladder wall, but it is important to remove all of the endometriotic implants and the vessels arising from neoangiogenesis that are supplying them. The choice between laser ablation and electrosurgical resection of focal disease is usually a matter of individual preference, but may be influenced by the range of equipment available and the location of the deposits concerned. The relative merits of these two techniques have been covered elsewhere.[15] In our center we tend to use carbon dioxide laser vaporization through a second cannula placed laterally (Figs 83.6, 83.7) with a rotating mirror delivery system, employing the laser in super- or ultrapulse mode for more effective cutting. Although an electrosurgical needle is the most common method of treatment for peritoneal disease, on occasions we use excision, especially if the uterosacral ligaments are involved.

While most clinicians are familiar with the use of lasers in the operating theater, and will have read papers describing the technique of laser ablation of endometriotic deposits, most would probably be surprised to learn that the first study subjecting this therapy to the rigors of

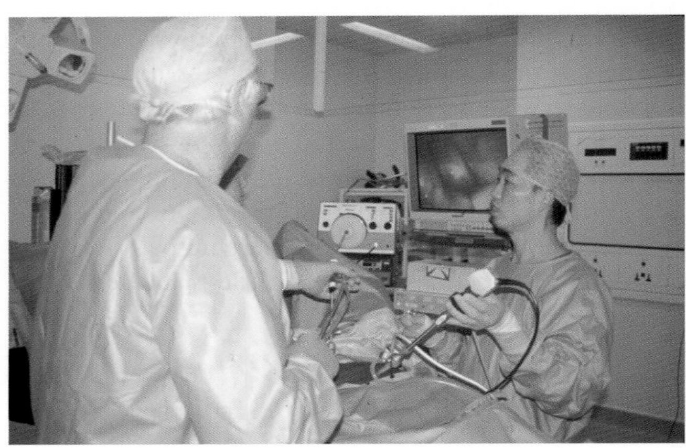

Figure 83.6. *Laparoscopic laser surgery using television monitors on either side of the operating table.*

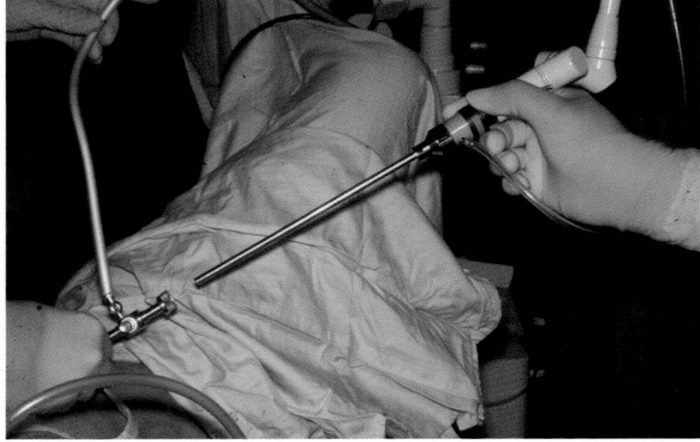

Figure 83.7. *CO_2 laser laparoscopy with the laser cannula inserted in the right or left iliac fossa.*

a prospective, randomized, double-blind study was not published until 1994. An earlier report described the use of laser ablation in the treatment of pelvic pain secondary to endometriosis followed up over 5 years by our unit at St Luke's Hospital, Guildford.[16] Of 228 consecutive patients treated for endometriosis, pelvic pain was improved in 126 of 181 women (69.6%) who suffered with it. Thirty-eight patients were no better and second look laparoscopy did not show any sign of endometriosis; however, most of these patients had other diagnoses such as irritable bowel syndrome. Only 17 had recurrent disease during the 5-year study and six were lost to follow-up (Fig. 83.8). The authors had some reservations about the design of this study because it was retrospective and therefore liable to all the biases inherent in this kind of study, particularly the ability of a surgeon to coerce the patient into saying she is better which often happens because of some innate wish to please the surgeon who performed the operation, whereas in reality she is really no better at all. Such biases can only be eliminated by a double-blind study where neither the patient nor the doctor or nurse following them up is aware of the treatment arm to which the patient had been allocated. Therefore, we consequently embarked on a prospective, double-blind, randomized trial.[17] Although the findings of this study have been well publicized, there are several interesting aspects that bear closer inspection.

The study examined patients with symptoms suggestive of endometriosis who were recruited and then randomized to receive either a diagnostic laparoscopy only, or laparoscopy combined with laser ablation of all visible deposits of endometriosis and uterine nerve transection. Of the patients eligible for analysis, 62.5% of those who received laser therapy reported that symptoms were better or improved. This finding was statistically different from the 22.6% who had improved in the group that received laparoscopy alone (Figs 83.9–83.12).

When the results were analyzed stage by stage, it was discovered that response rates were lowest amongst those with stage I disease; if these patients were excluded from the final analysis, then 73.7% of patients with mild or moderate disease obtained benefit. The authors suggested that endometriosis was in fact a chance finding in the group with minimal disease, and was not responsible for their symptoms. Some credence is given to this suggestion by the finding that three of the five women who did not derive benefit from laser ablation had no residual disease when they underwent a

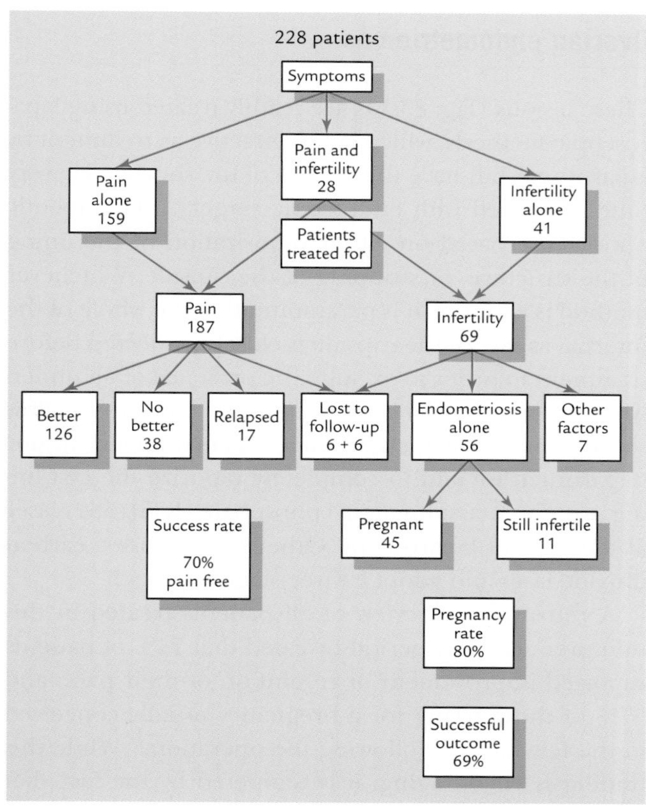

Figure 83.8. *Results of laser laparoscopy in patients with endometriosis.*

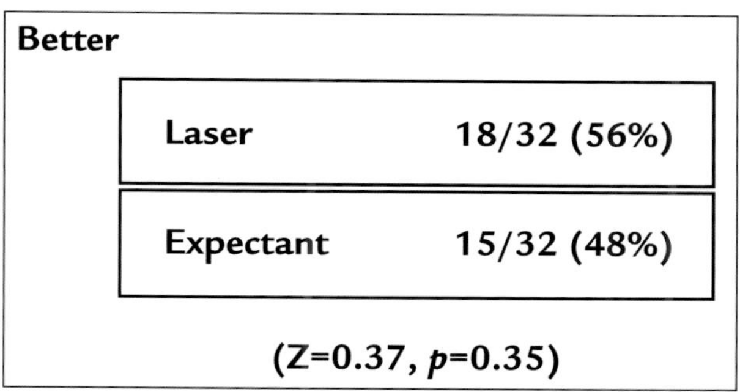

Figure 83.9. *Results of the Guildford trial of laser versus placebo showing very little difference at 3 months.*

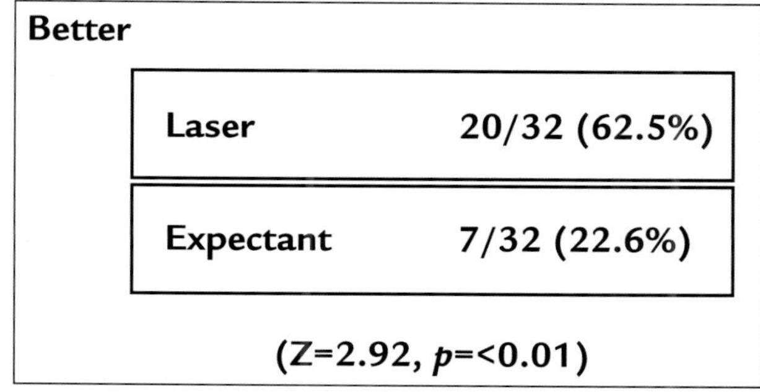

Figure 83.10. *Results of the Guildford trial of laser versus placebo showing statistically different results at 6 months.*

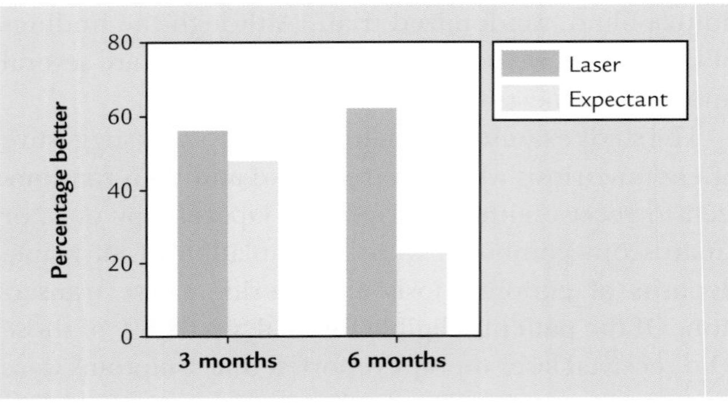

Figure 83.11. *Guildford double-blind trial of laser versus placebo at 3 and 6 months. Proportion of patients with pain symptom alleviation – all stages.*

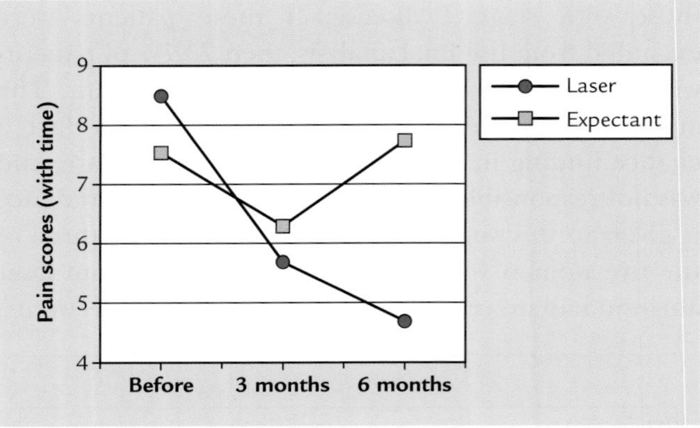

Figure 83.12. *Guildford double-blind randomized controlled trial of laser versus placebo. Median visual analog pain scores (with time). Note difference at 6 months.*

second laparoscopy. This obviously raises doubts about the pathology responsible for their symptoms. It is suggested that, in cases of minimal disease, the diagnosis of endometriosis, which was invariably based on the interpretation of vascular patterns, may have been incorrect. It was suggested that the affected areas should be biopsied at the time of treatment so that a histologic diagnosis is available to help further treatment planning, should the response to laser ablation be suboptimal. This is of more than just academic interest because a diagnosis of endometriosis can have far-reaching consequences for a woman.

The other aspect of the study that needs to be considered is that, in the two other patients who showed no improvement after laser laparoscopy, endometriosis had recurred but was not present at the site of previous laser treatment. This reminds us that endometriosis can be an aggressive and progressive condition, and that on some occasions laser surgery may need adjuvant medical therapy.

The patients were followed-up for 1 year after surgery and it is of some significance that, of those who responded initially, symptom relief was maintained in 90%.[18]

The main criticism directed at this study was that patients in the treatment arm received both laser ablation and uterine nerve transection, and it was therefore unclear which was responsible for the symptomatic benefit.[19] To clarify this issue, a second prospective, double-blind study was undertaken, in which patients were randomized to receive laser ablation either alone or in addition to uterine nerve transection. The results of this study were completely contrary to our expectations which shows the value of a double-blind study when the endpoint is improvement or otherwise of pelvic pain. The study showed that laparoscopic uterine nerve ablation (LUNA) did not add to the beneficial effects of ablation of the implants – in fact the results were almost identical to the earlier study.[20] This not only validated the earlier study but also demonstrated that, where pathology is encountered, the addition of a denervation procedure does not provide additional symptomatic relief. These findings were similar to another study by Vercellini et al.,[21] which was not double-blind but had larger numbers and a longer period of follow-up.

Ovarian endometriomas

These lesions (Fig. 83.13) are readily treated using laparoscopic methods, which are as effective as treatment by laparotomy, but have the benefit of the shorter recovery time associated with endoscopic surgery.[22] Therapeutic options are based on either vaporization of the lining of the structure, or stripping of the capsule. Whichever method is adopted, it is paramount that the whole of the internal aspect of the capsule is closely inspected before treatment in order to exclude the presence of an underlying malignancy. The use of multiple biopsies to allow subsequent histologic assessment is encouraged. In our department we aim to completely vaporize the cyst lining using a potassium titanyl phosphate (KTP/532) laser at the time of laparoscopy. Other centers use a carbon dioxide laser and adopt a three-stage approach.[23]

A retrospective review of all patients treated in this unit over a 10-year period revealed that 74% of patients reported improvement or resolution of their pain, and 57% of those trying for a pregnancy usually conceived in the few months following the operation.[24] While this finding is encouraging, it is tempered by the fact that the recurrence rate was 19% during the study period and subsequent 2-year follow-up.[25] Several facts need emphasizing, however:

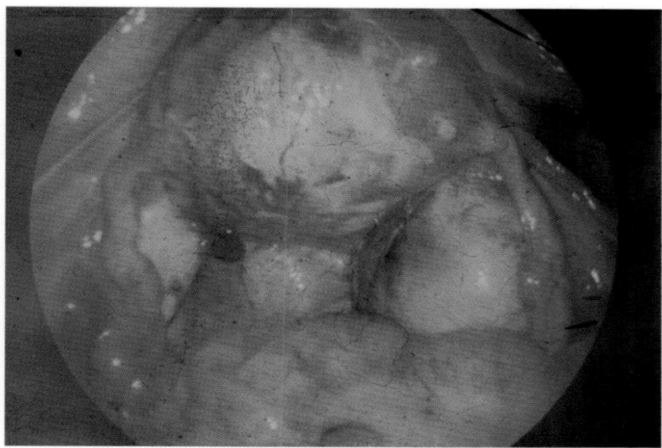

Figure 83.13. *Bilateral ovarian endometriomas firmly adherent to the pelvic sidewall.*

1. Not all the endometriomas occurred in the same site, nor indeed the same ovary;
2. This recurrence rate is in broad agreement with that of 11% quoted by others;
3. Lower rates of recurrence have also been quoted – 3.2% (1/31) – but follow-up extended to only 6 months in this study.[26]

The evidence therefore suggests that although laparoscopic treatment of ovarian endometriomas is possible, in common with peritoneal disease, there is a problem with recurrent disease. The incidence and delayed nature of recurrent disease should always be borne in mind when counseling patients prior to surgery, as well as those with a resurgence of symptoms.

Rectovaginal septum endometriosis

The presence of endometriosis in the rectovaginal septum is not only particularly painful, but is also difficult to treat. In some cases a retroperitoneal nodule (Fig. 83.14) will be seen at the time of laparoscopy, lying in the posterior fornix of the vagina and extending down into the septum. Unfortunately, in many cases a deeply infiltrating septal lesion is almost impossible to see at the time of laparoscopic assessment and may be missed (Fig. 83.15). These nodules are, however, palpable on combined rectovaginal examination, particularly at the time of menstruation. Although these patients will constitute a minority of those presenting to a gynecologic clinic with chronic pelvic pain, there are some important points to raise.

Most of these lesions are amenable to endoscopic laser or electrosurgery, as demonstrated in a series reported by Donnez et al.[27] employing the carbon dioxide laser. The

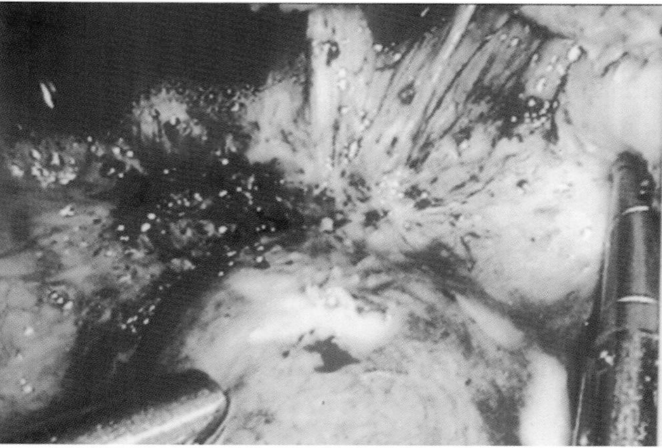

Figure 83.14. *Large nodule of deep infiltrating endometriosis (adenomyosis) on the anterior surface of the rectum going down into the rectovaginal septum.*

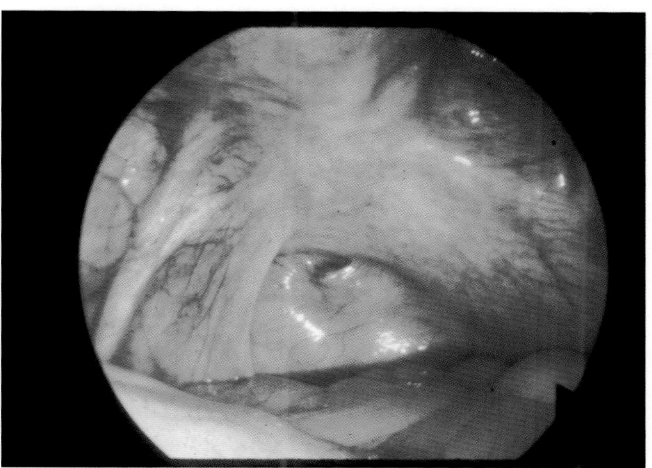

Figure 83.15. *The cul-de-sac may look normal to the inexperienced laparoscopist but closer inspection reveals a small dimple overlying a nodule in the rectovaginal septum and fibromuscular hyperplasia in the uterosacral ligaments and around the ureters.*

number of women with each of the presenting symptoms was not clearly defined, but it appears that most patients suffered from severe pelvic pain, severe dysmenorrhea, and severe dyspareunia. Of the 242 patients followed-up for more than 2 years, only 3.7% experienced recurrent severe dysmenorrhea and 1.2% dyspareunia. While the figures are not readily available, the impression is one of major symptomatic benefit.

The second issue arising from this study is that, although the surgeons were among the most experienced in the world, four out of 497 patients treated by laparoscopy suffered a rectal perforation. It is therefore only too clear that any woman suffering from this condition should be referred to a suitably qualified surgeon.

PELVIC DENERVATION PROCEDURES

As well as treating visible organic pathology at the time of laparoscopic assessment, the ability to interrupt several of the neural pathways responsible for the transmission of pain has also been used. Indeed, there are many who advocate the use of these methods when no pathology is demonstrable. There are two commonly used techniques: uterine nerve transection and presacral neurectomy (PSN).

Uterine nerve transection

The idea is to disrupt the course of pain fibers as they leave the uterus in an effort to decrease dysmenorrhea; this is not a new idea, having previously been described over 40 years ago.[28] The original paper reported that, by transecting the uterosacral ligaments close to their point of origin on the posterior aspect of the cervix (a technique that could be performed either abdominally or vaginally), it was possible to achieve complete pain relief in 86% of women with primary dysmenorrhea and 86.8% of women with secondary dysmenorrhea.

The advent of non-steroidal anti-inflammatory agents and the combined contraceptive pill tended to focus attention on the medical management of these conditions, rather than the surgical, and the technique became almost forgotten. The emergence of laparoscopic surgery and the ability to divide these nerves (Fig. 83.16) without the need for open surgery generated much interest in resurrecting this technique, which had produced such good results. The technique is now a common procedure in our unit as well as many others around the world. Two recent review articles have described the history, anatomic rationale, and the various methods of dividing the nerves that are currently employed in this technique.[29,30]

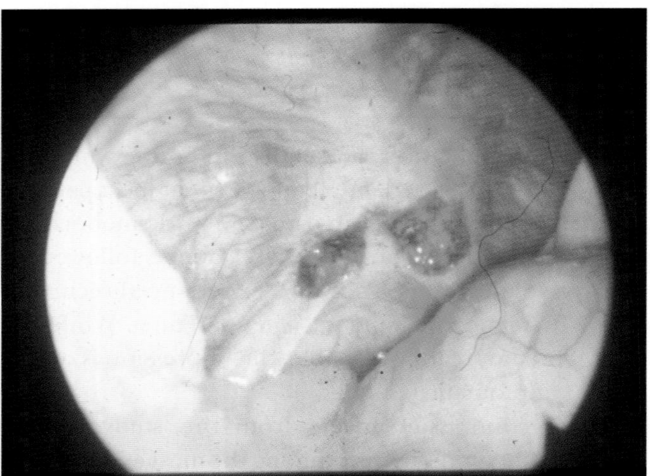

Figure 83.16. *Laparoscopic uterine nerve ablation dividing the uterosacral ligaments and the Lee–Frankenhauser plexus close to the point of insertion in the back of the cervix.*

It is of considerable relevance that in these times of evidence-based medicine, laser uterine nerve ablation (LUNA) has been subjected to the rigors of a prospective, randomized, double-blind study.[31] Although the numbers in this report were small, and the surgeons used electrosurgery rather than laser, the results still warrant mention. In women with severe dysmenorrhea but no obvious pathology, 81% of those undergoing LUNA reported almost complete relief of pain at 3 months, although this fell to 45% at 12 months. None of those in the control group reported any benefit. Another study investigating the outcome of patients with primary dysmenorrhea reported an improvement rate of 73%, whereas in the 100 patients with endometriosis, 86% reported an improvement in symptoms, mainly dysmenorrhea.[29] Other reported rates of improvement for primary dysmenorrhea range from 50 to 73%.[11,32–34] These differences may be due to differing patient subgroups, and perhaps the degree of demarcation of the uterosacral ligaments, since if they are poorly developed an incomplete procedure is often performed.[29]

The group of patients who find that their dysmenorrhea worsens after this operation is of particular interest. Daniell and colleagues[32–34] reported that 10% of their patients with primary dysmenorrhea experienced deterioration in symptoms after surgery. Because preoperative counseling includes an explanation of this potential development to the patient, it has been suggested that this may be a self-fulfilling prophecy, whereas it does not occur if you do not inform your patient of the possibility, as is the policy in our department.[29]

One publication[35] has provided evidence suggesting that the benefits of a LUNA procedure could be due to an entirely different mechanism. Nisolle et al.[35] demonstrated that, in patients with an apparently normal pelvis at the time of laparoscopy, histologic evidence of endometriosis may be found in biopsy samples of the uterosacral ligaments in 6% of cases. There is obviously considerable debate about the significance of this finding. If it transpires that these deposits are located laterally to the usual site of a LUNA procedure, this may help to explain why not all patients derive the same degree of benefit from this operation. The other explanation is that at second-look laparoscopy some of these LUNA procedures were very extensive, and may have removed much of the fibromuscular hyperplasia that is associated with deep infiltration of the uterosacral complex and is known to be associated with considerable pain.

The last area to be considered is that of safety. Although widely performed, LUNA is not without risks since the rectum, ureter, and uterine artery are all within the immediate vicinity. Two deaths due to postoperative hemorrhage[33] and two cases of severe uterine prolapse[36] have been reported. However, when one considers the many thousands of LUNA procedures performed, this is a very low complication rate and we have had no serious complications in over 8000 cases.

Presacral neurectomy

Interruption of the hypogastric plexus at the sacral promontory has been used for more than 60 years to provide relief from pelvic pain and dysmenorrhea. An early review of this topic showed that significant relief could be obtained from these symptoms in 80% of patients.[37] This procedure has been well described in three recent reviews.[30,38,39]

Rather than performing a traditional excisional neurectomy, some workers recommend a divisional neurotomy, which is far quicker and, in the short term at least, appears to be just as effective.[40]

While there have been several publications considering the role of LUNA in patients with pelvic pain and a negative laparoscopy, most of the literature relating to PSN combines it with other therapeutic procedures. However, Candiani et al.[41] have found that the addition of PSN made no difference to patient outcome. Seventy-one patients with stage III or IV endometriosis and pelvic pain were assigned to conservative surgery alone, or with the addition of PSN. Postoperatively there was no significant difference in the reduction of dysmenorrhea, dyspareunia or intermenstrual pain between the two study groups. The findings of this paper are contradicted by those of Tjaden et al.[42] which showed such overwhelming benefit from the addition of PSN that the trial was halted on the grounds that it would be unethical to continue because the response rate was so good. Unfortunately, the number of patients treated was hopelessly underpowered and merely demonstrated the folly of stopping a well-designed clinical trial far too early.

Perry and Perez[43] have raised the important issue of the reasons for failure of PSN. Although they reported a successful outcome in most of 103 women treated for pelvic pain or dysmenorrhea, the interest lies within a small subgroup. Of the patients in the study, 11 had previously undergone LUNA, without symptomatic benefit, yet all experienced alleviation of midline pain following PSN. The authors noted that the most common reason for PSN failing to improve midline pain was incomplete division of the presacral nerve. This is a reflection of operator experience and confidence, and is reflected in our own practice where we see patients referred for assessment of their pelvic pain, having previously undergone a LUNA procedure, only to find little evidence of this at the time of surgery. We would suggest that the above observation could also be applied to LUNA.

Several themes run through the literature on PSN, one being that patient assessment is paramount, especially with regard to the location of the pain. Reports have suggested that PSN is useful in the treatment of midline pain, but of no benefit when the pain is more lateral.[44] This is supported by a report revealing that out of 27 women undergoing PSN, midline pain was relieved in 22 and reduced in a further four; however, lateral pain remained in three of 12 cases.[45]

Another theme common to most of these publications is that PSN should be reserved for patients with midline pain in whom previous attempts at medical therapy have failed. It should also be remembered that there are many potential complications associated with this procedure. Immediate complications include damage to major vessels,[30,45] and long-term problems such as constipation are common.

In view of the above evidence, it seems prudent that patients are carefully assessed and counseled prior to this procedure, and that it is performed by a competent and experienced endoscopic surgeon. Since transection of the uterosacral ligaments is easier to perform and less dangerous than division of the presacral nerve, the suggestion that PSN should be reserved for patients who have undergone an adequate transection of the uterosacral ligaments but still have persistent pelvic pain and dysmenorrhea seems wise.[30]

ADHESIOLYSIS

Laparoscopic adhesiolysis crosses the boundary of gynecologic and general surgery. Adhesiolysis usually involves enterolysis – the release of adhesions involving the bowel – and a high degree of experience is required because of the risk of causing an intestinal perforation. Introduction of the trocar can be hazardous, and surgeons should be aware of the different methods by which this can be achieved and the various techniques available for enterolysis. These have been reviewed recently.[30,46]

As with the other causes of chronic pelvic pain, the relationship between adhesions and chronic pelvic pain is unclear, with several workers describing the presence of adhesions in 23–25% of patients with chronic pain, but also in 14–17% of women without pain.[7,47] Coupled with this are the observations that, of women with adhesions, 50% have no risk factors for their development,[30] and 66% have a completely normal abdominopelvic examination.[48] While there appears to be little correlation between the degree of the adhesions and the severity of the symptoms,[49] the pain does seem to be located at the site of the adhesions in most cases.[49,50] If adhesions are relatively common in the asymptomatic population, what is it that makes certain adhesions painful, and does dividing them make any difference?

Laparoscopic laser adhesiolysis was reported to produce pain relief in 76% of women;[51] the authors noted that success was usual in patients who had a thick adhesive band limiting the mobility of the small intestine. This finding is corroborated by an important randomized trial in which 48 patients with stage II–IV adhesions either underwent adhesiolysis via a midline laparotomy, or were merely clinically observed.[52] At 9–12 months follow-up there was no significant difference between the groups with regard to pelvic pain. More importantly, the improvement rate in the control group was 50%. A small subgroup of patients with severe, dense, vascular lesions involving the bowel did, however, show a significant improvement (89%) compared with the control group (17%).

A review of the efficacy of adhesiolysis quotes improvement rates that vary between 63 and 89%.[30] The design of these studies varied widely, however, and the period of review was only 1 month in some cases. Of interest is the fact that 4.7–23% of patients derive some initial benefit but then develop a recurrence of their symptoms; it has been suggested that this is due to reformation of adhesions.[53] This makes it mandatory to scrutinize the length of follow-up, since good results at 1 month may have deteriorated dramatically by 12 months. The improvement rates should also be interpreted in light of the 50% response rate in the control group described above.

Fayez and Clark[50] appear to report much better results than other studies. In this study, 156 patients with chronic pelvic pain associated with postoperative adhesions were treated with laser adhesiolysis. Complete relief, defined as disappearance of symptoms and an ability to carry on with normal daily activity during the 12-month follow-up period, was reported in 137 (88%) patients. The remaining 19 (12%) improved, but to a lesser degree. However, five of these 19 (3% overall) patients – in all of whom severe, dense adhesions had been divided – presented with a recurrence of their symptoms after only 4–6 months. These women underwent repeat surgery, which confirmed the presence of adhesions at the site of pain, and subsequently rendered them pain-free. It is not clear why the results should be so much better in this study than in others. However, the prevention of de novo adhesions at the time of initial surgery and of redevelopment after adhesiolysis are areas that are attracting considerable interest.

It is difficult to decide what recommendations can be made from the above data. However confusing the results may be, it seems sensible to attempt to prevent the initial formation of adhesions at the time of surgery. To this end, the use of laparoscopy for the initial surgery, which causes fewer postoperative adhesions than laparotomy, seems sensible.[54]

The main issue is the treatment that should be offered to patients with pelvic pain and adhesions. One study showed that adhesiolysis, combined with a second procedure in poor responders, gave excellent results,[50] whereas others have shown that improvement can be achieved in the majority, but that this is often little better than can be achieved by a conservative approach. Taking an evidence-based approach, it could be argued that adhesiolysis should be offered only to women with stage IV adhesions involving the bowel, and should not be offered to those with lesser pathology. This approach may need to be modified in light of the development of conscious pain mapping (discussed below); however, if it can be demonstrated unequivocally that the adhesion is the source of the pain, rather than an incidental finding, then adhesiolysis becomes a far more attractive option.

A more recent double-blind, randomized controlled trial involving surgical patients was reported by Swank and colleagues.[55] Of 116 patients enrolled for diagnostic laparoscopy for chronic abdominal pain attributed to adhesions, 100 were randomly allocated to either laparoscopic adhesiolysis (52) or no treatment (48). Patients and assessors were unaware of treatment, and pain was assessed at 1 year by visual analog score (VAS; scale 0–100), pain change score, use of analgesics, and quality of life score. Analysis was by intention to treat.

Both groups reported substantial pain relief and a significantly improved quality of life, but there was no difference between the groups (mean change from baseline of VAS score at 12 months: difference 3 points, p=0.53; 95% CI: 7–13).

This was an extremely well-designed study and a huge battery of investigations were performed to exclude other causes of chronic abdominal pain. Although this study concluded that laparoscopic adhesiolysis was no more effective than diagnostic laparoscopy alone, there was obvious improvement in both groups and similar studies have drawn attention to the enormous placebo effect in laparoscopy alone in diseases such as endometriosis.[17] Additionally, of the 52 patients who underwent adhesiolysis, 14 (27%) had incomplete adhesiolysis, and although there were no complications in the diagnostic group there were six major complications in five (10%) individuals in the adhesiolysis group, which could have skewed the results. Nevertheless, this is the best evidence-based study in the literature and calls into question whether laparoscopic adhesiolysis with its attendant risk of complications has any advantage over diagnostic laparoscopy alone.

CONSCIOUS PAIN MAPPING

Laparoscopy under general anesthesia allows a thorough evaluation of a patient's pelvis but does not permit the surgeon to assess the significance of these findings. The concept of performing an interactive procedure where the surgeon is able to probe a lesion to see if it is responsible for the symptoms is obviously an attractive one. However, equipment manufacturers have only recently produced small-diameter laparoscopes with high-quality resolution that have made the widespread use of microlaparoscopy a feasible prospect. For this procedure, a laparoscopy is performed with a 2 mm laparoscope under local anesthesia and intravenous sedation. The lack of general anesthesia allows a degree of surgeon–patient interaction, and means that the surgeon can gently probe all the pelvic organs or demonstrate pathology to ascertain if any significant discomfort is produced. In theory this should enable the surgeon to differentiate between symptomatic and asymptomatic incidental findings and, therefore, to tailor patient care more appropriately.

An early study on this subject compared the performance of office microlaparoscopy under local anesthetic (OLULA) in a group of patients with chronic pelvic pain, and a second group undergoing assessment for infertility.[56] The operation was well tolerated by 20 of the 22 patients; two procedures were terminated, one because of benzodiazepine-induced disorientation in a non-English-speaking patient, and one because of an intraoperative anxiety attack in a patient with a history of severe anxiety disorders. These two cases obviously give some useful information as to the future selection criteria for this technique.

This study produced two areas of interest in addition to the profound reduction in the cost of the procedure by avoiding expensive hospital charges. First, in three patients with chronic pelvic pain, an area of marked pain sensitivity was diagnosed. Two of these related to deposits of endometriosis but, importantly, both patients had other areas of endometriosis within the pelvis that did not produce increased pain sensitivity. In the third patient, the area of increased sensitivity related to a loop of bowel adherent to the anterior abdominal wall. This is of considerable interest because, as mentioned earlier, while adhesions are found in many patients with chronic pelvic pain, they are also found in 14–17% of asymptomatic patients. The use of OLULA could therefore potentially allow surgeons to discriminate between symptomatic and asymptomatic adhesions in a patient with chronic pelvic pain, so that adhesiolysis, a potentially dangerous procedure, can be restricted to the areas where it would be expected to be of some benefit.

The second interesting finding was that 10 of the 11 patients with chronic pelvic pain had a generalized visceral hypersensitivity to pain; this was not found in any of the patients being investigated for underlying infertility. The authors proposed several explanations for this finding and also suggest that, in the future, this may act as a marker for a certain subgroup of patients and may be of some prognostic significance.

A second paper on this topic[57] also demonstrated that this technique was highly acceptable to the patients, and reviewed the findings of 50 consecutive patients undergoing microlaparoscopy for chronic pelvic pain. Operative as well as diagnostic procedures were performed, and 14 of the 48 women who needed therapeutic procedures had these performed under local anesthesia. The incidence of significant adhesions was 62% (31 patients), and all of these were lyzed, irrespective of whether they were tender at the time of probing. Of these 31 women, 25 had pain on manipulation of their adhesions, but it is not clear whether their outcome was any better than that of the six women who had lysis of non-tender, perhaps asymptomatic, adhesions. This is obviously an important area of interest worthy of further work, a point noted by the authors. Thirteen of these women had a markedly tender appendix during their pain mapping, and all underwent appendicectomy, with subsequent symptomatic relief. Abnormal histologic findings were present in nine women, and seven women, including all those with normal histology, had severe periappendiceal adhesions. The authors made the critical point that although two of these appendices appeared distorted secondary to the presence of fecaliths, the others appeared macroscopically normal and would have been missed by performing a traditional laparoscopy on an unconscious patient; conscious pain mapping was the only technique capable of demonstrating this pathology.

An interesting extension of this technique has been introduced by Demco[58] who has shown that if conscious pain mapping is performed with a specially adapted xenon light source delivering blue light at a specific frequency, endometriotic lesions, particularly neoangiogenesis, can be seen (and confirmed by biopsy) in areas that appear visually normal when observed with a conventional white light source. This would also add credence to the earlier finding of Nisolle et al.[35] of biopsy-positive endometriosis in visually normal endometrium.

SUMMARY

At present it is not entirely clear what clinical features are required to make a diagnosis of chronic pelvic pain. Until that definitive statement is published and adhered to throughout the scientific and medical communities, it will continue to be difficult to compare one putative treatment with another. However, for the time-being, there are several aspects of this condition that can be critically reviewed.

- The investment of time with the patient during the initial consultation may well pay dividends. A thorough history may suggest other pathology such as irritable bowel syndrome, or an underlying unrelated anxiety disorder that may manifest as pelvic pain, and needs addressing before more invasive investigation of the pelvis. This degree of assessment may well prevent many patients undergoing unnecessary laparoscopy.
- Diagnostic laparoscopy will reveal pathology in a variable percentage of cases, and the rationale for treating these findings laparoscopically has been discussed above. It should be remembered that this treatment can often be performed at the same time as the initial diagnostic laparoscopy, and that other treatments are available for conditions such as endometriosis, notably medical management, hysterectomy, and bilateral oophorectomy.
- That pathology can be demonstrated and treated does not necessarily imply that symptomatic relief will follow. Indeed, it should not be forgotten that these lesions may not be causal or may return rapidly following treatment, especially when dealing with endometriosis and adhesions.
- In cases where pain persists, there is the option of performing one of the pelvic denervation procedures. It cannot be stressed too firmly, however, that these techniques have their limitations and, if they have any role at all, it is in patients with midline, not lateral, pain. One should not forget that procedures such as PSN can be highly dangerous and should only be performed in adequately investigated and counseled patients, and by suitably experienced surgeons.
- Finally, a negative laparoscopy does not imply that there is no organic cause for the pain. The widespread use of OLULA and conscious pain mapping in this subgroup of patients may lead to the demarcation of sensitive foci within the pelvis that may be of prognostic importance and amenable to treatment. Alternatively, it may indicate which areas of pathology are responsible for the symptoms when faced with multiple, possibly non-significant lesions. The possible benefits of this technique in assessing patients with chronic pelvic pain should not be underestimated, and it may be that this development is entirely responsible for a marked improvement in our comprehension of the pathophysiology of this poorly understood condition.

REFERENCES

1. Beard RW. Chronic pelvic pain. Br J Obstet Gynaecol 1998;105:8–10.
2. Stones RW. Chronic pelvic pain. Review 97/01. Personal Assessment in Continuing Education. London: Royal College of Obstetricians and Gynaecologists, 1997.
3. Mathias SD, Kupperman M, Liberman RF et al. Chronic pelvic pain: prevalence, health related quality of life and economic correlates. Obstet Gynecol 1996;87:321–7.
4. Zondervan KT, Yudkin PL, Vessey MP et al. The prevalence of chronic pelvic pain in women in the United Kingdom: a systematic review. Br J Obstet Gynaecol 1998;105:93–9.
5. Porpora MG, Gomel V. The role of laparoscopy in the management of pelvic pain in women of reproductive age. Fertil Steril 1997;68:765–79.
6. Collett BJ, Cordle CJ, Stewart CR. A comparative study of women with chronic pelvic pain, chronic nonpelvic pain and those with no history of pain attending general practitioners. Br J Obstet Gynaecol 1998;105:87–92.
7. Howard FM. The role of laparoscopy in the evaluation of chronic pelvic pain. Promises and pitfalls. Obstet Gynecol Surv 1993;48:117–18.
8. Kontoravdis A, Chryssikopoulos A, Hassiakos D et al. The diagnostic value of laparoscopy in 2365 patients with acute and chronic pelvic pain. Int J Gynaecol Obstet 1996;52:243–8.
9. Howard FM. Laparoscopic evaluation and treatment of women with chronic pelvic pain. J Am Assoc Gynecol Laparosc 1994;1:325–31.
10. Newham AP, van der Spuy ZM, Nugent F. Laparoscopic findings in women with chronic pelvic pain. S Afr Med J 1996;86:1200–3.
11. Wiborny R, Pichler B. Endoscopic dissection of the uterosacral ligaments for the treatment of chronic pelvic pain. Gynecol Endosc 1998;7:33–5.
12. Howard FM. The role of laparoscopy in the evaluation of chronic pelvic pain: pitfalls with a negative laparoscopy. J Am Assoc Gynecol Laparosc 1996;4:85–94.

13. Donnez J, Nisolle M, Casanas-Roux F. Three-dimensional architectures of peritoneal endometriosis. Fertil Steril 1992;57:980–3.
14. Martin DC, Hubert GD, Levy BS. Depth of infiltration of endometriosis. J Gynecol Surg 1989;5:55–60.
15. Redwine D. Non-laser resection of endometriosis. In: Sutton C, Diamond M (eds) Endoscopic Surgery for Gynaecologists. London: WB Saunders, 1993; 220–8.
16. Sutton CJG, Hill D. Laser laparoscopy in the treatment of endometriosis. A 5-year study. Br J Obstet Gynaecol 1990;97:181–5.
17. Sutton CJG, Ewen SP, Whitelaw N, Haines P. Prospective, randomised, double-blind, controlled trial of laser laparoscopy in the treatment of pelvic pain associated with minimal, mild, and moderate endometriosis. Fertil Steril 1994;62:696–700.
18. Sutton CJG, Pooley AP, Ewen SP et al. Follow-up report on a randomised controlled trial of laser laparoscopy in the treatment of pelvic pain associated with minimal to moderate endometriosis. Fertil Steril 1997;68:1070–4.
19. Reiter RC. Letter to the editor. Fertil Steril 1995;3:1355–6.
20. Sutton CJG, Dover RW, Pooley AP, Jones KD. Prospective, randomised, double-blind controlled trial of laparoscopic uterine nerve ablation in the treatment of pelvic pain associated with endometriosis. Gynecol Endosc 2001;10:217–22.
21. Vercellini P, Aimi G, Busacca M et al. Laparoscopic uterosacral ligament resection for dysmenorrhoea associated with endometriosis. Results of a randomised controlled trial. Fertil Steril 1997;68:3–5.
22. Bateman BG, Kolp LA, Mills S. Endoscopic versus laparotomy management of endometriomas. Fertil Steril 1994;62:690–5.
23. Donnez J, Nisolle M, Wayembergh M et al. CO_2 laser laparoscopy in peritoneal endometriosis and in ovarian endometrial cysts. In: Donnez J (ed) Laser Operative Laparoscopy and Hysteroscopy. Louvain, Belgium: Nauwelaerts, 1989; 53–78.
24. Sutton CJ. Endometriosis. Infertil Reprod Med Clin North Am 1995;6:591–613.
25. Sutton CJ, Ewen SP, Jacobs SA et al. Laser laparoscopic surgery in the treatment of ovarian endometriomas. J Am Assoc Gynecol Laparosc 1997;4:319–23.
26. Marrs RP. The use of potassium-titanyl-phosphate laser for laparoscopic removal of ovarian endometrioma. Am J Obstet Gynecol 1991;164:1622–8.
27. Donnez J, Nisolle M, Gillerot S et al. Rectovaginal septum adenomyotic nodules: a series of 500 cases. Br J Obstet Gynaecol 1997;104:1014–18.
28. Doyle JB. Paracervical uterine denervation by transection of the cervical plexus for the relief of dysmenorrhoea. Am J Obstet Gynecol 1955;70:1–16.
29. Sutton C, Whitelaw N. Laparoscopic uterine nerve ablation for intractable dysmenorrhoea. In: Sutton C, Diamond M (eds) Endoscopic Surgery for Gynaecologists. London: WB Saunders, 1993; 159–68.
30. Daniell JF, Lalonde CJ. Advanced laparoscopic procedures for pelvic pain and dysmenorrhoea. In: Sutton C (ed) Advanced Laparoscopic Surgery. London: Baillière Tindall, 1995; 795–808.
31. Lichten EM, Bombard J. Surgical treatment of dysmenorrhoea with laparoscopic uterine ablation. J Reprod Med 1987;32:37–42.
32. Daniell JF, Feste J. Laser laparoscopy. In: Keye WR (ed) Laser Surgery in Gynaecology and Obstetrics. Boston: GK Hall, 1985; 147–65.
33. Daniell JF. Fibreoptic laser laparoscopy. Baillières Clin Obstetr Gynecol Laparoscopic Surg 1989;3:545–62.
34. Daniell JF, Feste JR. Laser laparoscopy. In: Keye WR (ed) Laser Surgery in Gynecology and Obstetrics. Boston: GK Hall, 1985; 147–65.
35. Nisolle M, Paindevine B, Bourdon A et al. Histologic study of peritoneal endometriosis in infertile women. Fertil Steril 1990;53:984–8.
36. Good MC, Copas PR, Doody MC. Uterine prolapse after laparoscopic uterosacral transection. A case report. J Reprod Med 1992;37:995–6.
37. Black WT. Use of presacral sympathectomy in the treatment of dysmenorrhoea: a second look after 25 years. Am J Obstet Gynecol 1964;89:16–32.
38. Daniell E, Dover RW. Laparoscopic use of the argon beam coagulator. In: Sutton C (ed) Endoscopic Surgery for Gynaecologists, 2nd ed. London: WB Saunders, 1998; 105–10.
39. Biggerstaff ED, Foster SN. Laparoscopic surgery for dysmenorrhoea: uterine nerve ablation and presacral neurectomy. In: Sutton C (ed) Gynecological Endoscopic Surgery. London: Chapman and Hall, 1997; 63–83.
40. Daniell W, Kurtz BR, Gurley LD et al. Laparoscopic presacral neurectomy vs. neurotomy: use of the argon beam coagulator compared to conventional technique. J Gynecol Surg 1993;9:169–73.
41. Candiani G, Fedele L, Vercellini P et al. Presacral neurectomy for the treatment of pelvic pain associated with endometriosis: a controlled study. Am J Obstet Gynecol 1992;167:100–3.
42. Tjaden B, Schlaff WD, Kimball A et al. The efficacy of presacral neurectomy for the relief of midline dysmenorrhoea. Obstet Gynecol 1990;76:89–91.
43. Perry CP, Perez J. The role for laparoscopic presacral neurectomy. J Gynecol Surg 1993;9:165–8.
44. Nezhat C, Nezhat F. A simplified method of laparoscopic presacral neurectomy for the treatment of central pelvic pain due to endometriosis. Br J Obstet Gynaecol 1992;99:659–63.

45. Biggerstaff ED, Foster S. Presacral neurectomy for treatment of midline pelvic pain: laparoscopic approach with laparoscopic treatment of a single major complication. J Am Assoc Gynecol Laparosc 1994;1(S4):17.

46. Daniell JF, Dover RW. Laparoscopic enterolysis. In: Sutton C (ed) Endoscopic Surgery for Gynaecologists, 2nd ed. London: WB Saunders, 1998; 390–7.

47. Trimbos JB, Trimbos-Kemper GCM, Peters AAW et al. Findings in 200 consecutive asymptomatic women having a laparoscopic sterilisation. Arch Gynecol Obstet 1990;247:121–4.

48. Cunanan RG, Courey NG, Lippes J. Laparoscopic findings in patients with pelvic pain. Am J Obstet Gynecol 1983;146:589–91.

49. Stout AL, Steege JF, Dodson WC et al. Relationship of laparoscopic findings to self-report of pelvic pain. Am J Obstet Gynecol 1991;164:73–9.

50. Fayez JA, Clark RR. Operative laparoscopy for the treatment of localised chronic pelvic–abdominal pain caused by postoperative adhesions. J Gynecol Surg 1994;10:79–83.

51. MacDonald R, Sutton CJG. Adhesions and laser laparoscopic adhesiolysis. In: Sutton CM (ed) Lasers in Gynaecology. London: Chapman and Hall, 1992; 95–113.

52. Peters AAW, Trimbos-Kemper GCM, Admiraal C et al. A randomised clinical trial on the benefit of adhesiolysis in patients with intraperitoneal adhesions and chronic pelvic pain. Br J Obstet Gynaecol 1992;99:59–62.

53. Steege JF, Stout AL. Resolution of chronic pelvic pain after laparoscopic lysis of adhesions. Am J Obstet Gynecol 1991;165:278–83.

54. Lundorff P, Hahlin M, Kallfelt B et al. Adhesion formation after laparoscopic surgery in tubal pregnancy: a randomised study versus laparotomy. Fertil Steril 1991;55:911–15.

55. Swank DJ, Swank-Bordewizk SCG, Hop WCJ et al. Laparoscopic adhesiolysis in patients with chronic abdominal pain: a blinded randomised controlled multi-centre trial. Lancet 2003;361:1247-51.

56. Palter SF, Olive DL. Office microlaparoscopy under local anesthesia for chronic pelvic pain. J Am Assoc Gynecol Laparosc 1996;3:359–64.

57. Almeida OD, Val-Gallas M. Conscious pain mapping. J Am Assoc Gynecol Laparosc 1997;4:587–90.

58. Demco L. Laparoscopic spectral analysis of endometriosis [abstract]. 13th Congress of Gynecological Endocrinology (ISGE), Kuala-Lumpur, M1–2, 2004; 5.

84

Laparoscopic colposuspension and paravaginal repair

Rohna Kearney, Alfred Cutner

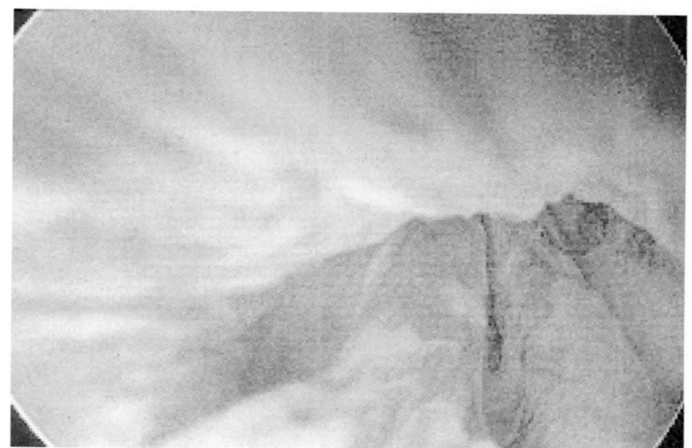

INTRODUCTION

Laparoscopic surgery should be considered the same as open surgery but carried out through smaller incisions with longer instruments. Although there is increased exposure and magnification deep in the pelvis, this is at the expense of less tactile feedback. Thus any discussion on laparoscopic colposuspension and paravaginal repair should be very similar to that of the open counterpart. However, the requirement to learn new surgical skills for the different operative environment results in a learning curve which has led some surgeons to develop 'short cut' surgery and hence new operations have been devised.[1] These are often given the same name as the traditional counterpart but must be assessed in their own right and should not be considered the same. Most alterations to the traditional approach are due to the difficulty that surgeons have had in learning suturing techniques.

Other problems in the early phase of laparoscopic surgery were in the limitations in the optical and instrumental technology. Advances in these areas enabled the surgeon to operate in a more dexterous manner. Syn-Optics launched the tube camera in 1978 and William Chang invented the first solid-state medical video camera in 1981. The first three-chip camera to be produced giving better clarity of vision arrived in 1989. The S-Video signal was developed in 1992 and the first digital zoom and digital enhancement capabilities were developed in 1999. This latest advancement in digital technology has been a further step forward in image clarity. Alongside this, instrumentation has advanced to be ergonomically more suitable, further aiding surgical movements. The development of robotic surgery may result in further advances (Fig. 84.1).

In this chapter we will first discuss colposuspension and then paravaginal repair. Techniques and outcomes, where available, will be discussed. The indications for the operation, as opposed to the route, will only be briefly mentioned as these are fully explained in the relevant other chapters of the book.

COLPOSUSPENSION

Although the Burch colposuspension was first described in 1961,[2] the Tanagho modification is now considered the standard method in which a colposuspension should be performed.[3] However, colposuspension is taken to be synonymous with Burch colposuspension, which is neither the case semantically, nor in the reporting of the literature. Colposuspension merely means elevating the 'colpos', i.e. the vagina.

The first report in the literature of a laparoscopic colposuspension was by Vancaille and Schuessler in 1991.[4] This was not in fact a Burch but rather a modification of the Marshall–Marchetti–Kranz procedure.[5] The authors suspended the vagina with two non-absorbable 2-0 sutures on either side to the pubic symphysis as they were unable to clearly visualize Cooper's ligaments. The first actual report of a laparoscopic modified Burch colposuspension was in 1993 by Liu and Paek.[6] They used two absorbable sutures to elevate the vaginal tissue to Cooper's ligaments. The various methods of colposuspension described in the literature are shown in Table 84.1.

Mesh technique

A technique using mesh to suspend the vagina to Cooper's ligaments has been described by several authors.[7,8] One or two pieces of Prolene mesh are inserted along the

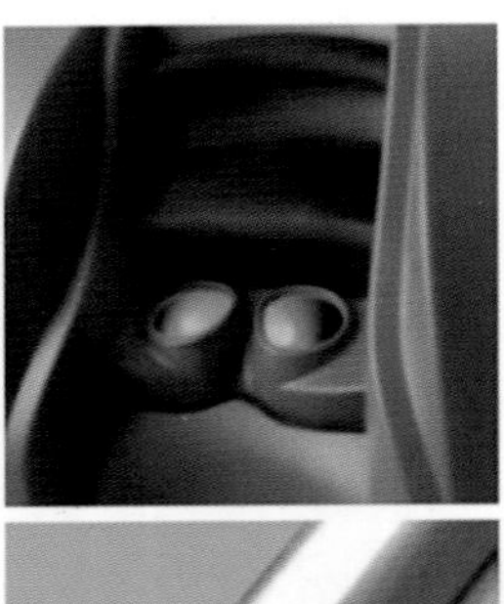

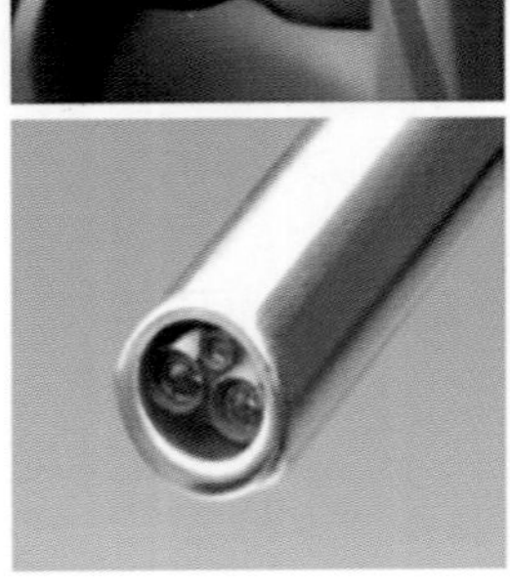

da Vinci®
Surgical
System

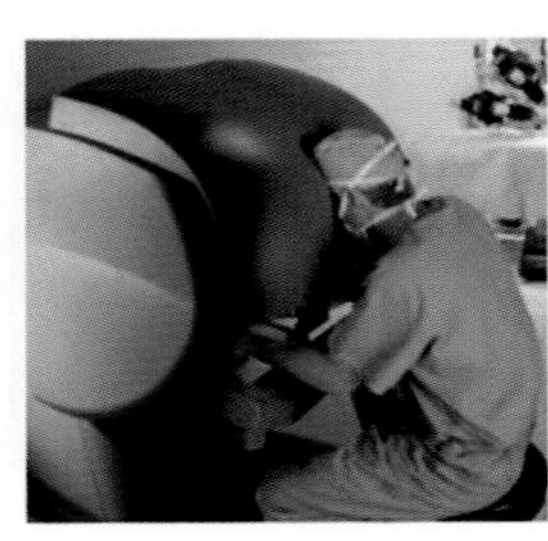

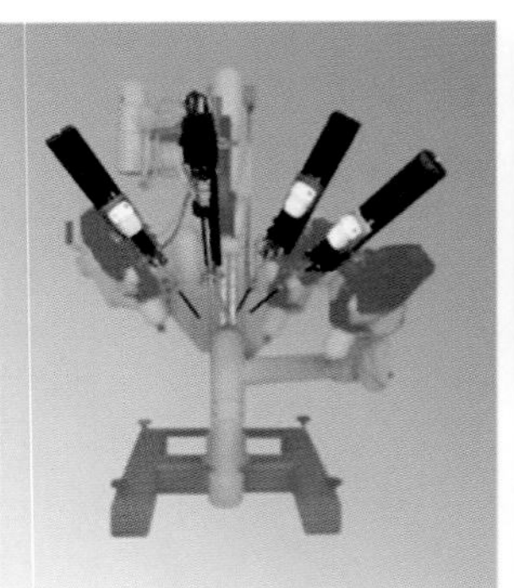

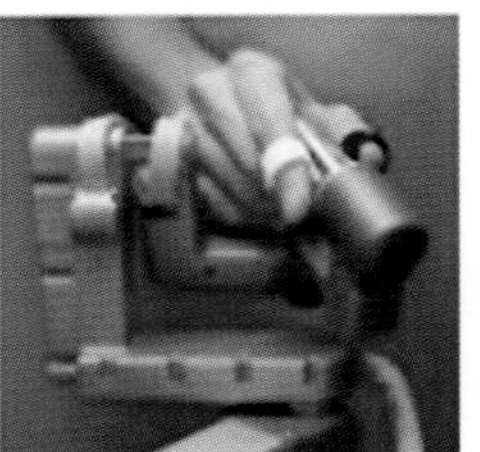

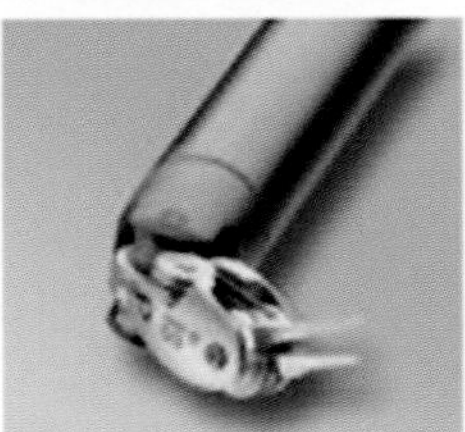

Figure 84.1. *The 'da Vinci' robotic surgical system.*

Table 84.1. ***Different methods used to suspend the vagina***

Author	Year	Method
Vancaille & Schuessler[4]	1991	Non-absorbable sutures to pubic symphysis
Liu & Paek[6]	1993	Absorbable sutures to Cooper's ligaments
Carter[10]	1996	Laparoscopic Stamey
Birken & Leggett[8]	1997	Mesh and staples
Breda et al.[9]	1996	Hand-held needle
Das[30]	1998	Bone anchors
Kiilholma et al.[65]	1995	Glue
Shoemaker & Wilkinson[11]	1998	Teleoscopy
El-Toukhy & Davies[48]	2001	Tacks
Zullo et al.[46]	2001	Staples
Ross et al.[12]	2002	Bipolar electrochemical energy

paravaginal fascia lengthwise, 2 cm lateral to the bladder neck on either side, and are fixed to Cooper's ligaments with staples or tacks. A combined laparoscopic and vaginal approach using a hand-held needle has been described.[9] This involves using one suprapubic port to create a pneumocavity in the space of Retzius. Two small suprapubic incisions are made on either side and a suture mounted on a specially designed hand-held needle is passed through Cooper's ligament and through the lateral fornix of the vagina. The needle is then withdrawn after taking a second bite of the vagina and the vagina is fixed to Cooper's ligaments with an extracorporeal knot.

Laparoscopic needle suspension

Carter described a laparoscopic Stamey procedure in 1996.[10]

Teleoscopy

Shoemaker and Wilkinson proposed using laparoscopy to examine the bladder after colposuspension.[11] They inserted a telescope through a 5 mm cannula into the dome of the bladder in 103 women following bladder neck suspension. They reported that sutures were found in the bladder in 8% of cases.

Bipolar electrochemical energy

Ross et al. describe using bipolar electrochemical energy to induce shrinkage of the paravaginal tissue causing bladder neck elevation in 94 women.[12] They found that this resulted in 30% shrinkage of the tissue.

Laparoscopy

Von Theobald et al. proposed using laparoscopy to assess women with recurrent stress urinary incontinence after previous colposuspension by laparotomy.[13] They reported their findings in five cases and advocated repeating the colposuspension if there was evidence of anatomic failure.

Technique of colposuspension

Currently there are two methods for carrying out a modified laparoscopic Burch colposuspension. They differ in the method of entry into the cave of Retzius. There are other variations including number and size of ports, type of ports, methods used for dissection, type of sutures, and method of knot tying. We will first describe in detail the method of transperitoneal laparoscopic Burch colposuspension as carried out in our unit.

Preoperative counseling includes a full explanation of the risks of the procedure and the advantages and disadvantages over the open procedure. The risks include those of laparoscopic entry and laparoscopic surgery, and those of the procedure itself. Preoperative bowel preparation is advised as it improves visualization of the operative field and reduces contamination in the event of a bowel injury.[14]

A single intravenous dose of prophylactic antibiotic is given. The patient is prepared for surgery, cleaned and draped. She is initially placed supine without any table tilt. The legs are placed in a lithotomy position at an angle of 30 degrees at the hips. A size 14 Foley catheter with 5 ml of water in the catheter balloon is placed in the bladder and left on free drainage.

We normally use a Veress needle to obtain a pneumoperitoneum. An incision is made in the umbilical region, as it is at this point that the layers of the rectus sheath and peritoneum are fused. The patient is placed supine with no tilt and the needle is first directed towards the sacral promontory and, when the characteristic clicks of passing through the layers are felt, the needle is then directed towards the pelvis. A water test is used to confirm entry into the correct space and the abdomen is insufflated. Insufflation ceases when the pre-set pressure of 20 mmHg is achieved. The main 11 mm trocar is then placed through the umbilical region.[15]

Where the patient is at high risk of bowel adhesions near the umbilicus from previous abdominal surgery, other sites are considered. We use Palmers point in high-risk cases (the left subcostal area in the mid-clavicular line)[16,17] (Fig. 84.2). Palpation to identify the spleen is carried out prior to insertion of the Veress needle, and a nasogastric tube is inserted to reduce the chance of perforating an inflated stomach (Fig. 84.3). Where the patient is very thin, a Hassan entry technique is used to reduce the risk of vascular injury.[18]

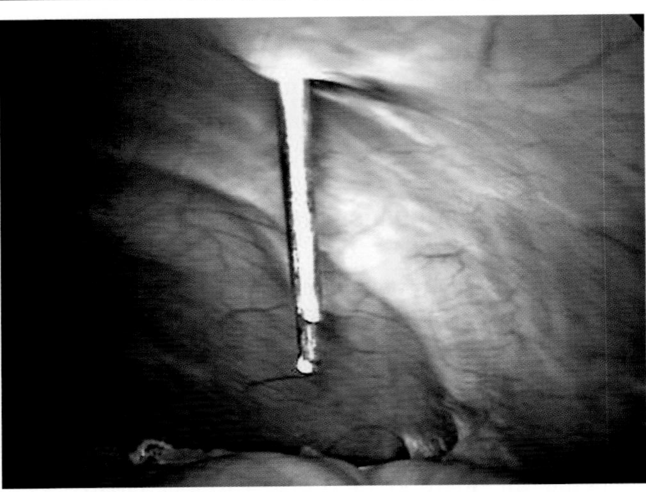

Figure 84.2. *Veress needle entry at Palmer's point.*

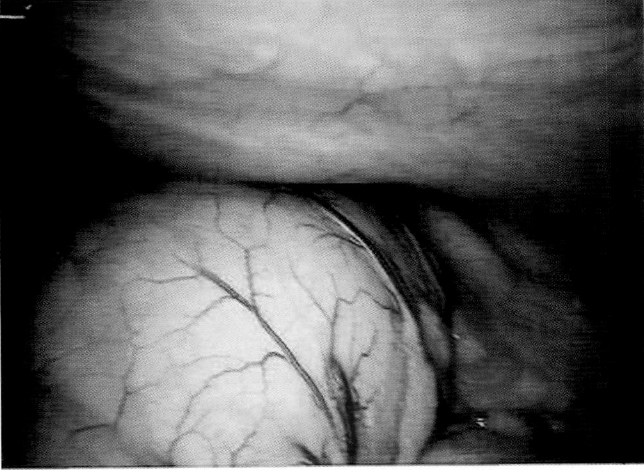

Figure 84.3. *Dilated stomach visible in the left subcostal region. To prevent injury to the stomach when inserting the Veress needle subcostally, a nasogastric tube is inserted to deflate the stomach.*

Once the laparoscope is inserted the abdominal contents are examined and the patient placed in a head-down tilt. The placement of additional ports is important. All additional ports must be placed under direct vision to avoid injury to viscera or vessels. Ports should be placed either very lateral or medial to avoid the inferior epigastric vessels.[19,20] They should be placed so that adequate dexterity can be achieved during the operation. For laparoscopic colposuspension we place two lateral 5 mm ports and one suprapubic 11 mm port. We use 11 mm ports with a variable top for ease of placing sutures through the ports. The lateral ports are placed at least 8 cm from the midline and inserted at a 90-degree angle to avoid the epigastric vessels. We do not use large ports laterally as these need to be formally closed to reduce the incidence of incisional hernias.[21,22] This closure increases postoperative discomfort.

Prior to the colposuspension, the abdominal cavity is assessed. If any additional surgery is required (such as hysterectomy or removal of an adnexa), this is carried out prior to the colposuspension. However, some additional procedures are carried out after the colposuspension.

The bladder is initially filled with 300 ml of blue saline to aid identification of the superior edge of the bladder dome. The obliterated median umbilical ligaments are used as markers for entry to the cave of Retzius. They are incised 2–4 cm cephalad to the bladder dome (Figs 84.4, 84.5). The cave of Retzius is dissected towards Cooper's ligaments. The bladder is then drained to enable better access to the paravaginal tissues (Fig. 84.6). Dissection is performed with monopolar scissors on 60 Watts coagulation. This enables the tissues to be dissected without much bleeding. The dissection should avoid the urethra and the dorsal vein to the clitoris in the midline and the obturator neurovascular bundle laterally. This dissection will expose the pubic symphysis and bladder neck in the midline, and Cooper's ligaments and the arcus tendineus fascia pelvis laterally.

The bladder is retracted medially to allow the colposuspension to be performed. A pledget on a grasper with a marker thread is used for blunt dissection (Fig. 84.7). Non-absorbable No. 0 Ethibond® sutures are used for the colposuspension. One suture is placed on either side at the level of the bladder neck. A second suture is then placed on each side in a slightly more cephalad position (Figs 84.8, 84.9). A double bite of the vagina is taken with each suture and the suture is then placed through the ipsilateral Cooper's ligament. Each suture is tied after insertion on limited tension using an extracorporeal surgical knot. A Redivac drain is left in the cave of Retzius

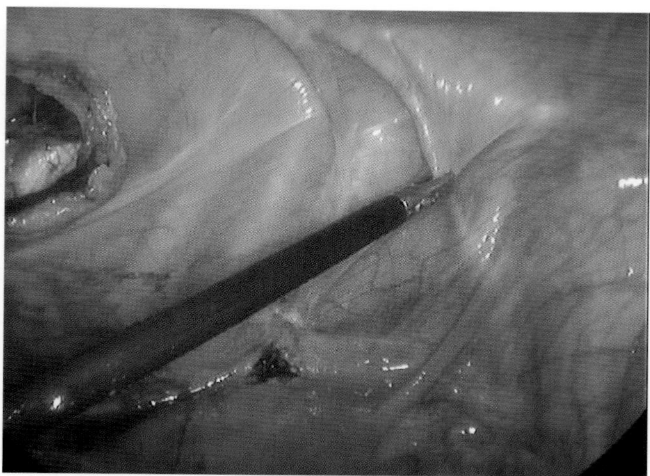

Figure 84.4. *The median umbilical ligament is grasped cephalad to the bladder dome after filling the bladder with 300 ml of saline.*

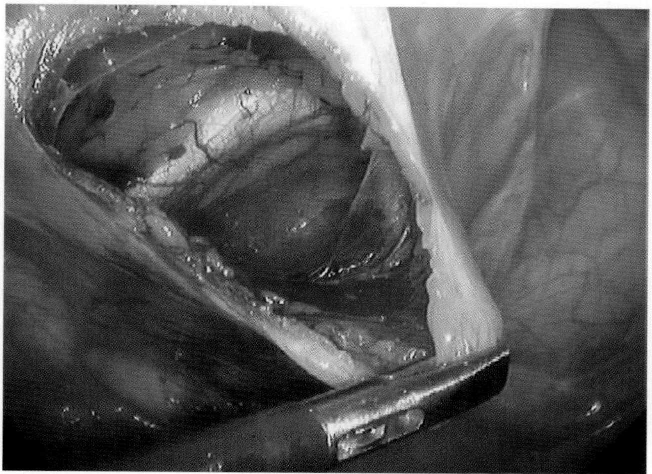

Figure 84.5. *An incision is made in the median umbilical ligaments cephalad to the bladder dome to gain access to the cave of Retzius.*

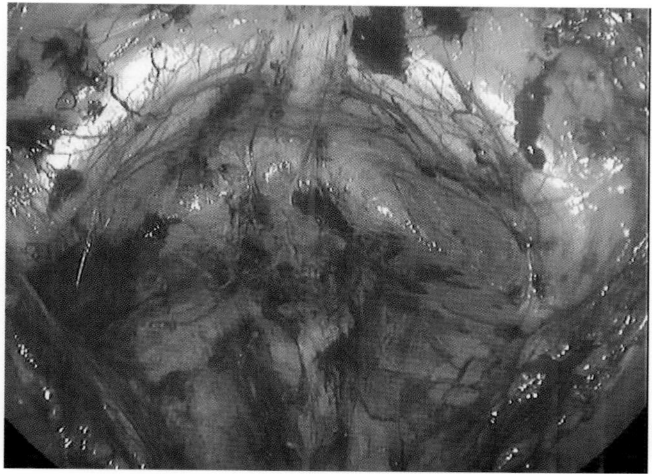

Figure 84.6. *The cave of Retzius is dissected, clearly demonstrating the pubic symphysis and Cooper's ligaments.*

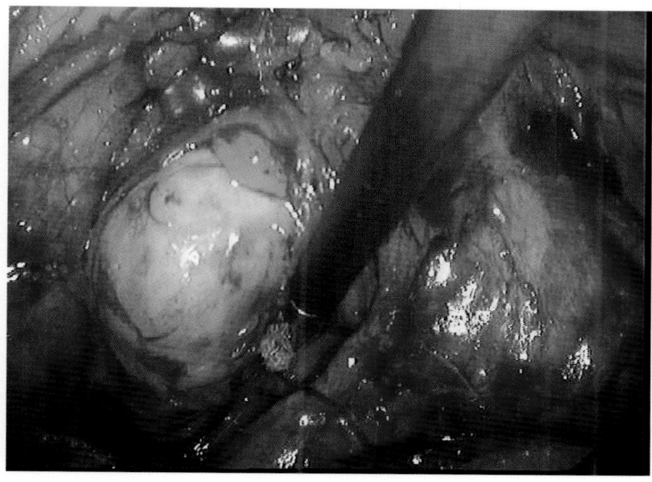

Figure 84.7. *A pledget is used to dissect the bladder medially to allow suture placement.*

for 48 hours. If there has been any difficulty with the procedure, a cystoscopy is performed with a 120-degree scope to identify any sutures inadvertently placed in the bladder and to verify that the ureters are patent.

If there appears to be a significant degree of uterine prolapse at the end of the procedure and the patient had not been considered for a hysterectomy, then a uterosacral plication is carried out at this stage. The uterosacral ligament is grasped medially and a lateral releasing peritoneal incision is performed to lateralize the ureter (Fig. 84.10). A 2-0 polydioxanone (PDS) suture is used to shorten each ligament and to approximate them in the midline (Fig. 84.11).[23] Care is taken not to constrict the rectum. Where there is a greater degree of prolapse, a suture hysteropexy using No. 0 Prolene to attach the right uterosacral ligament to the sacral promontory is performed. In addition, each ligament is shortened with a No. 0 Prolene suture.

An indwelling urethral catheter is left for 72 hours. After the catheter is removed, the post-void residual is measured with a bladder scanner after the second void. If the residual is more than 100 ml, a urethral catheter is reinserted for a further week. The patient is then discharged home and reviewed in the outpatient clinic in one week.

Variations in technique

The extraperitoneal approach involves accessing the preperitoneal space and dissecting into the cave of Retzius. Either a Veress needle can be placed in a suprapubic site

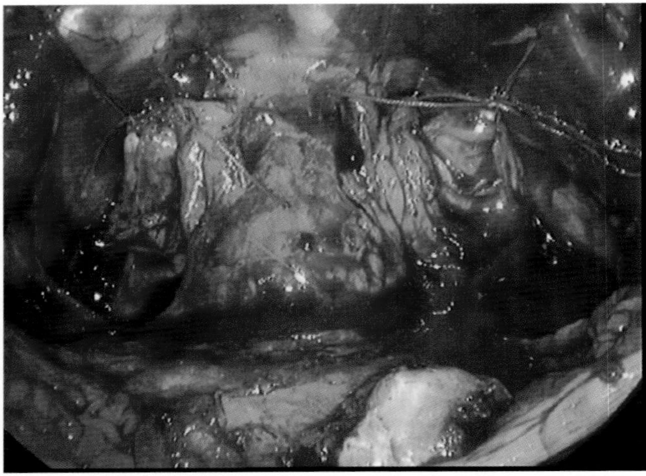

Figure 84.8. *The first suture is placed at the level of the bladder neck.*

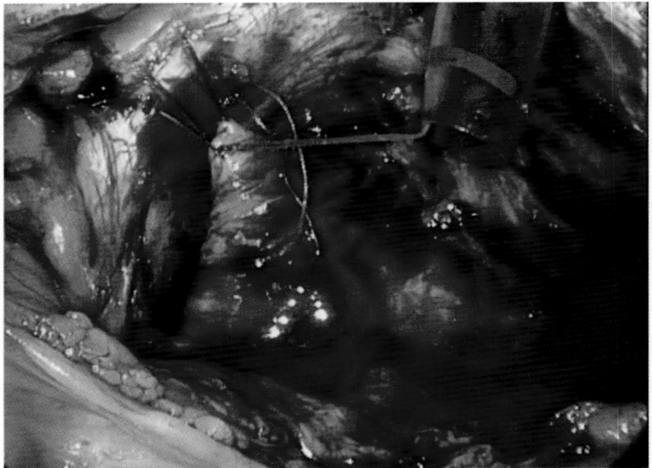

Figure 84.9. *The second suture is placed cephalad to the previously placed suture.*

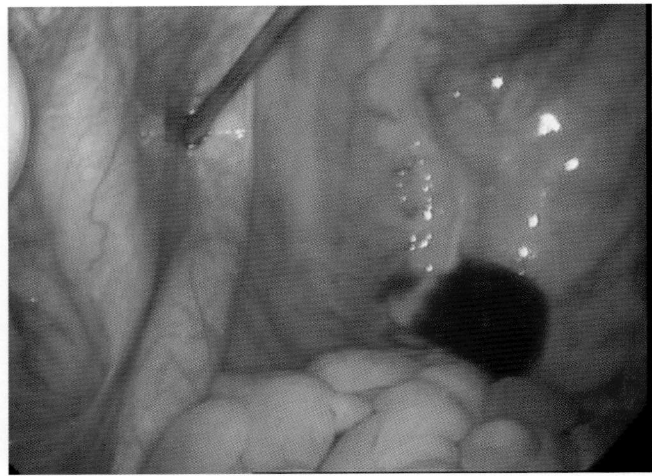

Figure 84.10. *The ureter is dissected lateral to the uterosacral ligaments.*

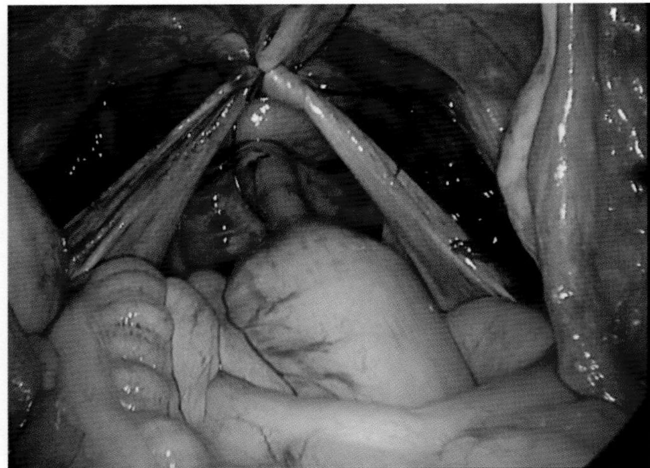

Figure 84.11. *Both uterosacral ligaments have been shortened and plicated together in the midline.*

to reduce the risk of accidental peritoneal cavity entry, or a cut-down technique with dissecting balloons can be used. In addition, a gasless laparoscopic colposuspension procedure using extraperitoneal balloon dissection followed by a mechanical abdominal wall retractor, has also been described.[24] Once a pneumo-Retzius has been obtained, the additional ports are inserted. Typically, two 11 mm trocars are used just above the hairline and close to either side of the midline. The colposuspension is then carried out in the same manner.

The advantage of the pre-peritoneal approach is reduced risk of injury to intra-abdominal organs and quicker dissection time. In particular, the incidence of bladder injury is reduced. However, it is not possible to inspect the abdominal contents or to carry out additional intraperitoneal procedures at the same time.

In addition, the reduced access of this approach and the close port placement makes suturing more difficult. Thus some authors adopting this approach changed to using mesh and tacks rather than sutures to carry out the colposupension.[25]

Apart from the approach to the cave of Retzius, the other variations in the literature relate to the type and number of sutures used and whether mesh is used. In addition, there are variations in the type of knots used to elevate the vagina but these are never expanded upon as it is assumed that they are all similar. However, it has been demonstrated in in-vitro studies that different methods of knot tying result in different strengths.[26,27] There are also reports of bone anchors, staples, and clips being used to attach the suture to Cooper's ligaments or the pubic ramus.[28–30]

Evaluation of success of laparoscopic colposuspension

The proposed advantages of the laparoscopic approach are better visualization of the anatomy, less postoperative pain, and an earlier return to normal activities.[31] However, many authors have advised caution with the laparoscopic approach due to concerns of higher complication rates with poorer results.[32,33] The Cochrane Database for Systemic Reviews was last updated on laparoscopic colposuspension in 2002 and includes eight studies up to April 2001.[34] It concluded that the long-term performance of laparoscopic colposuspension is still uncertain and may be worse than the open procedure. A systematic review published by the same authors in 2003 found a similar subjective cure rate for laparoscopic and open colposuspension with a higher urodynamic objective cure rate for the open approach.[35] However, the authors state that the evidence for the review is limited by small number of trials, low numbers of participants, and methodological problems. A review by Buller and Cundiff of laparoscopic surgeries for urinary incontinence evaluated 50 papers and found an 89% cure rate after 17 months with only 30% of papers reporting objective outcomes.[36] Table 84.2 shows the reported success rates for laparoscopic colposuspension in the literature where sutures were used to elevate the vagina.

When deciding what role laparoscopy has in the management of prolapse and incontinence, it is necessary to evaluate both the success rate and the complication rate of the laparoscopic approach. Previously many studies have compared laparoscopic colposuspension to open colposuspension with varying techniques and success rates reported. However, with the increasing use of tension-free vaginal tape (TVT) and other midurethral tapes, it is also necessary to compare laparoscopic colposuspension to these newer procedures.

Table 84.2. *Reported objective cure rates for laparoscopic colposuspension with sutures*

Author	No. of patients	Length of follow-up (months)	Cure rate (%)
Langebrekke et al.[66]	8	3	88
Gunn et al.[67]	15	4–9	100
Liu[68]	132	3–27	97.2
Burton[37]	30	12	73
Su et al.[39]	46	12	80.4
Persson & Wolner-Hanssen[45] (1 suture)	78	12	58
Persson & Wolner-Hanssen[45] (2 sutures)	83	12	83
Ross[69]	32	12	94
Ross[70]	35	12	91
Kung et al.[71]	31	14.4	97
Lam et al.[72]	107	16	98
Liu & Paek[73]	107	18	97.2
Liu & Paek[6]	58	22	94.8
Ross[74]	48	24	89
Papasakelariou & Papasakelariou[75]	32	24	90.6
Lee et al.[76]	48	26	93.8
Nezhat et al.[76]	40	30	91.9
Burton[41]	30	36	60
Fatthy et al.[38]	74	18	87.9
Üstün et al.[56]	23	18	82
Huang & Yang[44]	82	12	89
Zullo et al.[46]	30	12	89
Cheon et al.[40]	47	12	85

Laparoscopic colposuspension compared with open colposuspension

Table 84.3 shows the methodology of studies comparing the laparoscopic approach to open colposuspension. Of these, only four are prospective randomized trials that compare the same operation, differing only in the mode of abdominal access.[37–40] Burton randomized 60 women to laparoscopic or open colposuspension using two absorbable sutures on either side for both techniques. He reported a lower cure rate at 1 year with the laparoscopic approach compared to the open approach (60% versus 93%).[41] Similarly at 3-year follow-up the results of the laparoscopic group continued to be worse than the open group.[37] However, the author had only performed 10 laparoscopic procedures before the study and absorbable sutures were used. In addition, in the laparoscopic arm a 12 mm needle was used and this may have resulted in an inadequate bite of tissue for suspension.

Fatthy et al. showed a similar success rate for the two approaches, with the laparoscopic approach taking 17 minutes longer with 198 ml less blood loss, 40 hours less hospital stay, and return to light work 23 days earlier.[38] Su et al. investigated 92 women randomly assigned to the laparoscopic or the open route.[39] They included in the open group those patients who were unwilling to undergo the laparoscopic route after randomization. In addition, 14 women in the laparoscopic group had a laparotomy for hysterectomy immediately following colposuspension. They found less blood loss in the laparoscopy group, similar operating time but lower success rate at 1 year compared to the open group

Table 84.3. *Methodology of studies comparing laparoscopic colposuspension to open colposuspension*

Author	Year	Study design	No. of patients	Laparoscopic technique	Open	Follow-up period
Ankardal et al.[47]	2004	Prospective, randomized	240	Transperitoneal mesh and staples	2 non-absorbable sutures	1 year
Huang & Yang[44]	2004	Cohort	157	Transperitoneal 2 non-absorbable sutures	2 non-absorbable sutures	28 months laparoscopic group; 50 months open group
Cheon et al.[40]	2003	Prospective, randomized	90	Transperitoneal sutures		1 year
Fatthy et al.[38]	2001	Prospective, randomized	76	Extraperitoneal: *n*=34, 1 non-absorbable suture	1 non-absorbable suture	18 months
El-Toukhy & Davies[48]	2001	Prospective, non-randomized	87	Extraperitoneal and transperitoneal: Prolene mesh and titanium tacks	2 non-absorbable sutures	32 months
Das[30]	1998	Prospective, non-randomized	20	Bone anchors	2 absorbable sutures	30 months
Saidi et al.[43]	1998	Retrospective	157	Extraperitoneal: 1 non-absorbable suture	2 non-absorbable sutures	12.9 months laparoscopic group; 16.3 months open group
Miannay et al.[42]	1998	Retrospective	72	1 Non-absorbable suture	2 non-absorbable sutures	17 months laparoscopic group; 46 months open group
Burton[37]	1997	Prospective, randomized	60	2 Absorbable sutures	2 absorbable sutures	3 years
Su et al.[39]	1997	Prospective randomized	92	Transperitoneal: 1 or 2 non-absorbable sutures (rarely 2) followed by laparotomy in 14 women	2–3 non-absorbable sutures	3 months

(80.4% versus 95.6%). The follow-up period was only 3 months and in the majority of cases only one suture was placed in the laparoscopic group compared to two or three sutures in the open group. The complication rate in the open group was higher than in the laparoscopic group (17.4% versus 10.8%). This study was included in the systematic review by Moehrer et al.; however, when a separate analysis was performed, excluding it due to methodologic flaws, the higher objective cure rate reported with the open approach was no longer significant.[35] Cheon et al., in a randomized study of 90 women comparing open and laparoscopic colposuspension, reported similar objective cure rates at 1 year (86% versus 85%).[40]

Three further retrospective studies showed similar success rates at 1 year between the laparoscopic and open routes when non-absorbable sutures were used in both arms with less analgesia, shorter hospital stay, and earlier return to work seen in the laparoscopic group in two studies.[42,43] The third study compared the anatomic result of the two procedures by assessing the bladder neck position with postoperative ultrasound and found no difference in resting, straining bladder neck position, and urethral mobility at 1 year postoperatively.[44] Interestingly, one of these studies also showed a higher non-significant complication rate with the open procedure.[43] McDougall reports a 30% success rate at 45 months for laparoscopic colposuspension with a non-absorbable suture compared with 35% for needle suspension.[28] However, the suture was attached to Cooper's ligament by an absorbable clip. One randomized trial of 161 women undergoing laparoscopic colposuspension showed a higher objective success with two single-bite sutures on each side (83%) compared with one double-bite suture (58%).[45]

In the Medical Research Council colposuspension trial, 291 women were recruited in six centers in the UK. Of the 144 women allocated to laparoscopic surgery, 11 received open surgery and two had no operation. Of the 147 women allocated to open surgery, one had laparoscopic surgery and three had no operation. On intention-to-treat analysis at 2 years, the objective outcome (1-hour pad test) showed 80% cured in the laparoscopic group (85.4% data available), and 82% cured in the open group (79.6% data available); the subjective outcome ('perfectly happy/pleased' – Question 33 in the Bristol Female Urinary Tract Symptom Questionnaire) showed 55% cured in both the laparoscopic and the open group. These results demonstrate that, in the hands of experienced laparoscopic surgeons, laparoscopic surgery does not produce an inferior cure rate to open colposuspension.

Success rates of non-suture colposuspension

Table 84.1 demonstrated the different methods that have been used to carry out a colposuspension laparoscopically. Apart from the traditional suture method, the main method variation still adopted is the use of mesh and tacks to carry out the suspension.

One randomized trial of 60 women compared the two laparoscopic methods. The authors demonstrated a higher objective failure rate at 1 year of 26.9% with the mesh technique compared to 11.1% with sutures.[46] There are a further two studies in the literature that compare the laparoscopic route using mesh to the open procedure using sutures.[47,48] Both studies reported a lower success rate with the laparoscopic approach. However, these studies are in fact comparing two entirely different operative procedures and the results cannot therefore be interpreted as outcome data for all laparoscopic colposuspension procedures.

Complications

Major complications reported following laparoscopic colposuspension include urinary tract injury, bowel injury, major vascular injury requiring transfusion, and abscess in the space of Retzius. In the longer term, failure of the procedure requiring repeat surgery, de novo detrusor overactivity, voiding difficulty, pain, ureteral obstruction, fistula, or posterior compartment prolapse may occur as for the open procedure.

Buller and Cundiff, in their review of 1867 patients, report an overall complication rate of 10.3%.[36] The bladder dome was the most commonly injured site and was repaired laparoscopically in the majority of cases. The lower urinary tract is injured in 2–3% of cases of laparoscopic colposuspension and paravaginal repairs.[14,49] This is lower than the 10% reported with the open procedure.[50] Intraoperative diagnosis of urinary tract injury is the main factor associated with decreased morbidity.[51] Small bladder injuries can be managed by catheterization but if greater than 0.5 cm they should be closed laparoscopically in one or two layers with an absorbable suture.

Where mesh has been substituted for sutures, different additional complications can occur. Kenton et al. have reported two cases of women who presented with complications following laparoscopic colposuspension with Prolene mesh and tacks. Both women had tacks removed retropubically from the bladder and retropubic space and no tacks were seen in Cooper's ligament in either patient.[52] In both cases, postoperative cystoscopy was not performed at the time of the colposuspension.

Disadvantages

The main disadvantage of the laparoscopic approach is that the surgeon must possess adequate minimal access skills to perform the procedure competently. It would appear that the modifications introduced, designed to overcome the difficulty of suturing in the cave of Retzius, result in lower success rates. There is a steep learning curve in laparoscopic surgery and this has resulted in fewer laparoscopic colposuspensions being performed. However, as the field of minimal access expands, there will be more competent laparoscopic surgeons available to mentor trainees.

Cost

The laparoscopic approach consistently requires longer operating time than the open colposuspension or TVT. The other cited factor against the laparoscopic approach is the increased cost associated with minimal access procedures. Kohli et al. reported a retrospective 2-year cost analysis of laparoscopic colposuspension with sutures compared with open colposuspension[53]. They found that the laparoscopic approach was more expensive than the open approach ($4960 versus $4079). This reflected the high hourly operative room charges in North America as the laparoscopic group took on average 44 minutes longer operating time. The postoperative care costs were lower in the laparoscopic group. Persson et al. reported that a laparoscopic colposuspension is cheaper than a TVT in Sweden (E1273.4 versus E1342.8) despite the TVT procedure being performed in less time.[54] Differences in costs are difficult to assess as there is great variation in each country as to how long patients tend to stay in hospital following surgery and there are differing costs of operating time.

Laparoscopic colposuspension versus tension-free vaginal tape procedures

With the advent of midurethral tape procedures it is now pertinent to evaluate the performance of laparoscopic colposuspension compared with these newer minimally invasive procedures. The outcomes of two prospective randomized studies, comparing laparoscopic colposuspension to TVT, have been reported.[55,56] One study comparing a laparoscopic colposuspension using Prolene mesh and tacks to the TVT in 121 women found similar cure rates at 6 weeks following surgery, with the TVT arm taking less operative time, shorter hospital stay, and earlier return to work.[55] One patient in the laparoscopic group required a laparotomy to remove the tacks inadvertently placed in the bladder, as they were too difficult to remove laparoscopically. However, 1-year data from the same study showed that the success rate of the TVT as defined by a negative stress test was 85.7% but the laparoscopic colposuspension group success rate had fallen to 56.9%.[57] Of note, however, as discussed above, the mesh procedure is not synonymous with a standard colposuspension.

A second study compared the laparoscopic approach using two absorbable sutures to the TVT in 46 women and reported similar outcomes with both procedures after 18 months.[56] The TVT group required shorter operating time, shorter hospital stay, and less catheterization.

Most recently an abstract publication has compared 're-do' surgery where the patients were randomized to laparoscopic colposuspension or TVT and reported that the two procedures were equally effective in the medium term.[58] Thus, overall, the data comparing a standard laparoscopic colposuspension with TVT would suggest that they are largely equivalent. However, the data available are too few to draw any firm conclusions.

PARAVAGINAL REPAIR

The aim of a paravaginal repair is to assess the integrity of the lateral attachment of the anterior vaginal wall from the pubic symphysis to the ischial spine and to repair any defects in this attachment (Fig. 84.12). This procedure can be completed at the same time as laparoscopic colposuspension.

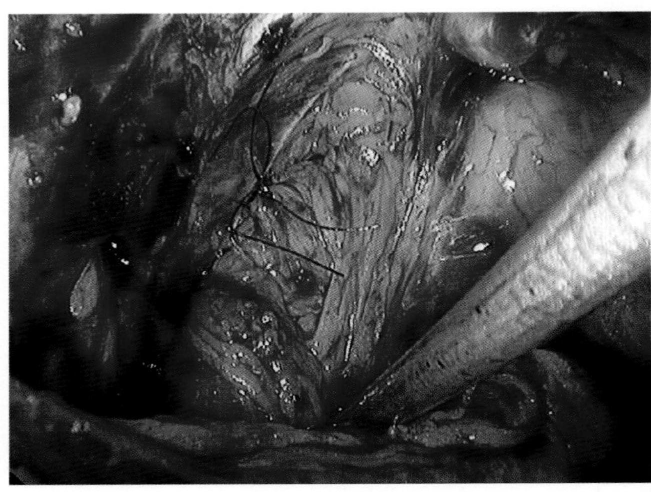

Figure 84.12. *Sutures have been placed to complete the paravaginal repair.*

Technique of paravaginal repair

The anterior vaginal wall is elevated and the pubocervical fascia is reattached to the ipsilateral obturator internus muscle and fascia around the arcus tendineus with non-absorbable 2-0 sutures tied extracorporeally.[14] A technique of stapling Prolene mesh to the vaginal margins and attaching it to Cooper's ligament has also been described.[59]

The advantage of laparoscopic paravaginal repair compared with vaginal paravaginal is direct visualization of the anatomy.

Complications

Vaginal paravaginal repair is associated with a high complication rate with a transfusion rate reported as high as 16%.[60] Mallipeddi et al. also reported a significant complication rate in 45 women undergoing vaginal paravaginal repair.[61] Complications included one case of bilateral ureteric obstruction, one hematoma requiring drainage, two vaginal abscesses, and two women were transfused.

A technique of vaginal paravaginal repair using Alloderm graft had an objective failure rate of 41% at 18 months postoperatively.[62] Speights et al. reported no complications in 18 women who had a laparoscopic paravaginal repair.[49]

CONCLUSION

Laparoscopic Burch colposuspension and paravaginal repair can be performed successfully with fewer complications than the open approaches. Current evidence suggests that laparoscopic colposuspension performed with sutures may be as effective as the open approach and the TVT procedures.

The laparoscopic approach is associated with lower morbidity than the open procedures. It also avoids placing a permanent tape under the urethra, thereby reducing concern about the possibility of future tape erosion. However, the laparoscopic approach requires the surgeon to be competent in minimal access skills as well as urogynecology. The use of mesh and tacks or staples appears to reduce the success rate.

Further studies are needed to evaluate the long-term outcome of the laparoscopic approach. As more surgeons become competent at operative laparoscopy, the long-term outcome of these procedures in more experienced hands will become evident.

REFERENCES

1. Gor M, McCloy R, Stone R, Smith A. Virtual reality laparoscopic simulator for assessment in gynaecology. Br J Obstet Gynaecol 2003;110:181–7.
2. Burch J. Urethrovaginal fixation to Cooper's ligament for correction of stress incontinence, cystocele and prolapse. Am J Obstet Gynecol 1961;81:281–90.
3. Tanagho EA. Colpocystourethropexy: the way we do it. J Urol 1976;116:751–3.
4. Vancaille T, Schuessler W. Laparoscopic bladder-neck suspension. J Laparoendosc Surg 1991;1:169–73.
5. Marshall V, Marchetti A, Krantz K. The correction of stress incontinence by simple vesicourethral suspension. Surg Gynecol Obstet 1949;88:509–18.
6. Liu C, Paek W. Laparoscopic retropubic colposuspension (Burch procedure). J Am Assoc Gynecol Laparosc 1993;1:31–5.
7. Ou C, Presthus J, Beadle E. Laparoscopic bladder neck suspension using hernia mesh and surgical staples. J Laparoendosc Surg 1993;3:563–6.
8. Birken R, Leggett P. Laparoscopic colposuspension using mesh reinforcement. Surg Endosc 1997;11:1111–14.
9. Breda G, Silvestre P, Gherardi L, Xausa D, Tamai A, Giunta A. Correction of stress urinary incontinence: laparoscopy combined with vaginal suturing. J Endourol 1996;10:251–3.
10. Carter J. Laparoscopic Burch procedure for stress urinary incontinence: the Carter modification. Keio J Med 1996;45:168–71.
11. Shoemaker E, Wilkinson P. Teleoscopy after bladder neck suspension. J Am Assoc Gynecol Laparosc 1998;5:445–6.
12. Ross J, Galen D, Abbott K, Albala D, Presthus J, Su-Ou C, Turk T. A prospective multisite study of radiofrequency bipolar energy for treatment of genuine stress incontinence. J Am Assoc Gynecol Laparosc 2002;9:493–9.
13. Von Theobald P, Barjot P, Levy G. Feasibility of and interest in laparoscopic assessment in recurrent urinary stress incontinence after Burch procedure performed by laparotomy. Surg Endosc 1997;11:468–71.
14. Miklos J, Kohli N. Laparoscopic paravaginal repair plus Burch colposuspension: review and descriptive technique. Urology 2000;56:64–9.
15. A consensus document concerning laparoscopic entry techniques: Middlesbrough, March 19–20, 1999. Gynaecol Endosc 1999;8:403–6.
16. Childers J, Brzechffa P, Surwit E. Laparoscopy using the left upper quadrant as the primary trocar site. Gynecol Oncol 1993;50:221–5.
17. Pasic R, Levine R, Wolf W. Laparoscopy in morbidly obese patients. J Am Assoc Gynecol Laparosc 1999;6:307–12.

18. Bowrey DJ, Blom D, Crookes PF et al. Risk factors and the prevalence of trocar site herniation after laparoscopic fundoplication. Surg Endosc 2001;15(7):663–6.

19. Hurd W, Bude R, DeLancey J, Newman J. The location of abdominal wall blood vessels in relationship to abdominal landmarks apparent at laparoscopy. Am J Obstet Gynecol 1994;171:642–6.

20. Balzer K, Witte H, Recknagel S, Kozianka J, Waleczek H. Anatomical guidelines for the prevention of abdominal wall haematoma induced by trocar placement. Surg Radiol Anat 1999;21:87–9.

21. Montz I, Holschneider C, Munro M. Incisional hernia following laparoscopy: a survey of American Association of Gynecological Laparoscopists. Obstet Gynecol 1994;84:881–4.

22. Coda A, Bossotti M, Ferri F et al. Incisional hernia and fascial defect following laparoscopic surgery. Surg Laparosc Endosc Percut Tech 1999;9:348–52.

23. Maher C, Carey M, Murray C. Laparoscopic suture hysteropexy for uterine prolapse. Obstet Gynecol 2001;97:1010–4.

24. Flax S. The gasless laparoscopic Burch bladder neck suspension: early experience. J Urol 1996;156:1105–7.

25. Batislam E, Germiyanoglu C, Erol D. Simplification of laparoscopic extraperitoneal colposuspension: results of two-port technique. Int Urol Nephrol 2000;32:47–51.

26. Kadirkamanathan SS, Shelton JC, Hepworth CC, Laufer JG, Swain CP. A comparison of the strength of knots tied by hand and at laparoscopy. J Am Coll Surg 1996;182(1):46–54.

27. Shettko DL, Frisbie DD, Hendrickson DA. A comparison of knot security of commonly used hand-tied laparoscopic slipknots. Vet Surg 2004;33(5):521–4.

28. McDougall E. Laparoscopic management of female urinary incontinence. Urol Clin North Am 2001;28:145–9.

29. Henley C. The Henley suture-staple technique for laparoscopic Burch colposuspension. J Am Assoc Gynecol Laparosc 1995;2:441–4.

30. Das S. Comparative outcome analysis of laparoscopic colposuspension, abdominal colposuspension and vaginal needle suspension for female urinary incontinence. J Urol 1998;160:368–71.

31. Cutner A, Rymer J. Patient recovery after laparoscopic colposuspension. Gynaecol Endosc 1998;7:307–8.

32. Bidmead J, Cardozo L. Short cut to incontinence? Lancet 2000;355:2183–4.

33. Das S. Laparoscopic surgery for female urinary incontinence: prudence shall prevail. J Soc Laparoendosc Surg 1999;3:273–7.

34. Moehrer B, Ellis G, Carey M, Wilson D. Laparoscopic colposuspension for urinary incontinence in women. Cochrane Database Syst Rev 2002;1:CD002239

35. Moehrer B, Carey M, Wilson D. Laparoscopic colposuspension for urinary incontinence: a systematic review. Br J Obstet Gynaecol 2003;110:230–5.

36. Buller J, Cundiff G. Laparoscopic surgeries for urinary incontinence. Clin Obstet Gynecol 2000;43:604–18.

37. Burton G. A three year prospective randomized urodynamic study comparing open and laparoscopic colposuspension. Neurourol Urodyn 1997;16:353–4.

38. Fatthy H, El Hao M, Samaha I, Abdallah K. Modified Burch colposuspension: laparoscopy versus laparotomy. J Am Assoc Gynecol Laparosc 2001;8:99–106.

39. Su TH, Wang KG, Hsu CY, Wei HJ, Hong BK. Prospective comparison of laparoscopic and traditional colposuspension in the treatment of genuine stress incontinence. Acta Obstet Gynecol 1997;76:576–82.

40. Cheon W, Mak J, Liu J. Prospective randomised controlled trial comparing laparoscopic and open colposuspension. Hong Kong Med J 2003;9:10–4.

41. Burton G. A randomised comparison of laparoscopic and open colposuspension. Neurourol Urodyn 1993;13:497–8.

42. Miannay E, Cosson M, Lavvin D, Querleu D, Crepin G. Comparison of open retropubic and laparoscopic colposuspension for treatment of stress urinary incontinence. Eur J Obstet Gynecol Reprod Biol 1998;79:159–66.

43. Saidi M, Gallagher S, Skop I, Saidi J, Sadler K, Diaz K. Extraperitoneal laparoscopic colposuspension: short-term cure rate, complications, and duration of hospital stay in comparison with Burch colposuspension. Obstet Gynecol 1998;92:619–21.

44. Huang W, Yang J. Anatomic comparison between laparoscopic and open Burch colposuspension for primary stress urinary incontinence. Urology 2004;63:676–81.

45. Persson J, Wolner-Hanssen P. Laparoscopic Burch colposuspension for stress urinary incontinence: a randomised comparison of one or two sutures on each side of the urethra. Obstet Gynecol 2000;95:151–5.

46. Zullo F, Palomba S, Piccione F, Morelli M, Arduino B, Mastrantonio P. Laparoscopic Burch colposuspension: a randomised controlled trial comparing two transperitoneal surgical techniques. Obstet Gynecol 2001;98:783–8.

47. Ankardal M, Ekerydh E, Crafoord K, Milsom I, Stjerndahl JH, Engh ME. A randomised trial comparing open Burch colposuspension using sutures with laparoscopic colposuspension using mesh and staples in women with stress urinary incontinence. Br J Obstet Gynaecol 2004;111:974–81.

48. El-Toukhy T, Davies A. The efficacy of laparoscopic mesh colposuspension: results of a prospective controlled study. BJU Int 2001;88:361–6.

49. Speights S, Moore R, Miklos J. Frequency of lower urinary tract injury at laparoscopic Burch and paravaginal repair. J Am Assoc Gynecol Laparosc 2000;7:515–18.

50. Stevenson K, Cholhan H, Hartmann D, Buchsbaum G, Guzick D. Lower urinary tract injury during the Burch procedure. Is there a role for routine cystoscopy? Am J Obstet Gynecol 1999;181:35–8.
51. Sadik S, Onoglu S, Mendilcioglu I, Sehirali S, Sipahi C, Taskin O, Wheeler J. Urinary tract injuries during advanced gynaecologic laparoscopy. J Am Assoc Gynecol Laparosc 2000;7:569–72.
52. Kenton K, FitzGerald MP, Brubaker L. Multiple foreign body erosions after laparoscopic colposuspension with mesh. Am J Obstet Gynecol 2002;187:252–3.
53. Kohli N, Jacobs P, Sze E, Roat T, Karram M. Open compared with laparoscopic approach to Burch colposuspension: a cost analysis. Obstet Gynecol 1997;90:411–15.
54. Persson J, Teleman P, Eten-Bergquist C, Wolner-Hanssen P. Cost analyses based on a prospective randomised study comparing laparoscopic colposuspension with a tension-free vaginal tape procedure. Acta Obstet Gynecol Scand 2002;81:1066–73.
55. Valpas A, Kivela A, Pentinnen J et al. Tension-free vaginal tape and laparoscopic mesh colposuspension for stress urinary incontinence. Obstet Gynecol 2004;104:42–9.
56. Üstün Y, Engin-Üstün Y, Gungor M, Tezcan S. Tension-free vaginal tape compared with Burch urethropexy. J Am Assoc Gynecol Laparosc 2003;10:386–9.
57. Valpas A, Kivela A, Pentinnen J et al. Tension-free vaginal tape and laparoscopic mesh colposuspension in the treatment of stress urinary incontinence: immediate outcome and complications – a randomised clinical controlled trial. Acta Obstet Gynecol Scand 2003;82:665–71.
58. Maher C, Qatawneh A, Baessler K, Cropper M, Schluter P. Laparoscopic colposuspension or tension-free vaginal tape for recurrent stress urinary incontinence and or ISD: a randomised controlled trial. Neurourol Urodyn 2004;5/6:Abstract 25.
59. Washington J, Somers K. Laparoscopic paravaginal repair: a new technique using mesh and staples. JSJL 2003;7:301–3.
60. Young S, Daman J, Bony L. Vaginal paravaginal repair: one year outcomes. Am J Obstet Gynecol 2001;185:1360–7.
61. Mallipeddi PK, Steele AC, Kohli N, Karram MM. Anatomic and functional outcome of vaginal paravaginal repair in the correction of anterior vaginal wall prolapse. Int Urogynecol J Pelvic Floor Dysfunct 2001;12(2):83–8.
62. Clemons J, Myers D, Aguilar V, Arya L. Vaginal paravaginal repair with an Alloderm graft. Am J Obstet Gynecol 2003;189:1612–18.
63. Liu C. Laparoscopic retropubic colposuspension (Burch procedure). A review of 58 cases. J Reprod Med 1993;38:526–30.
64. Das S, Palmer J. Laparoscopic colpo-suspension. J Urol 1995;154:1119–21.
65. Kiilholma P, Haarala M, Polvi H, Makinem J, Chancellor M. Sutureless colposuspension with fibrin sealant. Tech Urol 1995;1:81–3.
66. Langebrekke A, Dahlstrom B, Eraker R, Urnes A. The laparoscopic Burch procedure: a preliminary report. Acta Obstet Gynecol Scand 1995;74:153–5.
67. Gunn GC, Cooper RP, Gordon NS, Gragnon L. Use of a new device for endoscopic suturing in the laparoscopic Burch procedure. J Am Assoc Gynecol Laparosc 1994;2:65–70.
68. Liu C. Laparoscopic treatment of genuine urinary stress incontinence. Clin Obstet Gynecol 1994;8:789–98.
69. Ross JW. Laparoscopic Burch repair compared to laparotomy Burch for cure of urinary stress incontinence. Int Urogynecol 1995;6:323–8.
70. Ross JW. Two techniques of laparoscopic Burch repair for stress incontinence: a prospective randomized study. J Am Assoc Gynecol Laparosc 1996;3:351–7.
71. Kung R, Lie K, Lee P et al. The cost effectiveness of laparoscopic versus abdominal Burch procedures in women with urinary stress incontinence. J Am Assoc Gynecol Laparosc 1996;3:537–44.
72. Lam AM, Jenkins GJ, Hyslop RS. Laparoscopic Burch colposuspension for stress incontinence: preliminary results. Med J Aust 1995;162:18–22.
73. Liu C, Paek W. Laparoscopic retropubic colposuspension (Burch procedure). J Am Assoc Gynecol Laparosc 1993;1:31–5.
74. Ross J. Multichannel urodynamic evaluation of laparoscopic Burch colposuspension for genuine stress incontinence. Obstet Gynecol 1998;91:55–9.
75. Papasakelariou C, Papasakelariou B. Laparoscopic bladder neck suspension. J Am Assoc Gynecol Laparosc 1997;4:185–9.
76. Lee C, Yen C, Wang C, Huang K, Soong Y. Extraperitoneoscopic colposuspension using CO_2 distension method. Int Surg 1998;83:262–4.
77. Nezhat CH, Nezhat F, Nezhat CR et al. Laparoscopic retropubic cystocolposuspension. J Am Assoc Gynecol Laparosc 1994;1:339–49.

85

Laparoscopic sacralcolpopexy

Marcus P Carey

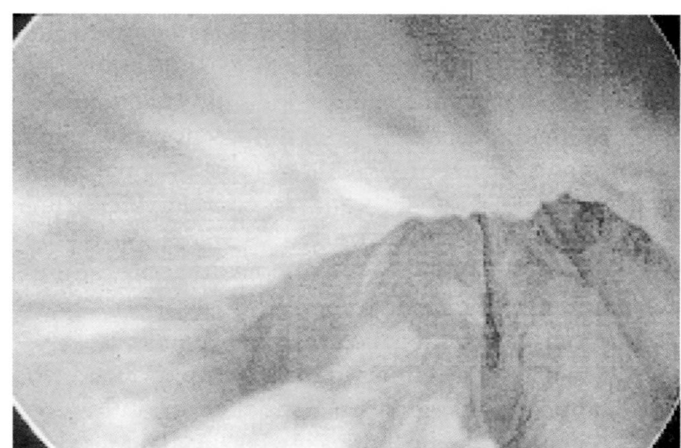

INTRODUCTION

The use of laparoscopy to treat pelvic organ prolapse has increased in recent years. In the United States the number of laparoscopic procedures performed for prolapse almost doubled in the period from 1979 to 1997 (1246 cases in 1979 and 2459 in 1997) against a small decline in the total number of operations performed for pelvic organ prolapse during this period.[1] The main limitation of laparoscopy for the treatment of pelvic organ prolapse is the relatively small number of surgeons with sufficient laparoscopic and reconstructive pelvic surgical skills to perform these procedures safely and successfully.

Approximately 200,000 women undergo surgery for pelvic organ prolapse in the United States each year.[1] In a study of women from a large United States health maintenance organization it was reported that, by the age of 80 years, 11.1% of women had undergone surgery for pelvic organ prolapse or urinary incontinence, or both.[2] Within 4 years of the primary surgical procedure, 29.2% of these women required repeat surgery for recurrent prolapse. Younger patients (age less than 60 years) and women with higher grades of prolapse (pelvic organ prolapse quantification [POPQ] stages 3 and 4) are more likely to experience recurrent prolapse after vaginal repair.[3,4] The prevalence of vaginal vault prolapse following hysterectomy is approximately 10%.[5] However, estimates of the prevalence of posthysterectomy vault prolapse vary markedly from 0.2% to 43%.[5–7] Vault prolapse occurs in equal numbers following abdominal and vaginal hysterectomy.[8,9]

The high rate of failure with vaginal surgery to treat vaginal vault prolapse led to the development of the abdominal sacrocolpopexy (ASC) procedure. This approach employs the retroperitoneal interposition of a suspensory prosthesis (synthetic, autologous, allograft or xenograft) between the vaginal apex and the sacrum. ASC was originally described by Huguier in 1957 and later by Lane in 1962.[10,11] Snyder and Krantz described attachment of the prosthesis along the full length of the rectovaginal septum.[12] Addison et al. described the broad attachment of the prosthesis to both the upper anterior and posterior vaginal walls.[13,14] Randomized trials comparing the ACS procedure with transvaginal sacrospinous ligament fixation to treat vaginal vault prolapse demonstrated a trend towards the ACS being the more effective procedure.[15–17] In addition to the high success rate reported with the ACS procedure, other advantages include preservation of vaginal capacity resulting in maintenance of coital function, use of synthetic material resulting in durable support, and the use of the synthetic graft on both anterior and posterior vaginal aspects providing for balanced support of the various vaginal sites and an acceptable vaginal axis. Significant problems associated with the ASC operation include de novo postoperative stress incontinence, intraoperative hemorrhage, dyspareunia, mesh erosion, and use of a laparotomy incision.[11,12,14,18,19]

Laparoscopic sacrocolpopexy (LSC) was first described by Nezhat et al. in 1994 although Wattiez et al. claim to have first performed this procedure in 1991.[20,21] The proposed advantages of the LSC over the ASC include the avoidance of a major laparotomy incision, less postoperative pain, shorter time in hospital, and a quicker return to normal activities. The laparoscopic approach provides the surgeon with an enhanced view of the pelvic and intra-abdominal anatomy compared to the abdominal approach.

The LSC takes advantage of the known high success rate of the traditional ASC combined with the benefits of laparoscopic surgery. The LSC should be performed in an identical manner to the ASC with the only difference being the smaller laparoscopic incisions.

ANATOMIC CONSIDERATIONS

Following hysterectomy, the upper third of the vagina (including the vault) is supported by two mechanisms:

1. *Direct* support for the vaginal vault is provided by the parametrium (cardinal and uterosacral ligaments) and paracolpium fibers. These fibers act like suspensory ligaments and arise from the fascia of the piriformis muscle, sacroiliac joint and lateral sacrum, and insert into the lateral upper third of the vagina.
2. *Indirect* support for the vaginal vault is provided by the levator plate, formed by the fusion of the right and left levator ani muscles between the rectum and coccyx.

Vaginal vault prolapse occurs as a consequence of failure of these direct and indirect supporting mechanisms. This is likely to involve weakness of the muscular pelvic floor and suspensory fibers of the parametrium and upper paracolpium.[22,23]

Recent work evaluating the fibromuscular composition of the vaginal wall in women with and without enterocele failed to demonstrate any focal ‘defect' of the vaginal muscularis.[24] Based on these anatomic considerations it is not surprising that a site-specific endopelvic fascial repair approach to the treatment of a vaginal apical defect is likely to carry an unacceptably high failure rate.[25,26]

For women with vaginal vault prolapse, surgical repair should generally be directed towards restoring vault support and a normal vaginal axis. These anatomic considerations lend credibility to the concept of the ASC and LSC procedures.

Anatomy of the sacral promontory

The presacral space is bounded superiorly by lumbosacral intervertebral disk and laterally by the right common iliac artery and left common iliac vein (Fig. 85.1). The right ureter is identified coursing in the right lateral aspect of the presacral space. The sacral promontory and presacral space are usually covered by the sigmoid colon. The sigmoid colon at this point is attached to the peritoneum, which is reflected over the left psoas major muscle and iliacus muscle. Once the sigmoid colon is retracted to the left side, the sacral promontory is easily identified. The presacral space and sacral promontory is accessed by gently lifting up the peritoneum directly over the sacral promontory and performing a midline longitudinal incision. This approach into the presacral space will avoid damage to the right common iliac artery and left common iliac vein. The middle sacral artery and vein are easily identified lying directly on the middle aspect of the sacrum. The middle sacral artery originates as a single branch from the posterior aspect of the aorta. The middle sacral vein arises from vessels emerging beneath the common iliac veins and drains into the inferior vena cava. Some women have an extensive venous plexus in the presacral space, and damage to these vessels can result in dramatic hemorrhage. The middle sacral artery gives off small branches that run laterally on the sacrum to either anastomose with the lateral sacral arteries or directly supply the ventral sacral nerve roots. Damage to these fine vessels can result in bleeding and ischemic injury to the ventral sacral nerve roots.

The hypogastric plexus of nerves descends into the pelvis anterior to the bifurcation of the aorta, enters the presacral space between the common iliac arteries, and is anterior to the middle sacral artery and vein. This plexus carries the autonomic nerves of the pelvic viscera. Extensive damage to this plexus of nerves may result in bladder, bowel, and sexual dysfunction. When performing a LSC procedure, meticulous dissection is recommended in order to reduce the risk of nerve damage. After entering the presacral space the anterior longitudinal ligament is exposed by gentle blunt dissection of the presacral tissues over the sacral promontory. Sharp dissection and the use of ablative techniques to access the anterior longitudinal sacral ligament should be avoided. When securing the prosthetic material to the sacral promontory the surgeon should avoid excessive use of sutures or stapling devices onto the sacral promontory. When performing a LSC procedure, the author uses only one or two sutures to secure the prosthesis onto the anterior longitudinal ligament on the sacral promontory, and has not encountered a case of mesh detachment from the sacral promontory with this approach.

CLINICAL ASSESSMENT AND PATIENT SELECTION

Clinical assessment is undertaken in the usual fashion. This includes obtaining a detailed history with particular emphasis on any symptoms associated with the vaginal vault prolapse, especially urinary, bowel, and coital symptoms. A detailed general and pelvic examination is undertaken. It is important for the clinician to identify all the vaginal defects accurately so that they can be corrected at the time of surgery. The patient should be examined for signs of stress incontinence with the pro-

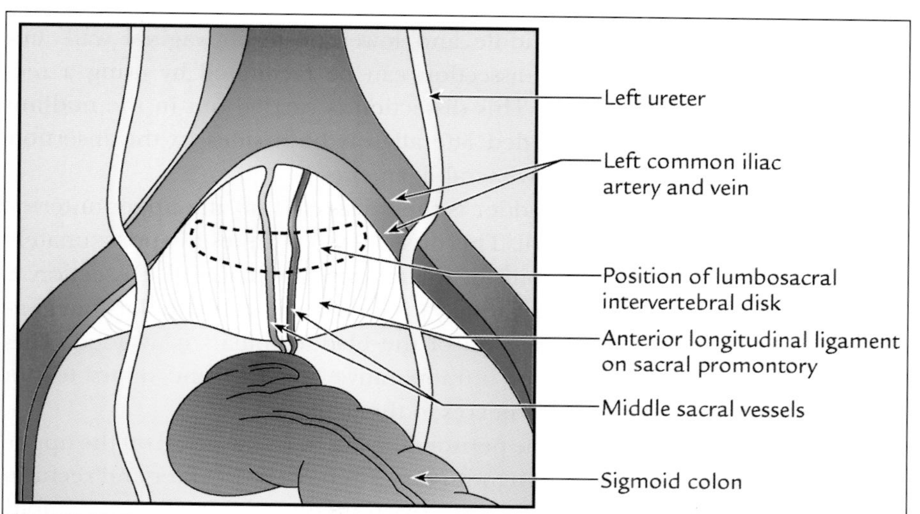

Figure 85.1. *The presacral space is bounded by the lumbosacral intervertebral disk above and laterally by the right common iliac artery and left common iliac vein. The middle sacral artery and vein course over the anterior longitudinal ligament on the sacral promontory.*

lapse present and reduced, and also for any anorectal pathology, including rectal prolapse.

Urodynamic studies should be made available to patients with associated urinary symptoms. Imaging of the pelvic floor and anorectal physiologic testing are recommended as indicated.

Indications

Currently, there is no consensus on the exact indications for both ASC and LSC procedures. The LSC is indicated for patients with symptomatic and significant prolapse of the vaginal vault who are considered appropriate candidates for an ASC. This approach is suitable for younger patients wishing to preserve coital function and in whom there are no contraindications to laparoscopic surgery. Gadonneix et al. reported that 89% of 46 consecutive patients presenting with multiple compartment prolapse could be treated by LSC.[27]

The LSC procedure should be made available to patients with significant vaginal vault prolapse with no contraindications to laparoscopy. Typically, these women have had a previous hysterectomy and an International Continence Society POPQ classification of stage 2 or greater prolapse at the vaginal vault site.[4] Patients with significant stage 1 vault prolapse are sometimes offered this approach. LSC can also be used in conjunction with a hysterectomy to treat marked uterine prolapse of stage 2 or greater in younger women.[10,26] LSC treats vaginal vault prolapse as well as high cystoceles and rectoceles when the mesh is extended onto the upper anterior and posterior vaginal walls.[29] On occasion, the LSC procedure with extension of mesh anteriorly and in combination with a laparoscopic paravaginal repair is offered to women with a recurrent cystocele, as this combination of procedures is very effective in treating recurrent high cystoceles.

LSC is a complex operation requiring both advanced laparoscopic and reconstructive pelvic surgery skills. Only surgeons competent in this operative technique should undertake this surgery.

Contraindications

Vaginal operations may be more appropriate for frail women who do not wish to preserve coital function. LSC is not indicated for women with minor degrees of vault prolapse. This procedure is also not suitable for patients who otherwise have a contraindication to laparoscopic surgery. In these women an ASC or vaginal surgery to treat the vault prolapse should be offered.

SURGICAL TECHNIQUE

A standardized technique for LSC does not exist. Surgery is performed under general anesthesia with muscle relaxation. A major challenge is the achievement and maintenance of adequate surgical exposure of the vaginal vault and sacral promontory. A steep Trendelenburg position, preoperative bowel preparation, avoidance of nitrous oxide anesthesia, and an adequate number of operating ports all facilitate good surgical exposure. Left lateral tilting of the patient can also be employed.[30] Laparoscopic bowel retractors appear to be of limited benefit. Following induction with general anesthesia the woman is placed in a low lithotomy position using Allen stirrups. Use of Allen stirrups allows the patient to be repositioned during surgery without the need to redrape. Repositioning may be required when concomitant vaginal surgery is undertaken.

Standard techniques are used to introduce a 10 mm operating laparoscope at the umbilicus. Under laparoscopic vision, two ports (for the right-handed surgeon a 10 mm port on the patient's left and a 5 mm port on the patient's right) are inserted through the anterior abdominal wall into the peritoneal cavity. In order to avoid injury to the inferior epigastric artery and vein and damage to the lateral cutaneous nerve to the thigh, these ports are sited two fingerbreadths above and two fingerbreadths medial to the anterior superior iliac spine. A further 5 mm port is introduced suprapubically in the midline under laparoscopic vision.

A vaginal probe is inserted to identify the vaginal vault. With the vagina elevated cranially using the vaginal probe (Fig. 85.2), the peritoneum is opened transversely at the vaginal apex. This dissection continues posteriorly into the rectovaginal septum so that the peritoneum is dissected off the upper half of the posterior vaginal wall. At around this point the rectovaginal septum is entered and the rectum is dissected off the middle and lower posterior vaginal wall. On occasion, dissection can be facilitated by using a rectal probe. This dissection is carried out in the midline and extended laterally on both sides to the insertion of the uterosacral ligaments.

The bladder is then dissected off the upper anterior vaginal wall. This dissection continues to approximately the midpoint of the anterior vaginal wall. Dissection is continued laterally towards both bladder pillars but generally dissection of the bladder pillars is avoided. This is to reduce intraoperative bleeding and injury to the autonomic nerves to the bladder.

Once the peritoneum has been dissected off the upper vagina, along with dissection of the bladder and rectum, the sacral promontory is identified. Usually the sigmoid

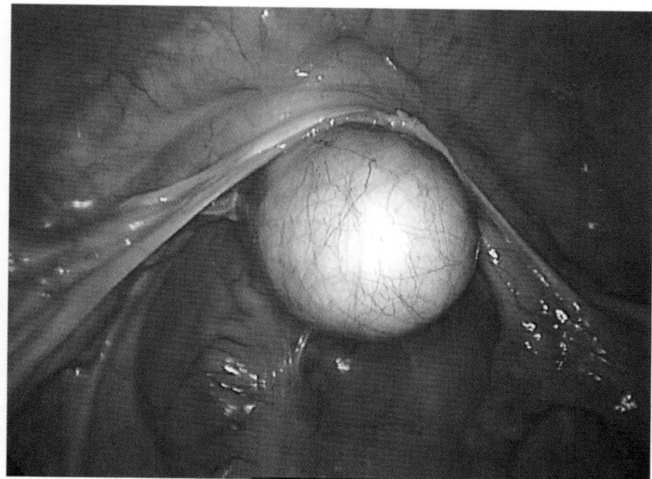

Figure 85.2. *The vagina is elevated using a vaginal probe. This facilitates the dissection of peritoneum, bladder and rectum off the upper vagina.*

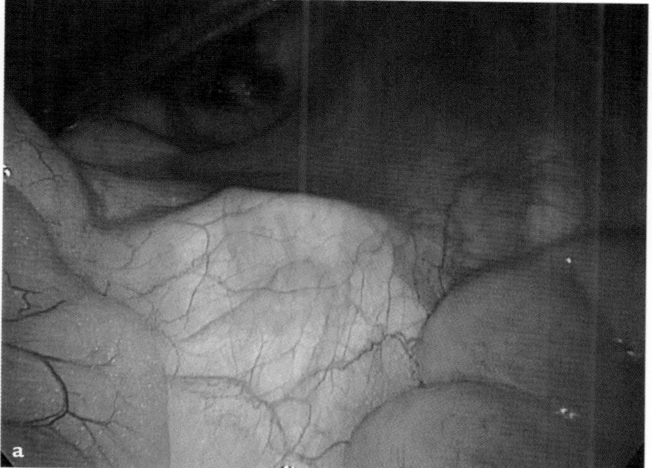

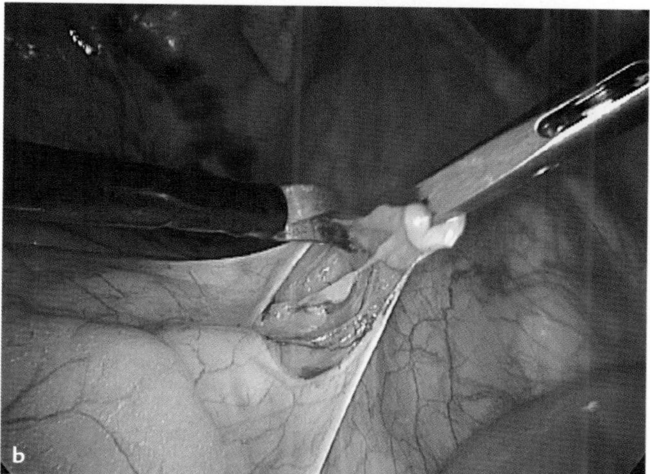

Figure 85.3. *(a) The sacral promontory is easily recognizable and accessible during laparoscopic sacral colpopexy. (b) The peritoneum over the sacral promontory is elevated and a vertical incision is made into the peritoneum in the midline to allow safe entry into the presacral space.*

colon obscures the sacral promontory and needs to be reflected to the patient's left. The sacral promontory is usually an easily recognizable and accessible structure (Fig. 85.3a). However, in obese patients the sacral promontory may be difficult to access. Prior to dissection in this region the right ureter should be carefully identified. The peritoneum over the sacral promontory is grasped and elevated. A vertical incision is made into the peritoneum in the midline to allow entry into the presacral space (Fig. 85.3b).

The peritoneum is further dissected in a caudal direction on the right of the rectum and sigmoid colon and below the right ureter into the cul-de-sac to join the posterior vaginal peritoneal dissection. Once this dissection is completed, the tissues in the presacral space over the sacral promontory are carefully reflected laterally so that the glistening white fibers of the anterior longitudinal ligament are exposed (Fig. 85.4a). At this point it is important to carefully identify any vascular structures on the sacral promontory in the midline so that injury to these structures can be avoided when the prosthesis is attached to the sacral promontory. Two rectangular pieces of mesh (e.g. Gynecare Gynemesh PS, a type 1 polypropylene mesh)[31] are then cut to size, the first being 15×3 cm and the second being 5×3 cm. The larger piece of mesh is used to support the posterior vaginal wall and vault and the smaller piece to support the anterior vaginal wall and vault. The larger mesh is introduced into the pelvis through the left 10 mm port. Using delayed absorbable monofilament sutures throughout, this mesh is attached to the posterior vaginal wall with four to six sutures. The smaller mesh is then introduced into the pelvis and attached to the upper anterior vaginal wall with four sutures. Two sutures are placed at the vaginal vault and through both anterior and posterior pieces of mesh.

The point of attachment of the mesh onto the sacral promontory is defined. The mesh is fixed to the sacral promontory without placing tension on the vagina. A permanent suture is passed in turn through the mesh and into the anterior longitudinal ligament in the middle of the sacral promontory, with care taken to avoid injury to any vessels at this site. Occasionally, a second bite into the anterior longitudinal ligament is taken (Fig. 85.4b). The suture is then passed again through the mesh and tied, anchoring the mesh onto the sacral promontory. Excess mesh above the knot is excised and removed from the abdomen (Fig. 85.5). The peritoneum is closed with a continuous delayed absorbable

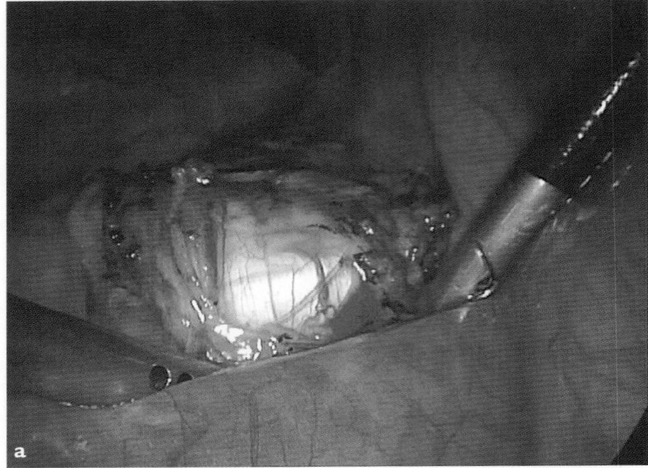

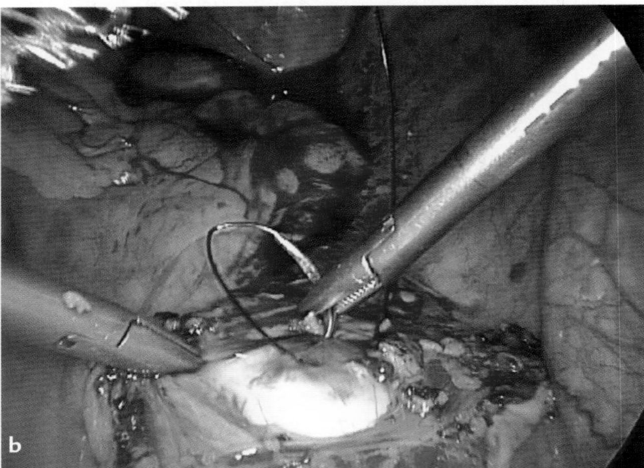

Figure 85.4. *(a) The tissues in the presacral space are carefully reflected laterally exposing the glistening, white fibers of the anterior longitudinal ligament on the sacral promontory. (b) A suture is passed in turn through the mesh and into the anterior longitudinal ligament on the sacral promontory in the midline.*

monofilament suture starting at the sacral promontory. Closure of the peritoneum completely isolates the prosthesis from intra-abdominal viscera and contributes to the obliteration of the pouch of Douglas. Occasionally the pouch of Douglas may remain deep on the left side in which case a left-sided Moschcowitz and Halban procedure can be performed to reduce the possibility of enterocele formation.

Types of prosthesis

Ideally, the prosthesis used for LSC should be durable over a patient's lifetime, user friendly, cost effective, and have a minimal risk of complications including erosion, infection, chronic inflammation, tissue contraction, pain, and dyspareunia. A variety of synthetic meshes and biologic grafts have been described for both ASC and LSC. There is insufficient research to provide surgeons with answers as to whether synthetic meshes are more durable than biologic grafts or whether specific meshes are superior to others with respect to clinical outcomes and complications.

Surgeons should base their selection of synthetic mesh used for LSC on a thorough understanding of the important biomechanical and biocompatible properties of each available mesh. There is an emerging consensus that lightweight, open-weave, monofilament polypropylene meshes are the most suitable of the existing meshes for use in surgery for pelvic organ prolapse. New generation meshes specifically designed for pelvic organ prolapse surgery will require appropriate animal and clinical evaluation before being recommended for use in prolapse surgery.

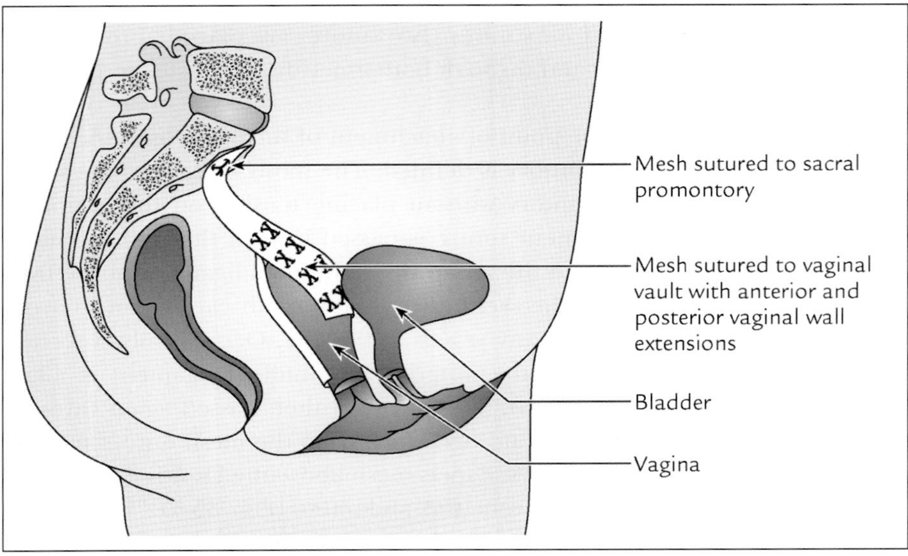

Figure 85.5. *Mesh is sutured to the vaginal vault with extension down the upper anterior and posterior vaginal walls. The mesh is then sutured to the sacral promontory with placing tension on the vaginal vault.*

Although biologic grafts are unlikely to erode, poor durability remains a major concern. FitzGerald et al. reported a high prevalence of prolapse recurrence following ASC using freeze-dried, irradiated donor fascia.[32] At 12-month median follow-up of 54 women after ASC, 43% experienced failure and this increased to 83% at 17 months. Of the 16 women who underwent repeat ASC with mesh, no graft material from initial ASC was identified in 13 (81%) cases, indicating a high rate of graft degradation and resorption. The authors concluded that the use of freeze-dried, irradiated donor fascia for ASC was associated with an unacceptably high failure rate.

Until more clinical information becomes available on the use of biologic grafts such as donor fascia, porcine small intestine submucosa, and porcine dermis for ASC and LSC procedures, these grafts should be reserved for specific indications. These indications might include extremely thin vaginal epithelium, replacement for mesh that has required removal, prior pelvic irradiation, and situations of high risk for mesh infection (e.g. bowel resection during combined surgery for genital and rectal prolapse). However, there remains a lack of evidence to support the use of biologic prostheses over mesh in these circumstances.

Sacral promontory fixation

Various methods of attaching the suspending prosthesis onto the sacral promontory at LSC have been reported. These include sutures, bone anchors, staples, and helical tacks.[9,27,29,30,33,34] There is a lack of research comparing the various methods of fixation of the prosthesis onto the sacral promontory. Due to the technical difficulties involved in laparoscopic suturing with LSC, some surgeons have preferred bone anchors and staples to sutures.

Surgeons have described attachment of the prosthesis to different points on the sacrum. Birnbaum advocated placement of the prosthesis at the level of S3–S4.[35] Sutton et al. advocated placement of the prosthesis at the level of S1–S2 in order to reduce the risk of massive sacral bleeding.[36] The author's preference has been to use the anterior longitudinal ligament on the sacral promontory and to attach the mesh with sutures. The sacral promontory is the most accessible point on the sacrum and is particularly well visualized at laparoscopic surgery. Mesh should not be fixed to the lumbosacral intervertebral disk because of the risk of discitis, hemorrhage, and pain from damage to the sensory nerve supply.[37] Superior visualization at the sacral promontory allows the surgeon to avoid damage to vascular structures more easily and to control excessive sacral bleeding than does the hollow of the sacrum. Use of the sacral promontory has no detectable negative effect on the vaginal axis.[36]

Robotic assistance

Elliot et al. reported on 20 patients treated by robotic-assisted LSC.[34] The mean operating time was 3.2 hours. The authors claim that robotic-assisted LSC is easier and quicker to perform than LSC using conventional laparoscopy. The major disadvantage of robotic-assisted LSC is the 'prohibitive' cost of the robotic system. No doubt robotic equipment will become cheaper and more widely available, and may eventually find an established role in LSC surgery.

Perioperative care

It is the author's practice that patients be administered a limited bowel preparation in the afternoon of the day prior to surgery. Patients should have an oral intake of clear fluids only during the 12-hour period prior to the commencement of fasting before surgery. Bowel preparation is used in order to improve surgical exposure rather than for anticipated bowel trauma. Intravenous broad-spectrum antibiotic therapy and subcutaneous thrombotic prophylaxis are administered with anesthesia induction and continued postoperatively. Handling of the mesh is kept to a minium. Maintaining hemostasis, liberal use of pelvic irrigation, evacuation of blood from the pelvis, and use of monofilament sutures to attach the mesh onto the vagina are all important measures undertaken to reduce the risk of mesh erosion. At the completion of surgery, cystoscopy may be undertaken to exclude ureteric or bladder injury. Digital rectal and vaginal examination should be performed to exclude the presence of perforating sutures.

Following discharge from hospital, patients should avoid strenuous activity for 3–4 weeks. By this time the mesh will have become incorporated into the tissues and patients can then resume activities of normal daily living. Patients should avoid sexual intercourse for at least 6 weeks following surgery. Pelvic floor exercises may be recommenced any time after surgery.[38]

CONCOMITANT ANTI-INCONTINENCE SURGERY

Urodynamic assessment is appropriate for women with symptomatic stress incontinence and vaginal vault prolapse. If urodynamic stress incontinence is demonstrated, then concomitant anti-incontinence surgery, in addition to the LSC operation, is indicated. Laparoscopic colposuspension or a midurethral tape procedure – for example, the tension-free vaginal tape (TVT) operation – can be employed. Occasionally, a transurethral bulking agent is indicated for women with a rigid urethra and, typically, previous failed anti-incontinence surgery. The simplicity and demonstrated effectiveness of the TVT procedure makes this an attractive option over the laparoscopic colposuspension procedure. Paraiso et al., in a randomized trial of 72 women, found the TVT procedure to result in significantly greater objective and subjective cure rates for stress incontinence than laparoscopic Burch colposuspension.[39] This finding was supported by Valpas et al.[40] Furthermore, the opposing vector effect of combining LSC with laparoscopic colposuspension may result in persistence of postoperative stress incontinence.

The role of anti-incontinence surgery for occult stress incontinence during surgery for pelvic organ prolapse remains the subject of ongoing debate. Nygaard et al. emphasized the clinical challenge of patients with occult stress incontinence and vault prolapse.[18] A systematic review by Maher et al. was unable to determine whether or not 'potential stress urinary incontinence detected on reduction of prolapse prior to surgery is best treated with formal continence surgery at the time of prolapse surgery, rather than being left untreated'.[17]

Based on current knowledge, the decision to offer concomitant anti-incontinence surgery during LSC is up to the clinical judgment of the surgeon after a careful discussion with the patient. The author gives patients the option of a concomitant TVT procedure or laparoscopic colposuspension during the LSC procedure when occult stress incontinence is present. Patients should always be warned of the possibility of persisting or de novo urinary incontinence developing following LSC, whether or not anti-incontinence surgery is also performed. The prevalence of de novo postoperative urinary incontinence is approximately 15–18%.[41]

RESULTS

To date, only a small number of studies on LSC have been reported (Table 85.1).[9,10,20,21,27–29,33,34,42] All studies report high success rates and low morbidity with the LSC procedure. However, the different study methodologies employed make the outcome data difficult to collate. It is difficult to draw any conclusions about the long-term outcomes for LSC due to a lack of a standardized technique, wide variation in the definition of outcomes, and lack of control for potential confounders, especially concomitant surgery. In some series the majority of subjects underwent laparoscopic sacral hysteropexy (LSH) rather than LSC.[10,27,29] However, the surgical outcomes in these studies did not differentiate between LSC and LSH.

Higgs et al. reported on 140 consecutive cases treated by LSC of whom 103 were available for long-term follow-up.[9] This is the largest case series of LSC reported to date with a median follow-up of 66 months. A prior vaginal hysterectomy had been performed in 48% of cases and prior abdominal hysterectomy in 52%. Prolene mesh was used in all cases and fixed to the sacrum by either sutures or staples. Concomitant surgeries included laparoscopic colposuspension (37.8%), paravaginal repair (19.4%),

Table 85.1. ***Effectiveness of laparoscopic sacral colpopexy***

Author	Year	*n*	Follow-up (months)	Objective success (%)	Subjective success (%)	Comments
Nezhat et al.[20]	1994	15	range 3–40	100	100	
Ross[42]	1997	19	12	100	–	
Wattiez et al.[21]	2001	125	32	93.4	100	
Cosson et al.[28]	2002	83	11	94	–	
Antiphon et al.[29]	2004	108	17	96.3	83.5	40 LSC, 68 LSH
Gadonneix et al.[27]	2004	46	24	83	95	7 LSC, 34 LSH, 5 conversions to open surgery
Sundaram et al.[33]	2004	10	16	90	–	
Elliot et al.[34]	2004	20	5.1	–	100	
Rozet et al.[10]	2005	363	14.6	98.9	96	97 LSC, 266 LSH
Higgs et al.[9]	2005	140	66	92%	62%	

LSC, laparoscopic sacral colpopexy; LSH, laparoscopic sacral hysteropexy.

vaginal repair (19.4%), rectopexy (3.8%), anal sphincter repair (1.9%), and transurethral collagen injection (1%). The average age of the patients was 58 years and the mean duration of surgery was 145 minutes overall and 107 minutes if LSC was the only procedure. Review was conducted independent of the surgeon. Of the 140 women, 66 were available for follow-up examination and 92% (objective success rate) of these demonstrated good long-term vault support. A total of 103 women completed follow-up questionnaires and the subjective success rate was 62% with 64 of the 103 women reviewed reporting no 'presence of a lump'.

Rozet et al. reported on a large case series of 363 women treated by either LSC or LSH with mesh interposition between 1996 and 2002.[10] Of the 363 cases, 97 (26.7%) underwent LSC (82 women had posthysterectomy vault prolapse and 12 underwent combined LSC and hysterectomy). The other 266 (73.3%) cases underwent LSH with mesh interposition. A polyester mesh, silicone coated on one side, was used with anterior and posterior mesh extensions. The mesh was sutured onto the sacral promontory and the peritoneum closed over the mesh. This study reported outcomes for the whole group and a subanalysis of patients who underwent LSC was not performed. A concomitant TVT procedure was performed in 163 (45%) cases, all of whom demonstrated the signs of stress incontinence preoperatively. The average age of the 363 subjects was 63 years and the average operating time 97 minutes. The prevalence of recurrent prolapse was only 4%.

COMPLICATIONS

Just over 3.7 million women underwent surgery for pelvic organ prolapse from 1979 to 1997 in the United States; this included 31,387 women with laparoscopically performed prolapse surgery. Complications in association with all the various procedures used to treat prolapse occurred in only 5.5% of cases. In women who underwent laparoscopic surgery to manage pelvic organ prolapse, complications were identified in only 6.6% of patients, which is comparable with other prolapse operations. Women treated laparoscopically had a significantly higher risk of pulmonary edema but a lower risk of urinary complications.[1]

Higgs et al. reported that immediate and short-term complications were rare.[9] However, the mesh erosion rate was high at 9%. When the mesh was introduced vaginally, the erosion rate was 20% but only 6% when introduced laparoscopically. The transvaginal introduction of the mesh was performed in 20 cases but abandoned in favor of laparoscopic introduction after the authors noticed a high erosion rate with this technique.

The main complications reported by Rozet et al. included eight conversions to ASC, three vaginal mesh erosions, two mesh infections, one bowel obstruction requiring bowel resection, and one case of spondylitis. No case of postoperative dyspareunia was reported.[10]

In the series reported by Cosson et al., conversion to ASC was required for six cases.[28] One rectal and two bladder injuries were reported. Reoperation for hemorrhage or hematoma was required in three women.

CONCLUSION

Posthysterectomy vaginal vault prolapse is a challenging clinical problem. The goals of surgery when treating vaginal vault prolapse are:

- the relief of patients' symptoms;
- the correction of vaginal vault prolapse by restoring the normal pelvic anatomy where feasible;
- the correction of coexisting urinary, coital, and lower bowel dysfunction;
- the avoidance of the development of urinary, coital, and lower bowel dysfunction;
- the achievement of a durable result, which in some cases may require the use of prosthetic materials.

The 'best' operation for treating vaginal vault prolapse remains the subject of ongoing debate. In treating vaginal vault prolapse, vaginal, abdominal, and laparoscopic approaches should not be viewed as competing procedures.[43] The choice of operation to treat vaginal vault prolapse depends on many factors: the surgeon's training and experience will influence the choice of surgery, and a recommendation for a specific operation can only be made after careful clinical assessment and after taking into consideration the patient's age, medical condition, coital activity, level of physical activity, and a history of failed prior surgery.

Systematic review of the surgical management of prolapse has demonstrated the ASC procedure to be associated with a lower recurrence of vault prolapse and less dyspareunia than vaginal approaches.[15–18] However, when compared to vaginal approaches, ASC required a longer operating time and patients were slower to return to activities of normal daily living. LSC should be performed in a similar fashion to ASC. Based on the reported experiences of many surgeons over the past 50 years,[18] and upon personal experience of ASC and LSC procedures, the following important principles of ASC and LSC are proposed:

- Careful patient selection;
- Appropriate level of surgical experience and expertise;
- Use of a biocompatible prosthesis;
- A broad area of prosthesis attachment to the vaginal vault, and upper anterior and posterior vagina;
- Fixation of the prosthesis to the anterior longitudinal ligament on the sacral promontory rather than to the sacral hollow;
- Placement of the prosthesis without tension to reduce the risk of postoperative urinary incontinence.

From the limited available data, LSC appears to be a highly effective procedure for the treatment of vaginal vault and marked uterovaginal prolapse. The LSC procedure combines the accepted effectiveness of ASC over vaginal operations for vault prolapse with the significant benefits of laparoscopic surgery. These benefits include superior surgical visualization, less pain, and quicker return to activities of normal daily living. The major limitation of LSC is the high degree of laparoscopic and reconstructive pelvic surgical skills required to perform this operation effectively and safely. With continued advances in laparoscopic equipment (including robotics) and more widespread training in advanced laparoscopic surgery, LSC is likely to gain in popularity. Currently, there is a paucity of data on the effectiveness, functional outcome, and safety of LSC. Further prospective studies, including comparative studies, are required to evaluate the role of the LSC procedure.

REFERENCES

1. Boyles SH, Weber AM, Meyn L. Procedures for pelvic organ prolapse in the United States, 1979–1997. Am J Obstet Gynecol 2003;188:108–15.
2. Olsen AL, Smith VJ, Bergstrom JO, Colling JC, Clark AL. Epidemiology of surgically managed pelvic organ prolapse and urinary incontinence. Obstet Gynecol 1997;89:501–6.
3. Whiteside JL, Weber AM, Meyn LA, Walters MD. Risk factors for prolapse recurrence after vaginal repair. Am J Obstet Gynecol 2004;19:1533–8.
4. Bump RC, Mattiasson A, Bo K et al. The standardization of terminology of female pelvic organ prolapse and pelvic floor dysfunction. Am J Obstet Gynecol 1996;175:10–17.
5. Marchionni M, Bracco GL, Checcucci V et al. True incidence of vaginal vault prolapse: 13 years of experience. J Reprod Med 1999;44:679–84.
6. Symmonds R, Williams T, Lee R, Webb M. Post hysterectomy enterocele and vaginal vault prolapse. Am J Obstet Gynecol 1981;140:852–9.
7. Toozs-Hobson P, Boos K, Cardozo L. Management of vaginal vault prolapse. Br J Obstet Gynaecol 1998;105:13–17.
8. Carey MP, Slack MC. Transvaginal sacrospinous colpopexy for vault and marked uterovaginal prolapse. Br J Obstet Gynaecol 1994;101:536–40.
9. Higgs PJ, Chua H-L, Smith ARB. Long term review of laparoscopic sacrocolpopexy. Br J Obstet Gynaecol 2005; in press.
10. Rozet F, Mandron E, Arroyo C et al. Laparoscopic sacral colpopexy approach for genito-urinary prolapse: experience with 363 cases. Eur Urol 2005;47:230–6.
11. Lane FE. Repair of posthysterectomy vaginal vault prolapse. Obstet Gynecol 1962;20:72–7.
12. Snyder TE, Krantz KE. Abdominal–retroperitoneal sacral colpopexy for the correction of vaginal prolapse. Obstet Gynecol 1991;77:944–9.
13. Addison WA, Livengood CH, Sutton GP, Parker RT. Abdominal sacral colpopexy with mersilene mesh in the retroperitoneal position in the management of posthysterectomy vaginal vault prolapse and enterocele. Obstet Gynecol 1985;153:140–6.
14. Addison WA, Timmons MC, Wall LL, Livengood CH. Failed abdominal sacral colpopexy: observations and recommendations. Obstet Gynecol 1989;74:480–3.
15. Bensen JT, Lucente V, McClellan E. Vaginal versus abdominal reconstructive surgery for the treatment of pelvic support defects: a prospective randomized study with long-term outcome evaluation. Am J Obstet Gynecol 1996;175:1418–22.
16. Maher CF, Qatawneh AM, Dwyer PL, Carey MP, Cornish A, Schluter PJ. Abdominal sacral colpopexy or vaginal sacrospinous colpopexy for vaginal vault prolapse: a prospective randomized study. Am J Obstet Gynecol 2004;190:20–6.
17. Maher C, Baessler K, Glazener C, Adams E, Hagen S. Surgical management of pelvic organ prolapse in women. Cochrane Database Syst Rev 2004;4:CD004014.
18. Nygaard I, McCreey R, Brubaker L et al. Abdominal sacrocolpopexy: a comprehensive review. Obstet Gynecol 2004;104:805–23.
19. Visco AG, Weidner AC, Barber MD et al. Vaginal mesh erosion after abdominal sacral colpopexy. Am J Obstet Gynecol 2001;184:297–302.
20. Nezhat CH, Nezhat F, Nezhat C. Laparoscopic sacral colpopexy for vaginal vault prolapse. Obstet Gynecol 1994;84:885–8.
21. Wattiez A, Mashiach R, Donoso M. Laparoscopic repair of vaginal vault prolapse. Curr Opin Obstet Gynecol 2003;15:315–19.
22. DeLancey JOL. Anatomic aspects of vaginal eversion after hysterectomy. Am J Obstet Gynecol 1992:166;1717–28.

23. Gosling JA. The structure of the bladder neck, urethra and pelvic floor in relation to female urinary incontinence. Int Urogynecol J 1996;7:177–8.
24. Tulikangas PK, Walters MD, Brainard JA, Weber AM. Enterocele: is there a histologic defect? Obstet Gynecol 2001;98:634–7.
25. Richardson AC. The anatomic defects in rectocele and enterocele. J Pelvic Surg 1995;1:214–21.
26. Miklos JR, Kohli N, Lucente V, Saye WB. Site-specific fascial defects in the diagnosis and surgical management of enterocele. Am J Obstet Gynecol 1998;179:1418–22.
27. Gadonneix P, Ercoli A, Salet-Lizee D et al. Laparoscopic sacrocolpopexy with two separate meshes along the anterior and posterior vaginal walls for multicompartment pelvic organ prolapse. J Am Assoc Gynecol Laparosc 2004;11:29–35.
28. Cosson M, Rajabally R, Bogaert E, Querleu D, Crepin G. Laparoscopic sacrocolpopexy, hysterectomy, and Burch colposuspension: feasibility and short-term complications of 77 procedures. J Soc Laparoendosc Surg 2002;6:115–19.
29. Antiphon P, Elard S, Benyoussef A et al. Laparoscopic promontory sacral colpopexy: is the posterior, recto-vaginal, mesh mandatory? Eur Urol 2004;45:655–61.
30. Paraiso MFR, Falcone T, Walters MD. Laparoscopic surgery for enterocele, vaginal apex prolapse and rectocele. Int Urogynecol J 1999;10:223–9.
31. Amid PK. Classification of biomaterials and their related complications in abdominal wall hernia surgery. Hernia 1997;1:15–21.
32. FitzGerald M, Edwards SR, Fenner D. Medium-term follow-up on use of freeze-dried, irradiated donor fascia for sacrocolpopexy and sling procedures. Int Urogynecol J Pelvic Floor Dysfunct 2004;15:238–42.
33. Sundaram CP, Venkatesh R, Landman J, Klutke CG. Laparoscopic sacrocolpopexy for the correction of vaginal vault prolapse. J Endourol 2004;18:620–3.
34. Elliot DS, Frank I, DiMarco DS, Chow GK. Gynecologic use of robotically assisted laparoscopy: sacrocolpopexy for the treatment of high-grade vaginal vault prolapse. Am J Surg 2004;188 (Suppl):52–6.
35. Birnbaum SJ. Rational therapy for the prolapsed vagina. Am J Obstet Gynecol 1973;115:411–19.
36. Sutton GP, Addison WA, Livengood CH, Hammond CB. Life threatening hemorrhage complicating sacral colpopexy. Am J Obstet Gynecol 1981;140:836–7.
37. Kapoor B, Toms A, Hooper P, Fraser AM, Cox CW. Infective lumbar discitis following laparoscopic sacral colpopexy. J R Coll Surg Edinb 2002;47:709–10.
38. Kannus P, Parkkari J, Jarvinen TLN, Jarvinen TAH, Jarvinen M. Basic science and clinical studies coincide: active treatment approach is needed after a sports injury. Scand J Med Sci Sports 2003;13:150–4.
39. Paraiso MF, Walters MD, Karram MM, Barber MD. Laparoscopic Burch colposuspension versus tension-free vaginal tape: a randomized trial. Obstet Gynecol 2004;104:1249–58.
40. Valpas A, Kivela A, Penttinen J et al. Tension-free vaginal tape and laparoscopic mesh colposuspension in the treatment of stress urinary incontinence: immediate outcome and complications – a randomised clinical trial. Acta Obstet Gynecol Scand 2003;82(7):665–71.
41. Bump RC, Hurt GW, Cotheofrastous JP et al. Randomized prospective comparison of needle colposuspension versus endopelvic fascia plication for potential stress incontinence prophylaxis in women undergoing vaginal reconstruction for stage 3 or 4 pelvic organ prolapse. Am J Obstet Gynecol 1996;175:326–35.
42. Ross JW. Techniques of laparoscopic repair of total vault eversion after hysterectomy. J Am Assoc Gynecol Laparosc 1997;4:173–83.
43. Carey MP, Dwyer PL. Genital prolapse: vaginal versus abdominal route of repair. Curr Opin Obstet Gynecol 2001;13:499–505.

86

Other laparoscopic support procedures

Peta Higgs

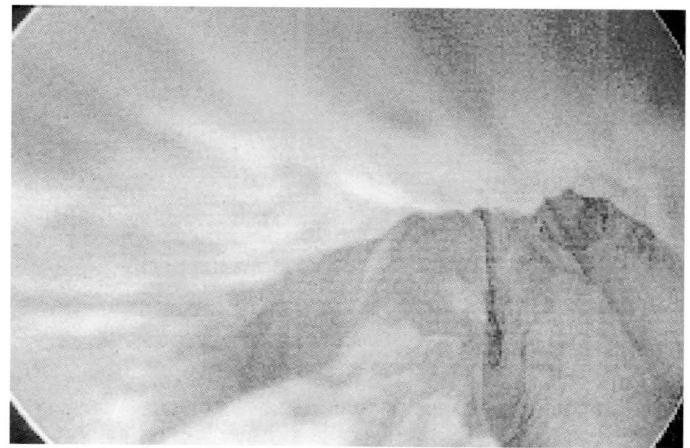

INTRODUCTION

Laparoscopic surgery has become popular in urogynecology and many treatments offered by the abdominal route have been described using the laparoscopic approach. There is, however, a paucity of data on this approach. The literature reveals descriptive techniques and case reports, often without results. There are no comparative studies between the laparoscopic and the abdominal or vaginal approach.

Nevertheless, laparoscopy may offer an enhanced view of the pelvis and improve recovery times. The role of these support techniques needs to be assessed by comparison to conventional surgery in robust clinical trials.

APICAL SUPPORT METHODS

Laparoscopic sacrocolpopexy

The best studied approach of laparoscopic apical support is laparoscopic sacrocolpopexy, discussed in Chapter 85. Other methods without the use of synthetic meshes and with uterine conservation are discussed here.

Laparoscopic uterosacral-ligament vault suspension

Vault suspension by the uterosacral ligaments has been described by a number of authors,[1–8] often in combination with an enterocele repair.

The technique involves peritoneal dissection to expose the vaginal apex. The uterosacral ligaments are then identified by elevating the vagina with a probe to stretch the ligaments. The course of the pelvic ureter must be identified to avoid damage. The uterosacral ligaments are then plicated proximally with non-absorbable sutures. Laterally, the vaginal fascia may be sutured to the cardinal ligaments. Anteriorly, the pubocervical fascia may be plicated to create a new 'vaginal cuff'. The vaginal vault is then sutured to the plicated uterosacral ligaments for support (Fig. 86.1).

At the end of the procedure the position of the ureters is checked. If there is excessive medial displacement, an incision into the pelvic peritoneum between the uterosacral ligament and the ureter is made.

Proponents of this technique feel that it offers a site-specific defect repair and anatomic alignment of the vaginal axis, without the use of synthetic materials.

Results of these techniques are presented in small case series with short follow-up times and are summarized in Table 86.1. The largest series is by Cook et al.[7] in which at least 71% of the women underwent concurrent prolapse repair at the time of surgery (see Table 86.1). The main apical support procedure was by enterocele

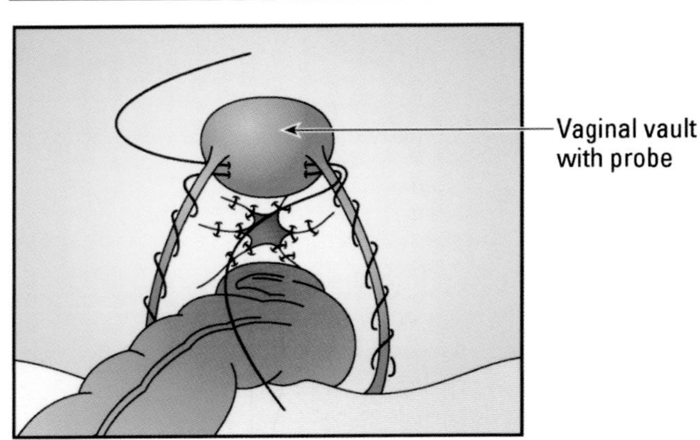

Figure 86.1. *Laparoscopic uterosacral ligament vault suspension.*

Table 86.1. *Laparoscopic uterosacral ligament vault suspension*

Author	No. of patients	Additional procedures	Follow-up (months)	Vault prolapse (%)
Ostrzenski[1]	15	–	6–24	0
Ostrzenski[2]	16 11	– Paravaginal repair	36+ Up to 42	31 9
Vancaillie & Butler[8]	17	Burch colposuspension, vaginal repair	3–12	0
Carter et al.[3]	8	Enterocele repair, 'multiple other defect repairs'	6–12	0
Miklos et al.[5]	17	Vaginal enterocele repair	6	12
Seman et al.[6]	10	Multiple*	8	0
Cook et al.[7]	44	Multiple*	Up to 36	7

* Additional procedures included laparoscopic enterocele repair, laparoscopic supralevator repair, laparoscopic adhesiolysis, laparoscopic paravaginal repair, laparoscopic Burch colposuspension, posterior colporrhaphy and anterior colporrhaphy.

repair with uterosacral ligament suspension. The follow-up time is not clearly stated. They found good vault support on pelvic organ prolapse quantification (POPQ) examination in 41 of 44 (93%) of women.

Major surgical complications have been described in 4.4% of patients, including enterotomy, rectal perforation, conversion to laparotomy, and vesicovaginal fistula.[6,7]

Laparoscopic vaginal suspension to anterior abdominal wall

Fedele et al.[9] describe a technique involving fixation of the vaginal vault with non-absorbable sutures to the anterior abdominal wall fascia. An initial enterocele repair is performed. The peritoneum over the vaginal vault is opened and two sutures placed in each corner of the vault. The sutures are passed subperitoneally and brought out of the trocars placed laterally 4–5 cm from the anterior iliac spine. The sutures are then fixed to the rectus sheath fascia.

In their series of 12 women, all 12 underwent an enterocele repair incorporating the uterosacral ligaments as part of the procedure and 11 women had a concurrent vaginal repair. They found no recurrent vault prolapse at 9–28 months follow-up.[9]

Tsin et al.[10] reported a similar technique using a synthetic mesh sutured to the cardinal ligament/uterosacral complex laparoscopically. Initial vaginal hysterectomy and McCall culdoplasty are performed. The mesh sling is tunneled from the round ligament insertion to the lateral pelvic wall to the skin incision. The mesh is then sutured to the rectus sheath fascia.

At 12 months follow-up in this series of 10 women there was no recurrent vault prolapse. Reported complications included infection of the mesh at the anterior abdominal wall in one in 10 (10%) and suture extrusion at the vaginal vault in one in 10 (10%).[10]

Laparoscopic extraperitoneal sacrospinous suspension

Lee et al.[11] reported this technique of sacrospinous suspension. The vaginal vault is suspended to the sacrospinous ligament similar to the vaginal approach. The retropubic space and the pararectal spaces are opened to identify the sacrospinous ligament. A non-absorbable suture is then placed from the sacrospinous ligament to the vaginal vault.

In their series of 12 women, one woman had recurrent vault prolapse at an average follow-up of 26 months. No surgical complications were reported.[11]

UTERINE PROLAPSE

Laparoscopic sacro colpohysteropexy

This technique is similar to sacrocolpopexy but allows for conservation of the uterus. It involves the use of synthetic mesh fixed from the cervix or uterosacral ligaments and the anterior vaginal wall to the sacral promontory for support.[12,13]

Rozet et al.[13] describes dissection of the peritoneum from the uterosacral ligaments and pouch of Douglas to open the rectovaginal space down to the level of the levator ani muscles. The mesh is then fixed to the levator ani muscles using absorbable sutures. The bladder is dissected from the anterior vaginal wall and the vesicovaginal space is opened. A second mesh is fixed to the anterior vaginal wall. The anterior mesh is then passed through the broad ligament on the right side of the uterus only. The peritoneum over the sacral promontory is incised and both meshes are then fixed to the sacral promontory with a non-absorbable suture. The peritoneum is then closed to cover the mesh (Fig. 86.2).

This technique can also be performed with the anterior mesh passed bilaterally through the broad ligaments and attached to either the posterior mesh or the

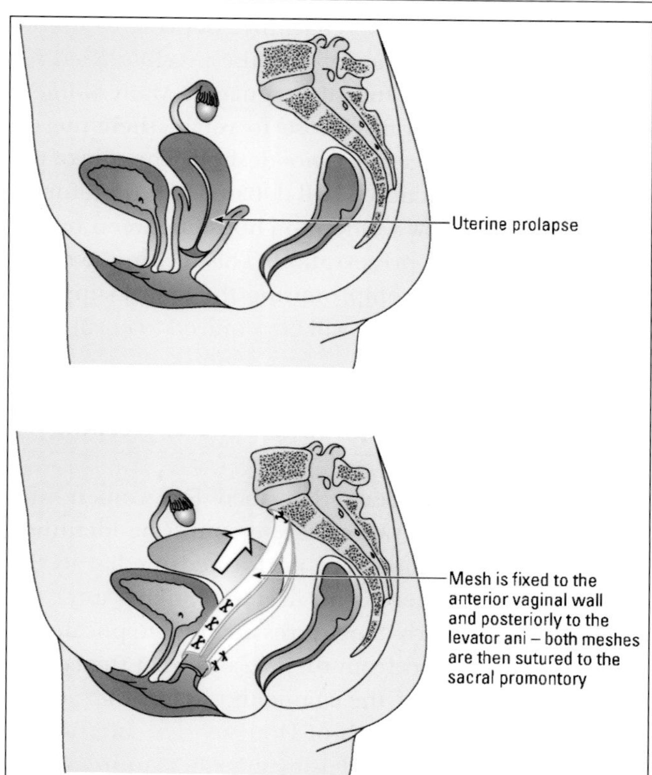

Figure 86.2. *Laparoscopic sacro colpohysteropexy.*

sacral promontory directly.[12] It can also be used with the mesh attached to the cervix alone if only level 1 support is required.

Rozet et al.[13] describes a series of 325 women, of whom 228 underwent laparoscopic sacro colpohysteropexy and 97 underwent laparoscopic sacrocolpopexy. Other procedures performed concurrently included Burch colposuspension, tension-free vaginal tape (TVT) and hysterectomy. Results include both the sacro colpohysteropexy and the sacrocolpopexy groups of women. They found prolapse recurrence in 13 of 325 (4%) of women with an average follow-up of 14.6 months. The prolapse recurred in the anterior compartment in 10 and in the posterior compartment in three. Excluded from analysis were eight women who were converted to laparotomy due to hypercapnia, extensive peritoneal adhesions, and bleeding.

Late complications included de novo urge incontinence (19), de novo stress incontinence (19%), intestinal obstruction requiring laparotomy and bowel resection (1), sacral spondylitis (1), port site hernia (1), mesh infection (2), mesh erosion (3), and urinary retention following TVT (2).

This technique offers a promising solution for women with apical support defects who wish to retain their uterus. Further pregnancies would be possible, although women should be warned of the likelihood of decreased fertility following surgery, recurrence of prolapse following a subsequent pregnancy, and the possible need for cesarean section in a future pregnancy. Many women, when given the option, choose to retain their uterus, even if future childbearing is not desired. The role of the cervix in sexual function is still debated and therefore it is preferable to allow women to choose between hysterectomy and uterine preservation. This technique offers this choice, without compromising the apical supports. Further longer term study will be required to ensure this support is lasting.

Uterosacral ligament plication and shortening

This technique has been described for women who desire uterine conservation. Ureters must be identified and peritoneal incisions are performed medial to the ureters to ensure there is no ureteric kinking after the plication. Non-absorbable sutures are used to plicate the uterosacral ligaments from their insertion at the cervix. Further sutures plicate the ligaments towards the sacrum and these close the pouch of Douglas. The uterosacral ligament is then shortened using a further suture placed from the cervical to the sacral end of the ligaments and tied[14] (Fig. 86.3).

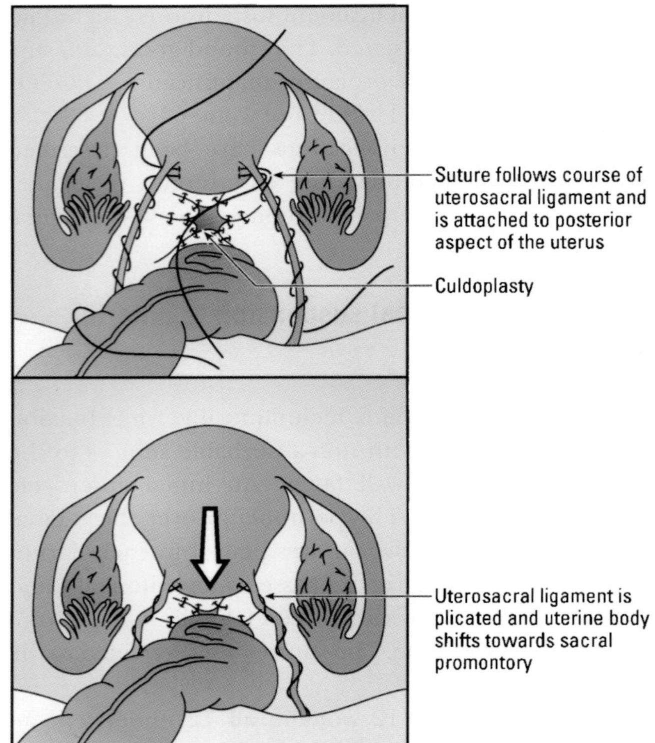
Suture follows course of uterosacral ligament and is attached to posterior aspect of the uterus
Culdoplasty
Uterosacral ligament is plicated and uterine body shifts towards sacral promontory

Figure 86.3. *Uterosacral ligament placation and shortening.*

The largest series for this procedure has been reported by Maher et al.[15] Forty-three women underwent the procedure, 41 of whom had concurrent procedures for prolapse including anterior and posterior vaginal repair, laparoscopic Burch colposuspension, and laparoscopic paravaginal repair. At an average follow-up of 12 months, nine (21%) women had recurrent uterine prolapse, with seven (16%) of the women having undergone further surgery for prolapse. The only surgical complication reported was one conversion to laparotomy for a uterine artery laceration. Two women had completed term pregnancies at the time of review.

Laparoscopic uterine suspension with round ligaments

The open technique is known to be unsuccessful when used for uterine prolapse. The round ligaments are suspended to or through the rectus sheath similar to the technique for a ventrosuspension. O'Brien and Ibrahim found this technique to be unsuccessful in eight of nine women who underwent the procedure.[16]

One case report has described this technique during pregnancy.[17] Surgery was performed at 13 weeks' gestation. No uterine prolapse was seen at 3 months postpartum.

ANTERIOR COMPARTMENT SUPPORT METHODS

This is covered in Chapter 84.

POSTERIOR COMPARTMENT SUPPORT METHODS

The posterior compartment is usually accessed via the vaginal route. Laparoscopic sacrocolpopexy may address posterior defects by extending the mesh down the posterior vaginal wall. This technique is discussed in Chapter 85.

Laparoscopic surgeons find that this compartment is usually well visualized; however, there is no clinical evidence to support the use of laparoscopic rectocele repair.

Laparoscopic enterocele repair

Laparoscopic enterocele repair can be performed in a number of different ways. The pressure created with the pneumoperitoneum of the laparoscopy aids identification of the enterocele sac.

The Moschcowitz procedure involves a purse-string non-absorbable suture to the peritoneum of the pouch of Douglas. The ureters must be observed after the procedure to ensure there is no kinking.[18]

The Halban procedure uses non-absorbable sutures placed in the sagittal plane from the posterior vagina to the inferior sigmoid serosa. Interrupted sutures are placed approximately 1 cm apart and tied as they are placed. Again the ureters must be identified at the end of the procedure.[18]

Alternatively, the enterocele is managed similar to a hernial sac. Upward traction with forceps in the vagina is used to identify the enterocele. The peritoneum is incised along the uterosacral ligaments and posterior vagina. The flap of excess peritoneum is then excised from the anterior rectum. The rectovaginal fascia is then plicated to close any fascial defects causing the enterocele. A synthetic mesh can be sutured over the posterior vaginal wall and uterosacral ligaments to close the fascial defect if required.[14]

Clinical results of the procedure alone are lacking as it is usually used in conjunction with other apical support procedures. Cadeddu et al.[19] reported on three women using a modified Moschcowitz procedure and found no recurrent enterocele after a mean follow-up of 10 months. In prolapse surgery the Moschcowitz procedure has generally fallen out of favor. In vaginal surgery, the McCall culdoplasty has been found to be superior to the Moschcowitz procedure in prevention of enterocele formation following vaginal hysterectomy. In a randomized study, after 3 years follow up, there were 0/32 enterocele formation in the McCall group compared to 6/33 in the Moschcowitz.[20]

Laparoscopic rectocele repair

This technique has been described using an absorbable mesh.[21] The rectovaginal septum is opened to the level of the perineal body. The mesh is attached to the perineal body and posterior surface of the vaginal vault. If the cervix is present, the mesh is attached to the cervix and uterosacral ligaments; if not, the uterosacral ligaments are sutured to the anterior and posterior vaginal fascia and the mesh attached to this complex.

Lyons and Winer[21] described a series of 20 women in whom they used this technique. Enterocele repair was performed laparoscopically in all women. Other concurrent procedures included laparoscopic Burch colposuspension, paravaginal repair, subtotal hysterectomy, sacrocolpopexy, rectopexy and perineorrhaphy. They reported an 80% subjective improvement at 1 year. No follow-up clinical examination was performed.

CONCLUSION

The evidence base for use of these laparoscopic support procedures is lacking. Studies to date are limited by small numbers, varied techniques, and short follow-up times.

The best studied are the apical support methods, especially laparoscopic sacro colpohysteropexy. This technique is similar to laparoscopic sacrocolpopexy but allows for conservation of the uterus. It would appear that the technique offers good support without 'shooting the messenger' as the uterus itself is not the cause of prolapse, but its lack of suspensory support at the level of the uterosacral and cardinal ligaments. If these supports can be recreated, then the choice of uterine conservation can be offered. Further long-term data are still required.

The nature of uterovaginal prolapse often requires that a number of the vaginal compartments need to be addressed simultaneously during surgery. This makes the analysis of one technique difficult. However, prospective trials with standardized examination techniques, such as the POPQ examination, with long-term follow-up would at least allow some comparison between different techniques.

Ultimately, clinical trials comparing the open and vaginal techniques with the laparoscopic approach are required to determine the best approach for women with prolapse.

ACKNOWLEDGMENTS

Illustrations by Bill Reid, ERC, Royal Children's Hospital, Melbourne, Australia.

REFERENCES

1. Ostrzenski A. Laser video-laparoscopic colpopexy. Ginkol Pol 1992;63:317–23.
2. Ostrzenski A. Laparoscopic colposuspension for total vaginal prolapse. Int J Gynecol Obstet 1996;55:147–52.
3. Carter J, Winter M, Mendehlsohn S, Saye W, Richardson A. Vaginal vault suspension and enterocele repair by Richardson-Saye laparoscopic technique: description of training technique and results. JSLS 2001;5:29–36.
4. Miklos J, Moore R, Kohli N. Laparoscopic surgery for pelvic support defects. Curr Opin Obstet Gynecol 2002;14:387–95.
5. Miklos J, Kohli N, Lucente V, Saye W. Site-specific fascial defects in the diagnosis and surgical management of enterocele. Am J Obstet Gynecol 1998;179:1418–23.
6. Seman E, Cook J, O'Shea R. Two-year experience with laparoscopic pelvic floor repair. J Am Assoc Gynecol Laparosc 2003;10:38–45.
7. Cook J, Seman E, O'Shea R. Laparoscopic treatment of enterocele: a 3-year evaluation. Aust N Z J Obstet Gynaecol 2004;44:107–10.
8. Vancaillie T, Butler D. Laparoscopic enterocele repair – description of a new technique. Gynecol Endosc 1993;2:211–6.
9. Fedele L, Garsia S, Bianchi S, Albiero A, Dorta M. A new laparoscopic procedure for the correction of vaginal vault prolapse. J Urol 1998;159:1179–82.
10. Tsin D, Whang G, Sequeira R, Mahmood D, Granato R. Laparo-vaginal treatment of uterine procidentia. J Laparoendosc Surg 1995;5:145–9.
11. Lee C, Wang C, Yen C, Soong Y. Laparoscopic extraperitoneal sacrospinous suspension for vaginal vault prolapse. Chang Gung Med J 2000;23:87–91.
12. Seracchioli R, Hourcabie J-A, Vianello F, Govoni F, Pollastri P, Venturoli S. Laparoscopic treatment of pelvic floor defects in women of reproductive age. J Am Assoc Gynecol Laparosc 2004;11:332–5.
13. Rozet F, Mandron E, Arroyo C et al. Laparoscopic sacral colpopexy approach for genito-urinary prolapse: experience with 363 cases. Eur Urol 2005;47:230–6.
14. Margossian H, Walters M, Falcone T. Laparoscopic management of pelvic organ prolapse. Eur J Obstet Gynecol Reprod Biol 1999;85:57–62.
15. Maher C, Carey M, Murray C. Laparoscopic suture hysteropexy for uterine prolapse. Obstet Gynecol 2001;97:1010–4.
16. O'Brien P, Ibrahim J. Failure of laparoscopic uterine suspension to provide a lasting cure for uterovaginal prolapse. Br J Obstet Gynaecol 1994;101:707–8.
17. Matsumoto T, Nishi M, Yokota M, Ito M. Laparoscopic treatment of uterine prolapse during pregnancy. Obstet Gynecol 1999;93:849.
18. Paraiso M, Falcone T, Walters M. Laparoscopic surgery for enterocele, vaginal apex prolapse and rectocele. Int Urogynecol J 1999;10:223–9.
19. Cadeddu J, Micali S, Moore R, Kavoussi L. Laparoscopic repair of enterocele. J Endourol 1996;10:367–9.
20. Cruikshank S, Kovac S. Randomized comparison of three surgical methods used at the time of vaginal hysterectomy to prevent posterior enterocele. Am J Obstet Gynecol 1999;180:859–65.
21. Lyons T, Winer W. Laparoscopic rectocele repair using polyglactin mesh. J Am Assoc Gynecol Laparosc 1997;4:381–4.

87

Prevention, recognition, and treatment of complications in laparoscopic pelvic floor surgery

Christopher Maher

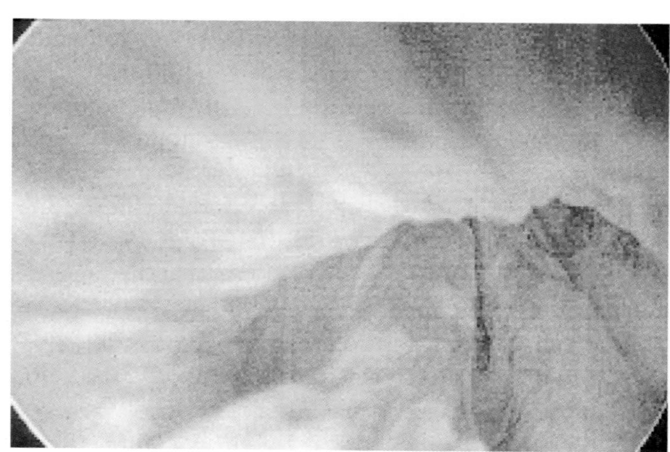

INTRODUCTION

Gynecologists have led the surgical specialties in recognizing the benefits to our patients of reduced postoperative pain, fewer hospital admissions and the quicker return to normal activities associated with laparoscopy. Improved optics, lighting, instrumentation and technology over the last 15 years have seen an explosion in operative general gynecology surgery previously performed via laparotomy. Over the next decade, as laparoscopic suturing techniques are mastered, the laparoscope is likely to play an increasingly important role in female pelvic floor reconstructive surgery. It is vital while laparoscopic pelvic floor surgery is in its infancy that we are competent in the prevention, recognition, and treatment of complications associated with this mode of access to the abdomen and pelvis.

In recent years the rate of complications from gynecologic laparoscopy has ranged from 4 to 8 per 1000[1–3] for diagnostic procedures and increased from 4 to 180 per 1000 operative gynecology surgeries.[3–7] Risk analysis has revealed that the important factors leading to gynecologic laparoscopic complications include establishing laparoscopic access,[5,6] concomitant laparoscopic hysterectomy[3,8] and surgeon inexperience.[4,9]

ACCESS COMPLICATIONS

At least 50% of all reported complications at laparoscopic surgery occur at time of entry to the abdomen.[5,6] The majority of gynecologists prefer the closed (Veress needle) technique to the open technique.[1,10] The major complications related to entry include vascular and bowel injuries and associated hernia formation.

Although entry-related complications using the closed approach are uncommon, they can be fatal and occur in 0.31–2.4/1000 procedures.[1,4,8,9,11] Chapron et al.[12] reported that major vascular injuries were reported five times more frequently following the closed technique as compared to the open approach. Of the 44 reported cases in the literature between 1982 and 1997, 82% followed the closed and 17% followed the open technique.[12]

A large Dutch review retrospectively compared open (12,444 patients) and closed (489,335 patients) access. They found the incidence of major vascular injury was 0.075% using the closed approach and 0% with the open approach ($p<0.05$). The incidence of visceral damage was 0.083% with the closed technique as compared to 0.048% with the open[13] ($p>0.05$).

In a randomized controlled trial (RCT), 150 subjects undergoing cholecystectomy were allocated to the open or the closed approach. Major complications were reported in 3/75 (4%) of the closed as compared to 1/75 (1.3%) of the open ($p<0.05$).[14] The open approach was also significantly faster to perform. In a smaller RCT of 50 patients undergoing laparoscopic surgery, no difference in complications were observed but the open approach took half the time of the closed approach to obtain access.[15]

In contrast, in a more recent questionnaire review of Dutch gynecologists, the complication rate in those undergoing open laparoscopy was significantly higher compared to those undergoing closed laparoscopy.[1] The complication rate amongst those undergoing open laparoscopy (579) was 1.38% as compared to 0.12% in the closed group (20,027) ($p=0.001$). While the rate of vascular injuries was the same in both groups, the rate of gastrointestinal injuries, wound infections and failed access was significantly greater in the open group. The rate of open laparoscopy among Dutch gynecologists was only 2% and was reserved for those with previous laparotomies, suspected adhesions, and the very obese or very thin. The authors concluded that the closed approach was safer than the open approach. An alternative message is that gynecologists should not perform procedures that they perform rarely in patients at high risk of complications. In my own tertiary referral urogynecology practice the open technique is used exclusively, but the literature only provides evidence that the risk of vascular injury is reduced with the open method.

It has been demonstrated that 50% of those with previous midline vertical incisions and 20% with low transverse incisions have some degree of periumbilical adhesions.[16] Studies have shown that employing counterpressure during gas insufflation of the peritoneal cavity produces a more consistent elevation of the anterior abdominal wall.[17] Although not proven, firm elevation of the anterior abdominal wall should make for safer insertion of laparoscopic ports, including the first port. When there is concern regarding the safety of blindly introducing the insufflating needle at the umbilicus, an alternative site of placement is the left upper quadrant 3 cm below the costal margin in the mid-clavicular line (Palmers point; Fig. 87.1b). In retrospective audits no significant complications have been reported with this approach.[18,19]

TROCAR-ASSOCIATED COMPLICATIONS

Primary trocars

In an attempt to minimize the risk associated with accessing the abdominal cavity, increased attention has been focused on trocar design. The traditional pyrami-

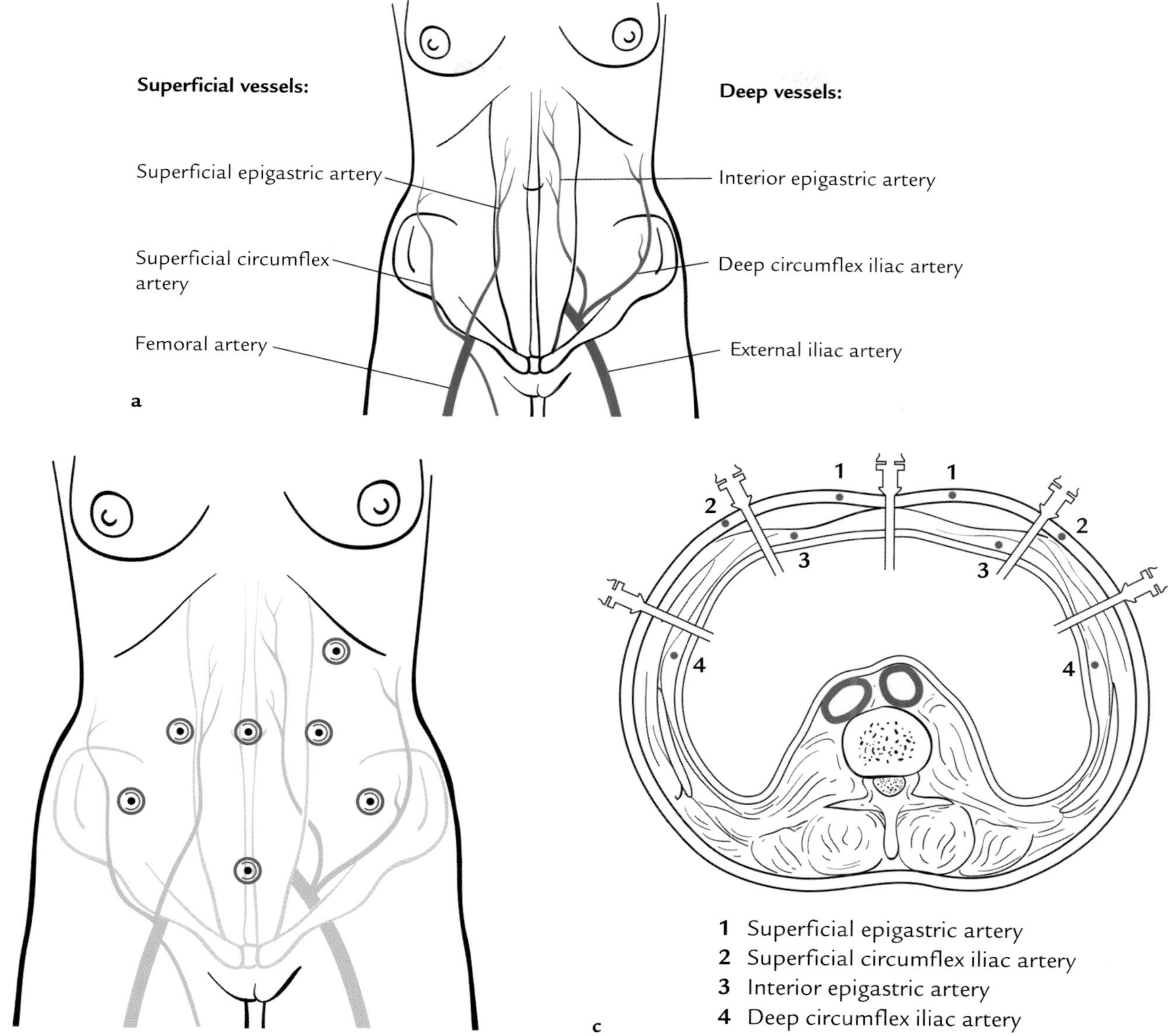

Figure 87.1. *Coronal view: (a) anterior abdominal wall vasculature; (b) trocar placement sites. (c) Transverse view: trocar placement sites in relation to vessels, just below the level of the umbilicus. (© Maher/Francis.)*

dal trocar (Fig. 87.2) cuts through the tissue, and safety shields (Fig. 87.2) have been added to try to reduce the risk to the abdominal wall or of perforation of intra-abdominal vessels or viscus. The cutting blade retracts into the plastic sleeve after the abdominal wall has been penetrated. Bhoyrul et al. reported that 87% of deaths from vascular injuries and 91% of bowel injuries at the time of entry involved trocars with safety shields.[20] They concluded that, despite the blade retracting soon after entry into the peritoneum, the momentary presence of the blade in the abdominal cavity as seen in Figure 87.3 is all that is required for injuries to occur. Surgeons should not overestimate the level of safety associated with this device.

Conical or blunt tip trocars have been designed to reduce the risk associated with bladed trocars (see Fig. 87.2). They dilate the fascia and muscular tissues, thus decreasing the potential trauma as the trocar enters the abdominal cavity. Conical tips require a greater entry force to the abdomen than sharper pyramidal trocars[21] and leave a defect approximately 50% narrower than the sharper pryamidal.[22] Leibl et al., in a non-randomized study, demonstrated that the reduced wound defect following the use of conical trocars was clinically relevant, with incisional hernia being reported 10 times more frequently after the pyramidal as compared to the conical trocar.[23] In a further study there were no reported injuries to blood vessels of the anterior abdominal wall

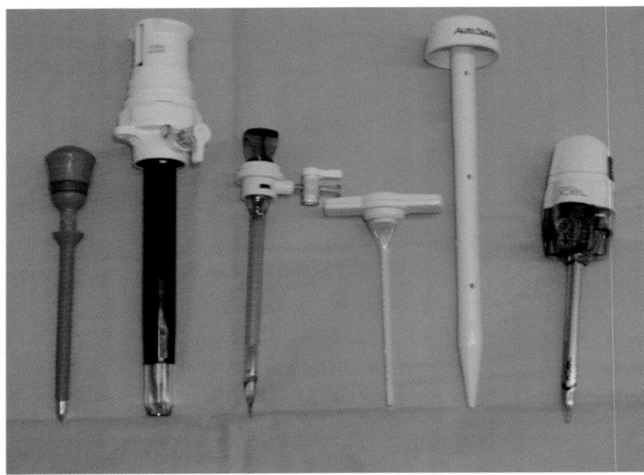

Figure 87.2. *A variety of trocar designs. From left to right: pyramidal trocar (E.M.T. Warriewood, N.S.W.); shielded trocar (Versaport, Tyco, Norwalk, CT); conical trocar (Seperator, Applied Medical, Santa Margarita, CA); conical trocar and obturator (Step, Tyco, Norwalk, CT); optical access trocar (Optiview, Ethicon Endo-surgery, Cincinnati, OH).*

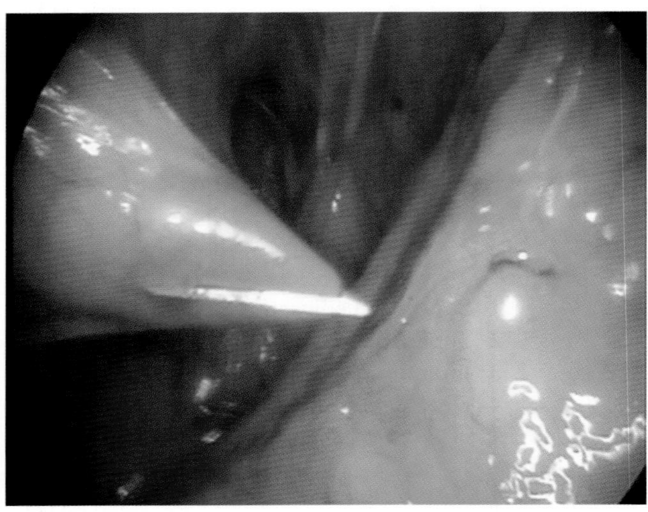

Figure 87.3. *The blade of a safety shield trocar, present momentarily prior to retracting, in an abdomen with adhesions.*

in the conical group as compared to 0.83% for the cutting trocar.

In more recent RCTs the radially expanding conical trocar had less cannula site bleeding, reduced pain, fewer wound complications and higher patient satisfaction compared to the pyramidal trocar.[24,25] Munro and Tarnay[26] recently demonstrated that the fascial and muscular defect from a 12 mm blunt trocar resulted in a fascial defect similar to the 8 mm pyramidal trocar and suggested that the fascial defects from 12 mm blunt trocars do not need closing, a view supported by others.[24,27]

Optical access trocars (see Fig. 87.2) are designed to decrease the injury to vessels and viscera by allowing the surgeon to visualize abdominal wall placement during entry. Two optical access systems are available – one utilizes a bladed trocar that strikes the fascia and peritoneum under vision, and the other utilizes a non-bladed trocar where a clear conical tip that is rotated under laparoscopic vision as it rotates through the layers. Sharp et al. describe 79 serious complications following optical access trocars, four of which were fatal and reported to the American Food and Drug Administration.[28] Only five of these were recorded in peer-reviewed literature. This report does not allow us to determine the incidence of these complications but more recent case series indicate an acceptable 0.3% entry-related complication rate using optical access trocars.[29,30]

An important advantage of laparoscopy over laparotomy is the lower rate of wound complications and hernias. In one study, the incidence of wound infection after open colposuspension was 11% as compared to 1% after the laparoscopic approach.[31] Magrina estimated that the incidence of trocar hernias after laparoscopic gynecology surgery was 10–100 times lower than laparotomy.[32] He found the incidence of hernia after laparoscopy ranged from 0.06 to 1% as compared to 13% 5 years after gynecologic laparotomy.

The incidence of incisional hernia increases to 3% with the use of 12 mm trocars.[33] It is largely accepted that while 5 mm trocars do not require fascial closure, when bladed trocars 10 mm or greater are utilized the defects should be closed to minimize the risk of bowel entrapment or incisional hernia. Preliminary studies have demonstrated that blunt trocars will significantly reduce the incidence of trocar site hernia[22] and many believe they do not need to be closed.[26,27]

Secondary trocars

Secondary trocars are required for operative laparoscopic surgery. The correct positioning of these trocars is vital to minimize damage to the vasculature of the anterior abdominal wall (see Fig. 87.1) and to allow laparoscopic suturing in a safe and biomechanically friendly position for the surgical team.

A thorough knowledge of the vasculature of the anterior abdominal wall is required to minimize and treat perforation of the vessels. The inferior epigastric artery arises from the external iliac artery and passes superior to the inguinal ligament, traveling superomedially just medial to the lateral edge of the rectus muscle. Its position deep to the rectus muscle and superior to the peritoneum allows for relatively easy laparoscopic localization (Fig. 87.4).

The superficial epigastric artery arises from the femoral artery near the inguinal ring and courses medially above the rectus muscle towards the midline. The smallest branch of the femoral artery, the superficial circumflex iliac artery, runs laterally to supply the skin and superficial fascia.

Perforation of the inferior epigastric artery will produce retroperitoneal or intraperitoneal bleeding; perforation of the superficial epigastric artery will result in intramuscular or subcutaneous bleeding. The deep circumflex iliac artery arises from the external iliac artery opposite the inferior epigastric artery and runs posterior to the inguinal canal to the anterior superior iliac spine where it anastomoses with a variety of vessels. Figure 87.1 demonstrates the course of the anterior abdominal wall vessels.

The surgeon can use transillumination for locating superficial abdominal wall vessels but intraperitoneal identification is required for the inferior epigastric artery. When the inferior epigastric artery is difficult to visualize, intra-abdominal landmarks can be helpful. It usually arises from the inguinal canal medial to the round ligament and travels cranially lateral to the obliterated umbilical arteries. The lower ports are placed as in Figure 87.1b and 87.1c lateral to the inferior epigastric and medial to the deep circumflex vessels. If further trocars are required they can be sited in the midline suprapubically or at the level of the umbilicus lateral to the edge of the rectus muscle. If a 10 mm trocar or greater is required for introducing mesh, the harmonic scalpel or the removal of pathology, this is placed either on the side of the surgeon or at the suprapubic site if utilized.

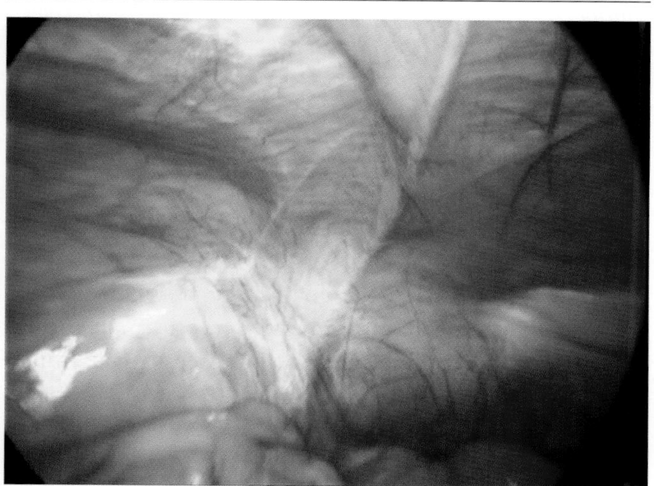

Figure 87.4. *Laparoscopic localization of the left inferior epigastric artery lateral to the obliterated umbilical artery.*

Even after these preventive measures are employed, experienced laparoscopic surgeons may still be faced with arterial bleeding from the inferior epigastric artery. The offending trocar should not be removed as this denotes the location of the artery that may become difficult to visualize as the hematoma spreads. If the bleeding is recognized early and the inferior epigastric artery can be identified, both ends of the transected vessel can be diathermied with bipolar forceps (Fig. 87.5a). If this is unsuccessful, a No. 12 Foley catheter can be passed through the 5 mm trocar and the Foley balloon inflated to 10–15 cm^3 with sterile water. The trocar is then removed over the catheter and firm traction secured with an umbilical cord clamp overnight (Fig. 87.5b). The following morning the clamp and catheter are removed. If this fails to secure the vessel, a CT-1 needle is passed through the abdominal wall into the abdomen and passed from inside the abdomen to the outside using laparoscopic needle holders and tied both cephalad and caudad to the trocar. The sutures are removed the following morning (Fig. 87.5c).

BOWEL INJURIES

The incidence of bowel injuries at gynecologic laparoscopy varies from zero to 5%.[7,34] Approximately 50% of these injuries occur during entry,[3,8,35] with the large and small bowel being equally involved.[4,36] As there appears to be no significant difference in the rate of bowel injuries with either the closed or open approach to entry, little can be done to minimize the occurrence of injury, although some surgeons believe that the damage may be more readily detected intraoperatively with the open technique.[37] After reviewing the literature, Magrina calculated that only 43% of bowel injuries at laparoscopic surgery were diagnosed intraoperatively.[32] The mortality rate from bowel injuries in gynecologic laparoscopy ranges from 2.5 to 5%[38] but this has been shown to increase to 21% in those with a delayed diagnosis of bowel injury.[39]

If there is a recognized Veress injury to the bowel at the time of surgery and there is no associated fecal spill, it is likely that the injury can be managed expectantly. Although no clear guidelines exist in nine cases of Veress injuries to the bowel treated expectantly, there were no complications.[1,8,35] Trocar damage to the small bowel mandates careful inspection of the whole bowel to ensure no through-and-through injuries have occurred. Simple small injuries to the small and large bowel should be repaired in one or two layers of inter-

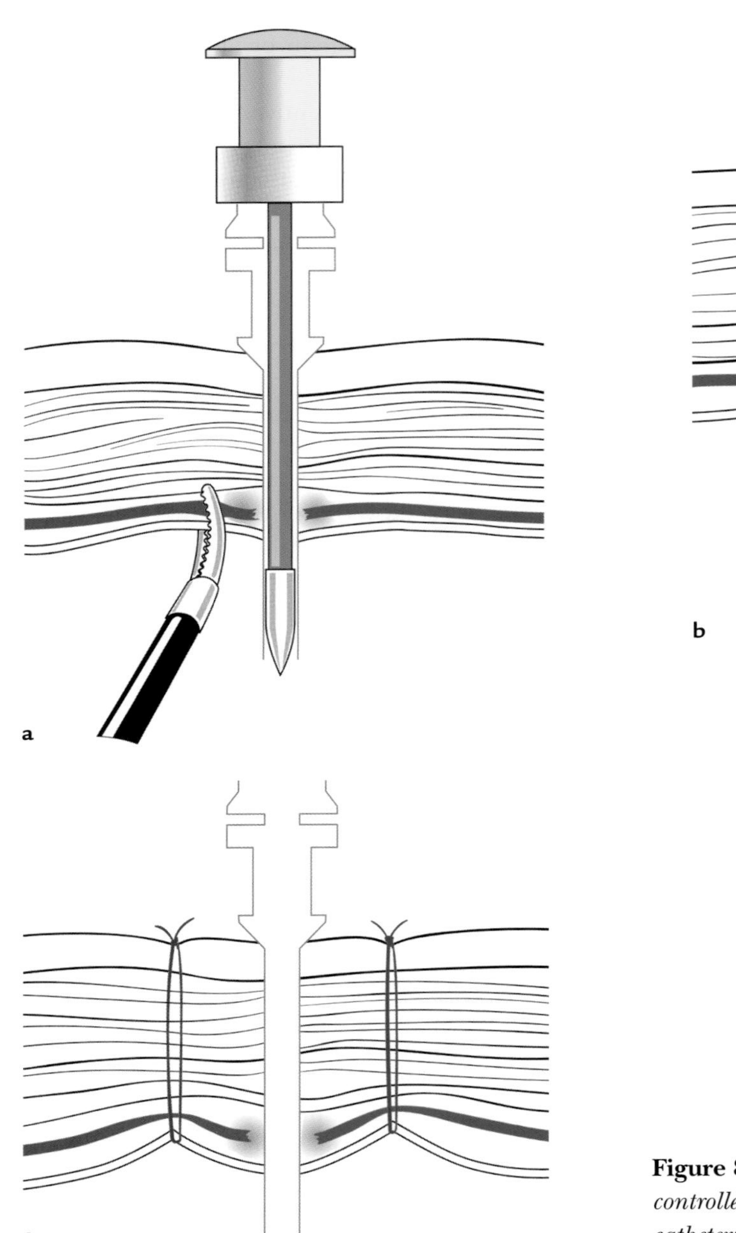

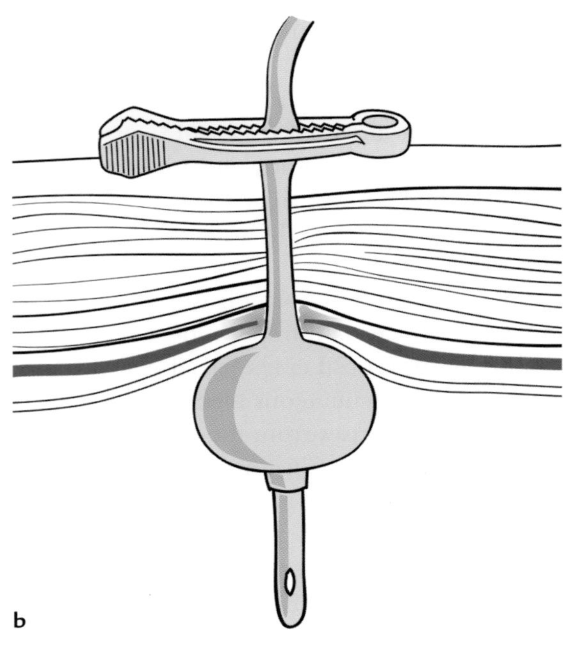

Figure 87.5. *Bleeding inferior epigastric artery: (a) controlled with bipolar diathermy; (b) tamponaded with Foley catheter; (c) sutured. (© Maher/Francis.)*

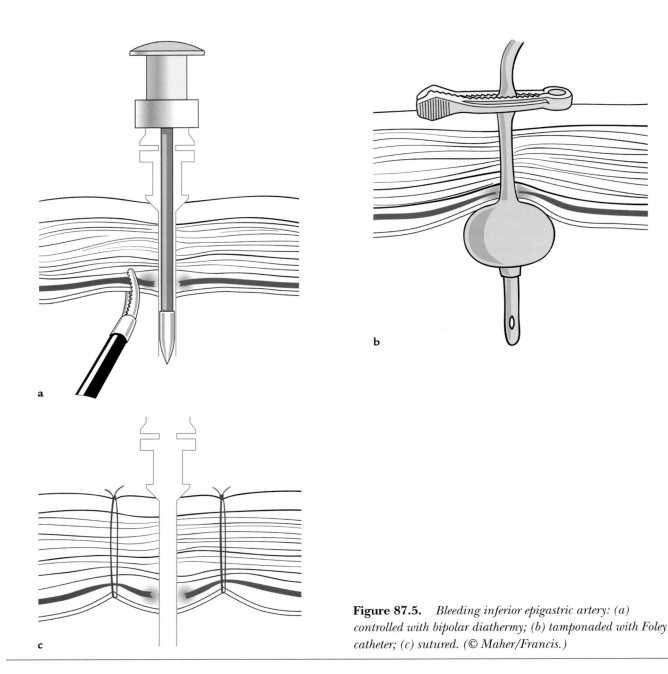

rupted sutures, the pelvis irrigated, and antibiotics commenced. Postoperatively, the patient is kept nil by mouth until flatus is passed.

Electrosurgical injuries are more commonly seen in bowel injuries that are diagnosed postoperatively. Brosens et al. estimated that the average time to diagnosis after needle or trocar injury to bowel was 1.3 days as compared to 10.4 days for electrosurgical burns.[39]

Electrical injuries to the intestine are not always diagnosed intraoperatively or their appearance leads the surgeon towards conservative treatment.[40] It is suggested that burns less than 5 mm in diameter can be treated expectantly.[41] If the area of blanching exceeds 5 mm it is estimated that thermal damage may exceed up to 5 cm from the apparent injury, and resection should be considered.[42]

In patients returning after discharge with bowel damage or bowel obstruction, pre- and intraoperative evaluation by a general surgical colleague is advisable. Damaged bowel must be repaired or resected with or without a temporary colostomy. All necrotic tissue should be removed to minimize the risk of abscess formation.

The most significant reduction in bowel complications during laparoscopic pelvic floor surgery will arise from preventing injury. The focus of attention should lie on careful adhesiolysis and enterolysis, and the detection of injuries intraoperatively rather than postoperatively. During adhesiolysis and enterolysis sharp dissection with minimal diathermy will be beneficial in preventing inadvertent bowel damage. Careful inspection of the bowel for hematoma or serosal damage that may suggest breaches of the mucosa, and the performance of the underwater test if there is any concern regarding the integrity of the bowel, are all useful in facilitating intraoperative rather than postoperative diagnosis of bowel damage. The underwater test involves holding any area of bowel suspected of damage under warmed saline to look for gas or bowel leakage. If the laparoscopic pelvic floor surgeon is faced with an abdomen of morbidly dense adhesions it may be prudent to remember that in a large prospective randomized controlled trial the vaginal approach to vault prolapse has been shown to be equally as effective as the abdominal route[43] and the conversion to the vaginal approach may be the safest approach. At laparoscopic sacral colpopexy four (1.5%) bowel injuries in 261 cases were reported. A rectal[44] and a colon[45] injury were repaired laparoscopically without sequelae and two small bowel injuries were diagnosed postoperatively and underwent subsequent laparotomy.[46]

Bowel preparation prior to surgery was utilized: 1) to remove the bulky intraluminal contents to improve surgical field vision and bowel handling; and 2) to decrease the risk of peritoneal and wound contamination if the bowel was inadvertently opened. Neither of these beliefs has been confirmed in randomized controlled trials in elective operative gynecology[47] or colorectal surgery.[48]

Finally, improving the laparoscopic experience of the surgeon may prove to be one of the simplest means of minimizing morbidity associated with bowel injuries at gynecologic laparoscopy. Brosens and Gordon reported that a gynecologist performing fewer than 100 laparoscopies a year had a five times higher rate of bowel injuries than those performing more than a 100 laparoscopies a year.[35] Skills can be improved in a variety of ways including training programs, skills workshops, and operating with colleagues.

INJURIES TO THE BLADDER

Inadvertent cystotomy has been reported in 4% of laparoscopic colposuspensions.[49] In 261 laparoscopic sacral colpopexies published, five (1.9%) inadvertent cystotomies were reported, all of which were repaired laparoscopically at the initial surgery without complication.[44–46] A gas-filled urinary bag or blood in the urine indicates bladder trauma until proven otherwise; this warrants careful laparoscopic inspection of the bladder distended to 300 ml and cystoscopy. Cystotomies should be repaired in two layers so that the bladder is watertight at 300 ml. Post-repair cystoscopy should be performed with the laparoscope in place, to ensure that there are no other unrecognized injuries and that the ureters are patent.

After a watertight cystotomy repair the catheter can safely be removed at 4 days.[46] If concomitant continence surgery is performed, nursing staff and the patient should be vigilant during the voiding trial to ensure that the bladder is not grossly overdistended.

Some surgeons believe that postoperative cystoscopy is vital to minimize lower urinary tract complications following pelvic floor surgery so that unrecognized cystotomy may be repaired to prevent vesicovaginal fistula.[50]

URETERIC INJURIES

Ureteric injuries following pelvic floor surgery are reported in 3% of cases.[51,52] The morbidity associated with ureteric injury can be dramatically reduced if identified intraoperatively using postoperative cystoscopy and intravenous indigo carmine.[51,52] If indigo carmine is not clearly visible following laparoscopic pelvic floor repair, the injury is likely to be related to kinking of the ureter in the lateral retropubic space or in relation to the uterosacral/cardinal ligament sutures during sacral colpopexy or vault suspending procedures. Lateral retropubic or vault suspending sutures should be removed one at a time until ureteric patency is obtained. The sutures are then replaced at a lower level and ureteric patency again confirmed. If patency is not confirmed with the removal of the sutures, retrograde dye studies and intraoperative urologic consultation is required.

Laparoscopic hysterectomy is associated with a 0.7–1.4% risk of ureteric injury[3,53] which is at least 10 times greater than at vaginal hysterectomy.[8] Most of these injuries are related to clamping, incision or diathermy damage. Ureteric injuries related to concomitant laparoscopic hysterectomy usually require ureteric reimplantation by urologic colleagues.

COMPLICATIONS RELATED TO PNEUMOPERITONEUM

Subcutaneous emphysema arises as carbon dioxide leaks into or is absorbed by subcutaneous tissue. Leaks to the extraperitoneal tissues can occur at entry, with opening of extraperitoneal spaces or through existing undetected herniae. The laparoscopic sacrocolpopexy involves significant retroperitoneal dissection, increasing the risk of subcutaneous emphysema that is usually quite innocuous. Significant or sudden subcutaneous emphysema around the face, neck, and chest must alert the physician to the possibility of mediastinal emphysema. This usually arises from a congenital defect of the diaphragm but can also occur after trauma associated with upper abdominal surgery.

Gas embolism can occur if gas enters the vascular system and usually occurs during or shortly after insufflation. The sudden development of hypotension, bradycardia or arrhythmias at this time should immediately raise the suspicion of gas embolism. While relatively rare, occurring in only 0.0014%,[13] the mortality rate is as high as 28%.[54] The pneumoperitoneum should be released and the procedure abandoned as soon as feasible.

ANETHESTIC COMPLICATIONS

The gynecologist must be aware of the cardiovascular changes associated with operative laparoscopy. Most of the changes are due to establishment and maintenance of pneumoperitoneum or Trendelenburg positioning. Carbon dioxide remains the most widely used distension medium but is rapidly absorbed from the peritoneum and may cause hypercarbia and acidosis. Hypercarbia is associated with arrhythmias, increased cardiac output, and decreased systemic vascular resistance. Hyperventilation minimizes the impact of hypercarbia.

Steep Trendelenburg may be required for posterior compartment or vault suspending procedures, and results in increased central venous pressure and decreased arterial pressure and cardiac output. Atelectasis and decreased pulmonary compliance can occur but are usually well controlled with general anesthesia, neuromuscular blockade, endotracheal intubation, and controlled ventilation. Both pneumoperitoneum and Trendelenburg positioning reduce femoral venous flow, increasing the risk of thrombotic complications.

CONCLUSION

Laparoscopic pelvic floor surgery affords the surgeon and the patient significant advantages; however, complications related to obtaining access, surgeon inexperience, and associated laparoscopic hysterectomy can occur. The judicious use of the open approach or access via the left upper quadrant may be beneficial in minimizing access-related complications. Newer bladeless trocars may also act to decrease morbidity associated with access.

Careful dissection during adhesiolysis and cautious and appropriate use of energy sources such as diathermy will decrease bowel injuries. Vigilance during surgery is required to detect and manage complications intraoperatively, rather than postoperatively.

Finally, experienced operating room staff – including assistants, scrub sisters, and anesthetists, who are well trained and enthusiastic in laparoscopic surgery – are vital to assist in avoiding complications associated with laparoscopic pelvic floor surgery.

REFERENCES

1. Jansen FW, Kolkman W, Bakkum EA et al. Complications of laparoscopy: an inquiry about closed- versus open-entry technique. Am J Obstet Gynecol 2004;190:634–8.
2. Miranda CS, Carvajal AR. Complications of operative gynecological laparoscopy. JSLS 2003;7:53–8.
3. Harkki Siren P, Sjoberg J, Kurki T. Major complications of laparoscopy: a follow-up Finnish study. Obstet Gynecol 1999;94:94–8.
4. Chapron C, Querleu D, Bruhat MA et al. Surgical complications of diagnostic and operative gynaecological laparoscopy: a series of 29,966 cases. Hum Reprod 1998;13:867–72.
5. Leonard F, Lecuru F, Rizk E, Chasset S, Robin F, Taurelle R. Perioperative morbidity of gynecological laparoscopy. A prospective monocenter observational study. Acta Obstet Gynecol Scand 2000;79:129–34.
6. MacCordick C, Lecuru F, Rizk E, Robin F, Boucaya V, Taurelle R. Morbidity in laparoscopic gynecological surgery: results of a prospective single-center study. Surg Endosc 1999;13:57–61.
7. Quasarano RT, Kashef M, Sherman SJ, Hagglund KH. Complications of gynecologic laparoscopy. J Am Assoc Gynecol Laparosc 1999;6:317–21.
8. Harkki Siren P, Kurki T. A nationwide analysis of laparoscopic complications. Obstet Gynecol 1997;89:108–12.
9. Jansen FW, Kapiteyn K, Trimbos Kemper T, Hermans J, Trimbos JB. Complications of laparoscopy: a prospective multicentre observational study. Br J Obstet Gynaecol 1997;104:595–600.
10. McMahon AJ, Baxter JN, O'Dwyer PJ. Preventing complications of laparoscopy. Br J Surg 1993;80:1593–4.
11. Tsaltas J, Healy DL, Lloyd D. Review of major complications of laparoscopy in a free standing gynaecologic day care hospital. Gynecol Endosc 1996;5:265–70.
12. Chapron CM, Pierre F, La Croix S, Querleu D, Lansac J, Dubuisson JB. Major vascular injuries during gynecologic laparoscopy. J Am Coll Surg 1997;185:461–5.
13. Bonjer HJ, Hazebroek EJ, Kazemier G, Giuffrida MC, Meijer WS, Lange JF. Open versus closed establishment of pneumoperitoneum in laparoscopic surgery. Br J Surg 1997;84:599–602.
14. Cogliandolo A, Manganaro T, Saitta FP, Micali B. Blind versus open approach to laparoscopic cholecystectomy: a randomized study. Surg Laparosc Endosc 1998;8:353–5.

15. Peitgen K, Nimtz K, Hellinger A, Walz MK. Open approach or Veress needle in laparoscopic interventions. Results of a prospective randomized controlled trial. Chirurg 1997;68:910–3.

16. Audebert AJ, Gomel V. Role of microlaparoscopy in the diagnosis of peritoneal and visceral adhesions and in the prevention of bowel injury associated with blind trocar insertion. Fertil Steril 2000;73:631–5.

17. Phillips G, Whittaker M, Garry R. The depth of the pneumoperitoneum determines the safety of primary cannula insertion. J Am Assoc Gynecol Laparosc 1996;3(Suppl 4): S39–40.

18. Parker J, Reid G, Wong F. Microlaparoscopic left upper quadrant entry in patients at high risk of periumbilical adhesions. Aust N Z J Obstet Gynaecol 1999;39:88–92.

19. Patsner B. Laparoscopy using the left upper quadrant approach. J Am Assoc Gynecol Laparosc 1999;6:323–5.

20. Bhoyrul S, Vierra MA, Nezhat CR, Krummel TM, Way LW. Trocar injuries in laparoscopic surgery. J Am Coll Surg 2001;192:677–83.

21. Bohm B, Knigge M, Kraft M, Grundel K, Boenick U. Influence of different trocar tips on abdominal wall penetration during laparoscopy. Surg Endosc 1998;12:1434–8.

22. Bhoyrul S, Mori T, Way LW. Radially expanding dilatation. A superior method of laparoscopic trocar access. Surg Endosc 1996;10:775–8.

23. Leibl BJ, Schmedt CG, Schwarz J, Kraft K, Bittner R. Laparoscopic surgery complications associated with trocar tip design: review of literature and own results. J Laparoendosc Adv Surg Tech A 1999;9:135–40.

24. Bhoyrul S, Payne J, Steffes B, Swanstrom L, Way LW. A randomized prospective study of radially expanding trocars in laparoscopic surgery. J Gastrointest Surg 2000;4:392–7.

25. Yim SF, Yuen PM. Randomized double-masked comparison of radially expanding access device and conventional cutting tip trocar in laparoscopy. Obstet Gynecol 2001;97:435–8.

26. Munro MG, Tarnay CM. The impact of trocar-cannula design and simulated operative manipulation on incisional characteristics: a randomized trial. Obstet Gynecol 2004;103:681–5.

27. Liu CD, McFadden DW. Laparoscopic port sites do not require fascial closure when nonbladed trocars are used. Am Surg 2000;66:853–4.

28. Sharp HT, Dodson MK, Draper ML, Watts DA, Doucette RC, Hurd WW. Complications associated with optical-access laparoscopic trocars. Obstet Gynecol 2002;99:553–5.

29. Thomas MA, Rha KH, Ong AM et al. Optical access trocar injuries in urological laparoscopic surgery. J Urol 2003;170:61–3.

30. String A, Berber E, Foroutani A, Macho JR, Pearl JM, Siperstein AE. Use of the optical access trocar for safe and rapid entry in various laparoscopic procedures. Surg Endosc 2001;15:570–3.

31. Lavin JM, Lewis CJ, Foote AJ. Laparoscopic Burch colposuspension: a minimum 2-year follow-up and comparison with open colposuspension. Gynaecol Endosc 1998;7:251–8.

32. Magrina JF. Complications of laparoscopic surgery. Clin Obstet Gynecol 2002;45:469–80.

33. Kadar N, Reich H, Liu CY, Manko GF, Gimpelson R. Incisional hernias after major laparoscopic gynecologic procedures. Am J Obstet Gynecol 1993;168:1493–5.

34. Mirhashemi R, Harlow BL, Ginsburg ES, Signorello LB, Berkowitz R, Feldman S. Predicting risk of complications with gynecologic laparoscopic surgery. Obstet Gynecol 1998;92:327–31.

35. Brosens I, Gordon A. Bowel injuries during gynaecological laparoscopy. A multinational survey. Gynaecol Endosc 2001;10:141–5.

36. Chapron C, Pierre F, Harchaoui Y et al. Gastrointestinal injuries during gynaecological laparoscopy. Hum Reprod 1999;14:333–7.

37. Perone A. Laparoscopy using a simple open technique: a review of 585 cases. J Reprod Med 1985;30:660–3.

38. Champault G, Cazacu F, Taffinder N. Serious trocar accidents in laparoscopic surgery: a French survey of 103,852 operations. Surg Laparosc Endosc 1996;6(5):367–70.

39. Brosens I, Gordon A, Campo R, Gordts S. Bowel injury in gynecologic laparoscopy. J Am Assoc Gynecol Laparosc 2003;10:9–13.

40. Levy BS, Soderstrom RM, Dail DH. Bowel injuries during laparoscopy: Gross anatomy and histology. J Reprod Med 1985;30:168–72.

41. Nezhat C, Siegler AM, Nezhat FR, Nezhat C, Seidman DS, Luciano AA. Operative Gynecology Laparoscopy: Principles, Techniques and Complications. New York: McGraw-Hill, 2000.

42. Wheeless CR. Gastrointestinal injuries associated with laparoscopy. In: Phillips JM (ed) Endoscopy in Gynecology. Baltimore: Williams and Wilkins, 1978.

43. Maher CF, Qatawneh AM, Dwyer PL, Carey MP, Cornish A, Schluter PJ. Abdominal sacral colpopexy or vaginal sacrospinous colpopexy for vaginal vault prolapse: a prospective randomized study. Am J Obstet Gynecol 2004;190:20–6.

44. Cosson M, Bogaert E, Narducci F, Querleu D, Crepin G. Promontofixation coelioscopique: resultats a court terme et complications chez 83 patientes. J Gynecol Obstet Biol Reprod (Paris) 2000;29:746–50.

45. Bruyere F, Rozenberg H, Abdelkader T. La promonto-fixation sous coelioscopie: une voie d'abord seduisante pour la cure des prolapsus. Prog Urol 2001;11:1320–6.

46. Antiphon P, Elard S, Benyoussef A et al. Laparoscopic

promontory sacral colpopexy: is the posterior, recto-vaginal, mesh mandatory? Eur Urol 2004;45:655–61.

47. Muzii L, Angioli R, Zullo MA, Calcagno M, Panici PB. Bowel preparation for gynecological surgery. Crit Rev Oncol Hematol 2003;48:311–5.
48. Miettinen RP, Laitinen ST, Makela JT, Paakkonen ME. Bowel preparation with oral polyethylene glycol electrolyte solution vs. no preparation in elective open colorectal surgery: prospective, randomized study. Dis Colon Rectum 2000;43:669–75.
49. Smith AR, Stanton SL. Laparoscopic colposuspension. Br J Obstet Gynaecol 1998;105:383–4.
50. Cook JR, Seman EI, O'Shea RT. Laparoscopic treatment of enterocele: a 3-year evaluation. Aust N Z J Obstet Gynaecol 2004;44:107–10.
51. Harris RL, Cundiff GW, Theofrastous JP, Yoon H, Bump RC, Addison WA. The value of intraoperative cystoscopy in urogynecologic and reconstructive pelvic surgery. Am J Obstet Gynecol 1997;177:1367–9.
52. Jabs CF, Drutz HP. The role of intraoperative cystoscopy in prolapse and incontinence surgery. Am J Obstet Gynecol 2001;185:1368–71.
53. Garry R, Fountain J, Brown J et al. EVALUATE hysterectomy trial: a multicentre randomised trial comparing abdominal, vaginal and laparoscopic methods of hysterectomy. Health Technol Assess 2004;8:1–154.
54. Cottin V, Delafosse B, Viale JP. Gas embolism during laparoscopy. A report of seven cases in patients with previous abdominal surgical history. Surg Endosc 1996;10:166–9.

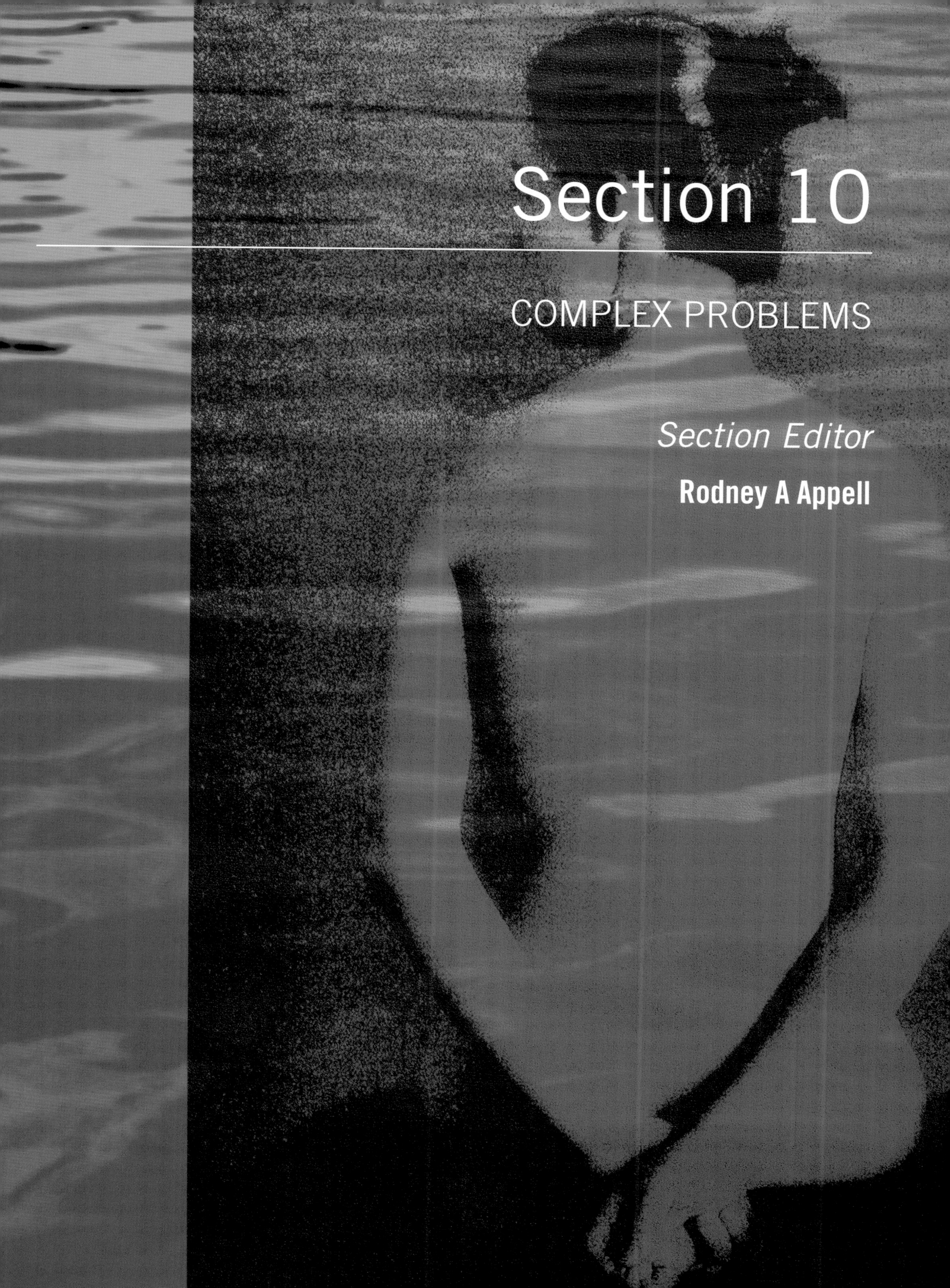

Section 10

COMPLEX PROBLEMS

Section Editor

Rodney A Appell

88

Urogenital fistulae – surgical

Paul Hilton

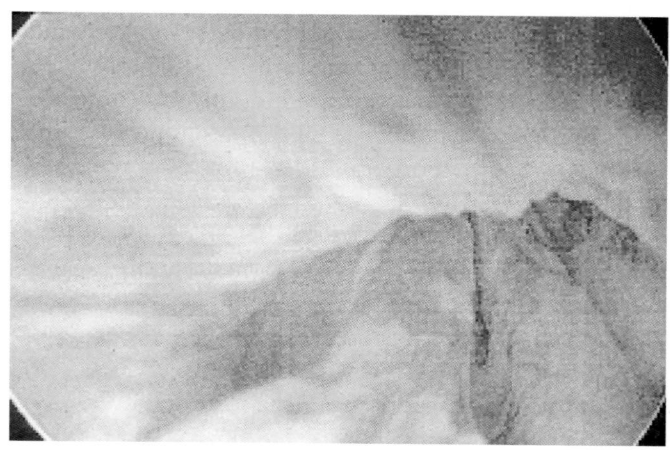

ETIOLOGY AND EPIDEMIOLOGY

Urogenital fistulae may occur congenitally, but are most often acquired from obstetric, surgical, radiation, malignant, and miscellaneous causes. In most third world countries over 90% of fistulae are of obstetric etiology,[1–4] whereas in the UK and USA over 70% follow pelvic surgery[5,6] (Table 88.1). Obstetric fistulae are covered in Chapter 89; this chapter deals primarily with surgical fistulae.

Urogenital fistulae may occur following a wide range of surgical procedures within the pelvis (Fig. 88.1). It is often supposed that this complication results from direct injury to the lower urinary tract at the time of operation. Certainly on occasions this may be the case; careless, hurried, or rough surgical technique makes injury to the lower urinary tract much more likely. However, of 233 urogenital fistulae referred to the author over the last 17 years, 156 (66.9%) have been associated with pelvic surgery, and 118 (50.6%) followed hysterectomy; of these only five (4.2%) presented with leakage of urine on the first day postoperatively. In other cases it is presumed that tissue devascularization during dissection, inadvertent suture placement, infection or pelvic hematoma formation developing postoperatively results in tissue necrosis, with leakage developing most usually between 5 and 14 days later. Overdistension of the bladder postoperatively may be an additional factor in many of these latter cases. It has been shown that there is a high incidence of abnormalities of lower urinary tract function in fistula patients;[7] whether these abnormalities antedate the surgery, or develop with or as a consequence of the fistula, is unclear. It is likely that patients with a habit of infrequent voiding, or those with inefficient detrusor contractility, may be at increased risk of postoperative urinary retention. If this is not recognized early and managed appropriately, the risk of fistula formation may be increased.

Although it is important to remember that the majority of surgical fistulae follow apparently straightforward hysterectomy in skilled hands, several risk factors may be identified, making direct injury more likely (Table 88.2). Obviously anatomic distortion within the pelvis by ovarian tumor or fibroid will increase the surgical difficulty, and abnormal adhesions between bladder and uterus or cervix following previous surgery, or associated with previous sepsis, endometriosis or malignancy, may make fistula formation more likely. Preoperative or early radiotherapy may decrease vascularity, and make the tissues in general less forgiving of poor technique.

Issues of training and surgical technique are also important. The ability to locate and if necessary dissect out the ureter must be part of routine gynecologic training, as should the first aid management of lower urinary tract injury when it arises. The use of gauze swabs to separate the bladder from the cervix at cesarean section or hysterectomy should be discouraged; sharp dissection with knife or scissors does less harm, especially where the tissues are abnormally adherent.

PREVALENCE

The prevalence of genital fistulae obviously varies from country to country and continent to continent as the main causative factors vary. Data from the Regional Health Authority Information Units in England and Wales suggests an average of 10 fistula repairs per health region per year over the last few years, and a national figure of approximately 152 repair procedures per year.[8]

The rate of fistula formation following hysterectomy in the UK has been variously estimated at between 1 in 640 operations[5] and 1 in 1300 operations (Lawson J, 1990, personal communication). Using the above figure of 152 fistula repair procedures per year, of which 50% can be assumed to follow hysterectomy, at a time when approximately 72,000 hysterectomies were undertaken annually in England and Wales, would indicate a fistula rate of approximately 1 in 950 hysterectomies. This is comparable with the figure reported from health insurance data from Finland.[9] Following laparoscopic assisted vaginal hysterectomy, the incidence of fistula development may approach 1%.[10–12] Figures of between 1 and 4% fistulae have been reported following radical hysterectomy,[13,14] with a similar incidence following radiation for gynecologic malignancies.[15] The incidence of fistula formation following pelvic exenteration may be as high as 10%.[16]

CLASSIFICATION

Many different fistula classifications have been described in the literature on the basis of anatomical site; these may include urethral, bladder neck, subsymphysial (a complex form involving circumferential loss of the urethra with fixity to bone), midvaginal, juxtacervical or vault fistulae, massive fistulae extending from bladder neck to vault, and vesicouterine or vesicocervical fistulae. While over 60% of fistulae in the third world are midvaginal, juxtacervical or massive (reflecting their obstetric etiology), such cases are relatively rare in Western fistula practice; by contrast, 50% of the fistulae managed in the UK are situated in the vaginal vault (reflecting their surgical etiology).[5] Cases are often subclassified into simple cases (where the tissues are healthy

Table 88.1. ***Etiology of urogenital fistulae in two series, from north-east of England (Hilton, unpublished) and from south-east Nigeria****

	NE England (*n*=233)		SE Nigeria (*n*=2389)[†]	
Etiology	%	*n*	%	*n*
obstructed labor		7		1918
cesarean section		11		165
ruptured uterus		8		119
forceps/ventouse		4		
breech extraction		1		
symphysiotomy		1		
placental abruption		1		
Obstetric	14.2	33	92.2	2202
abdominal hysterectomy		97		33
radical hysterectomy		13		
vaginal hysterectomy		4		25
LAVH		3		
cesarean hysterectomy		1		
cervical stumpectomy		2		
laparoscopic oophorectomy		1		
colporrhaphy		5		35
cystoplasty		3		
colposuspension		3		
sling		1		
needle suspension		1		
urethral diverticulectomy		11		
subtrigonal phenol injection		1		
nephroureterectomy		2		
lithoclast		1		
colectomy		5		
unknown surgery in childhood		1		
suture to vaginal laceration				12
Surgical	66.9	156	4.4	105
Radiation	8.6	20	0.0	0
Malignancy	0.0	0	1.8	42
foreign body		6		
uncertain		6		
vaginal pessary		4		
catheter associated		2		
trauma		2		11
infection		1		7
congenital		3		
coital injury				22
Miscellaneous	10.3	24	1.7	40
Total	100.0	233	100.0	2389

* Data from ref. 2.
† 2389 patients for whom notes could be examined, out of a total series of 2484 patients.
LAVH, laparoscopically assisted vaginal hysterectomy.

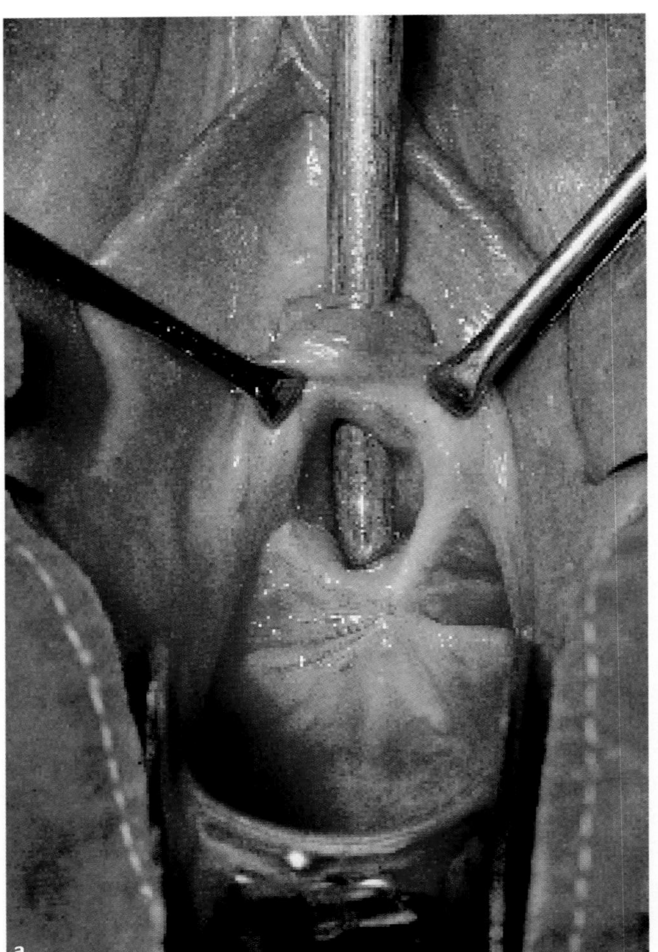

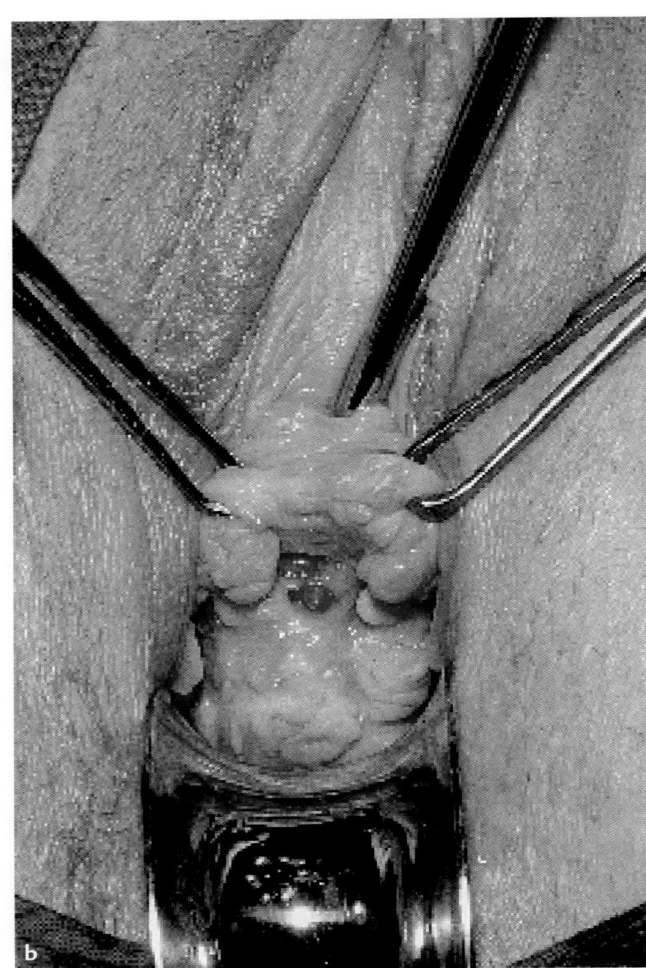

Figure 88.1. *Postoperative urogenital fistulae following: (a) anterior colporrhaphy; (b) urethral diverticulectomy.*

Table 88.2. ***Risk factors for postoperative fistulae***

Risk factor	Pathology	Specific example
Anatomical distortion		Fibroids Ovarian mass
Abnormal tissue adhesion	Inflammation	Infection Endometriosis
	Previous surgery	Cesarean section Cone biopsy Colporrhaphy
	Malignancy	
Impaired vascularity	Ionizing radiation Metabolic abnormality Radical surgery	Preoperative radiotherapy Diabetes mellitus
Compromised healing		Anemia Nutritional deficiency
Abnormality of bladder function		Voiding dysfunction

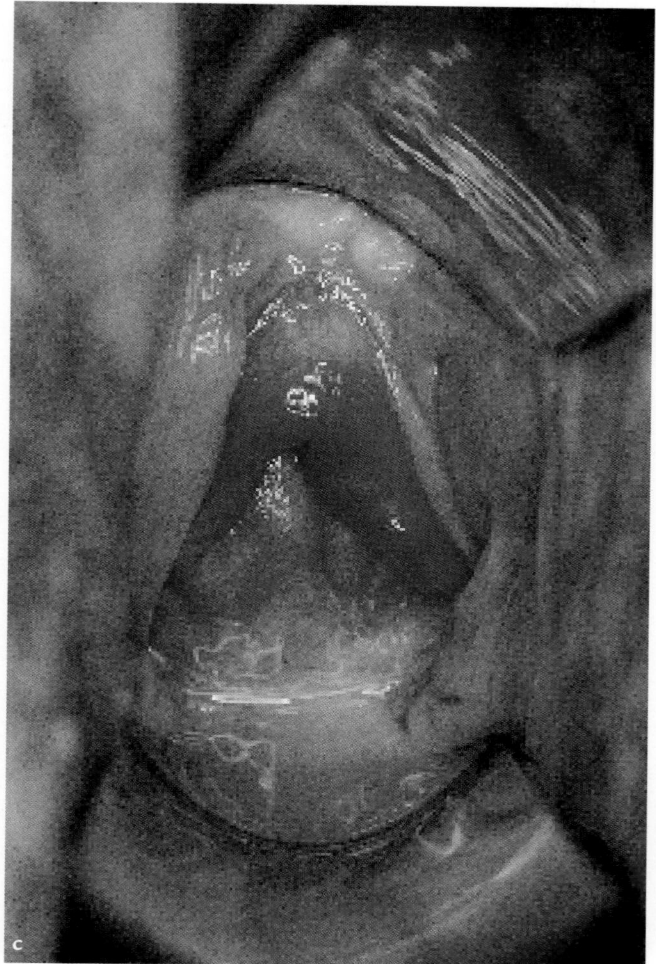

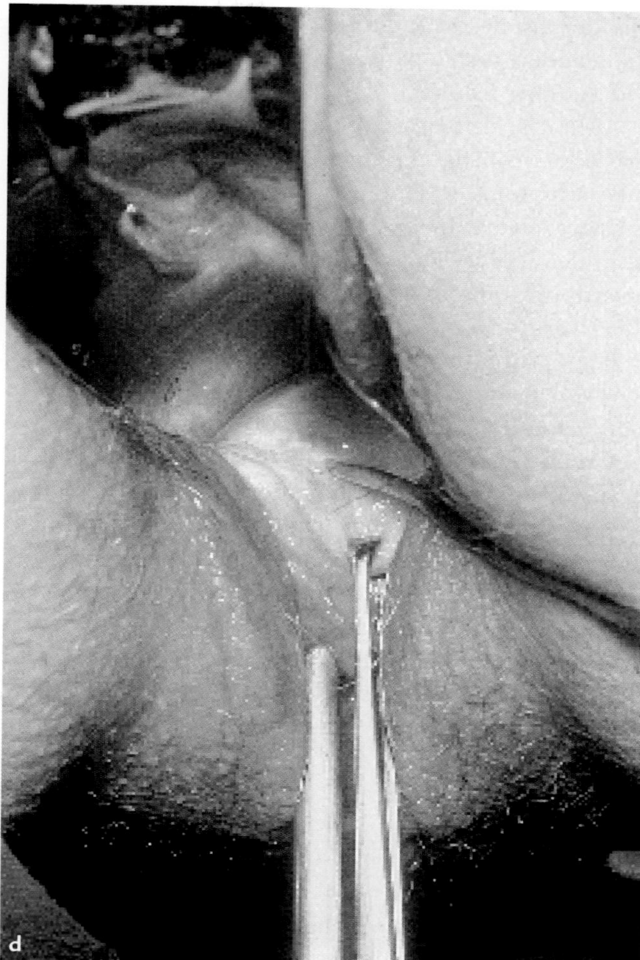

Figure 88.1. *Postoperative urogenital fistulae following (cont.): (c) radical hysterectomy; (d) colposuspension (the fistula in the latter case was fixed retropubically in the midline at the bladder neck, and the photograph shows the patient prone, in the reverse lithotomy position).*

and access good) or complicated (where there is tissue loss, scarring, impaired access, involvement of the ureteric orifices, or the presence of coexistent rectovaginal fistula). An alternative classification, based on the extent of sphincter involvement in longitudinal and circumferential aspects, has been proposed by Waaldijk;[17] this has the potential benefit of being more informative of both treatment and prognosis.

PRESENTATION

Fistulae between the urinary tract and the female genital tract are characteristically said to present with continuous urinary incontinence, with limited sensation of bladder fullness, and with infrequent voiding. Where there is extensive tissue loss, as in obstetric or radiation fistulae, this typical history is usually present, the clinical findings gross, and the diagnosis rarely in doubt. With postsurgical fistulae, however, the history may be atypical and the orifice small, elusive or occasionally completely invisible. Under these circumstances the diagnosis can be much more difficult, and a high index of clinical suspicion must be maintained.

Occasionally a patient with an obvious fistula may deny incontinence, and this is presumed to reflect the ability of the levator ani muscles to occlude the vagina below the level of the fistula. Some patients with a vesicocervical or a vesicouterine fistula following cesarean section may maintain continence at the level of the uterine isthmus, and complain of cyclical hematuria at the time of menstruation, or menouria.[18,19] In other cases patients may complain of little more than a watery vaginal discharge, or intermittent leakage which seems posturally related. Leakage may appear to occur specifically on standing or on lying supine, prone, or in left or right lateral positions, presumably reflecting the degree of bladder distension and the position of the fistula within the bladder; such a pattern is most unlikely to be found with ureteric fistulae.

Although in the case of direct surgical injury leakage may occur from day one, in most surgical and obstetric fistulae symptoms develop between 5 and 14 days after the causative injury; however, the time of presentation may be quite variable. This will depend to some extent on the severity of symptoms, but as far as obstetric fistulae in the third world are concerned, is determined more by access to health care. In a recent review of cases from Nigeria, the average time for presentation was over 5 years, and in some cases over 35 years, after the causative pregnancy.[2]

Urethrovaginal fistulae distal to the sphincter mechanism will often be asymptomatic, and require no specific treatment. Some may lead to obstruction, and are more likely to present with postmicturition dribbling than other types of incontinence; they can therefore be very difficult to recognize. More proximally situated urethral fistulae are perhaps most likely to present with stress incontinence, since bladder neck competence is frequently impaired.

INVESTIGATIONS

If there is suspicion of a fistula, but its presence is not easily confirmed by clinical examination with a Sims' speculum, further investigation will be necessary to confirm or fully exclude the possibility. Even where the diagnosis is clinically obvious, additional investigation may be appropriate for full evaluation prior to deciding treatment. The main principles of investigation therefore are:

- to confirm that the discharge is urinary;
- to establish that the leakage is extraurethral rather than urethral;
- to establish the site of leakage;
- to exclude multiple fistulae.

Biochemistry and microbiology

Excessive vaginal discharge or the drainage of serum from a pelvic hematoma postoperatively may simulate a urinary fistula. If the fluid is in sufficient quantity to be collected, biochemical analysis of its urea content in comparison to that of urine and serum will confirm its origin.

Urinary infection is surprisingly uncommon in fistula patients; however, especially where there have been previous attempts at surgery, urine culture should be undertaken and appropriate antibiotic therapy instituted.

Dye studies

Although other imaging techniques undoubtedly have a role (see below), carefully conducted dye studies remain the investigation of first choice. Phenazopyridine may be used orally, or indigo carmine intravenously, to stain the urine and hence confirm the presence of a fistula. The identification of the site of a fistula is best carried out by the instillation of colored dye (methylene blue or indigo carmine) into the bladder via a catheter with the patient in the lithotomy position. The traditional 'three swab test' has its limitations and is not recommended. The examination is best carried out with direct inspection, and multiple fistulae may be located in this way. If leakage of clear fluid continues after dye instillation, a ureteric fistula is likely, and this is most easily confirmed by a 'two dye test', using phenazopyridine to stain the renal urine, and methylene blue to stain bladder contents.[20]

Imaging

Excretion urography

Although intravenous urography is a particularly insensitive investigation in the diagnosis of vesicovaginal fistula, knowledge of upper urinary tract status may have a significant influence on treatment measures applied, and should therefore be looked on as an essential investigation for any suspected or confirmed urinary fistula. Compromise to ureteric function is a particularly common finding when a fistula occurs in relation to malignant disease or its treatment (by radiation or surgery).

Dilation of the ureter is characteristic in ureteric fistula, and its finding in association with a known vesicovaginal fistula should raise suspicion of a complex ureterovesicovaginal lesion (Fig. 88.2). While essential for the diagnosis of ureteric fistula, intravenous urography is not completely sensitive; the presence of a periureteric flare is, however, highly suggestive of extravasation at this site.

Retrograde pyelography

Retrograde pyelography is a more reliable way of identifying the exact site of a ureterovaginal fistula, and may be undertaken simultaneously with either retrograde or percutaneous catheterization for therapeutic stenting of the ureter.

Cystography

Cystography is not particularly helpful in the basic diagnosis of vesicovaginal fistulae, and a dye test carried out

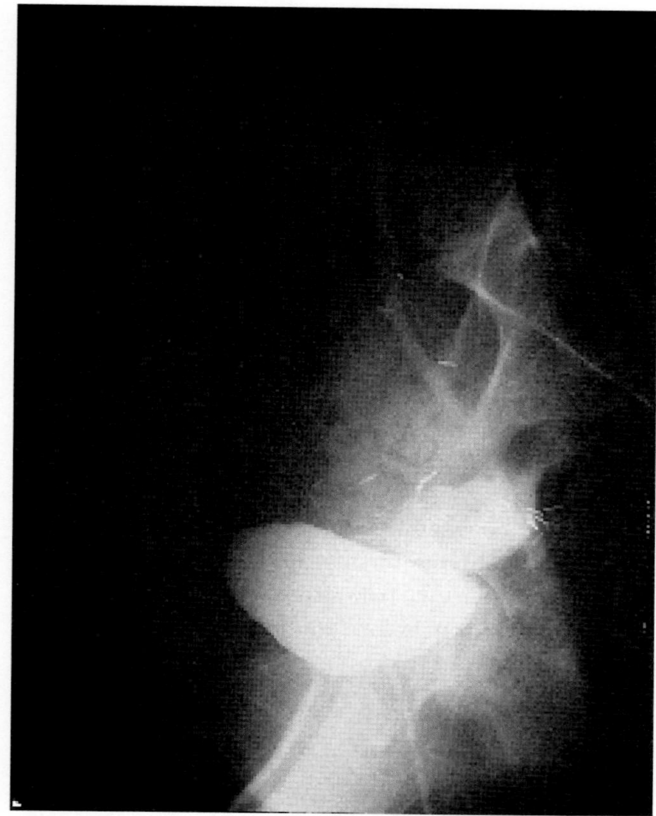

Figure 88.2. *Intravenous urogram (with simultaneous cystogram) demonstrating a complex surgical fistula occurring after radical hysterectomy. After further investigation including cystourethroscopy, sigmoidoscopy, barium enema, and retrograde cannulation of the vaginal vault to perform fistulography, the lesion was defined as a ureterocolovesicovaginal fistula.*

under direct vision is likely to be more sensitive. It may, however, occasionally be useful in achieving a diagnosis in complex or vesicouterine fistulae.

Ultrasound, computed tomography, and magnetic resonance imaging

Endoanal ultrasound and magnetic resonance imaging (MRI) are particularly useful in the investigation of anorectal and perineal fistulae. Although abdominal, vaginal, transperineal, and Doppler ultrasound have all been reported in known cases, the role of these techniques in the diagnosis or assessment of urogenital fistulae remains to be clarified.[21–25]

Examination under anesthesia

Careful examination, if necessary under anesthetic, may be required to determine the presence of a fistula, and is deemed by several authorities to be an essential preliminary to definitive surgical treatment.[5,26–29] It is important at the time of examination to assess the available access for repair vaginally, and the mobility of the tissues. The decision between the vaginal and the abdominal approach to surgery is thus made: when the vaginal route is chosen, it may be appropriate to select between the more conventional supine lithotomy position with a head-down tilt, and the prone (reverse lithotomy) with head-up tilt. This may be particularly useful in allowing the operator to look down onto the bladder neck and subsymphysial fistulae; it is also of advantage in some massive fistulae in encouraging the reduction of the prolapsed bladder mucosa.[30]

ENDOSCOPY

Cystoscopy

Although some authorities suggest that endoscopy has little role in the evaluation of fistulae, it is the author's practice to perform cystourethroscopy in all but the largest defects. In some obstetric and radiation fistulae the size of the defect and the extent of tissue loss and scarring may make it difficult to distend the bladder; nevertheless, much useful information is obtained. The exact level and position of the fistula should be determined, and its relationship to the ureteric orifices and bladder neck are particularly important. With urethral and bladder neck fistulae the failure to pass a cystoscope or sound may indicate that there has been circumferential loss of the proximal urethra, a circumstance which is of considerable importance in determining the appropriate surgical technique and the likelihood of subsequent urethral incompetence.[3,7]

The condition of the tissues must be carefully assessed. Persistence of substantial slough means that surgery should be deferred, and this is particularly important in obstetric and postradiation cases. Biopsy from the edge of a fistula should be taken in radiation fistulae if persistence of recurrent malignancy is suspected. Malignant change has been reported in a longstanding benign fistula, so where there is any doubt at all about the nature of the tissues, biopsy should be undertaken.[30] In areas of endemicity, evidence of schistosomiasis, tuberculosis, and lymphogranuloma may become apparent in biopsy material, and again it is important that specific antimicrobial treatment is instituted prior to definitive surgery.

PREOPERATIVE MANAGEMENT

Before epithelialization is complete, an abnormal communication between viscera will tend to close spontaneously, provided that the natural outflow is unobstructed. Bypassing the sphincter mechanisms by urinary catheterization may encourage closure. The early management is of critical importance, and depends on the etiology and site of the lesion. If surgical trauma is recognized within the first 24 hours postoperatively, immediate repair may be appropriate, provided that extravasation of urine into the tissues has not been great. The majority of surgical fistulae are, however, recognized between 5 and 14 days postoperatively, and these should be treated with continuous bladder drainage. It is worth persisting with this line of management in vesicovaginal or urethrovaginal fistulae for 6–8 weeks, since spontaneous closure in both surgical and obstetric cases may occur within this period.[31,32]

It is important to appreciate that some fistulae may be associated with few or no symptoms, and even if persistent these do not require surgical treatment. Small distal urethrovaginal fistulae, uterovesical fistulae with menouria, and some low rectovaginal fistulae may fall into this category.

Palliation and skin care

During the waiting period from diagnosis to repair, incontinence pads should be provided in generous quantities so that patients can continue to function socially to some extent. Fistula patients usually leak very much greater quantities of urine than those with urethral incontinence from whatever cause, and this needs to be recognized in terms of provision of supplies.

The vulval skin may be at considerable risk from urinary dermatitis, and liberal use of silicone barrier cream should be encouraged. Steroid therapy has been advocated in the past as a means of reducing tissue edema and fibrosis, although these benefits are refuted and there may be a risk of compromise to subsequent healing. Local estrogen has been recommended by some, and while empirically there may be benefit in postmenopausal women, or those obstetric fistula patients with prolonged amenorrhea, the evidence for this is lacking.

Antimicrobial therapy

Opinions differ on the desirability of prophylactic antibiotic cover for surgery, some avoiding their use other than in the treatment of specific infection, and some advocating broad spectrum treatment in all cases. The only randomized trial in this area failed to demonstrate benefit from antibiotic prophylactic treatment in obstetric fistula patients,[33] although the author's current practice is for single dose prophylaxis in patients undergoing repair of surgical fistulae.

Counseling

As surgical fistula patients are usually previously healthy individuals who entered hospital for what was expected to be a routine procedure, and end up with symptoms infinitely worse than their initial complaint, they are invariably devastated by their situation. It is vital that they understand the nature of the problem, why it has arisen, and the plan for management at all stages. Confident but realistic counseling by the surgeon is essential and the involvement of nursing staff or counsellors with experience of fistula patients is also highly desirable. The support given by previously treated sufferers can also be of immense value in maintaining patient morale, especially where a delay prior to definitive treatment is required.

GENERAL PRINCIPLES OF SURGICAL TREATMENT

Timing of repair

The timing of surgical repair is perhaps the single most contentious aspect of fistula management. While shortening the waiting period is of both social and psychological benefit to what are always very distressed patients, these issues must not be traded for compromise to surgical success. The benefit of delay is to allow slough to separate and inflammatory change to resolve. In both obstetric and radiation fistulae there is considerable sloughing of tissues, and it is imperative that this should have settled before repair is undertaken. In radiation fistulae it may be necessary to wait 12 months or more. In obstetric cases most authorities suggest that a minimum of 3 months should be allowed to elapse, although others have advocated surgery as soon as slough is separated.

With surgical fistulae the same principles should apply, and although the extent of sloughing is limited, extravasation of urine into the pelvic tissues inevitably sets up some inflammatory response. Although early repair is advocated by several authors, again most would agree that 10–12 weeks postoperatively is the earliest appropriate time for repair.

Pressure from patients to undertake repair at the earliest opportunity is always understandably great, but is never more so than in the case of previous surgical failure. Such pressure must, however, be resisted, and 8 weeks is the minimum time that should be allowed between attempts at closure.

Route of repair

Many urologists advocate an abdominal approach for all fistula repairs, claiming the possibility of earlier intervention and higher success rates in justification. Others suggest that all fistulae can be successfully closed by the vaginal route. Surgeons involved in fistula management must be capable of both approaches, and have the versatility to modify their techniques to select that most appropriate to the individual case. Where access is good and the vaginal tissues sufficiently mobile, the vaginal route is usually most appropriate (Fig. 88.3a,b). Access for vaginal repair may be improved by the use of unilateral or bilateral episiotomy, although where even this proves inadequate and the fistula cannot be brought down, the abdominal approach should be considered. Overall, more surgical fistulae are likely to require an abdominal repair than obstetric fistulae, although in the author's series of cases from the UK, and those reviewed from Nigeria, two-thirds of cases were satisfactorily treated by the vaginal route regardless of etiology.

Instruments

All operators have their own favored instruments, although those described in the treatise by Chassar Moir[26] and Lawson[30] are eminently suitable for repair by any route. The following are particularly useful:

- series of fine scalpel blades on the No. 7 handle, especially the curved No. 12 bistoury blade;
- Chassar Moir 30-degree angled-on-flat and 90-degree curved-on-flat scissors;
- cleft palate forceps;
- Judd-Allis, Stiles, and Duval tissue forceps;
- Millin's retractor for use in transvesical procedures, and Currie's retractors for vaginal repairs. The Lone Star™ ring retractor may give considerable advantage, particularly for vaginal procedures;
- Skin hooks to put the tissues on tension during dissection;
- Turner-Warwick double curved needle holder is particularly useful in areas of awkward access, and has the advantage of allowing needle placement without the operator's hand or the instrument obstructing the view.

Dissection

Great care must be taken over the initial dissection of the fistula, and the surgeon should probably take as long over this as over the repair itself. The fistula should be circumcised in the most convenient orientation, depending on size and access. All things being equal, a longitudinal incision should be made around urethral or midvaginal fistulae; conversely, vault fistulae are better handled by a transverse elliptical incision (Fig. 88.3c). The tissue planes are often obliterated by scarring, and dissection close to a fistula should therefore be undertaken with a scalpel or scissors (Fig. 88.3d). It must be recognized that, in many cases, particularly of obstetric fistulae, the defect in the bladder may be considerably larger than the visible defect in the vagina, and circumcision must be undertaken well away from the fistula edges. Sharp dissection is easier with countertraction applied by skin hooks, tissue forceps or retraction sutures. Blunt dissection with small pledgets may be helpful once the planes are established, and provided one is away from the fistula edge. Wide mobilization should be performed so that tension on the repair is minimized (Fig. 88.3e). Bleeding is rarely troublesome with vaginal procedures, except occasionally with proximal urethrovaginal fistulae. Diathermy is best avoided, with pressure or underrunning sutures preferred.

Suture materials

Although a range of suture materials have been advocated over the years, and a range of opinion still exists, the author's view is that absorbable sutures should be used throughout all urinary fistula repair procedures. Polyglactin (Vicryl) 2-0 suture on a 25 mm heavy tapercut needle is preferred for both the bladder and vagina, and polydioxanone (PDS) 4-0 on a 13 mm round-bodied needle is used for the ureter.

SPECIFIC REPAIR TECHNIQUES

Vaginal procedures

Dissection and repair in layers

There are two main types of closure technique applied to the repair of urinary fistulae: the classical saucerization technique described by Sims,[34] and the much more commonly used dissection and repair in layers. Sutures must be placed with meticulous accuracy in the bladder wall, care being taken not to penetrate the mucosa which should be inverted as far as possible. The repair should

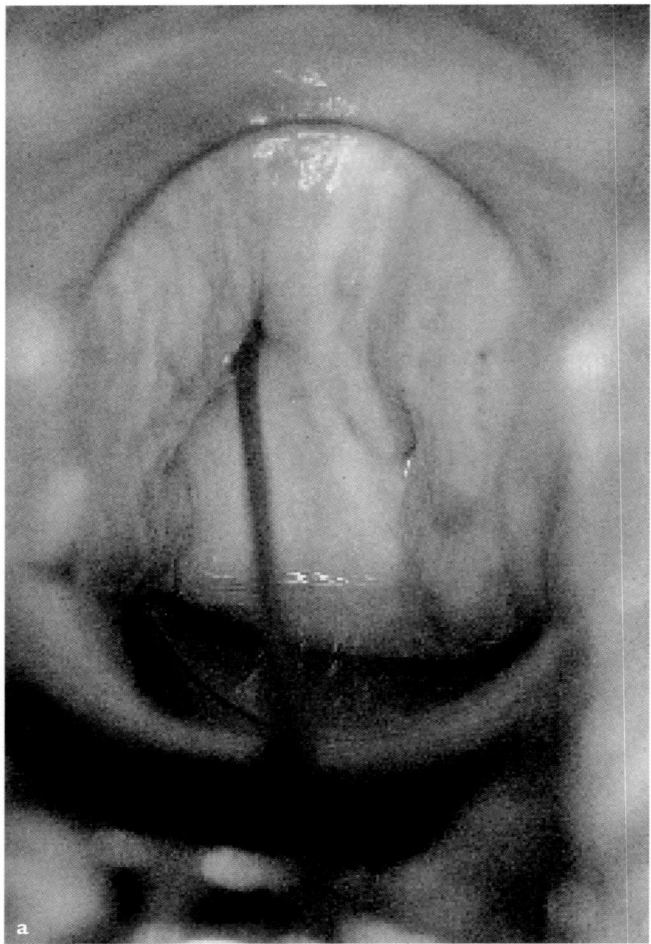

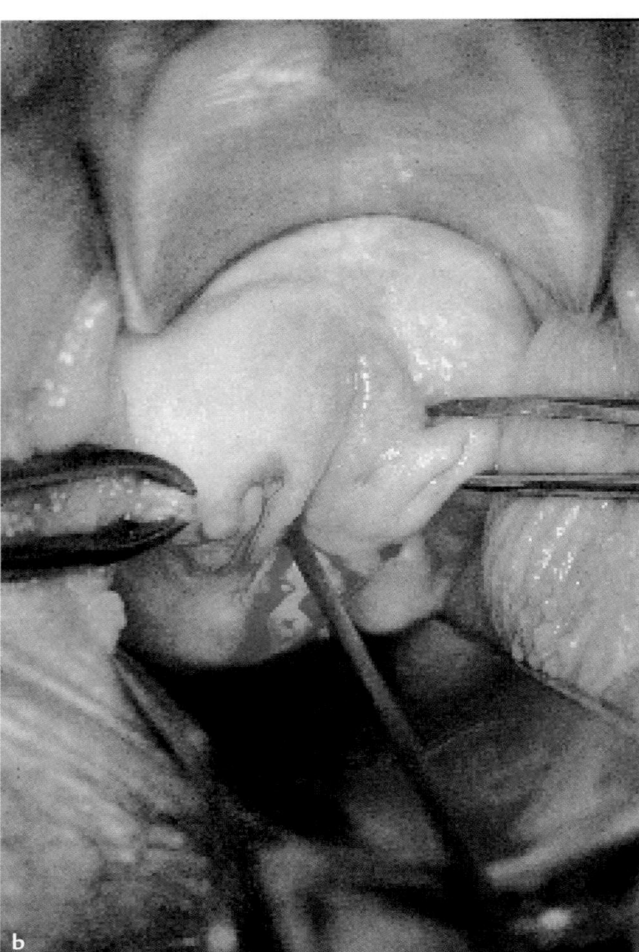

Figure 88.3. *Simple posthysterectomy vault vesicovaginal fistula, and steps in vaginal repair procedure by dissection and closure in layers: (a) fistula visible in vaginal vault; (b) tissue forceps applied illustrating tissue mobility, and ease of access for repair per vaginam.*

be started at either end, working towards the midline, so that the least accessible aspects are sutured first (Fig. 88.3g). Interrupted sutures are preferred and should be placed approximately 3 mm apart, taking as large a bite of tissue as feasible. Stitches that are too close together, or the use of continuous or purse-string sutures, tend to impair blood supply and interfere with healing. Knots must be secure with at least three hitches, so that they can be cut short, leaving the minimum amount of material within the body of the repair.

With dissection and repair in layers the first layer of sutures in the bladder should invert the edges; the second adds bulk to the repair by taking a wide bite of bladder wall, but also closes off dead space by catching the back of the vaginal flaps (Fig. 88.3h). After testing the repair (Fig. 88.3i) (see below), a third layer of interrupted mattress sutures is used to evert and close the vaginal wall, consolidating the repair by picking up the underlying bladder wall (Fig. 88.3j).

Saucerization

The saucerization technique involves converting the track into a shallow crater, which is closed without dissection of bladder from vagina using a single row of interrupted sutures. The method is applicable only to small fistulae and perhaps to residual fistulae after closure of a larger defect; in other situations the technique does not allow secure closure without tension.

Vaginal repair procedures in specific circumstances

The conventional dissection and repair in layers as described above is entirely appropriate for the majority of midvaginal fistulae, although modifications may be necessary in specific circumstances. In juxtacervical fistulae, or indeed vesicocervical fistulae, vaginal repair may be feasible if the cervix can be drawn down to provide access. Dissection should include mobilization of the bladder from the cervix. The repair should be

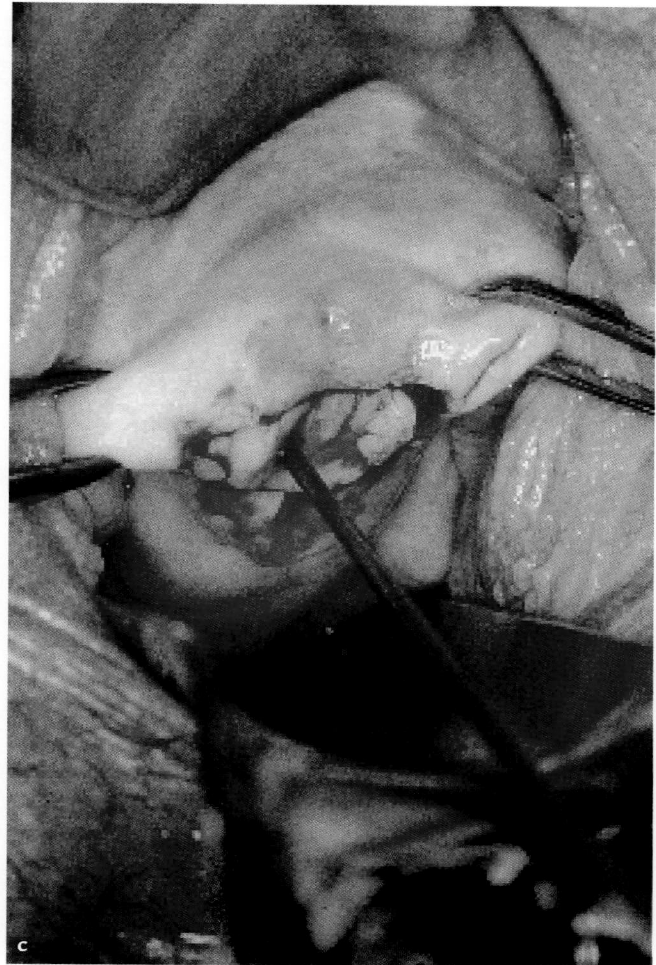

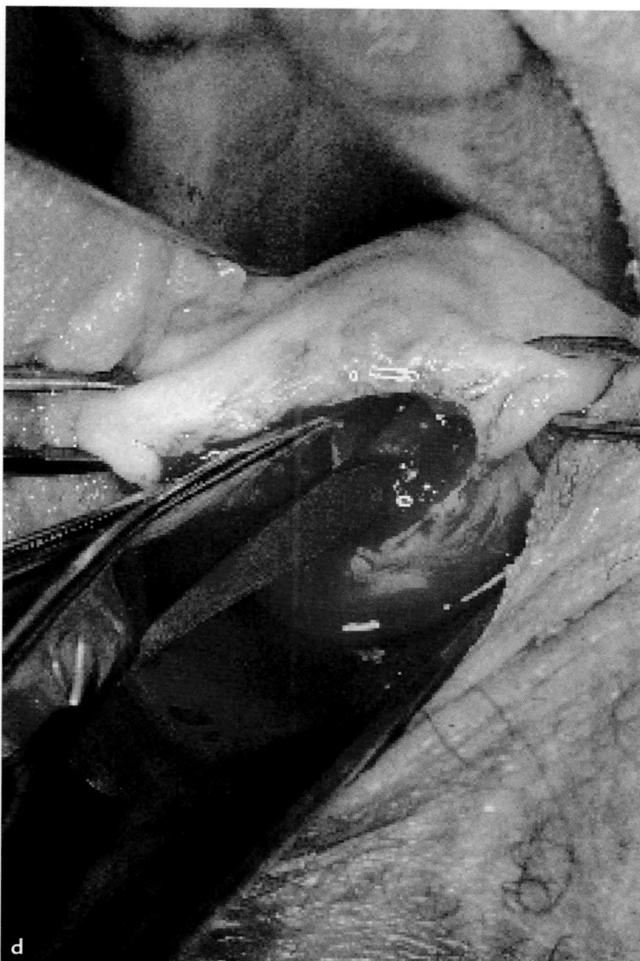

Figure 88.3. *Simple posthysterectomy vault vesicovaginal fistula, and steps in vaginal repair procedure by dissection and closure in layers (cont.): (c) fistula circumcised using No. 12 scalpel; (d) sharp dissection around fistula edge.*

undertaken transversely to reconstruct the underlying trigone and prevent distortion of the ureteric orifices.

Vault fistulae, particularly those following hysterectomy, can again usually be managed vaginally. The vault is incised transversely and mobilization of the fistula is often aided by deliberate opening of the pouch of Douglas.[35] The peritoneal opening does not require to be closed separately, but is incorporated into the vaginal closure.

With subsymphysial fistulae involving the bladder neck and proximal urethra as a consequence of obstructed labor, tissue loss may be extensive, and fixity to underlying bone a common problem. The lateral aspects of the fistula require careful mobilization to overcome disproportion between the defect in the bladder and the urethral stump. A racquet shape extension of the incision facilitates exposure of the proximal urethra. Although transverse repair is often necessary, longitudinal closure gives better prospects for urethral competence.

Where there is substantial urethral loss, reconstruction may be undertaken using the method described by Chassar Moir[26] or Hamlin and Nicholson.[36] A strip of anterior vaginal wall is constructed into a tube over a catheter. Plication behind the bladder neck is probably important if continence is to be achieved. The interposition of a labial fat or muscle graft not only fills up the potential dead space, but also provides additional bladder neck support and improves continence by reducing scarring between bladder neck and vagina.

With very large fistulae extending from bladder neck to vault, the extensive dissection required may produce considerable bleeding. The main surgical difficulty is to avoid the ureters. They are usually situated close to the superolateral angles of the fistula and, if they can be identified, they should be catheterized. Straight ureteric catheters passed transurethrally or double pigtail catheters may both be useful in directing the intramural

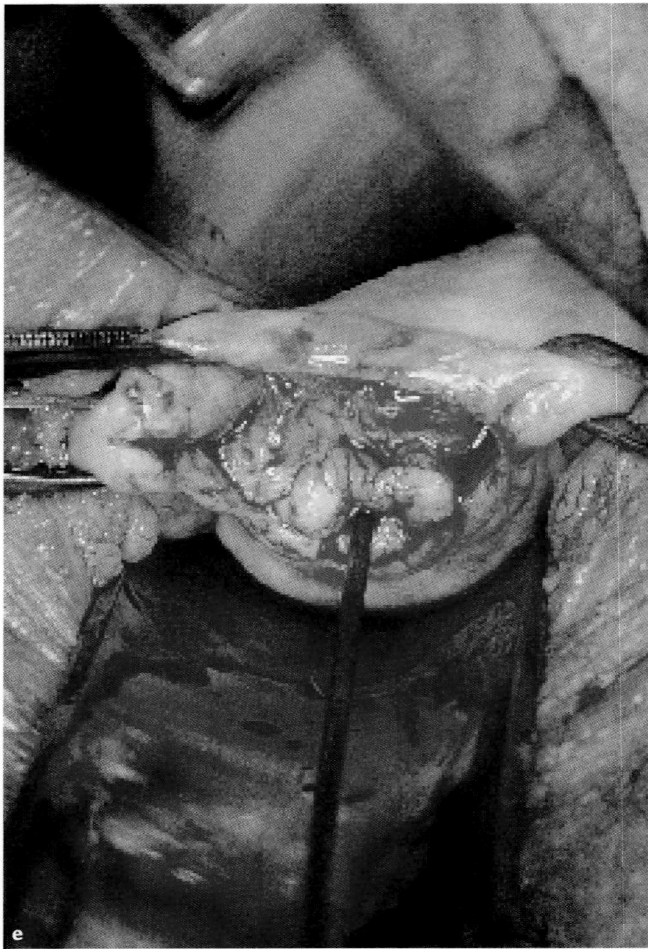

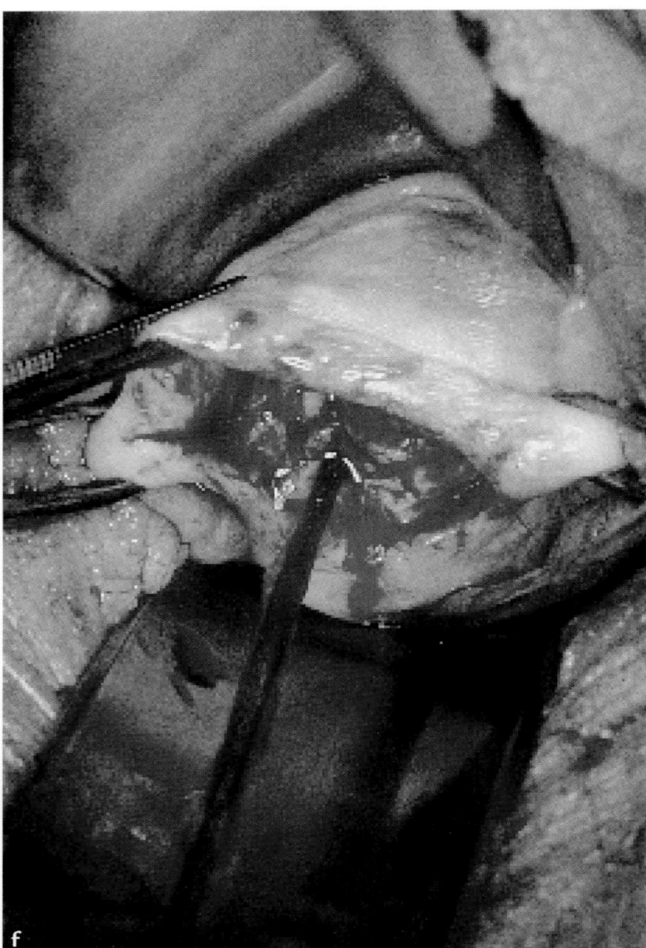

Figure 88.3. *Simple posthysterectomy vault vesicovaginal fistula, and steps in vaginal repair procedure by dissection and closure in layers (cont.): (e) fistula fully mobilized; (f) vaginal scar edge trimmed.*

portion of the ureters internally; nevertheless great care must be taken during dissection.

Abdominal procedures

Transvesical repair

Repair by the abdominal route is indicated when high fistulae are fixed in the vault and are inaccessible per vaginam. Transvesical repair has the advantage of being entirely extraperitoneal. It is often helpful to elevate the fistula site by a vaginal pack, and the ureters should be catheterized under direct vision. The technique of closure is similar to that of the transvaginal flap-splitting repair except that for hemostasis the bladder mucosa is closed with a continuous suture.

Transperitoneal repair

It is often said that there is little place for a simple transperitoneal repair, although a combined transperitoneal and transvesical procedure is favored by urologists and is particularly useful for vesicouterine fistulae following cesarean section. A midline split is made in the vault of the bladder and extended downwards in a racquet shape around the fistula. The fistulous track is excised and the vaginal or cervical defect closed in a single layer. The bladder is then closed in two layers.

Interposition grafting

Several techniques have been described to support fistula repair in different sites. In each case the interposed tissue serves to create an additional layer in the repair, to fill dead space, and to bring in new blood supply to the area. The tissues used include:

- *Martius graft* – labial fat and bulbocavernosus muscle passed subcutaneously to cover a vaginal repair; this is particularly appropriate to provide additional bulk in a colpocleisis and in urethral and bladder neck fistulae may help to maintain

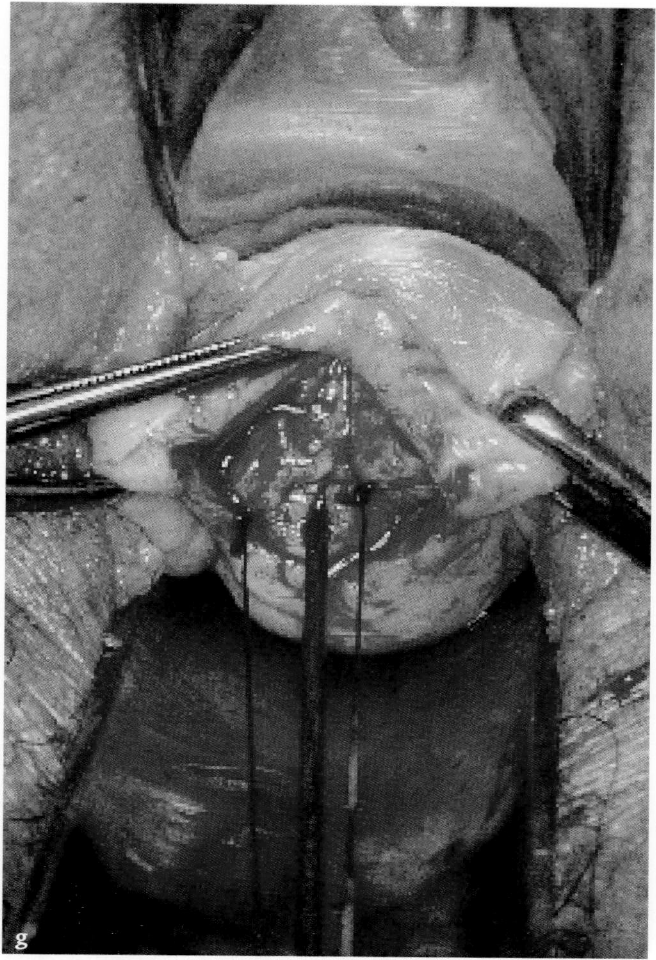

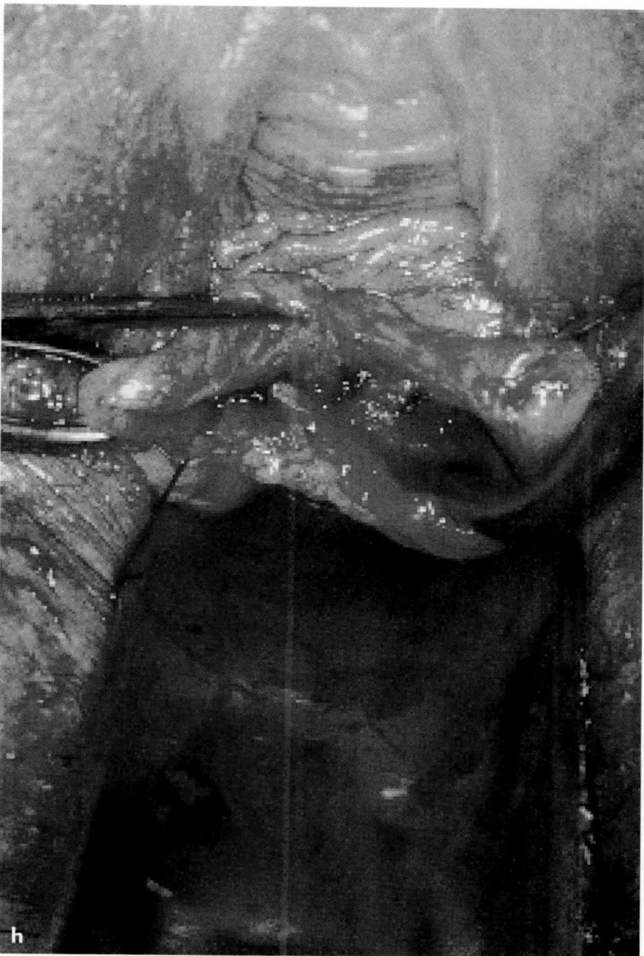

Figure 88.3. *Simple posthysterectomy vault vesicovaginal fistula, and steps in vaginal repair procedure by dissection and closure in layers (cont.): (g) first two sutures of first layer of repair in place lateral to the angles of the repair; (h) second layer completed, sutures catching the back of the vaginal flaps to close off dead space.*

competence of closure mechanisms by reducing scarring;[37]

- *Gracilis muscle* passed either via the obturator foramen or subcutaneously is used as above;[36]
- *Omental pedicle grafts* may be dissected from the greater curve of the stomach and rotated down into the pelvis on the right gastroepiploic artery. This may be used at any transperitoneal procedure, but has its greatest advantage in postradiation fistulae;[38,39]
- *Peritoneal flap graft* is an easier way of providing an additional layer at transperitoneal repair procedures, by taking a flap of peritoneum from any available surface, most usually the paravesical area.[27]

Testing the repair

The closure must be watertight and so should be tested at the end of vaginal repairs by the instillation of dye into the bladder under minimal pressure; a previously unsuspected second fistula is occasionally identified in this way. Testing after abdominal procedures is impractical.

POSTOPERATIVE MANAGEMENT

Fluid balance

Nursing care of patients who have undergone urogenital fistula repair is of critical importance, and obsessional postoperative management may do much to secure success. As a corollary, however, poor nursing may easily undermine what has been achieved by the surgeon. Strict fluid balance must be kept and a daily fluid intake of at least 3 liters, and output of 100 ml per hour, should be maintained until the urine is clear of blood. Hematuria is more persistent following abdominal than vaginal procedures, and intravenous fluid is therefore likely to be required for longer in this situation.

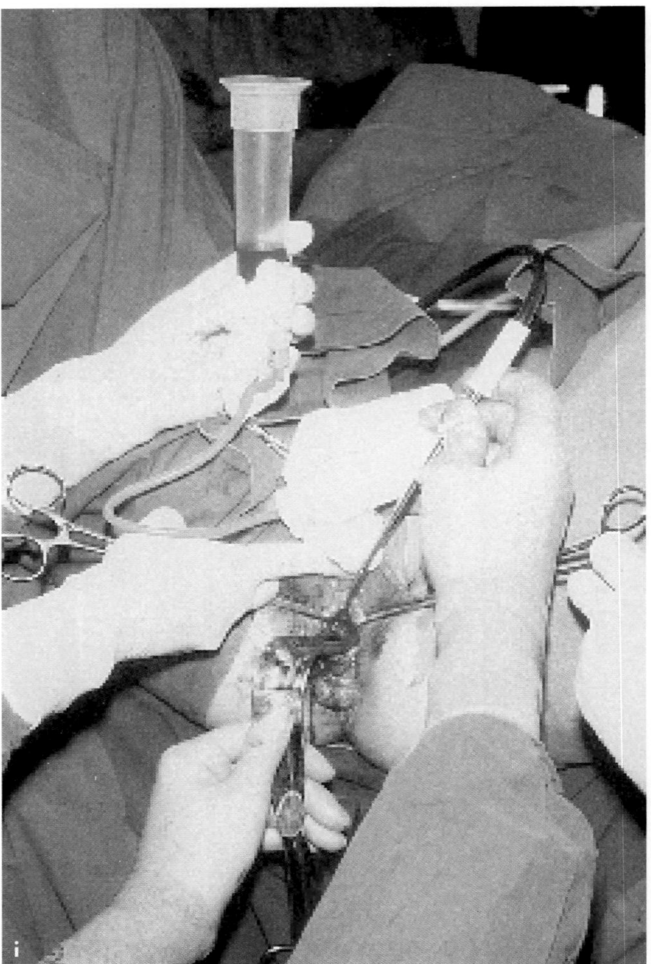

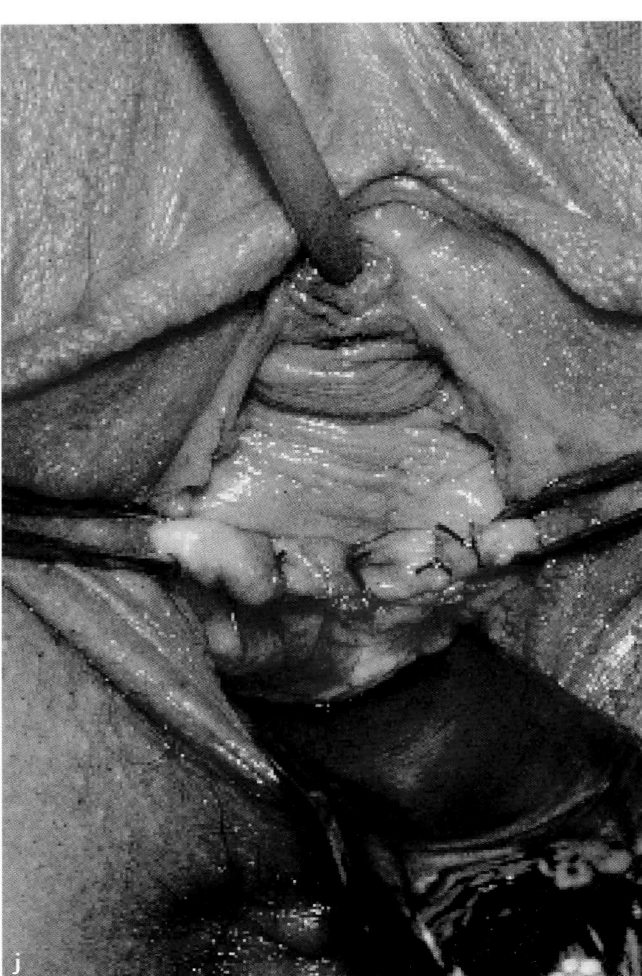

Figure 88.3. *Simple posthysterectomy vault vesicovaginal fistula, and steps in vaginal repair procedure by dissection and closure in layers (cont.): (i) testing the repair with methylene blue dye instillation; (j) final layer of mattress sutures in the vaginal wall. (Reproduced from ref. 8 with permission.)*

Bladder drainage

Continuous bladder drainage in the postoperative period is crucial to success, and nursing staff should check catheters hourly throughout each day to confirm free drainage and check output. Bladder irrigation and suction drainage are not recommended.

Views differ as to the ideal type of catheter. The caliber must be sufficient to prevent blockage, although whether the suprapubic or urethral route is used is to a large extent a matter of individual preference. The author's usual practice is to use a 'belt and braces' approach of both urethral and suprapubic drainage initially, so that if one becomes blocked, free drainage is still maintained. The urethral catheter is removed first, and the suprapubic retained, and used to assess residual volume, until the patient is voiding normally.[40]

The duration of free drainage depends on the fistula type. Following repair of surgical fistulae, 12 days is adequate. With obstetric fistulae up to 21 days' drainage may be appropriate, and following repair of radiation fistulae 21–42 days is required. Routine cystography is not advocated, although if there is any doubt about the integrity of the repair it is wise to carry out dye testing prior to catheter removal. Where a persistent leak is identified, free drainage should be maintained for 6 weeks.

Mobility and thromboprophylaxis

The biggest problem in ensuring free catheter drainage lies in preventing kinking or drag on the catheter. Restricting patient mobility in the postoperative period helps with this, and some advocate continuous bed rest during the period of catheter drainage. If this approach is chosen, patients should be looked on as being at moderate to high risk for thromboembolism, and prophylaxis must be employed.[41] If patients are restricted to bed following urogenital fistula repair, a laxative should be administered to prevent excessive straining at stool.

Subsequent management

On removal of catheters most patients will feel the desire to void frequently, since the bladder capacity will be functionally reduced having been relatively empty for so long. In any case it is important that they do not become overdistended, and hourly voiding should be encouraged and fluid intake limited. It may also be necessary to wake them once or twice through the night for the same reason. After discharge from hospital patients should be advised to gradually increase the period between voiding, aiming to be back to a normal pattern by 4 weeks postoperatively.

Tampons, pessaries, douching, and penetrative sex should be avoided until 3 months postoperatively.

PROGNOSIS

It is difficult to compare the results of treatment in different series, since the lesions involved and the techniques of repair vary so greatly, and definitions of cure are inconsistent. Cure rates are perhaps best considered in terms of closure at first operation, and vary from 60 to 98%.[2,5,6,36,42–48]

Stress incontinence has long been recognized to persist following fistula closure,[23] most commonly in obstetric fistula patients when the injury involves the sphincter mechanism, particularly if there is tissue loss,[49] although persistence of this and other functional abnormalities of the lower urinary tract have also been reported in a proportion of surgical fistulae involving the urethra or bladder neck.[7] We have recently investigated the persistence of urinary symptoms between 1 and 10 years following anatomically successful closure of surgical fistulae; while seriously bothersome symptoms were very uncommon, mild symptoms were reported in 75% of patients.[50]

Of the 233 patients in the author's series managed in the UK, 19 (8.2%) healed without operation, 10 declined surgery for various reasons, 4 (1.7%) underwent primary urinary diversion, and 3 patients with radiotherapy fistulae died without being operated upon – 2 from recurrent disease and 1 from cachexia without recurrence. Of the 178 patients who have undergone repair surgery, 170 (95.5%) were cured by the first operation; of the 105 fistulae following simple hysterectomy, 103 (98.1%) were cured at their first operation.

A law of diminishing returns is evident in fistula surgery as in many other forms of surgery. Although repeat operations are certainly justified, the success rate decreases progressively with increasing numbers of previous unsuccessful procedures. Surgical series are rarely large enough for this to be evident; in a series of 2484 largely obstetric fistulae the success rate fell from 81.2% for first procedures to 65.0% for those requiring two or more procedures.[2] It cannot be overemphasized that the best prospect for cure is at the first operation, and there is no place for the well-intentioned occasional fistula surgeon, be they gynecologist or urologist.[8]

REFERENCES

1. Danso K, Martey J, Wall L, Elkins T. The epidemiology of genitourinary fistulae in Kumasi, Ghana, 1977–1992. Int Urogynecol J Pelvic Floor Dysfunct 1996;7(3):117–20.
2. Hilton P, Ward A. Epidemiological and surgical aspects of urogenital fistulae: a review of 25 years experience in south-east Nigeria. Int Urogynecol J Pelvic Floor Dysfunct 1998;9:189–94.
3. Waaldijk K. The surgical management of bladder fistula in 775 women in Northern Nigeria. MD thesis, University of Utrecht, Nijmegen, 1989.
4. Zacharin R. Obstetric Fistula. Vienna: Springer-Verlag, 1988.
5. Hilton P. Urogenital fistulae. In: Maclean A, Cardozo L (eds) Incontinence in Women – Proceedings of the 42nd RCOG Study Group. London: RCOG, 2002; 163–81.
6. Lee R, Symmonds R, Williams T. Current status of genitourinary fistula. Obstet Gynecol 1988;71:313–9.
7. Hilton P. The urodynamic findings in patients with urogenital fistulae. Br J Urol 1998;81:539–42.
8. Hilton P. Debate: Post-operative urinary fistulae should be managed by gynaecologists in specialist centres. Br J Urol Int 1997;80(Suppl 1):35–42.
9. Harkki-Siren P, Sjoberg J, Tiitinen A. Urinary tract injuries after hysterectomy. Obstet Gynecol 1998;92:113–8.
10. Chapron CM, Dubuisson JB, Ansquer Y. Is total laparoscopic hysterectomy a safe surgical procedure? Hum Reprod 1996;11(11):2422–4.
11. Malik E, Schmidt M, Schneidel P. [Complications following 106 laparoscopic hysterectomies.] Zentralbl Gynakol 1997;119(12):611–5.
12. Price JH, Nassief SA. Laparoscopic-assisted vaginal hysterectomy: initial experience. Ulster Med J 1996;65(2):149–51.
13. Averette HE, Nguyen HN, Donato DM et al. Radical hysterectomy for invasive cervical cancer. A 25-year prospective experience with the Miami technique. Cancer 1993;71:1422–37.

14. Emmert C, Köhler U. Management of genital fistulas in patients with cervical cancer. Arch Gynecol Obstet 1996;259:19–24.
15. White A, Buchsbaum H, Blythe J, Lifshitz S. Use of the bulbocavernosus muscle (Martius procedure) for repair of radiation-induced rectovaginal fistulas. Obstet Gynecol 1982;60(1):114–8.
16. Bladou F, Houvenaeghel G, Delpero JR, Guerinel G. Incidence and management of major urinary complications after pelvic exenteration for gynecological malignancies. J Surg Oncol 1995;58:91–6.
17. Waaldijk K. Surgical classification of obstetric fistulas. Int J Gynaecol Obstet 1995;49(2):161–3.
18. Falk F, Tancer M. Management of vesical fistulas after Cesarean section. Am J Obstet Gynecol 1956;71:97–106.
19. Youssef A. 'Menouria' following lower segment Cesarean section: a syndrome. Am J Obstet Gynecol 1957;73:759–67.
20. Raghavaiah N. Double-dye test to diagnose various types of vaginal fistulas. J Urol 1974;112:811–2.
21. Abulafia O, Cohen HL, Zinn DL, Holcomb K, Sherer DM. Transperineal ultrasonographic diagnosis of vesicovaginal fistula. J Ultrasound Med 1998;17(5):333–5.
22. Adetiloye VA, Dare FO. Obstetric fistula: evaluation with ultrasonography. J Ultrasound Med 2000;19(4):243–9.
23. Huang WC, Zinman LN, Bihrle W 3rd. Surgical repair of vesicovaginal fistulas. Urol Clin North Am 2002;29(3):709–23.
24. Volkmer BG, Kuefer R, Nesslauer T, Loeffler M, Gottfried HW. Colour Doppler ultrasound in vesicovaginal fistulas. Ultrasound Med Biol 2000;26(5):771–5.
25. Yang JM, Su TH, Wang KG. Transvaginal sonographic findings in vesicovaginal fistula. J Clin Ultrasound 1994;22(3):201–3.
26. Chassar Moir J. The Vesico-vaginal Fistula, 2nd ed. London: Baillière, 1967.
27. Jonas U, Petri E. Genitourinary fistulae. In: Stanton S (ed) Clinical Gynecologic Urology. St Louis: Mosby, 1984; 238–55.
28. Lawson J. The management of genito-urinary fistulae. Clin Obstet Gynaecol 1978;6:209–36.
29. Lawson L, Hudson C. The management of vesico-vaginal and urethral fistulae. In: Stanton S, Tanagho E (eds) Surgery for Female Urinary Incontinence. Berlin: Springer-Verlag, 1987;193–209.
30. Lawson J. Injuries to the urinary tract. In: Lawson J, Stewart D (eds) Obstetrics and Gynaecology in the Tropics and Developing Countries. London: Edward Arnold, 1967; 481–522.
31. Davits R, Miranda S. Conservative treatment of vesico-vaginal fistulas by bladder drainage alone. Br J Urol 1991;68:155–6.
32. Waaldijk K. Immediate indwelling bladder catheterisation at postpartum urine leakage: personal experience of 1200 patients. Tropical Doctor 1997;27:227–8.
33. Tomlinson AJ, Thornton JG. A randomised controlled trial of antibiotic prophylaxis for vesico-vaginal fistula repair. Br J Obstet Gynaecol 1998;105:397–9.
34. Sims J. On the treatment of vesico-vaginal fistula. Am J Med Sci 1852;XXIII:59–82.
35. Lawson J. Vesical fistulae into the vaginal vault. Br J Urol 1972;44:623–31.
36. Hamlin R, Nicholson E. Reconstruction of urethra totally destroyed in labour. Br Med J 1969;2:147–50.
37. Martius H. Die operative Wiederherstellung der vollkommen fehlenden Harnrohre und des Schiessmuskels derselben. Zentralbl Gynakol 1928;52:480.
38. Kiricuta I, Goldstein A. The repair of extensive vesicovaginal fistulas with pedicled omentum: a review of 27 cases. J Urol 1972;108:724–7.
39. Turner-Warwick R. The use of the omental pedicle graft in urinary tract reconstruction. J Urol 1976;116:341–7.
40. Hilton P. Bladder drainage. In: Stanton SL, Monga AK (eds) Clinical Urogynecology. London: Churchill Livingstone, 2000.
41. Thromboembolic Risk Factors (THRIFT) Consensus Group. Risk of and prophylaxis for venous thromboembolism in hospital patients. Br Med J 1992;305:567–74.
42. Chassar Moir J. Vesico-vaginal fistulae as seen in Britain. J Obstet Gynaecol Br Commonw 1973;80:598–602.
43. Elkins TE, Drescher C, Martey JO, Fort D. Vesicovaginal fistula revisited. Obstet Gynecol 1988;72:307–12.
44. Goodwin WE, Scardino PT. Vesicovaginal and ureterovaginal fistulas: a summary of 25 years of experience. Trans Am Assoc Genitour Surg 1979;71:123–9.
45. Hudson C, Hendrickse J, Ward A. An operation for restoration of urinary continence following total loss of the urethra. Br J Obstet Gynaecol 1975;82:501–4.
46. Kelly J. Vesicovaginal fistulae. Br J Urol 1979;51:208–10.
47. O'Conor VJ. Review of experience with vesicovaginal fistula repair. J Urol 1980;123:367–9.
48. Turner-Warwick RT, Wynne EJ, Handley-Ashken M. The use of the omental pedicle graft in the repair and reconstruction of the urinary tract. Br J Surg 1967;54:849–53.
49. Waaldijk K. Step-by-Step Surgery for Vesico-vaginal Fistulas. Edinburgh: Campion, 1994.
50. Dolan L, Dixon W, Hilton P. Quality of life and urodynamic abnormality in patients following urogenital fistula repair [abstract]. Int Urogynecol J Pelvic Floor Dysfunct 2003;14:S42.

89

Urogenital fistulae – obstetric

Andrew Browning

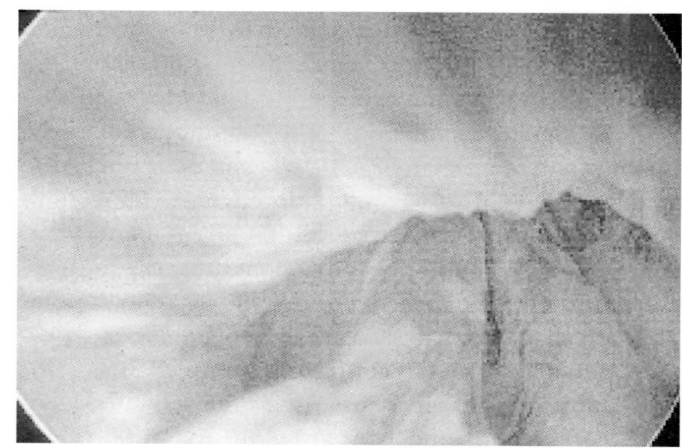

INTRODUCTION

The majority of women throughout the world still do not have access to medical attention for the delivery of their child. Maternal mortality is still unacceptably high throughout the developing world and paralleling this are high rates of maternal morbidity. One of the most feared consequences of a morbid delivery is the obstetric fistula – reducing a woman to a life of shame, isolation, and misery – a life which sometimes ends in suicide or at least the victim wishing she had died during that frightful labor.

ETIOLOGY AND EPIDEMIOLOGY

It is clear that the etiology of obstetric fistula is ischemic necrosis from an obstructed labor. The impacted presenting part compresses the pelvic tissues against the mother's bony pelvis. This connection was made a thousand years ago. The early medical text *Al Kanoun* by Avicenna who died in 1037 gave the warning of labor causing a tear in the bladder – a condition 'incurable and remains so until death'.[1] This accounts for the vast number of obstetric vesicovaginal fistulae seen throughout the world. Less common causes of obstetric fistulae include those iatrogenic in origin: from trauma during cesarean section, forceps delivery or manipulations, and cuttings from poorly trained health attendants. Vesicovaginal fistulae have been recorded after almost every pelvic surgery. Less common causes include advanced cervical cancer, sexual trauma, and infections (e.g. tuberculosis of the bladder, schistosomiasis, and lymphogranuloma venereum).

There have been numerous epidemiologic studies of obstetric fistula patients from various parts of the globe. Typically, the patient is primiparous (43–62.7%),[2,3] but a significant number are multiparous (up to 20–25% having had four or more deliveries),[2,4] presumably due to delivering larger children or malpresentations. Interestingly, a number of studies have shown these women to be short, often less than 150 cm tall, in Nigeria,[4] India,[5] Ethiopia,[6] and Niger.[7] Ampofo et al. showed them to be, on average, 7 cm shorter than the general female population.[8] The women are largely uneducated, more than 92% having had no formal education.[3,9,10] They are also young. Although it is difficult to get a true estimate of their age as it is often unknown, it is evident from their appearance that most are in their teens. If their age is asked and the answer relied upon, 42% are aged less than 20, with 65% being less than 25 years old.[3] Other studies confirm this trend.[9–11]

The majority have had home deliveries with no skilled attendant present and typically more than 50% have been divorced by their husbands due to their offences.[3] It has been noted in Nigeria that if the woman is childless, she is more likely to be divorced, whereas those women who have live children are more likely to be attending those children and the husband has remained with her.[10] What is unclear is the association of obstetric fistula and female genital cutting. The opinion of many fistula surgeons is that the obstructed labor occurs against the mother's bony pelvis and not against the scarred tissues resulting from a circumcision at the outlet. From the experience in Addis Ababa, fistula can result from an infundibulation indirectly when a traditional health attendant may cut the circumcision open during labor, cutting anteriorly, damaging the urethra, bladder neck, and bladder base.

The other factor that leads to some controversy is early or child marriage. It seems reasonable to assume that because adult height and sexual maturity are reached before the completion of pelvic growth, that early marriage and hence pregnancy may lead to an increase in obstructed labor and hence obstetric fistula.[12–14] This has not been concretely confirmed by studies in the field. Unfortunately, early marriage can also result in traumatic fistula, if the husband needs to enlarge the young girl's vagina to enable intercourse to take place. This is sometimes done, again by a traditional healer cutting open the vaginal tissues anteriorly and sometimes damaging the urethra and/or bladder in the process. This is similar to a 'gishiri' cut performed in some areas as a folk treatment for a variety of gynecologic ills.[9]

PREVALENCE

There are no accurate figures for the true prevalence of obstetric fistula. There have been no population-based studies to determine the scope of the problem. A large hospital-based study of over 22,000 patients gave the incidence of obstetric fistula as 0.35% of deliveries.[15] Knowing that the majority of women in the developing world deliver in their villages and not in a hospital, the true incidence is likely to be higher. That having been said, the World Health Organization (WHO) often quotes the incidence as 0.3%. Using this figure, throughout the world there are probably between 50,000 and 100,000 new cases of obstetric fistula each year and approximately 2 million women suffering from this condition.[16] Others have taken further calculations equating the obstetric fistula rate with maternal mortality. Knowing that for every maternal death 30 women suffer some morbidity of which obstetric fistula is one, Danso and colleagues proposed that the obstetric fistula rate would approximate the materal mortality rate. If this is the case, there would be approximately 500,000 new cases worldwide each year.[2]

SYMPTOMS AND SIGNS

The average length of labor that the patient has endured is 3.9 days and 98% end with a stillbirth. The woman is weak and shocked postdelivery and on average it takes a woman 26.1 days before she is strong enough to be able to walk unaided.[3]

The immediate course of the injury is that 3–10 days postdelivery a necrotic slough is extruded through the vagina and the vesicovaginal fistula is exposed, rendering her completely incontinent. If she has sustained similar injuries to the posterior vaginal wall she is also rendered incontinent of feces.

It is easy to think of obstetric fistula just as a hole in the bladder and perhaps the rectum. However, unlike iatrogenic surgical fistula which is usually a discrete injury, the pathology of the obstetric fistula is broader and the term 'field injury' has been coined to refer to the range of injuries caused.[17] The ischemic process not only affects the tissues of the bladder, vagina, and often the rectum and vagina, but also all the other tissues in the mother's pelvis. This results in primary conditions, i.e. those associated with the etiology of obstetric fistula. There are also secondary conditions – delayed conditions that arise later as a result of incontinence or scarring within the pelvis.

Primary conditions

Vesicovaginal fistula (Figs 89.1, 89.2)

The level of impaction during labor determines the site of injury. If the impaction occurs at the pelvic inlet, the vesicovaginal fistula may be juxta- or even intracervical.[18] If impaction occurs lower the urethra may be involved. The urethra is injured in 28% of cases, with 5% of patients having the urethra completely destroyed.[17] This has prognostic indications as the mechanisms for continence in the female have been destroyed.[17–20]

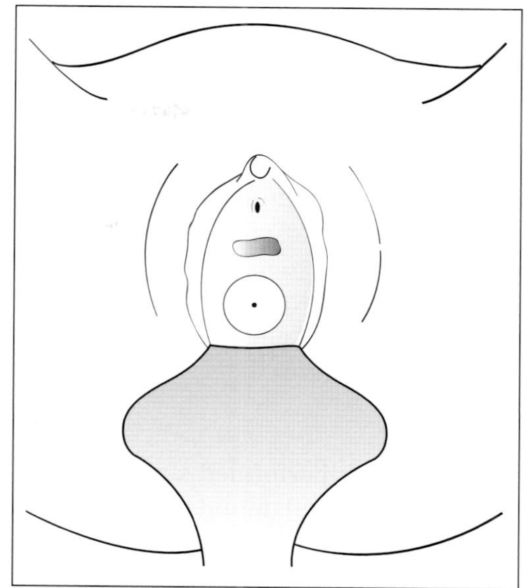

Figure 89.1. *Simple midvaginal vesicovaginal fistula.*

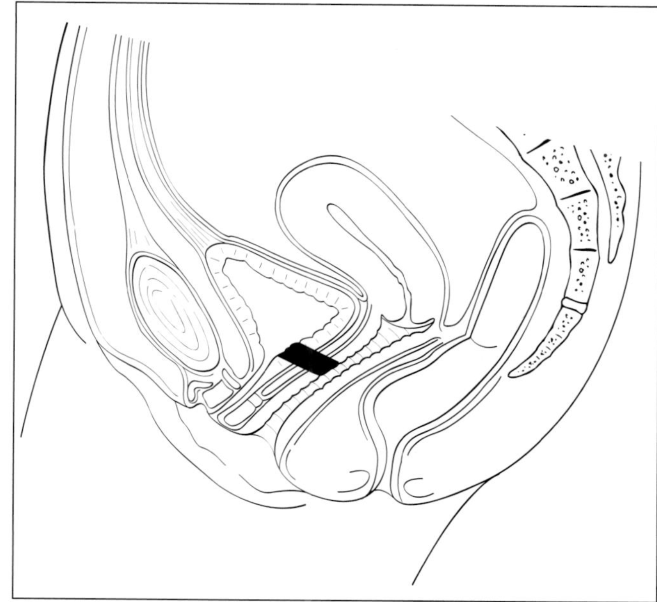

Figure 89.2. *Simple midvaginal vesicovaginal fistula in cross-section.*

Ureteric injury

In a small number of obstetric fistula cases the lower part of the ureter can be involved. The whole ureterovesical junction is necrosed and sloughed away, leaving the vesicovaginal fistula with the ureter draining outside of the bladder straight into the vagina.

Rectovaginal injuries

A rectovaginal fistula occurs if the presenting part is impacted against the sacrum during labor, causing ischemic necrosis of the rectovaginal septum. It has various reported prevalence, ranging from 6% (Hancock B, personal communication) to 22%.[3] If present, it usually occurs in conjunction with a vesicovaginal fistula; it rarely presents in isolation.[3] The status of the anal sphincter should always be noted as there may be residual flatal or fecal incontinence even after repair.[21] Neglected fourth degree tears are also common.

Reproductive tract

The tissues of the vagina are obviously injured, but in some cases the whole vagina has necrosed, leaving little or no identifiable remaining vaginal skin. Overall, approximately 28% of patients will need some form of vaginoplasty.[17] The cervix is often torn or partly necrosed and fistula surgeons testify that it is rare to see an uninjured cervix. Vesicouterine fistulae, although more uncommon, do occur when the uterus is affected.

Muscles

The muscles of the pelvic basin are often affected by a neuropathy, directly weakened by the ischemic process or even completely destroyed.

Bones

A series by Cockshott performed x-rays on 312 women with obstetric fistula and found that 32% had some radiographic abnormality, including bony resorption, bony spurs, obliteration or separation of the symphysis pubis.[22]

Nerves

It has been quoted that between 20 and 65% of obstetric fistula patients will have some form of peroneal neuropathy manifesting as bilateral or unilateral foot drop.[17,23] There are currently three theories as to its etiology: a prolapsed intervertebral disk, direct compression of the fetus on the lumbosacral trunk during labor, or impingement of the common peroneal nerve during prolonged squatting in labor as it transverses the head of fibula.[24,25] Waaldjik and Elkins commented that most patients do improve with time, although 13% still show some signs at 2 years.[23]

Secondary conditions

Social consequences

The consequences of complete incontinence for a woman in the developing world, where the status of women is usually low, is far reaching. Over half are divorced, because the husband realizes that his wife is now unable to fulfill her marital duties and is unable to bear children.[3]

Her incontinence has other consequences, as she is now in urine-soaked clothes, unable to clean herself or her attire. She is unable to interact socially, as others find her presence unacceptable. She cannot go to church to worship, to the market, or go to the well to draw water. She lives in isolation stripped of her dignity and place in society.

Mental health

Little has been researched into the mental health status of fistula sufferers although suicide has been reported. A recent series of mental health questionnaires revealed a 93% positive screening for depression (Goh JTW, unpublished work). In areas where there are almost no services to address mental health issues, this is a very pressing need indeed.

Limb contractures

There are often stories of patients being shut away in huts for months if not years. It is thought that, with time, disuse can cause limb contractures. This is seen in roughly 1–2% of patients in Ethiopia. It is occasionally so severe that the woman's legs are locked in the fetal position.

Malnutrition

Malnutrition results from isolation as the patient may be fed and cared for inadequately by a relative in a small room or hut. The average body mass index (BMI) from a small unpublished series from Ethiopia was 19 (Browning A, unpublished work). Cases of severe malnutrition with hypoproteinemia are not uncommon.

Upper renal tract damage

One study from Nigeria investigating intravenous pylorograms in women with fistula revealed 49% of patients sustained upper renal tract damage. The commonest damage was hydronephrosis (34%) but the damage extended all the way to non-functioning kidneys.[26] This is presumably due to scarring partially or totally occluding the lower ureter causing obstructive uropathy and partly due to repeated ascending infections.

Bladder stones

The constant leakage of urine leads many women to drink less water and hence pass less urine. The concentrated urine might collect in pockets of scar, vagina or bladder and, with time, form calculi, causing pain, infection, and increased odor. Occasionally the woman herself or perhaps a local healer will insert foreign bodies into the vagina to try to stem the flow. Such foreign bodies have included stones, rags or plant material, acting as a nidus for calculi formation.

Urine dermatitis (Fig. 89.3)

The leakage of urine, often concentrated, affects the skin. The ammonias and phosphates can encrust on the skin, causing excoriations, secondary infections, and areas of tender hyperkeratosis. Much thought has gone into how to treat this condition – coined 'urine dermatitis' – but the most expedient way is to ensure that the urine is not in contact with the skin, either by applying barrier ointments such as Vaseline or (better) by closing the fistula, rendering the patient continent.

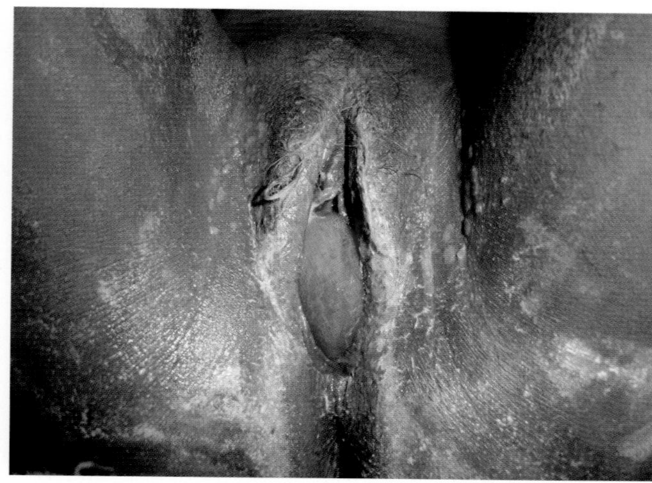

Figure 89.3. *Urine dermatitis. Note the reddened transitional epithelia of the bladder fundus inverting through the introitus.*

Reproductive outcomes

After fistula occurrence, up to 44–63% of women may suffer from amenorrhoea.[17,27] This has a multifactorial causality, most of which have not been clearly delineated. Surely some are due to stresses of the delivery and the resulting social isolation. Some patients do have their menses return following repair.[27] A low BMI is often found to be the cause. In addition, it is thought that some women will have focal anterior pituitary necrosis from shock during the long labor.[28] A small unpublished series by Dosu Ojengbede from Nigeria investigating the use of hysteroscopy showed that intrauterine scarring is common (Asherman's syndrome) (Wall LL, personal communication). Others will have cryptomenorrhea from an obstructed outflow tract which, with time, can cause a large hematometra.

If the patient does receive treatment, remarries or returns to her husband, the subsequent fertility rates are quite despondent. A number of studies have shown that as few as 19% achieve pregnancy[27,29,30] with perhaps a higher rate of prematurity and infant mortality.[31] Subsequent deliveries are hazardous. One small series following the pregnancies in women delivering post fistula repair showed an alarming 27% fistula recurrence rate with a supervised vaginal delivery.[29] It is commonly recommended that any further deliveries should be performed by cesarean section.

INVESTIGATIONS

The investigations of the fistula are kept simple, merely because most patients with obstetric fistulae present in areas where resources are limited.

The majority of obstetric fistula patients can be confidently diagnosed by history and examination alone – a history of a long labor (more than 1 day) with a stillborn child and complete incontinence of urine is the rule. Most obstetric fistulae can be diagnosed on simple vaginal examination – noting the site, size, and amount of scarring.

Some very small vesicovaginal fistulae can give symptoms of stress urinary incontinence and in these circumstances a dye test must be performed. The classical teaching for this is to place three clean swabs into the vagina and insert 50–100 ml of gentian violet diluted with distilled water or saline via a catheter into the bladder. The swabs are left in the vagina for some minutes and then removed. A fistula is confirmed by the presence of dye on the gauze, and – depending on which of the three gauzes is stained – reveals the approximate site of the fistula. However, it is common in many centers to visualize the fistula directly by examining the patient with the aid of a Sims speculum, retracting on the posterior vaginal wall to expose the anterior wall, instilling the dye and seeing where the dye leaks into the vagina. In some very small fistulae and some vesicouterine or vesicocervical fistulae the dye may take some minutes to find its way into the vagina. In these circumstances, it is best to insert a gauze into the vagina, instill 50–100 ml of dye into the bladder, remove the catheter and ask the patient to walk about for 15–30 minutes. It is surprising how many gauzes are stained with dye at the end of this time when the initial examination showed a negative test.

The posterior vaginal wall is examined digitally, again noting the site, size, and any scarring associated with a rectovaginal fistula. The status of the anal sphincter is noted as is the distance of the fistula margin to the sphincter. A small number of patients will complain of flatal incontinence with or without incontinence of diarrhea through the vagina, hinting that a small fistula, unrecognizable to the physician's palpation, is present. A dye test can also be performed by the instillation of dilute colored fluid into the rectum via a Foley catheter.

Routine urine tests, renal function tests or intravenous urography are not warranted as the results do not often influence management. Furthermore, not only are these tests very expensive, they are also unavailable in most units where fistula surgery is performed.

CLASSIFICATION

There are no standardized classifications for obstetric fistula. However, at a recent meeting of fistula surgeons hosted by the WHO, it was agreed that a classification system should include the main factors of site, size, and scarring. A three-tiered classification system with this in mind has been proposed by Goh and colleagues.[32] It is still awaiting validation, but holds promise for a reliable and useful tool for the future (Table 89.1).

TIMING OF REPAIR

It has been commonly taught that a surgeon should wait for roughly 3 months after the insult before attempting repair.[33] The rationale behind this is to allow the necrotic tissue to slough away and the often suboptimal tissue that remains to recover before attempting to operate. There has been one compelling paper advocating earlier repair – to repair as soon as the dead tissue has come away, with active debridement while waiting. This affords a good success rate and enables the woman to regain health more quickly, before she is made an outcast.[16] However, the tissues are much more difficult to handle at this stage, with the tissues tearing and sutures cutting out. This series was done by an extremely experienced fistula surgeon and the results are yet to be replicated in other units and with more inexperienced surgeons. It would be prudent for the inexperience fistula surgeon to rely on the traditional teaching of waiting.

IMMEDIATE MANAGEMENT

If a patient presents within the first few weeks of injury, while the tissues are still raw, a large gauge catheter should be inserted and kept on free drainage for up to 4 weeks. With this management, up to 20–40% of vesicovaginal fistulae will heal.[16] Greater success is usually seen with smaller fistulae.

ROUTE OF REPAIR

The route of repair – vaginal or abdominal – traditionally depends on the experience and training of the surgeon. Those with gynecologic training often favor the vaginal route while those with urologic training tend to favor the abdominal route. The abdominal route might be found easier with high vault, juxtacervical or vesico-

Table 89.1. *Proposed classification system for female genital fistula*

Type	Classification
Genitourinary fistula	
1	Distal edge of fistula >3.5 cm from the external urinary meatus
2	Distal edge of fistula 2.5–3.5 cm from the external urinary meatus
3	Distal edge of fistula 1.5–<2.5 cm from the external urinary meatus
4	Distal edge of fistula <1.5 cm from the external urinary meatus
a	Size <1.5 cm in the largest diameter
b	Size 1.5–3 cm in the largest diameter
c	Size >3 cm in the largest diameter
(i)	None or only mild fibrosis (around fistula and/or vagina) and/or vaginal length >6 cm, normal capacity
(ii)	Moderate or severe fibrosis (around fistula and/or vagina) and/or reduced vaginal length and/or normal capacity
(iii)	Special considerations, e.g. postradiation, ureteric involvement, circumferential fistula, previous repair
Genitoanorectal fistula	
1	Distal edge of fistula >3 cm from hymen
2	Distal edge of fistula 2.5–3 cm from hymen
3	Distal edge of fistula 1.5–<2.5 cm from hymen
4	Distal edge of fistula <1.5 cm from hymen
a	Size <1.5 cm in the largest diameter
b	Size 1.5–3 cm in the largest diameter
c	Size >3 cm in the largest diameter
(i)	None or only mild fibrosis around the fistula and/or vagina
(ii)	Moderate or severe fibrosis
(iii)	Special considerations, e.g. postradiation, inflammatory disease, malignancy, previous repair

vaginal/vesicouterine fistulae. Even these cases can be confidently managed vaginally with experience. This has obvious benefits postoperatively.

SURGICAL TREATMENT

Many surgical techniques have been described, including the open transvesical and transperitoneal or combined techniques, fibrin glue, laparoscopic techniques, partial colpocleisis, and cauterization. The most popular 'flap splitting' technique will be described here.

At a recent meeting of fistula surgery experts hosted by the WHO it was agreed that the flap splitting technique should follow the principles of:

1. exposure of the fistula and protection of the ureters;
2. wide mobilization of the bladder off the vagina/cervix/uterus and surrounding tissues;
3. tension-free closure of the bladder (single or double layer to the bladder);
4. dye test to confirm watertight closure of the bladder.

Exposure of the fistula and protection of the ureters

The patient is placed in the exaggerated lithotomy position with the patient's buttocks over the end of the operating table. The table is placed in steep Trendelenburg which will bring the anterior vaginal wall perpendicular to the surgeon's gaze.

In up to 28% of patients there is significant vaginal scarring that renders it impossible to insert a speculum. Lateral relaxing incisions are necessary to release the scar, expose the fistula and enable the speculum to be inserted for adequate exposure.

In all trigonal and supratrigonal fistulae except the very small, the ureters should be identified and catheterized (Fig. 89.4). This can be done through the fistula and the catheter ends advanced through the urethra. This is to prevent inadvertent injury during dissection and inadvertent suturing of the ureter during repair.

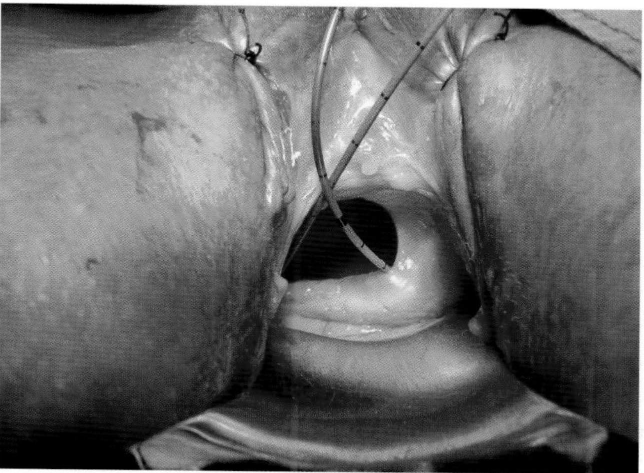

Figure 89.4. *Ureters catheterized through the vesicovaginal fistula.*

Wide mobilization of the bladder off the vagina/cervix/uterus and surrounding tissues

The secret of successful vesicovaginal fistula surgery is wide mobilization of the bladder, releasing it from scarred attachments to the surrounding structures and excision of scar tissue from the bladder and surrounds so that good viable tissue is approximated in the repair.

Tension-free closure of the bladder

Once successfully mobilized, the bladder is sutured together under no tension. If tension remains on the suture line, it runs the risk of disruption. The initial sutures secure the angles of the fistula. The bladder is closed with interrupted sutures (2-0 Vicryl) approximately 4 mm apart. Some surgeons place a second layer of sutures to the bladder. Wider mobilization may be necessary to achieve this but usually a one-layer closure of healthy bladder tissue should suffice.

Dye test to confirm watertight closure of the bladder

Between 50 and 100 ml of dilute colored fluid (gentian violet; some surgeons use milk if no dye is available) is instilled into the bladder to ensure that a watertight closure has been achieved (Fig. 89.5).

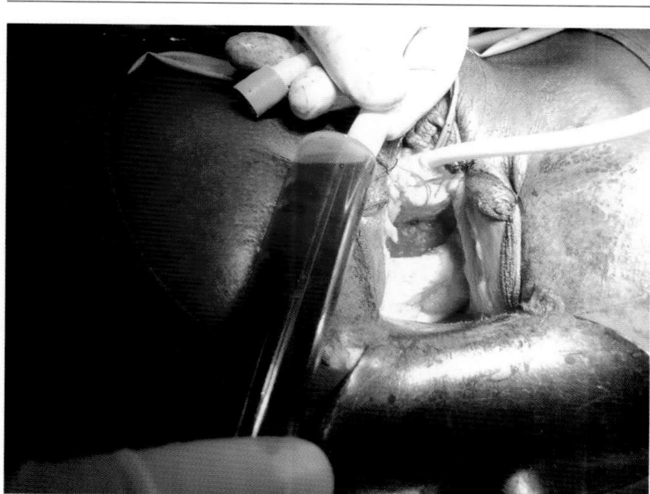

Figure 89.5. *Dye test ensuring a watertight closure of the fistula.*

Interpositional graft

A contentious issue in fistula surgery is whether to use an interpositional graft. It has been traditionally taught that this aids healing by bringing a fresh blood supply to these compromised tissues. It may also plug any undetected microleaks. One small study did show an increased success rate using this graft.[34] More experienced fistula surgeons now use grafts less often with no difference in rates of success; however, this is after accumulating experience with some thousands of vesicovaginal fistula repairs. Until further studies show otherwise, it is best to err on the side of caution and use a graft.

The most common graft used is the Martius fibrofatty graft harvested from the labia majora. Other grafts of gracilis muscle, peritoneum, omentum, and broad ligament have been described.

To form a Martius graft, an incision is made longitudinally along the bulge of the labia majora. The fat underneath is exposed and a flap of fat developed from anterior to posterior with the pedicle still being attached posteriorly. A tunnel is created into the vagina superficial to the inferior pubic ramus, beneath the bulbocavernosus and vaginal skin. The fat is introduced into the vagina and placed over the fistula repair with anchoring sutures.

The vaginal and labial skins are repaired, taking precautions to prevent hematoma formation.

Specific surgical problems

Absent urethra

About 5% of obstetric fistulae have the entire urethra sloughed, which poses one of the most difficult problems for the fistula surgeon[17,35] (Fig. 89.6). An anatomic closure may be quite possible, but a functioning closure is very difficult. Two methods are commonly used:

1. A new urethra may be created from the remaining paraurethral tissues. Initial incisions are made about 2.5–3 cm apart on either side of where the new urethra will lie (Fig. 89.7). Flaps are then created and sewn over a Foley catheter and this delicate structure is anastomosed to the bladder. A graft is placed to help support and nourish this frail construction. Although a gracilis graft has been described, the Martius graft is more commonly used.[36] The vaginal epithelia are drawn over the repair.
2. A new urethra may be created from an anterior flap of bladder tissue. A longitudinal flap is created after dissecting the bladder off the symphysis pubis and this is then advanced towards the urethral meatus. The flap is sewn into a tube over a Foley catheter, a graft placed and the vagina repaired.[37] However, this is often not possible with obstetric fistulae as these types of fistula often result in much loss of bladder tissue; this procedure will thus decrease the size of an already small bladder.

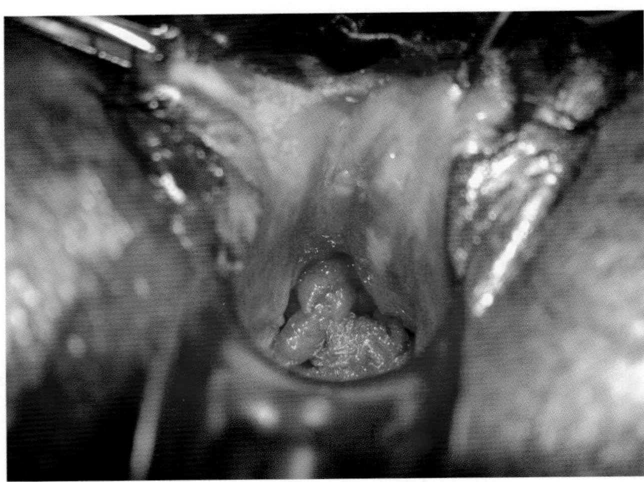

Figure 89.6. *Absent urethra.*

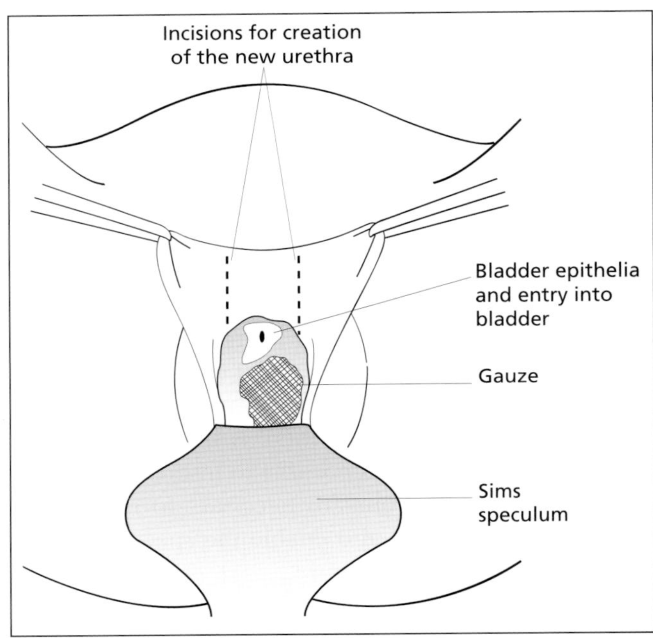

Figure 89.7. *Initial incisions for the creation of a new urethra.*

When a new urethra is created from the remaining paraurethral tissues, urethral strictures may form in the long term, resulting in urinary retention and voiding disorders. There is also a high rate of residual incontinence after repair – presumably stress urinary incontinence. To help reduce this, a sling of levator muscle can be used to support the repair, taking a flap of levator from the right and left (or scar tissue if there is no other tissue remaining) and sewing this in the midline.[20]

Circumferential fistula

A circumferential fistula occurs against the posterior pubic symphysis. In these cases, the bladder is completely detached from the remaining urethra (Figs 89.8, 89.9). The bladder needs to be mobilized not only off the vagina and surrounding structures, but also off the pubic symphysis, dissecting high into the cave of Retzius.

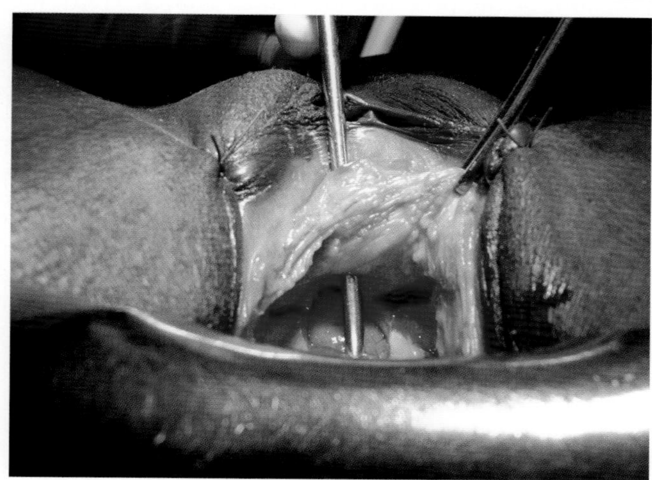

Figure 89.8. *Small circumferential fistula. The urethra has been detached from the bladder neck.*

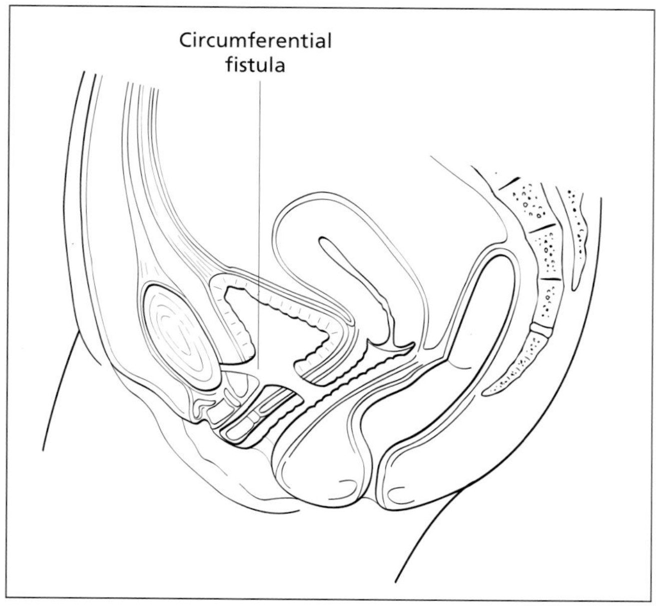

Figure 89.9. *Circumferential fistula in cross-section.*

The bladder is then advanced en masse to the urethra and anastomosed to it.

Again there is a high rate of residual urinary incontinence, presumably stress urinary incontinence. This can be improved by the use of a levator muscle sling employed at the time of repair.[20]

Rectovaginal fistula

The technique for repair is similar to that of the vesicovaginal fistula: flap splitting with wide mobilization, excision of scar tissue, repair of the fistula under no tension, and repair of vaginal epithelia. Grafts are rarely used for rectovaginal fistulae, but the Martius graft may be employed if a long enough pedicle is developed for it to reach the operative site. Rectovaginal fistulae can be comfortably repaired per vaginum but some surgeons may prefer to use the abdominal route for the high fistula adhered to the sacral promontory.

No vaginal tissue remaining

Approximately 28% of cases will need some form of vaginoplasty due to vaginal skin loss; after repair, dyspareunia and apareunia can result.[29] Vaginoplasty may be anything from a simple Fenton type procedure to release vaginal scarring to reconstruction of a new vagina from tissue flaps, anteriorly from the labia minora and majora and posteriorly with rotational flaps of gluteal skin. This does result in a scarred vagina. Other options are a neurovascular flap of tissue from the groin crease or a sigmoid neovagina.

POSTOPERATIVE CARE

The ureteric catheters can be removed upon completion of the operation if the ureteric orifices were far from the fistula margin. If they were close to or on the margin, they remain for 5–7 days to ensure that the ureters do not obstruct with postsurgical swelling. Occasionally, the ureters will need reimplanting; if so, the catheters remain in place for 10–14 days.

The Foley catheter remains on free drainage for 14 days postoperatively. This takes meticulous nursing as a full bladder will put pressure on the repair site and may even disrupt it.

A vaginal pack is usually placed at the end of the operation. This reduces the operative dead space and is removed 24–72 hours later.

The patient should mobilize as soon as she is able; however, it is important that the indwelling catheter be secured with either strong tape or a suture so that the balloon of the catheter does not pull on the fistula repair site while the patient is mobile.

A high fluid intake is encouraged to keep the bladder irrigated and a normal diet is encouraged. The stools should be kept loose in cases of rectovaginal fistula.

RESULTS

The fistula can be closed in up to 94% of cases with their first operation.[3] If a fistula is not closed successfully, repeat operations prove difficult. With the second operation, the success rate drops to 79% and, with the third, to 53% (Browning A, unpublished work). Successful closure, however, does not necessarily equate to a functional cure. Rates of postoperative incontinence, largely stress urinary incontinence, vary between 5.6 and 33%.[20,38] This rate reflects short-term follow-up, within the first few days of catheter removal. With time and with bladder retraining and strengthening of the pelvic floor muscles, this may improve. In northern Nigeria patients have been followed up over a period of 6 months and 15% of closed fistula patients still have some incontinence at time of final follow-up (Waaldjik K, personal communication). At the Addis Ababa Fistula Hospital patients are asked to return in 6 months if they are still experiencing leakage; 8% of patients do so (Browning A, unpublished work).

Rectovaginal fistula repair appears to have a lower initial success rate of 73%.[17] However, with subsequent operations it is almost always possible to get a successful closure although the patient may have some remaining anal flatal and/or stool incontinence from a poorly functioning sphincter.[21]

POSTOPERATIVE COMPLICATIONS

The most concerning complication of fistula surgery is residual incontinence. This is thought mainly to be stress urinary incontinence in type, but detrusor instability must also play a role. One study of 22 women with severe incontinence following fistula closure underwent urodynamic assessment and 41% had genuine stress incontinence (GSI), 14% had GSI and poor compliance, 41% had GSI and detrusor overactivity, and 4% had voiding disorder and overflow incontinence.[39]

There have been several corrective methods proposed, but the most successful to date is a sling described by Carey and colleagues in which urodynamically selected patients have a tension-free sling of rectus sheath inserted beneath the midurethra. This is performed with open dissection into the cave of Retzius and the sling inserted under direct vision. The open step is necessary due to the often dense retropubic scarring and high risk of bladder perforation if carried out as closed procedure with use of a trocar to pass the sling retropubically. A flap of omentum is inserted between the freed urethra and symphysis pubis to try to prevent further scarring. This procedure has a 66% cure rate at 14 months.[39]

FAILED REPAIRS

One study examined 71 failed repairs. All 71 cases had a fistula described as complicated, meaning that one or more of the following was present: excessive scarring, total destruction of the urethra, ureteric orifices outside the bladder or at the edge of the fistula, a small bladder, both recto- and vesicovaginal fistulae in conjunction, or the presence of bladder stones. There was a statistically significant association for a failed repair as compared to a cured patient if the patient had a ruptured uterus at the time of labor, if they had a previous failed repair, if they presented with limb contractures, presented malnourished or in poor health, if the fistula was described as complicated, and if a blood transfusion was required.[38]

The irreparable fistula

The term 'irreparable fistula' may be misleading, but some injuries are so severe that no bladder remains to be repaired. The only option for these women to have any quality of life is either to have a bladder augmentation or a urinary diversion operation.

Bladder augmentations are not without their problems. In patients with such severe injuries the urethra is often affected, so even with a good reservoir, they are still unable to hold their urine. If the urethra is intact, then self-catheterization may be needed to effect full drainage of the bladder. This may be unmanageable for a woman living in the developing world, far from a supply of catheters and clean equipment.

The diversional operations commonly used are direct ureterosigmoidostomy, Mainz II pouch or ileal conduit. The former two options require an intact anal sphincter and the woman to agree to pass urine through the anus. The Mainz II shows promise for women in developing nations as there are perhaps fewer long-term complications following this procedure.[40–42]

The ileal conduit restricts a patient to living near a service that can supply the conduit bags, which are often rare in the developing world. The patient also needs to be close to a health center that knows how to deal with any complications. The ureters and kidneys in these women are often dilated and compromised, and ascending infections can be common.

THE FUTURE

Obstetric fistula, like many morbidities suffered by women during labor, is preventable. This should be an attainable dream in the 21st century and this suffering placed in medical texts of yesteryear. The task, however, is immense, with up to 75,000 new obstetric units being required for Africa alone to supply adequate maternity care.[43] In tandem with this, roads need to be built, transport systems put in place and, most importantly, men and women educated. Until all this is achieved, the obstetric fistula patient will still need our caring attention.

REFERENCES

1. Zacharin RF. Obstetric Fistula. New York: Springer-Verlag, 1988.
2. Danso KA, Martley JO, Wall LL. The epidemiology of genitourinary fistulae in Kumasi, Ghana 1977–1992. Int Urogynecol J 1996;7:117–20.
3. Kelly J, Kwast BE. Epidemiological study of vesico-vaginal fistulas in Ethiopia. Int Urol J 1993;4:278–81.
4. Wall LL, Karshima JA, Kirschner C et al. The obstetric vesicovaginal fistula: characteristics of 899 patients from Jos, Nigeria. Am J Obstet Gynecol 2004;190:1011–19.
5. Bhasker Rao K. Genital fistula. J Obstet Gynaecol India 1975;25:58–65.
6. Bal JS. The vesico-vaginal and allied fistulae – a report on 40 cases. Med J Zambia 1975;9:69–71.
7. Docquier J, Sako A. Fistules recto-vaginales d'origine obstetricale. Med d'Afrique Noire 1983;30:213–15.
8. Ampofo K, Out T, Uchebo G. Epidemiology of vesico-vaginal fistulae in northern Nigeria. West Afr J Med 1990;9:98–102.
9. Tahzib F. Epidemiological determinants of vesicovaginal fistulas. Br J Obstet Gynaecol 1983;90:387–91.
10. Murphy M. Social consequences of vesico-vaginal fistula in Northern Nigeria. J Biosoc Sci 1981;13:139–50.
11. Ibrahim T, Sadiq AU, Daniel SO. Characteristics of VVF patients as seen in the specialist hospital, Sokoto, Nigeria. West Afr Med J 2000;19:59–63.
12. Moerman ML. Growth of the birth canal in adolescent girls. Am J Obstet Gynecol 1982;143:528–32.
13. Wall LL. Dead mothers and injured wives: the social context of maternal morbidity and mortality among the Hausa of Northern Nigeria. Stud Family Planning 1998;29:341–59.
14. Ampofo EK, Omotara BA, Out T et al. Rick factors of vesico-vaginal fistulae in Maiduguri, Nigeria: a case-control study. Tropical Doctor 1990;20:138–9.
15. Harrison KA. Childbearing, health and social priorities: a survey of 22,774 consecutive hospital births in Zaria, Northern Nigeria. Br J Obstet Gynaecol 1985;92(Suppl 5):1–119.
16. Waaldjik K. The immediate management of fresh obstetric fistulas with catheter and/or early closure. Int J Gynecol Obstet 1994;45:11–16.
17. Arrowsmith S, Hamlin EC, Wall LL. Obstructed labour injury complex: obstetric fistula formation and the multifaceted morbidity of maternal birth trauma in the developing world. Obstet Gynecol Surv 1996;51:568–74.
18. Mafouz N. Urinary fistula in women. J Obstet Gynaecol Br Emp 1957;64:23–34.
19. Hassim AM, Lucas C. Reduction in the incidence of stress urinary incontinence complicating a fistula repair. Br J Surg 1974;51:461–5.
20. Browning A. Prevention of residual urinary stress incontinence following successful repair of obstetric vesico-vaginal fistula using a fibro-muscular sling. Br J Obstet Gynaecol 2004;111:357–61.
21. Murray C, Goh JT, Fynes M et al. Urinary and faecal incontinence following delayed primary repair of obstetric genital fistula. Br J Obstet Gynaecol 2002;109:828–32.
22. Cockshott WP. Pubic changes associated with obstetric vesico-vaginal fistulae. Clin Radiol 1973;24:241–7.
23. Waaldjik K, Elkins TE. The obstetric fistula and peroneal nerve injury: an analysis of 974 consecutive patients. Int Urogynecol J 1994;5:12–14.
24. Reif ME. Bilateral common peroneal nerve palsy secondary to prolonged squatting in natural childbirth. Birth 1988;15:100–2.
25. Sinclair RSC. Maternal obstetric palsy. South Afr Med J 1952;26:708–14.
26. Langundoye SB, Bell D, Gill G et al. Urinary changes in obstetric vesico-vaginal fistulae: a report of 216 cases studied by intravenous urography. Clin Radiol 1976;27:531–9.
27. Aimaku VE. Reproductive functions after the repair of obstetric vesicovaginal fistulae. Fertil Steril 1974;25:586–91.
28. Bieler RW, Schnabel T. Pituitary and ovarian function in women with vesicovaginal fistula after obstructed and prolonged labour. South Afr Med J 1976;50:257–66.
29. Evoh NJ, Akinia O. Reproductive performance after the repair of obstetric vesico-vaginal fistulae. Ann Clin Res 1978;10:303–6.
30. Bhasker Rao K. Vesicovaginal fistula – a study of 269 cases. J Obstet Gynaecol India 1972;22:536–41.
31. Naidu PM, Krishna S. Vesico-vaginal fistulae and certain problems arising subsequent to repair. J Obstet Gynaecol Br Emp 1963;70:473–5.
32. Goh JTW. New classification for female genital tract fistula. Aust N Z J Obstet Gynaecol 2004;44:502–4.
33. Moir JC. The Vesico-vaginal Fistula. London: Baillière Tindall, 1967.

34. Rangnekar NP, Imdad AN, Kaul SA. Role of the Martius procedure in the management of urinary–vaginal fistulas. J Am Coll Surg 2000;191:259–63.

35. Ward A. Genito-urinary fistulae: a report on 1787 cases. Second International Congress on Obstetrics and Gynaecology, Lagos, Nigeria.

36. Hamlin RHJ, Nicholson EC. Reconstruction of urethra totally destroyed in labour. Br Med J 1969;1:147–50.

37. Elkins TE, Ghosh TS, Tagoe GA. Transvaginal mobilization and utilization of the anterior bladder wall to repair the vesicovaginal fistulas involving the urethra. Obstet Gynaecol 1992;79:455–60.

38. Kelly J, Kwast BE. Obstetric fistulas: evaluation of failed repairs. Int Urogynecol J 1993;4:271–3.

39. Carey MP, Goh JT, Fynes MM et al. Stress urinary incontinence after delayed primary closure of genitourinary fistula: a technique for surgical management. Am J Obstet Gynecol 2002;186:948–53.

40. Koo HP, Avolio L, Dickett JW Jr. Long-term results of ureterosigmoidostomy in children with exstrophy. J Urol 1996;156:2037–40.

41. Venn SN, Mundy AR. Continent urinary diversion using the Mainz-type ureterosigmoidostomy – a valuable salvage procedure. Eur Urol 1999;36:247–51.

42. D'elia G, Paherhink S, Fisch M et al. Mainz pouch II technique: 10 years' experience. BJU Int 2004;93:1037–42.

43. Waaldik K. Evaluation report XIV on VVF projects in Northern Nigeria and Niger. Katsin, Nigeria: Babbar Ruga Fistula Hospital; 1998.

90

Urethral diverticulum and fistula

Kenneth C Hsiao, Kathleen C Kobashi

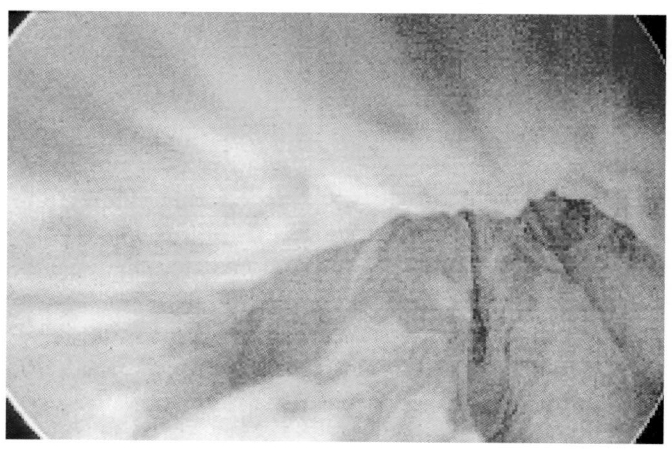

URETHRAL DIVERTICULUM

INTRODUCTION

Female urethral diverticulum (UD) has been a historically underdiagnosed condition. Novak[1] stated, 'This is a relatively rare condition and no gynecologist will see more than a few in a lifetime'. However, with higher clinical suspicion and improved diagnostic techniques, the frequency of diagnosis has increased.

History

The existence of UD has been known since at least the early 19th century, when Hey reported the first case in 1805.[2] In 1938, Hunner[3] reported three cases associated with calculi and commented on the rarity of the condition. In 1956, Davis and Cian[4] reported 50 cases, more than had been reported previously in the entire history of the Johns Hopkins Hospital. They also developed a double-balloon catheter to be used in conjunction with positive-pressure profilometry to facilitate diagnosis of UD.

Incidence and patient profile

The incidence of female UD is reported in the urologic literature as 0.6–6%[5,6] and in the gynecologic literature as 5%.[7] However, these numbers are probably an underestimate and, with increasing clinical suspicion, the true incidence may prove to be higher.[8]

Patients typically present in the third to sixth decades of life, with a mean age of 45 years.[9] Rarely, UD has been diagnosed in neonates and children.[10,11] A racial predilection has been suggested, with diagnosis in African–American women being two to six times that in white women;[12] however, Ganabathi et al.[9] found no racial differences. A concomitant UD[13] has been found in 1.4% of women diagnosed with stress urinary incontinence (SUI).

Etiology and pathophysiology

There are two main schools of thought regarding the etiology of UD: acquired and congenital. The most widely accepted theory is UD formation due to infection of the periurethral gland. The periurethral glands are tuboalveolar structures located posterolaterally beneath the periurethral fascia. They are found in the proximal two-thirds of the urethra and drain into the distal third.[14] Infection leads to obstruction of the glands, local abscess formation, and eventual rupture into the urethral lumen, as first described by Routh[15] in 1890.

Trauma secondary to childbirth or forceps delivery[16] remains a problem in developing countries, possibly contributing to UD formation.[17] However, with current obstetric technology, traumatic delivery is no longer a prevalent factor in developed nations. In fact, 15–20% of patients diagnosed with UD are nulliparous, thereby completely refuting this etiologic theory.[11]

A congenital etiology is doubtful, although there has been some evidence supporting this theory.[10] Faulty union of primordial folds, genesis from cell rests or Gartner's duct remnants, and müllerian remnants causing vaginal cysts have all been suggested as possible etiologies.[17] The discovery of mesonephric adenoma and adenocarcinoma has implicated Gartner's duct remnants. Paneth cell metaplasia lining a UD also supports a congenital basis.[18] Blind-ending ureters resulting from an aborted ureteral duplication may rarely lead to an anterior UD.[19] Other suggested etiologies of UD include high-pressure voiding against outlet obstruction, urethral calculi, instrumentation, and complications of previous anterior vaginal surgery.[17] Recently, a UD has been described following transurethral collagen injection therapy for stress urinary incontinence.[20] The authors hypothesize that the collagen injections caused obstruction of the periurethral glands, resulting in the gradual accumulation of glandular secretions and subsequent development of a non-communicating diverticulum.

Associated complications

Complications associated with UD include incontinence, infection, stones, and malignancy. Urinary incontinence is common in patients with UD. In fact, Ganabathi et al.[9] reported a 65% incidence of SUI among patients with UD (57% with SUI as the presenting complaint). These patients may also suffer from urge incontinence or 'paradoxical incontinence', in which urine stored in the UD is lost during stress.[5]

About 25–33% of patients present with recurrent urinary tract infections, including some who suffer from systemic infections. The most common infecting organisms of UD are *Escherichia coli*, Chlamydia and gonococcus; however, multiple organisms have been cultured.[17,21] Up to 13% of patients present with calculi in the UD, and this can be confirmed by plain radiograph.[22,23] Stones form secondary to stasis, infection and chronic inflammation in the UD.[6] Stones can be multiple and, in some cases, quite large. A 5 × 6 cm stone was discovered in the urethral diverticulum of an elderly woman during workup for a firm vaginal mass. Urethrovaginal fistula secondary to rupture of a UD is another potential complication.[24,25]

Approximately 200 cases of neoplasm within a UD have been reported in the world literature.[26–29,37–43] There have also been reports of 16 cases of nephrogenic adenoma, a benign metaplastic condition.[30–35] Malignancy must be considered whenever a UD is diagnosed, particularly when accompanied by hematuria, induration or firmness of a UD on physical examination, non-calcified filling defects within the UD on radiography, or a visible lesion on cystoscopic examination. Despite the fact that squamous epithelium lines most of the urethra, adenocarcinoma is by far the most common histopathologic condition demonstrated within UD.[31] This lends further support to the theory that urethral diverticula develop from glandular origins. More than 80% of the diverticular cancers seen are either adenocarcinoma (61%) or transitional cell carcinoma (27%).[36] Squamous cell carcinoma is rare, comprising only 12% of UD malignancies.[36] When identified within a urethral diverticulum, squamous cell carcinoma appears to be very aggressive, with a mortality rate of 78% at 3 years.[37]

Treatment of diverticular carcinoma includes wide local excision for localized disease.[28] Adjuvant radiation therapy or chemotherapy may also be indicated for extensive malignancy or for non-surgical candidates.[38,39] Survival is a function of stage[39] and grade[38] of the disease. Squamous cell carcinomas are typically diagnosed at an advanced stage, with all reported cases presenting at stage T2 or higher, and require a more aggressive treatment approach.[38,40–43] Because of the relative rarity of carcinoma in urethral diverticula, it has been difficult to develop a common definitive treatment strategy (Table 90.1). Among the 79 patients reviewed with variable lengths of follow-up between 6 months and 10 years, anterior pelvic exenteration appeared to offer the highest likelihood of prolonged disease-free interval (73%) and the lowest rate of local recurrence (4%).[37] Rates of death and metastasis were similar between the treatment modalities.[37]

PRESENTATION

Clinical symptoms

Patients found to have UD present with a variety of symptoms ranging from irritative voiding complaints to pelvic pain and dyspareunia (Table 90.2).[5] The classic triad of UD is known as the '3 Ds' – dysuria, dyspareunia, and dribbling. However, many patients are asymptomatic. Urinary urgency, frequency, and hematuria may also be associated with UD.[44] The diagnosis is often not straightforward and UD may mimic other pelvic floor disorders, resulting in diagnostic delay.[45] In a review of 46 consecutive cases of UD, the mean interval between onset of symptoms to diagnosis was 5.2 years.[45] Frequently, patients are given an initial, erroneous diagnosis for which a variety of treatments are attempted (Table 90.3). A high index of suspicion is required in order to diagnose UD because many patients may not be overtly symptomatic upon initial evaluation. In cases

Table 90.2. *Presenting symptoms in 627 women with urethral diverticula from published reports*

Symptom	*n* (%)
Frequency	351 (56)
Dysuria	345 (55)
Recurrent infection	251 (40)
Tender mass	219 (35)
Stress incontinence	201 (32)
Post-void dribbling	160 (26)
Urge incontinence	157 (25)
Hematuria	107 (17)
Dyspareunia	376 (16)
Pus per urethram	75 (12)
Retention	25 (4)
Asymptomatic	38 (6)

Data from ref. 5.

Table 90.1. *Frequency and outcome for treatment modalities used for carcinoma in a urethral diverticulum*

Treatment	Patients (*n*)	Disease-free (%)	Local recurrence (%)	Death/metastasis (%)	Follow-up
Diverticulectomy	27	9 (33)	13 (48)	5 (19)	9 months–7 years
Radiation	10	2 (20)	5 (50)	2 (20)	2–5 years
Diverticulectomy + radiation	16	8 (50)	5 (31)	3 (19)	1–10 years
Anterior exenteration	26	19 (73)	1 (4)	6 (23)	6 months–3 years

Data from ref. 37.

Table 90.3. *Most common initial diagnoses and subsequent treatments given to patients before identification of a urethral diverticulum*

Diagnosis	Treatment
Chronic cystitis trigonitis	Long- or short-term antibiotics
Stress urinary incontinence	Anti-incontinence surgery
Urge incontinence	Anticholinergics
Interstitial cystitis	Hydrodistension
Idiopathic pelvic pain syndrome	DMSO instillation Tricyclic antidepressants
Urethral syndrome	Urethral dilation
Vulvovestibulitis	Vaginal creams (antifungal/antibiotic)
Cystocele	Surgery
Sensory urgency	Anticholinergics
Psychosomatic disorder	Psychotherapy

Data from ref. 44.

of persistent irritative voiding symptoms, pelvic pain, and urinary incontinence unresponsive to therapy, UD should be kept in mind and excluded.[45]

Physical examination

Patients with UD most commonly have anterior vaginal wall tenderness, with or without a concomitant palpable suburethral mass.[45] Pressure on the mass may demonstrate expressible purulence or blood from the UD (Fig. 90.1), and firmness of the area may indicate a diverticular stone or neoplasm. Rarely, some patients are without any pertinent physical findings and workup is based only on clinical suspicion established by the patient's history. Importantly, the clinician must also examine patients for urethral hypermobility with or without SUI, which can be addressed at the time of repair of the UD if deemed necessary.

Differential diagnosis

The differential diagnosis of urethral and meatal/perimeatal masses (Figs 90.2, 90.3) is illustrated in Tables 90.4 and 90.5 respectively. Note that Table 90.5 includes conditions that occur in locations distal to the majority of UD; however, they should be considered in the differential diagnosis.[46]

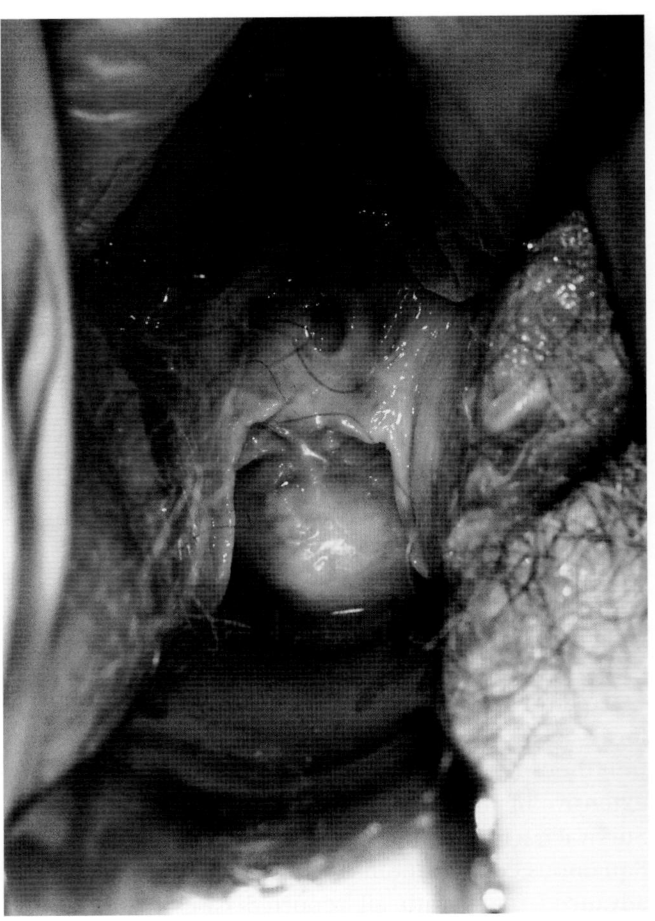

Figure 90.1. *Urethral diverticulum presenting as an anterior vaginal mass. (Reproduced from ref. 9 with permission.)*

Classification system

Leach and co-workers[51] created a system for classification of female UD known as the L/N/S/C3 system. This acronym represents Location, Number, Size, Configuration, Communication, and Continence. This system facilitates preoperative assessment of UD and standardizes the classification, thereby simplifying comparison between series. Table 90.6 illustrates the classification of 63 patients.

DIAGNOSIS

Endoscopic examination

A blunt-tip female urethroscope with a 0 or 30-degree lens is used. The anterior vaginal wall is compressed with a finger in the vagina, and the urethral lumen is inspected for any expression of pus from the floor or

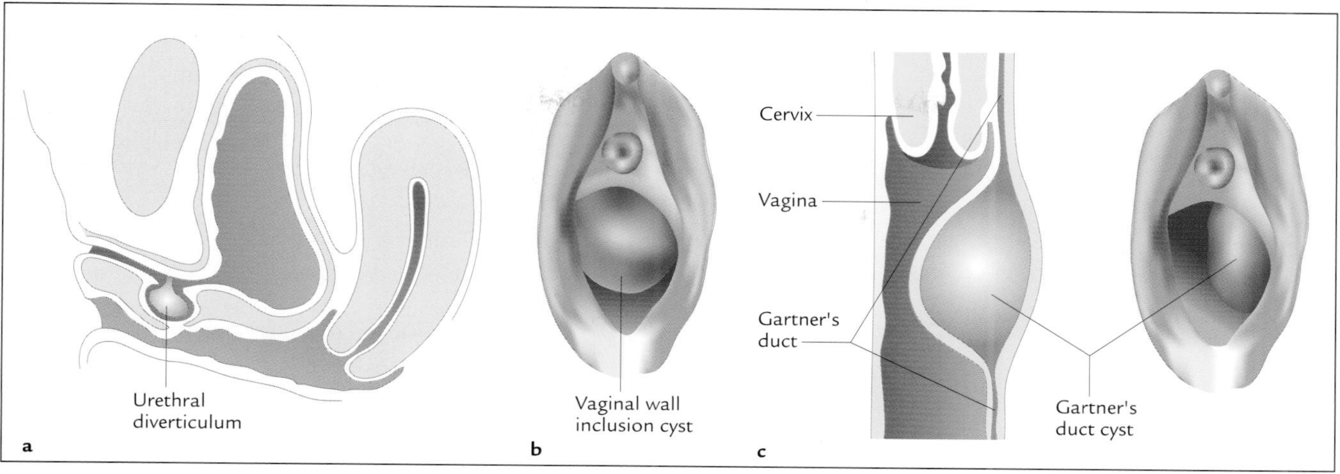

Figure 90.2. *Differential diagnosis of urethral and anterior vaginal wall masses: (a) urethral diverticulum; (b) vaginal wall inclusion cyst; (c) Gartner's duct cyst.*

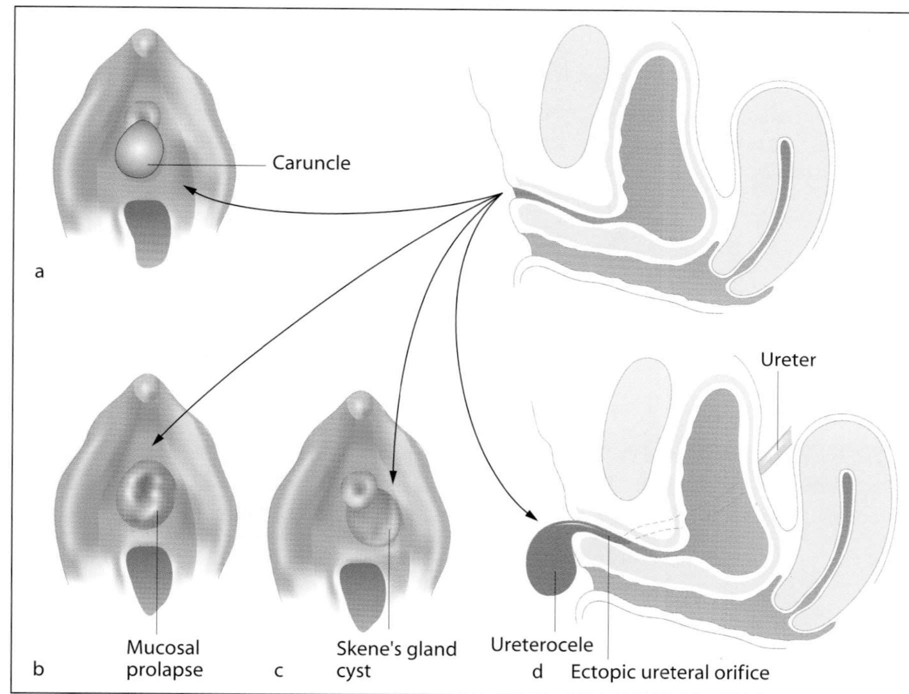

Figure 90.3. *Differential diagnosis of meatal and perimeatal lesions: (a) caruncle; (b) mucosal prolapse; (c) Skene's gland (or duct) cyst; (d) ureterocele.*

roof of the urethra (Fig. 90.4). In 50% of patients there will be multiple diverticula and more than half of the UD will communicate with the middle third of the urethra.[7] Cystoscopy is the only diagnostic tool that allows direct inspection of the urethra and bladder. In some cases, neoplasm or bladder stones may also be diagnosed; however, its value as a diagnostic tool has recently been questioned.[52] Often the diverticular neck is hidden between collapsed urethral folds, and non-communicating diverticula will not have a visible orifice.[53,54] Cystoscopy does not reveal any information regarding size, shape, or appearance of the diverticular wall.[54] In addition, cystoscopy is invasive and carries the risk of urinary tract infection. A negative finding on cystoscopy does not rule out the presence of a UD. Further evaluation including urodynamics or imaging studies should be performed as cystoscopy will frequently fail to diagnose UD.

Urodynamic evaluation

Urodynamic studies are not always required in the evaluation of all patients with UD. The indications include patients with symptoms of SUI or bladder dysfunction.[55–57] These symptoms may include urinary leakage with

Table 90.4. *Differential diagnosis of urethral and anterior vaginal wall lesions*

Lesion	Location	Symptoms/ physical exam	Cystoscopy/radiography	Comments
Urethral diverticulum	Anterior vaginal wall, midline	UTI, dysuria, dyspareunia, post-void dribbling, cystic mass	Orifice of diverticulum visible on urethral floor, VCUG opacifies lesion	May be multilocular
Vaginal wall cyst	Anterior vaginal wall, midline or eccentric	Cystic mass; may be loculated	None or extrinsic compression	–
Gartner's duct cyst	Anterolateral vaginal wall	Cystic mass	None or extrinsic compression; IVP may indicate ectopic ureteral drainage	Rule out ectopic ureter prior to excision
Müllerian remnant cyst	Midline	Cystic mass	None	–
Ectopic ureterocele[48]	Anywhere in bladder, urethra, vagina (upper third), uterus, fallopian tubes	Cystic mass	May be seen on IVP, US or cystoscopy	–
Leiomyoma, hamartoma	Vaginal wall	Solid mass	None or extrinsic compression	Rule out malignancy
Malignant urethral or vaginal neoplasms	Urethral or vaginal wall or hematuria	Solid mass; may have pain, may be seen on cystoscopy	None or extrinsic compression; ± adjuvant therapy, erythema, obvious lesion or tumor growing from the diverticulum into the urethral lumen	Wide local excision, radiation, combination, anterior pelvic exenteration

IVP, intravenous pyelography; US, ultrasonography; UTI, urinary tract infection; VCUG, voiding cystourethrogram. Adapted from ref. 47.

Table 90.5. *Differential diagnosis of meatal and perimeatal lesions*

Lesion	Location	Presentation	Comments
Caruncle	Inferior to meatus	Asymptomatic or dysuria/pain with atrophic or ischemic mucosal changes	Postmenopausal age group
Skene's gland cyst or abscess[49]	Inferior and lateral to meatus	Painful, orifice of duct visible at urethral meatus	
Mucosal prolapse	Circumferential mucosal prolapse with central meatus	Pain and dysuria, atrophic or ischemic mucosal changes	Young girls or postmenopausal women
Prolapsed ureterocele[50]	Submeatal, prolapsed through meatus	Glistening mucosa, may be fluid filled, may be ischemic, may be asymptomatic	IVP to evaluate upper tract status

IVP, intravenous pyelography. Adapted from ref. 47.

increased intra-abdominal pressure, urge incontinence, or spontaneous loss of urine, which may represent intrinsic sphincter deficiency, paradoxical incontinence (i.e. loss of urine that has 'pooled' in the UD), or detrusor instability. Identification of these problems is critical in proper surgical planning. If a patient has a workup indicative of SUI, appropriate correctional surgery can be considered at the time of diverticulectomy. The urodynamic findings in 55 women studied by Leach and Ganabathi[55] are noted in Table 90.7.

Radiologic studies

Voiding cystourethrogram

The voiding cystourethrogram (VCUG) is performed under fluoroscopic visualization with the patient stand-

Table 90.6. *L/N/S/C3 Classification system applied to 63 patients with urethral diverticula*

Location (L)	Number (N)	Size (S)	Configuration (C1)	Communication (C2)	Continence (C3)
Proximal, beneath bladder neck (9)	Single	0.2 × 0.2 cm to 6.0 × 4.5 cm	Multiloculated (22)	Proximal urethra (16)	Complete (26)
Proximal urethra (7)	Multiple		Single (41)	Midurethra (35)	SUI only (30)
Midurethra (36)			Saddle-shaped (14)*	Distal urethra (12)	Urge incontinence only (3)
Distal urethra (11)					SUI and urge incontinence (4)

* These patients are also included in the 'simple' or 'multiloculated' groups.
SUI, stress urinary incontinence. Adapted from ref. 51.

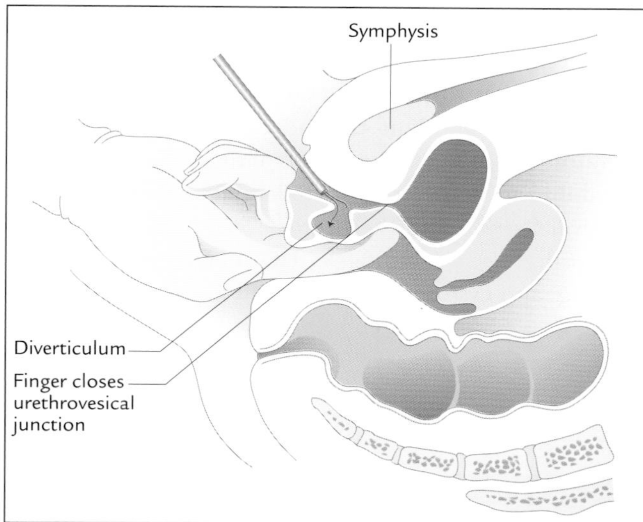

Figure 90.4. *The technique of endoscopic examination of the urethra while 'milking' the anterior vaginal wall and urethral roof.*

Table 90.7. *Urodynamic findings in 55 women with urethral diverticula*

Urodynamic finding	*n* (%)
Normal	22 (40)
SUI alone	18 (32.7)
SUI + DI	8 (14.5)
DI alone	5 (9)
Sensory urgency	1 (2)
Myogenic decompensation	1 (2)

DI, detrusor instability; SUI, stress urinary incontinence. Data from ref. 55.

ing (Fig. 90.5). Assessment of the bladder neck and proximal urethra as well as bladder neck competency is imperative to document incontinence that may be treated at the time of diverticulectomy. Filling defects

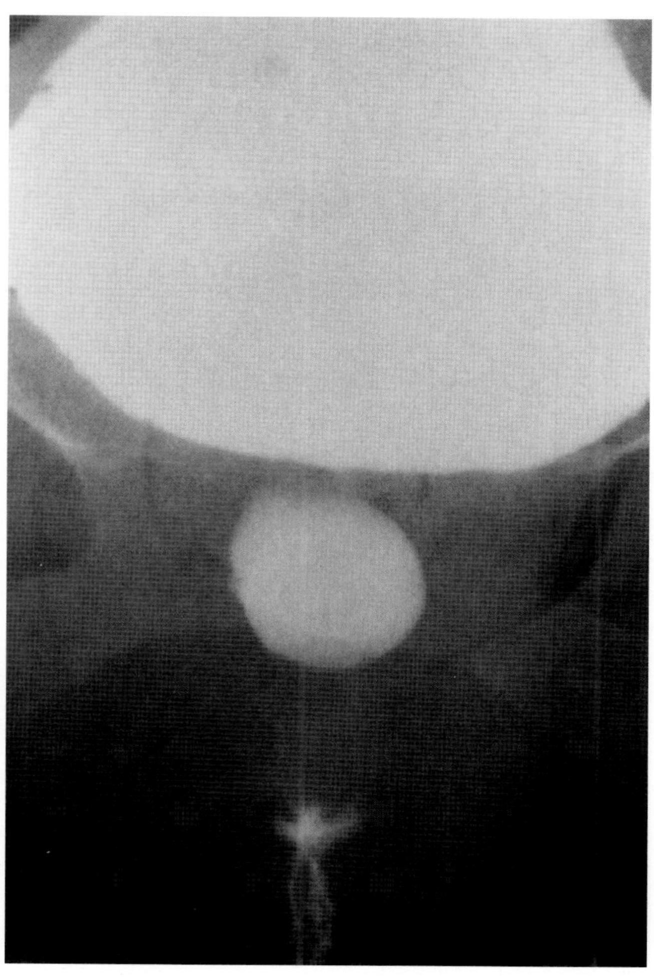

Figure 90.5. *A voiding cystourethrogram demonstrating a multiloculated diverticulum. (Reproduced from ref. 51 with permission.)*

within a UD may represent tumor or stones[5] (Fig. 90.6). An air–fluid level in the UD may indicate a UD that is much larger than it appears radiographically. In 50% of patients there will be multiple UD. Correct identification is critical to ensure complete excision of all components of the UD. Although VCUG has historically been considered the study of choice for the diagnosis of UD (Fig. 90.5), recent studies have begun to question the ability of VCUG to diagnose UD. A 3-year experience comparing VCUG to positive-pressure urethrography (PPUG) in the evaluation of UD found that the positive predictive value of VCUG after PPUG was only 60%.[53] VCUG will also fail to identify UD in up to 56% of cases.[58,59] Once considered the gold standard for diagnostic evaluation, VCUG is now used by many mainly as a screening test. Should it fail to adequately characterize or identify UD and there is still high suspicion that the entity exists, other imaging modalities should be applied.[53]

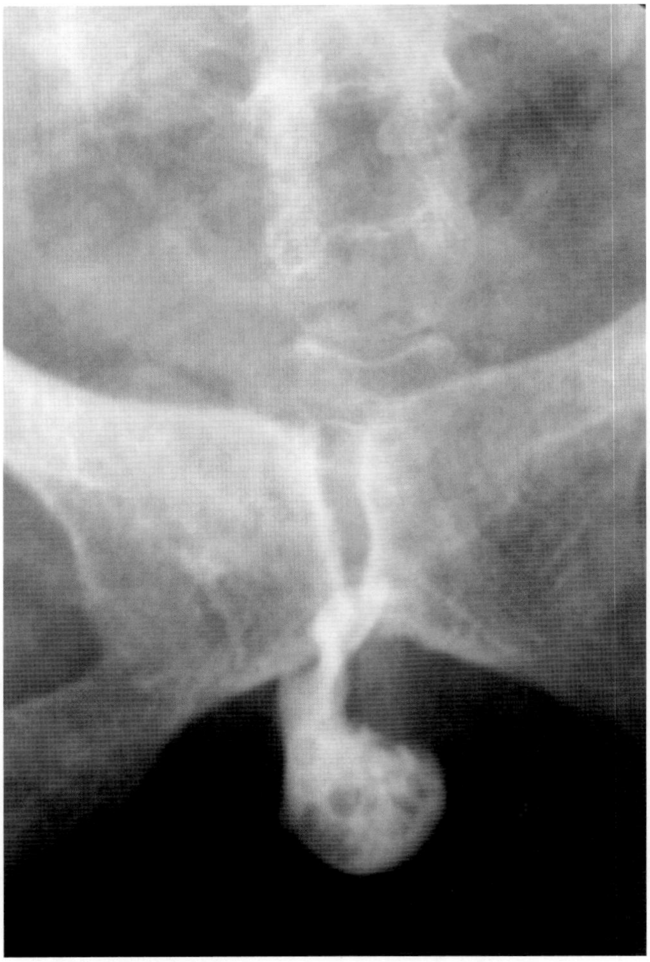

Figure 90.6. *A post-void film demonstrating filling defects within a urethral diverticulum suggestive of stones or tumor. (Reproduced from ref. 57 with permission.)*

Ultrasonography

Ultrasonography is used in the evaluation of the upper tracts or, occasionally, in conjunction with VCUG to confirm the number and size of diverticula, especially in those not completely filled during urethrography[23,60,61] (Fig. 90.7). Vargas-Serrano et al.[61] advocate transrectal ultrasonography (TRUS) as the most sensitive tool in the diagnosis of female UD. Keefe et al.[60] support transperineal or transvaginal sonography, stating 100% sensitivity in their small series and stressing the non-invasive nature of the technique. Multiple approaches to ultrasonography have been employed, including transvaginal,[62,63] translabial,[64] suprapubic,[60] perineal,[60] and TRUS.[61] Intraoperative endoluminal ultrasonography has been described for localization of the UD;[65,66] however, this is very difficult to perform. One limitation is that the modality is dependent on the technical skills of the operator. Advantages include real-time evaluation and the ability to clarify the spatial relationships between the diverticulum and the urethra.[52] Compared to other diagnostic tools including VCUG, magnetic resonance imaging, and cystoscopy, ultrasound is less expensive.[52]

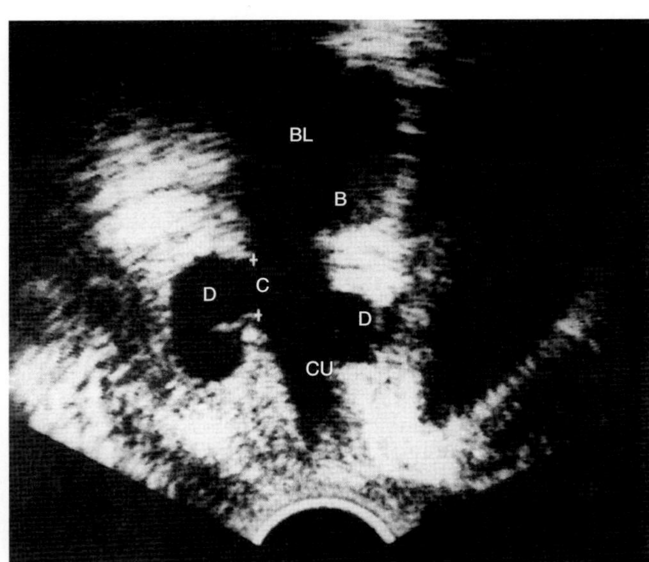

Figure 90.7. *Transvaginal ultrasonography demonstrating a multiloculated urethral diverticulum opening into the proximal urethra. B, Foley catheter balloon; BL, bladder; C, diverticular communication; CU, intraurethral Foley catheter; D, diverticulum. (Reproduced from ref. 9 with permission.)*

Intravenous pyelography

Intravenous pyelography (IVP) can be useful to evaluate the upper tracts and rule out an ectopic ureterocele.[67–69] Ectopic ureterocele may be considered when there is an abnormal protrusion into the urethra or from the meatus. It is important to obtain a low pelvic view in order to visualize the urethra completely (Fig. 90.8).

Magnetic resonance imaging

Magnetic resonance imaging (MRI) has recently been found to be a useful diagnostic tool with a high sensitivity for identifying fluid-filled cavities.[30,70–73] Endorectal and endovaginal coil MRI techniques differ from surface or body coil MRI because the coil is placed within the body cavity adjacent to the tissue of interest. This results in improved signal-to-noise ratio and higher resolution imaging of the urethra.[74] Kim et al.[75] reported 100% sensitivity of MRI in the detection of UD. The signal intensity of fluid is high on T2-weighted images and isointense on T1-weighted images (Fig. 90.9).

MRI is being advocated as helpful in defining the extent of a UD and differentiating it from other urethral or vaginal masses, such as malignancy, paraurethral cysts, and Gartner's duct cysts. Endorectal coil MRI can also be useful in the diagnosis of periurethral fibrosis and other periurethral pathology.[76] When compared to VCUG, MRI has been touted to have higher sensitivity and better characterization of size, location, and complexity of the diverticulum.[74] The superior imaging may also impact surgical planning by more accurately delineating the extent of the diverticulum. The high cost

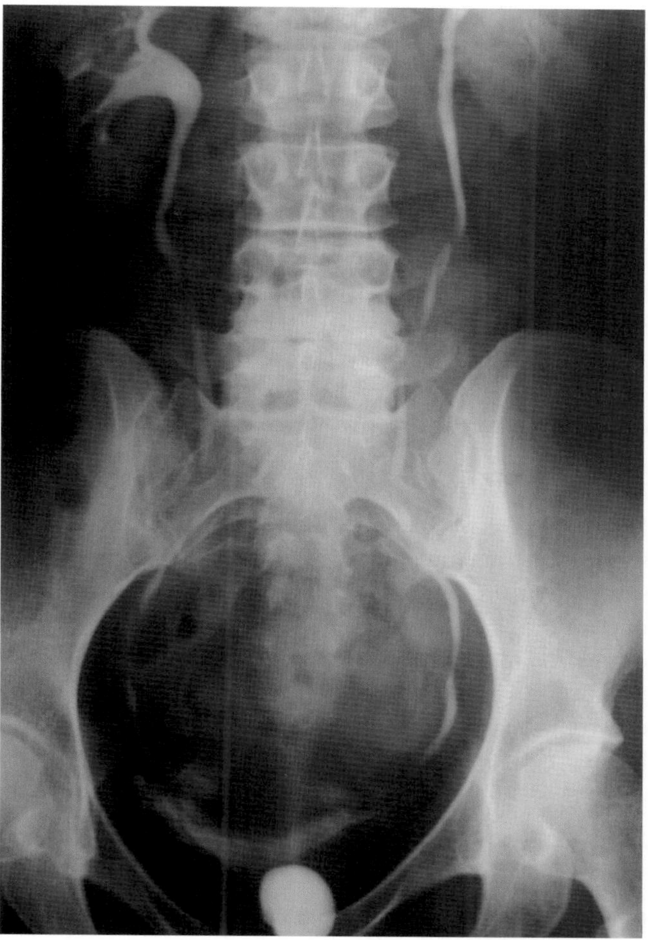

Figure 90.8. *Intravenous pyelogram demonstrates the urethral diverticulum and the upper tracts.*

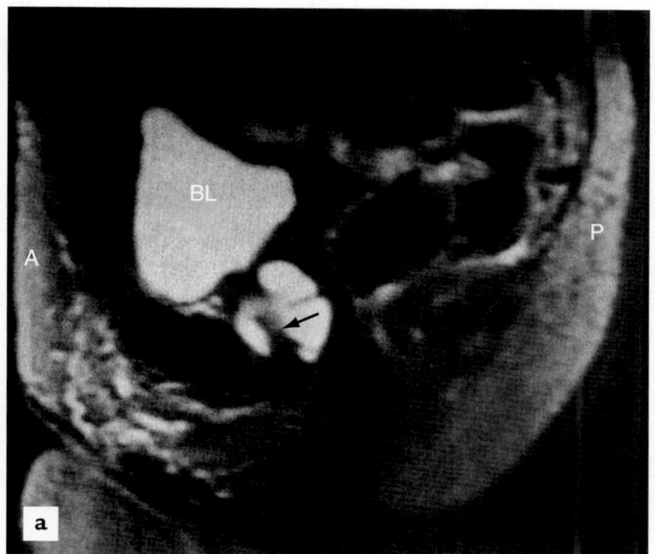

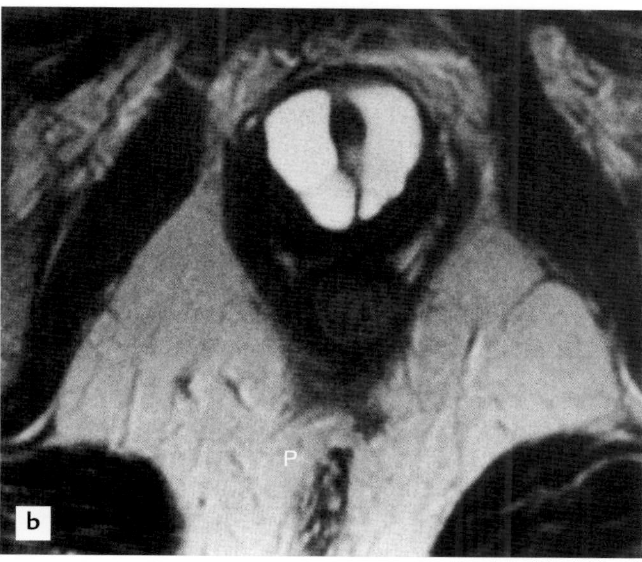

Figure 90.9. *T2-weighted magnetic resonance imaging illustrates a multiloculated diverticulum (arrow) posterolateral to the urethra; (a) sagittal view; (b) axial view. A, anterior; BL, bladder; P, posterior. (Reproduced from ref. 72 with permission.)*

of MRI is a detraction compared to other modalities. Endovaginal coil MRI may also be uncomfortable for the patient, but probably not any more so than VCUG or PPUG. The superior anatomic delineation provided by MRI makes it the present-day gold standard for imaging of UD.

Retrograde positive-pressure urethrography

Retrograde positive-pressure urethrography (PPUG) is reported by Robertson[7] to have a 90% accuracy. Additional studies have reported superior sensitivity of PPUG over VCUG for diagnosis of UD.[58,59] However, the authors rarely use this technique and, in urologic practice today, it is employed only as a last resort, when high-quality VCUG or MRI is not available. It is a painful procedure for patients, often necessitating anesthesia; it is also technically difficult to obtain an adequate study, requiring a special catheter known as the Davis or Tratner catheter[7,77] (Fig. 90.10). This catheter has a double balloon: one balloon is placed in the bladder; the distal (wedge-shaped) balloon slides to occlude the external meatus during injection of contrast via ports located between the balloons (Fig. 90.10).

THERAPY

History

Numerous techniques for identification and repair of UD have been described. Intradiverticular placement of a sound,[3,78] a Foley catheter,[79] a Fogarty catheter,[80] gauze,[81] silicone, or blood products[82] have been used to facilitate identification of the defect. Repair has been performed endoscopically and transvaginally by incision of the urethral floor with layered reconstruction,[34] marsupialization,[83,84] packing of the UD with various materials to obliterate the cavity,[85,86] and transvaginal flap creation with layered closure.[55,79,87,88]

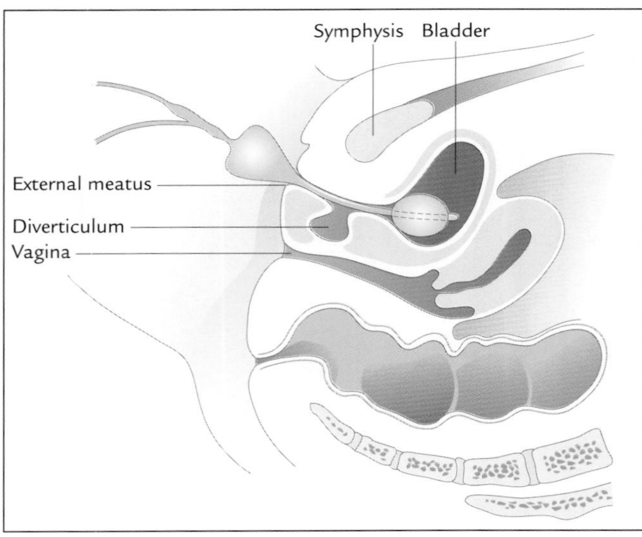

Figure 90.10. *Placement of a Tratner/Davis double-balloon catheter for positive-pressure retrograde urethrography.*

Observation

Surgical resection and reconstruction are frequently necessary in the treatment of UD. However, observation is an option in the asymptomatic or very small UD. Marshall[89] reported that UD in young girls might regress spontaneously; therefore, in this rare situation, observation may be a reasonable option.

Endoscopic treatment

Endoscopic treatment should be utilized only for distal UD to avoid injury to the proximally located continence mechanism. Transurethral saucerization with incision of the urethral floor[90,91] or of the anterior urethra overlying the UD[92] with a Collins' knife through a pediatric resectoscope can be performed with minimal risk of complication. The major risk is incontinence and can be avoided by limiting this technique to distal UD.[5] This risk also applies to transvaginal marsupialization (Fig. 90.11), an outpatient procedure often referred to as the Spence procedure.[7] One blade of the scissors is placed in the vagina, the other in the urethra to marsupialize the cavity.

Excision with vaginal flap technique

The authors prefer the transvaginal flap technique for all midurethral or proximal UD. This technique allows complete resection of the UD with a three-layer closure and no overlapping suture lines. Simultaneous needle bladder neck suspension (BNS) can easily be performed when deemed necessary (in cases of SUI or bladder neck/proximal urethral hypermobility).

Preoperative preparation

Preoperatively, the risks of diverticulectomy – including bleeding, infection, recurrence, urethrovaginal fistula formation, and incontinence – are explained to the patient in detail. Patients may benefit from a short course of oral antibiotics, and all receive perioperative intravenous antibiotics.

Diverticulum
a
b
c
Running stitch
Urethra
Urethra
Vagina
d
e
f

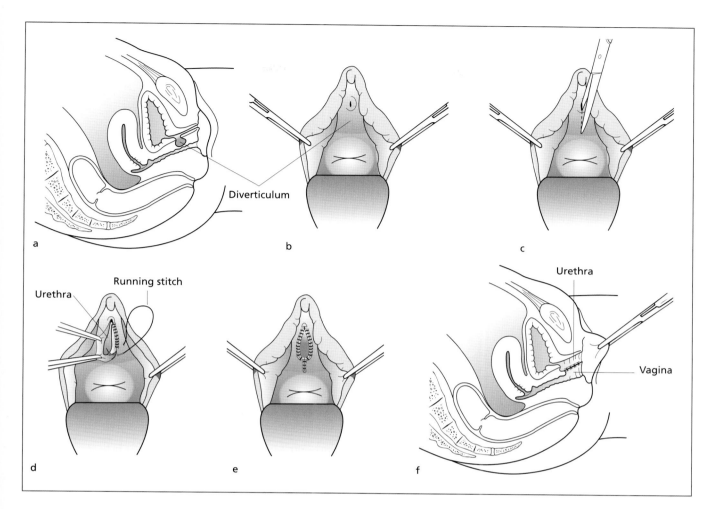

Figure 90.11. *The Spence technique for marsupialization of distal urethral diverticula (UD): (a) lateral and (b) surgical views of UD; (c) one blade of the scissors is inserted into the UD and the other into the vagina and a full thickness cut of the diverticular septum is performed; (d) a running absorbable suture promotes hemostasis; (e) and (f) the new urethral meatus is created.*

Surgical technique

The patient is placed in the lithotomy position, and a suprapubic tube (SPT) is placed. A 14 Fr urethral Foley catheter is passed and a weighted vaginal speculum and a Scott ring retractor facilitate exposure. The anterior vaginal wall (Fig. 90.12) is infiltrated with saline to facilitate dissection in the proper plane. A U-shaped incision is made with the apex located distal to the UD (Fig. 90.13).

If concomitant BNS is performed, the vaginal dissection is extended laterally beneath the vaginal wall to the pubic bone on each side. The suspension sutures should be placed prior to manipulation or decompression of the UD to avoid postoperative infection. The endopelvic fascia is perforated with the bladder completely emptied and the retropubic space is developed. Helical 1-0 Prolene

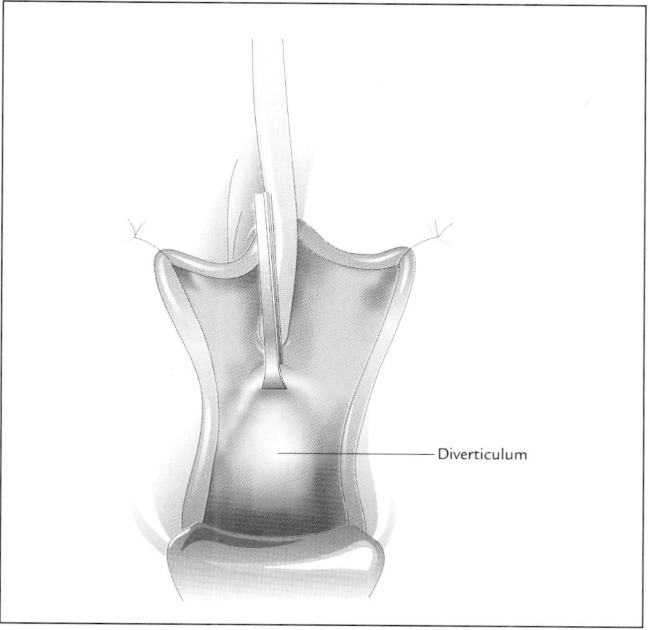

Figure 90.12. *Anterior vaginal wall and urethral diverticulum. (Reproduced from ref. 55 with permission.)*

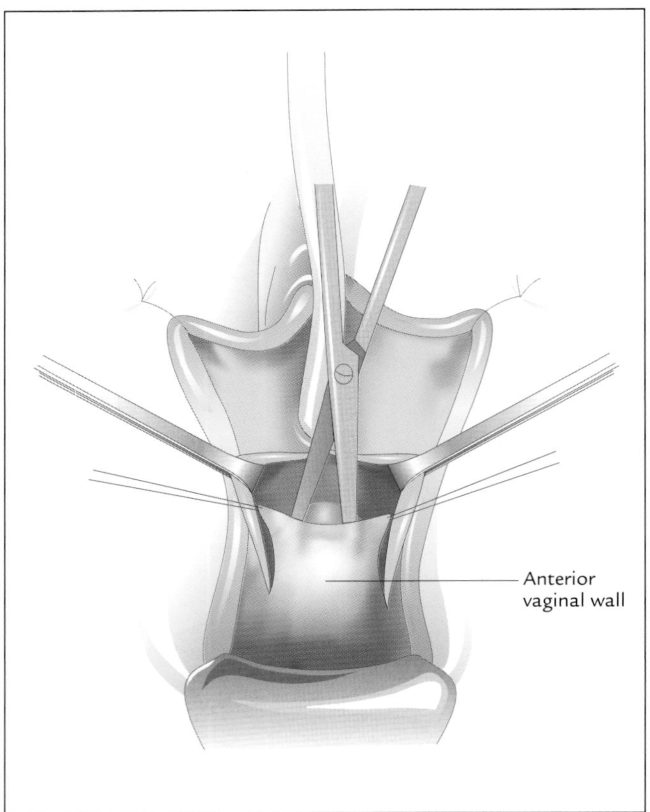

Figure 90.13. *An inverted U-incision is made in the anterior vaginal wall, and the vaginal wall is dissected off the underlying periurethral fascia.*

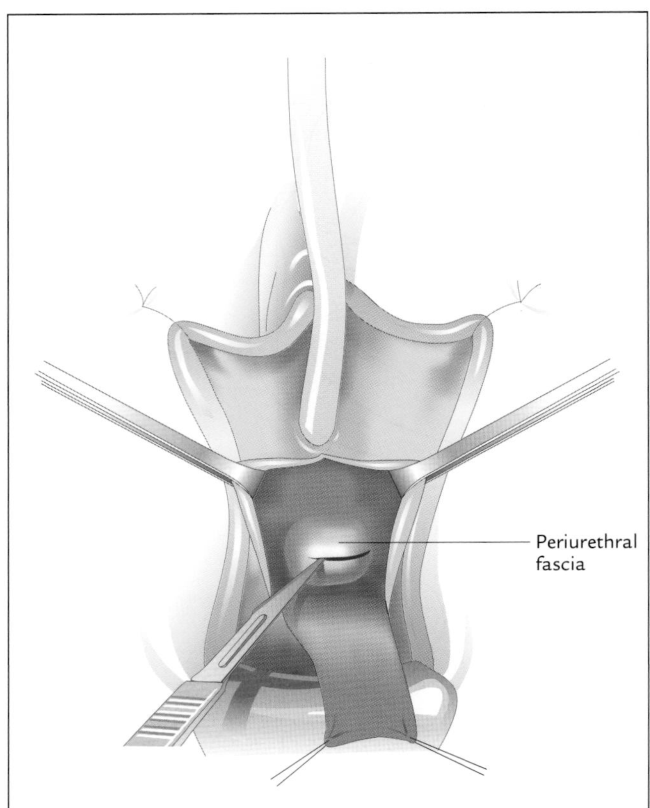

Figure 90.14. *The periurethral fascia is incised transversely.*

sutures are placed in the vaginal wall and directed with a Pereyra needle into the suprapubic incision. Cystoscopy is performed to ensure that no suture has passed into the bladder or urethra. *Care must be taken to avoid entry into the UD during suture placement. If the UD is large and/or proximally located, it may be difficult to avoid; in this situation, the BNS should be postponed.* The use of bone anchors for the BNS has been described;[87] however, the authors do not advocate this when diverticulectomy is being performed in view of the risk of infection. Additionally, Swierzewski and McGuire[93] have recommended a concomitant pubovaginal sling with diverticulectomy; however, the authors avoid the use of a concomitant sling procedure because of concerns of urethral erosion of the sling and breakdown of the reconstruction site.

The diverticulectomy is continued with creation of a vaginal flap with sharp dissection directly on the shiny white layer of the vaginal wall. *Dissection in the wrong plane can result in significant bleeding or inadvertent entry into the periurethral fascia or the UD, thereby rendering the remainder of the dissection very difficult.* Mobilization of the vaginal flap towards the bladder neck, followed by a transverse incision in the periurethral fascia (Fig. 90.14) exposes the UD, which lies directly beneath this layer. The periurethral fascia is then sharply dissected off the UD (Fig. 90.15), which is then exposed circumferentially until the diverticular neck is encountered (Fig. 90.16). *Difficulty in identification of the urethral communication site can result in incomplete resection of the UD and subsequent recurrence. Identification can be facilitated by insertion of a pediatric sound into the UD.*

Complete excision of both the UD and its neck can create a significant urethral defect (Fig. 90.17). Incomplete resection of the diverticulum can lead to recurrence. However, when the UD is large, extensive dissection beneath the trigone can endanger the ureters and bladder base, sometimes necessitating leaving the most proximal portion of the UD behind. In these cases, cautery to the inner epithelial surface will obliterate the cavity. The urethral defect is closed vertically over a 14 Fr catheter without tension using a full-thickness 4-0 Vicryl stitch, incorporating both urethral mucosa and the urethral wall (Fig. 90.18). The periurethral fascia is closed transversely with running 3-0 Vicryl (Fig. 90.19). Dead space should be obliterated beneath this layer. In cases in which there is insufficient tissue for closure of a second layer, or when the vaginal tissue is tenuous or fibrotic (such as secondary to previous surgery or radiation), a well-vascularized 8–12 cm Martius fat-pad graft may be placed between the vagina and urethra. The third and final layer is the vaginal wall, which is closed with 2-0 absorbable suture. The three layers of closure include the urethral wall vertically, the periurethral fascia transversely, and the vaginal U-inci-

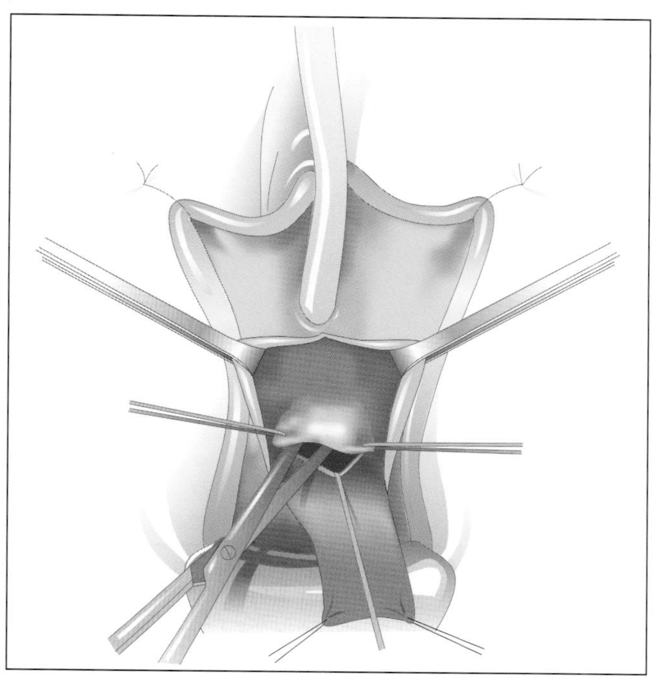

Figure 90.15. *The periurethral tissue is dissected from the diverticulum.*

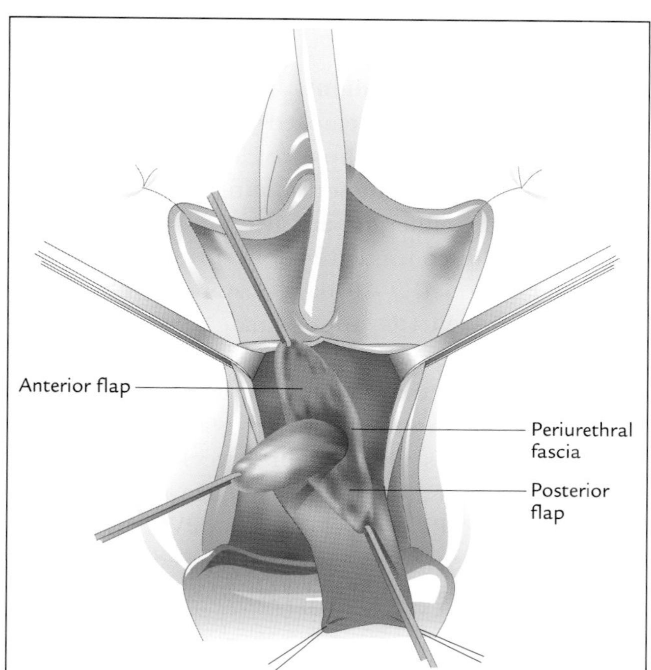

Figure 90.16. *The diverticulum is isolated and carefully dissected until the communication is identified.*

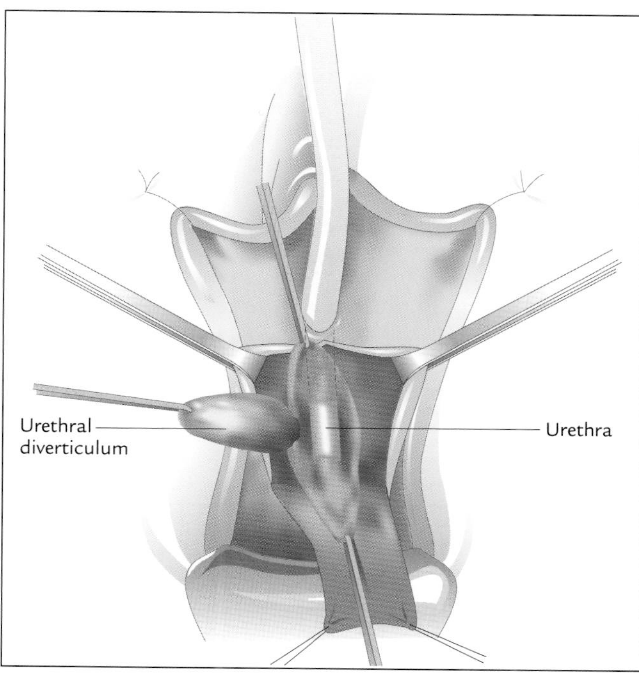

Figure 90.17. *The diverticulum is amputated at its communication site, thereby exposing the urethral Foley catheter and leaving a urethral defect.*

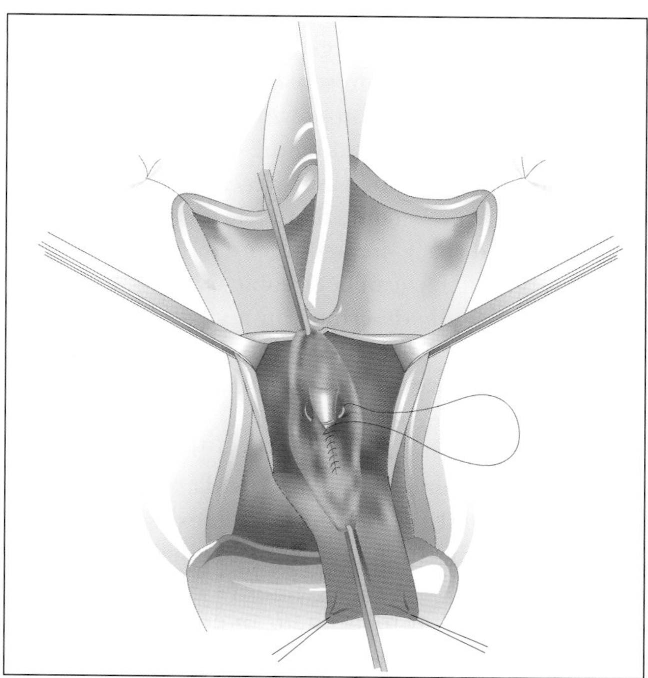

Figure 90.18. *The urethra is reapproximated longitudinally with 4-0 absorbable suture.*

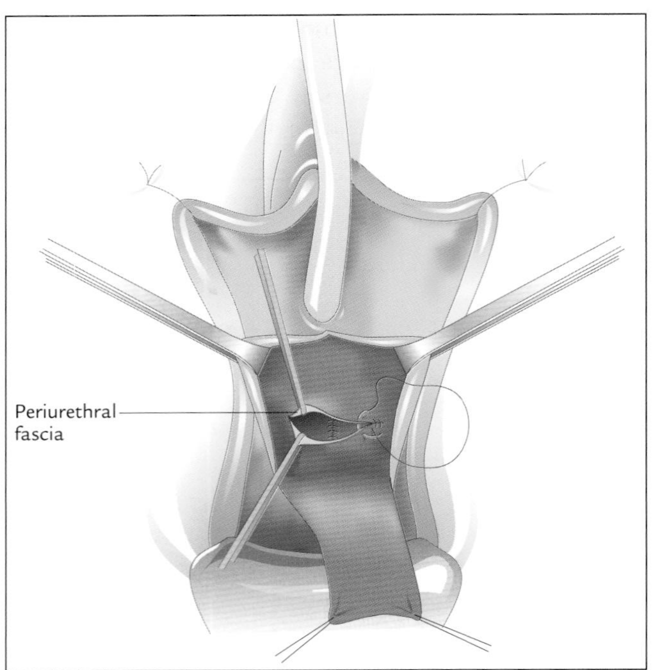

Figure 90.19. *The periurethral tissue is closed transversely with 3-0 absorbable suture.*

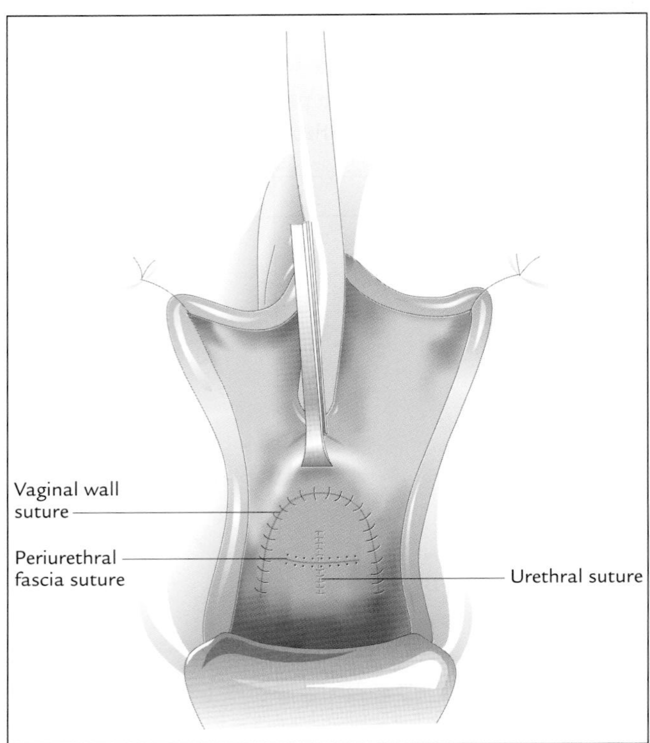

Figure 90.20. *The vaginal wall flap is closed, resulting in a three-layer closure with no overlapping suture lines.*

sion. The goal is to avoid overlapping suture lines (Fig. 90.20). Antibiotic- or estrogen-soaked vaginal packing is inserted, and the SPT and Foley catheter are placed to gravity drainage.

Anterior or dorsally located horseshoe-shaped and circumferential urethral diverticula present unique challenges to the pelvic surgeon. Because of their complexity, they frequently present as recurrent diverticula that have been operated on previously. The tissue planes may be obscured, complicating the dissection. The anterior location is also not easily accessed transvaginally. Anterior UD can become large, leading to difficulty filling the dead space created after excision. The subsequent urethral defect can be sizeable (>2 cm). Clyne and Flood have recently described an approach to anterior horseshoe-shaped UD using a suprameatal incision.[94] In addition, they utilize double wrapped porcine xenograft to aid in filling of dead space.

Retropubic approaches have also been described;[95] however, for circumferential diverticula, a separate vaginal incision would also be necessary to excise the ventral portion of the diverticulum. A parasagittal vaginal incision with detachment of the urethra from the inferior pubic ramus laterally to facilitate anterior dissection has recently been outlined.[96] Rovner and Wein have introduced a novel technique for excision and reconstruction of dorsal or circumferential UD by dividing the urethra to access the anterior portion of the diverticulum. Once excised, end-to-end urethroplasty or diverticular sac urethroplasty is performed.[97] Martius flap interposition was performed in nearly all patients to help with closure of dead space.

Postoperative management

The vaginal packing is removed on postoperative day 1. All patients receive 24 hours of intravenous antibiotics followed by oral antibiotics until the catheters are removed. Anticholinergics are given to relieve bladder spasms but are discontinued 24 hours prior to the VCUG, which is performed 7–10 days postoperatively. At the time of this first VCUG, approximately 50% of patients have some extravasation from the urethral reconstruction site.[5] When extravasation is evident, the SPT is left in place, but the urethral catheter is not reinserted. A follow-up VCUG is obtained in a week's time. When there is no extravasation, the SPT is clamped and a postvoid residual (PVR) is checked. If the PVR is 100 ml or less, the SPT is removed; if the PVR exceeds 100 ml, the SPT is left in place until this volume decreases.

RESULTS AND COMPLICATIONS

Potential complications following a urethral diverticulectomy include incontinence, UD recurrence,

Table 90.8. *Complications of urethral diverticulectomy*

Complication	Possible causes
Incontinence	Failure to identify SUI preoperatively New onset SUI DI Recurrent diverticulum leading to 'paradoxical incontinence' Urethrovaginal fistula
Recurrent diverticulum	Failure to identify multiple diverticula preoperatively Incomplete excision Faulty closure
Urethrovaginal fistula	Closure under tension Tenuous, unhealthy tissue Failure to close in layers Overlapping suture lines
Irritative symptoms	Urinary tract infection Bladder dysfunction (DI) Outlet obstruction
Urethral stricture	Extensive urethral wall excision Closure under tension

DI, detrusor instability; SUI, stress urinary incontinence.

Table 90.9. *Treatment modalities for 63 patients*

Operative treatment	56 (88.9%)
Diverticulectomy alone	29 (51.8%)
Diverticulectomy + BNS	27 (48.2%)
Martius fat-pad graft	7 (11.1%)
No operative treatment	7* (11.1%)

* In three cases surgery was refused; there were four cases of small asymptomatic diverticula not requiring surgery.
BNS, bladder neck suspension.
Reproduced, with modifications, from ref. 9 with permission.

Table 90.10. *Complications*

Recurrence (distal repair site)	2
Suprapubic tenderness*	1
Early urinary tract infection (none recurrent)	6
Urethrovaginal fistula†	1
Wound infection/urethral stricture	0

* Patient had concomitant bladder neck suspension.
† Required subsequent surgical repair.

urethrovaginal fistula, irritative symptoms, urethral stricture, and general postoperative complications (Table 90.8).[98]

Ganabathi et al.[9] evaluated 63 women who had been treated for UD between 1982 and 1992: 56 were treated operatively and seven were observed. The specific treatment modalities employed are shown in Table 90.9. Patients were followed-up for a mean of 70 months, with a range of 10–124 months. Table 90.10 reports the complications encountered. The two recurrences of the UD occurred distal to the initial repair site.

Overall continence status, shown in Table 90.11, indicates that the majority of patients were totally continent. A greater percentage of the patients who underwent diverticulectomy alone were reported as continent, than were those who underwent diverticulectomy with concomitant BNS (Table 90.12). It was reported that incontinence was more frequently secondary to SUI than to detrusor instability, despite the presumed increase in bladder neck support.

Incontinence may be secondary to persistent SUI that was present preoperatively. This situation can be avoided by a comprehensive preoperative evaluation so that it can be addressed at the time of diverticulectomy.[9,99,100] Incontinence can also be a result of urethrovaginal fistula, recurrent diverticulum with paradoxical loss of urine with stress, infection, persistent detrusor instability or new-onset SUI. The first two conditions may

Table 90.11. *Overall continence of 56 patients with mean follow-up of 70 months*

Incontinence	*n* (%)
Nil or moderate (dry or 0 pads/day)	45 (80.4)
Moderate (1–2 minipads/day)	10 (17.9)
Severe (several pads/day)	1 (1.8)

Table 90.12. *Continence status of 56 patients with mean follow-up of 70 months*

	Diverticulectomy alone (*n*=29)	Diverticulectomy and BNS (*n*=27)
Continent	25 (86.2%)	20 (74%)
Incontinent	4 (13.8%)	7 (26%)
DI	1 (3.4%)	1 (3.7%)
SUI	3 (10.3%)	6 (22.2%)

BNS, bladder-neck support; DI, detrusor instability; SUI, stress urinary incontinence.
Reproduced, with modifications, from ref. 9 with permission.

require surgical intervention. New-onset SUI may be a result of the urethral dissection, which may compromise urethral support, or secondary to dissection beneath the proximal urethra and bladder neck, which is often necessary when removing a large UD. Detrusor instability can be treated successfully in some cases with behavioral therapy, anticholinergic therapy or the addition of a tricyclic antidepressant such as imipramine; this not only increases bladder outlet tone but also decreases detrusor contractility.

Recurrent UD is often a result of failure to identify multiple UD preoperatively, secondary to lack of either suspicion or proper high-quality studies.[9,100] Incomplete excision of the diverticular neck, as well as faulty closure of the urethral defect, are also possible causes. This problem can be managed with interposition of a Martius fat-pad graft between the vagina and urethra.[9] For small, distal recurrences, endoscopic saucerization or Spence marsupialization may suffice;[5] however, caution must be exercised not to injure the proximally located continence mechanism. Urethrovaginal fistulae (UVF) formation, another potential complication, is managed in much the same manner and may be prevented by intraoperative Martius flap if tissues appear tenuous or under tension. UVF is discussed in more detail in the next section.

Finally, urethral stricture resulting from extensive excision of the urethral wall at the time of diverticulectomy can be prevented by a tension-free urethral closure over a 14 Fr catheter. If this is not possible, reconstruction using vaginal wall can be contemplated, again with consideration of a Martius labial fat-pad graft.

URETHROVAGINAL FISTULA

INTRODUCTION

Urethrovaginal fistula (UVF) is a rare condition. Fistulae range from small communications between the urethra and the vagina to total loss of the urethra and bladder neck.[5,101–103] A distal fistula may present with vaginal voiding or a splayed urinary stream. Midurethral or proximal fistulae can present with varying degrees of continence, depending upon fistulae location and bladder neck competence.[104,105] Urethral fistulae are most commonly caused by complications of previous surgery, such as anterior colporrhaphy or urethral diverticulectomy (see previous section). Urethral erosion of synthetic pubovaginal slings leading to fistulae formation is a relatively recent phenomenon. Its increased frequency is most likely due to the increased popularity of the procedure over the past few years.[106] A urethrovaginal fistula has also been reported following periurethral collagen injection.[107] Other causes include radiation therapy and birth trauma, although this is rare with modern obstetric techniques. Obstructed labor remains the most common cause of urethral injury in developing countries.[16]

DIAGNOSIS

The differential diagnosis of UVF includes SUI, intrinsic sphincter deficiency (ISD), or vaginal voiding due to other conditions.

A careful history and physical examination can help to differentiate between the above conditions. Careful history taking may reveal previous vaginal or pelvic surgery or symptoms of stress versus urge incontinence. Physical examination is important to assess urethral loss, location and size of the fistula, urethral and bladder neck mobility, and quality of vaginal tissue, including scarring and atrophy.

Studies that may aid in the diagnosis include cystourethroscopy, IVP to evaluate the upper tracts, renal ultrasonography, VCUG, and urodynamic studies. Cystoscopy is performed with a 20 Fr female urethroscope with a 0-degree lens. It is essential to examine the urethra, bladder neck, trigone, and quality of the tissue. A concomitant vesicovaginal fistula must be excluded. If identification of the UVF is difficult, simultaneous vaginal examination with a speculum may identify fluid spraying into the vagina through the communication.

Upper tract evaluation is essential when the trigone is involved and may be accomplished with IVP or renal ultrasonography. A standing fluoroscopic VCUG is often helpful in identification of the urethral defect and in excluding a vesicovaginal fistula. VCUG also aids in assessment of urethral hypermobility and/or leakage of urine across the bladder neck during stress. Finally, urodynamic studies may be of benefit in evaluation of bladder function and sphincter integrity when the UVF is in the distal third of the vagina.

TREATMENT

The goal of treatment of urethral fistulae is to create a competent neourethra of adequate length to permit unobstructed passage of urine while preserving urinary continence.[102] Additionally, urethrovaginal repair must be tension free. Distal fistulae may be managed with an extended meatotomy.[5] The postoperative incontinence rate may be as high as 50% if SUI is not considered at the time of fistula repair.[5] Some authors have suggested concomitant sling at the time of fistula repair.[102] Because of concerns about the risks of erosion of the sling at the time of mid- or proximal UVF repair, the authors avoid performing a sling simultaneously with UVF repair.

Operative technique

Preoperative preparation is similar to that for urethral diverticulectomy (see previous section). Estrogen is administered preoperatively, if indicated, to treat atrophic vaginitis. Urine culture is performed to ensure that the urine is sterile preoperatively. If necessary, a short course of oral antibiotics is given. All patients receive perioperative intravenous ampicillin and gentamicin, unless contraindicated.

Essentially, all types of urethral and bladder neck defects can be approached transvaginally, often in conjunction with a Martius fat-pad graft.[104,105,108] This includes simple fistula repair and vaginal flap total urethral reconstruction.

Our preferred approach for transvaginal fistulae closure and vaginal flap urethral reconstruction requires placement of the patient in the lithotomy position (Fig. 90.21). A 20–24 Fr SPT is placed and a 14 Fr urethral catheter is inserted. Postoperative self-catheterization of the neourethra must be avoided, hence the necessity of the SPT. The SPT also serves as a 'safety valve' if the urethral catheter becomes obstructed. The vaginal wall is infiltrated with saline to develop the proper plane, and an inverted U-incision is made. The apex of the incision is located just proximal to the fistula for fistulectomy and at the meatus for total urethral reconstruction. Dissection in the avascular plane exposes the shiny white surface of the interior vaginal wall. Excessive bleeding and bladder perforation are risks if dissection is too deep.

When concomitant BNS is necessary, lateral dissection and perforation of the endopelvic fascia is performed. The suspension sutures in the anterior vaginal wall and periurethral tissue are placed but not tied. The authors tend not to advocate routine simultaneous sling procedures, owing to the risk of erosion through the reconstructed urethra. However, if the decision to proceed with a concomitant sling is made, the authors

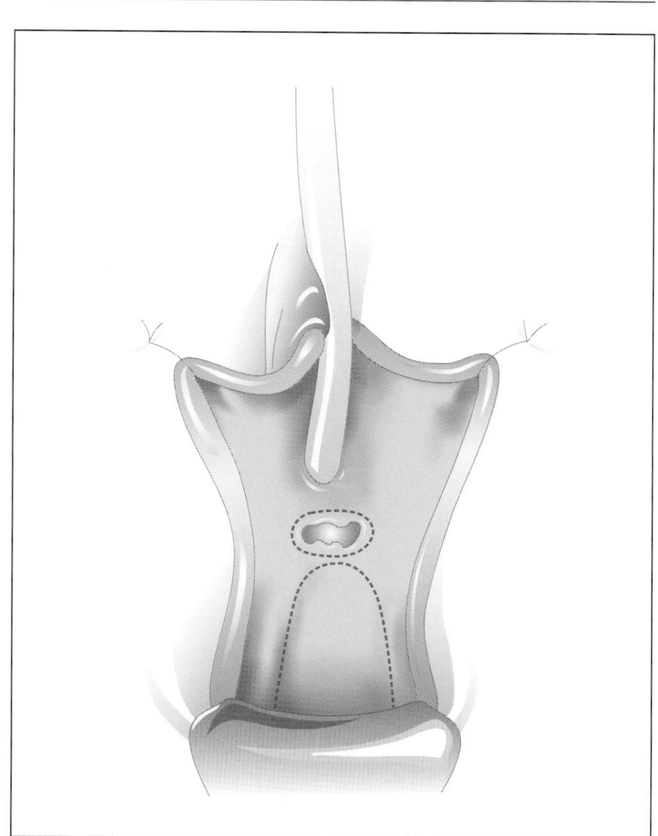

Figure 90.21. *An inverted U-incision is made in the vaginal wall with the apex just proximal to the fistula.*

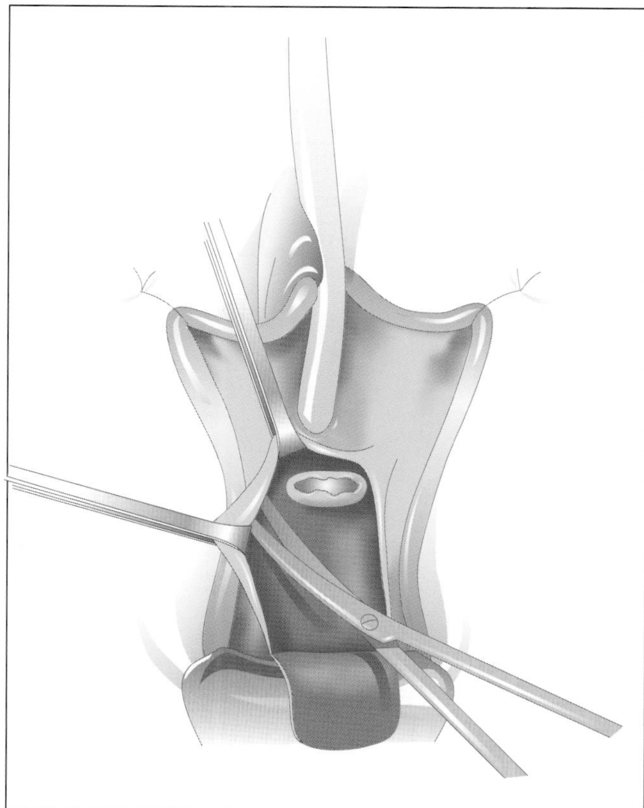

Figure 90.22. *The fistula is circumscribed but not excised. The avascular plane beneath the lateral vaginal wall is developed.*

would certainly recommend the use of autologous or allograft tissue. Flisser and Blaivas have reported good success using autologous fascia slings with Martius labial fat-pad graft in patients at risk of postoperative incontinence with few complications.[106] Leng et al. also endorse use of the autologous fascia sling in cases of urethrovaginal fistulae with type III SUI as it offers the advantage of dual function as a reinforcing layer and continence procedure.[109]

The fistula is circumscribed but not excised (Fig. 90.22). Scarred tissue margins are freed to allow a tension-free closure of the tract. A portion of the vaginal wall just distal to the fistula is then mobilized to create a flap. The fistula is closed with running locking absorbable suture (Fig. 90.23). For total reconstruction of the urethra, two vaginal wall incisions are made parallel to and on either side of the urethra to create medially based flaps (Fig. 90.24). The flaps are tubularized around a 14 Fr urethral catheter and approximated at the midline with 4-0 absorbable sutures (Fig. 90.25). For fistula repair, a second layer of running Lembert stitch with 3-0 absorbable suture is placed to complete a watertight closure. The third layer is the closure of the vaginal flap with a locked running stitch using absorbable suture. In this manner, overlapping suture lines are avoided (Fig. 90.26).

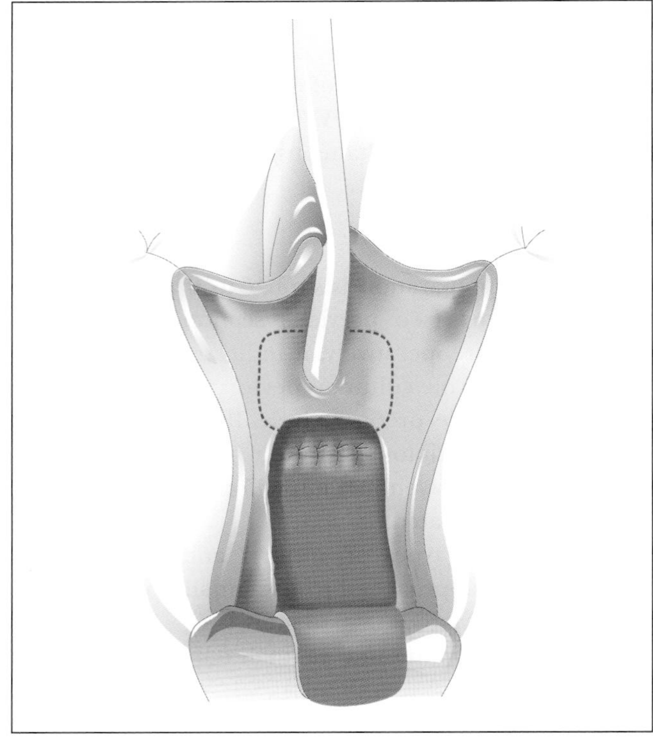

Figure 90.24. *Two longitudinal incisions are made to create medially based flaps.*

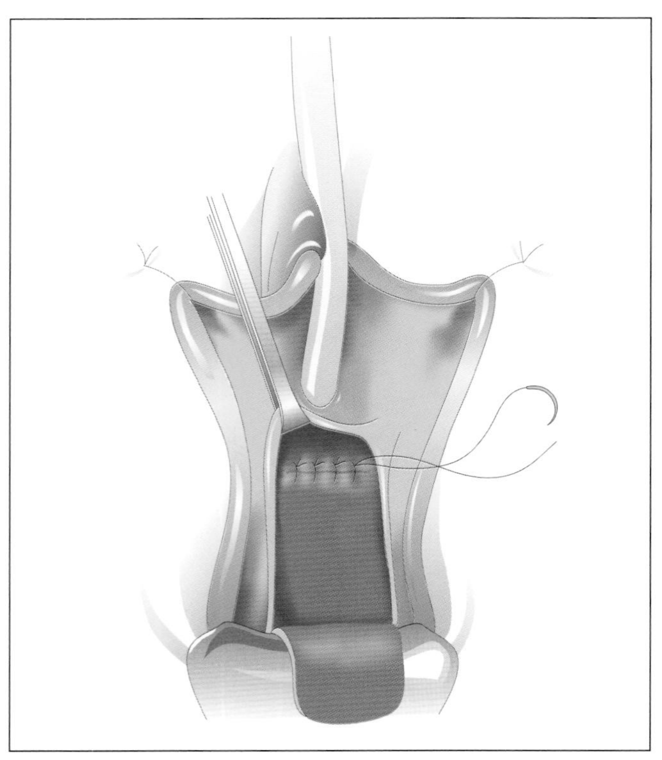

Figure 90.23. *The fistula is closed with absorbable suture.*

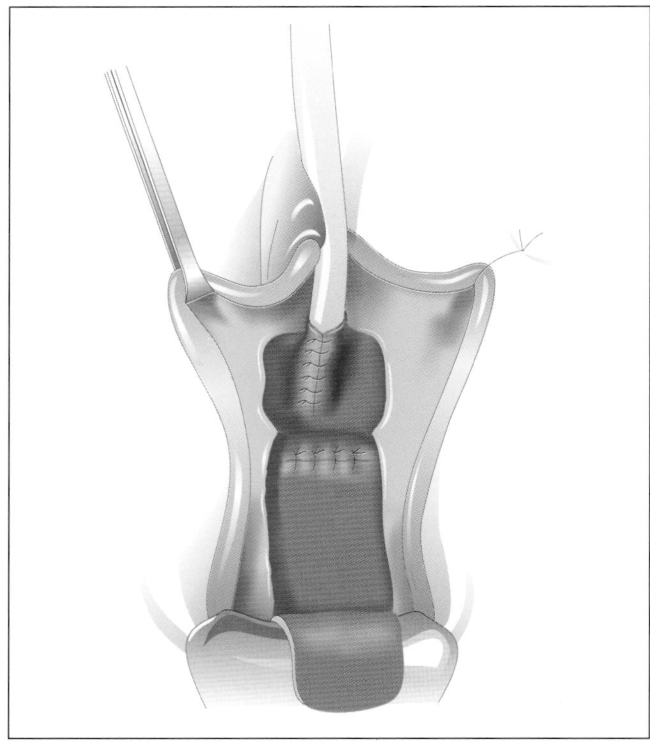

Figure 90.25. *The flaps are rolled over a 14 Fr urethral catheter.*

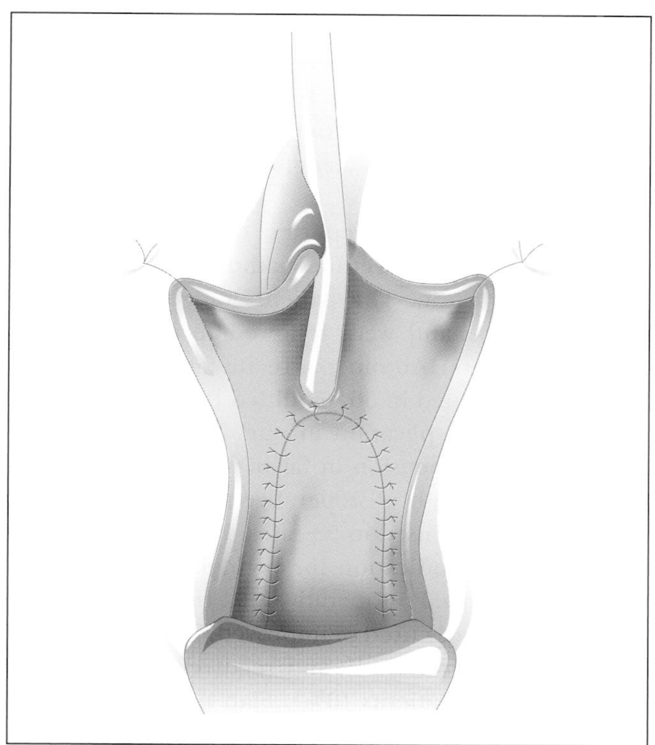

Figure 90.26. *The vaginal flap is closed with a running, locking absorbable suture.*

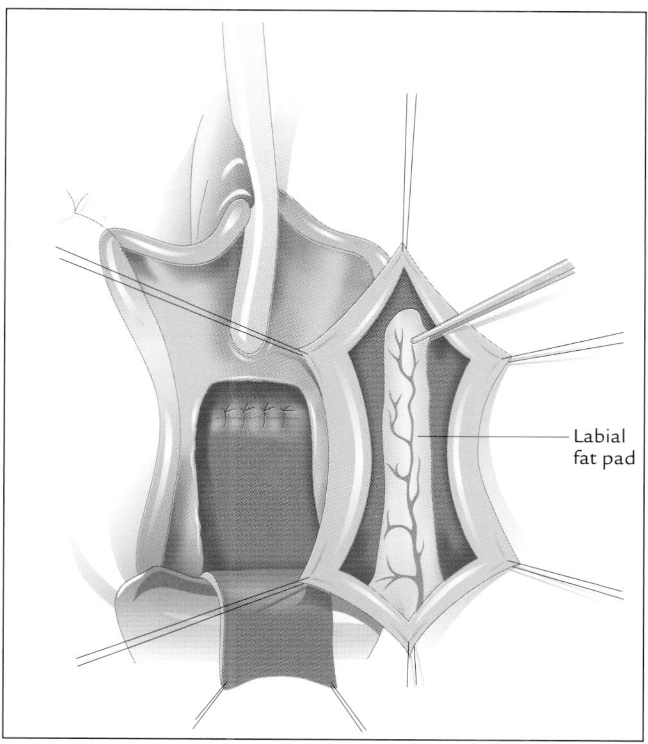

Figure 90.27. *The labium majus is incised, and the Martius fat-pad graft is mobilized with care to preserve the posteriorly located pudendal vessels.*

If the tissues are tenuous or inadequate, a Martius fat-pad graft may be interposed between the urethra and the vagina. The labium majus is incised to expose the underlying fat pad. The flap is mobilized, preserving the pudendal vessels, located posteriorly (Fig. 90.27). The fat pad is passed through a subcutaneous tunnel from the labium majus to the vagina and secured over the fistula repair site with absorbable sutures (Fig. 90.28). A ¼-inch Penrose drain is placed deep into the labial wound, and the labial incision is closed in layers. The vaginal flap (described above) is closed over the Martius flap (Fig. 90.29).

When a Martius fat-pad graft is not feasible, a meatal-based vaginal flap can be rotated distally (Fig. 90.30)[102] or a neourethra can be created from a cutaneous portion of the gracilis muscle or a perineal artery-based myocutaneous flap.[102] Finally, in selected cases, one may resort to closure of the bladder neck with creation of a catheterizable stoma or placement of a suprapubic catheter.[110]

The urethral Foley catheter and SPT are placed to gravity drainage, and an antibiotic- or estrogen-soaked vaginal pack is placed. Patients receive perioperative intravenous antibiotics, which are converted to oral medication on postoperative day 1. Anticholinergics are administered to prevent bladder spasm, and are dis-

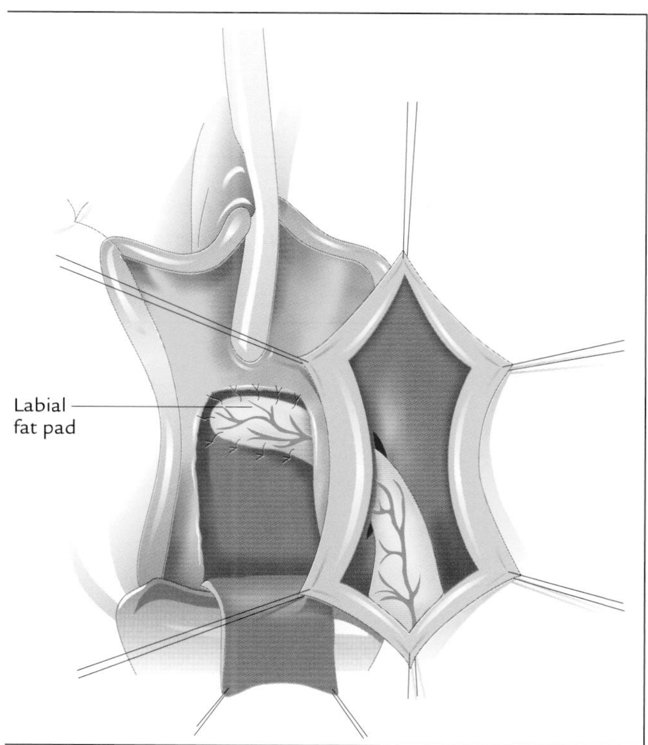

Figure 90.28. *The labial fat pad is passed through a medial tunnel and secured over the fistula repair site.*

continued at least 24 hours prior to the VCUG, which is performed between postoperative days 7 and 10. If extravasation is noted, the SPT is left to gravity and the urethral catheter is not replaced.

The VCUG is repeated after 1–2 weeks and the SPT is removed when there is no extravasation and PVRs are minimal (<100 ml).

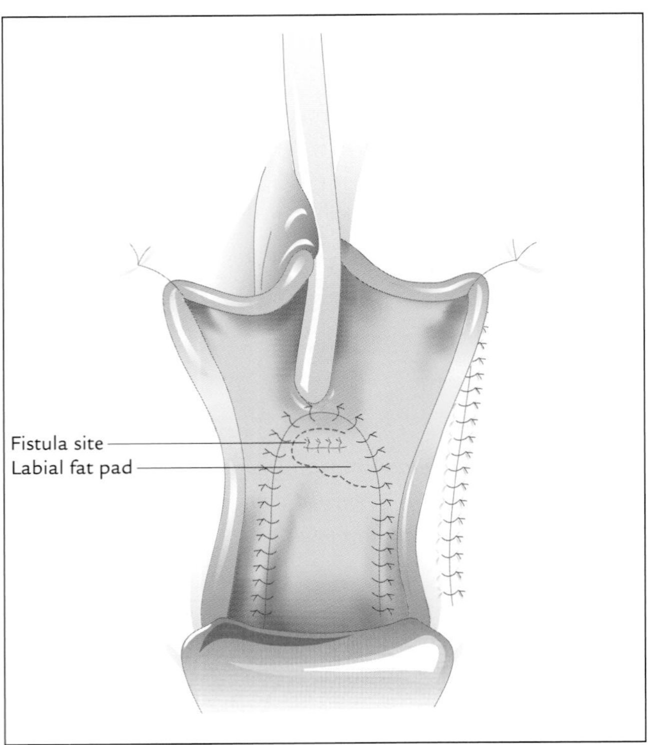

Figure 90.29. *The vaginal wall flap is advanced over the fat-pad graft, resulting in closure with no overlapping suture lines.*

RESULTS

Few series in the literature report the results of UVF repair. Most series include 10 or fewer patients, and continence rates range from 30 to 87%, including patients who underwent a single operation or multiple repairs.

Flisser and Blaivas[106] reported on their experience with 74 women with urethral pathology requiring surgical reconstruction. The patients ranged from 22 to 80 years of age and were followed-up for 1–15 years (median 1.5 years). Autologous rectus fascia pubovaginal sling was performed in 56, modified Pereyra procedure in five, and Kelly plication in one. The authors abandoned needle suspension in favor of pubovaginal sling after observing high postoperative incontinence rates. Martius flaps were used in 58 cases. Preoperative incontinence was the indication for vaginal flap reconstruction in 62 patients. Postoperatively 54 (87%) considered their incontinence cured or improved. The symptomatic obstruction rate was 1.3% and recurrent fistulae were reported in two patients (3%). Flap necrosis occurred in three patients, leading to continent urinary diversion in two patients and use of a gracilis flap in one patient. Intermittent catheterization was required in one woman for 6 months and less than 6 weeks in three others. The symptomatic obstruction rate was 1.3%. Postoperatively, 12 patients (16%) reported severe urinary urgency or urge incontinence.

Goodwin and Scardino[111] similarly reported a 70% success rate following one operation in 24 patients treated for vesicovaginal or urethrovaginal fistula. Their success rate was 92% following a second operation. Keetel et al.[112] reviewed their results in 24 patients with UVF and reported an overall success rate of 87.5%. Lee[105] claimed

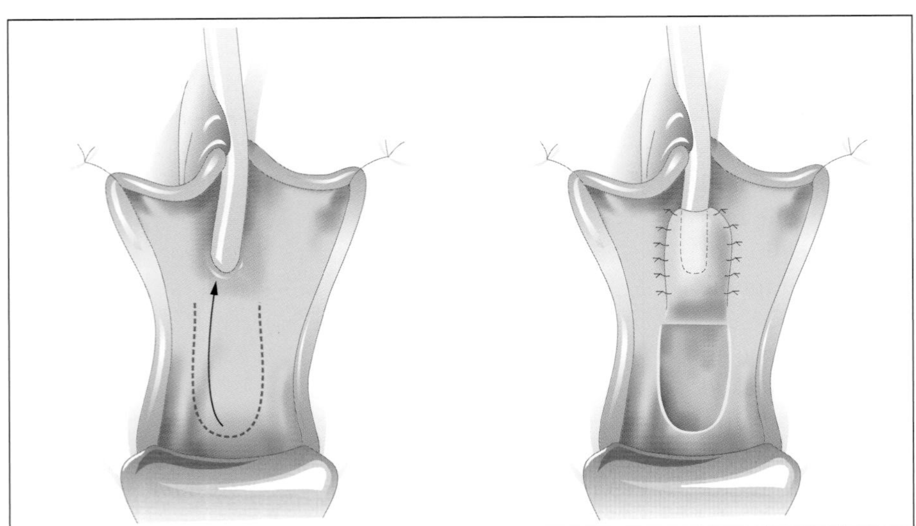

Figure 90.30. *A meatus-based vaginal flap is rotated distally.*

a 92% correction rate of UVF in 50 patients after one surgery and 100% success rate with two operations. Each of the series favored the vaginal approach over the abdominal approach: the vaginal approach generally involves a lower blood loss, shorter hospital stay and shorter operating time.[111,112]

COMPLICATIONS

Postoperative complications following urethral fistula repair may include urinary retention and urinary incontinence. High PVRs are not uncommon following urethral reconstruction, especially when performed with a simultaneous anti-incontinence procedure. Urinary retention usually resolves within a few weeks and can be managed by keeping the SPT in place until the PVRs reduce to 100 ml or less. If retention persists, the patient may be instructed on how to perform clean intermittent self-catheterization, which should not be initiated until the urethra has healed completely.

Urinary incontinence may be secondary to undetected preoperative SUI, new-onset SUI if extensive dissection has been performed, or urge incontinence due to detrusor instability. SUI may be managed with concomitant needle suspension or sling procedure following adequate healing of the urethra. Periurethral collagen may also be considered if hypermobility is not a major concern. Anticholinergic medications may be helpful in the treatment of detrusor instability.

CONCLUSION

Urethral diverticula in women represent a relatively rare entity that presents with a wide variety of symptoms. A high index of suspicion is necessary to establish the correct diagnosis, especially in patients with persistent lower urinary tract symptoms that have been refractory to conventional therapy. Advances in imaging techniques, including endoluminal MRI and transvaginal ultrasound, are capable of providing better characterization of the extent of some complex urethral diverticula.

The goals of surgery include complete excision of the diverticulum with reconstruction of the resultant urethral defect. Patients with preoperative incontinence are potential candidates for a concomitant pubovaginal sling procedure. A Martius flap interpositional graft should be considered in cases where the tissues appear tenuous or fibrotic from previous surgery or radiation. Because of the risk of postoperative complications, including recurrent diverticula, stricture, or urethrovaginal fistula, surgical intervention must be individualized to each patient.

In the modern era, with appropriate preoperative planning and strict adherence to the basic surgical principles of a tension-free, multilayered repair, urethral diverticula and urethrovaginal fistulae can be treated with excellent anatomic and functional outcomes.

REFERENCES

1. Novak R. Editorial comment. Obstet Gynecol Surv 1953;8:423.
2. Hey W. Practical Observations in Surgery. Philadelphia: J. Humphries, 1805.
3. Hunner GL. Calculus formation in a urethral diverticulum in women. Urol Cutan Rev 1938;42:336.
4. Davis HJ, Cian LG. Positive pressure urethrography: a new diagnostic method. J Urol 1956;75:753–7.
5. Leach GE, Trockman BA. In: Walsh PC, Retik AB, Vaughan ED, Wein AJ (eds) Campbell's Urology, 7th ed. Philadelphia: Saunders, 1997; 1141–51.
6. Wittich AC. Excision of urethral diverticulum calculi in a pregnant patient on an outpatient basis. J Am Osteopath Assoc 1997;97:461–2.
7. Robertson JR. Urethral diverticula. In: Ostergard DR (ed) Gynecologic Urology and Urodynamics: Theory and Practice, 2nd ed. Baltimore: Williams and Wilkins, 1985; 329–38.
8. Levinson ED, Spackman TJ, Henken EM. Diagnosis of urethral diverticula in females. Urol Radiol 1979–80;1:165–7.
9. Ganabathi K, Leach GE, Zimmern PE, Dmochowski RR. Experience with the management of urethral diverticulum in 63 women. J Urol 1994;152:1445–52.
10. Hesserdorfer E, Kuhn R, Sigel A. [Pathogenetic synopsis of diverticular disease of the female urethra] (abstract). Urologe 1988;27:343–7.
11. Lee RA. Diverticulum of the urethra: clinical presentation, diagnosis, and management. Clin Obstet Gynecol 1984;27:490–8.
12. Davis BL, Robinson DG. Diverticula of the female urethra: assay of 120 cases. J Urol 1970;104:850–3.
13. Aldridge CW, Beaton JH, Nanzig RP. A review of office urethroscopy and cystometry. Am J Obstet Gynecol 1978;131:432–7.
14. Huffman AB. The detailed anatomy of the paraurethral ducts in the adult human female. Am J Obstet Gynecol 1948;55:86–101.
15. Routh A. Urethral diverticula. Br J Urol 1890;1:361.
16. McNally A. Diverticula of the female urethra. Am J Surg 1935;28:177.
17. Raz S, Little NA, Juma S. Female urology. In: Walsh, PC, Retick AB, Stamey TA, Vaughan ED (eds) Campbell's Urology, 6th ed. Philadelphia: Saunders, 1992; 2782–8.

18. Niemic TR, Mercer LJ, Stephens JK et al. Unusual urethral diverticulum lined with colonic epithelium with Paneth cell metaplasia. Am J Obstet Gynecol 1989;260:186–8.
19. Silk MR, Lebowitz JM. Anterior urethral diverticulum. J Urol 1969;101:66–7.
20. Clemens JQ, Bushman W. Urethral diverticulum following transurethral collagen injection. J Urol 2001;166:626.
21. Peters WH, Vaughan ED. Urethral diverticulum in the female. Obstet Gynecol 1976;47:549–52.
22. Aragona F, Mangano M, Artibani W, Passerini GG. Stone formation in a female urethral diverticulum. Review of the literature. Int Urol Nephrol 1989;21:621–5.
23. Pavlica P, Viglietta F, Losinno F et al. [Diverticula of the female urethra. A radiological and ultrasound study] (abstract). Radiol Med 1988;75:521–7.
24. Ginsberg S, Genandry R. Suburethral diverticulum: classification and therapeutic considerations. Obstet Gynecol 1983;61:685–8.
25. Nielsen VM, Nielsen KK, Vedel P. Spontaneous rupture of a diverticulum of the female urethra presenting with a fistula to the vagina. Acta Obstet Gynecol Scand 1987;66:87–8.
26. Evans KJ, McCarthy MP, Sands JP. Adenocarcinoma of a female urethral diverticulum: case report and review of the literature. J Urol 1981;126:124–6.
27. Okubo Y, Fukui I, Sakano Y et al. [Mesonephric adenocarcinoma arising in the female urethral diverticulum] (abstract). Nippon Hinyokika Gakkai Zasshi 1996;87:1138–41.
28. Seballos RM, Rich RR. Clear cell adenocarcinoma arising from a urethral diverticulum. J Urol 1995;153:1914–5.
29. Srinivas V, Dow D. Transitional cell carcinoma in a urethral diverticulum with a calculus. J Urol 1983;129: 372–3.
30. Klutke CG, Akdmna EI, Brown JJ. Nephrogenic adenoma arising from a urethral diverticulum: magnetic resonance features. Urology 1995;45:323–5.
31. Materne R, Dardenne AN, Opsomer RJ et al. [Apropos of a case of nephrogenic adenoma in a urethral diverticulum in a woman] (abstract). Acta Urol Belg 1995;63: 13–8.
32. Medeiros LJ, Young RH. Nephrogenic adenoma arising in urethral diverticula. A report of five cases. Arch Pathol Lab Med 1989;113:125–8.
33. Paik SS, Lee JD. Nephrogenic adenoma arising in an urethral diverticulum. Br J Urol 1997;80:150.
34. Parks J. Section of the urethral wall for correction of urethrovaginal fistula and urethral diverticula. Am J Obstet Gynecol 1965;93:683–92.
35. Summit RL, Murrmann SG, Flax SD. Nephrogenic adenoma in a urethral diverticulum: a case report. J Reprod Med 1994;39:473–6.
36. Poore RE, McCullough DL. Urethral carcinoma. In: Gillenwater JY, Grayhack JT, Howards SS, Duckett JW (eds) Adult and Pediatric Urology, 3rd ed. Salem, MA: Mosby, 1996; 1846–7.
37. Shalev M, Mistry S, Kernen K, Miles BJ. Squamous cell carcinoma in a female urethral diverticulum. Urol 2002;59:773iii–773v.
38. Gonzalez MO, Harrison ML, Boileau MA. Carcinoma in diverticulum of female urethra. Urology 1985;26: 328–32.
39. Jimenez de Leon J, Luz Picazo M, Mora MM et al. [Intradiverticular adenocarcinoma of the urethra in women] (abstract). Arch Exp Urol 1989;42:L931–5.
40. Wishard WN, Nourse MH, Mertz J. Carcinoma in a diverticulum of a female urethra. J Urol 1960;104:409–13.
41. Huvos AG, Muggia FM, Markewitz M. Carcinoma of the female urethra. N Y State J Med 1970;69:2042–5.
42. Torres SA, Quattlebaus RB. Carcinoma in a urethral diverticulum. South Med J 1972;65:1374–6.
43. Olivia E, Young RH. Clear cell adenocarcinoma of the urethra: a clinicopathologic analysis of 19 cases. Mod Pathol 1996;9:513–20.
44. Aspera AM, Rackley RR, Vasavada SP. Contemporary evaluation and management of the female urethral diverticulum. Urol Clin North Am 2002;29:617–24.
45. Romanzi LJ, Groutz A, Blaivas JG. Urethral diverticulum in women: diverse presentations resulting in diagnostic delay and mismanagement. J Urol 2000;164:428–33.
46. Jensen LM, Aabech J, Lundvall F, Iversen HG. Female urethral diverticulum. Clinical aspects and a presentation of 15 cases. Acta Obstet Gynecol Scand 1996;75:748–52.
47. Dmochowski RR, Ganabathi K, Zimmern PE, Leach GE. Benign female periurethral masses. J Urol 1994;152: 1943–51.
48. Curry NS. Ectopic ureteral orifice masquerading as a urethral diverticulum. Am J Roentgenol 1983;41:1325–6.
49. Dias P, Hillard P, Rauh J. Skene's gland abscess with suburethral diverticulum in an adolescent. J Adolesc Health Care 1987;8:372–5.
50. Konami T, Wakabayashi Y, Takeuchi J, Tomoyoshi T. Female wide urethra masquerading as a urethral diverticulum in association with ectopic ureterocele. Hinyokika Kiyo 1988;34:1437–41.
51. Leach GE, Sirls LT, Ganabathi K et al. LNSC3: a proposed classification system for female urethral diverticula. Neurourol Urodyn 1993;12:523–31.
52. Gerrard ER, Lloyd LK, Kubricht WS, Koettis PN. Transvaginal ultrasound for the diagnosis of urethral diverticulum. J Urol 2003;169:1395–7.
53. Wang AC, Wang CR. Radiologic diagnosis and surgical treatment of urethral diverticulum in women. A reap-

praisal of voiding cystourethrography and positive pressure urethrography. J Reprod Med 2000;45:377–82.

54. Siegel CL, Middleton WD, Teefey SA, Wainstein MA, McDougall EM, Klutke CG. Sonography of the female urethra. Am J Roentgenol 1998;170:1269–74.

55. Leach GE, Ganabathi K. Urethral diverticulectomy. Atlas Urol Clin North Am 1994;2:73–85.

56. Leach GE, Bavenden TG. Female urethral diverticula. Urology 1987;30:407–15.

57. Reid RE, Gill B, Laor E et al. Role of urodynamics in management of urethral diverticulum in females. Urology 1986;28:342–6.

58. Jacoby K, Rowbotham RK. Double balloon positive pressure urethrography is a more sensitive test than voiding cystourethrography for diagnosing urethral diverticulum in women. J Urol 1999;162:2066–9.

59. Golomb J, Leibovitch I, Mor Y, Morag B, Ramon J. Comparison of voiding cystourethrography and double-balloon urethrography in the diagnosis of complex female urethral diverticula. Eur Radiol 2003;13:536–42.

60. Keefe B, Warshauer DM, Tucker MS, Mittelstaedt CA. Diverticula of the female urethra: diagnosis by endovaginal and transperineal sonography. Am J Roentgenol 1991;156:1195–7.

61. Vargas-Serrano B, Cortina-Moreno B, Rodriguez-Romero R, Ferreiro-Arguees I. Transrectal ultrasonography in the diagnosis of urethral diverticula in women. J Clin Ultrasound 1997;25:21–8.

62. Iula G, Stefano ML, Castaldi L, del Vecchio E. Post irradiation female urethral diverticula: diagnosis by voiding endovaginal sonography. J Clin Ultrasound 1995;23:63–5.

63. Mouritsen L, Bernstein I. Vaginal ultrasonography: a diagnostic tool for urethral diverticulum. Acta Obstet Gynecol Scand 1996;75:188–90.

64. Martensson O, Duchek M. Translabial ultrasonography with pulsed colour Doppler in the diagnosis of female urethral diverticulum. Scan J Urol Nephrol 1994;28:101–4.

65. Chancellor MB, Liu JB, Rivas DA et al. Intraoperative endo-luminal ultrasound evaluation of urethral diverticula. J Urol 1995;153:72–5.

66. Lopez Rasines G, Rico Guttierez M, Abascal F, Calbia de Diego A. Female urethral diverticula: value of transrectal ultrasound. J Clin Ultrasound 1996;24:90–2.

67. Blacklock ARE, Shaw RE, Geddes JR. Late presentation of ectopic ureter. Br J Urol 1982;54:106–10.

68. Boyd SD, Raz S. Ectopic ureter presenting in midline urethral diverticulum. Urology 1993;41:571–4.

69. Goldfarb S, Mieza M, Leiter E. Postvoid film of intravenous pyelogram in diagnosis of urethral diverticulum. Urology 1981;17:390–2.

70. Debaere C, Rigauts H, Steyaert L et al. MR imaging of a diverticulum in a female urethra. J Belg Radiol 1995;78:345–6.

71. Hricak H, Secaf E, Buckley DW et al. Female urethra: MR imaging. Radiology 1991;178:527–35.

72. Neitlich JD, Foster HE, Glickman MG, Smith RC. Detection of urethral diverticula in women: comparison of a high resolution fast spin echo technique with double balloon urethrography. J Urol 1998;159:408–10.

73. Siegelman ES, Banner MP, Ramchandani P, Schneall MD. Multicoil MR imaging of symptomatic female urethral and periurethral disease. Radiographics 1997;17:349–65.

74. Blander DS, Rovner ES, Schnall MD et al. Endoluminal magnetic resonance imaging in evaluation of urethral diverticula in women. Urology 2001;57:660–5.

75. Kim B, Hricak H, Tanagho EA. Diagnosis of urethral diverticula in women: value of MR imaging. Am J Roentgenol 1993;161:809–15.

76. Lorenzo AJ, Zimmern P, Lemack GE, Nureberg P. Endorectal coil magnetic resonance imaging for diagnosis of urethral and periurethral pathologic findings in women. Urology 2003;61:1129–34.

77. Greenberg M, Stone D, Cochran ST et al. Female urethral diverticula: double-balloon catheter study. Am J Roentgenol 1981;136:259–64.

78. Young HH. Treatment of urethral diverticulum. South Am J 1938;31:1043–7.

79. Moore TD. Diverticulum of the female urethra. An improved technique of surgical excision. J Urol 1952;68:611–6.

80. Wear JB. Urethral diverticulectomy in females. Urol Times 1976;4:2–3.

81. Hyams JA, Hyams MN. New operative procedures for treatment of diverticulum of female urethra. Urol Cutan Rev 1939;43:573–7.

82. Feldstein MS. Cryoprecipitate coagulum as an adjunct to surgery for diverticula of the female urethra. J Urol 1981;126:698–9.

83. Downs RA. Urethral diverticula in females: alternative surgical treatment. Urology 1987:2:201–3.

84. Spence HM, Duckett JW. Diverticulum of the female urethra: clinical aspects and presentation of a simple operative technique for cure. J Urol 1970;14:432–7.

85. Ellik M. Diverticulum of the female urethra: a new method of ablation. J Urol 1957;77:243–6.

86. Mizrahi S, Bitterman W. Transvaginal, periurethral injection of polytetrafluoroethylene (polytef) in the treatment of urethral diverticula. Br J Urol 1988;62:280.

87. Fall M. Vaginal wall bipedicled flap and other techniques in complicated urethral diverticulum and urethrovaginal fistula. J Am Coll Surg 1995;180:150–6.

88. Leach GE, Schmidbauer CP, Hadley HR et al. Surgical treatment of female urethral diverticulum. Semin Urol 1986;4:33–42.

89. Marshall S. Urethral diverticula in young girls. Urology 1981;17:243–5.

90. Lapides J. Transurethral treatment of urethral diverticula in women. J Urol 1979;121:736–8.

91. Vergunst H, Blom JH, De Spiegeleer AH, Miranda SI. Management of female urethral diverticula by transurethral incision. Br J Urol 1996;77:745–6.

92. Spencer WF, Streem SB. Diverticula of the female urethra roof managed endoscopically. J Urol 1987;138:157–8.

93. Swierzewski SJ, McGuire EJ. Pubovaginal sling for treatment of female stress urinary incontinence complicated by urethral diverticulum. J Urol 1993;149:1012–4.

94. Clyne OJ, Flood HD. Giant urethral diverticulum: a novel approach to repair. J Urol 2002;167:1796.

95. Gilbert D, Cintron F. Urethral diverticula in the female: review of the subject and introduction of a different surgical approach. Am J Obstet Gynecol 1954;67:616.

96. Vakili B, Wai C, Nihira M. Anterior urethral diverticulum in the female: diagnosis and surgical approach. Obstet Gynecol 2003;102:1179–83.

97. Rovner ES, Wein AJ. Diagnosis and reconstruction of the dorsal or circumferential urethral diverticulum. J Urol 2003;170:82–6.

98. Coddington CC, Knab DR. Urethral diverticulum: a review. Obstet Gynecol Surv 1983;38:357–64.

99. Bass JS, Leach GE. Surgical treatment of concomitant urethral diverticulum and stress urinary incontinence. Urol Clin North Am 1991;18:365–73.

100. Ganabathi K, Sirls L, Zimmern PE, Leach GE. Operative management of female urethral diverticulum. In: McGuire E (ed) Advances in Urology. Chicago: Mosby, 1994; 199–228.

101. Blaivas JG. Vaginal flap urethral reconstruction: an alternative to the bladder flap neourethra. J Urol 1989;141:542–5.

102. Blaivas JG. Treatment of female incontinence secondary to urethral damage or loss. Urol Clin North Am 1991;18:355–63.

103. Robertson JR. Urinary fistulas. In: Ostergard DR (ed) Gynecologic Urology and Urodynamics: Theory and Practice, 2nd ed. Baltimore: Williams and Wilkins, 1985; 323–8.

104. Leach GE. Urethrovaginal fistula repair with Martius labial fat pad graft. Urol Clin North Am 1991;18: 409–13.

105. Lee RA. Current status of genitourinary fistula. Obstet Gynecol 1988;72:313–9.

106. Flisser AJ, Blaivas JG. Outcome of urethral reconstructive surgery in a series of 74 women. J Urol 2003;169: 2246–9.

107. Carlin BI, Klutke CG. Development of urethrovaginal fistula following periurethral collagen injection. J Urol 2000;164:124.

108. Chassagne S, Haav F, Zimmern PE. [The Martius flap in vaginal surgery: technique and indications] (abstract). Prog Urol 1997;7:120–5.

109. Leng WW, Amundsen CL, McGuire EJ. Management of female genitourinary fistulas: transvesical or transvaginal approach. J Urol 1998;160(6 Pt 1):1995–9.

110. Zimmern PE, Hadley HR, Leach GE et al. Transvaginal closure of the bladder neck and placement of a suprapubic catheter for destroyed urethra after long-term indwelling catheter. J Urol 1985;134:554–7.

111. Goodwin WE, Scardino PT. Vesicovaginal and urethrovaginal fistulas: a summary of 25 years of experience. Trans Am Assoc GU Surg 1979;71:123–9.

112. Keetel WC, Schring FG, deProsse CA, Scott JR. Surgical management of urethrovaginal and vesicovaginal fistulas. Am J Obstet Gynecol 1978;131:425–31.

91

Electrical stimulation of the lower urinary tract

Firouz Daneshgari

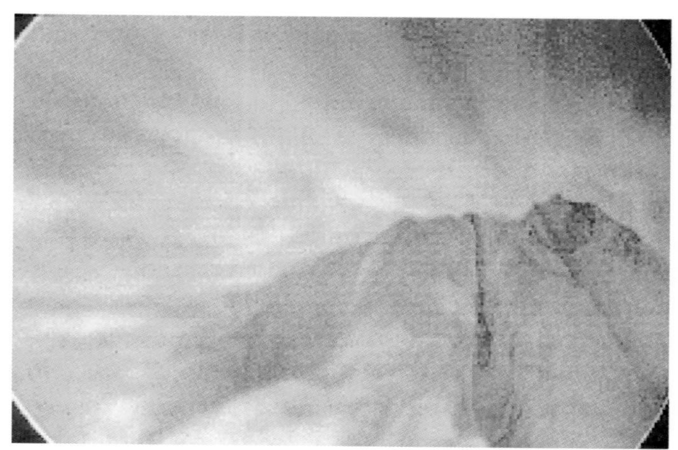

INTRODUCTION

The first attempt at electrical stimulation of the lower urinary tract (LUT) may date back to 1878, when the Danish surgeon Saxtorph treated patients with urinary retention by intravesical stimulation,[1] in which he inserted a special catheter with a metal electrode transurethrally.

In 1811 Bell was the first to conduct experiments on the spinal nerve roots.[2] His anatomic studies showed that manipulation of the intradural anterior fasciculus led to muscle convulsions of the back, whereas cutting across the posterior fasciculus of nerves resulted in no contractions.[3] However, Bell drew the conclusion that the anterior nerve roots, connected to the cerebrum, conduct sensory and motor impulses. In his concept, the posterior nerve roots were connected to the cerebellum and accounted for the vital functions. Magendie was the first to conduct a physiologic investigation of spinal nerve roots.[2] In radiculotomy studies on young puppies he found that cutting the posterior root extinguished sensation, although movement was still present,[4] whereas cutting the anterior root abolished movement, but sensation was still present. Hence, he postulated that nerve roots consist of an anterior, efferent motor portion and a posterior, afferent sensory portion. It was not until 1833 that Hall uncovered a distinct function of the spinal cord and medulla oblongata – that of reflex action.[5] These first perceptions formed the basis for further examinations of organ innervation by the autonomic nervous system.

However, it was not until the 1940s that further efforts were undertaken. The central question was: Which part of the neuromuscular pathway for micturition should be chosen to initiate voiding in urinary retention or to prevent voiding in incontinence? Numerous techniques were developed and may be classified according to the location of electrical stimulation as follows: transurethral bladder stimulation, direct detrusor stimulation, pelvic nerve stimulation, pelvic floor stimulation, spinal cord stimulation, and sacral root stimulation.[6]

After experimentation with various methods of simulating the bladder through the transurethral approach, direct detrusor stimulation,[7] pelvic nerve stimulation,[8] pelvic floor stimulation,[9] spinal cord stimulation,[10] with pioneering work of Tanagho and later Schmidt,[11–14] it was demonstrated that the stimulation of sacral root S3 generally induces detrusor and sphincter action.[15] Following two decades of experimentation with various approaches to sacral root stimulation, finally, in October 1997, sacral neuromodulation for treatment of refractory urge incontinence was approved by the Food and Drug Administration (FDA) in the United States. Since then and at the time of this writing, more than 20,000 Medtronic InterStim® systems have been implanted for three approved indications of sacral nerve stimulation (SNS) of the lower urinary tract.

In this chapter we will review the various aspects of the electrical stimulation of the bladder and its application in managementv of LUT dysfunctions.

MECHANISMS OF ACTION

Neuromodulation of LUT function can be explained by relatively simple spinal circuits mediating somatovisceral interactions within the sacral spinal cord. It is proposed that SNS activates or 'resets' the somatic afferent inputs that play a pivotal role in the modulation of sensory processing and micturition reflex pathways in the spinal cord (Fig. 91.1).[16] Urinary retention and dysfunctional voiding can be resolved by inhibition of the guarding reflexes. Detrusor hyperreflexia and the overactive bladder syndrome can be suppressed by one or more pathways, i.e. direct inhibition of bladder preganglionic neurons, as well as inhibition of interneuronal transmission in the afferent limb of the micturition reflex (Figs 91.2–91.4).

PATIENT SELECTION

The selection of patients for SNS begins with a careful history, physical examination, routine tests such as urinalysis and urine culture, and – most importantly – use

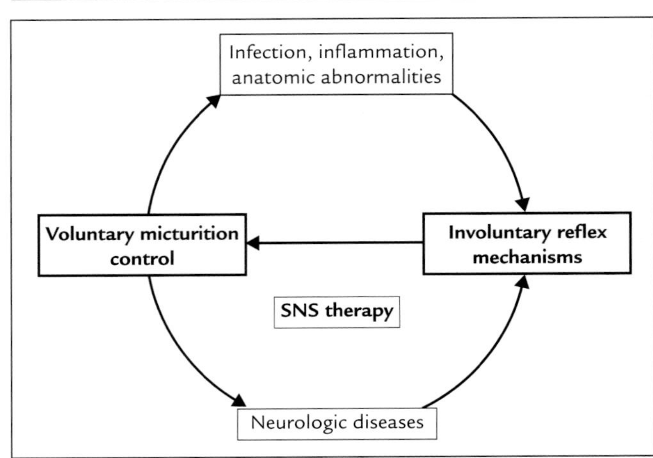

Figure 91.1. *The concept of sacral nerve stimulation (SNS) is to modulate the abnormal involuntary reflexes of the lower urinary tract and restore voluntary control. (Reproduced from ref. 16 with permission.)*

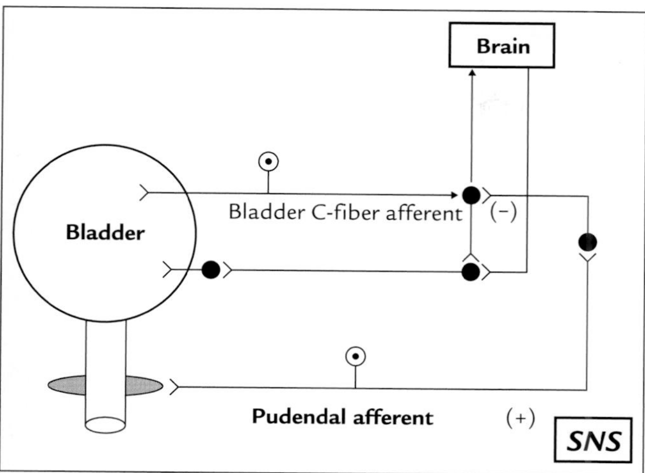

Figure 91.2. *Pudendal afferent nerve stimulation can inhibit the micturition reflex. (Reproduced from ref. 16 with permission.)*

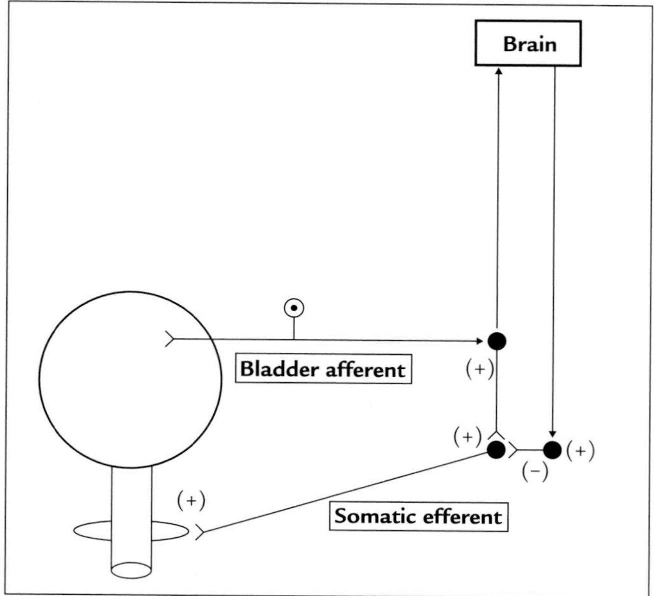

Figure 91.3. *The guarding reflex prevents urinary incontinence. When there is a sudden increase in intravesical pressure, such as during a cough, the urinary sphincter contracts via the spinal guarding reflex to prevent urinary incontinence. The spinal guarding reflex is turned off by the brain to urinate. (Reproduced from ref. 16 with permission.)*

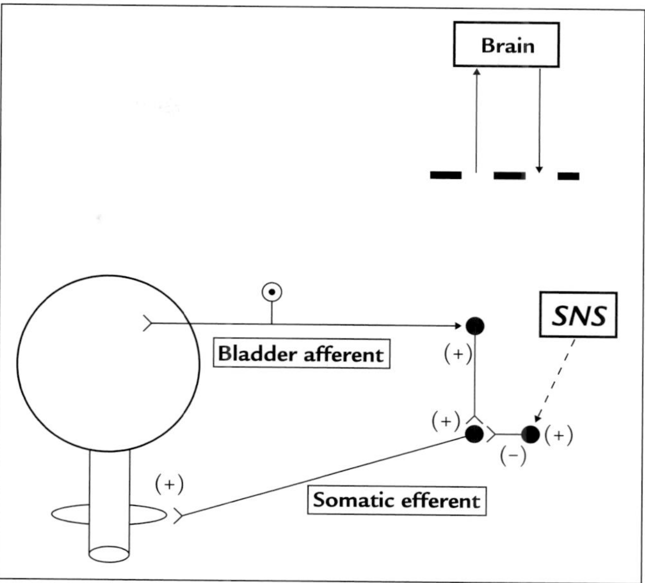

Figure 91.4. *The spinal guarding reflexes can be turned off by the brain to urinate. In neurologic disease, the brain cannot turn off the guarding reflex and retention can occur. However, SNS is capable of restoring voluntary micturition in cases of voiding dysfunction and urinary retention by inhibiting the spinal guarding reflex. (Reproduced from ref. 16 with permission.)*

of bladder diaries to objectively record voiding variables. Urodynamic examination is commonly used to identify patients with detrusor overactivity (DO) with or without urinary leakage or urinary retention. Some reports suggest the utility of urodynamics in identification of proper candidates to SNS.

History

The important elements of history focuses on the primary voiding variables such as the frequency and severity of urge incontinent episodes and the number of pads used per 24-hour period. For patients with refractory urgency frequency, the number of voids, the voided volumes and the degree of urgency are assessed; in patients who experience inefficient voiding or urinary retention, the amount voided versus catheterized volumes per 24 hours and the patient's sense of completeness of evacuation are fathomed. Associated symptoms such as pelvic pain and bowel and sexual symptoms are also assessed. As an extension of the history, a voiding diary is invaluable in order to document the patient's voiding habits and complaints objectively.

Physical examination

The physical examination should start with a neurourologic examination, checking for saddle sensation, sphincter tone, and bulbocavernosus reflex. Some investigators put emphasis on high pelvic tone noticed during the vaginal examination.[17] In addition to examination of the bladder, urethra, perineum and vagina, rectal examination is a key aspect of the physical examination of any patient with voiding dysfunction.

ANATOMIC LANDMARK AND SURGICAL TECHNIQUES OF SACRAL NEUROMODULATION

The S3 foramen is the desired anatomic landmark for placement of the leads for sacral neuromodulation. The techniques for S3 localization have included manual or fluoroscopic methods. The manual approach includes palpation of the sciatic notch, observation for the least curved portion of the sacrum, and measurement of approximately 11 cm from the caudal tip of the coccyx (Fig. 91.5). The manual method is more difficult with obese patients or in those without palpable landmarks, and in 2001 Chai et al. introduced the use of the 'cross-hair' fluoroscopic technique for S3 localization.[18] The intent of fluoroscopy was not meant to 'see' the S3 foramen, but rather to help the surgeon identify a specific region to start percutaneous access of the S3 foramen (Fig. 91.6). More importantly, the use of lateral imaging helped determine the depth required for implanting the S3 lead (Fig. 91.7). As surgeons, particularly urologists, were familiar with the use of fluoroscopy due to their work in stone surgery, the application of fluoroscopy to sacral neuromodulation surgery was quickly accepted. The widespread use of fluoroscopic localization of S3 later allowed the introduction of the tined S3 lead[19] and transformed the placement of a lead from an open procedure[20] to a completely percutaneous one.[21] The widely adopted percutaneous use of the tined lead approach superseded the need for fixation of the lead by methods such as bone anchors.

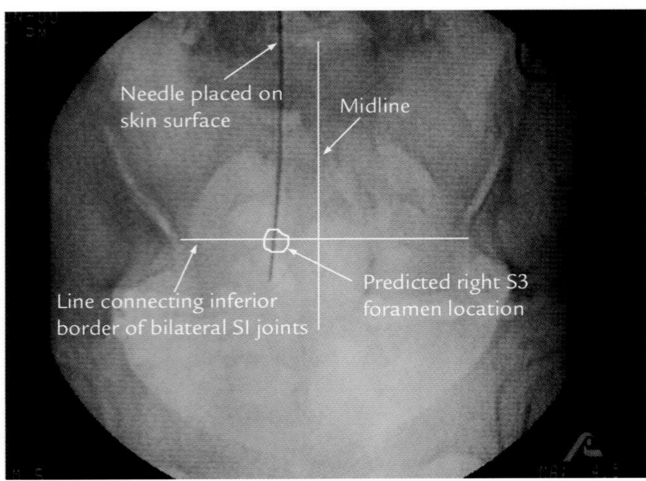

Figure 91.6. *Localization of the S3 foramen by the cross-hair technique. (Reproduced from ref. 16 with permission.)*

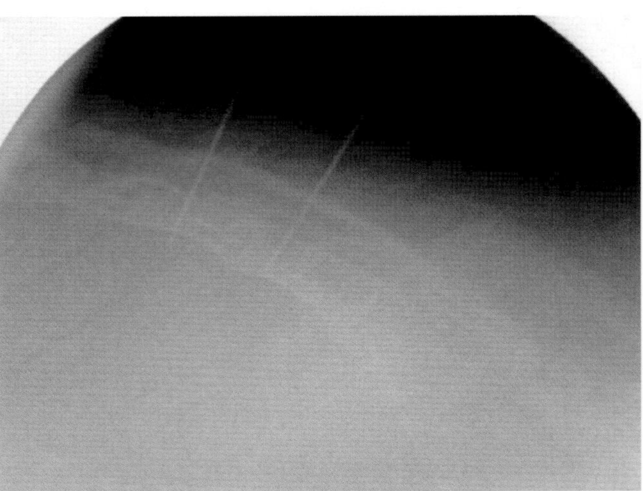

Figure 91.7. *Site of percutaneous placement of needle stimulations and stage I lead.*

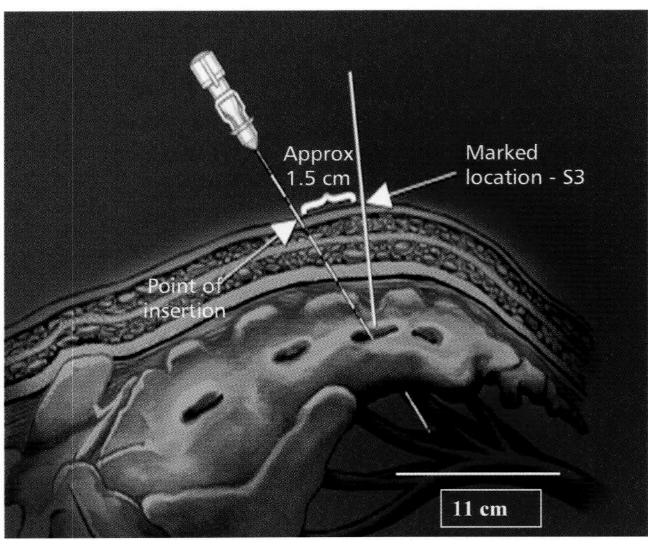

Figure 91.5. *Localization of the S3 foramen by anatomic landmarks.*

The original method of SNS – entitled percutaneous nerve examination (PNE) – followed two steps: testing of the patient's bladder response to sacral neurostimulation via a temporary lead placed into the S3 foramen, followed by possible simultaneous implantation of the chronic lead and the generator if the patient responded positively to the first step. Janknegt et al.[22] first described the staged implantation approach in which an implanted S3 lead, rather than the temporary lead, was used for initial testing. The staged technique bypassed the problems with PNE which included a high risk of lead migration and the fact the original response of the patient obtained by the temporary wire may not be reproduced by the permanent lead. Several reports later confirmed a higher positive response rate, and a lesser rate of lead migration obtained by the staged approach.

After placement of the lead, the following sensory and motor responses related to stimulation of the specific sacral root may be observed:

- S2:
  - clamp movement or twisting and pinching of the anal sphincter (pulling down the coccyx);
  - plantar flexion of the entire foot, lateral rotation.
- S3:
  - bellows movement of the pelvic floor;
  - plantar flexion of the great toe(s);
  - paresthesia in the rectum, perineum, scrotum or vagina.
- S4:
  - bellows motion of the pelvic floor;
  - no lower extremity activity;
  - sensing pulling in the rectum only.

The desired response and localization for electrical stimulation of the LUT should include S3 responses.

Surgical approach

Implantation of SNS consists of two steps: stage I and stage II.

Stage I – or the trial step – involves the placement of a stimulation lead next to the dorsal root of S3 for a test period of between 1 and 4 weeks. If the patient's symptoms under the existing indications for SNS improve more than 50%, then the patient is a candidate to undergo stage II (or permanent step) in which the permanent implantable pulse generator (IPG) unit is implanted in the soft tissue of the patient's buttock.

There is no consensus as to whether one or two implanted S3 leads should be performed as in stage I. Bilateral implantation allows for testing for both the left and right S3 nerve roots. At the time of stage II, the lead that is less efficacious can be removed or remain implanted for possible 'backup' in case the lead on the other side fails. Currently, there is no evidence that bilateral simultaneous stimulation has any added benefits to unilateral stimulation. Furthermore, it is not possible to stimulate both wires with one IPG because the IPG is not a dual channel stimulator. One would need to implant two IPGs for bilateral simultaneous stimulation. Nevertheless, bilateral implantation allows for a more complete evaluation and possibly offers the patient a higher chance of responding to sacral neurostimulation.

Stage I can be performed while the patient is under local anesthesia with conscious sedation (Fig. 91.8). After localization of the S3 foramen, the patient's sensory and motor response is elicited. The proper position of the needle stimulator could also be checked by fluoroscopy. It is not uncommon for two different needle stimulators to lodge into the same foramen despite their distance on the skin (Fig. 91.9). After confirmation of the proper placement of the needle, a nick is made in the skin to allow for easier passage of the wider introducer. In addition to the foramen needle, the set-up for stage I includes the directional guide and the introducer assembly (Fig. 91.10). The introducer, with the obturator in place, is inserted coaxially over the directional guide wire (Fig. 91.11). Lateral fluoroscopy is required to determine the depth to which to insert the introducer. Once at the correct depth, the obturator is removed, leaving the introducer sheath within the S3 foraminal canal. The tined lead, with four plastic collapsible projections, is inserted into the sheath under lateral fluoroscopic guidance

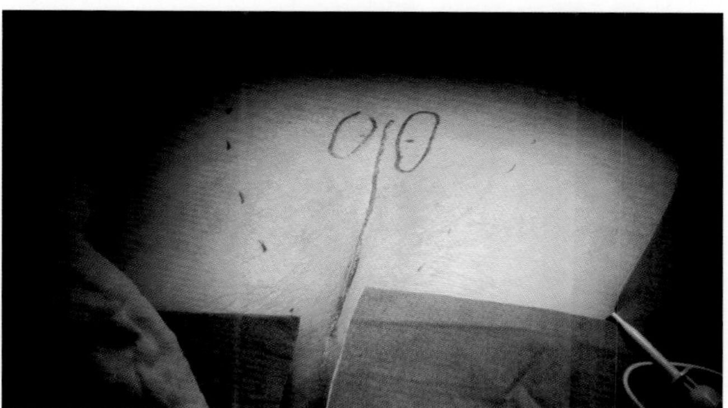

Figure 91.8. *Lateral fluoroscopy view shows the proper site of needle stimulation in the S3 and S4 foramen.*

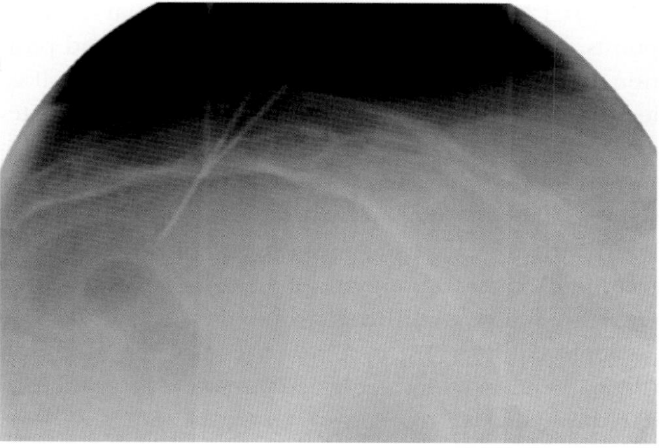

Figure 91.9. *Lateral fluoroscopy view shows convergence of two needles into the S3 foramen.*

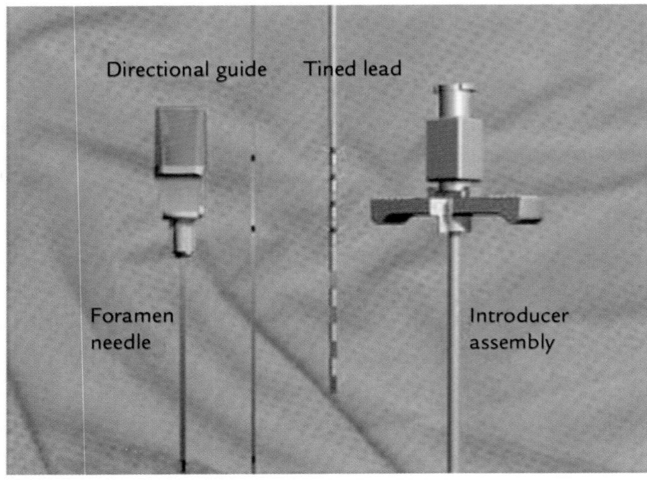

Figure 91.10. *Set-up for stage I sacral neuromodulation, including directional guide, tined lead, foramen needle, and introducer assembly.*

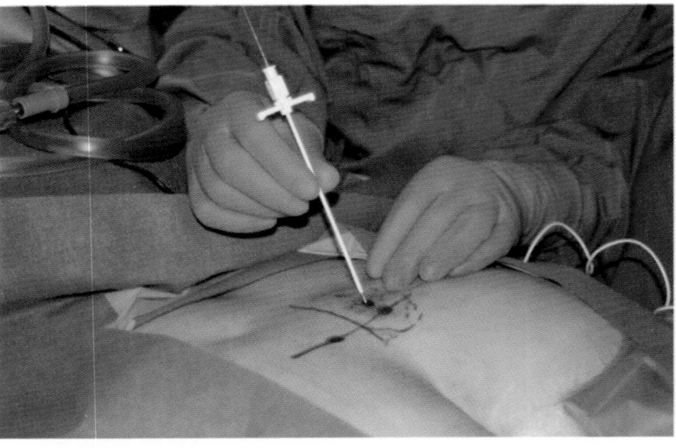

Figure 91.11. *Placement of introducer sheet over the directional guide. (Reproduced from ref. 21 with permission.)*

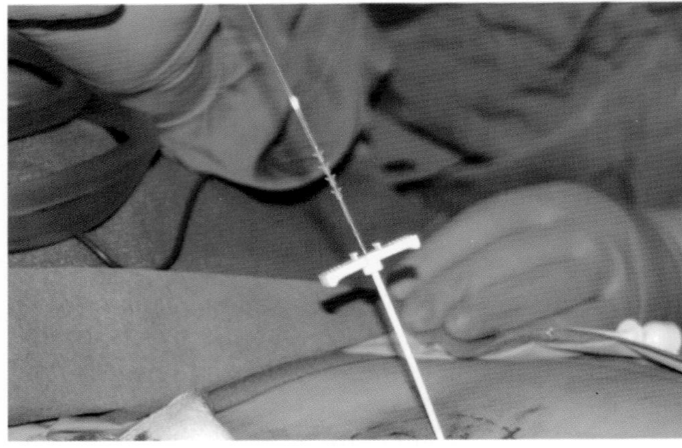

Figure 91.12. *Placement of quadripole chronic lead through the introducer sheet. (Reproduced from ref. 21 with permission.)*

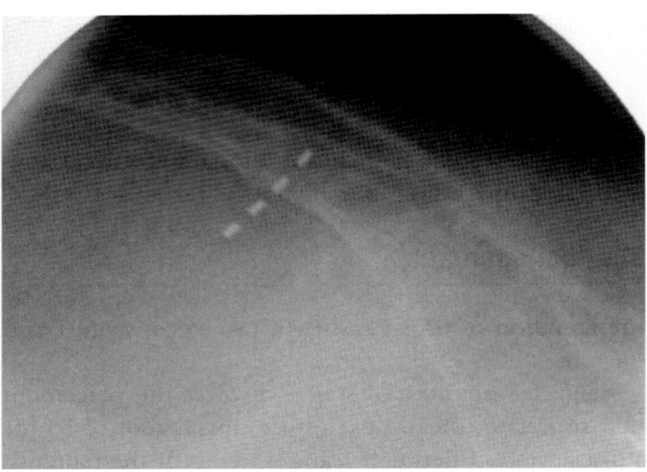

Figure 91.13. *The tined lead is in the proper position: two to three contact plates of the quadripole lead are resting on the S3 dorsal nerve root.*

(Fig. 91.12). The lead has four quadripolar contact points. The position for the lead is such that lead position 1 is 'straddling' the ventral S3 foramen, i.e. half of lead position 1 is anterior and the other half is posterior to the ventral sacral cortex (Fig. 91.13). To test for proper motor and sensory responses in the patient, the sheath will be moved back to a white line marked on the lead by the manufacturer to expose all quadripolar contact points, but without engaging the plastic projections. Once stimulation confirms proper sensory and motor responses, the sheath is removed completely, allowing the plastic projections to engage the soft tissues and thus anchor the lead.

Using a tunneler device supplied in the manufacturer's kit, the tunneler is passed from the exit point of the tined lead to the right upper buttock incision, and the proximal tip of the lead is connected to an extension cable. The connection is covered with a boot. The proximal tip of the extension cable is then passed subcutaneously to the contralateral buttock and is exited via a stab incision. Passing the extension wire to the contralateral side is performed in order to minimize the risk of infection. The incision sites are closed appropriately. Over the next 1–4 weeks, the patient is sequentially stimulated (one S3 at a time in case of bilateral implantation) via an external stimulator connected to the external extension to determine optimum bladder response (Fig. 91.14). The lead on the side giving the best response will be connected to the IPG during stage II surgery. In this step, the existing extension cable is removed and the proximal tip of the quadripole lead is connected to the IPG unit which is buried in the existing subcutaneous pocket

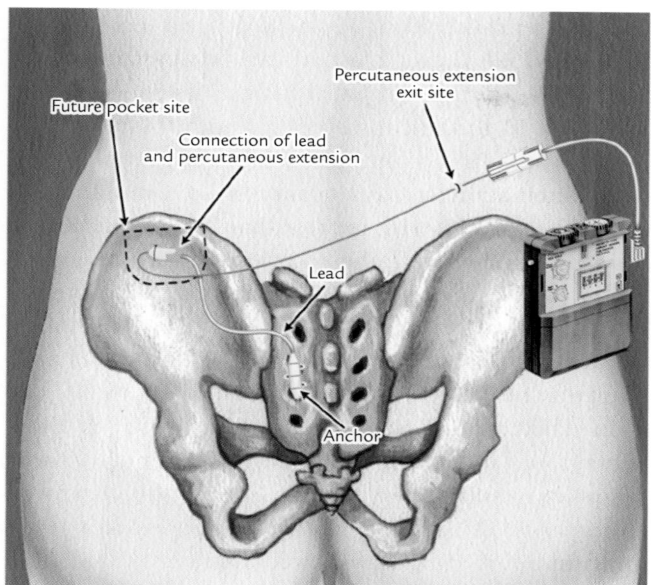

Figure 91.14. *Stage I sacral neuromodulation: the external stimulator is connected to the chronic lead for the test period.*

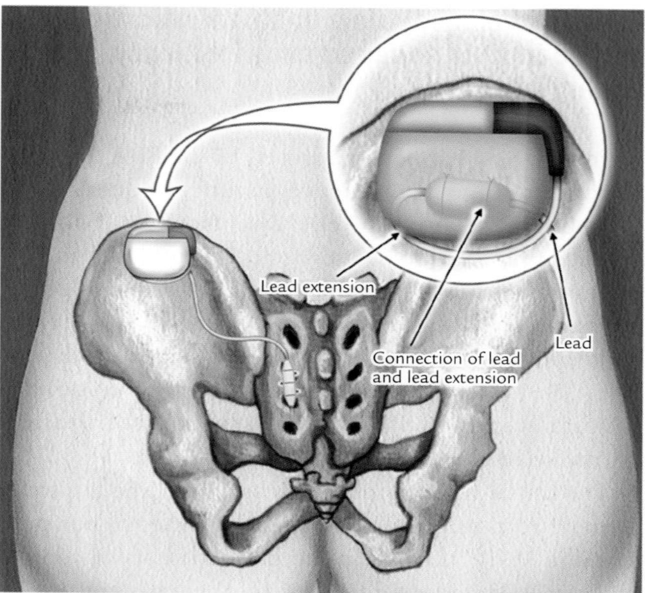

Figure 91.15. *Stage II sacral neuromodulation: the implantable pulse generator unit is placed in the subcutaneous pocket.*

(Fig. 91.15). The programming of the IPG unit can be done extracorporeally. A hand-held device also allows the patient to adjust the intensity of the IPG stimulation or control its on/off function (Fig. 91.16).

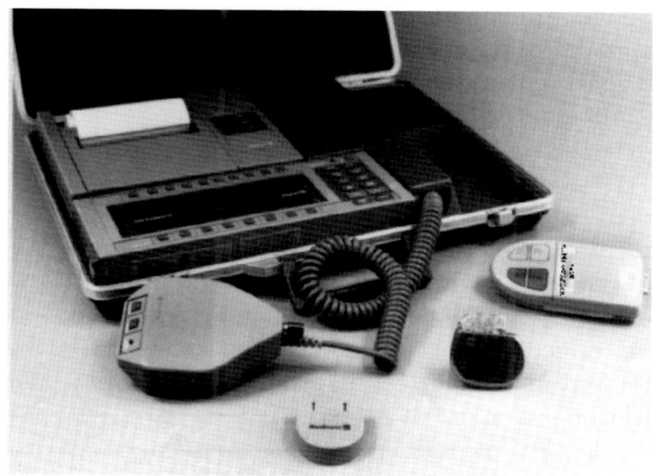

Figure 91.16. *The programming equipment for the implantable pulse generator unit.*

CLINICAL RESULTS

The reported outcomes of SNS usually include the response of patients to stage I (test stage) and to stage II (permanent implantation). The evidence reported in the medical literature is limited to data reported in clinical trials, specifically excluding expert opinion.

The International Consultation on Incontinence has adopted the Oxford level of evidence as the following categories:

1. *Level 1* – usually involves meta-analysis of randomized clinical trials (RCTs).
2. *Level 2* – includes 'low' quality RCTs or meta-analysis of good quality prospective 'cohort studies'. These may include a single group when individuals who develop the condition are compared with others from within the original cohort group. There can be parallel cohorts, where those with the condition in the first group are compared with those in the second group.
3. *Level 3* – evidence includes:
   - good quality retrospective 'case-control studies' where a group of patients who have a condition are matched appropriately (e.g. for age, sex, etc.) with control individuals who do not have the condition;
   - good quality 'case series' where a group of patients, all with the same condition/disease/ therapeutic intervention, are described, without a comparison control group.
4. *Level 4* – evidence includes expert opinion where the opinion is based not on evidence but on 'first principles' (e.g. physiologic or anatomic) bench research. The process can be used to give 'expert opinion' or greater authority.

Reports of clinical trials on three indications of urge incontinence, urgency frequency, and urinary retention

Currently, SNS has been approved by the FDA for three indications: urge incontinence, urgency frequency, and non-obstructive urinary retention. However, SNS has also been reported to be used for other 'off label' indications, such as neurogenic bladders in multiple sclerosis, interstitial cystitis, and chronic pelvic pain. There are also reports regarding the possible benefits of bilateral SNS. The majority of the reports on the non-formally indicated usages of SNS appear in the form of abstracts or case series.

The initial report on the efficacy of SNS in the treatment of refractory urinary urge incontinence was published in 1999[23] (Level 2, as no placebo or sham control was used). This study reported on the treatment of 76 patients with refractory urinary urge incontinence from 16 contributing worldwide centers. The patients were randomized either to immediate implantation or to a control group with delayed implantation for a 6-month period. At 6 months, the number of daily incontinence episodes, severity of episodes, and absorbent pads or diapers replaced daily due to incontinence was significantly reduced in the stimulation group compared to the delayed group. Of the 34 stimulation group patients, 16 (47%) were completely dry, and an additional 10 (29%) demonstrated a greater than 50% reduction in incontinence episodes. The interesting finding was that during the therapy evaluation, the group returned to the baseline level of incontinence when the stimulation was inactivated. Complications were site pain of the stimulator implantation in 16%, implant infection in 19%, and leak migration in 7%.

The use of SNS in urgency frequency was first reported in 2000.[24] Similar to the previous design, 51 patients from 12 centers were randomized into either an immediate stimulation group or a control group (25 and 26 patients, respectively) (Level 2, as no placebo or sham control was used). Patients were followed for 1, 2 and 6 months, and afterwards at 6-month intervals for up to 2 years. At the 6-month evaluation, the stimulation group showed improvement in the number of voiding dailies (16.9 ± 9.7 to 9.3 ± 5.1), volume per void (118 ± 74 to 226 ± 124 ml), and degree of urgency (rank 2.2 ± 0.6 to 1.6 ± 0.9). In addition, significant improvement in quality of life was demonstrated, as measured by the SF-36 questionnaire.

The first report on the use of SNS in urinary retention was published in 2001.[25] In this study 177 patients with urinary retention refractory to conservative therapy were enrolled from 13 worldwide centers between 1993 and 1998 (Level 2, as no placebo or sham control was used). Thirty-seven patients were assigned to treatment and 31 to the control group, with follow-up at 1, 2, 6, 12, and 18 months. The treatment group showed 69% elimination of catheterization at 6 months and an additional 14% with greater than 50% reduction in catheter volume per catheterization. Temporary inactivation of SNS therapy resulted in significant increases in residual volume, but the effectiveness of central nervous stimulation was sustained for 18 months after implantation.

In 2000, a follow-up report on some of these patients was published[26] (Level 3). This report showed follow-up results after 3 years in all the improved indications. Of 41 patients, 59% had urinary urge incontinence. Patients showed greater than 50% improvement, with 46% of patients being completely dry. After 2 years, 56% of the urgency frequency patients showed greater than 50% reduction in voids per day, and after 1–1.5 years, 70% of 42 retention patients showed greater than 50% reduction of catheter volume per catheterization.

Other studies, generally case series, have published results on the use of SNS following its initial approval (Table 91.1).

The results of the use of SNS in the US population were published in 2002[27] (Level 3). This publication showed the data collected from the US Patient Registry. The report included the use of SNS in 81 patients with all three indications: 27 for urgent continence, 10 with urgency frequency and 10 with urinary retention. In this report, 27 out of 43 patients with urge incontinence, 10 out of 19 with urgency frequency and 10 out of 19 with urinary retention showed improvement of more than 50%.

The results of an Italian registry were published in 2001[28] (Level 3). This report included the details of 196 patients – 46 males and 150 females – for idiopathic urinary retention. Fifty percent of patients stopped catheterization and another 13% catheterized once a day at 1 year after implantation. At 12-month follow-up, 50% of patients with hyperreflexia had less than one incontinence episode daily and the problem was completely solved in 66 patients. Of the patients with urge incontinence, 39% were completely dry and 23% had less than one incontinence episode daily.

In Norway, the results of users of this modality were published in 2002[29] (Level 3). The authors reported the first 3 years' experience with 53 patients: 45 women and 8 men. This study showed similar results to previous studies.

Table 91.1. ***Published reports of use of SNS in various conditions of lower urinary tract dysfunction***

		Patients with UI			Patients with U/F		Patients with UR		
Study	Total	Cured	>50%	Improved	>50%	Improved	>50%	Improved	Follow-up
US National Patient Register	81		27/43		10/19		10/19		
Amundsen & Webster[40]	12		12/12	2/12					
Hedlund et al.[29]	14		13/14	8/14					
Bosch & Groen[41]	45		27/45	18/45					
Shaker & Hassouna[42]	18		12/18	8/18					
Siegel et al.[26]	112		21/41	19/41	16/29	5/29	29/42	24/42	
Schmidt et al.[23]	34	16/34	10/34	26/34			16/34		18 m
Grunewald et al.[37]	39		13/18				18/21		
Jonas et al.[25]	29						20/29		18 m
Hassouna et al.[24]	25				14/25				12 m
Aboseif et al.[30]	32						18/20	2/20	24 m

UI, urinary incontinence; U/F, urgency frequency; UR, urinary retention.

Urinary retention

Aboseif et al.[30] reported on the use of SNS in functional urinary retention (Level 3). Thirty-two patients were evaluated and underwent temporary PNE. Those that had at least a 50% improvement in symptoms during the test period underwent permanent generator placement. All patients who went to permanent generator placement were able to void spontaneously. There was both an increase in voided volume (48–198 ml) and a decrease in post-void residual (315 to 60 ml), and 18 of 20 patients reported a greater than 50% improvement in quality of life.

Other indications

Use of SNS for other off-labeled applications has been reported for treatment of refractory interstitial cystitis, chronic pelvic pain, pediatric voiding dysfunction, and neurogenic lower urinary dysfunction seen in multiple sclerosis.[31] None of the reported case series (level 4) has led to new approved indications for SNS at the time of writing.

Peripheral nerve stimulation

In 1987, Stoller et al. reported that stimulation of the peripheral tibial nerve in pig-tailed monkeys was able to inhibit bladder instability[32] (Level 3). This initial work led to its use in patients with refractory overactive bladder. The Stoller afferent nerve stimulator (SANS) has been FDA approved for use in refractory overactive bladder (Fig. 91.17).

Method

A 34-gauge stainless steel needle is placed about 5 cm cephalad to the medial malleolus and the needle is advanced posterior to the tibia. Once in place, a ground pad is placed on the calcaneus. A stimulator is then

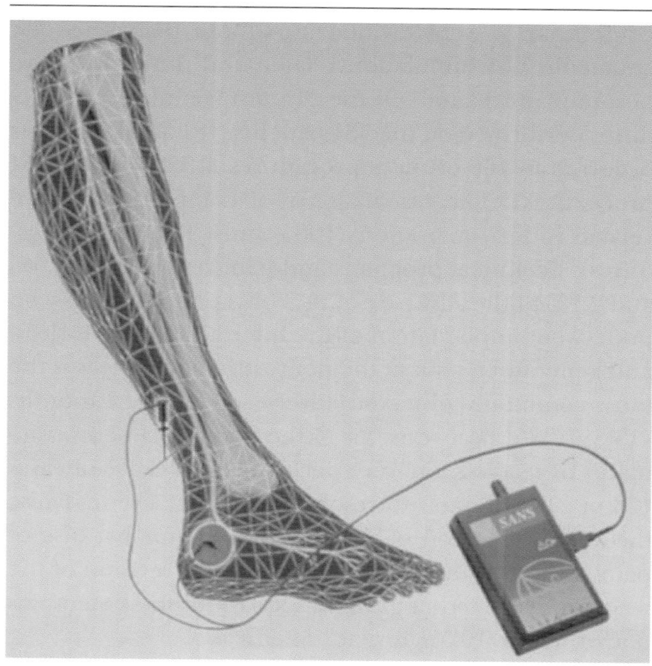

Figure 91.17. *SANS device for percutaneous neurostimulation.*

connected to the needle and the ground pad. With the stimulator on, flexion of the great toe indicates the correct needle position. Thirty-minute treatments then take place once a week for 10–12 weeks.

Results

In 2000, Klinger et al. performed a prospective trial on 15 patients with urgency frequency syndrome.[33] They underwent 12 stimulations with the SANS device (Level 3). Ten patients responded with a reduction in voiding frequency per day (16 to 4) and daily leakage episodes (4 to 2.4). The single complication was a hematoma at the puncture site.

Govier et al.,[34] in a multicenter study (Level 3), reported on the efficacy of SANS in 53 patients. All patients had refractory overactive bladder and were seen at five different sites in the US. After a 12-week stimulation, 71% of patients had at least a 25% decrease in daytime or night-time frequency. No adverse effects were noted.

COMPLICATIONS

A number of reports have been published on the complications of SNS.[23,25,26,35] The earlier reports describe the complications with PNE which is no longer used in the majority of centers in the US. Siegel et al. summarized the complications in patients with refractory urge incontinence, urgency frequency and urinary retention that were included in the original trials of SNS.[26] The complications were divided into those that were percutaneous test stimulation related and those that were post-implant related. Of the 914 test stimulation procedures performed on the 581 patients, 181 adverse events occurred in 166 of these procedures (18.2% of the 914 procedures). The vast majority of complications were related to lead migration (108 events, 11.8% of procedures). Technical problems and pain represented 2.6% and 2.1% of the adverse events. For the 219 patients who underwent implantation of the InterStim® system (lead and generator), pain at the neurostimulator site was the most commonly observed adverse effect at 12 months (15.3%). Surgical revisions of the implanted neurostimulator or lead system were performed in 33.3% of cases (73 of 219 patients) to resolve an adverse event. These included relocation of the neurostimulator because of pain at the subcutaneous pocket site and revision of the lead for suspected migration. Explant of the system was performed in 10.5% for lack of efficacy.[1]

Everaert et al. reported on complications related to SNS itself. Among the 53 patients who had undergone implantation of the quadripolar electrode (InterStim® Model 3886 or 3080) and subcutaneous pulse generator in the abdominal site (InterStim® Itrel 2, IPG) between 1994 and 1998, device-related pain was the most frequent problem, occurring in 18 of the 53 patients (34%), and occurred equally at all implantation sites (sacral, flank or abdominal).[36] Pain responded to physiotherapy in eight patients; no explantation was given for this pain. Current-related complications occurred in 11%. Fifteen revisions were performed in 12 patients. Revisions for prosthesis-related pain (n=3) and for late failures (n=6) were not successful.

Grunewald et al. reported their results after 4 years of use of SNS.[37] Complications requiring surgical revisions occurred in 11 of the 37 implanted patients (29.7%). They included infections in three cases (8.1%), lead migration in two cases (5.4%), pain at the site of the implanted pulse generator in three cases (8.1%), and a lead fracture, an electrode insulation defect and skin erosion at the site of the impulse generator in one case (2.7%).

Hijaz and Vasavada reported the complications of our group at the Cleveland Clinic Foundation (CCF).[35] Of the 180 stage I procedures performed for indications of refractory overactive bladder, idiopathic and neurogenic urinary retention, and interstitial cystitis, 130 (72.2%) proceeded to stage II implantation of the implantable pulse generator. In this group, 59 stage I leads were explanted (27.8%). The majority of lead explants were performed for unsatisfactory or poor clinical response (46/50; 92%), with the remainder being carried for infection (4/50; 8%). Stage I revisions comprised 22 of the 180 stage I (12.2%) procedures. Revisions were done for marginal response (13/22), frayed subcutaneous extension wire (6/22), lead infection (3/22) and improper localization of stimulus (1/22). Eleven (50%) of the revisions proceeded for stage II generator implant. When the revision was done for a marginal response (13/22), the response was ultimately clinically satisfactory in 5/13 (38.5%) and they proceeded to generator implant. For stage II complications, explants were performed in 16/130 (12.3%) of the CCF group. Explants were carried out for infection and failure to maintain response in 56.3% and 43.7% of cases, respectively. Revisions were performed for infection, and mechanical (generator related) and response causes. The revision rate with stage II was 20% (26/130).

In summary, stage I complications can lead to either explants or revision of the tined lead. The reasons for either cause could be related to patient response, mechanical failure or infection. Explants for response reasons should not truly be considered a complication as much as it is an integral part of the procedure. Stage

II complications are also seen for decay of response, mechanical or infection reasons. Table 91.2 summarizes the common complications of SNS reported in several series.

Hijaz and Vasavada have also presented algorithms for trouble-shooting of SNS problems.[35] When infection at the generator site is diagnosed, the best management would be explanation of the whole system. Despite attempts to salvage some of these patients, follow-up revealed that the infection persisted in all and eventual explant was inevitable. Trouble-shooting algorithms include search for causes of: 1) pocket (IPG site) discomfort; 2) recurrent symptoms; 3) stimulation occurring in the incorrect pelvic area; 4) no stimulation; and 5) intermittent stimulation.

THE BION® DEVICE

In search for a smaller, less invasive, and more selective electrical stimulation of the bladder, use of the BION® device in two forms – radiofrequency-activated BION® (RF BION®) and rechargeable BION® (BION-R®) – have been reported. The BION® device is a self-contained, battery-powered, telemetrically programmable, current-controlled mini-neurostimulator with an integrated electrode. It has a size of 27 × 3.3 mm and weighs only 0.7 g. It can be implanted adjacent to the pudendal nerve at Alcock's canal (Fig. 91.18).[38,39] The results of the BION® pilot studies indicate that a considerable reduction in the degree of detrusor overactivity incontinence can be obtained in severely refractory cases, including women who had failed sacral nerve neuromodulation. The described technique is well tolerated by the patients. It is minimally invasive and relatively simple. Clinical trials of the BION-R® device involving larger numbers of patients are currently underway in the US and Europe.

FUTURE DIRECTIONS

The initial success of SNS in treatment of some of the most bothersome conditions of the bladder has entered the electrical stimulation of the LUT into the therapeutic armamentarium of physicians dealing with those conditions. Subsequently, entry of this therapy has introduced new lines of research to enable us to answer many open and unresolved questions related to various issues of SNS in clinical practice. Daneshgari and Abrams compiled a list of the pertinent research questions that, in the opinion of several experts in the area of SNS, need to be addressed. These research questions include the following:

- Clinical predictors of responders: It is highly desirable to predict, with a reasonable level of accuracy, the potential response of patients to SNS, thus avoiding the test trial.

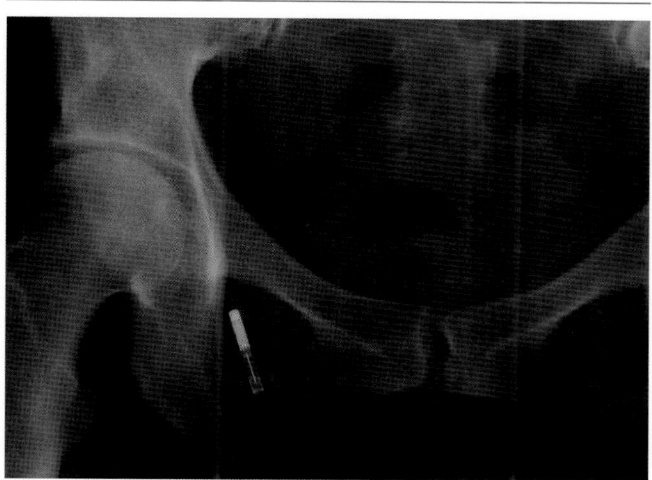

Figure 91.18. *BION® device. (Reproduced from ref. 16 with permission.)*

Table 91.2. ***Summary of common complications of SNS***

	Siegel et al.[26]	Everaert et al.[36]	Grunewald et al.[37]	Hijaz & Vasavada[35]
Number of patients	581	53	37	167
PNE – Overall	18.02%	N/A	N/A	N/A
Stage I – Overall	N/A	N/A	N/A	12.2%
Stage II – Overall	N/A	N/A	29.7%	20%
Pain at neurostimulator site	15.3%	34%	8.1%	N/A
Suspected lead migration	8.4%	N/A	5.4%	N/A
Infection	6.1%	N/A	8.1%	10.7%
Revision of permanent SNS	33.3%	23%	29.7%	20%

N/A, not applicable; PNE, peripheral nerve stimulation; SNS, sacral nerve stimulation.

- A comparison between the effects of continuous versus intermittent stimulation with the aim of improving the percentage of patients benefiting from SNS.
- Whether a unilateral versus a bilateral stimulation in either category of the current indications would lead to an improved and more durable response.
- Comparing the effects of direct pudendal nerve stimulation versus SNS in patients with refractory overactive bladder.
- Functional brain imaging of responders and failures after implant of SNS to study possible differences in CNS effects of SNS in these two groups.
- Animal models to better delineate mechanisms of action for neuromodulation (i.e. neurotransmitters).
- Longitudinal studies to better understand the interaction between genitourinary, gastrointestinal and gynecologic complaints.

As in other areas in medicine, we are looking for those sparks of success that will lead to creative fires of expanding knowledge. But we also need to respect the well-established integrity of our field by being true to our clinician-investigative tools such as properly designed clinical trials as we protect and explore the increasing territory of electrical stimulation of the lower urinary tract.

REFERENCES

1. Madersbacher H. [Conservative therapy of neurogenic disorders of micturition]. Urologe A 1999;38:24–9.
2. Cranefield P. Bibliography. Mount Kisco: Futura Publishing, 1974; 30.
3. Bell C. Idea of a new anatomy of the brain; submitted for the observations of his friends. London: Strahan and Preston, 1811; 136.
4. Magendie F. Expériences sur les fonctions des racines des nerfs rachidiens. Journal de Physiologie Expérimentale et Pathologique 1822;2:276.
5. Hall M. On the reflex function of the medulla oblongata and medulla spinalis. Phil Trans 1833; 635.
6. Fandel T, Tanagho EA. Neuromodulation in voiding dysfunction: a historical overview of neurostimulation and its application. Urol Clin North Am 2005;32:1–10.
7. Boyce WH, Lathem JE, Hunt LD. Research related to the development of an artificial electrical stimulator for the paralyzed human bladder: a review. J Urol 1964;91:41–51.
8. Dees JE. Contraction of the urinary bladder produced by electric stimulation. Preliminary report. Invest Urol 1965;15:539–47.
9. Caldwell KP. The electrical control of sphincter incompetence. Lancet 1963;2:174–5.
10. Nashold BS Jr, Friedman H, Boyarsky S. Electrical activation of micturition by spinal cord stimulation. J Surg Res 1971;11:144–7.
11. Nashold BS Jr, Friedman H, Glenn JF et al. Electromicturition in paraplegia. Implantation of a spinal neuroprosthesis. Arch Surg 1972;104:195–202.
12. Schmidt RA, Bruschini H, Tanagho EA. Sacral root stimulation in controlled micturition. Peripheral somatic neurotomy and stimulated voiding. Invest Urol 1979;17:130–4.
13. Tanagho EA, Schmidt RA. Bladder pacemaker: scientific basis and clinical future. Urology 1982;20:614–9.
14. Tanagho EA, Schmidt RA. Electrical stimulation in the clinical management of the neurogenic bladder. J Urol 1988;140:1331–9.
15. Tanagho EA, Schmidt RA, Orvis BR. Neural stimulation for control of voiding dysfunction: a preliminary report in 22 patients with serious neuropathic voiding disorders. J Urol 1989;142:340–5.
16. Leng WL, Chancellor MB. How sacral nerve stimulation neuromodulation works. Urol Clin North Am 2005;32:11–18.
17. Siegel SW. Selecting patients for sacral nerve stimulation. Urol Clin North Am 2005;32:19.
18. Chai TC, Mamo GJ. Modified techniques of S3 foramen localization and lead implantation in S3 neuromodulation. Urology 2001;58:786–90.
19. Spinelli M, Giardiello G, Gerber M et al. New sacral neuromodulation lead for percutaneous implantation using local anesthesia: description and first experience. J Urol 2003;170:1905–7.
20. Hohenfellner M, Schultz-Lampel D, Dahms S et al. Bilateral chronic sacral neuromodulation for treatment of lower urinary tract dysfunction. J Urol 1998;160:821–4.
21. Chai TC. Surgical techniques of sacral implantation. Urol Clin North Am 2005;32:27–35.
22. Janknegt RA, Hassouna MM, Siegel SW et al. Long-term effectiveness of sacral nerve stimulation for refractory urge incontinence. Eur Urol 2001;39:101–6.
23. Schmidt RA, Jonas U, Oleson KA et al. Sacral nerve stimulation for treatment of refractory urinary urge incontinence. Sacral Nerve Stimulation Study Group. J Urol 1999;162:352–7.
24. Hassouna MM, Siegel SW, Nyeholt AA et al. Sacral neuromodulation in the treatment of urgency-frequency symptoms: a multicenter study on efficacy and safety. J Urol 2000;163:1849–54.
25. Jonas U, Fowler CJ, Chancellor MB et al. Efficacy of sacral nerve stimulation for urinary retention: results 18 months after implantation. J Urol 2001;165:15–9.

26. Siegel SW, Catanzaro F, Dijkema HE et al. Long-term results of a multicenter study on sacral nerve stimulation for treatment of urinary urge incontinence, urgency-frequency, and retention. Urology 2000;56:87–91.

27. Pettit PD, Thompson JR, Chen AH. Sacral neuromodulation: new applications in the treatment of female pelvic floor dysfunction. Curr Opin Obstet Gynecol 2002;14:521–5.

28. Spinelli M, Bertapelle P, Cappellano F et al. Chronic sacral neuromodulation in patients with lower urinary tract symptoms: results from a national register. J Urol 2001;166:541–5.

29. Hedlund H, Schultz A, Talseth T et al. Sacral neuromodulation in Norway: clinical experience of the first three years. Scand J Urol Nephrol Suppl 2002;210:87–95.

30. Aboseif K, Tamaddon K, Chalfin S et al. Sacral neuromodulation in functional urinary retention: an effective way to restore voiding. BJU Int 2002;90:662–5.

31. Bernstein AJ, Peters K. Expanding indications for neuromodulation. Urol Clin North Am 2005;32:59–63.

32. Stoller M, Copeland S, Millard R. The efficacy of acupuncture in reversing the unstable bladder in pig-tailed monkeys [abstract]. J Urol 1987;137:104A.

33. Klinger H, Pycha A, Schmidbauer J, Marberger M. Use of peripheral neuromodulation for treatment of detrusor overactivity: a urodynamic-based study. Urology 2000;56:766.

34. Govier FE, Litwiller S, Nitti V et al. Percutaneous afferent neuromodulation for the refractory overactive bladder: results of a multicenter study. J Urol 2001;165:1193–8.

35. Hijaz A, Vasavada S. Complications and trouble shooting of sacral neuromodulation therapy. Urol Clin North Am 2005;32:65–9.

36. Everaert K, De Ridder D, Baert L et al. Patient satisfaction and complications following sacral nerve stimulation for urinary retention, urge incontinence and perineal pain: a multicenter evaluation. Int Urogynecol J Pelvic Floor Dysfunct 2000;11:231–5.

37. Grunewald V, Hofner K, Thon WF et al. Sacral electrical neuromodulation as an alternative treatment option for lower urinary tract dysfunction. Restor Neurol Neurosci 1999;14:189–93.

38. Bosch R. Treatment of refractory urge urinary incontinence by a novel minimally invasive implantable pudendal nerve mini-stimulator. J Pelvic Med Surg 2003;9:310.

39. Grill WM, Craggs MD, Foreman RD et al. Emerging clinical applications of electrical stimulation: opportunities for restoration of function. J Rehabil Res Dev 2001;38:641–53.

40. Amundsen CL, Webster GD. Sacral neuromodulation in an older, urge-incontinent population. Am J Obstet Gynecol 2002;187(6):1462–5; discussion 1465.

41. Bosch JLHR, Groen J. Sacral nerve neuromodulation in the treatment of patients with refractory motor urge incontinence: long-term results of a prospective longitudinal study. J Urol 2000;163:1219–22.

42. Shaker HS, Hassouna M. Sacral nerve root neuromodulation: an effective treatment for refractory urge incontinence. J Urol 1998;159(5):1516–9.

92

Complex reconstructive surgery

Christopher R Chapple, Richard T Turner-Warwick

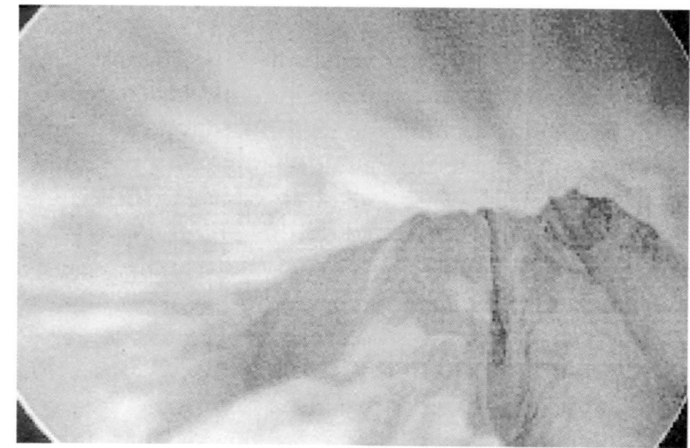

INTRODUCTION

Complex reconstructive surgery may be more appropriately considered as surgical restoration of lower urinary tract function. Preoperative evaluation relies upon accurate functional assessment and hence knowledge and understanding of the principles and practice of urodynamic investigation. An appreciation of lower urinary tract anatomy and pelvic surgery with some understanding of both gynecologic and urologic pathology is essential. The basic surgical principles are those underlying any form of successful surgical reconstruction, namely an understanding of anatomy and function with attention to excision of ischemic tissue, obliteration of dead space, interposition of vascularized tissue, avoidance of infection and hematoma, and tension-free anastomosis.

The term 'reconstructive surgery' inspires images of difficult and esoteric surgical practice best confined to specialist centers. While there is no doubt that subspecialization increases the success of such surgery, the basic underlying principles are fundamental to the practice of all surgery, namely:

1. a detailed knowledge of normal anatomy and a clear definition of abnormal radiology;
2. comprehensive and appropriate assessment of upper and lower urinary tract function;
3. good surgical technique, with good access and exposure, and a full appreciation of available surgical techniques.

In this brief exposition on the subject, it is the intention to consider areas in urogynecologic practice where functional and anatomic reconstruction is important; for example, where there is damage to the ureter, the bladder or urethra, and the important area of surgical resolution of severe detrusor overactivity which has proved resistant to conventional therapy.

URETERIC INJURY

The ureter is an elastic and well-protected structure lying in the retroperitoneal space. Injury from external trauma is therefore uncommon, the majority of injuries being iatrogenic in origin. Although ureteral injuries account for only a small proportion of all urologic pathology, being the sole conduit from the kidney, ureteric integrity is essential for normal renal function. Such injuries therefore demand careful appraisal and timely intervention.

Iatrogenic ureteric injury

As a number of iatrogenic ureteric injuries may never become clinically apparent, the true incidence of injury is therefore difficult to estimate. The incidence of clinical ureteric injury in routine gynecologic surgery has been reported to vary from 0.2 to 1.5% in retrospective studies.[1–5] This rises to 2.5% for prospective studies where postoperative urograms are carried out and up to 30–35% when radical pelvic surgery is involved.[6–10]

In a large study by Goodna et al., the incidence of ureteric injuries involving 4665 surgical operations was noted to be 0.4%, a figure which has not changed significantly over the years.[2,11] In most series, gynecologic surgery accounts for about two-thirds of iatrogenic ureteral injuries. Most are related to abdominal, radical or vaginal hysterectomy, ovarian tumor surgery, and incontinence surgery. Non-gynecologic causes of iatrogenic injuries include colorectal surgery (15%), ureteroscopic surgery (2–17%), vascular surgery (6%), laminectomy/spinal fusion (1%), bladder neck suspension procedures (3%), appendicectomy (1%), and cesarean section (1%).[12] Rare causes of ureteral injury following procedures such as open herniorrhaphy, CT-guided chemical sympathectomy, termination of pregnancy, and Kirschner wire application for hip dislocation in a child have also been reported.[13–16]

In recent years, with the development and proliferation of new laparoscopic techniques, there has been a significant increase in associated injuries, especially in gynecology, where laparoscopy now accounts for 25% of all gynecologic injuries to the ureter.[17] This rise parallels the rise of ureteral injuries associated with a similar expansion in endoscopic approaches to complex ureteric problems in urologic practice. In a recent review by Selzman and Spirnak of 165 ureteric injuries, urologic surgery accounted for 42% of the total compared with 34% for gynecologic surgery and 24% for general surgery. The bulk of injuries to the ureter in this series followed endoscopic urologic surgery (79%) compared to gynecologic surgery and general surgery where the majority of ureteral injuries occurred during open procedures.[18]

Risk factors for iatrogenic ureteric injuries

Previous surgery, bulky or invasive tumors, ureteric duplication and ectopic ureters, endometriosis, retroperitoneal fibrosis and inflammatory conditions such as chronic pelvic infection all predispose to iatrogenic ureteric injury. Situations when life is threatened due to hemorrhage, or during emergency cesarean section when speed becomes critical, can also predispose to iatrogenic ureteric injury.

Types of iatrogenic injury

1. *Avulsion*: Avulsion occurs when forceful retraction is used, especially when tissues are soft as a result of infection or necrosis.
2. *Transection*: This is caused by the scissors or scalpel, especially when the ureters are enveloped within tumor or fibrous tissue. Common sites of such injuries during gynecologic surgery include:
   - the pelvic brim where the vascular pedicle to the ovary is in close proximity to the ureter;
   - the broad ligament where the ureter is crossed by the uterine artery;
   - the ureteric canal in the cardinal ligament, 1 cm lateral to the supravaginal cervix and 1 cm above the lateral vaginal fornix.

   In surgery of the rectum and sigmoid colon, the left ureter is more commonly involved in iatrogenic ureteric injury. Invasive tumor, dense fibrosis, and inflammatory conditions all contribute to ureteric trauma, even in the hands of experienced surgeons. Retrocecal appendicitis has been known to result in similar iatrogenic ureteric injuries on the right.

   During vascular surgery, ureteric injury can occur with aortoiliac and aortofemoral bypass. Predisposing factors include retroperitoneal fibrosis, radiation exposure, long-term ureteral stents, graft infections or graft dilation.
3. *Ligation*: This occurs when the ureters are mistaken for bleeding vessels. It can also occur during vaginal hysterectomy when the uterine arteries are being ligated, and in procidentia when the ureters prolapse with the uterus.
4. *Crushing*: This may occur when clamps are used blindly to control hemorrhage and is seen at sites similar to transection injury, especially during radical hysterectomy for cancer. Necrosis and ultimately stricture or fistula formation can result.
5. *Devascularization*: This occurs when extensive or overenthusiastic dissection of the ureter is performed. The ureter is supplied in 80% of individuals by a single artery along its entire length with anastomotic feeding vessels at each end and in the middle. Devascularization results in ischemic necrosis which ultimately leads to fistula or stricture.
6. *Perforation*: This is commonly caused by ureteroscopy and associated endoscopic manipulation for ureteric stones. Edematous tissue surrounding the stone and tissue traumatized by lithotripsy are predisposing factors. Needle injury during open surgery may result in perforation but is rarely a cause of problems in healthy tissues.
7. *Fulguration*: This can occur during transurethral resection of bladder cancers resected close to the ureteric orifices and then extensively diathermied. Laparoscopic diathermy and laser treatment of endometriotic lesions are an increasingly important cause of thermal injury to the urinary tract that has seen an increase in parallel with the rise of laparoscopic surgery in gynecology.
8. *Fistula formation*: This can follow transection, ischemic necrosis or perforation if the distal end of the ureter is not in continuity or is obstructed. Urine will then discharge from the vagina, operative wound or drain site, or into the peritoneal cavity or retroperitoneal space.
9. *Stricture formation*: This can follow any of the above injuries and ultimately lead to obstruction of the ureters, hydronephrosis, and renal damage.

Non-iatrogenic ureteric injury

Non-iatrogenic ureteric injuries are uncommon, but are found in 2.3–17% of cases of penetrating abdominal trauma, most commonly gunshot or stab wounds.[19] Associated injuries to the colon, duodenum, pancreas, and great vessels make such injuries potentially life threatening.

Blunt or avulsion injuries are very rare, most commonly occurring after a fall from a height or being thrown from a car. Severe compression injuries such as those related to the steering wheel and seat belts can also cause ureteric injuries which may even present with a soft non-tender abdomen. Most blunt trauma involves the pelviureteric junction and often presents late with a ureteric fistula or urinoma as a result of an avulsion injury.[20,21]

Radiation injury to the ureters is rare and can occur in radiotherapy for cervical, bladder, rectal, and other pelvic tumors. Most post-irradiation ureteric strictures, however, are due to recurrent tumor. Presentation may be from 3 months up to 10 years, usually with a long thread-like stenotic lesion or a localized constriction about 4–6 cm from the bladder. These are thought to be due to endarteritis obliterans resulting from radiotherapy. Subsequent surgery on such poor quality tissues also predisposes to a higher complication rate involving the ureters.[22]

Presentation

Approximately 15–25% of iatrogenic ureteric injuries during open surgery are discovered intraoperatively. The majority present postoperatively, delays in diagnosis being the rule rather than the exception. Delays can vary from 2 days to 12 years.[23–27] Early signs of ureteral injuries are subtle and usually missed, the injury being discovered several days or weeks later when a complication occurs. In urologic surgery, however, where injury is most commonly associated with ureteroscopic procedures for stone disease, 77% are diagnosed intraoperatively. Of these ureteric injuries, 91% occur in the lower third, 7% in the middle third and 2% in the upper third.

Penetrating injuries involving the ureter usually present with associated injuries and in most cases are identified intraoperatively during exploration of the wound. Gross hematuria is present in approximately one-third of the patients, whereas about another third do not have any blood on urinalysis at all.[20,21,28,29]

Diagnosis

Ureteric injuries recognized intraoperatively and repaired immediately carry a better prognosis of cure than those which become manifest postoperatively as a result of complications.[18,23,25,30] In a recent review of 165 ureteral injuries by Selzman and Spirnak, the number of procedures required to repair urologic injuries was 1.2 for those diagnosed intraoperatively compared to 1.6 for those diagnosed postoperatively.[18] Seventy-seven percent of urologic injuries were diagnosed intraoperatively compared to 16% in gynecologic surgery and 56% in general surgery. This difference is due mainly to the different procedures that cause such injuries in these specialties in addition to the greater familiarity with ureteric anatomy amongst urologists.

A high index of suspicion is required for the diagnosis of iatrogenic ureteric injury in the immediate postoperative period, especially in non-urologic operations. Fever is a common feature after any surgery; however, if persistent, it may be a sign of urinary sepsis which occurs in 10% of those with ureteric obstruction. Flank pain occurs in 36–90% of cases of hydronephrosis.[25,27,31] Fistulae of the vagina and skin tend to present 7–10 days after surgery with urinary leakage.[23–25,27,31] Those involving the peritoneum may leak urine from the wound or drains. An abdominal and pelvic mass, urinoma or pelvic abscess may also result. Malaise and gastrointestinal upset or ileus are often accompanying features. These do not settle spontaneously and an abdomen distended as a consequence of ileus and supposed 'ascites' should raise the suspicion of urinary leakage. Excessive wound drainage or leakage per vaginam may be collected, analyzed, and its electrolytes compared with those in the patient's urine to establish the likely origin of this fluid. Inevitably, ureteric injuries must first be suspected if they are to be detected.

An intravenous urogram (IVU) is mandatory whenever ureteric injury is suspected. This will usually demonstrate the site of injury as well as associated pathology such as hydronephrosis and ureteric fistulation. Should an IVU be inconclusive, cystoscopy and retrograde pyelogram or antegrade nephrostogram is often useful; higher concentrations of contrast in these studies allow demonstration of leakage and establish the diagnosis in most cases.

Following penetrating trauma, the ureters should be explored if injury is suspected. IVUs using high doses of contrast have not been helpful and, in a series of 12 patients with penetrating injuries of the ureter, only 25% were diagnosed on IVU.[19] Features such as extravasation of contrast, ureteral obstruction, deviation, dilation or non-visualization are diagnostic. In 75% of such cases, IVU demonstrated only kidney presence and function.[19–21] Conversely, direct exploration of the ureter and the use of indigo carmine dye intraoperatively provided the diagnosis in 83% of cases.[19] CT scans are of limited value in demonstrating ureteral injuries per se but may be helpful when extravasation is seen or when urinomas have developed. The primary role of CT remains in the assessment of other associated abdominal and pelvic injuries. The absence of hematuria in a third of ureteral injuries and a negative IVU in about three-quarters of penetrating ureteral injuries implies that, in such cases – even in the presence of a negative preoperative diagnostic radiology – the suspicion of ureteric injury warrants exploration.[20,21,28]

Following blunt trauma, delays in diagnosis are relatively common due to the lack of early characteristic features and the association of other severe life-threatening injuries warranting more immediate attention.

Prevention

Iatrogenic injuries are best managed by preventive rather than corrective measures. Avoidance of ureteric injury is invariably the principle of all good surgical practice and begins with a thorough knowledge of the course of the ureters, the nature and site of potential ureteric injuries, and adequate preoperative evaluation. This may include an IVU or contrast-enhanced CT scans to define anatomy if major pelvic or retroperitoneal surgery is planned. A preoperative IVU allows for comparative studies should a postoperative IVU become necessary. However, preoperative IVUs have not been shown to be of value prior to routine hysterectomy and cannot substitute for good surgical technique and identification of anatomic landmarks.[32,33]

Congenital anomalies, ectopic ureters, and ureteric duplications should be recognized in advance and may be defined on preoperative imaging. Where radical surgery is being carried out and the ureters are involved or displaced by the pathology, their course should be mapped and the necessary precautions taken. Preoperative, or more commonly intraoperative placement of ureteric catheters may facilitate their identification during difficult anatomic dissection. Such maneuvers should not induce complacency since injuries are known to occur despite the presence of a ureteric catheter.[34] Nevertheless, identification of the length of ureter within the operative field should significantly reduce the risk of damage. The ureters are recognized by the glistening appearance of their sheaths, peristalsis on stimulation, and characteristic feel on palpation. Dissection of the ureters may be necessary, especially when in close proximity to resection margins. Sharp dissection along the line of the ureter, incorporating a generous cuff of periureteric adventitia, should reduce the risk of ischemic injury.

The close relationship of the uterine artery and the last 3 cm of the ureter makes it vulnerable to injury when mass ligature and blind clamping of an injured artery occurs. Proper identification and isolation of the uterine artery before ligation and digital compression of the internal iliac artery to control hemorrhage can avoid the need for blind clamping. Most unexpected hemorrhage can be controlled by suitable compression of the bleeding point until the ureter is identified.

If ureteric injury is suspected during open surgery, indigo carmine dye may be useful in identifying the presence and site of the lesion. Contrast solution with intraoperative imaging is more useful during ureteroscopic procedures. Most ureteroscopic injuries occur during stone extraction and fragmentation. The experience of the urologist has also been shown to be an important risk factor.[35] Other important principles in the prevention of ureteroscopic injuries include careful patient selection, availability of good endoscopic instrumentation and the use of intraoperative fluoroscopy. Large and high stones may be better managed by open surgery.

Management of ureteric injury

The management of a ureteral injury depends on its extent and location, its etiology, associated injuries, and the time of its discovery.

Timing of surgery

Ureteral injuries discovered intraoperatively and repaired immediately have excellent results, probably due to the absence of sequelae following urine leak and complications such as infection.[18,36] If the injury is incurred during a ureteroscopic procedure, an internal stent placed retrogradely across the defect may be all that is required. Small perforations usually heal within 1–2 weeks, whereas larger defects and thermal injuries require up to 6 weeks of internal stenting. If immediate stenting is impossible, initial percutaneous nephrostomy and subsequent antegrade placement of the ureteral stent is indicated.[17]

Injuries diagnosed postoperatively may initially be managed conservatively using nephrostomy drainage and/or subsequent ureteric stenting if the ureteric defect is short (<2.5 cm) and a stent can be passed across the defect, either retrogradely or antegradely.[26] About half of all ureteric injuries can be treated by such endoscopic stenting whereas the remainder will require an open procedure for definitive repair. In a series of 165 iatrogenic ureteric injuries, 49% were treated with 6 weeks of internal stenting, 89% showing no evidence of obstruction on follow-up lasting 1–20 years (mean of 8.5 years).[18] A further series of 50 ureteric injuries found that endoscopic treatment performed for defects of less than 2 cm required less operating time, had fewer complications, and shorter hospital stays compared with those undergoing open surgery.[37] No recurrences were noted over a 2-year follow-up period. However, 14 of the 30 patients selected for endoscopic treatment failed ureteric catheterization and subsequently required open repair (all were ureteric injuries diagnosed after 3 weeks). The authors concluded that endoscopic management of ureteric injuries should be carried out only in those with defects less than 2 cm in length diagnosed within 3 weeks of injury. In a further series of 27 patients, it was reported that percutaneous nephrostomy alone or in conjunction with ureteral stenting was successful in treating 11 (65%) of the 17 ureteral injuries considered suitable for endoscopic stenting.[24] As reported by Cormio et al.,[37] only one of 20 attempted retrograde ureteric catheterizations was successful in those with delayed diagnoses. All ureteric fistulae required ureteric stenting for healing and percutaneous nephrostomy was successful only in those with demonstrable ureteric obstruction. These cases presumably represent ligation or crush injuries requiring time for dissolution of sutures and tissue healing. Ureteric obstruction persisting after 8 weeks of percutaneous drainage will require open exploration and repair.[24] In a series of 20 patients with ureteric injuries who had percutaneous nephrostomy with or without a stent as a primary procedure, 80% had spontaneous recovery of the injured ureter without further intervention. Morbidity and re-operation rates were reduced compared with 24 ureteric injuries treated by immediate open ureteric repair.[38]

For those that require open surgical correction, immediate repair is increasingly shown to have similar if not better results compared with the traditional approach of waiting for 6 weeks to 3 months before definitive repair. A number of series support early surgical intervention within 3 weeks.[23,25,26,29,30,39,40] Selzman and Spirnak also found that complications were five times higher in the group treated by delayed compared with immediate repair for urologically injured ureters.[18]

Open surgical management

Ureteral transection is best repaired by immediate spatulated ureteroureterostomy. This should be carried out with a tension-free anastomosis using interrupted absorbable sutures. Sutures should not be too close together in an attempt to achieve a watertight anastomosis, as ischemia and subsequent stricture formation may result. A double 'J' stent is often used as a splint and removed between 2 and 6 weeks. Ligation injuries are simply de-ligated but crush injuries may be of greater extent due to ischemia and must be handled carefully.[31] If doubt exists as to the viability of the ureter, partial excision and spatulated re-anastomosis may be required (Fig. 92.1).

For injuries at or below the pelvic brim, an antireflux ureteroneocystostomy is the treatment of choice, for which various methods have been described. In the event of a gap between the end of the ureter and bladder, extra length can be obtained with a psoas hitch.[41] Alternatively a Boari flap may be employed to achieve a tension-free anastomosis[42,43] (Fig. 92.2). A graft length to width ratio of 3:2 is necessary, using a vascular pedicle based on the superior vesical artery. As the tubularized flap has no functional activity, the tube should be open-mouthed for adequate drainage.[44] The theoretical advantage of the psoas hitch is the better preservation of the blood supply which may be more precarious in the Boari flap. Other practical advantages include the relative ease of closure of the incision in thick-walled bladders. The incision is relatively smaller to produce an equivalent length of tube, thereby facilitating a non-refluxing reimplantation, and the subsequent ureteric positioning facilitates ureteroscopy.

For ureteric defects above the pelvic brim, additional length of ureter of a few centimeters can be obtained by

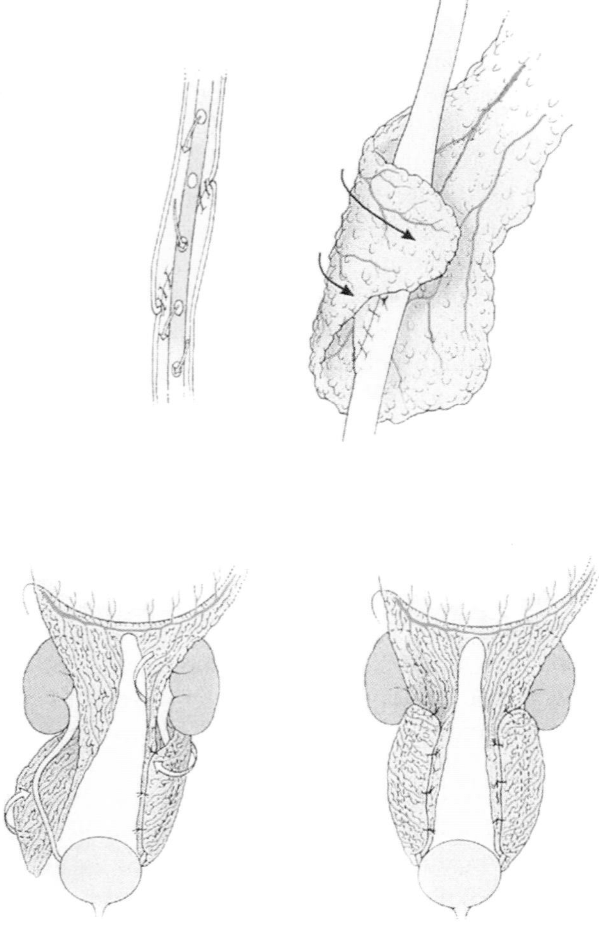

Figure 92.1. *The principle of end-to-end spatulated anastomosis of the ureter with omental wrap around to provide support to the repair.*

mobilization of the kidney, allowing spatulated uretero-ureterostomy. Other options to foreshorten the ureteric course include calicoureterostomy, transureterostomy, and autotransplantation.[45–47] If all else fails, nephrectomy is a final resort which, although previously an acceptable form of management for such injuries, is now less acceptable given the other available options.

A number of non-biologic ureteral substitutes have been investigated with limited and generally short-lived success. The ileal ureter has proved the most reliable ureteric replacement to date.[48,49] The main drawbacks to the use of bowel, as in other bowel replacement surgery, relates to the production of mucus (which can cause obstruction), inadequate peristalsis, anastomotic stricture, and reabsorption of excretory waste products. Consequently, contraindications to ileoureteric substitution include uncorrected bladder outlet obstruction and impaired renal function. Recurrent urinary tract infection and subsequent renal impairment are potential

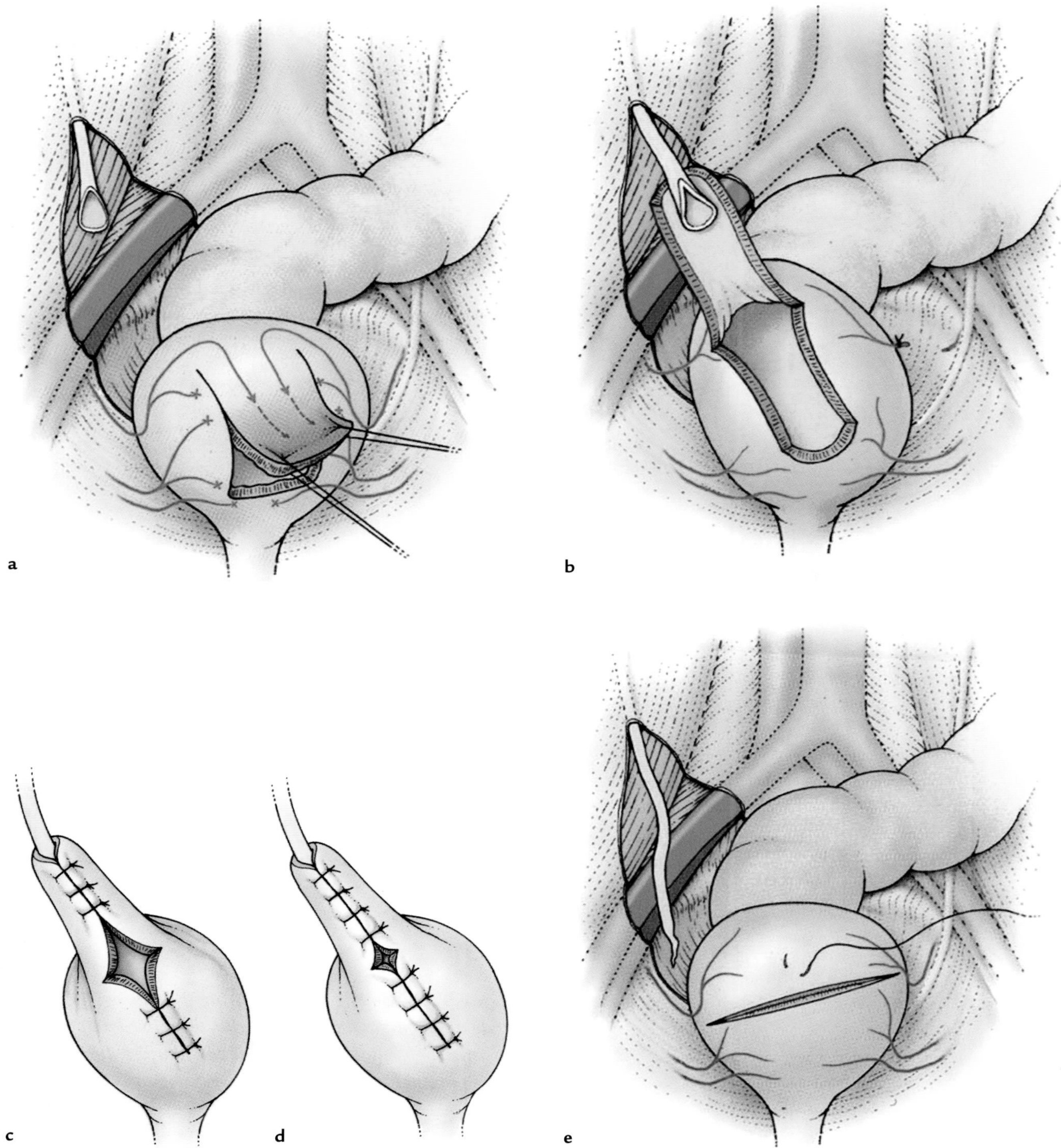

Figure 92.2. *(a) With the formation of a Boari flap, a flap of bladder is raised; note the ischemic nature of the apex. (b) The ureter is anastomosed. (c, d) The flap is completed. (e) Forming a bladder elongation flap.*

complications.[44] The appendix is an alternative biologic substitute but is of limited length.[50] The fallopian tube has been employed but is limited by its relatively small caliber.

Postoperative care and follow-up

Postoperative care following surgery for ureteric injuries requires close monitoring of renal function with appro-

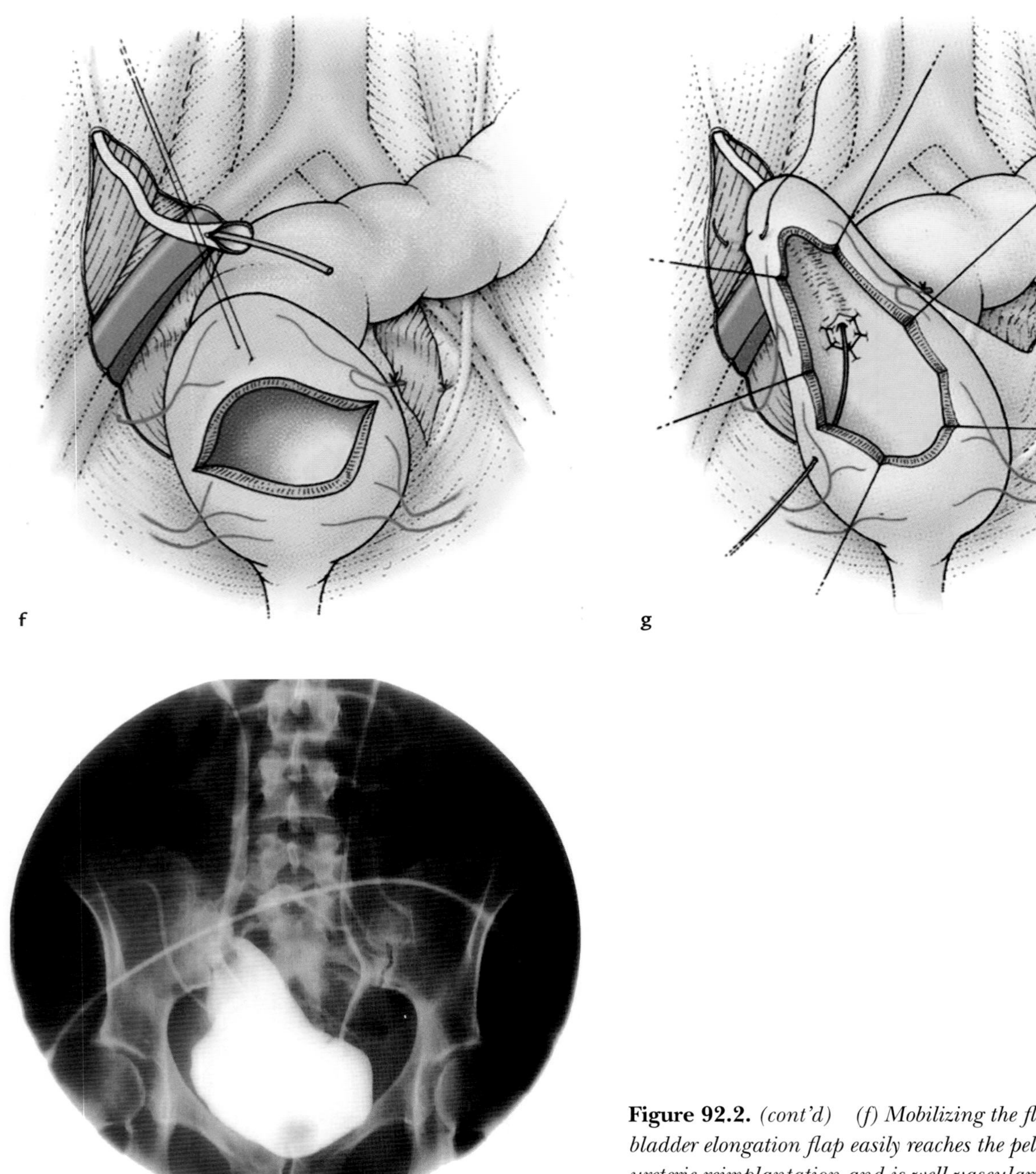

Figure 92.2. *(cont'd) (f) Mobilizing the flap. (g) The bladder elongation flap easily reaches the pelvic brim, allowing ureteric reimplantation and is well vascularized. It is secured to the psoas muscle. (h) Postoperative cystogram.*

priate fluid and electrolyte replacement, especially in the presence of postobstruction diuresis. Adequate antibiotic cover, wound care, and prophylaxis against deep vein thrombosis follow standard surgical practice. Meticulous care of catheters and drains is critical, given the dependence of renal function and uneventful postoperative recovery on these devices.

Common complications include urinary leakage, infection and hematoma, and complications related to drains and catheters. Percutaneous nephrostomy tubes may kink or become displaced due to their awkward locations in the flank. Proper anchoring techniques and after-care are therefore essential. Chronic and recurrent infections can also result from the use of long-term nephrostomy drainage. Alternatively, the use of internal stents may avoid such complications but often causes irritative symptoms and, in the long term, may become encrusted if not changed every 4–6 months. Vesicoureteric reflux may occur following reimplantation and may present with recurrent infection and dilation of the pelvicalyceal system.

Monitoring of wound drainage and contrast radiography immediately after placement of stents or drains is essential. Tube nephrostograms are useful for diagnostic purposes. A repeat IVU following stent removal and long-term follow-up (including IVU at 6 weeks, and possibly longer) are recommended

Conclusions

It is evident that it is important to diagnose ureteral injury as soon as possible and, if identified at the time of surgery, to carry out ureteral stenting (if possible) during endoscopic surgery or direct repair during open surgery. Failing this, a number of open surgical options to foreshorten the course of the ureter are available. If this is not possible, either ureteral substitution or autotransplantation should be considered.

Definitive management of ureteric injury diagnosed postoperatively depends on the level and the extent of ureteric loss, its etiology, associated injuries or complications, and time to discovery. The functional status of the kidneys, and the age, condition, and prognosis of the patient are similarly important. Most injuries below the pelvic brim can be treated with a neoureterocystostomy employing a bladder elongation procedure. Mid and upper ureteric injuries above the pelvic brim, however, are more challenging. Small defects above the pelvic brim can be repaired with a spatulated ureteroureterostomy. In cases of extensive ureteral loss, measures such as mobilizing the kidney, transureteroureterostomy, renal autotransplantation, and ureteral substitution using small bowel may be required.

Although reconstruction should be attempted whenever possible, in rare situations, based on the general condition of the patient, the function of both kidneys, and the degree of damage to the ureter, nephrectomy may represent the most appropriate management.

LOWER URINARY TRACT FISTULAE

Fistulous communications between the bladder or urethra and adjacent structures can be a cause of great distress to the patient. Few patients are more anxious to be cured of their affliction, or are more grateful when this has been accomplished. The vast majority of such fistulae occur in women and follow gynecologic or obstetric trauma – most commonly urinary vaginal fistulae involving the bladder, ureter and, rarely, the urethra. Vesicointestinal communications usually occur as a complication of inflammatory or malignant bowel disease, with the exception of the rare case of the radiation-damaged 'frozen-pelvis' following treatment of gynecologic malignancy. Urethrorectal and urethrocutaneous fistulae are the only group that occurs most commonly in men.

The subdivision of fistulae into 'simple' and 'complex' introduces further nomenclature. At first sight this might be considered to unnecessarily complicate matters – but serves a useful purpose in defining the most appropriate surgical approach. Simple fistulae can usually be resolved by a simple closure in layers. More complex cases with associated tissue devascularization, previous failed surgical repair attempts or irradiation, extensive tissue loss or persistence of a focus of infection or malignancy, may require the use of adjunctive procedures. Fistulae arising from a diverse range of etiologies – whether traumatic, surgical, inflammatory, neoplastic or radiation-induced – are almost invariably amenable to surgical repair.

Urinary vaginal fistulae

> Whatever may be the cause of this distressing affection, it is a matter of serious importance to both surgeon and patient that it be rendered susceptible of cure.
>
> Sims 1852.[51]

Fistulae involving the vagina in undeveloped societies are most commonly associated with obstetric trauma and, as such, have from ancient times represented an important cause of severe morbidity and mortality in young women. In developed countries urinary vaginal fistulae occur most commonly between the bladder and vagina, sometimes involve the ureter, and usually follow gynecologic surgery, occasionally complicating the management of gynecologic malignancy.

Diagnosis

The classic symptom of a urinary vaginal fistula is continuous involuntary incontinence following a hysterectomy or other pelvic operation. Nevertheless, where the fistula is small, the presentation may be far less florid, comprising no more than a watery vaginal discharge accompanied by normal voiding. Definition of the precise anatomic abnormality is of paramount importance when planning the most appropriate management of a fistula. The combined use of imaging modalities and a careful examination under anesthetic are essential elements of this process, since in many cases more than one structure (e.g. both the bladder and ureter) is involved. In addition, the demonstration of associated functional abnormalities and the presence of malignant disease are important contributory factors which must be considered and investigated prior to undertaking definitive surgery.

All patients should have an IVU to assess the number of ureters and to look for the presence of dilation or extravasation from a ureter which would be suggestive of its involvement in the fistula (Fig. 92.3).

A voiding cystourethrogram may demonstrate the presence of a fistula and will document any associated vesicoureteric reflux, bladder base prolapse, and stress incontinence which may either relate to the patient's symptomatology or could be usefully corrected at the time of surgical repair of the fistula.

The 'three-swab test' (Fig. 92.4) can be helpful in the preoperative assessment. The identification of individual swabs is facilitated by the use of identifying sutures on their 'tails'. Aqueous methylene blue dye is instilled into the bladder: the demonstration of dye staining of only the swab placed high in the vagina occurs with a vesicovaginal fistula; staining of the lowermost swab alone occurs with urethral leakage, either stress incontinence or a urethrovaginal fistula. Conversely if the uppermost swab is wet but not stained by dye and the lower two are dry, a ureteric fistula is likely. Obviously this test will not delineate the presence of a ureteric fistula in association with a vesical fistula.

Cystoscopy, vaginoscopy, and examination under anesthesia (EUA) are essential in all cases and will often demonstrate small fistulae not demonstrated using other modalities. Where doubt remains as to the exact diagnosis, even at the time of an EUA, the synchronous use of the three-swab test can again provide helpful additional information. Similarly, CO_2 insufflation of the vagina in the presence of a fistula produces a stream of air bubbles which can be seen at cystoscopy. A biopsy should be taken from the edges of the fistula in all cases where there is any history of pelvic malignancy. If ureteric damage is suspected, ascending bulb ureterograms can be carried out, and this can be followed by the insertion of double 'J' stents.

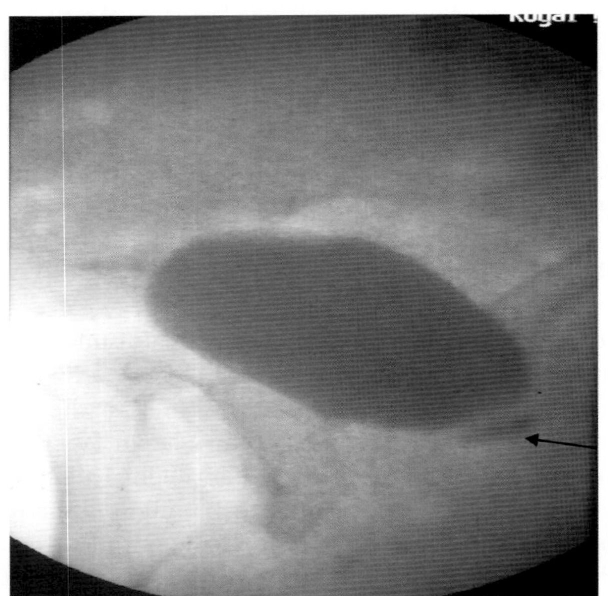

Figure 92.3. *Cystogram demonstrating leakage at the bladder base due to vesicovaginal fistula.*

Conservative management

What are the indications for surgery versus conservative treatment? In a proportion of patients with small 'simple' vesicovaginal and ureterovaginal fistulae, conservative therapy may result in resolution of the fistula. In such patients the use of continuous drainage with a urethral catheter or internal splintage with a double 'J' stent, respectively, may be considered. It must be borne in mind that there is a low incidence of spontaneous closure in many series; Marshall reported only one case in a series of 92 patients.[52] Following all nonsurgical management it should be remembered that the majority of fistulae will fail to heal spontaneously, a fact which must be balanced against the near certainty of surgical success, particularly if there is an iatrogenic etiology.

A number of adjunctive measures can be used in addition to drainage:

- Local or systemic estrogen therapy;[53]
- Antibiotic prophylaxis;[54]
- Cystoscopic fulguration of the fistula;[55]
- Corticosteroid therapy.[56]

Both estrogen therapy in the postmenopausal patient and antibiotic prophylaxis are likely to be helpful by improving the quality of the tissues and aiding subsequent surgery. Cauterization of fistulae was described as of limited benefit except in small fistulae by Sims,[51] a sentiment reiterated by O'Conor who reported success with six patients.[55] It seems unlikely that corticosteroid therapy has much to recommend it since, although it will reduce edema, it will also impair healing.

Timing of surgery

It is an essential requirement prior to surgery to have accurate knowledge of the patient's vaginal and urinary

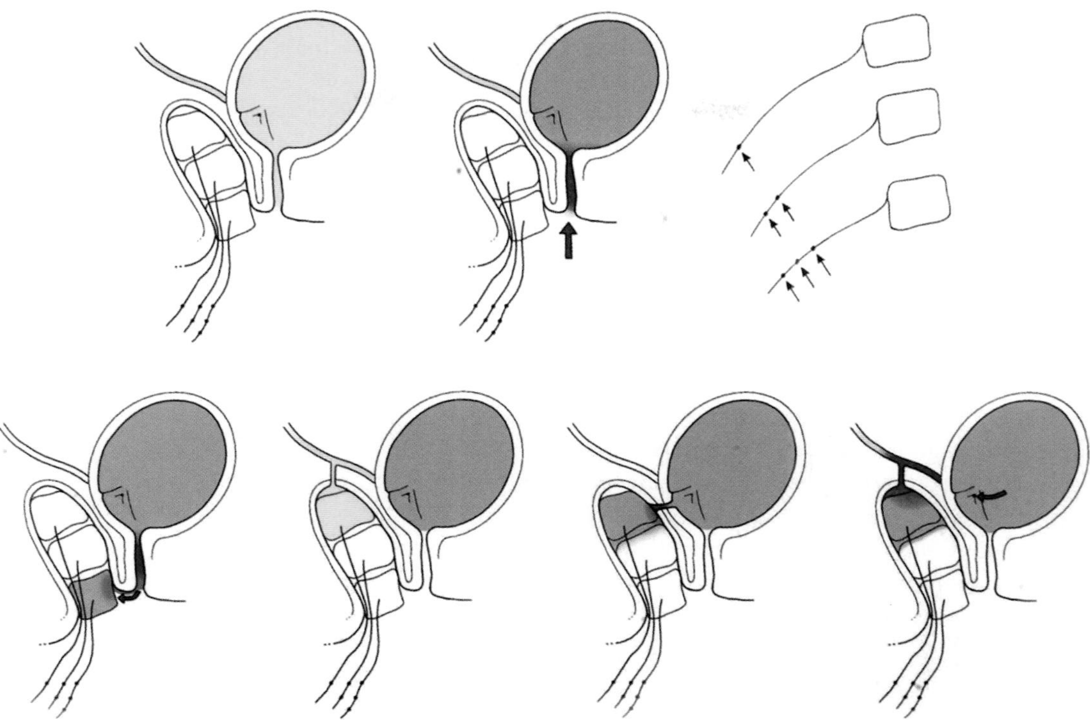

Figure 92.4. *Three-swab test showing the importance of identifying individual swabs, and the way in which this can localize a site of leakage. Bottom right: false-positive result due to reflux up the ureter and leakage from a ureterovaginal fistula.*

tract bacteriology, so that any pathogens can be eradicated by appropriate antimicrobial therapy; antibiotic prophylaxis should be used routinely. It is difficult to generalize as to the appropriate timing of surgical intervention for every case, since this will depend upon the systemic and local factors influencing the healing potential of the local tissues in the individual case. In the otherwise uncomplicated simple postoperative fistula, it is almost invariably possible to resolve the problem by early exploration within a few weeks, before the processes of inflammation and repair render surgery difficult. The majority of evidence suggests that if this window of opportunity is missed it is wise to defer surgery for at least 3 months.[52,57] It is clearly inappropriate to carry out a surgical procedure which would potentially be rendered more complex and extensive and where morbidity is likely to be higher.

In more complex fistulae where tissue healing is dependent on the interposition of a pedicled flap of vascularized tissue such as omentum, this timing is less critical to healing of the fistula. Although some workers have advocated repair between 3 and 12 weeks, it must be remembered that these cases all included interposed flaps of peritoneum or omentum.[58,59] It is salutary to note that in a reported series of 11 'early' repairs of vesicovaginal fistulae, 10 were successfully treated before 3 weeks had elapsed after injury; the remaining case, however, repaired by simple layered closure at 35 days, recurred on the fifth postoperative day.[60]

Choice of approach

The decision as to the best surgical approach for an individual case will be considerably biased by an individual surgeon's preference and training. It will also depend upon the etiology, position, and size of the vesical fistula and the coexistence of associated ureteric or urethral damage. Adequate surgical access is crucial, not only for direct repair of the fistula itself, but also to allow additional procedures such as urethral repair, ureteric reimplantation or the interposition of pedicle flaps, essential to a successful outcome, to be undertaken. These requirements should be the most important factor in the selection of surgical approach.

A vaginal approach provides limited access but avoids the morbidity associated with abdominal procedures; it is ideally suited to closure of the low simple fistula, and can be combined with the use of an interposed pedicled flap of labial/scrotal tissue or gracilis muscle for more complex fistulae. The abdominal approach is more invasive but is indicated for the repair of high or complex fistulae and lends itself to the concomitant interposition of a pedicled omental flap in the repair. The most logical approach is to have the available expertise to utilize all of these procedures as necessary;[61,62] preparing the patient for a synchronous perineoabdominal procedure at the outset of an operation, thereby facilitating the progression from one to the other if required.[57]

Repair technique

The plethora of reports and techniques reported in the literature bear witness not only to the variation in the success of the different surgical methods in the hands of individual surgeons, but also to the diversity of available procedures. Surgical repair will succeed provided that it removes any predisposing etiologic cause for a fistula and reconstitutes the defect by the approximation of healthy, well-vascularized tissue. These criteria are easily achieved in simple fistulae by the trimming and tension-free approximation of adjacent wound edges. In more complex cases where the fistulous defect is large or fibrosis (resulting from infection, surgery or irradiation) compromises tissue healing, the interposition of a pedicled flap of well-vascularized tissue markedly increases the chances of success. In these cases it must be remembered that if the tension-free apposition of an epithelial defect is not possible, migration of epithelial cells will occur over an interposed vascularized pedicled flap. It is therefore acceptable to leave such defects provided that they are adequately covered by the flap.

Vaginal repair of vesicovaginal fistula

Exposure

The patient is placed on the operating table in the prone position slightly head-down, hips flexed to 30 degrees and legs widely abducted. The use of the prone position has the disadvantage that should vaginal repair prove difficult, progression to a synchronous abdominal approach is difficult or impossible. This is more than compensated for by the principal advantage of the position which places the fistula on the 'floor' of the vagina, in front of the operating surgeon.

Optimal exposure to the fistula is achieved by the use of a Parkes anal retractor (Fig. 92.5), often combined with a ring retractor. In the presence of a narrowed introitus, exposure can be improved by a posterolateral episiotomy prior to insertion of the retractor.

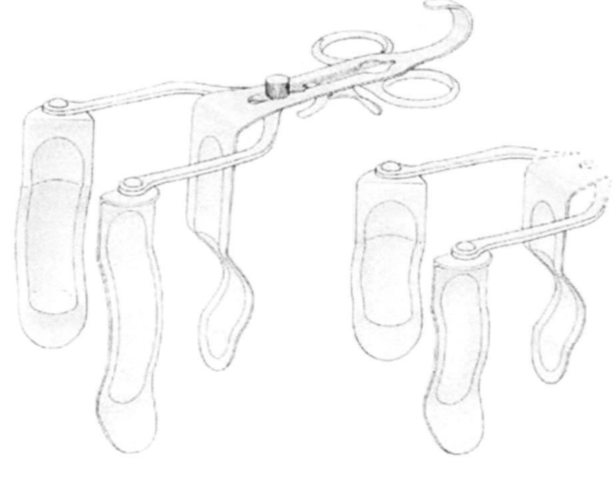

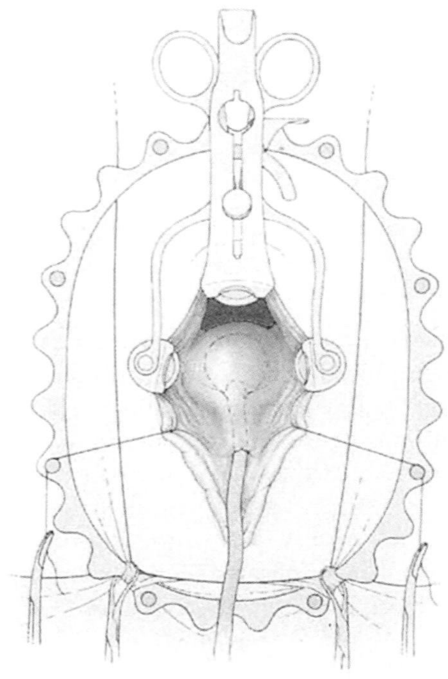

Figure 92.5. *Use of a Parkes self-retaining retractor for fistula surgery.*

Dissection

The vaginal epithelial margin of the fistula is circumcised. This can be facilitated by upward retraction on a Foley catheter passed through the fistula into the bladder. In the uncomplicated case, excision of the fistulous tract is usually contraindicated since it will enlarge the size of the fistula, thereby making the repair more difficult. The tissue plane between vagina and bladder is developed and these structures are separated. These steps are important, since the success of any fistula repair depends upon the excision of damaged and devascularized tissues and tension-free closure in layers with meticulous attention to the integrity and positioning of the subcutaneous tissues.

Closure

It is important that the tissues used in the closure should be well vascularized and, wherever possible, suture lines which are in contact should be offset or placed at 180 degrees to each other. Absorbable sutures of interrupted 3-0 Vicryl/Monocryl are recommended.

A rim of vaginal epithelium may be excised from around the fistula allowing repair by colpocleisis using a double or triple layer closure of the subcutaneous tissues.[63] A modification reported by Twombly and Marshall[64] involves the preservation of a flap of vaginal epithelium which is then used as the first layer closure of the defect. These techniques do produce some shortening of the vagina but are reported to produce little interference with sexual activity.[63,65] They are most suitable for the postmenopausal patient, particularly if there is a deep vagina and a vault fistula and can, in experienced hands, be applicable to a wide range of different fistulae.[66]

Postoperative care

It is important to provide a postoperative milieu that promotes satisfactory healing of the surgical repair. Careful review of urine bacteriology should be undertaken. The urinary tract should be drained continuously under low pressure. The synchronous use of both urethral and suprapubic drainage of adequate caliber (18 Fr) reduces the likelihood that blockage of a single catheter will result in overdistension and disruption of the surgical repair. Catheters should be left on free drainage for at least 10 days and the integrity of the repair confirmed at this juncture by the use of contrast studies; if there is any contrast leakage, the catheters should be left on drainage for a further week and radiologic re-evaluation repeated at that time.

Vaginal repair of the complex fistula

In some cases the local vaginal tissues are damaged to the extent that a simple layered closure of the vagina is felt to be potentially precarious; such a situation may result from tissue loss or fibrosis produced by infection, radiation or previous surgery. In this situation it is necessary to augment the operation by the interposition of a vascularized flap between the two layers of the repair, filling dead space and bringing in a much needed blood and lymphatic supply. Many of these fistulae can be repaired using a vaginal procedure.

A number of techniques have been described for the mobilization and deployment of adjacent soft tissue structures. These include the transposition of the medial fibers of the levator ani, the use of a gracilis muscle flap or a gracilis myocutaneous flap, and the use of a pedicle flap of vulval fat and bulbocavernosus muscle.[67–72] While the use of procedures utilizing the gracilis may be invaluable for the repair of extensive defects, the majority of cases can be satisfactorily resolved by the use of a Martius flap[72] and hence this procedure will be described in detail here.

A vertical incision is made in either labium majus allowing a posteriorly based pedicled vascularized flap of labial tissue to be raised. The size of the flap is determined by the size of the fistula and can be increased by anterior extension of the incision into the mons. The flap is mobilized, taking care not to damage the blood supply from the inferior hemorrhoidal vessels which enter posteriorly. Next a tunnel is made beneath a vulval skin bridge to the site of fistula closure. The labial flap is secured in position as part of the final layer closure (Fig. 92.6).

A less common problem is that of a urethrovaginal fistula. The majority of patients with a distal urethrovaginal fistula are continent and asymptomatic provided that the bladder neck mechanism is competent.[73] Vaginal repair of such a fistula is easily carried out. An associated urethral mucosal defect can be replaced by a suitable flap of adjacent vaginal mucosa supported by a Martius flap. Alternatively, a modification of the Martius procedure can be used whereby the urethral repair is facilitated by a suitably positioned skin island left on the labial pedicle.[74] If the fistula is more proximal and a more extensive repair of urethra is likely to be necessary, or if it is associated with a vesicovaginal fistula, then a combined transvesical and abdominal approach is preferable.

Abdominal repair of urinary tract fistulae

Exposure

The patient is placed in the lithotomy position. A midline incision should always be used for the abdominal approach to a fistula repair because it is often necessary to extend this up to the xiphisternum to provide the necessary access for mobilization of the omentum. A more cosmetic result can be achieved, particularly in those patients who have recently undergone a gynecologic procedure via a Pfannenstiel incision, by reopening the transverse skin incision and making a vertical incision through the abdominal wall musculature. An additional upper midline incision may be necessary to aid omental mobilization (Fig. 92.7).

Dissection

A combined transperitoneal transvesical approach to a vesicovaginal fistula is to be preferred over the conventional anterior transvesical approach first described by

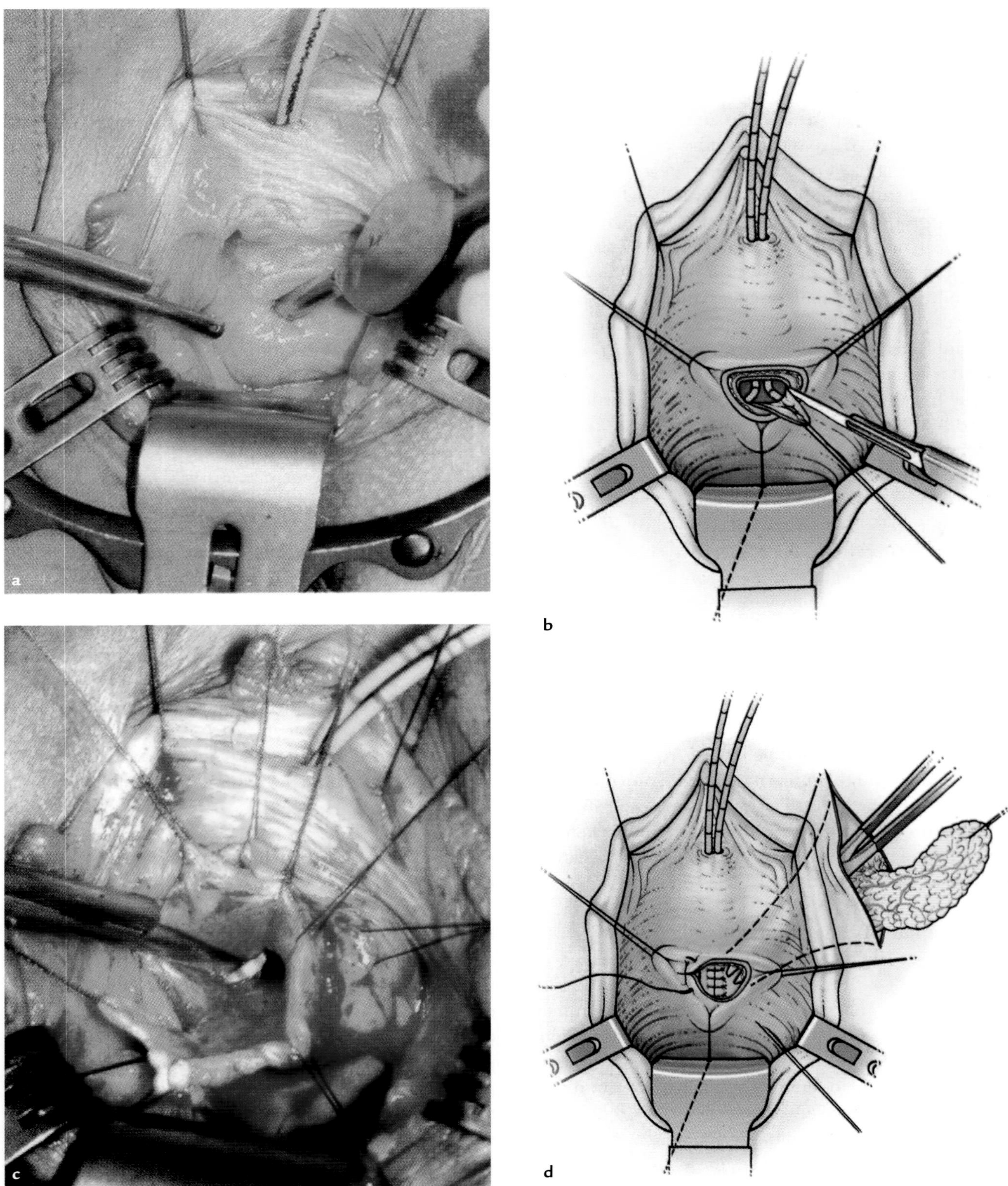

Figure 92.6. *(a) Sound through a vesicovaginal fistula. (b) Having catheterized the ureters, the fibrotic margins of the fistula are excised. (c) Operative view of Figure 92.6d showing the importance of stay sutures. (d) Having closed the fistula, the deployment of a Martius flap.*

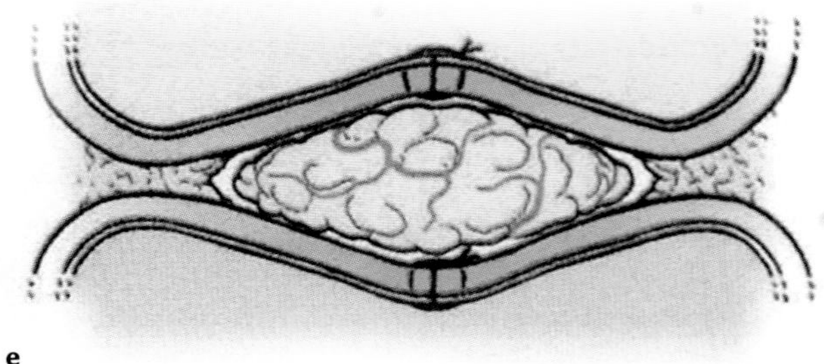

e

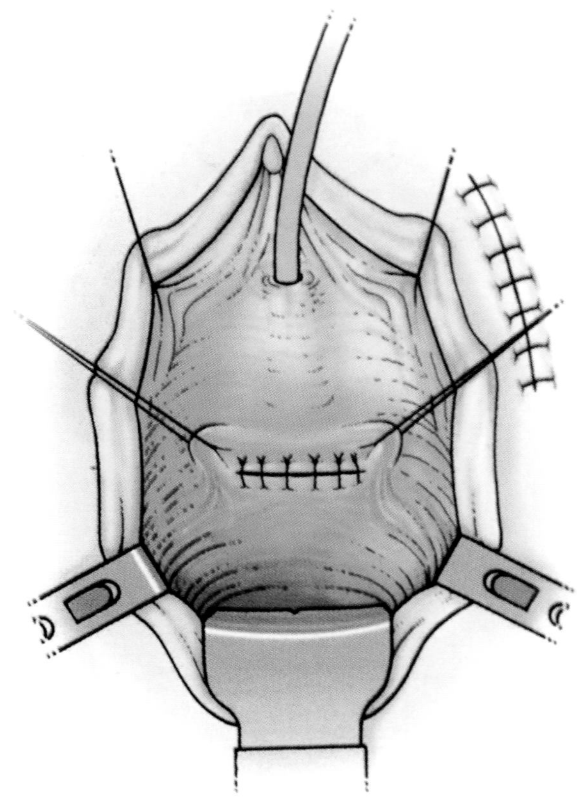

f

Figure 92.6. *(e) showing the importance of the deployed tissue as a sandwich between the two closure layers. (f) Final closure.*

Trendelenburg in 1890[75] and subsequently modified.[76] This allows good access to the area of the fistula and facilitates separation of the bladder from the vagina with the formation of an abdominoperineal tunnel and good extravesical exposure of the terminal ureters.[77] An initial incision is made in the vesicovaginal peritoneal fold and the posterior wall of the bladder opened in the midline down to the fistula.

Separation of the vaginal vault from the bladder is facilitated by an orientating finger placed within the vagina (Fig. 92.8a). A three fingerbreadths space is completed in the plane between bladder and vagina. It is important to create adequate space to allow the tension-free interposition of a suitable bulk of omentum. In difficult cases, in particular those where previous surgery has been attempted, the abdominal dissection can be combined with a subsequent vaginal dissection to produce an abdominoperineal tunnel, thereby allowing linear deployment of the omentum along the whole length of the vagina[77,78] (Fig. 92.8b–e).

Closure

The vagina is closed with an absorbable 3-0 suture.

The bladder is closed with a similar absorbable suture and adequate drainage ensured by the use of combined urethral and suprapubic drainage, the repair being wrapped in omentum. This surgical technique is applicable to a wide variety of fistulae and provides virtually guaranteed success.[79] At the end of the procedure a colposuspension may be carried out if necessary, to reposition the proximal urethra and bladder neck, optimizing the transmission of intra-abdominal pressure and thereby mitigating against the development of stress incontinence.[80]

The use of pedicled interposition flaps

The interposition of well-vascularized tissue, such as omentum as described above, brings in a good blood supply and fills dead space. While this acts as an added safeguard for a successful result in simple fistulae, it is essential to the closure of complex fistulae.

A number of techniques have been described in the literature. These include the use of peritoneal interposition, first described by Bardescu in 1900,[81,82] the use of island myocutaneous and fasciocutaneous flaps,[83,84] bladder mucosa,[85] and omentum, first reported by Walters in 1935[78] and popularized in the last three decades.[86,87] The omentum should be the tissue of first choice, as it is readily available and easy to mobilize, reaching down to the perineum in most cases. It has a good blood and lymphatic supply, and sufficient bulk to fill dead space without producing marked fibrosis during healing, which may compromise lower urinary tract function and render subsequent surgery more difficult. In contrast, peritoneum – while being readily available – does not possess these other properties and is commonly involved in local pathology or in the irradiated field. Bladder mucosal grafts can be used in a manner analogous to the techniques using vaginal epithelium, but carry the same potential disadvantages as suggested for peritoneum. Other flap procedures are an important part of the armamentarium but require particular expertise.

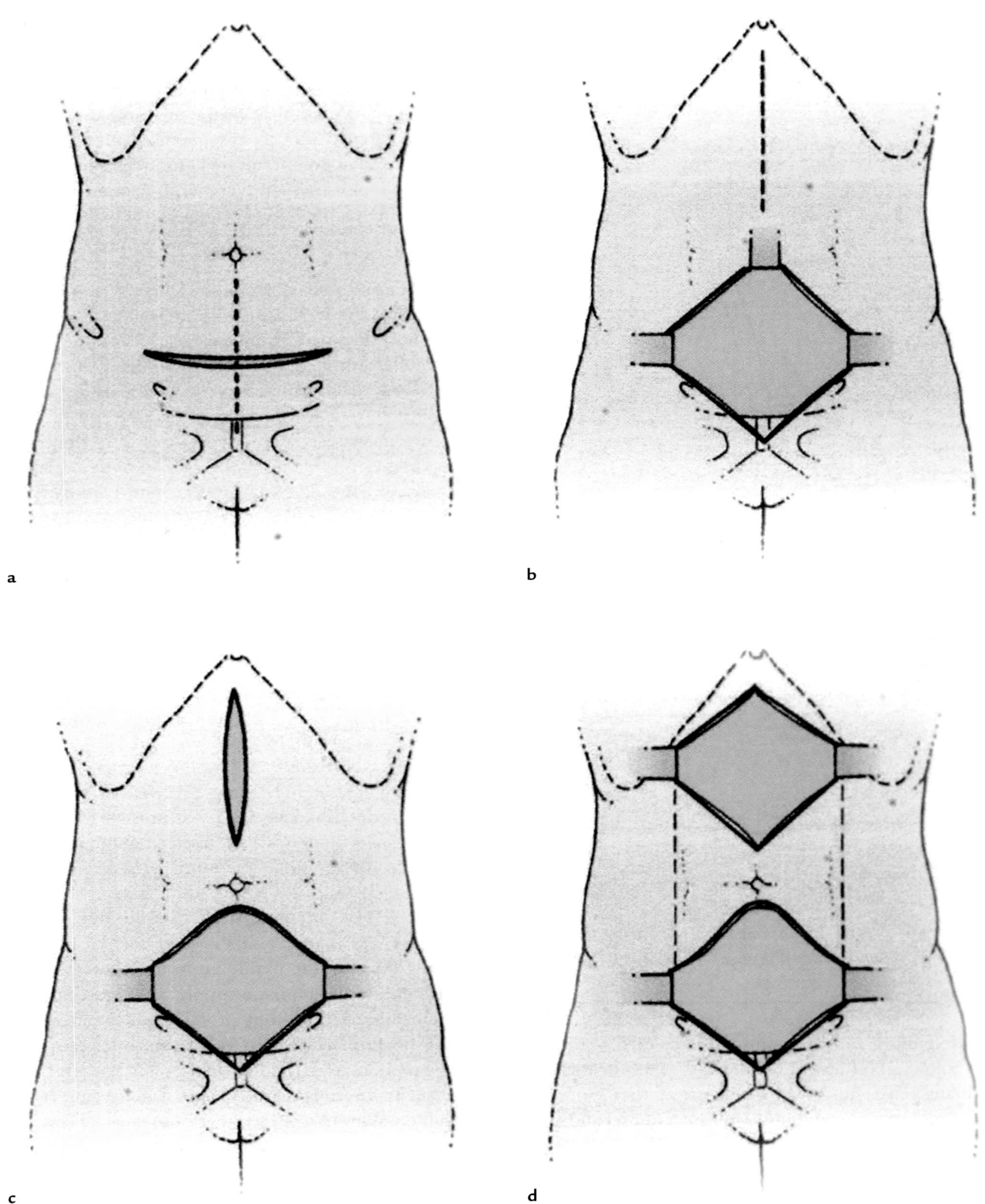

Figure 92.7. *(a) A midline incision via a Pfannenstiel skin incision. (b) Retractors in place allowing access to the abdomen as per a midline incision. (c, d) Occasionally, to allow full mobilization of the omentum, an upper midline incision may be necessary.*

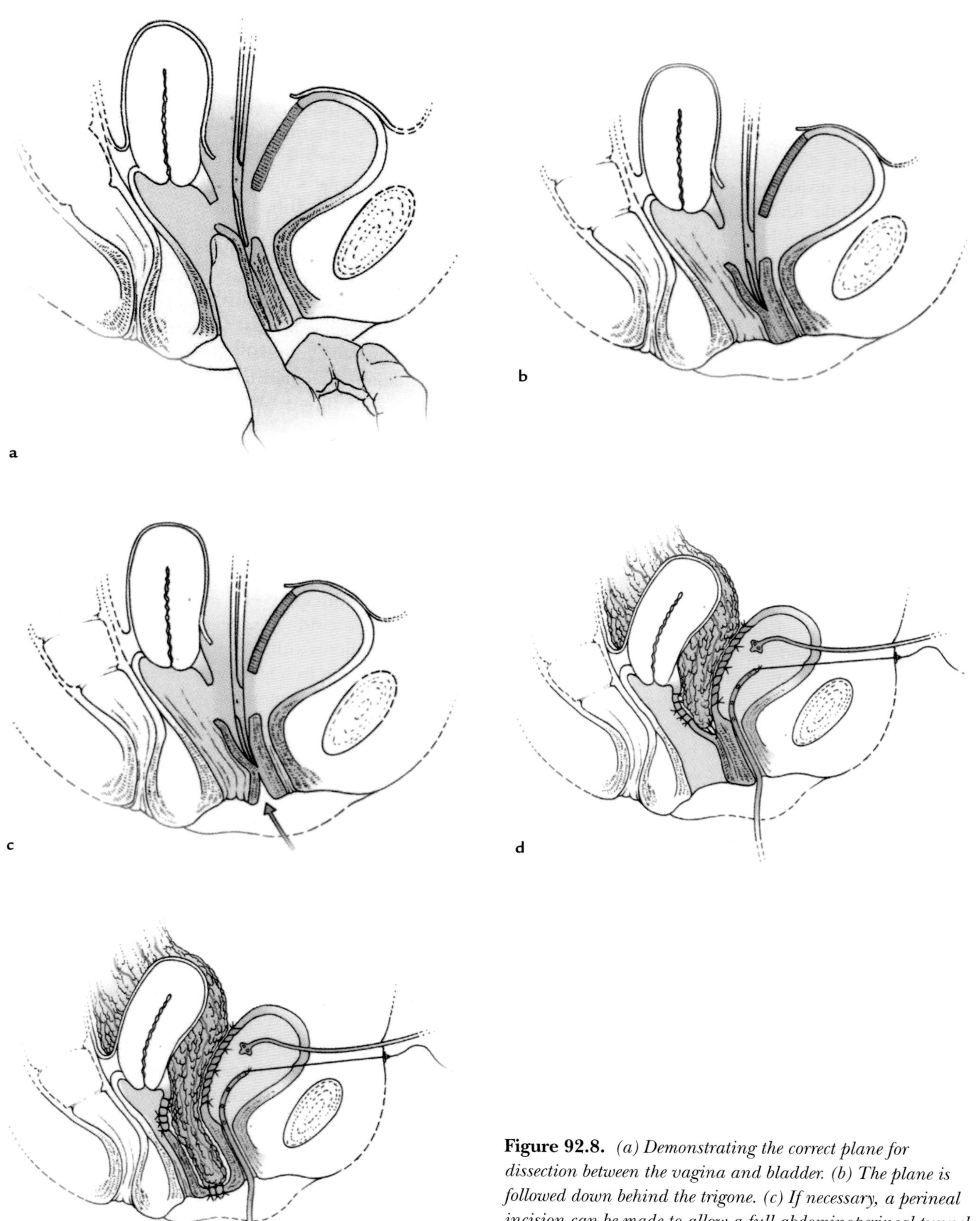

Figure 92.8. *(a) Demonstrating the correct plane for dissection between the vagina and bladder. (b) The plane is followed down behind the trigone. (c) If necessary, a perineal incision can be made to allow a full abdominoperineal tunnel to be developed. (d, e) Showing the fistula closed and omentum interposed.*

The omentum should always be separated from its attachment to the transverse colon and mesocolon since postoperative distension of the bowel may otherwise disrupt its relationship with the repair.

The lower margin of the omental apron will reach the perineum without additional mobilization in 30% of cases. In a further 30%, some degree of mobilization of the omentum by division of part of its vascular pedicle is necessary. While Kiricuta and Goldstein suggested that the omentum should be mobilized on the left gastroepiploic pedicle,[86] Turner-Warwick et al. raised the important technical point that the gastroepiploic arch becomes increasingly small towards its left extremity and suggested that the omental flap should be based on the right gastroepiploic pedicle for a more reliable blood supply.[87] In approximately 30% of cases, sufficient elongation is achieved by division of the left gastroepiploic pedicle and those of the direct left lateral vessels to the omentum. In the remaining cases, full mobilization of the omentum is required, based on the right gastroepiploic vessel as far as its gastroduodenal origin to prevent undue traction on individual short gastric vessels which might result in shearing and postoperative hemorrhage. Individual ligation of short gastric vessels is necessary using an absorbable suture. The resultant slender pedicle of this omental flap is protected by relocating it behind the mobilized descending colon. Mobilization of the omentum from the stomach does result in a mild ileus and it is therefore appropriate to institute gastric suction for a few days postoperatively. Insertion of a gastrostomy tube is a humane alternative to a nasogastric tube, particularly as the stomach is suitably exposed.

Repair of complex fistulae

In our experience, the repair of complex vesicovaginal fistulae is most satisfactorily tackled via the abdominoperineal approach with omental interposition as described above.[79] Certain additional points are, however, worthy of comment.

If radiotherapy is implicated in the etiology of the fistula, the wall of the bladder is usually rendered more rigid and inflexible than is normally the case. In this situation, an oblique incision in the bladder wall is often preferable to one in the midline as this facilitates subsequent bladder closure by the rotation of a broad-based bladder flap. In those patients with radiation-induced fibrosis and necrosis the surgical procedure must be considered to consist of two separate stages. It is first necessary to excise all macroscopically abnormal tissue. If residual malignancy is suspected, this can be confirmed by frozen section. The presence of malignancy per se, unless extensive, should not preclude a reconstructive procedure, but will clearly lead to more radical excision. The second stage of this operation involves a functional restoration of the integrity of the rectum, bladder, and vagina as far as this is feasible, filling the dead space within the inevitably ischemic pelvis with omentum and/or a cecolovaginoplasty.[80]

If there is an extensive defect then it may not be possible to obtain satisfactory apposition of the edges of the bladder wall without compromising its functional capacity. Closure of the bladder defect can be carried out with the additional use of an augmentation cystoplasty. Alternatively, the bladder defect can be left and the omentum used to patch it; animal studies have demonstrated that such a defect is covered within 2–3 weeks by new transitional epithelium, with the subsequent formation of a new smooth muscle layer within the omentoplasty, in continuity with the detrusor muscle at the margins of the defect.[88,89] Clinical experience over the last 25 years has confirmed the efficacy of this technique in the clinical setting.[87,90,91]

SURGERY FOR DETRUSOR OVERACTIVITY

Detrusor overactivity can result in considerable morbidity in patients with idiopathic detrusor overactivity (DO) and also those with neurogenic detrusor overactivity (NDO). In patients with DO, marked bladder overactivity leads to disabling frequency and incontinence, whereas in NDO, renal impairment may result from voiding dysfunction and back pressure on the upper tracts in association with high pressure phasic detrusor contractions and detrusor sphincter dyssynergia. In both conditions the cornerstone of the pharmacotherapy is still anticholinergic agents, often combined with bladder retraining. In the context of neurogenic bladder dysfunction, the clinical picture is complicated by an admixture of other functional problems associated with the bladder overactivity including uncoordinated detrusor contraction and varying degrees of bladder outflow obstruction.

The aim of surgical therapy directed at the detrusor in both these conditions is to increase functional bladder capacity and decrease the amplitude of detrusor contractions, thereby preventing incontinence and protecting the upper tracts in patients with NDO.

In recent years the mainstay of contemporary therapy for bladder overactivity has been augmentation cystoplasty, most usually using the 'clam' technique.[92] Two further options have been recently explored: bladder autoaugmentation[93] and sacral neuromodulation.[94]

While a number of surgical techniques for the treatment of detrusor overactivity have been described, it is now widely accepted that procedures such as detrusor transection and transtrigonal phenol injection produce unpredictable and temporary improvement with potentially serious side effects. Their routine use can therefore no longer be supported. More recently, botulinum toxin injection therapy into the bladder has become more popular and is being increasingly used. Definitive comments as to its efficacy will, however, await the results of adequately conducted long-term studies.[95]

Augmentation cystoplasty

The principle underlying augmentation cystoplasty is that by bivalving a functionally overactive bladder and introducing a segment of detubularized intestine a low pressure bladder with an increased functional capacity will result.

The two commonly used intestinal segments are ileum and sigmoid colon. The sigmoid is usually used in patients where a short small bowel mesentery renders the use of ileum difficult. Ileum is preferred as it produces lower reservoir pressures and better compliance. The original technique described for clam cystoplasty is still widely used but modifications to this include opening the bladder in the sagittal plane which appears to be equally effective, or opening the bladder as a 'star'.[96] This specific modification can be particularly useful in patients with NDO where the bladder is small and thick walled. An alternative surgical technique popularized by McGuire is his modification of the hemi-Koch procedure. This utilizes a transverse 'smile' incision (looking posteriorly) which is fashioned 3 cm above the ureteral orifices, creating an anteriorly based detrusor flap.[97] Most workers find coronal or sagittal bivalving of the bladder to be effective and acceptable, provided that adequate opening of the bladder is performed right down to the ureteral orifices, both to adequately open the bladder and to prevent 'diverticulation' of the cystoplasty segment.

A number of studies attest to the efficacy of augmentation cystoplasty in children, adolescents, and adults with DO and NDO:[98–103]

- Mundy and Stephenson reported a series of 40 cases in whom 90% were cured at a mean follow-up of 1 year.[98] Mean functional bladder capacity was increased from 280 to 440 ml, reduced compliance was improved in 70% of patients, and detrusor overactivity abolished in 50%, the remainder having low pressure detrusor overactivity.
- In a series of 26 adolescents undergoing enterocystoplasty, of whom 19 had a 'clam' cystoplasty, results were satisfactory in all three males but poor in five out of the 16 females. In three patients, difficulty was experienced with intermittent self-catheterization.[99]
- In a series of 39 children with spina bifida, bladder capacity at safe storage pressures of less than 29 cm of saline was achieved in all patients with a reduction in upper tract distension in 91.7% of kidneys.[100] A satisfactory result was achieved in all but one patient.
- Singh and Thomas reviewed 67 patients who underwent augmentation cystoplasty.[101] Of these, 47 had an ileal segment and 20 a sigmoid segment. These data are presented in combination with a further 11 patients who had an ileocecal cystoplasty. Fifty-two patients had an artificial sphincter, nine had a colposuspension and one had both. Acceptable continence was achieved in 93.6% of patients.
- Hasan et al. reported on 48 patients who underwent augmentation cystoplasty for DO (n=35) or NDO (n=13).[102] Mean follow-up was 38 months, with 83% achieving a good outcome, 15% a moderate outcome, and 2% an unsatisfactory result.
- Flood et al. reported on 122 augmentation cystoplasties.[103] It must, however, be borne in mind that the 'McGuire' technique used was different from the standard clam procedure reported for all the other series described above, and this was a very mixed group of patients: 67% had an ileal augmentation, 30% a detubularized cecocystoplasty, and 3% sigmoid. In 19 patients this procedure was related to undiversion and 17% had interstitial cystitis, 7% radiation cystitis, 13% miscellaneous conditions and the remainder were either NDO or DO. Mean follow-up was 37 months. Bladder capacity was increased from a preoperative mean of 108 ml to 438 ml and, of 106 successful patients, 75% had an excellent result, 20% were improved and 5% had major, persistent problems.

The above literature would support augmentation cystoplasty as being an effective therapy with a low operative morbidity and satisfactory long-term results, although most of the reported series have a follow-up of less than 5 years. It must be remembered that this is major surgery and despite adequate preoperative counseling, many patients take some months to adapt to their new bladder and to learn to void effectively by abdominal straining. It is important to monitor postoperative residual urine volumes. Intermittent self-catheterization (ISC) is necessary for a number of these patients, particularly those with NDO. Interestingly, the reported incidence of ISC varies from 15% up to 85% of cases.[98] It is evident that a number of factors contribute to the need for ISC. These include the level of residual deemed acceptable by the supervising urologist and the concomitant use of procedures directed at the bladder outflow – either urethral dilation (rebalancing) or treatments for stress incontinence. A particular debate centers on the treatment of coexisting stress incontinence at the time of clam cystoplasty; contemporary opinion remains divided on this matter since measures designed to treat stress incontinence will generally increase the need for ISC.

Other problems encountered with augmentation cystoplasty include persistent mucus production, recurrent or persistent urinary tract infections, and metabolic disorders which are usually mild and subclinical. Provided that patients are counseled preoperatively, this is rarely a problem. Persistent urinary infection can be troublesome, particularly in female patients, and has been reported in up to 30% of cases, often requiring long-term antibiotic therapy. Long-term bowel dysfunction occurs in up to a third of patients and is thought to be related to the interruption of the normal enterohepatic circulation.[101,102,104] Bladder perforations have been reported in up to 10% of patients.[100] At present, lifelong follow-up of these patients is recommended, not only because of the above complications, but also in view of the suggestion that augmentation cystoplasty predisposes to the subsequent development of malignancy.[105] However, there remains no convincing evidence to support an association with tumor in the absence of other predisposing factors such as previous tuberculosis or chronic urinary stasis such as that associated with paraplegia.

Augmentation cystoplasty is an effective management option in contemporary practice in patients with intractable DO or NDO resistant to conventional therapy. In addition, cystoplasty can be used as part of an undiversion procedure. Although a proportion of patients are not significantly improved by this procedure, one series found a 'good to moderate' outcome in only 58% of patients with DO.[102] It must be borne in mind that up to 30% of patients experience increased frequency and looseness of bowel motions and a tendency to incontinent episodes, with a significant number of patients requiring long-term ISC. With these observations in mind, alternative therapies have been explored, in particular bladder autoaugmentation.[93]

Bladder autoaugmentation

In 1989, Snow and Cartwright initially reported a technique which they named bladder autoaugmentation.[106] This procedure involves the excision of the detrusor muscle over the entire dome of the bladder, leaving the underlying bladder urothelium intact. A large epithelial 'bulge' is created which functions by augmenting the storage capacity of the bladder and this is referred to as autoaugmentation.

Following initial studies in six dogs, this technique was extended to seven patients aged 4–17 years, all of whom had poorly compliant bladders documented on pressure flow urodynamics. Following excision of the dome detrusor muscle, the lateral margins of the detrusor were fixed bilaterally to the psoas muscles. Patient follow-up was short. A subsequent report by these workers after studying a total of 19 patients concluded that, with a follow-up of between 3 months and 4 years, 80% of patients were continent and another 10% were significantly improved. A significant increase in bladder capacity of greater than 50 cc occurred in only 40% of patients, with minimal change in 35%; 25% actually had a decrease in capacity. The procedure was, however, accompanied by improved continence and reduced rates of hydronephrosis.[106]

In 12 pediatric patients with low capacity bladders and demonstrable detrusor overactivity (aged 4–14 years, 10 with NDO), 6 months following autoaugmentation the mean increase in bladder capacity was 40% with a 33% decrease in mean leak point pressure.[107] Postoperative complications were minor. A modification of the previous technique was used whereby a vesicomyotomy was used rather than vesicomyectomy with no fixation of the bladder laterally to the psoas muscles. A subsequent preliminary report in five adult patients, with the follow-up ranging from 12 to 82 weeks, reported an increase in bladder capacity which varied from 40% up to 310%; this was measured at an intravesical pressure of 40 cmH_2O.

Stohrer et al. reported a series of 29 patients aged 14–64 years with an average age of 35 years. Of these patients, 24 were felt likely to have NDO.[108,109] All patients underwent preoperative urodynamic evaluation. The technique reported by these authors is based on the original one described by Snow and Cartwright with an extraperitoneal approach filling the bladder to 200–250 ml. A 7–8 cm diameter section of the detrusor around the urachus is dissected completely and removed leaving the mucosa intact. The detrusor is not fixed to the psoas muscle and all bands of detrusor overlying the urothelium are removed. The authors now have follow-up to 7 years and while they find that 50% of patients can void without significant residuals, up to half require ISC. They found an improved compliance and increasing capacity of 130–600 ml.

An alternative surgical approach which has been explored in case reports is laparoscopic-assisted autoaugmentation but comment on this cannot be made in the absence of adequate numbers of patients and no significant follow-up.[110] It is recognized that spontaneous perforation of an augmentation cystoplasty bladder is a potential risk, occurring in up to 10% of cases. This may be due to high intravesical pressure[111] and can usually be managed successfully by conservative measures.[112] Patients may be at even greater risk of perforation following autoaugmentation because of the thinness of the mucosa in the bulging 'diverticulum' produced by the operation. Evidence in support of this is provided by animal studies where autoaugmentation resulted in higher risk of perforation at lower pressures than augmentation cystoplasty.[113] To date this complication has yet to be reported in clinical series, possibly because of ingrowth of fibrous tissue around the mucosal diverticulum with time, which may also account for the limited increase in capacity seen following the procedure. This phenomenon, if progressive, may limit the durability of this operation.

At present, while autoaugmentation has a number of attractive features, it is clear that the resultant increase in bladder capacity and reduction in detrusor overactivity are far less pronounced than following augmentation cystoplasty. The number of cases reported in the literature is small with relatively short follow-up. It is questionable whether the associated benefits adequately compensate for the limited long-term efficacy of the procedure. The search for less invasive techniques therefore continues.

URINARY DIVERSION

Urinary diversion may be either temporary or permanent. All surface diversions are simple surgical endeavors to correct the urinary waste disposal problems of patients who are unfortunate enough to have either lost, or never to have actually achieved, normal bladder function.

While clearly 'diversion is diversion' and 'cystoplasty is cystoplasty' the development of so-called 'continent diversion' has confused this distinction – the surgical principles and the procedures that are used to create the urinary reservoir of this diversion are identical to those for a total cystoplasty. Because the only difference between these is the mechanism of their emptying, we would suggest a more rational terminological distinction, i.e. 'stoma-cystoplasty' and 'sphincter-cystoplasty'.

The two key components of the creation, or recreation, of a naturally functioning bladder are bladder-base sensation and a sufficiency of functional sphincter muscle. These are irreplaceable but, all too often, one or both are sacrificed at the time of a urinary diversion.

Even a small area of urothelium that has normal sensation can make all the difference when it is available for inclusion in a functional reconstruction because the sensation of bladder fullness avoids the need to time its emptying. Similarly, the remnants of an incompetent sphincter mechanism can sometimes be made to function satisfactorily. Thus it is important to preserve every bit of the functional tissue that might be important to a future reconstruction – even if one cannot envisage either the possibility of an undiversion or that it could subserve a useful purpose. The opportunity of restoration of sphincteric function 'today' has often been denied by the excisions of 'yesterday'.

Similar considerations apply to rectal sensation and the sphincteric control of defecation. An anal mechanism, or even its apparently useless remnants, should never be excised needlessly – many patients have lost their chance of anorectal continence as a result of an unnecessarily extensive routine abdominoperineal resection.

The options for urinary tract diversion and reconstruction

A consideration of the range of procedure options available for urinary diversion, some of which are no longer advocated, summarizes the practical experience upon which the evolution of current preferences are based. These options can be conveniently considered in four distinct categories.

1. *Free-draining surface diversion of the upper urinary tract*: This naturally requires the collection of continuously draining urine. The need for this may be temporary; however, it may be permanent if the surgical retrieval of the reservoir function of the lower urinary tract is not possible.
2. *Incontinence surface diversion of the lower tract*: This is often required for the management of voiding difficulties; when these are irremediable this may be a long-term arrangement. An indwelling urethral catheter may be either drained continuously into a bag or intermittently released. Intermittent emptying of the natural bladder reservoir can also be achieved by intermittent catheterization of the urethra or a leak-proof suprapubic conduit (Fig. 92.9).
3. *'Cystoplastic reconstruction' of a urinary reservoir that is emptied either by sphincter control or by stomal catheterization*: A total substitution cystoplasty may be appropriate when the whole bladder has to be removed; however, many bladder abnormalities

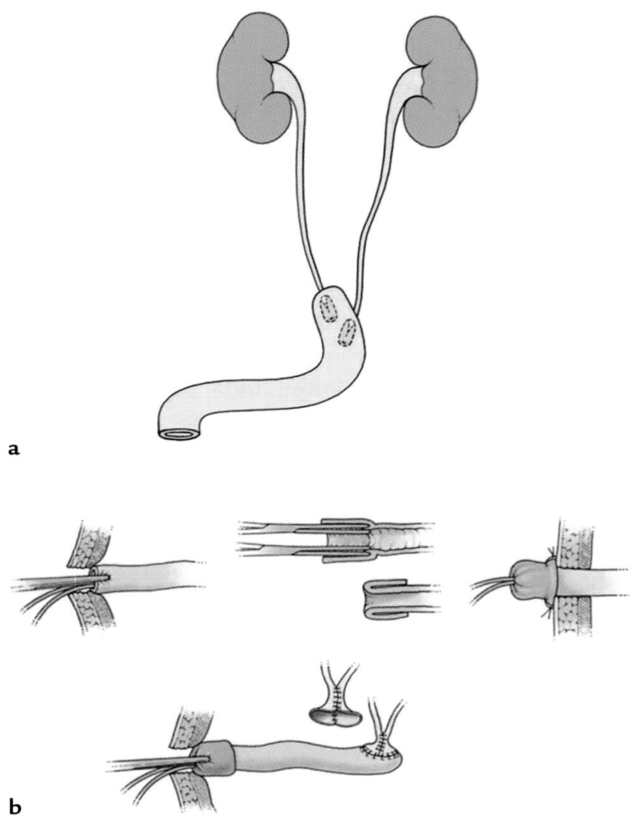

Figure 92.9. *(a) An ileal conduit. (b) Formation of the ileal conduit.*

require only a readjustment or a partial cystoplastic substitution. A reconstructed cystoplastic reservoir, partial or total, may be controlled by the sphincter mechanism – *'sphincter-cystoplasty'* – or it may be emptied by intermittent catheterization of a leak-proof conduit – *'stoma-cystoplasty'* (Fig. 92.10)

4. *Internal urinary diversion controlled by the anal sphincter – ureterosigmoidoscopy*: For some patients a rectosigmoid urinary diversion is a preferable alternative to surface diversion when the circumstances are appropriate. For nephrologic and carcinogenic reasons this procedure fell into disrepute for a number of years but procedural developments have addressed some of the potential problems: these include the limitation of renal damage and the early detection of malignant change (Fig. 92.11).

When satisfactory sphincteric control of a cystoplasty is irretrievable, many alternative procedures such as catheterizable stoma cystoplasty reservoirs enable patients to achieve a reasonably acceptable quality of urologic life.

'Cystoplasty', 'stoma-cystoplasty' and 'sphincter-cystoplasty' – a perspective of urinary reservoirs that are emptied intermittently

The surgical procedures of 'cystoplasty' and of 'continent diversion' have evolved as a result of the great endeavors and contributions of numerous colleagues over the years — whole textbooks have been written about them. However, the value of the terminological distinction between 'cystoplasty' and 'continent diversion' is questionable because the functional requirements and the surgical principles of creating their reservoirs are essentially similar.

'Cystoplasty' is a generic term for a reconstructive procedure (plasty) to recreate the functional capacity of a bladder reservoir (cysto). Like the term 'urodynamics', 'cystoplasty' is commonly used, understood, and misunderstood to mean different things. This adds additional confusion to the already complex field of the retrieval and the construction of functional urinary reservoirs.

Some 'simple' cystoplasty operations restore the natural functional reservoir capacity of the bladder without involving any substitution procedure and not all substitution procedures involve the use of bowel. However, the term 'cystoplasty' is commonly used somewhat loosely, as a 'semi-specific shorthand' to denote the substitution of the bladder reservoir, partial or total, generally with the tacit assumption that bowel is used for the substitution and also that the functional control of the outlet is the natural urethral sphincter mechanism.

Developments in the surgical retrieval of the natural bodily function of 'intermittent urinary waste disposal' often involve the creation of catheterizable leak-proof abdominal stoma conduits that are used for the intermittent emptying, either of normal bladders when the urethra is irremediably dysfunctional, or of substitution urinary reservoirs that are either partially or totally reconstructed. Thus an integrated reconsideration of the practical principles of cystoplasty and diversion seems appropriate, together with an integrated reconsideration of terminology.

In this section, we use simple descriptive terminological exactitudes.

A *urethra-cystoplasty* is a reconstructed urinary reservoir, the outlet of which is the urethra. When this is controlled by the sphincter it is a *sphincter-cystoplasty*; if it is emptied by self-catheterization it is a simple *urethra-cystoplasty*. The reservoir of a sphincter-cystoplasty may be either a partial or a total substitution of the bladder. If bowel is used for the substitution it can be optionally identified as an 'ileal sphincter-cystoplasty' or a 'colonic sphincter-cystoplasty' – as opposed to an 'omental ure-

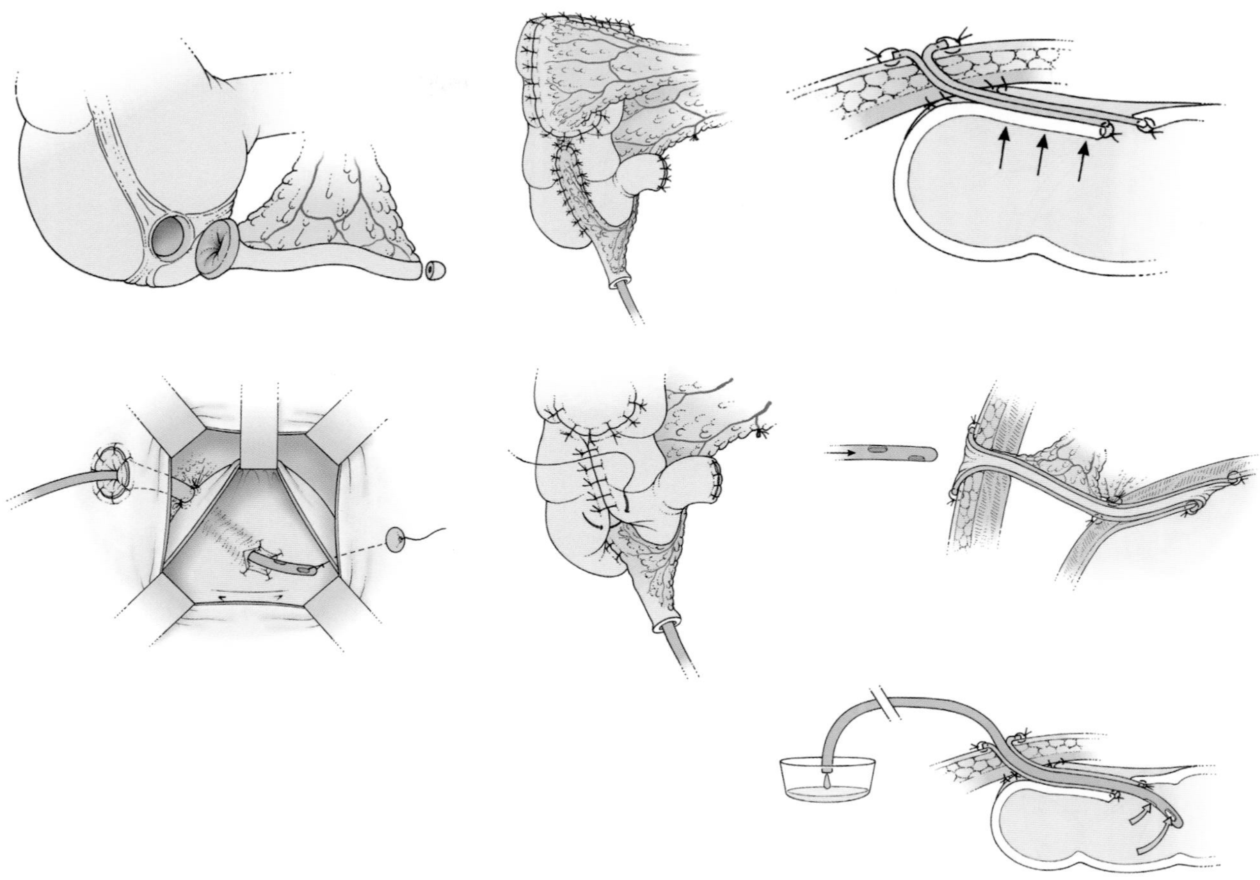

Figure 92.10. *Formation of a pouch with a catheterizable stoma.*

thra-cystoplasty'. A urethro-cystoplasty is a different entity because it denotes reconstruction of both the bladder *and* the urethra.

A *stoma-cystoplasty* is a urinary reservoir with an abdominal stoma-conduit outlet. Its 'continence' is usually maintained by a valved leak-proof conduit that can be catheterized intermittently. The reservoir may be the native bladder – a partial substitution in situ – or a total substitution that is either in situ or ex situ. Alternatively, a stoma-cystoplasty can be less precisely described as a 'continent diversion'.

The functional characteristics and the principles involved in the construction of the bowel substitution urinary reservoirs of both a stoma-cystoplasty and a sphincter-cystoplasty are essentially similar, the difference is simply the mechanism of their evacuation.

A leak-proof stoma conduit is a mechanistic construction specifically designed for emptying the reservoir by catheterization. The reliable sphincteric control of a sphincter-cystoplasty is often dependent upon a careful urodynamic assessment and appropriate surgical adjustment and management: this requires quite separate consideration.

Whether or not this terminology will be generally adopted, time will tell; it seems preferable to the ill-defined 'continent diversion'. A particular advantage is that it facilitates an independent analytical consideration of the three separate component procedure principles of cystoplastic reconstruction:

1. The creation of a urinary reservoir that has low pressure and reflux-proof ureteric implantations – these requirements are common to the reservoirs of both a sphinctercystoplasty and a stoma-cystoplasty.
2. The intricate mechanistic construction of a valved leak-proof stoma conduit that is required for the evacuation of the reservoir of a stoma-cystoplasty by self-catheterization.
3. A functionally orientated urodynamically controlled adjustment is often required to ensure the voiding efficiency and sphincteric control of a sphincter-cystoplasty.

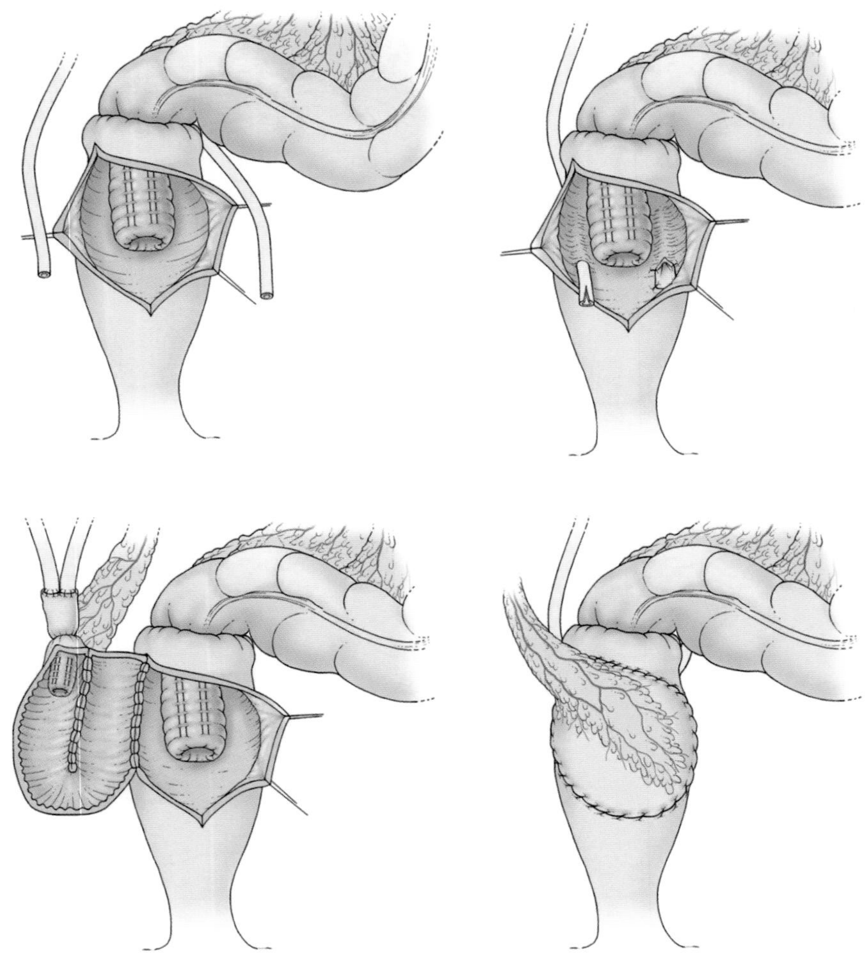

Figure 92.11. *Formation of a ureterosigmoid pouch of the Mainz 2 type.*

REFERENCES

1. Daly JW, Higgins KA. Injury to the ureter during gynaecological surgical procedures. Surg Gynaecol Obstet 1988;167:19–22.
2. Goodna JA, Powers TW, Harris VD. Ureteral injury in gynecology surgery. A ten year review in a community hospital. Am J Obstet Gynecol 1995;172(6):1817–20.
3. Amirikia H, Evans TN. Ten year review of hysterectomies trends, indications, risks. Am J Obstet Gynecol 1979;134:431–4.
4. Newell QU. Injury to the ureters during pelvic operations. Ann Surg 1939;109:981–6.
5. Benson RC, Hinman F. Urinary tract injuries in obstetrics and gynaecology. Am J Obstet Gynecol 1956;70:467–85.
6. St Martin EC, Trichel BE, Campbell JH, Locke CH. Ureteral injuries in gynaecologic surgery. J Urol 1953;70:51–7.
7. Solomons E, Levin EJ, Bauman J, Baron J. A pyelographic study of ureteric injuries sustained during hysterectomy for benign conditions. Surg Gynaecol Obstet 1960;111:41–8.
8. Gangai MP, Agee RE, Spence CR. Surgical injury to ureter. Urology 1976;8(1):22–7.
9. Mattsson T. Frequency and management of urological and some other complications following radical surgery for carcinoma of the cervix uteri, stages I and II. Acta Obstet Gynecol Scand 1975;54:271–80.
10. Underwood PB, Wilson WC, Kreutner A, Miller MC, Murphy E. Radical hysterectomy: a critical review of twenty-two years' experience. Am J Obstet Gynecol 1979;134(8):889–98.
11. Thompson JD. Operative injuries to the ureter: prevention, recognition and management. In: Telinde's Operative Gynecology, 7th ed. Philadelphia: JB Lippincott, 1992; 749–83.
12. Lezin MA, Stoller ML. Surgical ureteral injuries. Urology 1991;38(6):497–506.
13. Spence HM, Boone T. Surgical injuries to the ureter. JAMA 1961;176:1070.

14. Trigaux JP, Decoene B, Van Beers B. Focal necrosis of the ureter following CT-guided chemical sympathectomy. Cardiovasc Intervent Radiol 1992;15(3):180–2.

15. Meyer NL, Lipscomb GH, Ling FW. Ureteral injury during elective pregnancy termination. A case report. J Reproduct Med 1994;39(9):743–6.

16. Altin MA, Gundogdu ZH. Ureteral injury due to Kirschner wire in a five-year-old girl. A case report. Turkish J Pediatr 1994;36(1):77–9.

17. Assimos DG, Patterson LC, Taylor CL. Changing incidence and etiology of iatrogenic ureteral injuries. J Urol 1994;152:2240–6.

18. Selzman AA, Spirnak JP. Iatrogenic ureteral injuries: a 20 year experience in treating 165 injuries. J Urol 1996;155:878–81.

19. Brandes SB, Chelsky MJ, Buckman RF, Hanno PM. Ureteral injuries from penetrating trauma. J Trauma 1994;36(6):766–9.

20. Presti JC, Carroll PR, McAninch JW. Ureteral and renal pelvic injuries from external trauma: diagnosis and treatment. J Trauma 1989;29:370–4.

21. Campbell EW, Filderman PS, Jacobs SC. Ureteral injury due to blunt and penetrating trauma. Urology 1992;40:216–20.

22. Brady LW. Ureteral injury as a consequence of radiation treatment. In: Bergman H (ed) The Ureter. New York: Springer-Verlag, 1981.

23. Witters S, Cornelissen M, Vereecken R. Iatrogenic ureteral injury: aggressive or conservative treatment. Am J Obstet Gynecol 1986;155:582–4.

24. Dowling RA, Corriere JN, Sandler CM. Iatrogenic ureteral injury. J Urol 1986;135:912–5.

25. Hoch WH, Kursh ED, Persky L. Early, aggressive management of intraoperative ureteral injuries. J Urol 1975;114:530–2.

26. Badenoch DF, Tiptaft RC, Fowler CG, Blandy JP. Early repair of accidental injury to the ureter or bladder following gynaecological surgery. Br J Urol 1987;59:516–8.

27. Higgins CC. Ureteral injuries. JAMA 1967;199(2):82–8.

28. Walker JA. Injuries of the ureter due to external violence. J Urol 1969;102:410–3.

29. Bright TC 3rd, Peters PC. Ureteral injuries due to external violence: 10 years experience with 59 cases. J Trauma 1977;17:616–20.

30. Flynn JT, Tiptaft RC, Woodhouse CRJ, Paris AMI, Blandy JP. The early and aggressive repair of iatrogenic ureteric injuries. Br J Urol 1979;51:454–7.

31. Zinman LM, Libertino JA, Roth RA. Management of operative ureteral injury. Urology 1978;12(3):290–303.

32. Larson DM, Malone JM Jr, Copeland LJ et al. Ureteral assessment after radical hysterectomy. Obstet Gynecol 1987;69:612–6.

33. Piscitelli JT, Simel DL, Addison WA. Who should have intravenous pyelograms before hysterectomy for benign disease? Obstet Gynecol 1987;69:541–5.

34. Guerriero WG. Ureteral injury. Urol Clin North Am 1989;16(2):237–48.

35. Weinberg JJ, Ansong K, Smith AD. Complications of ureteroscopy in relation to experience: Report of survey and author experience. J Urol 1987;137:384–5.

36. Fry DE, Milholen L, Harbrecht PJ. Iatrogenic ureteral injury. Arch Surg 1983;118:454–7.

37. Cormio L, Battaglia M, Traficante A, Selvaggi FP. Endourological treatment of ureteric injuries. Br J Urol 1993;72:165–8.

38. Lask D, Abarbanel J, Luttwak Z, Manes A, Mukamel E. Changing trends in the management of iatrogenic ureteral injuries. J Urol 1995;154:1693–5.

39. Belande G. Early treatment of ureteral injuries found after gynaecological surgery. J Urol 1977;118(1):25–7.

40. Blandy JP, Badenoch DF, Fowler CG, Jenkins BJ, Thomas NWM. Early repair of iatrogenic injury to the ureter or bladder after gynaecological surgery. J Urol 1991;146:761–5.

41. Turner-Warwick RT, Worth PHL. The psoas bladder-hitch procedure for the replacement of the lower third of the ureter. Br J Urol 1969;41:701–9.

42. Spies JW, Johnson CE, Wilson CS. Reconstruction of the ureter by means of bladder flaps. Proc Soc Exp Biol Med 1933;30:425.

43. Ockerblad NF. Reimplantation of the ureter into the bladder by a flap method. J Urol 1947;57:845.

44. Benson MC, Ring KS, Olsson CA. Ureteral reconstruction and bypass: experience with ileal interposition, Boari flap-psoas hitch and autotransplantation. J Urol 1990;143:20–3.

45. Hodges CV, Barry JM, Fuchs EF, Pearse HD, Tank ES. Transureteroureterostomy: 25 year experience with 100 patients. J Urol 1980;123:834–8.

46. Hendren WH, Hensle TW. Transureteroureterostomy: experience with 75 cases. J Urol 1980;123:826–33.

47. Bodie B, Novick AC, Rose M, Straffon RA. Long-term results with renal autotransplantation for ureteral replacement. J Urol 1986;136:1187–9.

48. Thorne ID, Resnick MI. The use of bowel in urologic surgery: a historical perspective. Urol Clin North Am 1986;13:179–91.

49. Boxer RJ, Fritzsche P, Skinner DG et al. Replacement of the ureter by small intestine: clinical application and results of the ileal ureter in 89 patients. J Urol 1979;121:728–31.

50. Mesrobian HG, Azizkhan RG. Pyeloureterostomy with appendiceal interposition. J Urol 1989;142:1288–9.

51. Sims JM. On the treatment of vesicovaginal fistula. Am J Med Sci 1852;23:59–83.

52. Marshall VF. Vesicovaginal fistulas on one urological service. J Urol 1979;121:25–9.

53. Collins CG, Pent D, Jones FB. Results of early repair of vesicovaginal fistula with preliminary cortisone treatment. Am J Obstet Gynecol 1960;80:1005–12.

54. Lawson J. The management of genitourinary fistulae. Clin Obstet Gynecol North Am 1978;5:209–36.

55. O'Conor VJ. Review of experience with vesicovaginal fistula repair. Trans Am Assoc Genitourin Surg 1979;71:120–2.

56. Jonas U, Petri E. Genitourinary fistulae. In: Stanton SL (ed) Clinical Gynaecologic Urology. St Louis: Mosby, 1984.

57. Turner-Warwick RT. Repair of urinary vaginal fistulae. In: Rob C, Smith R (eds) Operative Surgery, 3rd ed. London: Butterworths, 1977; 206–18.

58. Persky L, Herman G, Guerrier K. Non-delay in vesicovaginal fistula repair. Urology 1979;13:273–5.

59. Badenoch DF, Tiptaft RC, Thakar DR, Fowler CG, Blandy JP. Early repair of accidental injury to the ureter or bladder following gynaecological surgery. Br J Urol 1987;59:516–8.

60. Cruikshank SH. Early closure of posthysterectomy vesicovaginal fistulas. South Med J 1988;81:1525–8.

61. Roen PR. Combined vaginal and transvesical approach in successful repair of vesicovaginal fistula. Arch Surg 1960;80:628–33.

62. Weyrauch HW, Rous SN. Transvesical–transvaginal approach for surgical repair of vesicovaginal fistulae. Surg Gynecol Obstet 1966;123:121–5.

63. Latzko W. Post-operative vesicovaginal fistulas. Am J Surg 1942;58:211–28.

64. Twombly GH, Marshall VF. Repair of vesico-vaginal fistula caused by radiation. Surg Gynec Obstet 1946;83:348.

65. Rader ES. Post-hysterectomy vesicovaginal fistula: treatment by partial colpocleisis. J Urol 1975;112:811–2.

66. Blaikley JB. Colpocleisis for difficult vaginal fistulae of bladder and rectum. Proc R Soc Med 1965;58:581–6.

67. Douglass M. Operative treatment of urinary incontinence. Am J Obstet Gynecol 1936;31:268–79.

68. Garlock JH. The cure of an intractable vesico-vaginal fistula by the use of a pedicled muscle flap. Surg Gynec Obstet 1928;47:255–60.

69. Ingleman-Sundberg A. In: Meigs JV (ed) Surgical Treatment of Carcinoma of the Cervix. London: Heinemann, 1954; 419.

70. Hamlin RHJ, Nicholson EC. Reconstruction of urethra totally destroyed in labour. Br Med J 1969;2:147–150.

71. McCraw JB, Massey FM, Shanklin KD, Horton CE. Vaginal reconstruction with gracilis myocutaneous flaps. Plast Reconstr Surg 1976;58:176–83.

72. Martius H. Die Operative Wiederherstellung der volkommen fehlenden Harnrohre und der Schliessmuskels derselben. Zentbl Gynak 1928;52:480–6.

73. Spence HM, Duckett JW. Diverticulum of the female urethra: clinical aspects and presentation of a simple operative technique for cure. J Urol 1970;104:432–7.

74. Turner-Warwick RT. The use of pedicle grafts in the repair of urinary tract fistulae. Br J Urol 1972;44:644–56.

75. Zacharin RF. Grafting as a principle in the surgical management of vesico-vaginal and recto-vaginal fistulae. Aust N Z J Obstet Gynaecol 1980;20:10–17.

76. O'Conor VJ, Sokol JK, Bulkley GJ, Nanninga JB. Suprapubic closure of vesicovaginal fistula. J Urol 1973;109:51–4.

77. Turner-Warwick RT. Urinary fistula in the female. In: Harrison ED, Gittes RF, Perlmutter AD (eds) Campbell's Urology. Philadelphia: Saunders, 1979; Ch. 85.

78. Walters W. Transperitoneal repair of a vesico-vaginal fistula. Proc Staff Meetings Mayo Clin 1935; 375–7.

79. Chapple CR, Turner-Warwick RT. Traumatic lower urinary tract fistulae – abdominoperineal repair with pedicled omental interposition. J Urol 1990;143:328A.

80. Turner-Warwick RT. The omental repair of complex urinary fistulae. In: Gingell C, Abrams P (eds) Controversies and Innovations in Urological Surgery. London: Springer-Verlag, 1988; Ch. 26.

81. Bardescu N. Ein neues verfahren fur die operation der tiefen blasen-uterus-scheidenfisteln. Centralbl f Gynak 1900;24:170.

82. Eisen M, Jurkovic K, Altwein JE, Schreiter F, Hohenfellner R. Management of vesicovaginal fistulas with peritoneal flap interposition. J Urol 1974;112:195–8.

83. Robertson CN, Riefkohl R, Webster GN. Use of the rectus abdominis muscle in urological reconstructive procedures. J Urol 1986;135:963–5.

84. McCraw JB, Arnold PG. Atlas of Muscle and Myocutaneous Flaps. Norfolk, VA: Hampton Press, 1986.

85. Coleman JW, Albanese C, Marion D et al. Experimental use of free grafts of bladder mucosa in canine bladders: successful closure of recurrent vesicovaginal fistula utilising bladder mucosa. Urology 1985;25:515–7.

86. Kiricuta I, Goldstein AMB. Epiplooplastia vezicala, metoda de tratament curativ al fistulelor vezico-vaginale. Obstetrica si Ginecologia Buceresti 1956;2:163.

87. Turner-Warwick RT, Wynne EJC, Handley-Ashken M. The use of the omental pedicle graft in the repair and reconstruction of the urinary tract. Br J Surg 1967;54:849–53.

88. Goldstein MB, Dearden LC. Histology of omentoplasty of the urinary bladder in the rabbit. Invest Urol 1966;3:460–9.

89. Helmbrecht LJ, Goldstein AMB, Morrow JW. The use of

pedicled omentum in the repair of large vesicovaginal fistulas. Invest Urol 1975;13:104–7.

90. Kiricuta I, Goldstein AMB. The repair of extensive vesicovaginal fistulas with pedicled omentum. J Urol 1972;108:724–7.

91. Chapple CR, Turner-Warwick RT. Surgical salvage of radiation induced fibrosis – the 'frozen pelvis'. J Urol 1990;143:349A.

92. Bramble FJ. The treatment of adult enuresis and urge incontinence by enterocystoplasty. Br J Urol 1992;54:693–6.

93. Cartwright PC, Snow BW. Bladder autoaugmentation: early clinical experience. J Urol 1989;142:505–7.

94. Schmidt RA. Advances in genitourinary neurostimulation. Neurosurgery 1986;18:1041–4.

95. Reitz A, Stohrer M, Kramer G et al. European experience of 200 cases treated with botulinum-A toxin injections into the detrusor muscle for urinary incontinence due to neurogenic detrusor overactivity. Eur Urol 2004;45(4):510–5.

96. Keating MA, Ludlow JK, Rich MA. Enterocystoplasty: the star modification. J Urol 1996;155:1723–5.

97. Weinberg AC, Boyd SD, Lieskovsky G et al. The hemi-Koch ileocystoplasty: a low pressure anti-refluxing system. J Urol 1988;140:1380–4.

98. Mundy AR, Stephenson TP. 'Clam' ileocystoplasty for the treatment of refractory urge incontinence. Br J Urol 1985;57:641–6.

99. Woodhouse CRJ. Reconstruction of the lower urinary tract for neurogenic bladder: lessons from the adolescent age group. Br J Urol 1992;69:589–93.

100. Krishna A, Gough DC, Fishwick J, Bruce J. Ileocystoplasty in children: assessing safety and success. Eur Urol 1995;27:62–6.

101. Singh G, Thomas DG. Enteroplasty in neuropathic bladder. Neurourol Urodyn 1995;14:5–10.

102. Hasan ST, Marshall C, Robson WA, Neal DE. Clinical outcome and quality of life following enterocystoplasty for idiopathic detrusor instability and neurogenic bladder dysfunction. Br J Urol 1995;76:551–7.

103. Flood HD, Malhotra SJ, O'Connell HE et al. Long-term results and complications using augmentation cystoplasty in reconstructive urology. Neurourol Urodyn 1995;14:297–309.

104. Barrington JW, Fern-Davies H, Adams RJ et al. Bile acid dysfunction after clam enterocystoplasty. Br J Urol 1995;76:169–71.

105. Barrington JW, Fulford S, Griffiths D, Stephenson TP. Tumors in bladder remnant after augmentation enterocystoplasty. J Urol 1997;157(2):482–6.

106. Snow BW, Cartwright PC. Bladder autoaugmentation. Urol Clin North Am 1996;23(2):323–31.

107. Stothers L, Johnson H, Arnold W et al. Bladder autoaugmentation by vesicomyotomy in the pediatric neurogenic bladder. Urology 1994;44(1):110–3.

108. Stohrer M, Kramer A, Goepel M et al. Bladder auto-augmentation – an alternative for enterocystoplasty: preliminary results. Neurourol Urodyn 1995;14:11–23.

109. Kramer G, Stoher M. Neurourology. Curr Opin Urol 1996;6(4):176–83.

110. McDougall EM, Clayman RV, Figenshau RS, Pearle MS. Laparoscopic retropubic auto-augmentation of the bladder. J Urol 1995;153:123–6.

111. Anderson PAM, Rickwood AMK. Detrusor hyperreflexia as factor in spontaneous perforation of augmentation cystoplasty for neuropathic bladder. Br J Urol 1991;67:210–2.

112. Slaton JW, Kropp KA. Conservative management of suspected bladder rupture after augmentation enterocystoplasty. J Urol 1994;152:713–5.

113. Rivas DA, Chancellor MB, Huang B, Epple A, Figueroa TE. Comparison of bladder rupture pressure after intestinal bladder augmentation (ileocystoplasty) and myomyotomy (autoaugmentation). Urology 1996;48:40–6.

93

Gynecologic developmental abnormalities

Melissa C Davies, Sarah M Creighton

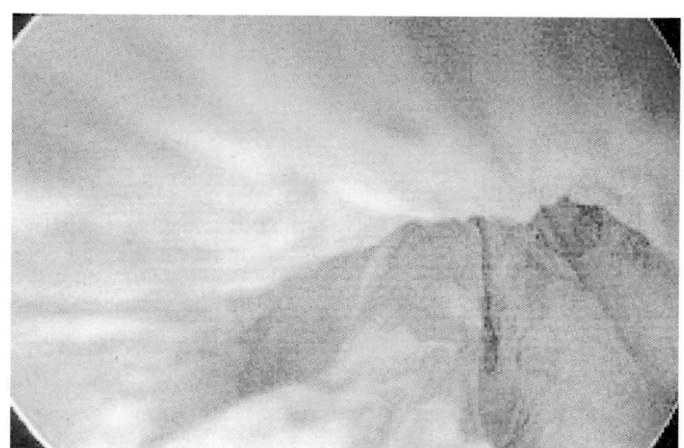

INTRODUCTION

The müllerian system develops from the sixth week of life and it is estimated that the prevalence of congenital abnormalities, both major and minor, is approximately 5%.[1–3] These anomalies may occur in isolation or in conjunction with other congenital malformations or as part of a syndrome. Many patients with simple anomalies will remain asymptomatic and may be diagnosed incidentally while being investigated for other problems or undergoing routine gynecologic/obstetric procedures. The others will present in a variety of ways depending upon the abnormality present. The most common presentations are primary amenorrhea, obstructed uterus or vagina, dyspareunia, and on investigation for infertility or recurrent miscarriage. Those diagnosed as neonates will usually be patients in whom there are associated major anomalies of the genitourinary and alimentary tracts such as persistent cloacal anomalies and anorectal malformations, or when urgent life-saving treatment is required (e.g. salt-wasting congenital adrenal hyperplasia).

DEVELOPMENT OF THE MÜLLERIAN TRACT

An understanding of the embryologic development of the urogenital system is essential to the diagnosis and management of developmental abnormalities. This subject is covered in detail in Chapter 00. What follows is a brief summary.

Primordial gonads (genital ridges) appear during the sixth week of embryogenesis. Associated ducts – the müllerian or wolffian ducts – also develop. The fate of these undifferentiated ducts depends upon the genetic sex of the embryo. In XY embryos, the SRY gene (sex determining region of the Y chromosome) stimulates testicular differentiation. The developing testes produce androgens and anti-müllerian hormone (AMH), which cause virilization and regression of müllerian structures. Therefore, in XX individuals, absence of the SRY gene allows the gonads to develop into ovaries, and the subsequent lack of AMH allows the müllerian ducts to develop into a uterus, fallopian tubes and vagina.

The müllerian ducts grow in a caudal and medial direction and fuse in the midline to form the primitive uterus. These ducts form the right and left fallopian tubes, and midline fusion of these structures produces the uterus, cervix, and proximal two-thirds of the vagina. This rudimentary vagina fuses with the posterior urethra at week 7 to form the urogenital sinus. Fusion of the müllerian ducts also brings together the lateral peritoneal folds that form the broad ligaments. The vagina develops from a combination of the müllerian tubercles and the urogenital sinus. Cells proliferate from the upper portion of the urogenital sinus to form structures called the sinovaginal bulbs. These fuse to form the vaginal plate which extends from the müllerian ducts to the urogenital sinus. This plate begins to canalize, starting at the hymen, and proceeds upwards to the cervix (Fig. 93.1). This process is not complete until 21 weeks of gestation.[4]

The external genitalia in females consist of the genital tubercle, the urogenital sinus, and the urethral and labioscrotal folds.[5] The genital tubercle becomes the clitoris, the urethral folds develop into the labia minora, and the labioscrotal folds become the labia majora. By week 12 of development these structures are recognizably female. These structures are sensitive to androgens and form the penis and scrotum in normal male development.

Imaging

Accurate imaging is pivotal to the diagnosis of many of the conditions described below. Ultrasound is routinely

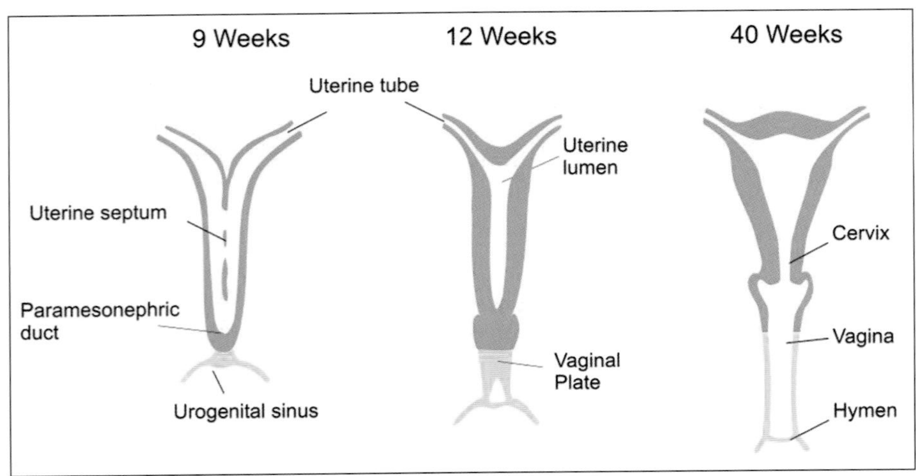

Figure 93.1. *Embryologic development of the müllerian system.*

used as the primary mode of investigation. Recent developments in this field have allowed better assessment of uterine anomalies, particularly with the introduction of high-resolution transvaginal ultrasound probes. Unfortunately, this may not be appropriate in children or young teenagers or in those whose problem is vaginal absence. More recently, three-dimensional (3-D) ultrasound has been employed in the diagnosis of uterine anomalies. Its benefits include the fact that it is non-invasive and allows for more accurate diagnosis compared with conventional ultrasound.[6] Ultrasound has the benefit of being safe in pregnancy which is useful given that the subjects are nearly all young fertile women; it also allows concomitant assessment of neighboring structures such as the urinary tract.

Magnetic resonance imaging (MRI) is an extremely useful tool in assessing these complex malformations,[7,8] particularly where there is no vaginal cavity in which to put an ultrasound probe, or in children or adolescents who have not engaged in sexual activity (Fig. 93.2). There are no studies as yet comparing the accuracy of MRI with 3-D ultrasound.

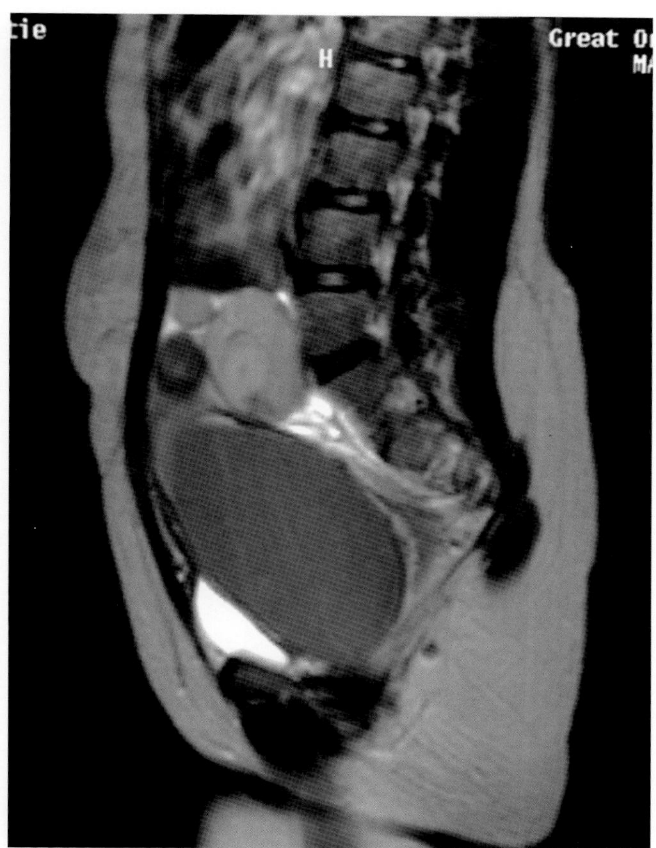

Figure 93.2. *MRI of an obstructed uterus in a young girl with cloaca.*

Other imaging modalities may give useful information:

- *Hysterosalpingography* (HSG) gives information about the internal contour of the uterus, and allows an assessment of the size and extent of uterine septa. However, it does not provide sufficient information to discern between a septate and a bicornuate uterus. It has two main drawbacks: 1) many patients consider it to be an uncomfortable procedure; and 2) it may be complicated by pelvic inflammatory disease.
- *Hysteroscopy* is of particular use in diagnosing uterine anomalies and has the benefit of allowing treatment in some cases, particularly in septate and arcuate uterus.[9] As hysteroscopy does not provide any information on the outer surface of the uterus, it may be difficult to distinguish between a septate and a bicornuate uterus.

Investigative laparoscopy should be undertaken only in cases where all other imagining modalities have failed, and the potential for combining this with laparoscopic treatment should also be considered. Nevertheless, it is considered to be the gold standard in the investigation of gynecologic anomalies.[10]

SIMPLE/ISOLATED ANOMALIES

Imperforate hymen

The hymen is the embryologic septum between the sinovaginal bulbs above and the urogenital sinuses below. The incidence of imperforate hymen is estimated to be 1 in 1000 live female births.[11] Hymen malformations are not usually associated with other müllerian or uterine anomalies. Failure of this septum to perforate in the embryo or in early childhood may present at adolescence with obstructed menstrual flow. The history is usually of several months of cyclical abdominal pain in an adolescent without menstruation. A pelvic mass may be palpated or found on ultrasound scan. On inspection of the vulva it is sometimes possible to see a bulging vaginal membrane. The treatment for these patients is a simple cruciate incision with excision of a quadrate of hymeneal tissue to allow drainage of the vagina and uterus. Wide excision of the hymen too close to the vaginal mucosa may result in stenosis at the introitus.[12]

There have been reports of familial cases of imperforate hymen, usually between siblings, suggesting a recessive mode of inheritance.[13] There has also been a report of imperforate hymen in two generations of the same family,[14] which suggests a possible dominant mode of transmission. There may be a case for assessing all female family members of affected individuals.

Transverse vaginal septum

This uncommon condition occurs in approximately 1 in 70,000 females[15] due to a failure of the müllerian ducts and urogenital sinus to canalize. These septa are most commonly found at the junction of the middle to upper two-thirds of the vagina. In cases of a complete transverse septum, associated uterine anomalies are common; one series reports the rate to be as high as 95%.[16] Most presentations of this condition are in young girls after the menarche with cyclical pelvic pain as a result of hematocolpos, which may be complicated by hematometra, bilateral hematosalpinges and possibly endometriosis. It can rarely occur before puberty when the presentation is with pelvic pain, the obstruction in this case thought to be due to a build-up of mucous secretions from the cervical glands.

In one interesting case expectant management was employed, where the thickness of the septum and volume of the dilated vagina were monitored regularly using ultrasonography. The thickness of the vaginal septum decreased from 26 to 8 mm over a period of 5 years, thus allowing a less complicated surgical procedure in a more mature patient.[17] The thinning of the septum was felt to be due to a pressure effect of the hematocolpos. However, in the majority of cases the treatment is surgical excision without delay. If the septum is thin and low it may be possible to remove it using a vaginal approach.[18] Care must be taken to ensure that the septum is entirely removed as vaginal stenosis may result if the procedure is incomplete. Thick transverse septa or those located higher up in the vagina will require an abdominoperineal approach. In those cases where the distance between the margins is too great, then some form of skin or intestinal graft may be required.

Longitudinal vaginal septum

Longitudinal septa are often asymptomatic and may not be apparent until the patient is sexually active (when it presents with dyspareunia) or in some cases during labor, where there may be a delay in the second stage.[19] They result as a failure of reabsorption of the vaginal septum during embryogenesis. The septum may be complete, and extend from the cervix to the introitus, or partial, which may be of any length along the course of the vagina. Management for the majority of these is usually surgical resection if symptomatic. Care must be taken to resect the septum right up to the cervix or dyspareunia will continue.

Rarely, one hemivagina is obstructed, with the other functioning normally. This may cause an unusual clinical picture of apparently normal menstruation from the unaffected side associated with pelvic pain. Vaginal examination may reveal a unilateral swelling due to hematocolpos. As menstruation appears initially normal, this results in delayed diagnosis of obstruction which would normally be made much quicker in the absence of any menstrual flow. Also, as this is an uncommon condition presenting in young females, the patient may attend a pediatrician rather than a gynecologist, especially as she is having what appear to be normal periods. Further investigation of these patients may demonstrate uterine anomalies. The imaging modality of choice in these cases would normally be MRI.[8] One large study of 20 women found that 87.8% of cases had an associated uterine malformation, the commonest of which was a complete uterine septum.[16] These more complex müllerian anomalies will be discussed in more detail later.

Surgical treatment of simple vaginal longitudinal septa is generally uncomplicated and is approached vaginally. As the vagina is a vascular structure, care should be taken with hemostasis. As with transverse septa and imperforate hymen, postoperative vaginal stenosis should be looked for and treated if necessary.

Uterine anomalies

Uterine anomalies are present in 0.5–2.0% of women;[20,21] this rate is higher in women who are infertile and who have had repeated miscarriages.[20] Attempts have been made to classify uterine anomalies. Perhaps the most widely accepted classification system for uterine anomalies is from the American Fertility Society.[22] This classification organizes the anomalies into six major uterine anatomic types (Fig. 93.3).

The resulting anomalies can be considered to be due to one of four events:[23]

1. Failure of one or more of the müllerian ducts to develop – *agenesis, unicornuate uterus without rudimentary horn*;
2. Failure of the ducts to canalize – *unicornuate uterus with rudimentary horn*;
3. Failure of or abnormal fusion of the ducts – *uterus didelphys, bicornuate uterus*;
4. Failure of the reabsorption of the midline uterine septum – *septate uterus, arcuate uterus.*

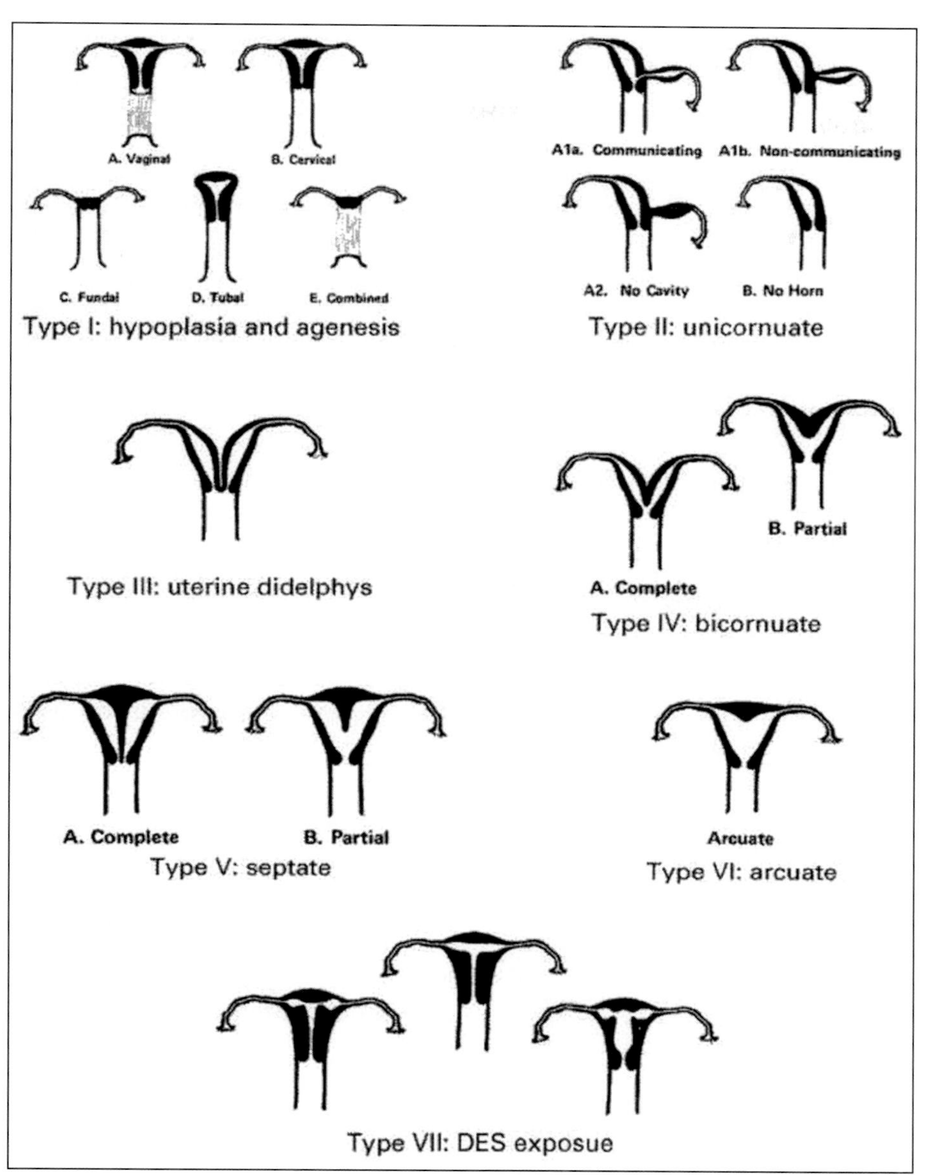

Figure 93.3. *The American Fertility Society classification of müllerian anomalies.*

Septate uterus

The commonest of these anomalies appears to be septate uterus which accounts for approximately 35% of all uterine anomalies.[23] The extent of the septum varies and may be partial or complete. It is known to result in early pregnancy loss and infertility, and this is how the majority of these patients present. However, septa can also be found by chance in women with an uncomplicated obstetric past history and so the decision on treatment can be complex. If treatment is recommended, then the most appropriate treatment for septate and arcuate uterus is resection of the septum; this can be achieved via hysteroscopic metroplasty, thus avoiding the need for a laparotomy and an incision in the uterus. It is known that metroplasty improves reproductive outcomes in these women.[24]

Bicornuate uterus

Bicornuate uterus accounts for 25% of uterine anomalies.[23] These patients also have recurrent miscarriage, premature delivery, and infertility. There have also been reported neonatal risks, including low Apgar scores and small-for-date infants. Surgical options for these patients are limited. Pregnancies do occur and these women should be carefully monitored throughout. This is complicated further if there are multiple pregnancies, and twin pregnancies in bicornuate uteri have been reported.[25,26]

Unicornuate uterus

Unicornuate uterus results from normal differentiation of only one müllerian duct. This may present with miscarriage or preterm delivery. One study demonstrated a preterm delivery rate of 25% and early miscarriage rate of 37.5%.[27] Non-communicating rudimentary horns with functional endometrium usually present with pain; this necessitates the removal of the horn, which may be carried out laparoscopically (Fig. 93.4).[28] Removal of the horn is essential as pregnancy may occur within the horn.[29] There have been reports of removal of pregnant uterine horns, and in this situation the risks are greater as the pregnant uterus is a more vascular structure. It is essential to obtain renal imaging such a preoperative intravenous pyelogram (IVP) as up to 30% will have associated renal tract anomalies.[30]

It is suggested that the standard treatment of these cases should include feticide and methotrexate as this, in addition to gonadotrophin-releasing hormone, would allow a safer approach to the laparoscopic removal of the uterine horn. The obstetric outcomes in subsequent pregnancies in this group of patients are largely unknown, although it is likely that they would result in premature labor. There have been case reports of full term labor after laparoscopic removal of a rudimentary horn with an ectopic pregnancy.[31] In those cases where there is no functional endometrium in the uterine horn, the issue of removal is debatable as there is no risk of pregnancy and its consequences.

Didelphic uterus

Didelphic uterus is often associated with a hemivagina, or a vaginal septum of varying degree, and possible duplicated kidneys or renal agenesis. It is thought to account for 10% of all uterine anomalies.

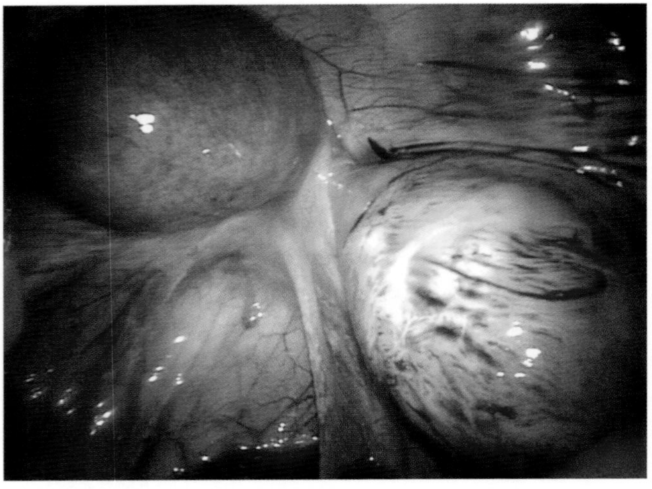

Figure 93.4. *Laparoscopic view of an obstructed uterine horn.*

Absent cervix

Congenital absence of the cervix is a rare condition and occurs in 1 in 80,000 to 100,000 births.[32] It is known to be associated with vaginal aplasia, both partial and complete, and renal anomalies. In a recent retrospective review of 18 patients, 39% had associated vaginal aplasia.[33] Presentation is usually with primary amenorrhea and cyclical lower abdominal pain. Endometriosis or pelvic infection may result from the chronic hematometra. The differential diagnosis includes high transverse vaginal septum and in some cases the actual diagnosis may not be clear until surgery.

The management of this condition has changed in recent years with the advances in reproductive technology. Previously, patients with cervical atresia were offered a total hysterectomy as complications of recanalizing the cervix were common and a viable pregnancy was unlikely.[19,34] Now the recommended treatment options consist of either suppression of menses with preservation of the uterus for pregnancy with reproductive assistance, or uterovaginal anastomosis. There are very few data on outcomes following uterovaginal anastomosis, the largest study published stating that the postoperative complication rate was low with only 22% requiring further surgery. Furthermore, they report six spontaneous pregnancies in four of their patients.[33] Despite these encouraging results it is important to realize that the possibility of serious complications exists and postoperative sepsis after uterovaginal anastomosis has resulted in septic shock and death.[35]

Reproductive technology has advanced to allow these patients an opportunity to become pregnant with the assistance of in vitro fertilization. There have been case reports of implanting embryos transmyometrially which have resulted in a viable pregnancy.[36,37] In the latter case report the patient underwent uterovaginal canalization using amniotic membrane at the time of cesarean section.[37]

One of the difficulties of these techniques is the management of miscarriage should it occur. Cervical dilation and curettage is often not an option as there may be no obvious cervix, or a small scarred cervix. Therefore most cases would require a laparoscopic or open removal of the remnants of pregnancy. One case report has used a conservative approach of observation where the patient's β-human chorionic gonadotropin levels were monitored with ultrasound examination of the uterus.[32]

COMPLEX ANOMALIES

Complex anomalies can be considered in two groups: anatomic and endocrine. This allows distinction based on the underlying cause rather than the system affected. Complex anatomic anomalies include the Mayer–Rokitansky–Kuster–Hauser syndrome.

Congenital absence of the vagina

Agenesis of the vagina occurs in approximately 1 in 5000 to 30,000 live female births.[38,39] It is commonly referred to as Mayer–Rokitansky–Kuster–Hauser syndrome (MRKH). In the majority of suffers there is no discernable vagina present, whereas approximately 25% will have a short blind-ending pouch. This is almost always associated with an absent or rudimentary uterus. There are normal ovaries and 46,XX karyotype. Anomalies of the urinary tract are present in an estimated 34% of patients, and spinal anomalies are found in 12%.[40] There is thought to be a genetic basis for this syndrome and currently possible implicated genes include HNF1b and members of the Wnt gene family.[41,42]

Treatment usually involves formation of a vagina. The preferred method for this is non-surgical with the use of pressure dilation therapy.[43] This involves the use of graded dilators applied to the perineum at the point where the vagina would normally be sited (Fig. 93.5). In most patients, while there is no vagina, there is often a vaginal 'pit' which acts as a guide to the site where the patient should apply pressure. Success of this treatment is limited to motivated patients and it is recommended that they are seen regularly during this treatment and offered psychological support to improve outcomes.

For those in whom dilation has not worked, or is not possible, then surgical construction is necessary. The timing of this procedure should be carefully considered, as many of those who have surgery will need to use some form of pressure dilation to maintain the vagina. Numerous forms of vaginoplasty have been employed in the treatment of these patients. They range from simple skin grafting to more complex intestinal vaginoplasties, The use of bowel segments for vaginoplasty was reported in the literature as early as 1907;[44] segments of rectum, ileum and sigmoid colon may be employed. Stenosis (apart from at the introitus) is rare, and the vagina remains moist and of appropriate caliber. However, a vagina constructed from intestine will be relatively insensitive, and may have excess mucus production requiring the patient to wear pads permanently. There have been reports of diversion colitis with colovaginoplasty and this can be difficult to treat.[45] This seems to be less common with ileal vaginoplasty. Vaginal malignancy has also been reported following both intestinal and skin graft vaginoplasty,[46] with a mean length of time to diagnosis of carcinoma of approximately 17 years.[47] More recent reports of laparoscopic techniques that have become available include laparoscopic Davydov and Vecchietti procedures[48,49] (Fig. 93.6).

Psychological preparation is essential both before and after surgery. The maintenance of the neovagina postoperatively often requires regular dilation until regular sexual intercourse occurs. This is of particular importance in skin graft vaginas. The patient should be emotionally well adjusted and mature.[50]

Fertility options for these patients are limited, but as they have normal functioning ovaries then surrogacy is an option. There have been reports of successful surrogacy treatment in patients with Rokitansky syndrome.[51–53]

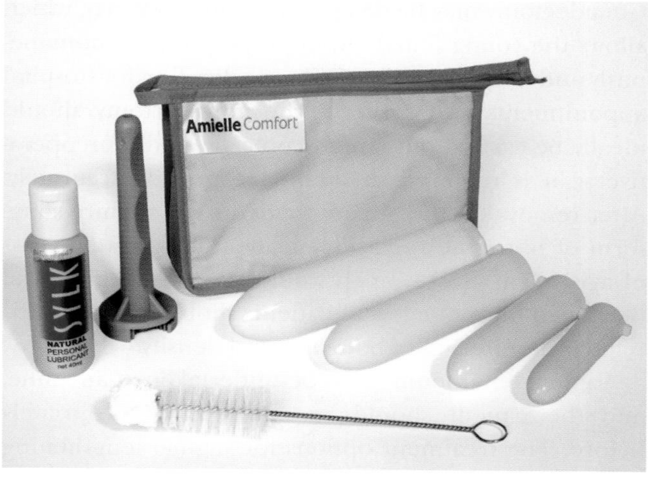

Figure 93.5. *Amielle dilators.*

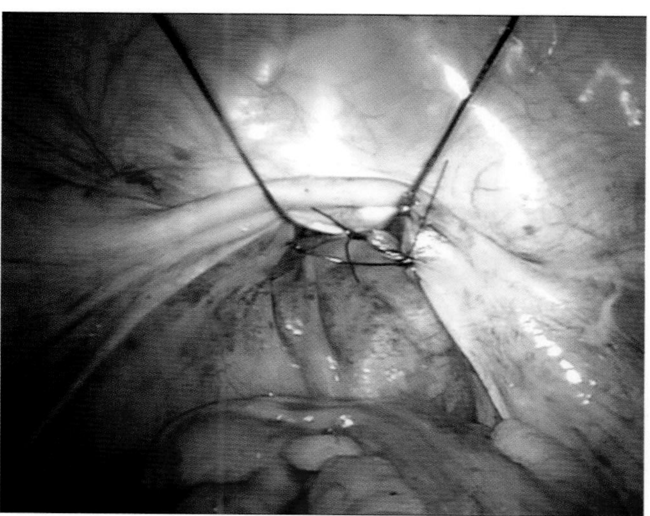

Figure 93.6. *Laparoscopic Vecchietti.*

Congenital adrenal hyperplasia

Congenital adrenal hyperplasia (CAH) is the most common cause of ambiguous genitalia and occurs in approximately 1 in 14,000 births in the UK. The pathogenesis in the majority of cases is 21-hydroxylase deficiency. The lack of this enzyme leads to a decrease in the level of cortisol, which in turn causes an increase in adrenocorticotropic hormone (ACTH) secretion. This causes an increase in the levels of cortisol precursors which are forced along the androgen pathway. In its most severe form, aldosterone levels will also be low, which may lead to salt wasting, volume depletion, hypotension, reduced renal blood flow, and raised renin activity. The aim of treatment in these patients is to replace the aldosterone with fludrocortisone and replace glucocorticoid to suppress the ACTH overactivity

Presentation differs depending upon the form of disease, and ranges from neonatal salt wasting crisis to adult onset of virilization. The majority of cases are diagnosed in children or neonates who are noted to have ambiguous or masculinized genitalia at birth. Virilization of the female genitalia occurs to a varying degree, causing labial fusion, clitoromegaly, and a confluence of the vagina and distal urethra (Fig. 93.7).[54] Current standard practice includes corrective genital surgery to separate the labia, reduce the size of the clitoris and separate vagina and urethra.[55] The aims of this are to create a feminine appearance, allow passage of menses, preserve sexual function, and prevent subsequent urinary tract complications.[56] This is usually performed as a 'one-stage' procedure in infancy, although many patients require further surgery in adolescence to facilitate menstrual flow and allow penetrative sexual intercourse. There has been increasing recent controversy amongst clinicians and patient peer support groups as to the need for and timing of feminizing genital surgery. Genital surgery is associated with damage to sensory innervation of the clitoris and is associated with loss of sexual sensation and an increased risk of sexual dysfunction.[57] Long-term data are, however, scanty and at present no consensus has been reached.

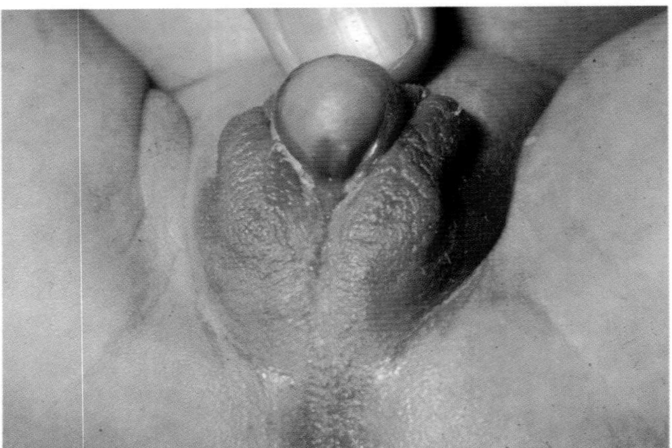

Figure 93.7. *Newborn with congenital adrenal hyperplasia.*

Androgen insensitivity – complete and partial

Androgen insensitivity syndrome, due to a defect in the androgen receptor (AR), has an incidence thought to be somewhere in the region of 1 in 13,000 to 40,000 live births.[39,58] It is an X-linked recessive disorder where affected individuals have a normal male karyotype (XY) with a spectrum of clinical manifestations, and is generally subdivided into complete and partial. All patients have testes and normal testosterone production and metabolism, with either a female or ambiguous phenotype. There are usually no müllerian structures present.

Patients with partial androgen insensitivity are diagnosed at birth, as there is ambiguity of the genitalia, and a decision regarding the sex of rearing needs to be made. This is a difficult and sensitive issue and should be handled in a specialist centre with a full multidisciplinary team of experts available, including a psychologist, pediatric urologist and endocrinologist. Those with complete androgen insensitivity (CAIS) may present later in life with primary amenorrhea or in some cases with inguinal hernia. The incidence of CAIS in females presenting with inguinal hernia is estimated to be in the region of 0.8–2.4%,[59] and some would suggest that all girls presenting with inguinal herniae should be investigated for androgen insensitivity.[60]

Recommended treatment for these patients includes removal of gonads, as there is a potential for malignant change, and lengthening of the vagina if necessary. Gonadectomy may be delayed until after puberty, which allows the young female to undergo puberty spontaneously and minimizes disruption to schooling for hospital appointments and surgery. The gonadectomy should ideally be carried out laparoscopically, and a preoperative scan is required to locate the gonads accurately. After removal of the gonads, patients will require some form of hormone replacement, typically until 50 years of age, when most women would experience a natural decline in hormone levels. Patients should also undergo regular monitoring of bone mineral density.

Vaginal lengthening may be undertaken at any time, and the patient should be counseled appropriately before. The treatment options for vaginal lengthening are as for MRKH, with dilation therapy as the first line choice of treatment.

ASSOCIATED WITH OTHER ANOMALIES OR AS PART OF A SYNDROME

Anorectal malformation and cloaca

Many patients with gynecologic developmental abnormalities may have other anomalies and the converse is also true. Females born with a persistent common cloacal channel will not only require reconstruction to separate the common cavity into three distinct structures (vagina, urethra and rectum) but there are also a significant percentage of these patients with associated gynecologic anomalies. The commonest of these is a duplicate vagina.[61] In patients with a persistent cloaca the rate is quoted as being as high as 50%.[62] Yet many of these patients are not routinely investigated for gynecologic developmental anomalies. In one recent study, 36% of female patients born with a cloacal anomaly presented with an obstructed uterus in puberty, all of whom required surgery.[63] Any surgery required is more difficult in these patients as they have often undergone multiple surgical procedures as young children. Furthermore, fertility issues are also complicated by the fact that these women, once pregnant, will need to deliver via cesarean section with an experienced surgeon present.

Turner's syndrome

Turner's syndrome (TS) is the most common sex chromosome disorder in females, and occurs in 1 in 2000 live female births.[64] It is the result of a complete or partial X chromosome monosomy. The syndrome is phenotypically characterized by short stature, webbed neck, wide carrying angle, and low posterior hair line.

Ovarian dysgenesis is documented as occurring in 95% of TS sufferers.[65] Ovarian failure occurs in the first few months or years of life. Therefore, these patients are not able to undergo a spontaneous puberty, and amenorrhea and minimal breast development are the norm, though not inevitable. One study has shown 16% of its Turner's population to have undergone spontaneous puberty.[66] However, few patients with Turner's syndrome are fertile and spontaneous pregnancy occurs in approximately 5%,[66] usually in patients who have mosaicism. Furthermore, those who mange to become pregnant have documented poor outcomes, with a 29% miscarriage rate, 7% perinatal death rate, and a 20% chance of having offspring with a chromosomal abnormality (e.g. Down's syndrome, Turner's syndrome).[67]

Initial management of these patients includes an echocardiogram and renal tract ultrasound as there are a significant percentage of associated cardiac and renal anomalies. Growth hormone therapy should be considered in childhood to try to increase final height. Estrogen replacement is also necessary to induce a normal puberty. After puberty nearly all TS patients will require long-term hormone replacement to prevent the onset of osteoporosis and atherosclerosis.[68] Due to the complex nature of this disease it is best managed by a multidisciplinary team where appropriate advice and counseling can be given.

CONCLUSION

As these conditions are rare, the diagnosis is often missed or delayed, causing much anxiety for both the patient and her family. The key to managing these patients is thoroughness and attention to detail, and it is imperative to provide as accurate a diagnosis as possible.

Many of these conditions have adverse implications for fertility or sexual function. Psychological input is crucial and should be offered to the family as a whole. Support will need to be ongoing in many cases through childhood and adolescence. Full information about the diagnosis and its implications must be made available to the family and should be explained clearly so that the patients and their parents can fully appreciate what the problem is and what the future holds for them.

Other helpful resources that are available to these patients include patient support groups which exist for some of the conditions discussed above. These can provide useful additional information for the patients, often of a more practical nature, and also reinforce the idea that the patient is not alone in her suffering. Details of such organizations should be available in the clinics where these patients are seen. Another useful tool in aiding patients' understanding of what are often quite difficult concepts is written literature, which should be in clear, easy-to-understand terms, and up to date.

Such complex and rare conditions need the input of a multidisciplinary team comprising at the very least a psychological, surgical, and endocrinologic component. Specialized back-up services such as imaging, biochemistry, and genetics are also essential. Patients with complex developmental anomalies should be referred to specialized clinics which can provide the services required.

REFERENCES

1. Cooper JM, Houck RM, Rigberg HS. The incidence of intrauterine abnormalities found at hysteroscopy in patients undergoing elective hysteroscopic sterilization. J Reprod Med 1983;28(10):659–61.
2. Jurkovic D, Gruboeck K, Tailor A, Nicolaides KH. Ultra-

sound screening for congenital uterine anomalies. Br J Obstet Gynaecol 1997;104(11):1320–1.

3. Simon C, Martinez L, Pardo F, Tortajada M, Pellicer A. Müllerian defects in women with normal reproductive outcome. Fertil Steril 1991;56(6):1192–3.
4. Kim HH, Laufer MR. Developmental abnormalities of the female reproductive tract. Curr Opin Obstet Gynecol 1994;6(6):518–25.
5. Cameron F, Smith C. Embryology of the female genital tract. In: Balen AH (ed) Paediatric and Adolescent Gynaecology. Cambridge: Cambridge University Press, 2004; 3–8.
6. Woelfer B, Salim R, Banerjee S, Elson J, Regan L, Jurkovic D. Reproductive outcomes in women with congenital uterine anomalies detected by three-dimensional ultrasound screening. Obstet Gynecol 2001;98(6):1099–103.
7. Troiano RN, McCarthy SM. Mullerian duct anomalies: imaging and clinical issues. Radiology 2004;233(1):19–34.
8. Minto CL, Hollings N, Hall-Craggs M, Creighton S. Magnetic resonance imaging in the assessment of complex Müllerian anomalies. BJOG 2001;108(8):791–7.
9. Grimbizis G, Camus M, Clasen K, Tournaye H, De Munck L, Devroey P. Hysteroscopic septum resection in patients with recurrent abortions or infertility. Hum Reprod 1998;13(5):1188–93.
10. Pellerito JS, McCarthy SM, Doyle MB, Glickman MG, DeCherney AH. Diagnosis of uterine anomalies: relative accuracy of MR imaging, endovaginal sonography, and hysterosalpingography. Radiology 1992;183(3):795–800.
11. Stelling JR, Gray MR, Reindollar RH. Endocrinology and molecular biology of the female genital tract in utero to puberty. In: Gidwani G, Falcone T (eds) Congenital Malformations of the Female Genital Tract: Diagnosis and Management. Philadelphia: Lippincott, Williams and Wilkins, 1999; 21–40.
12. Joki-Erkkila MM, Heinonen PK. Presenting and long-term clinical implications and fecundity in females with obstructing vaginal malformations. J Pediatr Adolesc Gynecol 2003;16(5):307–12.
13. Usta IM, Awwad JT, Usta JA, Makarem MM, Karam KS. Imperforate hymen: report of an unusual familial occurrence. Obstet Gynecol 1993;82:655–6.
14. Stelling JR, Gray MR, Davis AJ, Cowan JM, Reindollar RH. Dominant transmission of imperforate hymen. Fertil Steril 2000;74(6):1241–4.
15. Banerjee R, Laufer MR. Reproductive disorders associated with pelvic pain. Semin Pediatr Surg 1998;7(1):52–61.
16. Haddad B, Louis-Sylvestre C, Poitout P, Paniel BJ. Longitudinal vaginal septum: a retrospective study of 202 cases. Eur J Obstet Gynecol Reprod Biol 1997;74(2):197–9.
17. Beyth Y, Klein Z, Weinstein S, Tepper R. Thick transverse vaginal septum: expectant management followed by surgery. J Pediatr Adolesc Gynecol 2004;17(6):379–81.
18. MacDougall J, Creighton SM. Surgical correction of vaginal and other anomalies: a multidisciplinary approach. In: Balen AH (ed) Paediatric and Adolescent Gynaecology. Cambridge: Cambridge University Press, 2004; 120–30.
19. Hampton HL. Role of the gynecologic surgeon in the management of urogenital anomalies in adolescents. Curr Opin Obstet Gynecol 1990;2(6):812–18.
20. Acien P. Incidence of Müllerian defects in fertile and infertile women. Hum Reprod 1997;12(7):1372–6.
21. Heinonen PK. Clinical implications of the didelphic uterus: long-term follow-up of 49 cases. Eur J Obstet Gynecol Reprod Biol 2000;1(2):183–90.
22. The American Fertility Society. Classifications of adnexal adhesions, distal tubal occlusion, tubal occlusion secondary to tubal ligation, tubal pregnancies, mullerian anomalies and intrauterine adhesions. Fertil Steril 1988;49(6):944–55.
23. Grimbizis GF, Camus M, Tarlatzis BC, Bontis JN, Devroey P. Clinical implications of uterine malformations and hysteroscopic treatment results. Hum Reprod Update 2001;7(2):161–74.
24. Pabuccu R, Gomel V. Reproductive outcome after hysteroscopic metroplasty in women with septate uterus and otherwise unexplained infertility. Fertil Steril 2004;81(6):1675–8.
25. Barmat LI, Damario MA, Kowalik A, Kligman I, Davis OK, Rosenwaks Z. Twin gestation occupying separate horns of a bicornuate uterus after in-vitro fertilization and embryo transfer. Hum Reprod 1996;11(10):2316–18.
26. Narlawar RS, Chavhan GB, Bhatgadde VL, Shah JR. Twin gestation in one horn of a bicornuate uterus. J Clin Ultrasound 2003;31(3):167–9.
27. Raga F, Bauset C, Remohi J, Bonilla-Musoles F, Simon C, Pellicer A. Reproductive impact of congenital Müllerian anomalies. Hum Reprod 1997;12(10):2277–81.
28. Nezhat F, Nezhat C, Bess O, Nezhat CH. Laparoscopic amputation of a noncommunicating rudimentary horn after a hysteroscopic diagnosis: a case study. Surg Laparosc Endosc 1994;4(2):155–6.
29. Falcone T, Gidwani G, Paraiso M, Beverly C, Goldberg J. Anatomical variation in the rudimentary horns of a unicornuate uterus: implications for laparoscopic surgery. Hum Reprod 1997;12(2):263–5.
30. Cutner A, Saridogan E, Hart R, Pandya P, Creighton S. Laparoscopic management of pregnancies occurring in non-communicating accessory uterine horns. Eur J Obstet Gynecol Reproductive Biology 2004;113(1):106–9.
31. Adolph AJ, Gilliland GB. Fertility following laparoscopic removal of rudimentary horn with an ectopic pregnancy. J Obstet Gynaecol Can 2002;24(7):575–6.
32. Suganuma N, Furuhashi M, Moriwaki T, Tsukahara S, Ando T, Ishihara Y. Management of missed abortion in

a patient with congenital cervical atresia. Fertil Steril 2002;77(5):1071–3.

33. Deffarges JV, Haddad B, Musset R, Paniel BJ. Utero-vaginal anastomosis in women with uterine cervix atresia: long-term follow-up and reproductive performance. A study of 18 cases. Hum Reprod 2001;16(8):1722–5.

34. Rock JA, Schlaff WD, Zacur HA, Jones HW Jr. The clinical management of congenital absence of the uterine cervix. Int J Gynaecol Obstet 1984;22(3):231–5.

35. Casey AC, Laufer MR. Cervical agenesis: septic death after surgery. Obstet Gynecol 1997;90(4 Pt 2):706–7.

36. Anttila L, Penttila TA, Suikkari AM. Successful pregnancy after in-vitro fertilization and transmyometrial embryo transfer in a patient with congenital atresia of cervix: case report. Hum Reprod 1999;14(6):1647–9.

37. Lai TH, Wu MH, Hung KH, Cheng YC, Chang FM. Successful pregnancy by transmyometrial and transtubal embryo transfer after IVF in a patient with congenital cervical atresia who underwent uterovaginal canalization during Caesarean section: case report. Hum Reprod 2001;16(2):268–71.

38. Aittomaki K, Eroila H, Kajanoja P. A population-based study of the incidence of müllerian aplasia in Finland. Fertil Steril 2001;76(3):624–5.

39. Blackless M, Charuvastra A, Derryck A, Fausto-Sterling A, Lauzanne K, Lee E. How sexually dimorphic are we? Review and synthesis. Am J Human Biol 2000;12(2):151–66.

40. Griffin JE, Edwards C, Madden JD, Harrod MJ, Wilson JD. Congenital absence of the vagina. The Mayer–Rokitansky–Kuster–Hauser syndrome. Ann Intern Med 1976;85(2):224–36.

41. Lindner TH, Njolstad PR, Horikawa Y, Bostad L, Bell GI, Sovik O. A novel syndrome of diabetes mellitus, renal dysfunction and genital malformation associated with a partial deletion of the pseudo-POU domain of hepatocyte nuclear factor-1β. Hum Mol Genet 1999;8(11):2001–8.

42. Biason-Lauber A, Konrad D, Navratil F, Schoenle EJ. A WNT4 mutation associated with Müllerian-duct regression and virilization in a 46,XX woman. N Engl J Med 2004;351(8):792–8.

43. ACOG committee opinion. Nonsurgical diagnosis and management of vaginal agenesis. Number 274, July 2002. Committee on Adolescent Health Care. American College of Obstetrics and Gynecology. Int J Gynaecol Obstet 2002;79(2):167–70.

44. Baldwin JF. Formation of an artificial vagina by intestinal transplantation. Ann Surg 1907;40:398–403.

45. Syed HA, Malone PS, Hitchcock RJ. Diversion colitis in children with colovaginoplasty. BJU Int 2001;87(9):857–60.

46. Lawrence AA. Vaginal neoplasia in a male-to-female transsexual: case report, review of the literature, and recommendations for cytological screening. Int J Transgenderism 2001;5(1). (Online.)

47. Steiner E, Woernle F, Kuhn W et al. Carcinoma of the neovagina: case report and review of the literature. Gynecol Oncol 2002;84(1):171–5.

48. Langebrekke A, Istre O, Busund B, Sponland G, Gjonnaess H. Laparoscopic assisted colpoiesis according to Davydov. Acta Obstet Gynecol Scand 1998;77(10):1027–8.

49. Veronikis DK, McClure GB, Nichols DH. The Vecchietti operation for constructing a neovagina: indications, instrumentation, and techniques. Obstet Gynecol 1997;90(2):301–4.

50. Templeman C, Hertweck SP. Vaginal agenesis: an opinion on the surgical management. J Pediatr Adolesc Gynecol 2000;13(3):143–4.

51. Beski S, Gorgy A, Venkat G, Craft IL, Edmonds K. Gestational surrogacy: a feasible option for patients with Rokitansky syndrome. Hum Reprod 2000;15(11):2326–8.

52. Van Waart J, Kruger TF. Surrogate pregnancies in patients with Mayer–Rokitansky–Kustner–Hauser syndrome and severe teratozoospermia. Arch Androl 2000;45(2):95–7.

53. Esfandiari N, Claessens EA, O'Brien A, Gotlieb L, Casper RF. Gestational carrier is an optimal method for pregnancy in patients with vaginal agenesis (Rokitansky syndrome). Int J Fertil Womens Med 2004;49(2):79–82.

54. Hughes IA. Management of congenital adrenal hyperplasia. Arch Dis Child 1988;63(11):1399–404.

55. de Jong TP, Boemers TM. Neonatal management of female intersex by clitorovaginoplasty. J Urol 1995;154(2 Pt 2):830–2.

56. Consensus statement on 21-hydroxylase deficiency from the Lawson Wilkins Pediatric Endocrine Society and the European Society for Pediatric Endocrinology. J Clin Endocrinol Metab 2002;87(9):4048–53.

57. Crouch NS, Minto CL, Laio LM, Woodhouse CR, Creighton SM. Genital sensation after feminizing genitoplasty for congenital adrenal hyperplasia: a pilot study. BJU Int 2004;93(1):135–8.

58. Bangsboll S, Qvist I, Lebech PE, Lewinsky M. Testicular feminization syndrome and associated gonadal tumors in Denmark. Acta Obstet Gynecol Scand 1992;71(1):63–6.

59. Gans SL, Rubin CL. Apparent female infants with hernias and testes. Am J Dis Child 1962;104:82–6.

60. Viner RM, Teoh Y, Williams DM, Patterson MN, Hughes IA. Androgen insensitivity syndrome: a survey of diagnostic procedures and management in the UK. Arch Dis Child 1997;77(4):305–9.

61. Metts JC III, Kotkin L, Kasper S, Shyr Y, Adams MC, Brock JW III. Genital malformations and coexistent urinary tract or spinal anomalies in patients with imperforate anus. J Urol 1997;158(3 Pt 2):1298–300.

62. Pena A. The surgical management of persistent cloaca: results in 54 patients treated with a posterior sagittal approach. J Pediatr Surg 1989;24(6):590–8.

63. Warne SA, Wilcox DT, Creighton S, Ransley PG. Long-term gynecological outcome of patients with persistent cloaca. J Urol 2003;170(4 Pt 2):1493–6.
64. Gravholt CH, Juul S, Naeraa RW, Hansen J. Prenatal and postnatal prevalence of Turner's syndrome: a registry study. BMJ 1996;312(7022):16–21.
65. Saenger P, Wikland KA, Conway GS et al. Recommendations for the diagnosis and management of Turner syndrome. J Clin Endocrinol Metab 2001;86(7):3061–9.
66. Pasquino AM, Passeri F, Pucarelli I, Segni M, Municchi G. Spontaneous pubertal development in Turner's syndrome. Italian Study Group for Turner's Syndrome. J Clin Endocrinol Metab 1997;82(6):1810–13.
67. Tarani L, Lampariello S, Raguso G et al. Pregnancy in patients with Turner's syndrome: six new cases and review of literature. Gynecol Endocrinol 1998;12(2):83–7.
68. Elsheikh M, Bird R, Casadei B, Conway GS, Wass JA. The effect of hormone replacement therapy on cardiovascular hemodynamics in women with Turner's syndrome. J Clin Endocrinol Metab 2000;85(2):614–18.

94

Pediatric urogynecology

Andrew J Kirsch, Howard M Snyder

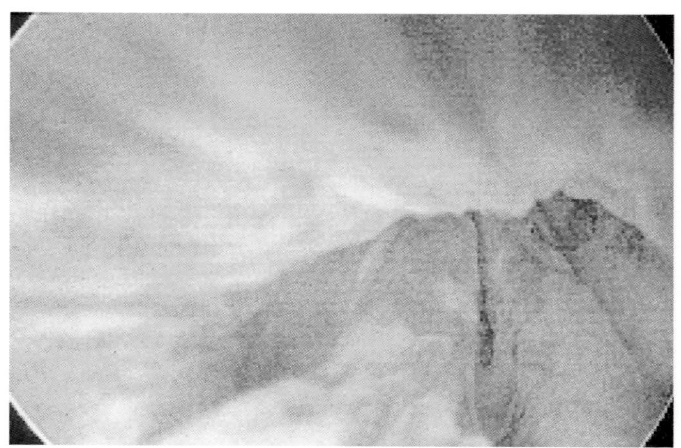

INTRODUCTION

The wide spectrum of anomalies of female embryogenesis results in problems related to the development of the urinary and genital tracts. Many of the clinical disorders seen in girls and young women that appear to involve the genitalia alone may be the harbinger of related urinary tract disorders. Abnormalities presenting in infancy may be easy to recognize secondary to an abnormal antenatal ultrasonographic or physical examination in the newborn period. Many urogenital malformations, however, are elusive and may become evident only when a clinical problem arises.

The most common urogynecologic disorders prompting childhood evaluation focus on problems of urinary continence and introital abnormalities. Interlabial masses, often included in the differential diagnosis of urinary incontinence, as well as difficulties with appropriate gender identification in genetic and phenotypic females, are discussed in this chapter. As congenital abnormalities result from abnormal embryogenesis, it is appropriate to begin with a brief overview of normal female embryology (see also Chapter 9).

FEMALE EMBRYOLOGY

Congenital abnormalities commonly involve both the urinary and genital tracts. An understanding of normal embryogenesis is a prerequisite for understanding congenital abnormalities. A detailed discussion of the embryology of the lower urinary tract is provided by Marshall[1] and by Stephens et al.[2]

The divergence of normal sexual differential into male and female phenotypes begins in week 9 of gestation. If no Y chromosome is present, the ovaries develop whereas the testes and Sertoli cells do not. As a result, the wolffian system regresses (absence of androgen production) and the müllerian ducts form the fallopian tubes, uterus, and proximal part of the vagina (absence of müllerian inhibiting factor). The embryologic origins and adult counterparts of the female genital tract are shown in Figure 94.1 and described in Table 94.1.

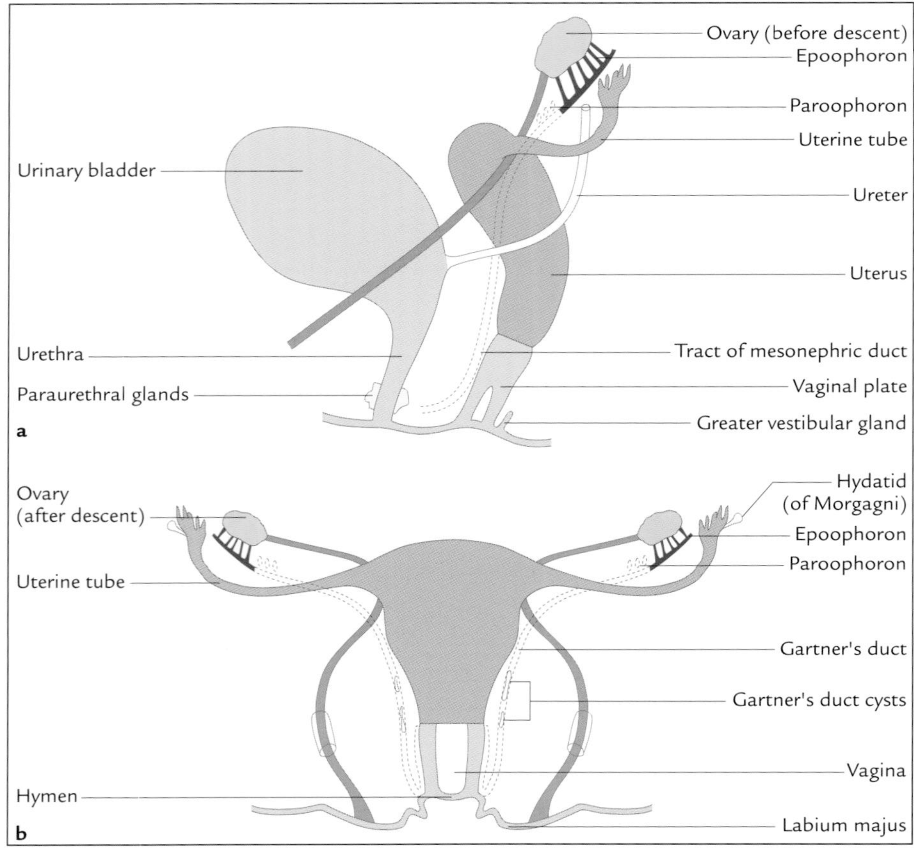

Figure 94.1. *Embryology and development of the female genital tracts: (a) a 12-week fetus; (b) a newborn female (▢ urogenital sinus; ■ mesonephric duct; ▢ paramesonephric duct).*

Table 94.1. *Female embryology*		
Weeks of gestation	Embryonic structure/event	Adult counterpart
7–8	Genital ridge transformed	Ovary
9–10	Müllerian ducts fuse distally	Fallopian tubes, uterus, cervix, proximal vagina
12–20	Sinovaginal bulbs elongate, form vaginal plate; canalization of plate at urogenital sinus	Distal vagina
	Genital tubercle elongates Urethral folds do not fuse Labial swellings enlarge Urogenital groove remains	Clitoris, hymen Labia minora Labia majora Introitus
	Mesonephric ducts	Ureters
	Vestigial structures: Mesonephric duct Proximal end	Appendix vesiculosa, paroöphoron and epoöphoron
	Distal end	Gartner's duct/cysts

URINARY INCONTINENCE IN GIRLS

Etiology

Urinary incontinence in females may have functional or neurogenic causes, or may be secondary to congenital abnormalities of the lower urinary tract. The most common cause of severe urinary incontinence in children is related to a neurologic deficit. The leading causes of neurogenic incontinence include myelomeningocele (spina bifida), sacral agenesis, and vertebral or spinal cord lesions. In these conditions, changes within the spinal cord may occur over time, making careful evaluation and close follow-up essential.

In all children presenting with urinary incontinence, urinalysis should be performed to assess the presence of infection, hematuria, proteinuria, glucosuria or renal concentrating defect (early morning specific gravity, 1.022). Chronic night-time wetting, polyuria or nocturia may indicate renal failure or diabetes and requires thorough medical evaluation.

Incontinence can be broadly divided between that requiring surgical intervention and that requiring medical or behavioral therapies. In general, incontinence related to primary nocturnal enuresis or infrequent voiding tends to resolve with time and does not require surgery. The following sections address the clinical presentation, evaluation, and treatment of lower urinary tract abnormalities associated with urinary incontinence in girls.

FUNCTIONAL CAUSES OF URINARY INCONTINENCE

Functional causes of urinary incontinence include primary nocturnal enuresis, dysfunctional voiding, and pseudo-incontinence (e.g. vaginal voiding).

Nocturnal enuresis

Primary nocturnal enuresis is defined as persistent night-time wetting past the age of 5 years. Nocturnal enuresis occurs in approximately 20% of 5-year-old children and is more common in boys than girls.[3] Daytime wetting, urinary urgency and frequency are more common in girls. Diagnosis and treatment of nocturnal enuresis is multifactorial, relying on both the pathophysiology and psychological analysis of the patient. Treatment using desmopressin, bedwetting alarm or combination therapy is often successful. Daytime symptoms such as enuresis, urgency and frequency may be treated with anticholinergic medications.

Dysfunctional voiding

Children with dysfunctional voiding have difficulty relaxing their pelvic floor musculature, which comprises the external urethral sphincter and which is traversed by the rectum. As a result, day- and night-time wetting, urinary frequency or infrequency, urgency, urinary tract infections, and constipation or encopresis are common.

It is helpful if patients and their families keep an elimination diary to ascertain the child's specific toileting habits. For example, many parents are not aware that their child has constipation unless specifically queried as to the frequency and caliber of the stool. Simple treatment of constipation with stool softeners (e.g. mineral oil, Kondremul) or laxatives (e.g. Milk of Magnesia or Dulcolax) permit better overall toileting behavior. Voiding dysfunction may be treated by behavior modification or pharmacologic agents and does not require surgical intervention. A list of common pharmacotherapeutic agents for neurovesical dysfunction is provided in Table 94.2.

Table 94.2. *Pharmacotherapy for neurovesical dysfunction*

Drug	Action	Dose/frequency
Bethanechol	Cholinergic	0.6 mg/kg/day 3–4 times daily
Dicyclomine	Anticholinergic	5–10 mg 3–4 times daily
Oxybutynin	Anticholinergic	0.2 mg/kg 2–4 times daily
Propantheline	Anticholinergic	1.5 mg/kg/day 3–4 times daily

Vaginal voiding

Vaginal voiding is often confused with true urinary incontinence. Micturition into the vagina results in leakage when the child stands upright, allowing efflux of urine from the vaginal vault. Simple maneuvers to direct the urinary stream more accurately by separating the legs further during voiding, and waiting a few minutes after micturition to allow efflux into the toilet, usually solve the problem (Fig. 94.2).

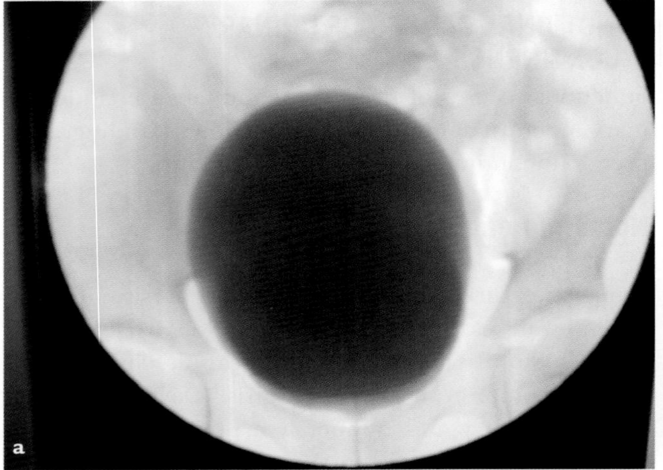

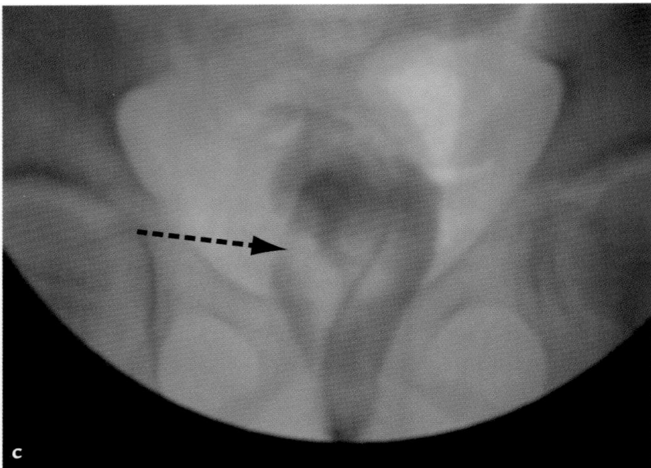

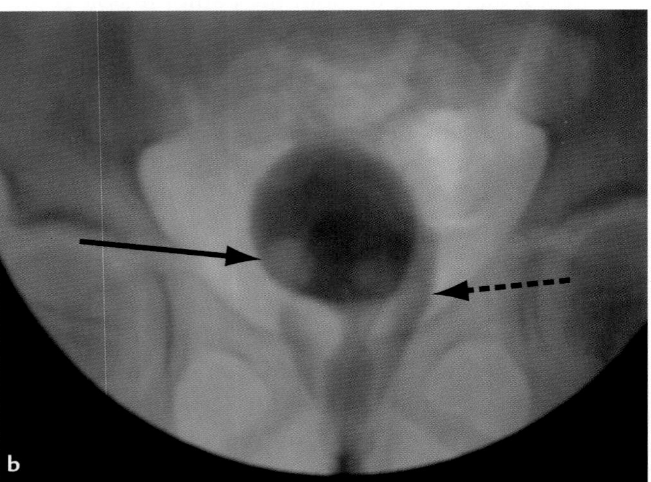

Figure 94.2. *A 4-year-old girl with bilateral vesicoureteral reflux and daytime 'dampness' was treated with endoscopic implantation of Deflux. A voiding cystourethrogram 3 months later shows cure of reflux, but the presence of vaginal voiding. (a) Bladder filling; (b) voiding phase showing absence of reflux, the presence of filling defects in bladder base (Deflux implants, solid arrow), and beginning of vaginally voided contrast (dashed arrow); (c) postmicturition film shows the presence of dense contrast within the vagina (dashed arrow) and nearly empty bladder.*

CONGENITAL ABNORMALITIES CAUSING INCONTINENCE

Congenital anomalies may cause incontinence by interfering with the function of the sphincter mechanisms or the storage function of the bladder, or by anatomically bypassing normal sphincter mechanisms (Table 94.3).

Imaging studies are essential to define the anatomic abnormalities causing the incontinence. The first studies obtained are usually renal and bladder ultrasonography and the voiding cystourethrogram (VCUG). The plain abdominal scout film of the VCUG assesses bony abnormalities and the presence or absence of fecal impaction. An intravenous pyelogram is useful to identify ectopic ureters, duplication anomalies, and ureteroceles, as well as providing useful information regarding renal function. Urodynamic studies are often useful in detecting sphincteric, storage, and urinary flow abnormalities, and are essential in all patients with neurogenic incontinence.

The goals of treatment for congenital abnormalities of the female urogenital tract are restoration of physical appearance and function, preservation of renal function, and achievement of manageable urine storage and continence.

Abnormal storage

Bladder exstrophy

Bladder exstrophy (Fig. 94.3) has an incidence of 1/30,000 live births and is less common in females than in males. Debate continues about the development of the bladder wall and matrix proteins. Why some children develop normal bladder capacities while others go on to develop small and poorly compliant bladders is incompletely understood. Treatment involves bladder closure within the first days of life. Bladder enhancement or diversion are surgical options later on. Bladder neck reconstruction may be performed at the time of bladder closure or afterward. Continence rates range from 43 to 87%.

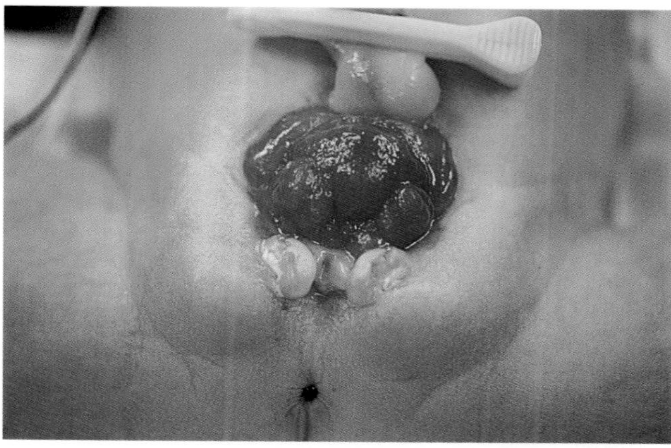

Figure 94.3. *A newborn girl with bladder exstrophy. Note separation of the labia and clitoris, and the normal vagina.*

Cloacal exstrophy

Cloacal exstrophy (Fig. 94.4) has an incidence of 1:200,000 and is much less common in females. Cloacal exstrophy is much more complex than bladder exstrophy and requires extensive evaluation for associated abnormalities of the nervous system, upper urinary tract, and gastrointestinal tract.

The treatment of storage abnormalities of the bladder usually involves bladder augmentation with intestinal segments. Clean intermittent catheterization (CIC) may also be required to maintain urinary continence.

Myelomeningocele

In the pediatric population, myelomeningocele (Fig. 94.5) is a common cause of neurogenic bladder leading to problems with urinary storage, sphincteric function, and elimination. In the United States, the prevalence

Table 94.3. *Mechanisms of incontinence in congenital genitourinary anomalies**

Abnormal storage	Abnormal sphincter	Bypass sphincter
Bladder exstrophy	Epispadias	Ectopic ureters
Cloacal exstrophy	Urogenital sinus	Vesicovaginal fistulae
Bladder agenesis	Ectopic ureteroceles	
Bladder duplication	Neurogenic†	
Neurogenic†		

* Multiple mechanisms for incontinence often coexist in a given patient.
† Abnormalities of storage or sphincteric function may be seen with neurogenic bladders (e.g. spina bifida) and may be related to detrusor hypo- or hyperactivity, or from secondary changes within the detrusor muscle, resulting in stiff (non-compliant) or floppy (very compliant) bladders.

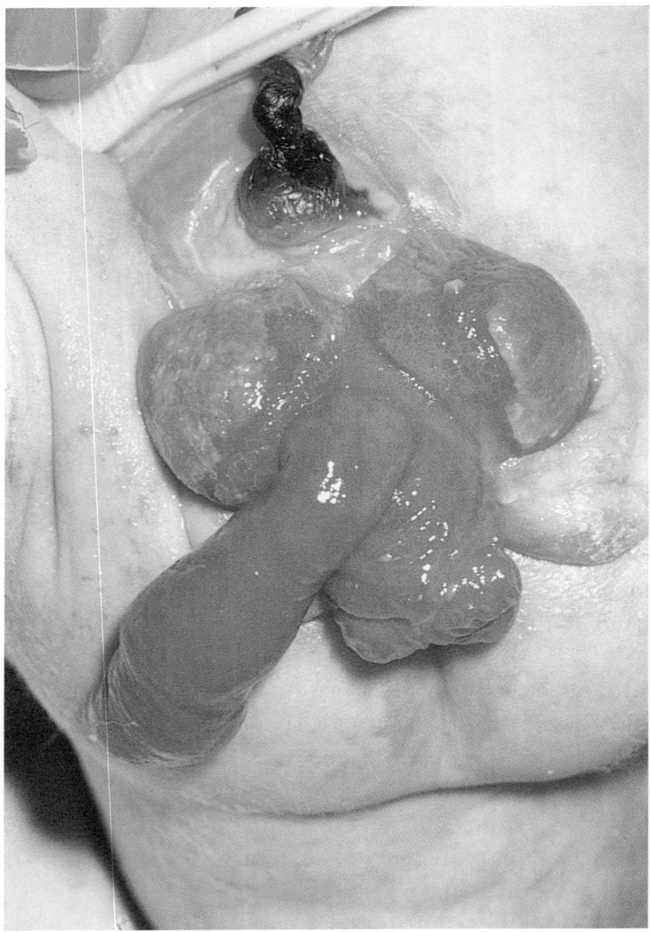

Figure 94.4. *Newborn with cloacal exstrophy illustrating separation of bladder halves, herniation of the hindgut and prolapse of the ileocecal segment.*

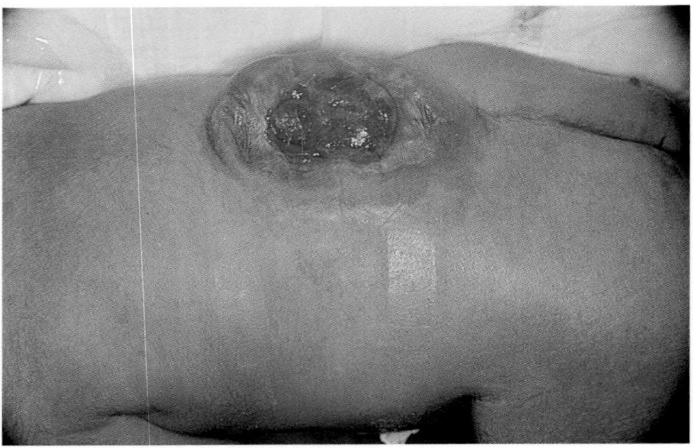

Figure 94.5. *A newborn with characteristic appearance of myelomeningocele protruding from the lower back.*

is approximately 1/1000 births. CIC in conjunction with anticholinergic medication has brought about a dramatic improvement in the management of patients with myelomeningocele. The use of CIC has been shown to promote continence, preserve renal function, and decrease the incidence of symptomatic pyelonephritis.[4] McGuire and co-workers[5] determined that a leak-point pressure (LPP) greater than 40 cmH_2O was predictive of renal deterioration over time. CIC serves to keep bladder pressure low, avoiding high LPP.

Abnormal sphincter

Anatomic abnormalities may impede normal development of the bladder neck. Incompetence of the bladder neck may result in primary urinary incontinence and is seen in conditions such as female epispadias, urogenital sinus, bilateral ureteral ectopia, and ectopic ureteroceles. Conservative measures to improve sphincteric function are limited and a surgical approach is needed. The surgical options focus on creation of an increase in bladder outlet resistance or of a new sphincter mechanism.

Female epispadias

Female epispadias (Fig. 94.6) may result in a variable presentation, depending on the severity of the urethral defect. In complete epispadias, incontinence results secondary to: 1) a foreshortened and widened urethra; 2) a partially absent external urethral sphincter; and 3) a poorly developed bladder neck. Treatment is directed at reconstruction of these deficient structures and ureteral reimplantation proximal to the reconstructed bladder neck region.[6,7] Persistent incontinence may be treated with collagen injection at the bladder neck.

Urogenital sinus anomalies

The persistence of a urogenital sinus may result in the urethra emptying into the vaginal vault. This may not be readily apparent unless the urethra is not seen during attempts at catheterization. Infants may present with a dilated vagina, possibly resulting in an abdominal mass, if the posterior lip of the hymen causes partial obstruction at the orifice of the urogenital sinus (Fig. 94.7). Retained urine in the vagina (urocolpos) and uterine canal may increase to enormous volumes. Drainage of urine with vaginal catheterization followed by a vaginogram showing contrast within the cervical canal and uterus, and possibly into the peritoneal cavity, is diagnostic. Treatment involves endoscopic division of the posterior hymenal lip. Further reconstructive surgery will usually be required.

Duplicated ectopic ureters

An ectopic upper pole ureter may join the lower end of the remnant mesonephric duct system comprising Gartner's ducts. These ureters are associated with non-function of

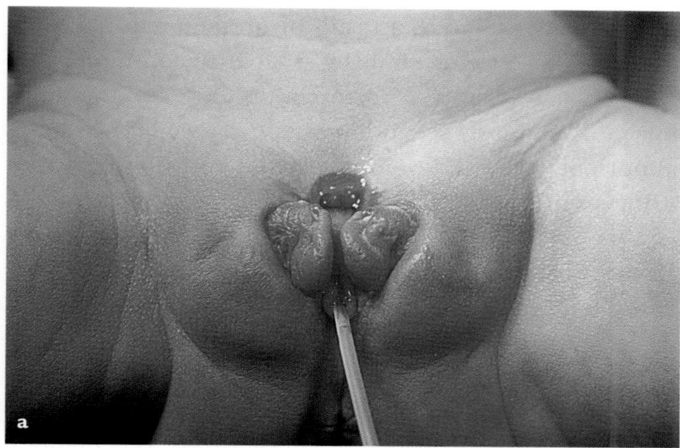

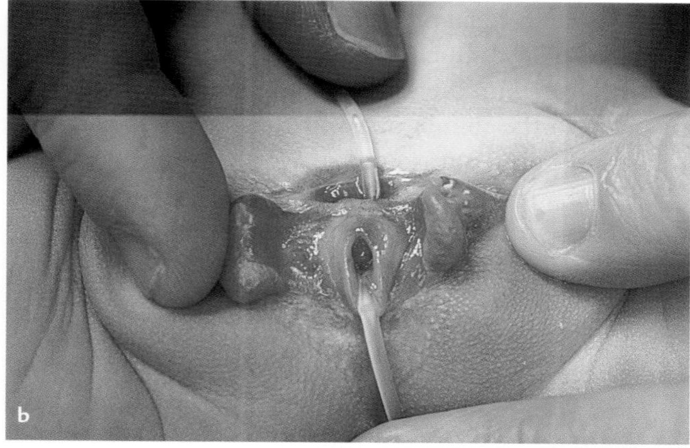

Figure 94.6. *Appearance of a newborn girl with epispadias (a); note the open bladder neck with a catheter introduced superior to a normal catheterized vagina, and separation of the labia and clitoris (b).*

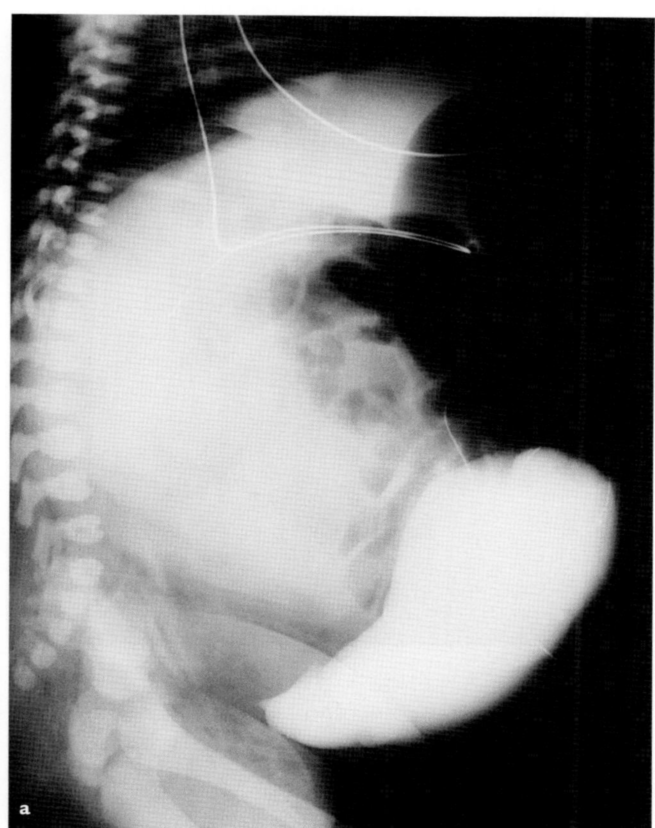

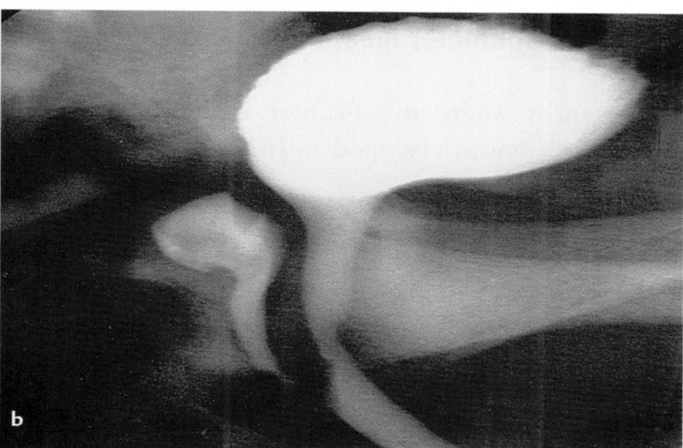

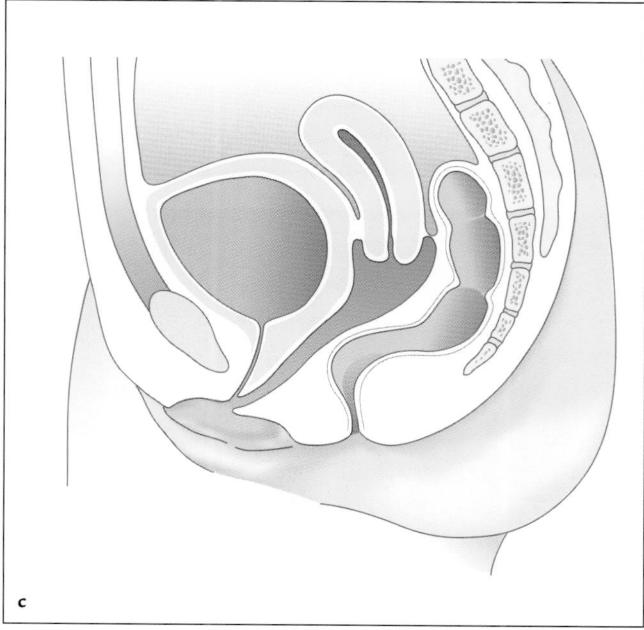

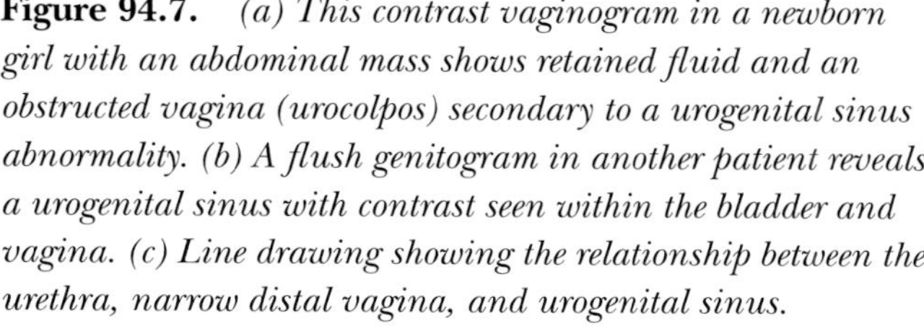

Figure 94.7. *(a) This contrast vaginogram in a newborn girl with an abdominal mass shows retained fluid and an obstructed vagina (urocolpos) secondary to a urogenital sinus abnormality. (b) A flush genitogram in another patient reveals a urogenital sinus with contrast seen within the bladder and vagina. (c) Line drawing showing the relationship between the urethra, narrow distal vagina, and urogenital sinus.*

the associated renal moiety and may result in cystic dilation of Gartner's duct with eventual rupture of the cyst and drainage into the vaginal opening. Drainage of fluid or pus into the vagina prompts further investigation. A renal and pelvic ultrasound scan may show a dilated or abnormal upper pole renal moiety, and a cystic structure may be seen in the pelvis or vaginal area. Computed tomography scanning or magnetic resonance imaging are helpful in further delineating the anatomy, while retrograde fluoroscopic studies are diagnostic if the often elusive ectopic orifice can be identified (Fig. 94.8).

The appropriate treatment of ectopic ureters depends on whether the ureter is ectopic or bilateral and whether it drains into the genital or urinary tracts. Ectopic ureters to the genital tracts may be treated by simple upper pole nephrectomy; ectopia to the urinary tract usually involves ureterectomy in addition to hemi-nephrectomy in order to prevent postoperative urinary reflux and infection (Fig. 94.9).

Bypass of sphincter mechanism

In instances where the bladder neck and sphincter mechanism have developed normally, urinary incontinence may develop as a result of ureteral ectopia distal to the continence mechanism. The most common cause of this abnormality is ectopic ureters. Incontinence may not be purely secondary to a bypass mechanism, as abnormal urethral development may contribute to poor urinary control.

Bilateral single ectopic ureters

Ectopic ureters result when a ureteric bud develops more cranially than usual from the mesonephric duct. In females, ectopic ureters usually open into the urethra, the vestibule or the vagina. Incontinence is a common complaint in girls with ectopic ureter(s). Bilateral ectopic ureters may enter the urethra just distal to the bladder neck. Because of the inadequacy of urethral length associated with this condition, incontinence may result. In single ectopic ureters, a cyclic VCUG may demonstrate vesicoureteral reflux when the bladder neck relaxes upon micturition; reflux is often not demonstrated during bladder filling when the bladder neck is in a contracted state. Treatment involves ureteral reimplantation and bladder neck reconstruction for bilateral single ectopic ureters, and upper pole partial nephrectomy and lower pole reimplantation for duplicated

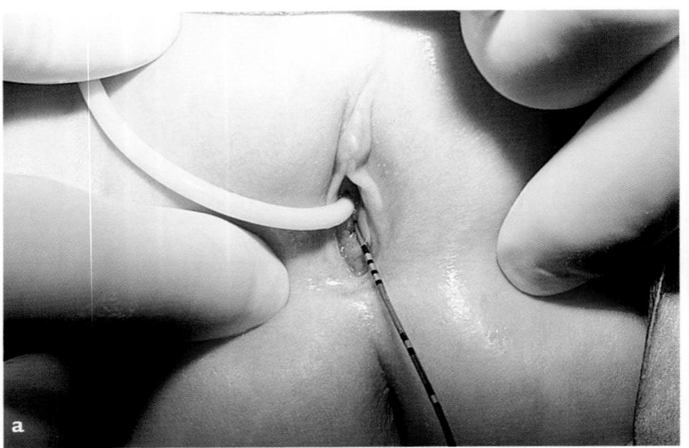

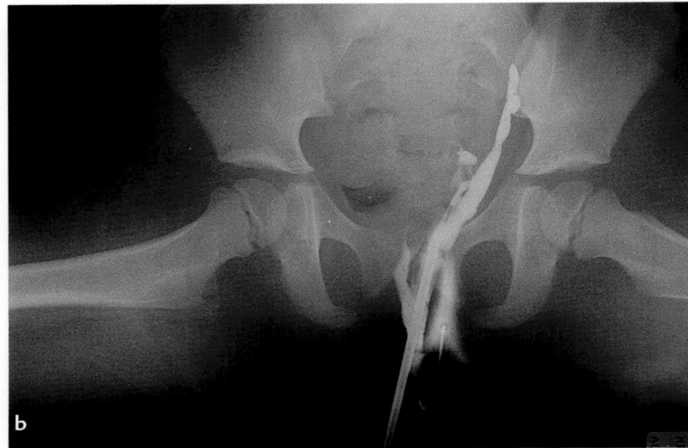

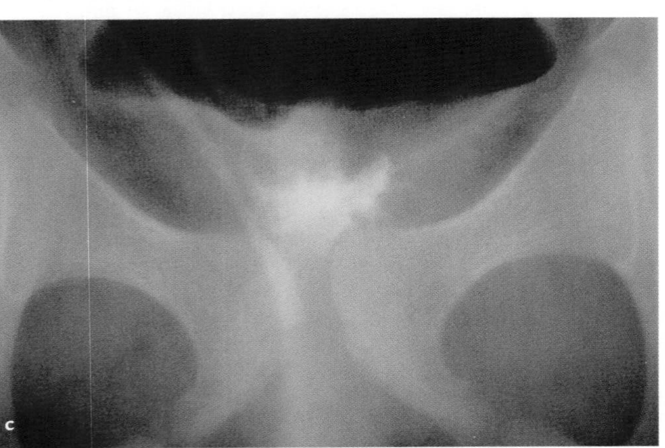

Figure 94.8. *A young girl with continuously damp underpants was found to have ureteral ectopia to her vagina: (a) The vagina showing a ureteral stent placed within the ectopic ureter and a Foley catheter within the urethra; (b) retrograde pyelogram shows contrast within the ectopic ureter. (c) An intravenous urogram in another patient reveals an ectopic ureter of an upper pole moiety terminating beyond the bladder neck and into the vaginal introitus.*

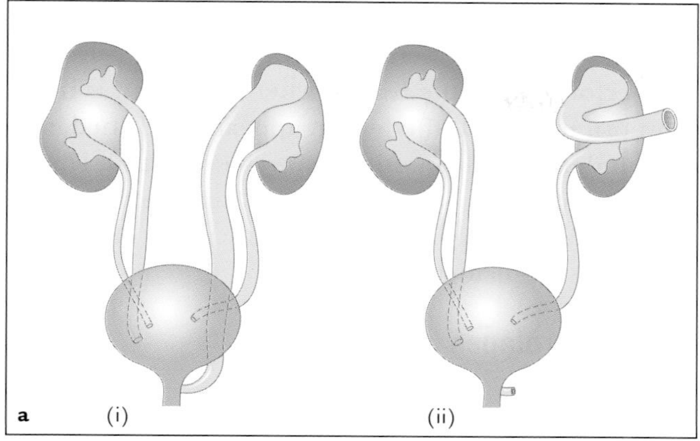

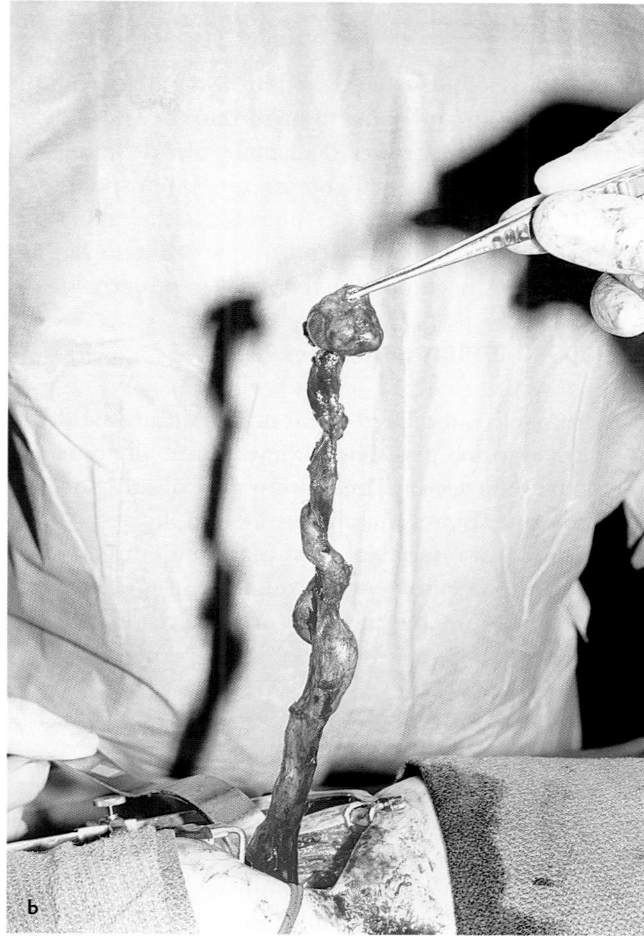

Figure 94.9. *(a) Illustration of nephroureterectomy: (i) preoperatively and (ii) postoperatively; (b) nephroureterectomy specimen from the patient in Figure 94.7.*

ectopic ureters. In unsuccessful cases, use of a continent catheterizable channel (e.g. appendicovesicostomy) or continent urinary diversion may be considered.

INTERLABIAL MASSES

Masses within the vagina presenting in infants and young girls are generally referred to as interlabial masses. Although many of these lesions arise within the introitus, those arising in the urethra or bladder must be recognized to afford proper management. Many patients with masses within the vaginal area complain of leakage of fluid (e.g. urine, pus, transudate). A thorough physical examination of the introitus is part of the complete evaluation of urinary incontinence.

Skene's glands (paraurethral glands)

The tubular Skene's glands (Fig. 94.10) arise from the urethral epithelium and are the counterparts to the male prostate gland. In females, these glands may end up in the urethral meatus and hymen. Cysts (tense, yellow, thin-walled) partially arising within the urethral meatus but mostly external to it may resemble a bulging hymen associated with hydrometrocolpos, or a prolapsing ureterocele (fleshy, compressible, protruding through the urethra).

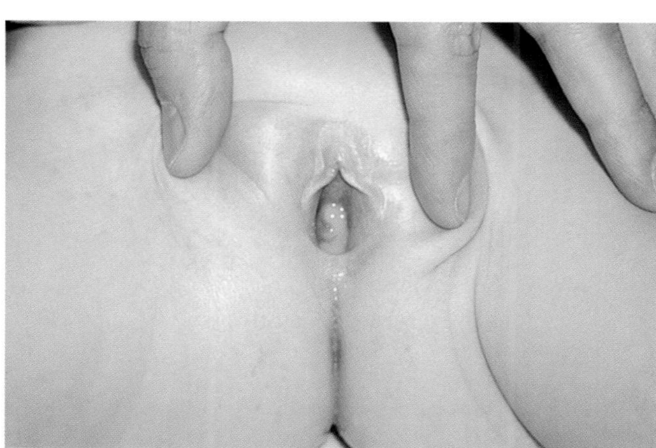

Figure 94.10. *Skene's glands in a newborn girl.*

Bartholin's glands

The major vestibular glands of Bartholin arise from the urogenital sinus and come to open into the vestibule on either side of the hymen. The main glands lie against the ischiopubic ramus deep to the bulbospongiosus muscle and cavernous tissue. Blockage of the main ducts of Bartholin's glands may lead to cystic dilation at any age, but rarely become infected prior to puberty.[1]

Prolapsed ureterocele

A ureterocele is a dilated distal ureter within the detrusor muscle which may extend beyond the bladder neck (ectopic ureterocele). These ureters are often associated with an upper pole renal moiety of a duplicated collecting system.[8] An interlabial mass may be identified if the ectopic ureterocele extends through the urethral meatus. Treatment is directed at ureterocele excision, bladder neck reconstruction, and ureteral reimplantation.

Hydro(metro)colpos

Circulating maternal estrogen in the newborn girl may result in an increase in the production of cervical mucus. Hydrocolpos and hydrometrocolpos result when mucus collects in the vaginal vault and uterus, respectively (Fig. 94.11). In these instances, the vaginal orifice may be blocked secondary to an imperforate hymen, within a urogenital sinus, anatretic rectocloacal canal, or vaginal/uterine atresia. Hydrometrocolpos, by virtue of its abdominal extension, may compress the urethra, rectum, and ureters.

Treatment of hydro(metro)colpos secondary to a normally located imperforate hymen may involve simple perforation of the hymen when the infant is in the newborn nursery. If the hymen appears thickened, incision under general anesthesia may be required. Higher obstruction involves a more formal approach to treat the associated urogenital abnormalities (e.g. urogenital sinus, atresia, rectocloacal canal).

Urethral prolapse

Eversion of the distal urethral mucosa through the urethral meatus results in a circumferential interlabial lesion (Fig. 94.12). The lesion may be painful or may bleed or weep serosanguinous fluid, prompting medical attention; however, such lesions do not lead to urinary incontinence. On examination, urethral prolapse appears edematous or necrotic, with the urethral meatus seen within its center. This lesion should be distinguished from neoplasms of the vagina or bladder (see below). A prolapsed urethra associated with mild edema without necrosis or significant pain may reasonably be treated conservatively with sitz-baths and estrogen cream over a 2- to 3-week period. More significant lesions should be excised.[9]

Rhabdomyosarcoma of the vagina

Rhabdomyosarcoma of the vagina and bladder (Fig. 94.13) may present as a grape-like interlabial lesion associated with vaginal bleeding.[10] Because of the propensity of these lesions to spread, a complete endoscopic and radiographic evaluation is indicated to confirm the diag-

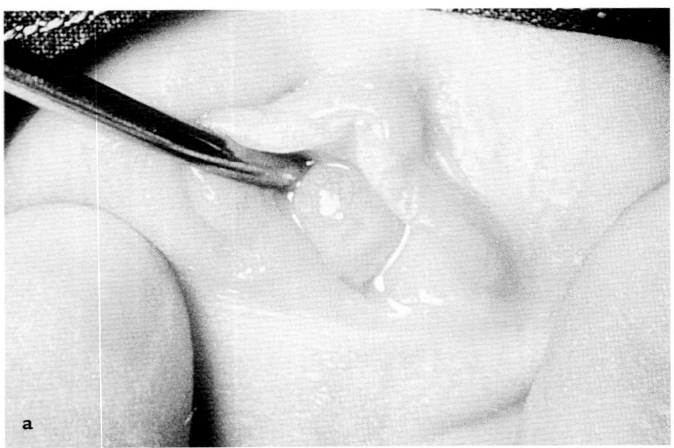

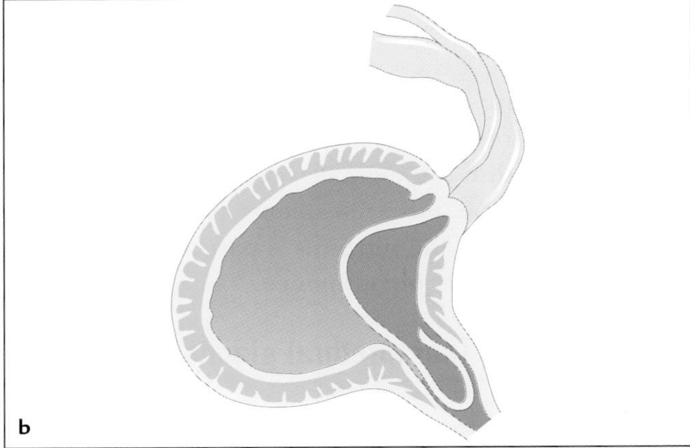

Figure 94.11. *A newborn girl with urinary obstruction: (a) external appearance of the prolapsing ectopic ureterocele; (b) illustration depicting the ectopic ureterocele with extension into the urethra.*

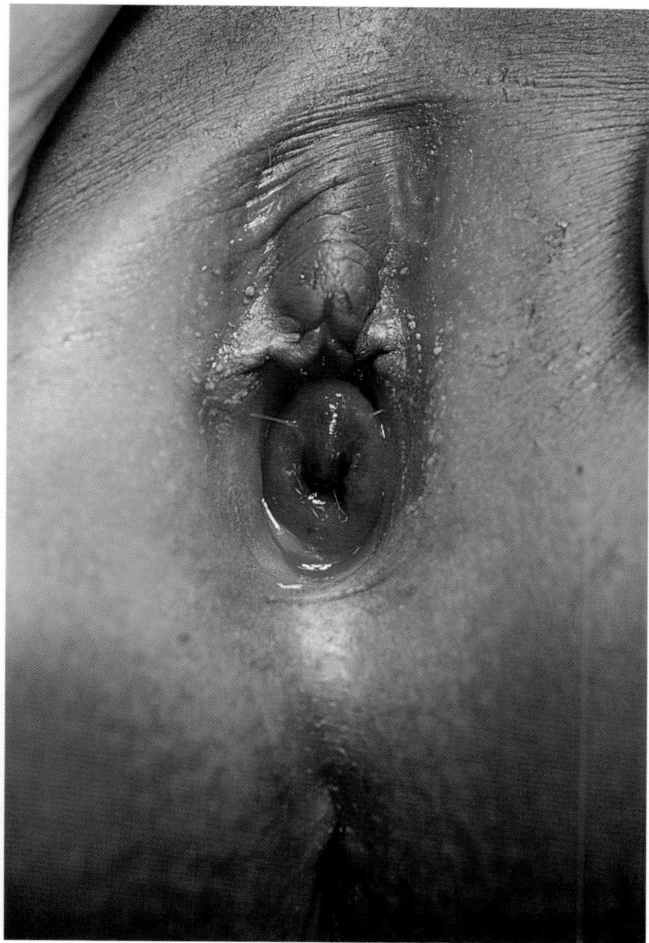

Figure 94.12. *An 8-year-old African–American girl with urethral prolapse presented with 'vaginal' pain and blood spotting.*

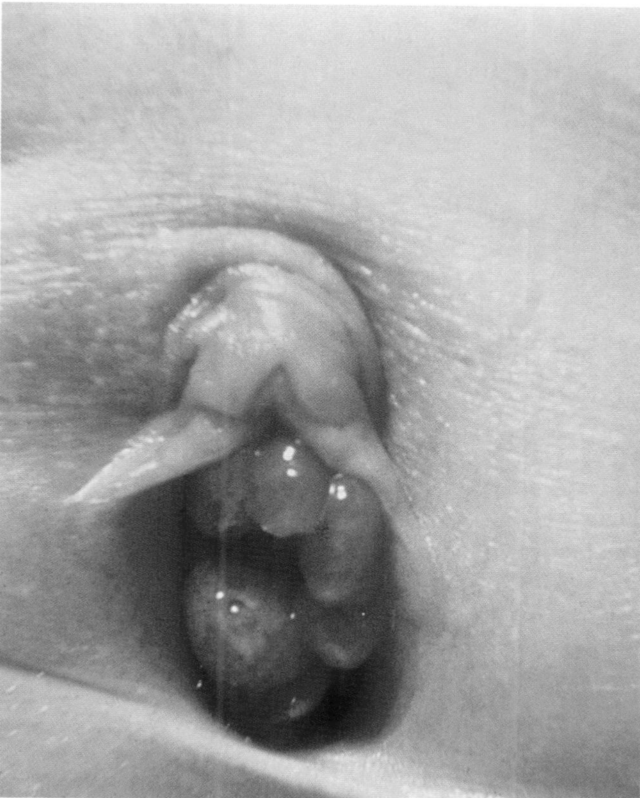

Figure 94.13. *A 5-year-old girl with rhabdomyosarcoma of the vagina (sarcoma botryoides) presented with blood spotting and dysuria.*

nosis and rule out local extension and distant lesions. Primary chemotherapy has resulted in better bladder salvage and can cure metastatic disease.[11] Surgical excision, with or without radiation therapy, is reserved for postchemotherapy biopsy-proven residual masses.

Introital hemangiomas

Hemangiomas of the female genitalia are rare lesions. In most cases, hemangiomas are congenital and may involve any part of the genitalia. Cavernous hemangiomas (angioma cavernosum, cavernoma) are similar to strawberry hemangiomas but are more deeply situated. They may appear as a red–blue spongy mass of tissue filled with blood. Some of these lesions disappear on their own, usually as a child approaches school age. In some cases, the hemangiomas can be quite large and may be confused with tumors, or – if involving the clitoris – may appear as clitoromegaly similar to that seen in cases of congenital adrenal hyperplasia (Fig. 94.14). Treatment may be by steroid injection, potassium-titanyl-phosphate (KTP) laser ablation and/or excision, depending on the size and location.

Urethral polyps

Urethral polyps are rare anomalies, characterized as benign urothelial-lined masses attached to a fibrovascular stalk, and may lead to symptoms by obstructing the ureter or bladder neck by a ball–valve mechanism. Some of these polyps, diagnosed later in life, may represent acquired lesions. Polyps may occur anywhere along the urinary tract. Primarily they are composed of connective tissue covered by epithelium. Additionally, smooth muscles and islands of glandular cells and even nerve tissue have been found. Treatment is by endoscopic ablation or excision, depending on the origin. Fibroepithelial polyps may present as interlabial masses and may lead to bleeding or dysuria when located in the urethral meatus (Fig. 94.15).

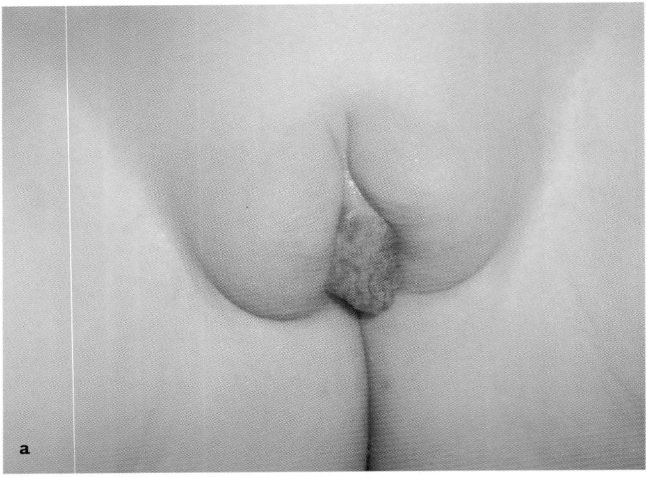

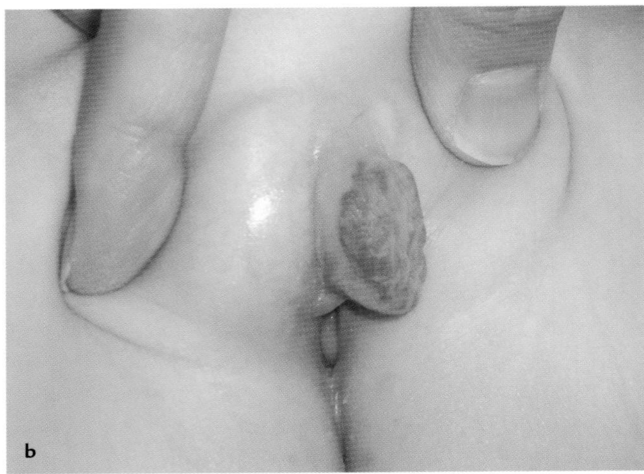

Figure 94.14. *(a, b) A 1-year-old girl presenting with an enlarging introital mass revealing a large cavernous hemangioma of the clitoris.*

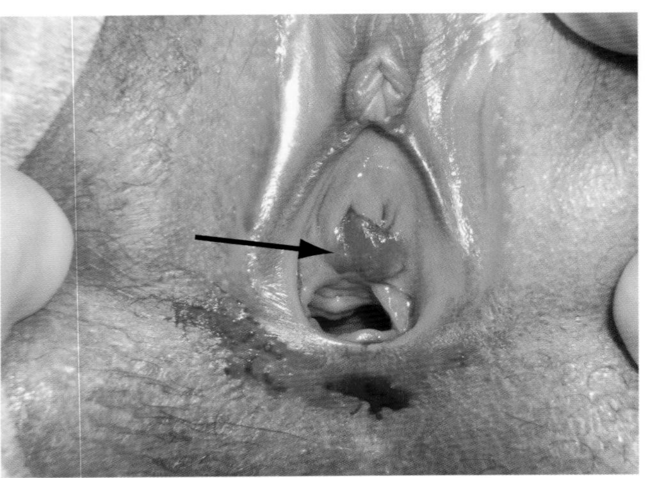

Figure 95.15. *A 6-year-old girl presenting with blood spotting in underwear and dysuria. Arrow shows urethral polyp.*

DISORDERS OF THE FEMALE GENITALIA

Intersex disorders

A complete description of the array of intersex disorders is beyond the scope of this chapter. However, urologists and gynecologists must be familar with the more common intersex disorders whereby gender assignment and rearing is along female lines. These conditions include girls of normal appearance who are genetically male (male pseudohermaphrodites) and genetic females appearing as males (female pseudohermaphrodites).

Female pseudohermaphroditism

Female pseudohermaphrodites are genetic females (XX karyotype) but may appear as males without testes (Fig. 94.16). The most common cause of female pseudohermaphroditism is congenital adrenal hyperplasia (21-hydroxylase deficiency in >90%). In this disorder, the absence of 21-hydroxylase results in the overproduction of androgens and results in a wide spectrum of genital abnormalities, ranging from mild masculinization of the clitoris (clitoromegaly) to complete masculinization. The labioscrotal folds are rugated and hyperpigmented, giving the physical appearance of severe hypospadias with cryptorchidism. In all cases, however, the internal female anatomy is normal. After the diagnosis is established, surgical treatment involves feminizing genitoplasty (reduction clitoroplasty, vaginoplasty, and labioplasty).

Male pseudohermaphroditism

Male pseudohermaphrodites are genetic males (XY karyotype) but may appear as normal females. Testicular feminization is the most common cause of male pseudohermaphroditism and results from the lack of androgen receptors at the cell surface of all tissues. The diagnosis should be suspected in all girls with inguinal hernias – the hernia sacs may be found to contain testes. The diagnosis should always be suspected in adolescent girls with normal development and primary amenorrhea. Development and sexual identity is female. Treatment involves bilateral orchidectomy. Testes left in place will produce testosterone, which is converted to estradiol, allowing spontaneous breast development. Testes should be removed because of the risk of gonadoblastoma. Estrogen must be replaced at puberty in girls who

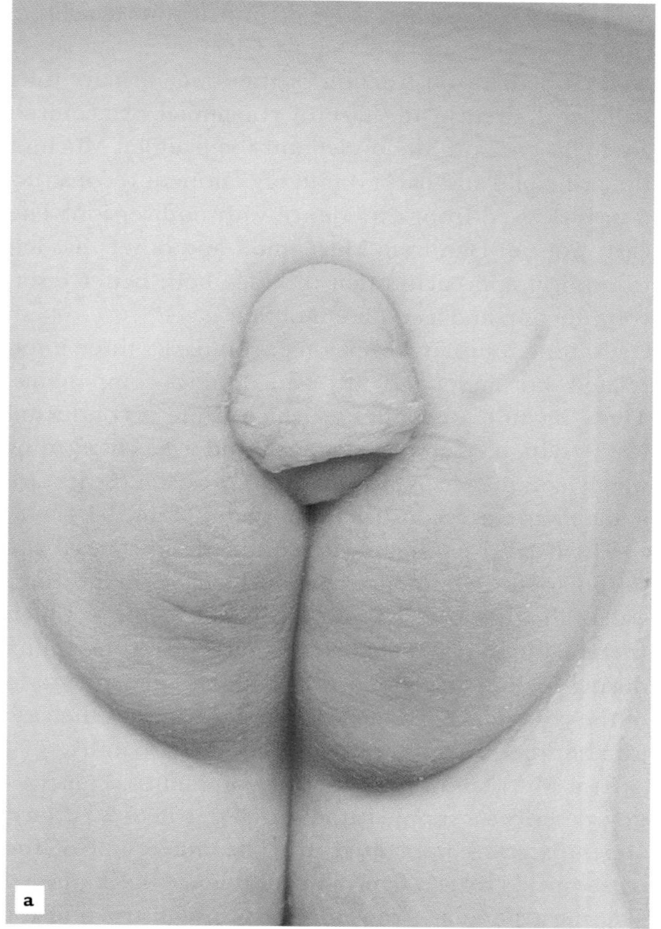

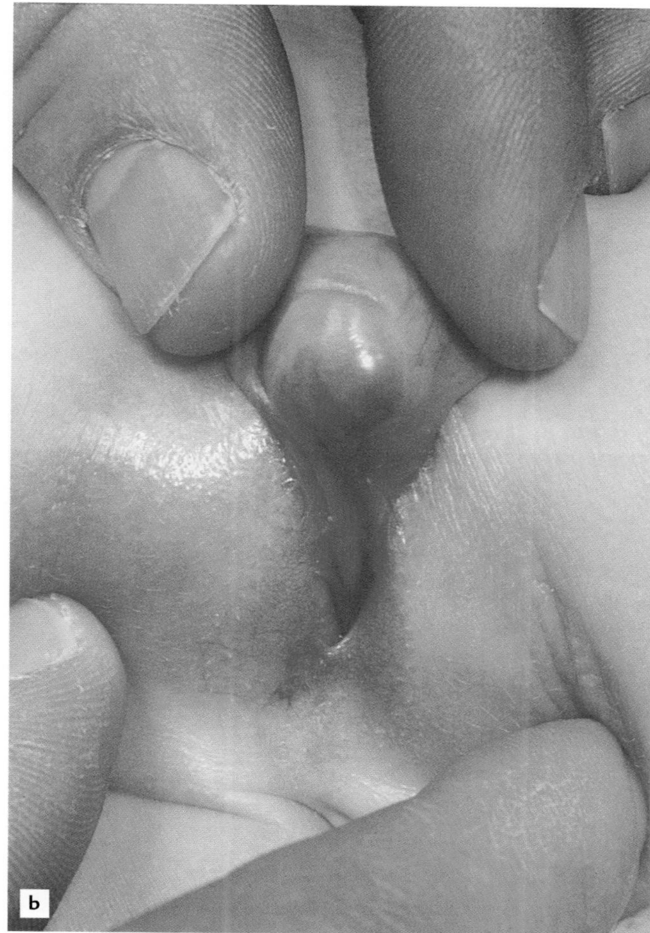

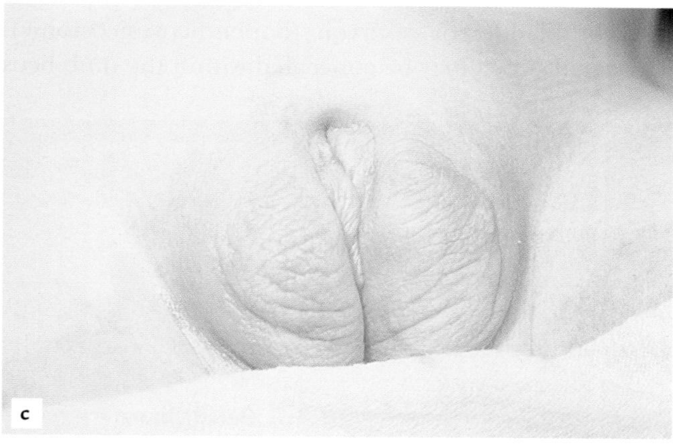

Figure 94.16. *This newborn with ambiguous genitalia, elevated 17-hydro-oxyprogesterone and XX chromosomes was diagnosed with congenital adrenal hyperplasia (21-hydroxylase deficiency): (a) preoperative appearance showing phallic structure and non-palpable gonads; (b) prominent scrotal folds and clitoromegaly; (c) appearance 6 months after reduction clitoroplasty and scrotoplasty.*

have undergone prepubertal orchidectomy, which is the standard treatment when the diagnosis is made.

Vaginal agenesis and the Mayer–Rokitansky syndrome

Agenesis of the vagina in genetic females (Fig. 94.17) may be accompanied by various other defects in the genitourinary tract. Most patients present in adolescence with amenorrhea or pain, but this condition may also present in young girls with urinary tract infection or hydrocolpos. Genital defects range from vaginal agenesis alone to agenesis of the uterus and fallopian tubes. These genital defects are associated with (ipsilateral) renal agenesis.[12] Some patients present after having urethral intercourse and stress urinary incontinence. Treatment of the Mayer–Rokitansky syndrome includes vaginoplasty or neovaginal reconstruction with bowel.

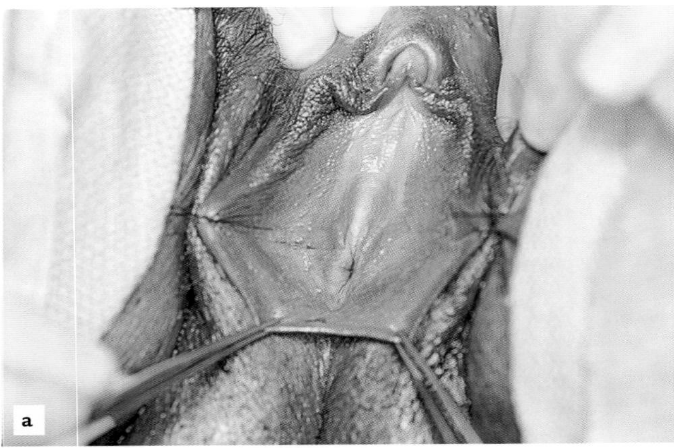

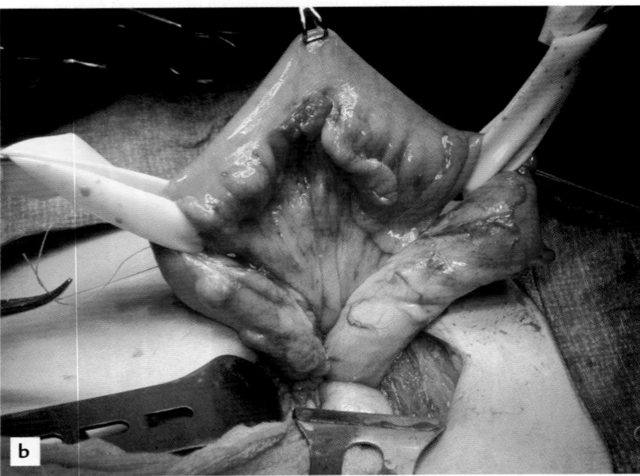

Figure 94.17. *(a) Vaginal agenesis in a 16-year-old with Mayer–Rokitansky syndrome. The sexually active patient engaged in urethral coitus. (b) The sigmoid colon (8–10 cm) is isolated on its mesentery and will be mobilized to the vaginal introitus to create a neovagina. The colonic mucus allows for natural lubrication during coitus.*

URINARY TRACT RECONSTRUCTION

Lower urinary tract reconstruction

Since 1950, bowel segments have been used to replace entirely a diseased or dysfunctional bladder. The current success in reconstruction of the lower urinary tract reflects our improved understanding of the physiologic principles involved in bladder and urethral function.[13–18] Spontaneous voiding can occasionally be achieved with a quite abnormal lower urinary tract. This, of course, is provided that the pressure gradient between the bladder and distal urethra is low. It follows, then, that even in cases where the bladder is replaced in part (intestinal cystoplasty) or entirely (neobladder), patients may still be able to empty their bladders satisfactorily. Many patients require bladder neck reconstruction[19] to achieve continence and most will require CIC.[20]

Continent reconstruction of the lower urinary tract is often desired in the face of congenital or acquired anomalies of both the outlet and the bladder. Much of the principles and background of continent reconstruction is derived from experience with undiversion. The early work of Hendren, Mitrofanoff and others has led to surgical approaches that produce both better reservoir function and a continent outlet.[21]

Continent urinary diversion encompasses three interrelated but independently functioning components. These include a channel by which urine is conducted to the skin, a reservoir or pouch, and a mechanism by which continence is achieved.[22] A host of tissues are available to the reconstructive surgeon (Table 94.4).

The flap valve principle for continence dictates that a portion of the continence channel be fixed on the inner wall of the reservoir. This is the same principle by which ureteral tunneling in the bladder muscle prevents reflux during voiding. In general, a 5:1 length-to-diameter ratio of the continence structure is required. This is the case whether the structure is ureter, ileum or appendix.

The Mitrofanoff principle of continent reconstruction describes a supple catheterizable structure (ureter, appendix, etc.) implanted into the inner wall of the reservoir to create a flap valve continence mechanism.[23] The most popular form of flap valve construction for urinary continence is the use of appendix implanted into the bladder or reservoir (appendicovesicostomy). The small stoma may be concealed within the umbilicus

Table 94.4. *Tissues available for lower urinary tract reconstruction**

External conduit	Urinary reservoir	Continence mechanism
Appendix	Bladder	Anal sphincter
Fallopian tube	Cecum	Artificial urinary sphincter
Ileum	Colon	Benchekroun (hydraulic valve)
Ileal tube	Ileum	Ileocecal valve
Skin tube	Rectum	Koch (nipple valve)
Stomach	Stomach	Mitrofanoff (flap valve)
Urethra		Urethral sphincter
Ureter		

In general, three components are required for continent diversion: 1) conduit from the reservoir to the skin; 2) a pouch or reservoir; and 3) a mechanism by which continence is attained.

(Fig. 94.18). Assurance of complete bladder emptying is essential, as this type of continence channel is very effective in its ability to withstand very high intraluminal pressure. In the non-compliant patient, pouch rupture or upper tract injury may result from failure to empty the reservoir regularly.

Urinary tract reconstruction and pregnancy

Future pregnancy must be kept in mind when reconstructing the genitourinary tract. Pregnancy may be complicated and requires care by both the obstetrician and urologist. Renal obstruction and incontinence may result as the uterus enlarges. Neobladder reconstruction has a good outcome, but chronic bacteriuria is frequent and occasionally requires an indwelling catheter in the third trimester.[24] Similarly, when suprapubic catheterizable continent stomas have been constructed, indwelling catheterization through the stoma during the third trimester may be needed to avoid serious urinary tract infections.[25]

Successful pregnancies and deliveries have been reported after both continent and loop urinary diversions.[26–28] The mode of delivery should be guided by obstetric indications,[27] although vaginal delivery has been successful in the majority of cases. Alternatively, if the bladder neck has been reconstructed it is usually advisable for delivery to be by cesarean section to avoid damage to the bladder neck reconstruction. The urologist should be available to the obstetric team for consultation if cesarean section is deemed necessary, especially if a bladder augmentation with bowel has been carried out, in order to avoid injury to the vascular pedicle to the bowel segment.

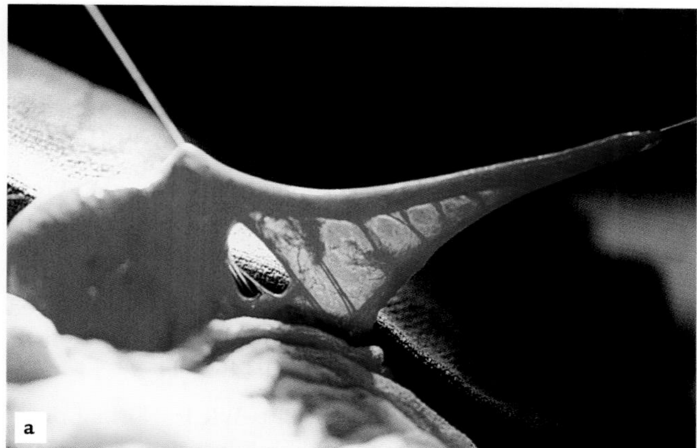

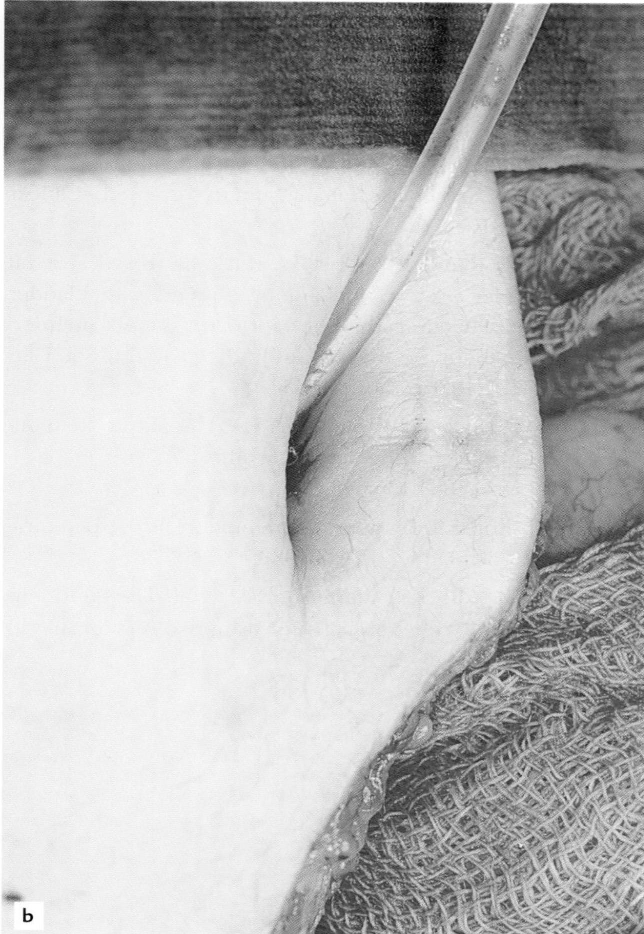

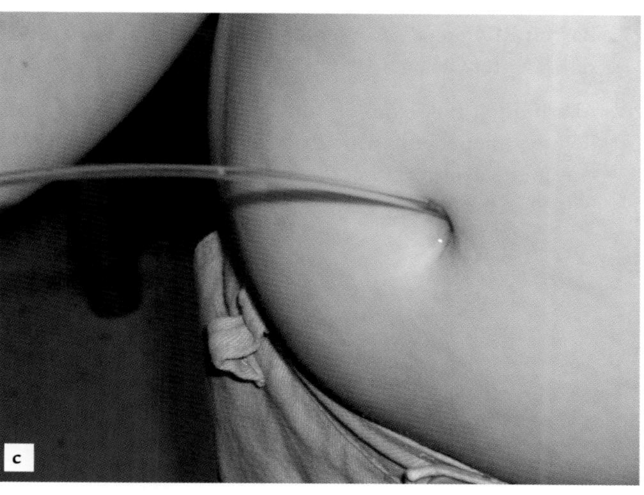

Figure 94.18. *In the Mitrofanoff procedure, the appendix is mobilized with its blood supply as illustrated in (a) and reimplanted into the bladder in a tunneled non-refluxing fashion. The proximal appendix may be brought out to the umbilicus for clean intermittent catheterization (b). Same patient 2 years after appendicovesicostomy performing self-catheterization (c).*

REFERENCES

1. Marshall FF. Embryology of the lower genitourinary tract. Urol Clin North Am 1978;5:3–15.
2. Stephens FD, Smith ED, Hutson JM. Congenital Abnormalities of the Urinary and Genital Tracts. Oxford: Isis Medical Media, 1996.
3. Miller FJW. Children who wet the bed. In: Kolvin I, MacKeith RC, Meadow SR (eds) Bladder Control and Enuresis. London: Heinemann Medical Books, 1973; 47–52.
4. Scott JE, Deegan S. Management of neuropathic urinary incontinence in children by intermittent catheterization. Arch Dis Child 1982;57:253–8.
5. McGuire EJ, Woodside JR, Borden TA et al. Prognostic value of urodynamic testing in myelodysplastic patients. J Urol 1981;126:205–9.
6. Geahart JP, Peppas DS, Jeffs RD. Complete genitourinary reconstruction in female epispadias. J Urol 1993;149: 1110–3.
7. Mollard P, Basset T, Mure PY. Female epispadias. J Urol 1997;158:1543–6.
8. Mandell J, Colodny AH, Lebowitz R et al. Ureteroceles in infants and children. J Urol 1980;123:921–6.
9. Jerkins GR, Verheeck K, Noe HN. Treatment of girls with urethral prolapse. J Urol 1984;132:732–3.
10. Hays DM. Pelvic rhabdomyosarcomas in childhood: diagnosis and concepts of management reviewed. Cancer 1980;45:1810–4.
11. Hays DM, Raney RB, Crist W et al. Improved survival and bladder preservation among patients with bladder – prostate rhabdomyosarcoma primary tumors in Intergroup Rhabdomyosarcoma Study III. Proc Am Soc Clin Oncol 1991;10:318 (abstract 1119).
12. Tarry WF, Duckett JW, Stephens FD. The Mayer–Rokitansky syndrome: pathogenesis, classification and management. J Urol 1986,136:648–57.
13. Kass EJ, Koff SA. Bladder augmentation in the pediatric neuropathic bladder. J Urol 1983;129:552–5.
14. Koch NG, Norlen L, Phillipson BM et al. The continent ileal reservoir (Koch pouch) for urinary diversion. World J Urol 1985;3:146–51.
15. Koff SA. Guidelines to determine the size and shape of intestinal segments used for reconstruction. J Urol 1988;140:1150–1.
16. Hinman F Jr. Selection of intestinal segments for bladder substitution: physical and physiological characteristics. J Urol 1988;139:519–23.
17. McDougal WS. Metabolic complications of urinary intestinal diversion. J Urol 1992;147:1199–1208.
18. Hall MC, Koch MO, McDougal WS. Metabolic consequences of urinary diversion through intestinal segment. Urol Clin North Am 1991;18:725–35.
19. Kropp KA, Angwafo FF. Urethral lengthening and reimplantation for neurogenic incontinence in children. J Urol 1986;135:533–6.
20. Lapides J, Dionko AC, Silber SJ et al. Clean intermittent catheterization in the treatment of urinary tract disease. J Urol 1972;107:458–61.
21. Hendren WH. Urinary tract refunctionalization after long-term diversion. Ann Surg 1990;212:478–95.
22. Kirsch AJ, Snyder HM. Trends in continent reconstruction of the lower urinary tract. Contemp Urol 1997;9:61–9.
23. Duckett JW, Snyder HM. Use of the Mitrofanoff principle in urinary reconstruction. World J Urol 1985;3:191–3.
24. Creagh TA, McInerney PD, Thomas PJ, Mundy AR. Pregnancy after lower urinary tract reconstruction in women. J Urol 1995,154:1323–4.
25. Hatch TR, Steinberg RW, Davis LE. Successful term delivery by Cesarean section in a patient with a continent ileocecal urinary reservoir. J Urol 1991:146:1111–2.
26. Greenberg M, Vaughan ED Jr, Pitts WR Jr. Normal pregnancy and delivery after ileal conduit urinary diversion. J Urol 1981;125:172–3.
27. Barrett RJ, Peters WA. Pregnancy following urinary diversion. Obstet Gynecol 1983;62:582–6.
28. Akerlund S, Bokstrom H, Jonson O et al. Pregnancy and delivery in patients with urinary diversion through the continent ileal reservoir. Surg Gynecol Obstet 1991;173: 350–2.

95

Complications of surgery for stress incontinence

Walter Artibani, Maria Angela Cerruto, Giacomo Novara

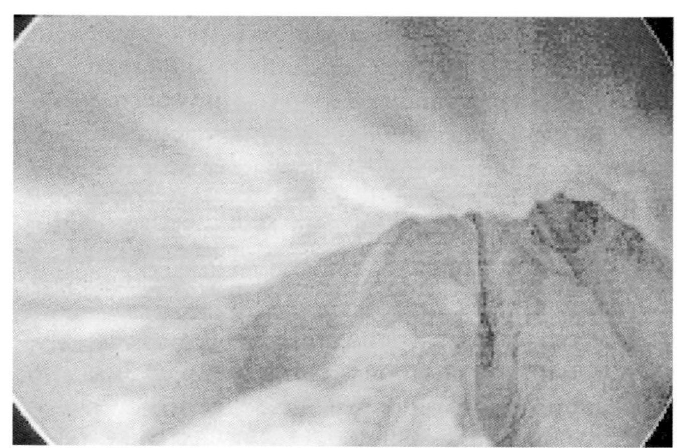

INTRODUCTION

There are two main types of treatment available for women with stress urinary incontinence (SUI): conservative (lifestyle interventions, treatments aimed at improving pelvic floor muscle outcomes, and drugs) and surgical. When conservative therapy fails, or in cases of severe SUI, surgery might be effective in improving this condition. Several surgical procedures have been described in the literature – indicating that none is entirely satisfactory. The main surgical interventions currently available with increasing invasiveness, efficacy, and complications are:

- periurethral or transurethral bulking injections;
- anterior colporrhaphy;
- needle suspensions (Pereyra, Stamey, and Raz procedures);
- sling procedures (classic sling and tension-free vaginal tape procedures);
- open and laparoscopic colposuspensions;
- artificial urinary sphincter (AMS 800).

The choice of surgical procedure should depend on the cause of SUI – bladder neck/urethral hypermobility (UH) and/or intrinsic sphincter deficiency (ISD) – and the assessment of postoperative outcomes should be based on the patient's clinical symptoms and signs, urodynamic evaluation, and short- and long-term results as well as immediate and delayed complications.

COMPLICATIONS OF SUI SURGERY

Chaliha and Stanton[1] comprehensively reviewed the literature on the complications of surgery for genuine stress incontinence. They identified studies assessing outcome by means of both an electronic and a hand search of the Medline Database from 1966 to 1997 of all English language articles, including randomized controlled trials, non-randomized trials, prospective and retrospective cohort studies, and case-control studies. A recently published French paper gave an exhaustive literature review up to 2003.[2]

SUI surgery consequences and complications may be conveniently classified as follows:

- immediate complications (within 24 hours);
- short-term complications (24 hours to 6 weeks);
- long-term complications (6 weeks onwards);
- impact on quality of life (QoL).

Immediate complications

Significant bleeding

A severe hemorrhage needing a transfusion may occur after a direct lesion of the perivesical venous plexus during different surgical procedures accessing the space of Retzius. The mean bleeding volume during colporrhaphy is 200 ml,[3] and 260 ml during Burch colposuspension.[4–6] No significant difference has been found between primary and secondary Burch colposuspension in terms of bleeding.[4] Only one case of massive hemorrhage in a series of 180 Burch colposuspensions has been reported.[5] The amount of perioperative bleeding after laparoscopic colposuspension is usually very low.[4,7,8] After a Marshall–Marchetti–Kranz (MMK) procedure the mean bleeding volume is 142 ml (range 20–500 ml)[9–11] and after needle suspension is 53 ml (range 10–150 ml).[12–14] After a polytetrafluoroethylene (Teflon) suburethral sling procedure the mean bleeding volume is 153 ml.[15]

A severe hemorrhage needing surgical drainage has been reported in up to 2.1% of cases after pubovaginal sling procedures.[16–20] Bleeding after a tension-free vaginal tape (TVT) procedure usually originates from veins of the pelvic floor or epigastric vessels. A perioperative hemorrhage after TVT may occur in 0.5–17% of cases,[21–27] and lesions of the iliac vessels, although very uncommon, have been reported.[24,28–30] A retrospective study[26] on 241 women having a previous TVT at six Canadian institutions detected a blood loss >500 ml in six patients (2.5%), none requiring transfusion. These data are consistent with those in the literature.[23,31–33]

Operative complications following transobturator suburethral tape (TOT) procedures are very few, and significant bleeding is rare.[34] Hematomas in the space of Retzius range from 0.2 to 2% after direct colposuspension,[9,12] and from 5 to 7% after needle colposuspension.[9,13,14] This complication has been reported in less than 2% of cases after TVT,[35,36] and very few cases needed surgical drainage.[23,26,29] Abouassaly et al. reported pelvic hematomas in four patients (1.9%), often diagnosed when retention was accompanied by prolonged suprapubic or pelvic pain.[26] Table 95.1 shows an overview of significant bleeding rates following SUI surgery.

Case: Two weeks after a TVT procedure performed for stress urinary incontinence in a different hospital, a 58-year-patient arrived at our outpatient clinic complaining of lower abdominal pain, which had started 3 days after surgery. The severity of the symptom required the use of an oral non-steroidal anti-inflammatory drug. At physical examination, the lower abdomen was tender and

Table 95.1. ***Significant bleeding following stress urinary incontinence surgery***

Complication	Authors	Operation	No. of patients treated	No. of complications (%)
Significant bleeding	Van Geelen et al.[3]	Anterior colporrhaphy	56	2 (3.6)
	Alcalay et al.[4]	Burch	109	8 (7.3)
	Stanton & Cardozo[5]	Burch	180	1 (0.6)
	Wee et al.[6]	Burch	99	3 (3)
	Green et al.[9]	MMK	21	2 (10)
	Riggs[10]	MMK	490	10 (2)
	Mainprize & Drutz[11]	MMK	2712	7 (0.3)
	Peattie & Stanton[13]	Needle suspension	44	3 (6.8)
	Varner[14]	Needle suspension	20	2 (10)
	Morgan et al.[16]	Sling	281	6 (2.1)
	Amundsen et al.[17]	Sling	104	1 (0.9)
	Young et al.[18]	Sling	200	3 (1.5)
	Carbone et al.[19]	Sling + bone anchor	70	1 (1.4)
	Crivellaro et al.[20]	Sling + bone anchor	253	3 (1.3)
	Wang & Lo[22]	TVT	70	11 (16)
	Meschia et al.[23]	TVT	404	2 (0.5)
	Ward & Hilton[24]	TVT	170	3 (1.7)
	Levin et al.[25]	TVT	313	4 (1.3)
	Abouassaly et al.[26]	TVT	241	6 (2.5)
	Rafii et al.[27]	TVT ± other procedures	186	2 (1)
	Krauth et al.[34]	TOT	604	7 (1.1)

MMK, Marshall–Marchetti–Kranz; TOT, transobturator suburethral tape; TVT, tension-free vaginal tape.

painful. Mild lower urinary tract symptoms of the filling phase were elicited. No other symptoms were present. On general practitioner request, the patient had undergone an abdominal ultrasound scan 7 days previously, which showed a 6 cm round liquid lesion in the Retzius space. A further ultrasound scan was immediately performed, which demonstrated the enlargement of the pelvic lesion up to 12 cm in diameter. Hemoglobin was 9.5 g/dl but the patient was hemodynamically stable. A contrast CT scan was immediately carried out, which confirmed the presence of a large pelvic hematoma in the space of Retzius, dislodging the bladder posteriorly, without any contrast leakage, even in the late scans (Fig. 95.1).

Once the available therapeutic options were explained, surgical drainage of the hematoma was performed. Through a midline infraumbilical prepubic incision, a large hematoma of the space of Retzius was drained, evacuating more than 800 ml of clots and blood. No source of active bleeding was found. The postoperative course was uneventful and the patient was discharged on the fourth postoperative day. The 2-month follow-up ultrasound scan was normal, and the patient remained continent and free of symptoms.

Urinary tract injuries

A bladder lesion may occur during colposuspension, sling, and TVT procedures[5,6,9,11,13,20,22–27,31,37–40] (Table 95.2). Lower urinary tract (LUT) injuries have been reported in 1–7% of cases after needle colposuspensions,[9,13,41,42] and in 6.3% of cases after slings.[38] Bladder perforation by TVT trocars is a common intraoperative complication reported in 0.8–21% of cases.[22,35,36,39,43–46] To avoid

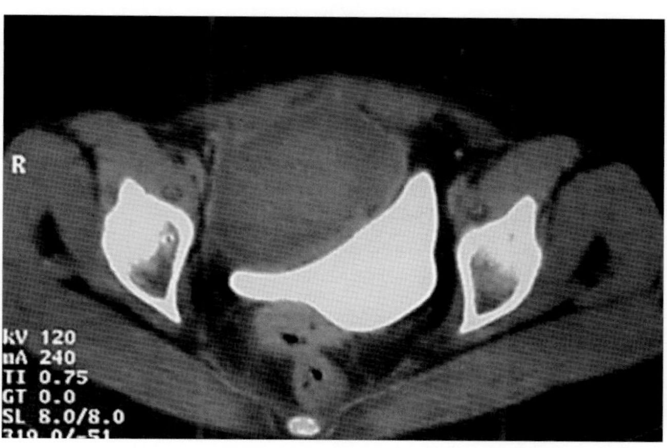

Figure 95.1. *CT scan of a large pelvic hematoma in the space of Retzius.*

intravesical misplacement of the tape, a careful cystoscopic examination must be performed to exclude any violation of the bladder mucosa. If any sign of bladder perforation is evident, correcting trocar placement is mandatory, prolonging catheter drainage for at least 3 days.[45]

When a primary bladder lesion has been missed, resulting in transvesical or submucosal tape placement with a secondary erosion, there is no possibility of correcting the position of the tape and it must be removed surgically. A synthetic suture or tape running through the bladder may promote bladder stone formation, recurrent urinary tract infections (UTIs), and severe voiding LUT symptoms.[47–50] Abouassaly et al. reported 14/241 (5.8%) cases of bladder perforation during TVT.[26]

Bladder and urethral lesions after Burch colposuspension have been reported in up to 6% of cases;[3,5,37] misdiagnosis of such lesions may lead to a urethrovaginal fistula.[51] In about 1% of cases it is possible to detect an underestimated ureteral lesion after this procedure.[9]

Laparoscopy implies a higher risk of LUT injury, occurring in up to 10% of cases.[7,52,53] After AMS 800 implant, urethral as well as anterior and posterior cervical lesions may be found in 3.7%, 11%, and 3.7% of cases, respectively.[54]

Visceral injuries

Before the advent of TVT, intestinal perforations were exceptional and usually occurred after suprapubic catheterization used during SUI surgery.[55–57] To date, approximately 15 cases of bowel perforation after TVT have been reported to the manufacturer, and only a few cases have been reported in the literature[31,58–62] (see Table 95.2). Potential predisposing risk factors for intestinal injury include previous intraperitoneal and retroperitoneal surgery, and abnormal bowel adhesion to the bladder and pelvic peritoneum. A case of small intestine erosion by AMS 800 reservoir tubing has been recently reported.[63]

Complications due to intraoperative patient position

A prolonged gynecologic position (>3 hours) may be responsible for a compartment syndrome. Protracted

Table 95.2. *Urinary tract and visceral injury during stress urinary incontinence surgery*

Complications	Authors	Operation	No. of patients treated	No. of complications (%)
Urinary tract injury	Green et al.[9]	Needle suspension	29	1 (3.4)
	Peattie & Stanton[13]	Needle suspension	44	1 (2)
	Stanton & Cardozo[5]	Burch	180	2 (1.1)
	Pow-Sang et al.[37]	Burch	38	2 (5.3)
	Van Geelen et al.[3]	Burch	34	1 (2.9)
	Wee et al.[6]	Burch	99	1 (1)
	Ward et al.[24]	Colposuspension	146	3 (2)
	Mainprize & Drutz[11]	MMK	2712	34 (1.3)
	Summitt et al.[38]	Sling	48	3 (6.3)
	Crivellaro et al.[20]	Sling + bone anchor	253	5 (2.1)
	Wang & Lo[22]	TVT	70	3 (4.3)
	Soulie et al.[39]	TVT	52	6 (11.5)
	Nilsson & Kuuva[31]	TVT	161	6 (3.7)
	Meschia et al.[23]	TVT	404	24 (6)
	Ward & Hilton[24]	TVT	170	20 (11.7)
	Tsivian et al.[40]	TVT	55	4 (7.3)
	Abouassaly et al.[26]	TVT	241	14 (5.8)
	Levin et al.[25]	TVT	313	313
	Rafii et al.[27]	TVT ± other procedures	186	18 (9.6)
	Krauth et al.[34]	TOT	604	15 (2.5)
Visceral injury	Peyrat et al.[58]	TVT	N/A	1
	Meschia et al.[59]	TVT	N/A	1
	Leboeuf et al.[60]	TVT	N/A	1
	Amna et al.[61]	TVT	N/A	1
	Castillo et al.[62]	TVT	N/A	1
	Yuan et al.[63]	Artificial sphincter	N/A	1
	Crivellaro et al.[20]	Sling + bone anchor	253	2 (0.9)

MMK, Marshall–Marchetti–Kranz; N/A, not applicable; TOT, transobturator suburethral tape; TVT, tension-free vaginal tape.

extrinsic lower limb compression could be responsible for impaired microcirculation with consequent edema compressing the nerves and affecting lower limb function. The involved nerves include the femoral, sciatic, and external sciatic–popliteus. Whenever a compartment syndrome is suspected, immediate treatment with long-lasting physiotherapy is mandatory.[64,65]

Short-term complications

Infections

Overall infections have been reported in up to 13% of cases after anterior colporrhaphy,[66] in up to 7% of infections after periurethral injection therapy,[67] and in 1–10% after retropubic colposuspension[5,6,12,24,66–68] (Table 95.3). Synthetic tapes increase the risk of infection, with sling erosion rates of up to 21% being reported.[69–74]

Osteomyelitis is the most feared complication of bone anchor procedures.[75] This complication requires removal of the anchor and prolonged antibiotics. Leach[76] reported five cases of infected anchor removal after implantation of 7000 anchors. Schultheiss et al.[77] described the removal of two anchors after a Vesica procedure: one for infection and one for a painful granuloma. From 1994 to 1998 there were eight confirmed cases of osteomyelitis in over 30,000 Boston Scientific anchors placed via the suprapubic route.[78]

Infections arising after periurethral and/or transurethral injection therapy may result in abscesses and granuloma formation.[79] Infections after AMS 800 implant may occur in up to 9.5% of cases.[80,81] The risk of postoperative UTIs after TVT ranges from 3.9 to 22%.[24,82] The incidence of postoperative UTIs is directly related with modality and duration of bladder drainage used to resolve bladder emptying problems.[83] A prolonged indwelling catheter is associated with a high risk of bacteriuria,[84] which increases by 6–7.5% per day with time.[85] Hence, to drain the bladder postoperatively, intermittent (self)-catheterization [I(S)C] appears to be more suitable, having less morbidity.[84]

Osteitis pubis

Osteitis pubis is a non-infectious, painful, inflammatory condition affecting periosteum, cartilage, and ligaments of the symphysis pubis, which may worsen in osteomyelitis. Its symptoms include severe pelvic pain, a tender suprapubic area, and a waddling gait. Its incidence is difficult to ascertain because of a lack of consensus about its definition. Its treatments range from conservative to aggressive, including anti-inflammatory agents, body-cast immobili-

Table 95.3. *Short-term complications of surgery for stress urinary incontinence (excluding transient voiding dysfunction)*

Complications	Authors	Operation	No. of patients treated	No. of complications (%)
Infections	Peters & Thornton[66]	Anterior colporrhaphy	294	38 (12.9)
	Muznai et al.[67]	Periurethral injections	98	7 (7.1)
	Lotenfoe et al.[68]	Needle suspension	27	1 (3.7)
	Stanton & Cardozo[5]	Burch	180	1 (0.6)
	Wee et al.[6]	Burch	99	2 (2)
	Ward & Hilton[24]	Colposuspension	146	10 (6.8)
	Peters & Thornton[66]	MMK	102	10 (9.8)
	Bryans[69]	Sling	69	4 (5.8)
	Beck et al.[70]	Sling	170	8 (4.7)
	Young et al.[18]	Sling	200	5 (2.5)
	Crivellaro et al.[20]	Sling + bone anchor	253	1 (0.8)
	Ward & Hilton[24]	TVT	241	1 (0.4)
	Abouassaly et al.[26]	TVT	170	4 (2.3)
Osteitis pubis	Green et al.[9]	Needle suspension	29	1 (3.4)
	Mainprize & Drutz[11]	MMK	2712	68 (2.5)
	Goldberg et al.[87]	Anchor suspension	225	3 (1.3)
Urogenital fistulae	Beck et al.[89]	Anterior colporrhaphy	519	2 (0.4)
	Guam et al.[90]	Needle suspension	60	1 (1.7)
	Mainprize & Drutz[11]	MMK	2712	7 (0.3)
	Kersey[91]	Sling	105	1 (0.9)
Nerve injury	Miyazaki & Shook[93]	Needle suspension	402	7 (1.7)
	Young et al.[18]	Sling	200	1 (0.5)
	Meschia et al.[23]	TVT	404	1 (0.2)

MMK, Marshall–Marchetti–Kranz; TVT, tension-free vaginal tape.

zation, surgical debridement, and pubectomy.[86] Its natural course usually leads to spontaneous recovery, with operative procedures needed in only 5–10% of cases.

Osteitis pubis represents the fourth major complication following MMK colposuspension and 2.5% of all complications after such a procedure.[11] It has been reported in 3.4% of cases after needle suspension,[9] and in up to 1.3% after bladder neck suspension using bone anchors, culminating in osteomyelitis.[87] Only one case of pubic osteitis after periurethral collagen injection has been reported in the literature.[88]

A possible explanation for this complication is nicking of the pubic periosteum during blind periurethral injection, followed by subperiosteal collagen migration initiating an acute inflammatory reaction and venous obstruction of the pubic bone.

Urogenital fistulae

A urogenital fistula is an uncommon complication of SUI surgery, usually occurring within the first 10 days after the operation. It may arise primarily as a result of infection or secondary to the erosion of synthetic material placed on a mistaken or poorly repaired lesion. It has been reported in 0.4% of cases after anterior colporrhaphy,[89] in 0.3% after MMK procedure,[11] and in 2% after needle suspension.[90] A case of vesicovaginal fistula (1%) has been reported by Kersey in a series of 105 patients who previously underwent sling procedures.[91] Figure 95.2 shows a case of urethrovaginal fistula after removal of an infected heterologous sling.

Nerve injuries

Femoral nerve injury may occur indirectly due to the abduction and flexion of the thigh in the lithotomy position during SUI surgery. After needle suspension the following nerves may be involved: common peroneal, sciatic, obturator, femoral, saphenous, and ilioinguinal.[92] Seven cases of ilioinguinal nerve entrapment following 402 needle suspension procedures have been described,[93] two of which were treated successfully with suture removal. Theoretically, the incidence of nerve entrapment should be minimal with anchor placement, as the anchor allows for more stable fixation medially on the pubic bone. To date, transvaginal placement of the anchors has not been associated with nerve entrapment.[75] Few cases of nerve injury have been described after TVT[23] or sling procedures.[18]

Transient voiding dysfunction

A potential complication of all anti-incontinence procedures is iatrogenic outlet obstruction leading to voiding dysfunction. This may result in voiding symptoms with partial or total urinary retention, recurrent UTIs, or in severe storage symptoms such as frequency, urgency, and urge incontinence.

In the early postoperative course, transient urinary retention occurred in up to 19.7% of patients after a TVT procedure,[26] and in up to 100% after colposuspension.[24] After resolution of postoperative edema and pain, temporary bladder drainage with I(S)C allows normal voiding to be regained. In patients who do not improve, conservative modalities such as prolonged I(S)C and pharmacologic therapy may be tried. If symptoms persist, surgical intervention may be required. Table 95.4 shows a literature overview of transient voiding dysfunction rates after SUI surgery.[6,11,19,20,24,26,27,34,39,71,89,92,94–96]

Long-term complications

Persistent voiding dysfunction

The incidence of permanent obstruction, urinary retention and/or voiding dysfunction after anti-incontinence procedures varies from 2.3 to 25%.[4,17–20,23–28,31,40,96–102] This variability depends on the different definitions of urinary

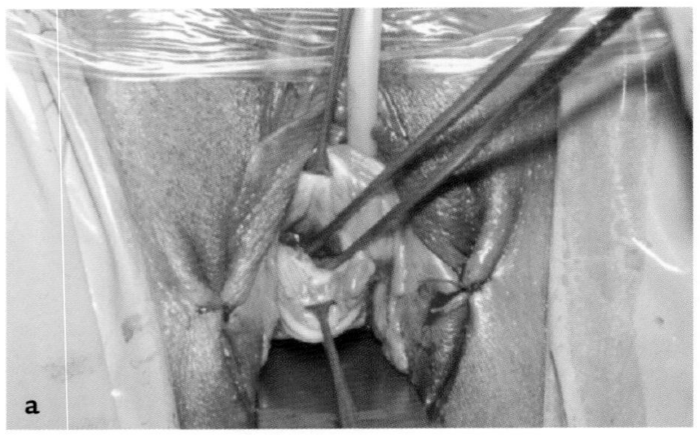

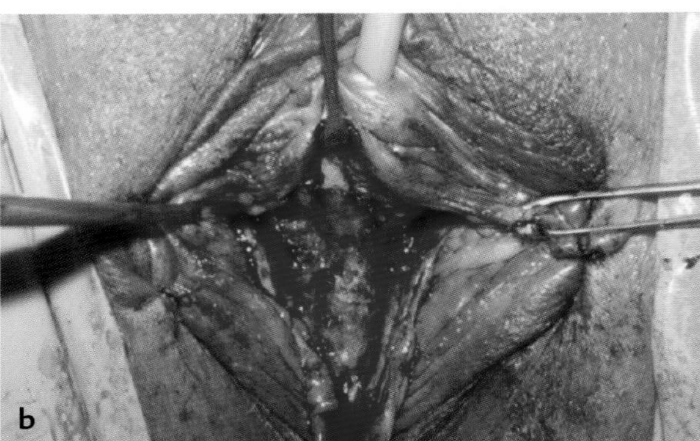

Figure 95.2. *(a) Urethral erosion due to an infected heterologous sling; (b) appearance of urethrovaginal fistula after sling removal.*

Table 95.4. *Transient voiding dysfunction after stress urinary incontinence surgery*

Complication	Authors	Operation	No. of patients treated	No. of complications (%)
Transient voiding dysfunction	Beck et al.[89]	Anterior colporrhaphy	519	3 (0.6)
	Karram et al.[92]	Needle suspension	93	14 (15)
	Galloway et al.[94]	Burch	50	8 (16)
	Lose et al.[95]	Burch	80	20 (25)
	Wee et al.[6]	Burch	99	13 (13.1)
	Ward & Hilton[24]	Colposuspension	146	146 (100)
	Mainprize & Drutz[11]	MMK	2712	98 (3.6)
	Chin & Stanton[71]	Sling	88	2 (2.3)
	Crivellaro et al.[20]	Sling + bone anchor	253	20 (8.5)
	Carbone et al.[19]	Sling + bone anchor	70	10 (14)
	Soulie et al.[39]	TVT	52	9 (17)
	Ward & Hilton[24]	TVT	170	64 (38)
	Abouassaly et al.[26]	TVT	241	47 (19.7)
	Rafii et al.[27]	TVT ± other procedures	186	30 (16)
	Delorme et al.[96]	TOT	32	6 (18.7)
	Krauth et al.[34]	TOT	604	17 (2.8)

MMK, Marshall–Marchetti–Kranz; TOT, transobturator suburethral tape; TVT, tension-free vaginal tape.

retention. There is a lack of consensus in the literature regarding the appropriate evaluation and management of this distressing problem.[103] Specific diagnosis is often difficult, and its management represents a challenge for specialists.

Persistent urinary retention is uncommon after injectable therapy. Voiding dysfunction rates vary from 5 to 7% after needle suspension,[12] 4–10% after pubovaginal slings,[104] 2–4% after TVT,[101] 5–20% following a MMK procedure,[105,106] and 4–22% following Burch colposuspension.[107] The incidence of voiding dysfunction after bone anchor procedures is minimal, and almost all series showed a low incidence of prolonged urinary retention[19,75,77] (Table 95.5).

Table 95.5. *Long-term complications of surgery for stress urinary incontinence (persistent voiding dysfunction and recurrent urinary tract infections)*

Complications	Authors	Operation	No. of patients treated	No. of complications (%)
Persistent voiding dysfunction	Ward & Hilton[24]	Colposuspension	146	11 (8)
	Amundsen et al.[17]	Sling	91	1 (1)
	Young et al.[18]	Sling	200	7 (3.5)
	Arunkalaivanan & Barrington[97]	Sling	74	11 (1.4)
	Carbone et al.[19]	Sling + bone anchor	70	9 (12.8)
	Crivellaro et al.[20]	Sling + bone anchor	253	5 (2.1)
	Meschia et al.[23]	TVT	404	16 (4)
	Nilsson & Kuuva[31]	TVT	161	7 (4.3)
	Ward & Hilton[24]	TVT	146	5 (3)
	Arunkalaivanan & Barrington[97]	TVT	68	23 (3.4)
	Tsivian et al.[40]	TVT	55	2 (3.6)
	Abouassaly et al.[26]	TVT	241	10 (4.1)
	Levin et al.[25]	TVT	313	20 (8.3)
	Rafii et al.[27]	TVT ± other procedures	186	7 (3.7)
	Delorme et al.[96]	TOT	32	5 (15.6)
Recurrent urinary tract infections	Nilsson & Kuuva[31]	Colposuspension	161	10 (6.1)
	Ward & Hilton[24]	TVT	170	38 (22.3)
	Ward & Hilton[24]	TVT	146	46 (31.5)
	Levin et al.[25]	TVT	313	2 (0.6)

TOT, transobturator suburethral tape; TVT, tension-free vaginal tape.

Surgical relief of voiding dysfunction may be accomplished by two main surgical approaches: transvaginal and transabdominal. There is no universal consensus as to which technique is better, but most surgeons prefer the transvaginal approach because of its lower morbidity. Foster and McGuire[108] reported that success rates following traditional urethrolysis varied according to the prior anti-incontinence procedure. Prior retropubic urethropexy had the highest success rate (71%), followed by needle suspension (63%), and pubovaginal sling (50%). The lowest success rates in the sling group can be attributed to the traditional urethrolysis technique, leaving the sling intact. More recently, surgeons preferred cutting or lyzing slings in the midline to improve the urethrolysis success rate.[109] Klutke et al.[102] stated that 17/600 patients (2.8%) who developed urinary retention after TVT required tape release; simple TVT release under local anesthesia resulted in normal voiding function in all 17.

In 2000, a survey regarding urethrolysis was mailed or e-mailed to the members of the American Urogynecology Society. Of the 262 respondents, 84% stated that they performed urethrolysis.[103] To evaluate postoperative voiding dysfunction they strongly recommended the following studies: pressure-voiding study (84%), cystoscopy (82%), and urodynamics (79%). Most surgeons chose a vaginal approach to urethrolysis (74%) and a significant number of physicians did not routinely re-suspend the bladder neck following urethrolysis (82%).

Although physical examination, urodynamics, and cystoscopy are crucial in the evaluation of postoperative voiding dysfunction, it may still be difficult to diagnose. The only absolute selection criterion for offering urethrolysis might be a clear temporal relationship of voiding dysfunction following anti-incontinence surgery. Overall, urethrolysis success rates are good, with both transvaginal and transabdominal approaches. Success rates are comparable following transvaginal urethrolysis with (77%) or without (68%) re-suspension of the bladder neck. Moreover, the incidence of postoperative SUI is acceptably low with (4%) or without (5.6%) re-suspension of the urethra following transvaginal urethrolysis.[103]

De novo overactive bladder

Women with SUI show an overactive bladder (OAB) in 30–50% of cases.[110] Treating SUI often means a resolution of OAB.[111,112] Unfortunately, in up to 40% of cases, there is a persistence of OAB after SUI surgery.[113,114]

Persistent OAB complicates 8–25% of all sling procedures performed,[73] 7.6–12% of TVT and 1.4–16.6% of retropubic urethropexy.[4,115,116] Moreover, in 7–21% of

Table 95.6. *Long-term complications of surgery for stress urinary incontinence (de novo overactive bladder)*

Complication	Authors	Operation	No. of patients treated	No. of complications (%)
De novo overactive bladder	Beck et al.[89]	Anterior colporrhaphy	436	28 (6.4)
	Hilton[119]	Needle suspension	10	1 (10)
	Raz et al.[120]	Needle suspension	206	11 (5.3)
	Cardozo et al.[118]	Burch	92	17 (18.4)
	Alcalay et al.[4]	Burch	109	16 (14.7)
	Ward & Hilton[24]	Colposuspension	146	11 (7.5)
	McGuire et al.[121]	Sling	82	5 (6.1)
	Chin, 1995[71]	Sling	80	22 (27.5)
	Amundsen et al.[17]	Sling	91	14 (15)
	Kuo[122]	Sling	50	7 (14)
	Young et al.[18]	Sling	200	12 (8.8)
	Barnes et al.[123]	Sling	38	2 (5.2)
	Arunkalaivanan & Barrington[97]	Sling	74	4 (6)
	Crivellaro et al.[20]	Sling + bone anchor	253	13 (5.5)
	Carbone et al.[19]	Sling + bone anchor	70	3 (4.2)
	Nilsson & Kuuva[31]	TVT	161	5 (3.1)
	Ward & Hilton[24]	TVT	170	10 (5.8)
	Arunkalaivanan & Barrington[97]	TVT	68	4 (9)
	Abouassaly et al.[26]	TVT	241	36 (15)
	Rafii et al.[27]	TVT ± other procedures	186	54 (29)
	Delorme et al.[96]	TOT	32	2 (6.2)
	Krauth et al.[34]	TOT	131	2 (1.5)

TOT, transobturator suburethral tape; TVT, tension-free vaginal tape.

cases a de novo OAB may occur[95,113,117,118] (see also complication rates in Table 95.6). Possible risk factors include misdiagnosed preoperative OAB, bladder wall thickness, bladder neck dissection, patient age, and postoperative cervicourethral obstruction.[117] Voiding dysfunction (2–27%) and de novo OAB (8–27%) are the most frequent complications after both open and laparoscopic colposuspension.[8,24,124,125] Abouassaly et al.[26] reported de novo OAB in 15% of cases after TVT. At 1-year follow-up after TVT, de novo AOB decreased up to 5.9%.[31,99,126]

De novo pelvic organ prolapse

After colposuspension, de novo pelvic organ prolapse (POP) may occur in up to 30% of cases.[4] At a mean follow-up of 9 years, Burch[127] detected enterocele in 8% of cases and cystocele in 3% after colposuspension. At a 5-year follow-up, Wiskind et al.[128] described POP secondary to Burch colposuspension needing reintervention in 26.7% of cases. At a mean follow-up of 17 months after needle suspension, Nitti et al. detected enterocele in 6.5%, rectocele in 3%, and uterine prolapse in 2% of cases.[129] Recently, Neuman[130] found de novo POP after TVT in 0.3% of cases (Table 95.7). A rare case of urethral prolapse has been reported after periurethral Teflon injection.[131]

Sexual dysfunction

Transvaginal SUI surgery may be responsible for sexual activity impairment[132–134] (Table 95.8). Information about this complication is difficult to obtain because 8–13% of women complain of dyspareunia with aging.[139,140] POP seems to negatively affect sexual activity and total sexual function more than SUI. Nevertheless, overall sexual satisfaction depends on both these conditions.[141] A combination of Burch colposuspension and posterior colporrhaphy may be associated with a more frequent occurrence of dyspareunia,[136] but overall sexual function and satisfaction seem to improve or do not change in most women after surgery for either prolapse or urinary incontinence, or both. Although Maaita et al.[142] did not find any significant modification of sexual function and activity after TVT, more recently sexual impairment of 20% (14.5% de novo dyspareunia and 5.4% of libido loss) has been reported following this procedure.[134]

Chronic pain

The incidence of dyspareunia and chronic pain after SUI surgery is difficult to detect because it is rarely reported in the literature (see Table 95.8). Dyspareunia has been reported in 0.4% of cases after a MMK procedure[11] and in up to 4% of cases after Burch colposuspension.[94] The so-called ‘postcolposuspension syndrome’ is characterized by more than 1-year suprapubic or ilioinguinal chronic pain. It has been reported in up to 12% of cases after colposuspension.[94] Only few isolated cases of ‘postcolposuspension syndrome’ after a TVT procedure have been reported in the literature.[143] Recently, persistent suprapubic discomfort after TVT has been reported in up to 7.5% of cases.[26]

Chronic pain after needle suspension may be due to direct nerve binding or to a peri-nervous inflammation secondary to a suture placed too closely to the nerves.[12] Up to 5% of patients who underwent this procedure needed suture ablation to soothe their persistent pain.[144]

Table 95.7. *Long-term complications of surgery for stress urinary incontinence (de novo pelvic organ prolapse)*

Complications	Authors	Operation	No. of patients treated	No. of complications (%)
De novo pelvic organ prolapse	Galloway et al.[94]	Burch	50	4 (8)
	Amundsen et al.[17]	Sling	91	1 (1)
	Neuman[130]	TVT	314	1 (0.3)
Vault/uterine prolapse	Raz et al.[120]	Needle suspension	206	2 (1)
	Neuman[130]	TVT	314	1 (0.3)
Cystocele	Raz et al.[120]	Needle suspension	206	4 (2)
	Neuman[130]	TVT	314	1 (0.3)
Rectocele	Wiskind et al.[128]	Burch	131	29 (22.1)
	Alcalay et al.[4]	Burch	109	28 (25.7)
	Neuman[130]	TVT	314	1 (0.3)
Enterocele	Raz et al.[120]	Needle suspension	206	7 (3)
	Wiskind et al.[128]	Burch	131	29 (22.1)
	Alcalay et al.[4]	Burch	109	5 (4.6)
Urethral prolapse	Kiilholma et al.[131]	Teflon injection	22	1 (4.5)

TVT, tension-free vaginal tape.

Table 95.8. *Long-term complications of surgery for stress urinary incontinence (sexual dysfunction, dyspareunia, and chronic pain)*

Complications	Authors	Operation	No. of patients treated	No. of complications (%)
Sexual dysfunction	Mazouni et al.[134]	TVT	71	4 (5.4)
Dyspareunia	Kursh et al.[135]	Needle suspension	142	1 (0.7)
	Raz et al.[120]	Needle suspension	206	3 (1.5)
	Galloway et al.[94]	Burch	50	2 (4)
	Van Geelen et al.[3]	Burch	34	1 (0.3)
	Weber et al.[136]	Burch + posterior	21	8 (38)
	Mainprize & Drutz[11]	colporrhaphy	2712	10 (0.4)
	Carbone et al.[19]	MMK	70	4 (5.7)
	Crivellaro et al.[20]	Sling + bone anchor	253	20 (7.9)
	Mazouni et al.[134]	Sling + bone anchor	7	10 (14.5)
		TVT		
Chronic pain	Galloway et al.[94]	Burch	50	6 (12)
	Wheelahan[137]	Burch	102	27 (26)
	Griffith-Jones &	Needle suspension	17	1 (5.9)
	Abrams[137]	Needle suspension	206	7 (3.4)
	Raz et al.[120]	TVT	241	18 (7.5)
	Abouassaly et al.[26]	Sling + bone anchor	253	11 (4.7)
	Crivellaro et al.[20]			

TVT, tension-free vaginal tape.

Recurrent urinary tract infections

Pelvic surgery represents one of the main risk factors for recurrent UTIs together with age, menopause, genital and LUT dysfunction and abnormalities, and sexual activity[145] (see Table 95.5). Predisposing conditions include preoperative recurrent UTIs, postoperative chronic retention, voiding dysfunction, and synthetic material erosion. Recurrent UTIs (see rate details in Table 95.4) may also hide other bladder diseases such as stones or tumors that should be investigated.

Complications due to biomaterials

Intraurethral injection therapy is the least invasive surgical procedure for SUI, showing a continuous success rate decline over time. Repeat injections are often required to maintain efficacy, and the surgeon is unable to determine material quantity needed for each patient and the occurrence of side effects when using injection materials (migration, foreign body reaction, immunologic effects).[146,147] Overall, urgency, UTIs, and urinary retention occur to a minimal extent after injectables.

Many different bulking agents are available, including autologous fat, glutaraldehyde cross-linked bovine (GAX) collagen, silicone, carbon beads, microballoons, hyaluronic acid, and dextranomer microspheres. Teflon periurethral injection may elicit a foreign body local reaction, resulting in periurethral abscess or granuloma formation[131,148] (Table 95.9). Moreover, there is a potential risk of particle migration with lymphatic and visceral embolism.[131] For all these reasons Teflon has not achieved universal acceptance and has never been approved by the United States Food and Drug Administration (FDA) for periurethral injections in female patients. Periurethral injections of autologous fat[149] may cause hematomas and ecchymosis at the fat collecting site. Less than 1% of the patients reported pain or hematoma formation at the injection site.[150]

Glutaraldehyde cross-linked collagen is a sterile non-pyrogenic material dispersed in a phosphate-buffered physiologic saline. This cross-linking process increases the time before degradation takes place and reduces its immunogenic potential.[150] This material should not elicit any foreign body local inflammation, and only one case of distal migration of collagen along the urethra has been reported, creating a periurethral pseudocyst.[151] Adverse reactions and complications from this procedure are rare. The most important immediate complication of collagen is the risk of allergic reaction due to pre-existing hypersensitivity to collagen, seen in 1–4% of patients.[150] To select suitable patients, it is advisable to perform an intradermic injection of collagen 1 month before the anti-incontinence procedure.

Urinary retention develops in less than 8% of cases and most episodes are transient, requiring I(S)C for 24–36 hours.[150] UTIs have been seen in up to 6% of patients, hematuria in 3%, and hematoma at the injection site in 2%.[150] A prospective study[152] comparing fat and collagen injection reported immediate postopera-

Table 95.9. ***Common and uncommon complications due to biomaterials employed***

Complications	Authors	Operation	No. of patients treated	No. of complications (%)
Tape erosion	Young et al.[18] Kuo[122] Ward & Hilton[24] Levin et al.[25] Tsivian et al.[40] Abouassaly et al.[26]	Mersilene sling Polypropylene sling TVT TVT TVT TVT	200 50 170 313 55 241	8 (4) 1 (2) 1 (0.6) 4 (1.3) 3 (5.4) 1 (0.4)
Vaginal stenosis	Young et al.[18]	Mersilene sling	200	5 (2.5)
Periurethral abscess	Kiilholma et al.[131]	Teflon injection	22	1 (4.5)
Urethral diverticulum	Kiilholma et al.[131]	Teflon injection	22	1 (4.5)
Periurethral granuloma	Kiilholma et al.[131]	Teflon injection	22	1 (4.5)

TVT, tension-free vaginal tape.

tive retention in up to 60% of patients with no significant difference between the two groups. Four patients (two in each group) required I(S)C for 2 weeks postoperatively. Other complications included postoperative UTIs in eight patients, transient voiding symptoms in seven and a subcutaneous abdominal wall hematoma in one patient from the fat group, without any local complications at the injection site. No patient had de novo OAB.

Desirable qualities of sling materials are availability, durability, affordability, lack of immune response, resistance to infection, and no potential risk of disease transmission. Autologous materials offer biocompatibility and durability, and appear to be associated with higher cure rates and fewer complications than synthetic materials.[153] Nevertheless, a second operative field is necessary with an attendant increase in postoperative pain and infection risk. Various cadaveric fascia allografts avoid this kind of morbidity but have questionable success rates (up to >20% failure)[154] and secondary vaginal erosion (up to 25%).[155] Usually, sling failure occurs within the first 6 months because of degeneration of fascia or failure of anchoring sutures.

Repliform acellular human dermal allograft consists of human cryopreserved allogenic dermis from which the epidermal and dermal cellular components have been removed, leaving the basement membrane complex, which is rapidly revascularized following placement. It is biologically inert and less likely to induce an immune response, without any disease transmission to recipient patients to date. This material offers the possibility of using a single piece of graft for concomitant pubovaginal sling placement and anterior POP repair.[20,156] The use of Repliform processed human cadaveric allograft skin for the transvaginal sling procedure for SUI appears to be effective and safe at a mean follow-up of 18 months. A prospective study[20] on a series of 253 patients with SUI treated with a transvaginal sling using a Repliform cadaveric human dermal allograft and bone anchor fixation reported the following immediate and early operative complications: bladder injury (2.1%), bowel injury (0.9%), significant bleeding (1.3%), transient urinary retention (8.5%), and perirectal abscess (0.8%). The perirectal abscess was due to spontaneous defecation during surgery and developed in a patient who underwent a transvaginal sling, anterior and posterior repair, vaginal hysterectomy, and sacrospinous suspension. Late complications included transient dyspareunia in 8.5% of cases, pain in 4.7%, constipation in 0.9%, voiding symptoms in 2.1%, de novo OAB in 5.5%, and slow vaginal wall healing associated with vaginal infection in 1.7%. Predisposing factors to the last complication include obesity, diabetes, and immunodeficiency. Since chronic inflammation of the tape is the main cause of altered wound healing, vaginal resection of the periurethral parts of the tape is mandatory.

The advantages of synthetic materials over autologous grafts for the surgical treatment of SUI are the avoidance of an additional incision to harvest fascia lata or rectus muscle fascia, a decrease in operating time, consistent material strength, high cure rates, and decreased postoperative pain.[157]

While cure rates and durability seem promising, several serious complications are of concern. The most frequent complications are voiding dysfunction with retention (1–4%), de novo OAB (6–14%), and synthetic sling rejection or erosion in the bladder, urethra, and vagina.[18,97,122,124]

The average reported erosion rate of synthetic grafts used for urethral slings is 7.3% (range 3–34%).[158] Teflon slings have erosion and infection rates as high as 23%.[159] The ProteGen sling was associated with infection or erosion and was voluntarily recalled.[160] More recently, polypropylene material has been used in tension-free sling procedures, such as TVT and TOT. While short-term follow-up studies show high success with a low complication rate, several complications not fully reported in the literature have been identified. A search through the FDA Adverse Event Reporting Program at www.fda.gov/medwatch revealed notable TVT complications, including erosion, retention, bladder perforation, and major complications of vascular and bowel injuries, sepsis and, rarely, death.

While these complications are probably not material related, caution is necessary in the use of TVT. It is important to bear in mind that the reported low morbidity of TVT as performed by experienced urologists and gynecologists does not reflect the real morbidity of this technique when performed by all practitioners. Bladder perforation is the most frequent intraoperative complication, occurring in around 1/25 procedures.[24,31,161] Voiding dysfunction (3–5%), UTIs (6–22%), and de novo OAB (3–9%) can occur postoperatively.[24,31,97,162,163] In up to 5% of cases, a retropubic hematoma can occur.[162] Complications related to the tape (e.g. erosion into vagina or urinary tract) may rarely occur.[161] Tsivian et al.[40] reported 14 cases of tape-related complications, 12 of them occurring among the 200 women who previously underwent the TVT procedure at their department for SUI. One woman had intravesical tape erosion with encrustation and stone formation on the tape, four had vaginal tape erosion, eight had an obstructed urethra and one had concomitant vaginal erosion and an obstructed urethra. A total of 12 patients required partial tape removal or tape incision, which was done transvaginally in 11. The remaining patient underwent cystotomy and excision of the intravesical part of the eroded tape. One patient was awaiting corrective surgery and one with asymptomatic vaginal erosion was only being observed.

There have been several recent reports in the literature on tape erosion into the urethra[164–166] and vagina.[146,148,149] The recommended treatment is foreign body removal.[167–169]

Aimed at reducing TVT complication rates, a tension-free transobturator modality (TOT outside-in) to place the polypropylene tape was proposed.[170,171] The TOT outside-in promoters stated that there might be no risk to bladder, urethra or bowel, and no vascular or nerve damage. Despite that, LUT injury has been reported in six patients, three of whom subsequently developed a urethral fistula.[172] A recent retrospective study,[34] assessing the morbidity related to TOT outside-in, reported a number of operative complications: 0.5% bladder perforations, 0.3% vaginal perforations, no urethral wounds, 0.8% 200–300 ml hemorrhage, and two perineal hematomas (0.33%). Short-term complications included 1.5% transient retention, 2.3% transient pain, 2.5% UTIs, and 1.3% transient voiding dysfunction, with a 1.5% rate of de novo voiding symptoms and urgency after 1-year follow-up.

To further reduce TOT complication rates, de Leval proposed a TOT inside-out procedure,[173] which was performed in 107 consecutive patients. No bladder or urethral injuries, or vascular or neurologic complications were encountered. Minor vaginal erosion was noted in one patient, and three women (2.8%) complained of complete retention, successfully treated by releasing the tape. Twenty-seven patients (15.9%) complained of transient moderate pain or discomfort in the thigh folds. The authors did not provide de novo OAB rates owing to the short follow-up time.

Mechanism failure after artificial urinary sphincter implant is common, even with today's sophisticated and very expensive devices. There is a mean expected revision rate due to mechanical and non-mechanical failure of 7.6% and 9%, respectively, with an average rate of both infection and erosion of 3.4%.[174] A recent meta-analysis carried out on 2606 patients showed an overall revision rate of 32% with mechanical and non-mechanical failure rates of 14% and 17%, respectively. Urethral erosion occurred in up to 11.7% of cases and infections in up to 4.5%.[81] Uncommon reservoir-related complications include small intestine erosion,[63] migration into the bladder,[175] and infection causing peritonitis.[176]

Impact on quality of life

Urinary incontinence negatively affects quality of life (QoL) of suffering women. Hence, any means to relieve this condition should theoretically improve patients' physical, social, and psychological well-being. Black et al.[177] found that 7% of 442 patients surgically treated for SUI reported a deterioration of their general health status 1 year after the intervention. Moreover, 25% of them reported worse mental health, reflecting the disappointing cure rate of only 28%. In that series, postoperative recovery was longer than anticipated, with 24% of women still on sick leave or left unpaid.

The main instruments to measure patients' QoL after SUI surgery are the Incontinence Impact Questionnaire (IIQ-7) and the Urogenital Distress Inventory (UDI-6).

Scores for both systems appear to improve after SUI surgery in patients showing a subjective cure; on the other hand, only UDI-6 scores appear to improve in patients with an objective cure.[178] Vassallo et al.,[179] using the abovementioned QoL measurement tools, demonstrated an objective and significant improvement in quality of life in patients who previously underwent TVT alone or with associated POP surgery, reporting an improvement of 81% and 85% in IIQ and UDI scores, respectively. This improvement was constant and independent of preoperative SUI severity. Morgan et al.[112] analyzing the measurements of QoL scores of patients previously treated with pubovaginal sling, detected a satisfaction rate of 92% at a 4-year follow-up. These patients showed a very low UDI score, an expression of the good clinical results achieved. On the other hand, those patients with postoperative storage symptoms were the most dissatisfied with surgery.

CONCLUSIONS

In the last century, more than 150 different surgical procedures have been reported for the treatment of SUI, indicating that there is no operation showing satisfactory results for all patients or reference standard treatment. Knowledge of the functional consequences and complications of these procedures may play a role in the choice of a particular operation, together with other factors that influence this choice, such as anatomic defects and both the surgeon's and patient's preferences.

It is crucial to monitor all new techniques. The complications outlined in the case reports highlight the need to consistently reassess why a patient does not do well after a supposedly less morbid procedure. Hence, the surgeon's mastery of all techniques and complications is mandatory for comprehensive patient information, and the choice of treatment must be determined case by case.

REFERENCES

1. Chaliha C, Stanton SL. Complications of surgery for genuine stress incontinence. Br J Obstet Gynaecol 1999;106:1238–45.
2. Ayoub N, Chartier-Kastler E, Robain G et al. Functional consequences and complications of surgery for female stress urinary incontinence. Prog Urol 2004;14(3):360–73.
3. Van Geelen JM, Theeuwes AG, Eskes TK et al. The clinical and urodynamic effects of anterior vaginal repair and Burch colposuspension. Am J Obstet Gynecol 1988;59:137–44.
4. Alcalay M, Monga A, Stanton M. Burch colposuspension: a 10–20 year follow-up. BJOG 1995;102:740–5.
5. Stanton SL, Cardozo LD. Results of the colposuspension operation for incontinence and prolapse. BJOG 1979;86:693–7.
6. Wee HY, Low C, Han HC. Burch colposuspension: review of perioperative complications at a women's and children's hospital in Singapore. Ann Acad Med Singapore 2003;32(6):821–3.
7. Liu CY, Paek W. Laparoscopic retropubic colposuspension (Burch procedure). J Am Assoc Gynecol Laparosc 1993;1:31–5.
8. Moehrer B, Carey M, Wilson D. Laparoscopic colposuspension: a systematic review. BJOG 2003;110:230–5.
9. Green DF, McGuire EJ, Lytton B. A comparison of endoscopic suspension of the vesical neck versus anterior urethropexy for the treatment of stress urinary incontinence. J Urol 1986;136:1205–7.
10. Riggs JA. Retropubic cystourethropexy: a review of two operative procedures with long-term follow-up. Obstet Gynecol 1986;68:98–105.
11. Mainprize TC, Drutz HP. The Marshall–Marchetti–Krantz procedure: a critical review. Obstet Gynecol Surv 1988;43:724–9.
12. Spencer JR, O'Conor VJ Jr, Schaeffer AJ. A comparison of endoscopic suspension of the vesical neck with suprapubic vesico-urethropexy for treatment of stress urinary incontinence. J Urol 1987;137:411–5.
13. Peattie AB, Stanton SL. The Stamey operation for correction of genuine stress incontinence in the elderly woman. BJOG 1989;96:983–6.
14. Varner RE. Retropubic long-needle suspension procedures for stress urinary incontinence. Am J Obstet Gynecol 1990;63:551–7.
15. Horbach NS, Blanco JS, Ostergard DR et al. A suburethral sling procedure with polytetrafluoroethylene for the treatment of genuine stress incontinence in patients with low urethral closure pressure. Obstet Gynecol 1988;71(4):648–52.
16. Morgan JE, Farrow GA, Stewart FE. The Marlex sling operation for the treatment of recurrent stress urinary incontinence: a 16-year review. Am J Obstet Gynecol 1985;151:224–6.
17. Amundsen CL, Visco AG, Ruiz H et al. Outcome in 104 pubovaginal slings using freeze dried allograft fascia lata from a single tissue bank. Urology 2000;56(Suppl 6A):2–8.
18. Young SB, Howard AE, Baker SP. Mersilene mesh sling: short- and long-term clinical and urodynamic outcomes. Am J Obstet Gynecol 2001;185:32–40.
19. Carbone A, Palleschi G, Ciavarella S et al. Experience with bone anchor sling for treating female stress

urinary incontinence: outcome at 30 months. BJU Int 2004;93:780–8.

20. Crivellaro S, Smith JJ, Kocjancic E et al. Transvaginal sling using acellular human dermal allograft: safety and efficacy in 253 patients. J Urol 2004;172:1374–8.

21. Groutz A, Gordon D, Wolman I et al. Tension-free vaginal tape for stress urinary incontinence: is there a learning curve? Neurourol Urodyn 2002;21:470–2.

22. Wang AC, Lo TS. Tension-free vaginal tape. A minimally invasive solution to stress urinary incontinence in women. J Reprod Med 1998;43:429–34.

23. Meschia M, Pifarotti P, Bernascone F et al. Tension-free vaginal tape: analysis of outcomes and complications in 404 stress incontinent women. Int Urogynecol J Pelvic Floor Dysfunct 2001;12:S24–S27.

24. Ward K, Hilton P. Prospective multicentre randomised trial of tension-free vaginal tape and colposuspension as primary treatment for stress incontinence. BMJ 2002;325:67–73.

25. Levin I, Groutz A, Gold R et al. Surgical complications and medium-term outcome results of tension-free vaginal tape: a prospective study of 313 consecutive patients. Neurourol Urodyn 2004;23(1):7–9.

26. Abouassaly R, Steinberg JR, Lemieux M et al. Complications of tension-free vaginal tape surgery: a multi-institutional review. BJU Int 2004;94:110–3.

27. Rafii A, Paoletti X, Haab F et al. Tension-free vaginal tape and associated procedures: a case control study. Eur Urol 2004;45(3):356–61.

28. Kuuva N, Nilsson CG. A nation-wide analysis of complications associated with the tension-free vaginal tape (TVT) procedure. Acta Obstet Gynecol Scand 2002;81:72–7.

29. Vierhout ME. Severe hemorrhage complicating tension-free vaginal tape (TVT): a case report. Int Urogynecol J Pelvic Floor Dysfunct 2001;12:139–40.

30. Primicerio M, De Matteis G, Montanino Oliva M et al. Use of the TVT (tension-free vaginal tape) in the treatment of female urinary stress incontinence. Preliminary results. Minerva Ginecol 1999;51:355–8.

31. Nilsson CG, Kuuva N. The tension-free vaginal tape procedure is successful in the majority of women with indications for surgical treatment of urinary stress incontinence. Br J Obstet Gynecol 2001;108:414–9.

32. Rezapour M, Falconer C, Ulmsten U. Tension-free vaginal tape (TVT) in stress incontinent women with intrinsic sphincter deficiency (ISD) – a long-term follow-up. Int Urogynecol J Pelvic Floor Dysfunct 2001;12(Suppl 2): S12–S14.

33. Rezapour M, Ulmsten U. Tension-free vaginal tape (TVT) in women with mixed urinary incontinence – a long-term follow-up. Int Urogynecol J Pelvic Floor Dysfunct 2001;12(Suppl 2):S15–S18.

34. Krauth JS, Rasoamiaramanana H, Barlett H et al. Suburethral tape treatment of female urinary incontinence. Morbidity assessment of the trans-obturator route and a new tape (I-STOP®): a multi-centre experiment involving 604 cases. Eur Urol 2005;47(1):102–7.

35. Ulmsten U, Falconer C, Johnson P et al. A multicenter study of tension-free vaginal tape (TVT) for surgical treatment of stress urinary incontinence. Int Urogynecol J Pelvic Floor Dysfunct 1998;9:210–3.

36. Jacquetin B. Use of TVT in surgery for female urinary incontinence. J Gynecol Obstet Biol Reprod 2000;29: 242–7.

37. Pow-Sang JM, Lockhart JL, Suarez A et al. Female urinary incontinence: preoperative selection, surgical complications and results. J Urol 1986;136:831–3.

38. Summitt RL, Bent AE, Ostergard DR et al. Suburethral sling procedure for genuine stress incontinence and low urethral closure pressure: a continued experience. Int Urogynecol J 1992;3:346–52.

39. Soulie M, Cuvillier X, Benaissa A et al. Tension-free transvaginal tape procedure in the treatment of female urinary stress incontinence: a French prospective multicentre study. Eur Urol 2001;39:709.

40. Tsivian A, Kessler O, Mogutin B et al. Tape related complications of the tension-free vaginal tape procedure. J Urol 2004,171:762–4.

41. Backer MH Jr, Probst RE. The Pereyra procedure. Favorable experience with 200 operations. Am J Obstet Gynecol 1976;125(3):346–52.

42. Pereyra AJ, Lebherz TB, Growdon WA et al. Pubourethral supports in perspective: modified Pereyra procedure for urinary incontinence. Obstet Gynecol 1982;59:643–8.

43. Klutke JJ, Carlin BI, Klutke CG. The tension-free vaginal tape procedure: correction of stress incontinence with minimal alteration in proximal urethral mobility. Urology 2000;55(4):512–4.

44. Niemczyk P, Klutke JJ, Carlin BI et al. United States experience with tension-free vaginal tape procedure for urinary stress incontinence: assessment of safety and tolerability. Tech Urol 2001;7:261–5.

45. Lebret T, Lugagne PM, Herve JM et al. Evaluation of tension-free vaginal tape procedure. Its safety and efficacy in the treatment of female stress urinary incontinence during the learning phase. Eur Urol 2001;40:543–7.

46. Jomaa M. Combined tension-free vaginal tape and prolapse repair under local anaesthesia in patients with symptoms of both urinary incontinence and prolapse. Gynecol Obstet Invest 2001;51:184–6.

47. Borgaonkar SS, Hackman BW. Neodymium:YAG laser removal of stone formed on nonabsorbable suture used previously in colposuspension. J Urol 1996;156(2 Pt 1):472.

48. Zderic SA, Burros HM, Hanno PM, Dudas N, Whitmore KE. Bladder calculi in women after urethrovesical suspension. J Urol 1988;139(5):1047–8.

49. Evans JW, Chapple CE, Ralph DJ et al. Bladder calculus formation as a complication of the Stamey procedure. Br J Urol 1990;65(6):580–2.

50. Zderic SA, Burros HM, Hanno PM et al. Bladder calculi in women after urethrovesical suspension. J Urol 1988;139:1047–8.

51. Zimmern P, Schmidbauer CP, Leach GE et al. Vesicovaginal and urethrovaginal fistulae. Semin Urol 1986;4: 24–9.

52. Radomski SB, Herschorn S. Laparoscopic Burch bladder neck suspension: early results. J Urol 1996;15:515–8.

53. Vancaillie TG, Schuessler W. Laparoscopic bladder neck suspension. J Laparoendosc Surg 1991;1:169–73.

54. Costa P, Mottet N, Elsandid M et al. The use of an artificial urinary sphincter in women with type III incontinence and a negative Marshall test. J Urol 2001;165:1172–6.

55. Drutz HP, Khosid HI. Complications with Bonanno suprapubic catheters. Am J Obstet Gynecol 1984;149(6):685–6.

56. Loughlin KR, Whitemore WF 3rd, Gittes RF et al. Review of an 8-year experience with modifications of endoscopic suspension of the bladder neck for female stress urinary incontinence. J Urol 1990;143:44–5.

57. Noller KL, Pratt JH, Symmonds RE. Bowel perforation with suprapubic cystostomy. Report of two cases. Obstet Gynecol 1976;48:67S–69S.

58. Peyrat L, Boutin JM, Bruyere F et al. Intestinal perforation as a complication of tension-free vaginal tape procedure for urinary incontinence. Eur Urol 2001;39:603–5.

59. Meschia M, Busacca M, Pifarotti P et al. Bowel perforation during insertion of tension-free vaginal tape (TVT). Int Urogynecol J Pelvic Floor Dysfunct 2002;13:263–5.

60. Leboeuf L, Tellez CA, Ead D et al. Complication of bowel perforation during insertion of tension-free vaginal tape. J Urol 2003;70:1310–1.

61. Amna MB, Randrianantenaina A, Michel F. Colic perforation as a complication of tension-free vaginal tape procedure. J Urol 2003;170:2387.

62. Castillo OA, Bodden E, Olivares RA et al. Intestinal perforation: an infrequent complication during insertion of tension-free vaginal tape. J Urol 2004;172(4 Pt 1):1364.

63. Yuan X, Mudge BJ, Raezer DM. Small intestine erosion by artificial urinary sphincter reservoir tubing. J Urol 2004;172(4 Pt 1):1363.

64. Adler LM, Loughlin JS, Morin CJ et al. Bilateral compartment syndrome after a long gynecologic operation in the lithotomy position. Am J Obstet Gynecol 1990;62: 1271–2.

65. Fowl RJ, Akers DL, Kempczinski RF. Neurovascular lower extremity complications of the lithotomy position. Ann Vasc Surg 1992;6:3567–9.

66. Peters WA, Thornton WN. Selection of the primary operative procedure for stress urinary incontinence. Am J Obstet Gynecol 1980;137:923–30.

67. Muznai D, Carrill E, Dubin C et al. Retropubic vaginopexy for the correction of urinary stress incontinence. Obstet Gynecol 1991;78:1011–8.

68. Lotenfoe R, O'Kelly JK, Helal M et al. Periurethral polytetrafluoroethylene paste injection in incontinent female subjects: surgical indications and improved surgical technique. J Urol 1993;149:279–82.

69. Bryans FE. Marlex gauze hammock sling operation with Cooper's ligament attachment in the management of recurrent urinary stress incontinence. Am J Obstet Gynecol 1979;133:292–4.

70. Beck RP, McCormick S, Nordstrom L. The fascia lata sling procedure for treating recurrent genuine stress incontinence of urine. Obstet Gynecol 1988;72:699–703.

71. Chin YK, Stanton SL. A follow-up of silastic sling for genuine stress incontinence. BJOG 1995;102:143–7.

72. Hom D, Desautel MG, Lumerma JH et al. Pubovaginal sling using polypropylene mesh and vesical bone anchors. Urology 1998;51:708–13.

73. Weinberger MW, Ostergard DR. Long term clinical and urodynamic evaluation of the polytetrafluoroethylene sub-urethral sling for treatment of genuine stress incontinence. Obstet Gynecol 1995;86:92.

74. Yamada J, Arai G, Masudo H et al. The correction of type 2 stress incontinence with polytetrafluoroethylene patch sling: 5 year follow-up. J Urol 1998;160:746.

75. Winters JC, Scarpero HM, Appell RA. Use of bone anchors in female urology. Urology 2000;56(Suppl 6A):15–22.

76. Leach G. Local anesthesia for urologic procedures. Urology 1996;48:284–8.

77. Schultheiss D, Hofner K, Oelke M et al. Does bone anchor fixation improve the outcome of percutaneous bladder neck suspension in female stress urinary incontinence? Br J Urol 1998;82:192–5.

78. Savageau D. Urology: bone anchoring without a drill. Surg Products 1998;17:27–31.

79. Beckingham IJ, Wemyss-Holden G, Lawrence WT. Long-term follow-up of women treated with periurethral Teflon injections for stress incontinence. Br J Urol 1992;69(6):580–3.

80. Scott FB. The artificial urinary sphincter. Experience in adults. Urol Clin North Am 1989;16:105–17.

81. Hajivassiliou CA. A review of the complications and results of implantation of the AMS artificial urinary sphincter. Eur Urol 1999;35(1):36–44.

82. Olsson L, Kroon U. A three-year postoperative evaluation of tension-free vaginal tape. Gynecol Obstet Invest 1999;48:267–9.

83. Bhatia NN, Bergman A. Urodynamic predictability of voiding following incontinence surgery. Obstet Gynecol 1984;63(1):85–91.

84. Warren JW. Catheter-associated urinary tract infections. Infect Dis Clin North Am 1987;1:823–54.

85. Foucher JE, Marshall V. Nosocomial catheter associated urinary tract infections. Infect Surg 1983;2:43.

86. Hanson PG, Algelvine MK, Luhl JH. Osteitis pubis in sports activities. Phys Sports Med 1978;6:111–4.

87. Goldberg RP, Tchetgen MB, Sand PK et al. Incidence of pubic osteomyelitis after bladder neck suspension using bone anchors. Urology 2004;63(4):704–8.

88. Matthews K, Govier FE. Osteitis pubis after periurethral collagen injection. Urology 1997;49(2):237–8.

89. Beck RP, McCormick S, Nordstrom L. A twenty five year experience with 519 colporrhaphy procedures. Obstet Gynecol 1991;78:1011–8.

90. Guam L, Ricciotti NA, Fair WR. Endoscopic bladder neck suspension for stress urinary incontinence. J Urol 1984;132:1119–21.

91. Kersey J. The gauze hammock sling operation in the treatment of stress incontinence. Br J Obstet Gynaecol 1983;90:945–9.

92. Karram MM, Angel O, Koonings P et al. The modified Pereyra procedure; a clinical and urodynamic review. Br J Obstet Gynaecol 1992;99:655–8.

93. Miyazaki F, Shook G. Ilioinguinal nerve entrapment during needle suspension for stress incontinence. Obstet Gynecol 1992;80(2):246–8.

94. Galloway NTM, Davies N, Stephenson TP. The complications of colposuspension. Br J Urol 1987;60(2):122–4.

95. Lose G, Jorgensen L, Mortensen SO et al. Voiding difficulties after colposuspension. Obstet Gynecol 1987;69:33–8.

96. Delorme E, Droupy S, de Tayrac R et al. Transobturator tape (Uratape): a new minimally-invasive procedure to treat female urinary incontinence. Eur Urol 2004;45: 203–7.

97. Arunkalaivanan AS, Barrington JW. Randomised trial of porcine dermal sling (Pelvicol implant) vs. tension-free vaginal tape (TVT) in the surgical treatment of stress incontinence: a questionnaire-based study. Int Urogynecol J Pelvic Floor Dysfunct 2003;14:17–23.

98. Nitti VW, Raz S. Obstruction following anti-incontinence procedures: diagnosis and treatment with transvaginal urethrolysis. J Urol 1994;152:93–8.

99. Moran PA, Ward KL, Johnson D et al. Tension-free vaginal tape for primary genuine stress incontinence: a 2-centre follow-up study. BJU Int 2000;36:39–42.

100. Ulmsten U, Johnson P, Rezapour M. A three-year follow-up of tension free vaginal tape for surgical treatment of female stress urinary incontinence. Br J Obstet Gynaecol 1999;106:345–50.

101. Rackley RR, Abdelmalak JB, Tchetgen MB et al. Tension-free vaginal tape and percutaneous vaginal tape sling procedures. Tech Urol 2001;7:90–100.

102. Klutke C, Siegel S, Carlin B et al. Urinary retention after tension-free vaginal tape procedure, incidence and treatment. Urology 2001;58:697–701.

103. Dunn JS Jr, Bent AE, Ellerkman RM et al. Voiding dysfunction after surgery for stress incontinence: literature review and survey results. Int Urogynecol J 2004;15:25–31.

104. Horbach NS. Suburethral sling procedures. In: Ostergard DR, Bent AE (eds) Urogynecology and Urodynamics: Theory and Practice, 4th ed. Baltimore: Williams and Wilkins, 1996; 569–79.

105. Zimmern PB, Hadley HR, Leach GE et al. Female urethral obstruction after Marshall–Marchetti–Krantz operation. J Urol 1987;138:517–20.

106. McDuffie RW Jr, Litin RB, Blundon KE. Urethrovesical suspension (Marshall–Marchetti–Krantz). Experience with 204 cases. Am J Surg 1981;141:297–8.

107. Maher C, Dwyer P, Carey M et al. The Burch colposuspension for recurrent urinary stress incontinence following retropubic continence surgery. Br J Obstet Gynaecol 1999;106:719–24.

108. Foster HE, McGuire EJ. Management of urethral obstruction with transvaginal urethrolysis. J Urol 1993;150: 1448–51.

109. Nitti VW, Carlson KV, Blaivas JG et al. Early results of pubovaginal sling lysis by midline sling incision. Urology 2002;59(1):47–52.

110. Swami SK, Abrams P. Urge incontinence. Urol Clin North Am 1996;23:417–25.

111. Griffiths D. Clinical aspects of detrusor instability and the value of urodynamics: a review of the evidence. Eur Urol 1998;34(Suppl 1):13–5.

112. Morgan JO, Westney OL, McGuire EJ. Pubovaginal sling: 4-year outcome analysis and quality of life assessment. J Urol 2000;163:1845–8.

113. Langer R, Ron-El R, Newman M et al. Detrusor instability following colposuspension for urinary stress incontinence. Br J Obstet Gynaecol 1988;95:607–10.

114. Sand PK, Bowen LW, Ostergard DR et al. The effect of retropubic urethropexy on detrusor stability. Obstet Gynecol 1988;71:818–22.

115. Langer R, Lipshitz Y, Halperin R et al. Long-term (10–15 years) follow-up after Burch colposuspension for urinary stress incontinence. Int Urogynecol J 2001;12:323–7.

116. Demirci F, Yucel O, Eren S et al. Long-term results of Burch colposuspension. Gynecol Obstet Invest 2001;51:243–7.

117. Bombieri L, Reeman RM, Perkins EP et al. Why do women have voiding dysfunction and de novo detrusor instability after colposuspension? BJOG 2002;109(4):402–12.

118. Cardozo LD, Stanton SL, Williams JE. Detrusor instability following surgery for genuine stress incontinence. Br J Urol 1979;51:204–7.

119. Hilton P. A clinical and urodynamic study comparing the Stamey bladder neck suspension and suburethral sling procedures in the treatment of genuine stress incontinence. Br J Obstet Gynaecol 1989;96:213–20.

120. Raz S, Sussman EM, Eriksen DB et al. The Raz bladder neck suspension: results in 206 patients. J Urol 1992;148:845–50.

121. McGuire EJ, Bennett CJ, Konnak JA et al. Experience with pubovaginal slings for urinary incontinence at the University of Michigan. J Urol 1987;138:525–6.

122. Kuo HC. Anatomical and functional results of pubovaginal sling procedure using polypropylene mesh for the treatment of stress urinary incontinence. J Urol 2001;166:152–7.

123. Barnes NM, Dmochowski RR, Park R et al. Pubovaginal sling and pelvic prolapse repair in women with occult stress urinary incontinence: effect on postoperative emptying and voiding symptoms. Urology 2002;59(6):856–60.

124. Smith T, Daneshgari F, Dmochowski RR et al. Surgical treatment of incontinence in women. In: Abrams P, Cardozo L, Khoury S, Wein A (eds) Incontinence, 2nd ed. Plymouth: Health Publication, 2002; 823–63.

125. Bidmead J, Cardozo L, McLellan A et al. A comparison of the objective and subjective outcomes of colposuspension for stress incontinence in women. BJOG 2001;108: 408–13.

126. Wang AC. An assessment of the early surgical outcome and urodynamic effects of the tension-free vaginal tape (TVT). Int Urogynecol J Pelvic Floor Dysfunct 2000;11:282–4.

127. Burch JC. Cooper's ligament urethrovesical suspension for stress incontinence. Nine years' experience – results, complications, technique. Am J Obstet Gynecol 1968;100(6):764–74.

128. Wiskind AK, Creighton SM, Stanton SL. The incidence of genital prolapse after Burch colposuspension. Am J Obstet Gynecol 1992;167:399–404.

129. Nitti VW, Bregg KJ, Sussman EM et al. The Raz bladder neck suspension in patients 65 years old and older. J Urol 1993;149:802–7.

130. Neuman M. Low incidence of post-TVT genital prolapse. Int Urogynecol J Pelvic Floor Dysfunct 2003;14(3): 191–2.

131. Kiilholma PJ, Chancellor MB, Makinen J et al. Complications of Teflon injection for stress urinary incontinence. Neurourol Urodyn 1993;12:131–7.

132. Creighton SM, Stanton SL. The surgical management of vaginal vault prolapse. Br J Obstet Gynaecol 1991;98(11):1150–4.

133. Drutz HP, Cha LS. Massive genital and vaginal vault prolapse treated by abdominal–vaginal sacropexy with use of Marlex mesh: review of the literature. Am J Obstet Gynecol 1984;149(6):685–6.

134. Mazouni C, Karsenty G, Bretelle F et al. Urinary complications and sexual function after the tension-free vaginal tape procedure. Acta Obstet Gynecol Scand 2004;83(10):955–61.

135. Kursh ED, Angell AH, Resnick MI. Evolution of endoscopic urethropexy: seven year experience with various techniques. Urology 1991;37:428–31.

136. Weber AM, Walters MD, Piedmonte MR. Sexual function and vaginal anatomy in women before and after surgery for pelvic organ prolapse and urinary incontinence. Am J Obstet Gynecol 2000;182:1601–5.

137. Wheelahan JB. Long-term results of colposuspension. Br J Urol 1990;65:329–32.

138. Griffith-Jones MD, Abrams PH. The Stamey endoscopic bladder neck suspension in the elderly. Br J Urol 1990;65:170–2.

139. Diokno AC, Brown MB, Herzog AR. Sexual function in the elderly. Arch Intern Med 1990;150(1):197–200.

140. Osborn MK, Hawton K, Gath D. Sexual dysfunction among middle aged women in the community. Br Med J 1988;296:959–62.

141. Barber AG, Visco JF, Wyman JA et al. Sexual function in women with urinary incontinence and pelvic organ prolapse. Obstet Gynecol 2002;99(2):281–9.

142. Maaita M, Bhaumik J, Davies AE. Sexual function after using tension-free vaginal tape for the surgical treatment of genuine stress incontinence. BJU Int 2002;90:540–3.

143. Barrington JW, Arunkalaivanan AS, Swart M. Post-colposuspension syndrome following a tension-free vaginal tape procedure. Int Urogynecol J Pelvic Floor Dysfunct 2002;13(3):187–8.

144. Jarvis GJ. Surgery for genuine stress incontinence. BJOG 1994;101:371–4.

145. Dwyer PL, O'Reilly M. Recurrent urinary tract infection in the female. Curr Opin Obstet Gynecol 2002;14(5):537–43.

146. Appell RA. Intra-urethral injection therapy. In: Cardozo L, Staskin D (eds) Textbook of Female Urology and Urogynaecology. London: Martin Dunitz, 2001; 479–91.

147. Pickard R, Reaper J, Wyness L et al. Periurethral injection therapy for urinary incontinence in women (Cochrane Review). In: The Cochrane Library. Chichester: Wiley, 2003; 4.

148. Politano VA, Small MP, Harper JM et al. Periurethral Teflon injection for urinary incontinence. J Urol 1974;111:180–3.

149. Gonzales Garibay S, Jimeno C, York M et al. [Endoscopic autotransplantation of fat tissues in the treatment of urinary incontinence in the female.] J Urol (Paris) 1989;95:363–6.

150. Winters JC, Appell RA. Periurethral injection of collagen in the treatment of intrinsic sphincter deficiency in the female patient. Urol Clin North Am 1995;22:673–7.

151. Wainstein MA, Klutke CG. Periurethral pseudocyst following cystoscopic collagen injection. Urology 1998;51(5):835–6.

152. Haab F, Zimmern PE, Leach GE. Urinary stress incontinence due to intrinsic sphincter deficiency: experience with fat and collagen periurethral injections. J Urol 1997;157:1283–6.

153. Bidmead J, Cardozo L. Sling techniques in the treatment of genuine stress incontinence. Br J Obstet Gynaecol 2000;107:147–56.

154. Fitzgerald MP, Mollenhauer J, Brubaker L. Failure of allograft suburethral slings. BJU Int 1999;84:785–8.

155. Kammerer-Doak DN, Rogers RG, Bellar B. Vaginal erosion of cadaveric fascia lata following abdominal sacrocolpopexy and suburethral sling urethropexy. Int Urogynecol J Pelvic Floor Dysfunct 2002;13:106–9; discussion 109.

156. Chung SY, Franks M, Smith CP et al. Technique of combined pubovaginal sling and cystocele repair using a single piece of cadaveric dermal graft. Urology 2002;59:538–41.

157. Kaplan SA, Santarosa RP, Te AE. Comparison of fascial and vaginal wall slings in the management of intrinsic sphincter deficiency. Urology 1996;47:885–9.

158. Iglesia CB, Fenner DE, Brubaker L. The use of mesh in gynecologic surgery. Int Urogynecol J Pelvic Floor Dysfunct 1997;8:105–15.

159. Bent AE, Ostergard DR, Zwick-Zaffuto M. Tissue reaction to expanded polytetrafluoroethylene suburethral sling for urinary incontinence: clinical and histologic study. Am J Obstet Gynecol 1993;169:1198–204.

160. Kobashi KC, Dmochowski R, Mee SL et al. Erosion of woven polyester pubovaginal sling. J Urol 1999;162:2070–2.

161. Cody J, Wyness L, Wallace S et al. Systematic review of the clinical effectiveness and cost-effectiveness of tension-free vaginal tape for treatment of urinary stress incontinence. Health Technol Assess 2003;7:1–189.

162. Karram MM, Segal JL, Vassallo BJ et al. Complications and untoward effects of the tension-free vaginal tape procedure. Obstet Gynecol 2003;101:929–32.

163. Petri E. Retropubic cystourethropexies. In: Cardozo L, Staskin D (eds) Textbook of Female Urology and Urogynaecology. London: Martin Dunitz, 2001; 513–24.

164. Sweat SD, Itano NB, Clemens JQ et al. Polypropylene mesh tape for stress urinary incontinence: complications of urethral erosion and outlet obstruction. J Urol 2002;168:144–6.

165. Madjar S, Tchetgen MB, Van Antwerp A et al. Urethral erosion of tension-free vaginal tape. Urology 2002;59:601.

166. Pit MJ. Rare complications of tension-free vaginal tape procedure: late intraurethral displacement and early misplacement of tape. J Urol 2002;167(2 Pt 1):647.

167. Volkmer BG, Nesslauer T, Rinnab L et al. Surgical intervention for complications of tension-free vaginal tape procedure. J Urol 2003;169(2):570–4.

168. Boublil V, Ciofu C, Traxer O et al. Complications of urethral sling procedures. Curr Opin Obstet Gynecol 2002;14:515–20.

169. Clemens JQ, DeLancey JO, Faerber GJ et al. Urinary tract erosions after synthetic pubovaginal slings: diagnosis and management strategy. Urology 2000;56:589–94.

170. Delorme E. La bandelette transobturatrice: un procédé mini-invasif pour traiter l'incontinence urinaire de la femme. Prog Urol 2001;11:1306–13.

171. de Tayrac R, Droupy S, Delorme E. Transobturator urethral support for female GSI: a new surgical procedure with one-year outcome. Int Urogynecol J Pelvic Floor Dysfunct 2002(Suppl 1);13:20.

172. Hermieu JF, Mesas A, Delmas V et al. Plaie vévicale après bandelette trans-obturatrice. Prog Urol 2003;13:115–7.

173. de Leval J. Novel surgical technique for the treatment of female stress urinary incontinence: transobturator vaginal tape inside-out. Eur Urol 2003;44:724–30.

174. Petrou SP, Elliott DS, Barrett DM. Artificial urethral sphincter for incontinence. Urology 2000;56(3):353–9.

175. Bartoletti R, Gacci M, Travaglini F et al. Intravesical migration of AMS 800 artificial urinary sphincter and stone formation in a patient who underwent radical prostatectomy. Urol Int 2000;64(3):167–8.

176. De Stefani S, Liguori G, Ciampalini S et al. AMS 800 artificial sphincter: an unusual case of circumscribed peritonitis due to prosthetic reservoir infection. Arch Esp Urol 1999;52(4):412–5.

177. Black NA, Bowling A, Griffiths LM et al. Impact of surgery for stress incontinence on the social lives of women. Br J Obstet Gynaecol 1998;105(6):605–12.

178. Fitzgerald MP, Kenton K, Shott S et al. Responsiveness of quality of life measurements to change after reconstructive pelvic surgery. Am J Obstet Gynecol 2001;185:20–4.

179. Vassallo BJ, Kleeman SD, Segal JL et al. Tension-free vaginal tape: a quality-of-life assessment. Obstet Gynecol 2002;100:518–24.

96

The effect of hysterectomy (simple and radical) on the lower urinary tract

Heinz Koelbl

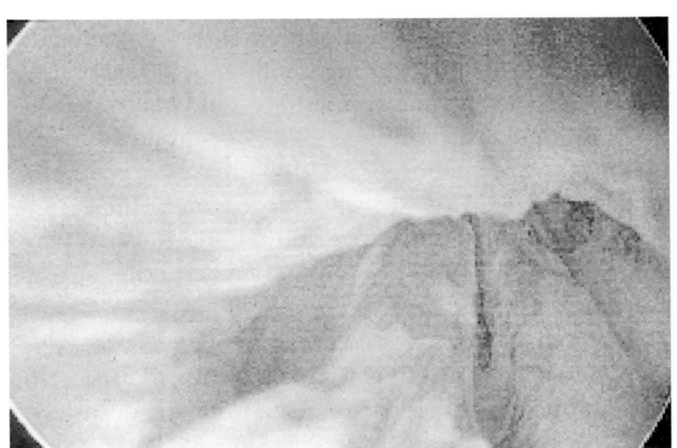

INTRODUCTION

Altered bladder function is a commonly recognized feature of pelvic surgery. This includes difficulty in voiding, high residual volumes (including distension of the upper urinary tract), recurrent urinary tract infections, loss of bladder sensation, stress urinary incontinence, and the development of urinary fistulae. The extent of postoperative complications is related to the degree of tissue disruption.

SYMPTOMS

Voiding disorders are often encountered in patients postoperatively. There is increasing evidence that even simple hysterectomy may cause vesicourethral dysfunction which appears neuropathic in origin. However, the risk of persistent damage is only slight because the bulk of the pelvic plexus lies below the cardinal ligaments. There is a growing body of evidence that hysterectomy is not associated with an increased risk of urge or stress urinary incontinence at long-term follow-up.[1]

Clinical studies of bladder function after a radical pelvic operation are conflicting. At least a portion of the confusion involves the timing of evaluation postoperatively. Causes of bladder dysfunction after pelvic surgery include nerve injury (either direct or by traction), direct vesical trauma, traumatic aseptic pericystitis, loss of bladder base support and/or tumor invasion of nerves. Other factors contributing to dysfunction postoperatively are stretch injuries (urinary retention), irradiation, and infection. Radical pelvic surgery may alter bladder function through many processes, not least because the sympathetic pathways are highly susceptible to injury. On the one hand, parasympathetic decentralization results in adrenergic hyperinnervation of the detrusor; on the other, clinical studies suggest that bladder compliance changes may be seen frequently, but only temporarily, after a radical pelvic operation, and that detrusor motor denervation occurs in only a small number of patients. Rectal or extensive parametrial resection or traction during mobilization may cause direct injury to the parasympathetic nerves and part of the pelvic plexus, resulting in bladder areflexia in up to 7.7%.[2] Sympathetic in addition to parasympathetic nerve injury may occur in patients with higher stage disease after dissection in the vicinity of the cardinal ligaments and in those who require extensive vaginal cuff removal.[3]

Techniques such as nerve-sparing radical hysterectomy have been introduced into radical surgical gynecologic oncology to avoid bladder function disorders. However, comparative trials are lacking.[4,5]

Various patterns of bladder dysfunction may occur after radical hysterectomy:[6]

1. decreased bladder capacity (low compliance) and incompetent bladder neck due to sympathetic denervation;
2. bladder areflexia with decreased proprioception sensation and increased bladder capacity due to parasympathetic denervation;
3. a combination of 1 and 2.

Voiding difficulty has been defined as a condition of abnormally slow or incomplete micturition. When severe, increasing amounts of urine are retained (chronic retention) which can cause urinary tract infection or upper urinary tract damage. In the extreme condition, a complete inability to void occurs (acute retention). Voiding difficulty and retention present a spectrum of progressive inefficiency of bladder emptying.

The postoperative development of stress incontinence de novo is related to a reduction in the urethral closure pressure. This is due to radical dissection of the paraurethral tissue, irritation or destruction of the sympathetic nerves of the urethral branch of the pudendal nerve. Radical hysterectomy and extensive anterior vaginal repair, pelvic exenteration, and urethral resection at vulvectomy are the procedures that typically have a detrimental impact on urethral closure function.

PREVENTION

Women with a diagnosis of voiding difficulty prior to planned pelvic surgery should be carefully counseled regarding the possibility of exacerbating the problem of retention postoperatively. Discussion must include the options of intermittent self-catheterization after surgery.

ASSESSMENT

An accurate assessment of residual urine volume is essential, either by catheterization or ultrasound. Repeated measurements are recommended when volumes of more than 50 ml occur.[7]

Urodynamic evaluation in patients undergoing radical pelvic surgery is important to exclude preoperative bladder outlet obstruction, infiltration of the tumor into the pelvic neuroplexus, and to assess the pattern of voiding dysfunction, which may change markedly postoperatively or even resolve.

THERAPY

Catheterization will be a part of therapy for all forms of urinary retention. Where the cause of urinary retention is detrusor failure, bladder drainage will often allow detrusor function to recover. If the cause is outflow obstruction, catheterization will provide temporary relief until spontaneous or surgical cure is obtained. Catheterization can be continuous or intermittent.

After radical pelvic surgery, the bladder should be drained immediately, either with a suprapubic catheter or with clean intermittent catheterization. This period of drainage should continue for 2–4 weeks. If the patient suffers bladder dysfunction, urodynamic studies should be performed.

In patients with impaired urethral closure function, a thorough assessment – including urodynamics and imaging to rule out complex disorders – is mandatory.

REFERENCES

1. de Tayrac R, Chevalier N, Chauveaud-Lambling A et al. Risk of urge and stress urinary incontinence at long-term follow-up after vaginal hysterectomy. Am J Obstet Gynecol 2004;191:90–4.
2. Gerstenberg TC, Nielsen ML, Clausen S. Bladder function after abdomino-perineal resection. Ann Surg 1980;191:81–6.
3. Ralph G, Winter R, Michelitsch L et al. Radicality of parametrial resection and dysfunction of the lower urinary tract after radical hysterectomy. Eur J Gynaecol Oncol 1991;12:27–30.
4. Hockel M, Horn LC, Hentschel B et al. Total mesometrial resection: high resolution nerve-sparing radical hysterectomy based on developmentally defined surgical anatomy. Int J Gynecol Cancer 2003;13:791–803.
5. Trimbos JB, Maas CP, Deruiter MC et al. A nerve-sparing radical hysterectomy: guidelines and feasibility in Western patients. Int J Gynecol Cancer 2001;11:180–6.
6. Benedetti-Panici P, Zullo MA, Plotti F et al. Long-term bladder function in patients with locally advanced cervical carcinoma treated with neoadjuvant chemotherapy and type 3-4 radical hysterectomy. Cancer 2004;100:2110–7.
7. Fischer W, Koelbl H. Urogynäkologie in Klinik und Praxis. Berlin: DeGruyter, 1995; 159–74.

97

Recognition and management of urologic complications of gynecologic surgery

Kevin R Loughlin

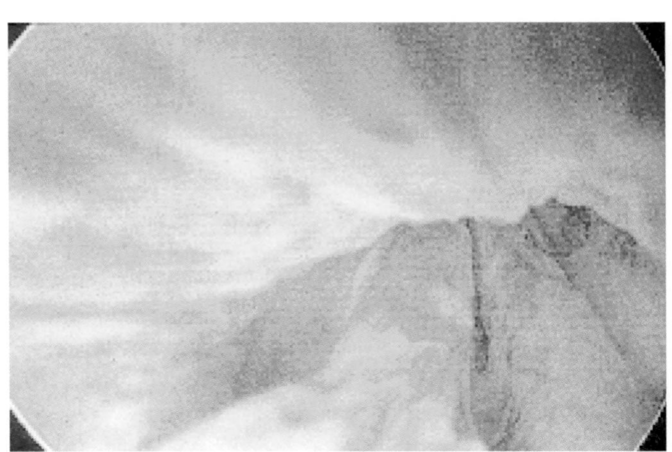

INTRODUCTION

The management of urologic injuries during gynecologic surgery represents a challenging problem to the surgeon. In this chapter, the methods of operative repair that are necessary to manage these injuries are reviewed. First, the female pelvic anatomy is described; the techniques necessary to manage these iatrogenic injuries (whether they are recognized intraoperatively or postoperatively) are then discussed.

FEMALE PELVIC ANATOMY AND ITS RELATIONSHIP TO THE URINARY TRACT

Ureteral injuries are less likely to occur if the operating surgeon has a thorough knowledge of the female pelvic anatomy and its relationship to the urinary tract. To that end, some of the female pelvic anatomy as it relates to ureteral injuries is reviewed briefly here.

The ureters cross over the pelvic brim and enter the pelvis in close proximity to the ovarian vessels. This is one of the three most common sites of urologic injury during gynecologic surgery.[1] The ureter then courses medially into the lower and medial portions of the broad ligament. At this juncture, the ureter is crossed by the uterine artery and this is the second area of the ureter that is commonly injured during gynecologic operations.[2] The ureter then continues its medial course and enters the bladder in the deep pelvis. The ureterovesical junction is the third common site of ureteral injury during female pelvic surgery. An outline of female pelvic anatomy and its relationship to the urinary tract appears in Figure 97.1.

Laparoscopic surgery and repeat pelvic surgery are associated with a higher risk of ureteral injury. In such circumstances, placement of ureteral stents prior to surgery is an option.

URETERAL INJURIES – INTRAOPERATIVE RECOGNITION AND REPAIR

Ureteral injuries occur in 0.5–2.5% of routine pelvic operations and in as many as 30% of radical pelvic procedures performed for malignancy.[3] However, less than one-third of these injuries are identified intraoperatively.[4] Ideally, the ureters should be identified and isolated prior to any extensive pelvic dissection. A useful maneuver is to identify the ureters as they cross the iliac vessels and then place Vascu-ties (vesiloop) around each ureter for later reference as the operation proceeds. Most ureteral injuries occur when there is extensive bleeding, or when the anatomy is distorted from previous surgery or radiation treatment. If the surgeon encounters extensive bleeding or there is a question of ureteral injury, the gynecologist or urologic consultant

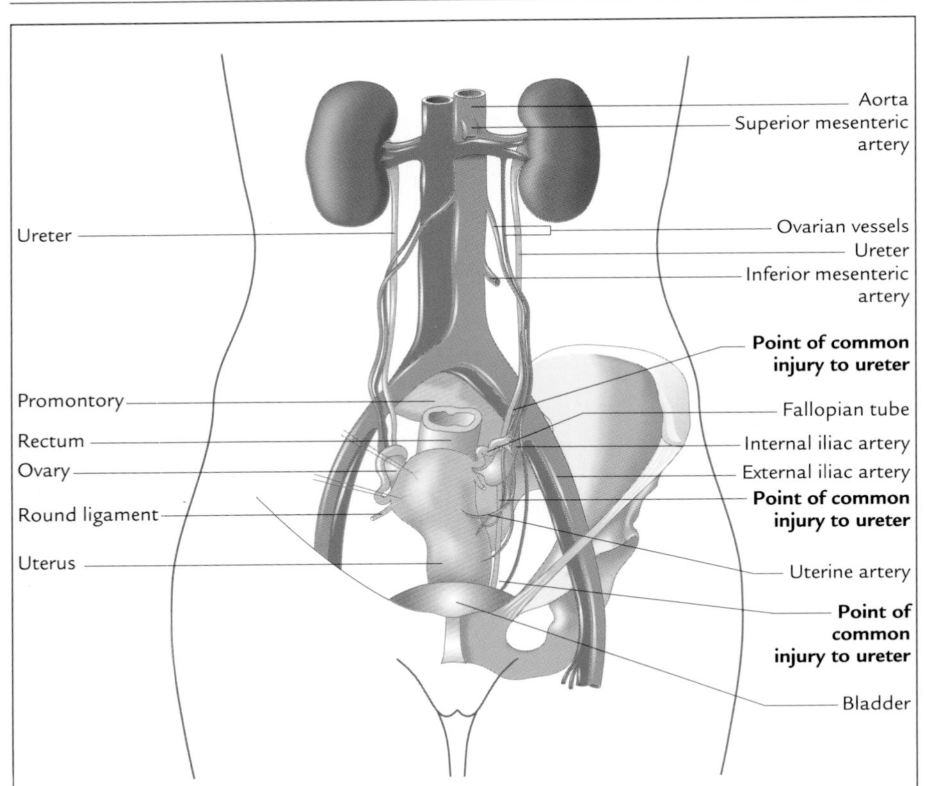

Figure 97.1. *An overview of the course of the ureters in the pelvis. The three most common sites of injury are at the pelvic brim near the ovarian vessels, at the point where the uterine artery crosses the ureter, and at the ureterovesical junction.*

should identify the ureter from above and trace out its course to the bladder.

THE ROLE OF THE UROLOGIC CONSULTANT

When the urologist is called to the operating room for consultation on a possible urologic injury, he should do several things before scrubbing up. First, he should read the chart for any relevant history that may affect the patient's urologic status. Second, he should ask if any preoperative radiologic studies, such as an intravenous pyelogram (IVP), are available for review. It is my practice to take a 'urology bag' with me when called for an intraoperative consultation. This bag contains ureteral stents, infant feeding tubes, Malecot catheters, and three-way urethral catheters, which are often unfamiliar to non-urologic nurses.

After scrubbing up, the urologist should assess the situation. If exposure is poor, there should be no reluctance about repositioning retractors or extending the surgical incision, if necessary. In addition, if hemostasis is inadequate, the urologist should ensure a relatively dry surgical field before proceeding. The ureter should be identified and traced out above and below the area of concern. The urologist should be aware that, if a ureter has been injured, the contralateral ureter or bladder might also have been injured; depending on the circumstances, these structures should also be examined intraoperatively. Indigo carmine or methylene blue may be given intravenously to aid in checking the integrity of the ureters; these dyes may be instilled via a urethral catheter to help identify or confirm bladder injuries.

INTRAOPERATIVE REPAIR – BLADDER INJURIES

Most bladder injuries are relatively straightforward to repair. They usually occur during a hysterectomy and usually involve the anterior bladder wall. Most bladder injuries are satisfactorily repaired with two layers of absorbable suture. Occasionally, the bladder wall will need to be debrided before closure. If a Foley catheter is not in place, one should be inserted and either indigo carmine or methylene blue can be injected to verify the adequacy of the closure. The urologist should remember the caveat of associated ureteral injuries. If there is uncertainty about a ureteral injury at the time of a bladder injury, 5 Fr or 8 Fr infant feeding tubes can be inserted into the ureteral orifices prior to closure of the bladder. This often makes identification of the ureters easier.

Bladder injuries associated with cesarean section are more difficult to manage. These bladder injuries are often more posterior and frequently are near the vaginal wall. Such injuries are difficult to close because the exposure is awkward and these injuries carry an increased risk of postoperative vesicovaginal fistula formation. It is often prudent, when faced with a posterior bladder wall repair, to interpose omentum between the bladder repair and vaginal wall to decrease the likelihood of postoperative fistula formation. All bladder injuries should be drained with an indwelling bladder catheter and either a closed or an open drainage system from the space of Retzius. The customary postoperative regime is to remove the drain from the space of Retzius on postoperative day 2 or 3 and to perform a cystogram about a week postoperatively to confirm satisfactory bladder repair before discontinuing the urethral catheter.

INTRAOPERATIVE REPAIR – LOWER URETER

Injuries to the distal 4 cm of the ureter can be handled in one of three ways, outlined below.

Ureteroureterostomy

If the ureteral injury is within 3–4 cm above the ureterovesical junction it can often be repaired by a primary ureteral anastomosis. It is important to resect a small portion of both the proximal and distal ureteral segments to ensure that viable tissue is being anastomosed. It is preferable to spatulate either end of the ureter that is being repaired and to use interrupted, absorbable sutures (Fig. 97.2). Whether to stent the anastomosis is best left to the discretion of the surgeon, but all anas-

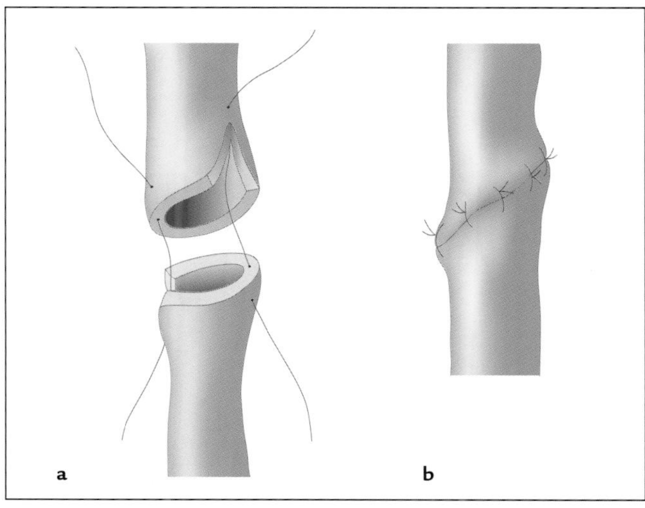

Figure 97.2. *A primary ureteroureterostomy is best performed after each ureteral segment has been resected back to viable tissue and with each end spatulated.*

tomoses should be drained. Non-transecting injuries of the ureter, such as ureteral tears or inadvertent ureteral clamping, are also best left to the judgment of the individual surgeon; however, in most cases, such injuries are best excised and a ureteral anastomosis performed to complete the repair.

Ureteral implant

When the ureteral injury is quite low – in the distal 2 cm – primary ureteral repair is usually difficult. In these situations, a ureteral reimplant is usually preferable. I prefer to utilize the Leadbetter–Politano technique of ureteral reimplantation (Fig. 97.3), but any method of reimplantation with which the surgeon feels comfortable is acceptable. A non-refluxing reimplantation is preferable in women who are in the age group where sexual activity is likely. Whether to stent the reimplanted ureter is, again, best left to the individual surgeon's judgment; however, all ureteral reimplants should be drained.

Psoas hitch

If the primary ureteroureterostomy or ureteral implant cannot be performed with a tension-free anastomosis, then a psoas hitch is a very good solution for lower ureteral injuries.[5–7] The techniques used for performing the psoas hitch have been described previously; below, I describe the technique that I have used over the years.[8,9]

Bladder mobilization is important in order to provide a tension-free ureteral reimplantation. It is usually necessary to mobilize the bladder bilaterally, not just on the side of the ureteral injury. The cystostomy should be made on the anterior wall of the bladder, away from the dome. This enables the surgeon's fingers to be placed in the bladder dome, thus aiding mobilization of the bladder as well as placement of the anchoring stitches in the psoas muscle (Fig. 97.4). My own preference is to use non-absorbable stitches to anchor the bladder to the psoas muscle. During this maneuver, care should be taken to avoid injury to the genitofemoral nerve or inad-

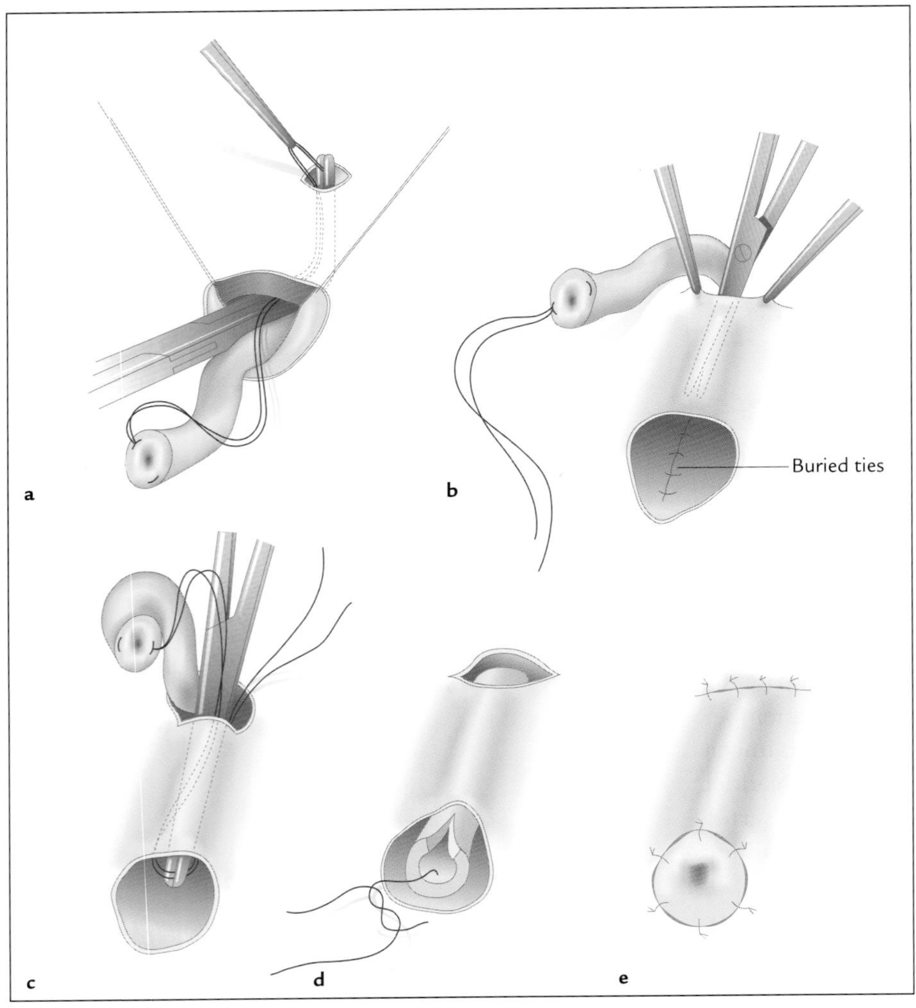

Figure 97.3. *The Leadbetter–Politano ureteral reimplantation technique.*

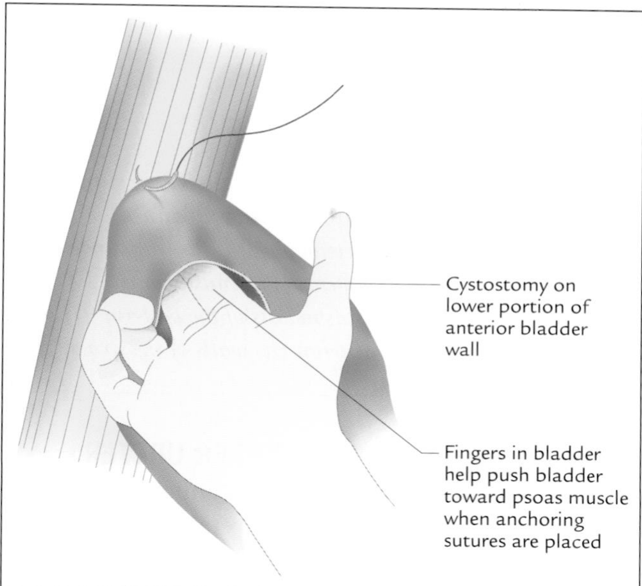

Figure 97.4. *The cystostomy should be made on the interior portion of the anterior bladder wall to permit the surgeon's finger to aid in bladder mobilization and guide in the anchoring stitches to the psoas muscle.*

vertent incorporation of the nerve within the sutures. In most cases I use the Leadbetter–Politano technique for ureteral reimplantation and, in these cases, I find it preferable to leave an indwelling ureteral stent (Fig. 97.5). The cystostomy is closed in the usual manner. A urethral catheter is left in place and a suprapubic tube is usually not necessary. An external drain is left near the reimplantation site.

INTRAOPERATIVE REPAIR – MIDURETER

Midureteral injuries that are not extensive can be repaired with a ureteroureterostomy, as described above. However, when a primary repair is not possible, other operative techniques are useful.

Transureteroureterostomy

The technique of transureteroureterostomy was first described in 1934 by Higgins to manage persistent unilateral ureteral reflux.[10] Since that time it has been used to treat unilateral ureteral injuries.[6,9,10] However, the concern has been that, if a complication occurs following a transureteroureterostomy, then both ureters are jeopardized.[11,12] A history of stone disease is a contraindication to this procedure.

The technique of transureteroureterostomy is straightforward. Both the donor and recipient ureters should be mobilized to prepare for a tension-free anastomosis. Under no circumstances should the recipient ureter be angulated in order to reach the donor ureter. My own preference is to spatulate the donor ureter and then to place stay sutures in the recipient ureter and perform the ureteroureterostomy between the stay sutures (Fig. 97.6a). I prefer to use 4-0 chromic sutures for the anastomosis: I perform a running suture line, with the knots on the outside on the posterior wall, and use interrupted sutures on the anterior wall (Fig. 97.6b). Because stenting a transureteroureterostomy is usually an awkward procedure, in most cases the anastomosis is left unstented; however, an external drain is always used.

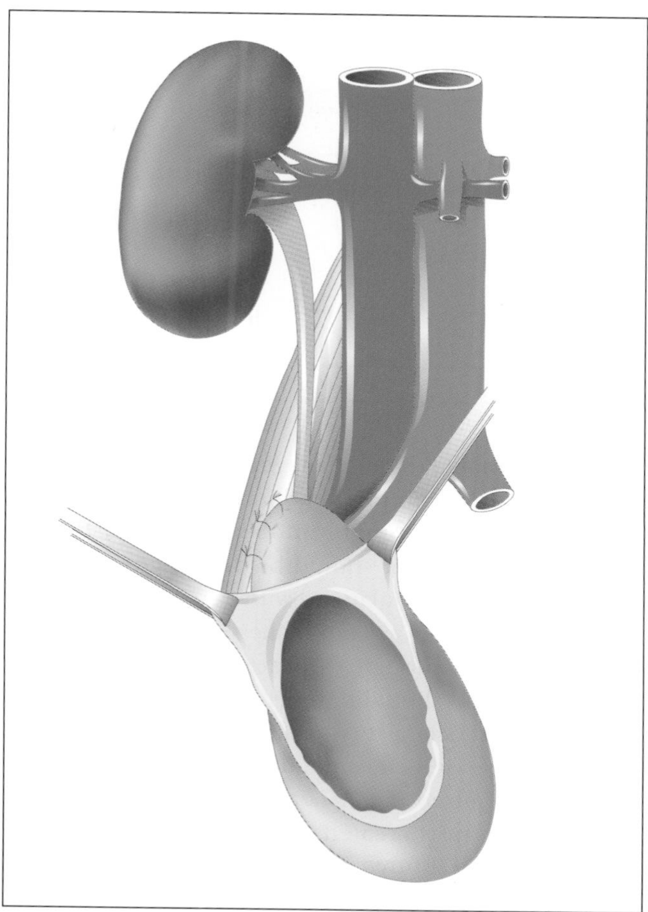

Figure 97.5. *Completed psoas hitch and ureteral implant.*

Boari flap

The Boari flap is an attractive solution for repair of extensive midureteral injuries. Boari first described his operative technique for ureteral replacement in a canine model in 1894.[13] Subsequently, the Boari flap has been incorporated into clinical practice and is par-

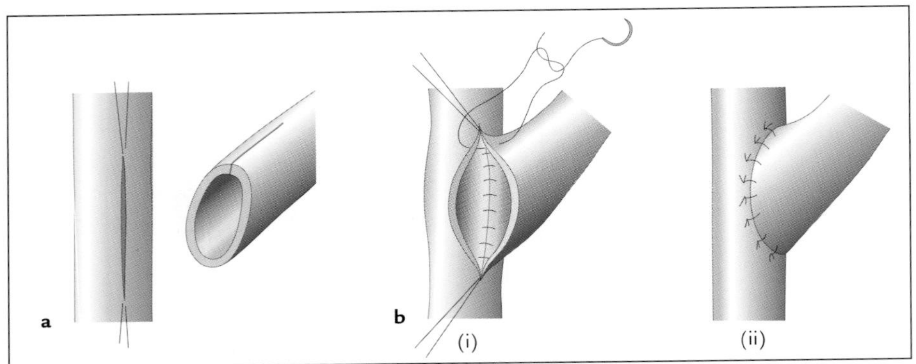

Figure 97.6. *(a) Stay sutures mark the area of planned ureterotomy; (b) the transuretero-ureterostomy anastomosis: anastomosis of the posterior (i) and anterior (ii) walls of the ureter.*

ticularly adaptable to the management of injuries to the midureter.[14–17] As with preparation for a psoas hitch, the bladder must be thoroughly mobilized. Before the flap is created, the bladder should be distended with saline and the flap carefully planned with a sterile marker. The most critical maneuver is to make sure that the base of the flap is wide enough to prevent distal ischemia in the flap: the flap should have its blood supply based on the superior vesicle artery; usually, the base of the flap should be at least 4 cm wide, depending on the length of the flap required (Fig. 97.7a).

After the flap is created, it is tubularized with running absorbable sutures. The distal ureter is then anastomosed to the flap (Fig. 97.7b) in the standard fashion. These anastomoses are preferably stented and all are drained. A urethral catheter is left indwelling to drain the bladder and a suprapubic tube is used at the surgeon's discretion.

INTRAOPERATIVE REPAIR – UPPER URETER

Injuries to the upper ureter that cannot be repaired with a straightforward ureteroureterostomy can be problematic. In most cases, a Boari flap will not reach an upper ureteral injury; therefore, the choices usually include autotransplantation, ileal ureter or nephrectomy.

Autotransplantation

Autotransplantation of the kidney is a formidable procedure and should not be undertaken if other options exist.[16,18,19] It is usually considered when the contralateral kidney is absent or poorly functioning. The kidney is harvested with maximal vessel length and the vascular anastomoses to the iliac vessels are performed in the standard fashion. The upper ureter or renal pelvis can then be anastomosed directly to the bladder.

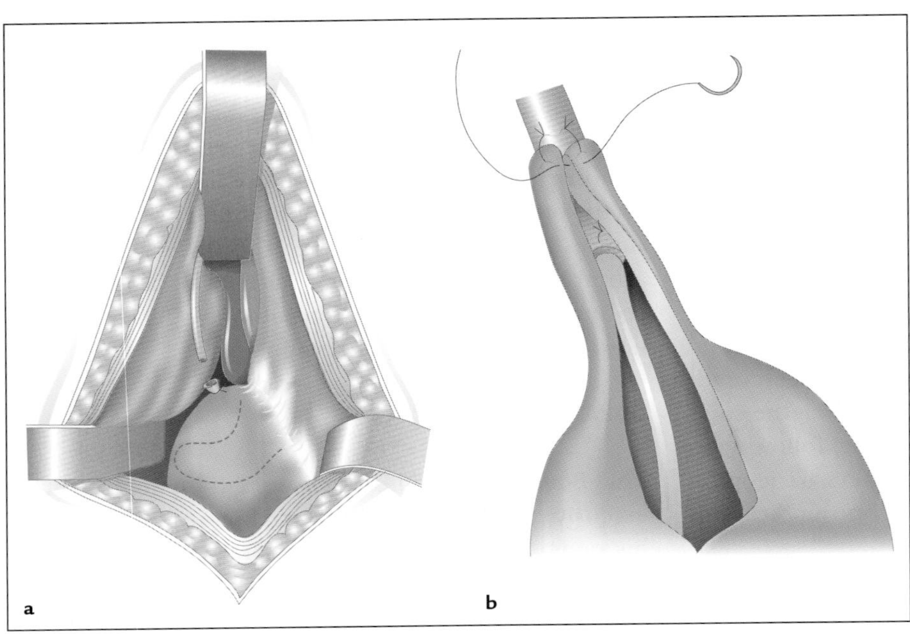

Figure 97.7. *(a) The Boari flap is planned out on the distended bladder wall; (b) the proximal ureter is anastomosed to the tubularized Boari flap.*

Ileal ureter

The use of ileal interposition for extensive upper ureteral injuries has also been reported.[6,16,20] As with autotransplantation, ileal interposition should be considered only when simpler alternatives are not practical. It is preferable to create an ileal ureter in patients who have had thorough preoperative bowel preparation; in emergency situations, however, an ileal segment can be isolated without such preparation. The techniques used for creation of an ileal ureter are similar to those used in an ileal conduit. The proximal and distal ureteral segments should be fully mobilized and the ureteral–ileal anastomoses are performed with absorbable sutures (Fig. 97.8). No stents are utilized and an external drain is necessary.

Nephrectomy

When a normal contralateral kidney is present, a simple nephrectomy should be considered as an expeditious solution to extensive upper ureteral injury.[6,21] A nephrectomy is often attractive because it obviates the postoperative complications, such as urinary leak or infection, that can be seen with other techniques used to manage upper ureteral injuries.

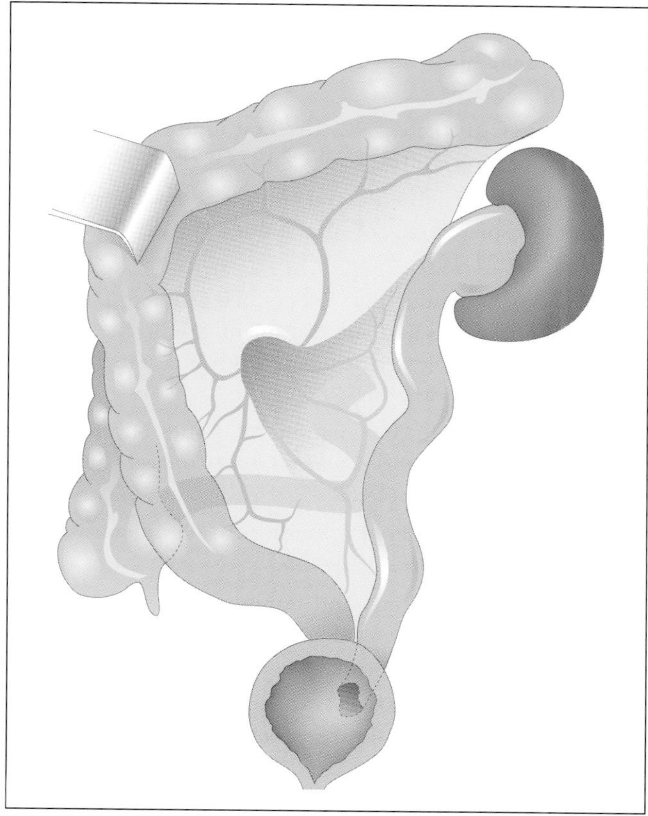

Figure 97.8. *Completed ileal ureter.*

POSTOPERATIVE PROCEDURES

Postoperative recognition of bladder injuries

Postoperative symptoms associated with delayed recognition of bladder injuries include fever, abdominal pain, abdominal distension, infection, decreased urine output, and rising serum creatinine. The management of these cases should be individualized, since the patient's overall condition is an important consideration. In general, however, extraperitoneal injuries can be managed with a trial of catheter drainage, whereas intraperitoneal injuries merit surgical exploration and repair. The most direct way to diagnose the presence and location of a bladder injury is a cystogram.

Postoperative recognition of ureteral injuries

Postoperative symptoms of ureteral injuries may include flank pain, fever, sepsis, decreased urine output, abdominal mass, elevated creatinine or urinary fistula. However, ureteral injuries can also be asymptomatic. If a ureteral injury is suspected, an IVP is the diagnostic study of choice,[21,22] although an abdominal ultrasound or computed tomography scan may also be helpful.

Once a diagnosis of ureteral injury is suspected or confirmed, a retrograde pyelogram can give more information regarding the precise location of the injury. There is genuine debate as to whether stent placement should be attempted at the time of a retrograde pyelogram. Dowling and associates[21] found that, in 19 of 20 patients, a retrograde stent could not be placed beyond the site of the urologic injury. However, others feel that, if a stent can be negotiated through the area of injury, in some cases this will promote satisfactory ureteral healing and avoid the need for open surgery.[23]

When ureteral stent placement is not possible, nephrostomy tube placement is an option.[21,24] Nephrostomy tube placement has two potential benefits. First, if the patient is septic or in other ways not ideally suitable for surgical re-exploration, the nephrostomy tube can temporize until the patient's condition improves to the point where surgery is a more realistic alternative. Second, some cases of ureteral obstruction secondary to suture entrapment have been reported to resolve successfully with nephrostomy tube drainage alone.[25] Again, which cases can be adequately managed with nephrostomy tube drainage can best be judged by the individual surgeon.

Conservative management of ureteral injuries recognized in the postoperative period can, in some cases, be successful. Ku et al. reported successful management in 11 of 17 patients treated with nephrostomy tube, stent, or both, following ureteral injury. However, the management of such cases must be individualized.[26]

If conservative measures are unsuccessful, and surgical re-exploration is required, the options available are identical to those mentioned previously for the management of injuries recognized intraoperatively.

Postoperative management

The urologic consultant should always dictate a separate operative note. Following the operation, the urologist should meet the family members and explain the urologic part of the surgery. The urologist should also make postoperative visits to the patient and be the only physician to order urologic radiographic studies or the removal of tubes. In general, suprapubic tubes are removed on postoperative day 2 or 3, or when the urine is clear. Urethral catheters are removed after a cystogram shows no leak – this is usually on about postoperative day 7. Internal stents and nephrostomy tubes are ordinarily removed later, about 2–3 weeks postoperatively, and after either an IVP or a nephrostogram has confirmed good healing of the surgical repair.

CONCLUSIONS

Bladder and ureteral injuries during gynecologic surgery present a difficult challenge to both the gynecologist and urologist. If the guidelines reviewed above – together with good judgment and good technique – are employed, most of these injuries can be resolved successfully.

REFERENCES

1. Tarkington MA, Detjer SW, Bresette JF. Early surgical management of extensive gynecologic ureteral injuries. Surg Gynecol Obstet 1991;173:17–21.
2. Gangi MP, Agee RE, Spence CR. Surgical injury to ureter. Urology 1976;8:22–7.
3. Neuman M, Eidelman A, Langer R et al. Iatrogenic injuries to the ureter during gynecologic and obstetric operations. Surg Gynecol Obstet 1991;173:268–72.
4. Turner-Warwick R, Worth PHL. The psoas bladder hitch procedure for the replacement of the lower third of the ureter. Br J Urol 1969;41:701–9.
5. Gross M, Peng B, Waterhouse K. Use of the mobilized bladder to replace the pelvic ureter. J Urol 1969;101:40.
6. Zinman LM, Libertino JA, Ruth RA. Management of operative ureteral injury. Urology 1978;12:290–303.
7. Ehrlich RM, Melman A, Skinner DG. The use of vesico-psoas hitch in urologic surgery. J Urol 1978;119:322–5.
8. Matthews R, Marshall FF. Versatility of the adult psoas hitch ureteral reimplantation. J Urol 1997;158:2078–82.
9. Hodges CV, Moore RJ, Lehman TH, Benham AM. Clinical experiences with transuretero-ureterostomy. J Urol 1963;90:552–62.
10. Smith IB, Smith JC. Transuretero-ureterostomy: British experience. Br J Urol 1975;47:519–23.
11. Ehrlich RM, Skinner DG. Complications of transuretero-ureterostomy. J Urol 1975;113:467–73.
12. Sandoz IL, Paull DP, MacFarlane CA. Complications with transuretero-ureterostomy. J Urol 1977;117:39–42.
13. Boari A. Chirurgia dell uretere, con pretazience de Dott: I. Albarran, 1,900 contribute sperementale alla plastica delle uretere. Atti Accad Med Ferrara 1894;14:444.
14. Konigsberg H, Blunt KJ, Muecke EC. Use of Boari flap in lower ureteral injuries. Urology 1975;5:751–5.
15. Colimbu M, Block N, Morales P. Ureterovesical flap operation for middle and upper ureteral repair. Invest Urol 1973;10:313–7.
16. Benson MC, Ring KS, Olsson CA. Ureteral reconstruction and bypass: experience with ileal interposition, the Boari flap–psoas hitch and renal autotransplantation. J Urol 1990;143:20–3.
17. Bright TC III, Peters PC. Ureteral injuries secondary to operative procedures. Urology 1977;9:22–6.
18. Hardy JD. High ureteral injuries: management by autotransplantation of the kidney. J Am Med Assoc 1963;184:97–101.
19. Novick AC, Stewart BH. Experience with extracorporeal renal operations and autotransplantation in the management of complicated urologic disorders. Surg Gynecol Obstet 1981;153:10–8.
20. McCullough DL, McLaughlin AP, Gittes RF, Kerr WS. Replacement of the damaged or neoplastic ureter by ileum. J Urol 1977;118:375–8.
21. Dowling RA, Corriere JN, Sandler CM. Iatrogenic ureteral injury. J Urol 1986;135:912–15.
22. Mann WJ. Intentional and unintentional ureteral surgical treatment in gynecologic procedures. Surg Gynecol Obstet 1991;172:453–6.
23. Mitty HA, Train JS, Dan SJ. Antegrade ureteral stenting in the management of fistulas, strictures and calculi. Radiology 1983;149:433–8.
24. Persky L, Hampel N, Kedia K. Percutaneous nephrostomy and ureteral injury. J Urol 1981;125:298–300.

25. Harshman MW, Pollack HM, Banner MP, Wein AJ. Conservative management of ureteral obstruction secondary to suture entrapment. J Urol 1982;127:121–3.

26. Ku JH, Kim ME, Jeon YS, Lee NK, Park YH. Minimally invasive management of ureteral injuries recognized late after obstetric and gynecologic surgery. Injury 2003;34(7):480–3.

98

Cosmetic vaginal surgery

James Balmforth, Linda Cardozo

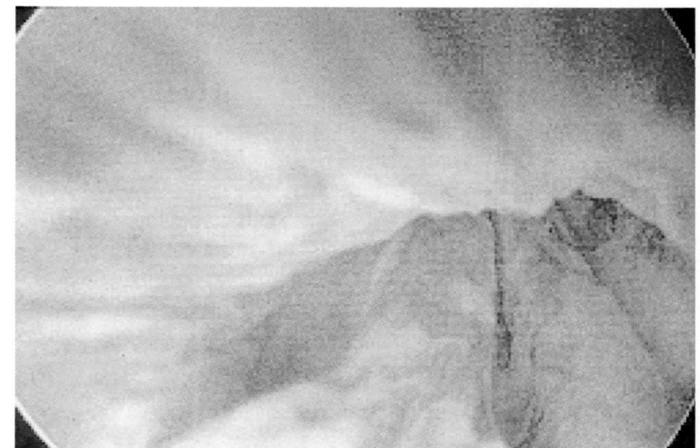

INTRODUCTION

In recent years there has been growing interest in the subject of cosmetic vaginal surgery, which parallels the ever-increasing public awareness of cosmetic surgery generally. Despite the large number of articles in the popular press on the subject of 'designer vaginas', there is very little evidence in the peer-reviewed medical literature to guide clinicians on possible surgical procedures and their indications, risks, and benefits. Reconstructive pelvic surgery for congenital developmental abnormalities of the female genital tract such as the Mayer–Rokitansky–Kuster–Hauser syndrome (congenital absence of the vagina)[1–4] or ambiguous genitalia in childhood[5] is a well-established area of adolescent gynecology. However, the largely patient-driven demand for purely esthetic vaginal surgery in adulthood is a more recent phenomenon.

The principal driving forces behind the rise in the number of requests for such procedures are the increasing consumerism of medical practice, greater willingness to undergo esthetic surgery generally and more widespread discussion of this subject in the popular media (Table 98.1). The last 3 years have seen articles published on cosmetic vaginal surgery in over 75 different women's magazine titles in Europe and North America as the number of women undergoing all forms of cosmetic surgery increases year on year. The gulf between reporting in the lay and professional literature is starkly made by the contrasting results of electronically searching for evidence on cosmetic gynecologic surgery. An internet search using the Google search engine yields several thousand matches for enquiries on topics such as 'cosmetic vaginal surgery', 'designer vagina', 'esthetic vaginal surgery' or 'laser labiaplasty', whereas Pub-med and Medline yield fewer than 50 relevant papers. There is therefore very scant medical evidence to guide the clinician confronted by a women seeking cosmetic vaginal surgery. Even the evidence that exists is mostly derived from the more 'mainstream' management of vaginal laxity and pelvic organ prolapse. This is mostly observational, non-randomized and employs 'doctor-orientated' outcome measures rather than 'patient-centred' quality of life measures. However, as public interest in this type of gynecologic surgery is increasing it is important that doctors keep abreast of current trends and developments.

Table 98.1. *Reasons behind the rise of consumer demand in gynecologic practice*

1. Increased access to information
   - Popular media
   - Internet
2. Society becoming more egalitarian
3. Delivery of healthcare becoming a partnership between the patient–consumer's 'wishes' and the doctor's 'professional opinion'
4. Most gynecologic disorders are not lethal and therefore qualitative outcome is increasingly important
5. Emergence of 'quality of life' as an important treatment outcome
6. 'Bothersomeness' of a condition is perceived by the patient within their own psychosocial context. This may be different from the 'doctor-centered' view of the condition

A wide variety of surgical procedures can be included under the term 'cosmetic vaginal surgery' ranging from purely esthetic operations like labiaplasty, hymenoplasty and 'vaginal rejuvenation' to the more conventional gynecologic reconstructive procedures like vaginal pelvic floor repair, which aim to restore function as well as enhance appearance (Table 98.2).

The labia minora of the vulva are two cutaneous–mucosal refolds located between the labia majora, the internal aspect of which is separated by the interlabial cleft. Relatively enlarged labia minora may be attributable to several factors. They are most commonly congenital but may also rarely be due to chronic irritation, exogenous androgenic hormones, or stretching with weights. Although some women require surgical reduction for functional reasons, most seek reduction of their labia minora because of psychological concerns relating to body image. Reduction labiaplasty is the most commonly performed esthetic surgical procedure and is usually undertaken on a day case basis. This is frequently suggested for so-called 'hypertrophic' labia minora. In fact, as any practicing gynecologist knows, there is a wide range of naturally occurring sizes and shapes of perfectly normal labia minora.

The effect of body image on psychological well-being and sexual behavior is comprehensively described in the literature. Ackard et al.[6] reported on the relationship between body image, self-worth, and sexual behaviors in 3627 women. They found that women who were more 'satisfied' with their body image reported more sexual activity, orgasms, and initiating sex, together with greater comfort undressing in front of their partner, having sex with the lights on or trying new sexual behaviors, than those who were 'dissatisfied'. Positive body image was inversely related to self-consciousness and importance of physical attractiveness, and positively related to relationships with others and overall satisfaction. As we move further towards a 'culture of physical perfection', many social commentators have suggested that increased dissatisfaction with physical aspects of our appearance is likely to lead to increased demand for esthetic surgery.

Table 98.2. *Range of cosmetic vaginal procedures*

Procedure	Description
Reduction labiaplasty	There is a wide variety of different techniques to alter the size and contour of external female genitalia[7–9]
Augmentation labiaplasty	Esthetically enhances labia majora to give a supposedly 'more youthful' appearance
Vulvar lipoplasty	Removal of unwanted fat from mons pubis and labia to alter cosmetic appearance
Reversal of female genital mutilation (FGM)	Exact technique is dependent upon the original extent of the FGM
Hymenoplasty	Partial or complete reconstruction of the hymen
G-spot amplification	Injectable bulking agent into Grafenberg spot on anterior vaginal wall
Perineal reconstruction	To restore perineal length following childbirth trauma or previous surgery
Pelvic floor repair	To restore normal vaginal contour and repair prolapse
Z-plasty or incision of constriction ring[10]	To resolve iatrogenic narrowing of vagina
Use of myocutaneous flaps[11]	In cases where more extensive reconstruction needs to be undertaken in order to restore function

Esthetically, asymmetric or enlarged labia minora cause self-consciousness sexually and when wearing tight underwear or clothing. They can also occasionally interfere with micturition, leading to voiding difficulties, 'anatomic entrapment' of urine, and poor hygiene. Most commonly, reduction labiaplasty is performed either by amputation of the protuberant segment and oversewing the edge or by a wedge excision and reapproximation of labial tissue. Choi and Kim[7] suggest that these techniques remove the natural contour and color of the edge of the labia, and offer an alternative method to preserve the contour and anatomy of the labia minora by simply reducing its central width through bilateral de-epithelialization and reapproximation of the central portion with preservation of the neurovascular supply to the edge.

In the largest reported series of reduction labiaplasty operations reported, 163 women who underwent surgical reduction of the labia minora were followed up over a 9-year period to determine whether they were satisfied with the procedure.[9] The women's age ranged from 12 to 67 years (median = 26 years) and the principal motives for requesting surgery were esthetic concerns (87%), discomfort in clothing (64%), discomfort with exercise (26%), and entry dyspareunia (43%). No significant surgery-related complications were reported. Anatomic results were satisfactory from the doctor's perspective in 93% of cases. Eighty-nine percent of the women found the results of surgery to be satisfactory from an esthetic standpoint and 93% were happy with the functional outcome; 4% of women said they would not undergo the same procedure again.

An exciting new technology that was originally developed for use in correcting major congenital vaginal anomalies and cloacal malformations that require extensive surgical reconstruction is in vivo tissue engineering of vaginal epithelial and smooth muscle cells.[12] In time, as these tissue engineering techniques become more widespread, they are likely to be used in the field of cosmetic surgery.

Vaginal epithelial and smooth muscle cells can be grown, expanded in culture, and characterized immunocytochemically before being seeded on polymer scaffolds to form vascularized vaginal tissue that has phenotypic and functional properties similar to those of normal vaginal tissues. The contractile properties of the tissue-engineered vagina constructs respond to electrical field stimulation in a similar way to normal, host vaginal tissue. This technology is being actively pursued to achieve the engineering of large sheets of immunologically comparable vaginal tissue in vivo for use in clinical applications.

CAN SURGERY IMPROVE FEMALE SEXUAL FUNCTION?

As well as purporting to restore normal anatomic relationships following the effects of childbirth and aging, some surgeons offer the promise of enhanced sexual gratification as a result of these procedures. Many of the claims made in the advertising literature of clinics that offer this type of surgery are unsubstantiated by clinical trial evidence, or indeed anything other than client testimonials. There is currently no objective evidence to support the idea that esthetic genital surgery leads to subjective or objective improvement in sexual function (Table 98.3). Indeed, most of the published literature on reconstructive pelvic surgery suggests that repeated vaginal surgery risks causing scarring, loss of sensation, and

Table 98.3. ***Claims made for cosmetic vaginal surgery***

Claim	Evidence
Enhanced esthetic appearance	Possibly
Increased sexual gratification	No evidence to support this

decreased sexual function.[13,14] If sexual dysfunction is the primary reason for seeking surgical intervention, then it is often more appropriate to consider other avenues of treatment first, including psychosexual counseling and pelvic floor muscle training.

In 1966, Masters and Johnson[15] described four classic phases in female sexual response: excitement, plateau, orgasm, and resolution. More recent theories stress the role of psychological components such as 'desire', together with physical sexual stimulus, leading to arousal, and modified by situational variables. Most studies looking at vaginal surgery and sexual function report a deterioration of frequency and increased discomfort associated with reconstructive vaginal surgery. This is particularly so for trials reporting the use of prosthetic mesh to augment intrinsically weak tissues. Milani et al.[16] reported a fall in sexual activity of 12% and an increase in dyspareunia of 63% in women undergoing anterior or posterior vaginal prolapse repair with Prolene mesh augmentation, despite an impressive 'anatomic' success rate of 94%. This and other similar studies involving the use of prosthetic materials underline the difference between functionally and anatomically successful surgical reconstruction.

'Traditional' levator plication posterior vaginal repairs are also associated with very high rates of sexual dysfunction. A retrospective review[13] of 231 women undergoing posterior repair found an increase in sexual dysfunction (18–27%), increased constipation (22–33%), and increased fecal incontinence (4–11%) despite a good rate of anatomic defect correction.

Helstrom and Nilsson[17] studied the effect of vaginal surgery for urinary incontinence and prolapse on sexual function and quality of life. In a questionnaire study of 118 women they found that sexual function deteriorated postoperatively and the mean frequency of sexual intercourse was reduced. Although pelvic floor disorders are known to impair sexual function, there was no improvement in sexuality after surgery to correct them. On the contrary, sexual function deteriorated and dyspareunia worsened after vaginal surgery. The explanation offered for this was vulnerability to disturbance of the nerve and blood supply of the vaginal wall resulting in impaired sexual arousal and lubrication.

Tunuguntla and Gousse[18] recently reviewed the mechanisms by which vaginal surgery affects female sexual function and related pathophysiology to potential causes. Altered anatomy, neurovascular supply of the clitoris and introitus, and pelvic innervation are all important factors. The vast majority of the literature on this subject supports the idea that, at best, surgery does not always harm sexual function, but rarely improves it.

ETHICAL CONSIDERATIONS

Female genital mutilation affects over 130 million women worldwide, mostly from just 28 African countries. However, it is increasingly encountered by healthcare workers in the developed world because of the influx of political and economic refugees.

Female genital mutilation is mostly performed on young girls and the World Health Organization estimates that 2 million girls are at risk each year. As consent is usually not given, it constitutes assault. Therefore, in the UK and in most of the developed world, female genital mutilation is unlawful – not only when performed on minors, but also when performed on adult women. It is interesting to contrast the banning of female genital mutilation – even for competent, consenting women – with cosmetic surgery, towards which the law takes a very permissive stance. There are those that argue that this legal dichotomy is ethically unsustainable:[19] that either the ban on female genital mutilation or the law's permissive attitude towards cosmetic surgery is unjustified as no woman could 'validly' consent to either practice as they involve the intentional infliction of injury. This argument contends that people in countries where female genital mutilation is practiced resent references to 'barbaric practices imposed on women by male-dominated primitive societies', especially when they look at the developed world and see women undergoing their own potentially hazardous 'feminization rites' intended to increase sexual desirability.

Other authors[20] have also juxtaposed the trend in cosmetic vaginal surgery in the West with the implications of the laws governing female genital mutilation, and highlighted the double morality of the situation. It is important to maintain the legal principle of equality before the law with respect to 'alterations' of the female genitalia. In essence the argument comes down to the principal of informed consent: that an adult woman can decide to request that a surgical procedure be undertaken, and as long as she can find a doctor who is willing to perform that procedure, then it is legal. If consent is not given, then it constitutes assault.

The other area of practice that arouses ethical debate is surgical hymen repair (hymenorrhaphy). This is predominantly requested by women from some African and Mediterranean cultures, where the suggestion of premarital sex places women from these cultures at risk of violence or being ostracized. The question then arises as to whether this makes hymenorrhaphy morally more justified than purely cosmetic surgery or whether, by performing such surgery, it is perpetuating a belief system that is degrading to women.

In considering how best to restore normal pelvic anatomy and function, it is important to consider all three pelvic organ systems – urinary, genital, and gastrointestinal. Appropriate preoperative assessment of function and the degree to which normal pelvic floor support has been lost is important in planning the most suitable type of surgical procedure. As well as the traditional methods of 'doctor-centered' assessment, there is currently an increased awareness of the need to formally evaluate the mental and physical impact of any condition on the patient's quality of life (QoL). Condition-specific sexual dysfunction QoL questionnaires have been designed and validated for this purpose.[21]

In order to provide women with realistic expectations, a thorough preoperative discussion about the aims and likely outcomes of any planned surgery is invaluable (Table 98.4). This may sometimes need to include a careful psychological assessment of their motivations in requesting surgery over more conservative treatments. Women should be made aware that while cosmetic vaginal surgery is not specifically directed towards correction of bladder or bowel function, it can adversely affect it. Postoperative urinary retention, voiding difficulties, urinary incontinence and altered sexual sensation are possible sequelae of all vaginal operations. Urinary retention is often a temporary effect of anterior vaginal surgery caused by edema, pain, and mild obstruction. It will generally be alleviated by time, but may need a short-term indwelling transurethral or suprapubic catheter or clean intermittent bladder drainage. Urinary incontinence can be unmasked when there is occult stress incontinence due to kinking of the urethra with a major anterior vaginal wall prolapse. Objective urodynamic assessment is therefore advisable as an aid to preoperative decision making and counseling in anyone undergoing any significant degree of vaginal reconstruction, as opposed to more local vulval surgery. An additional procedure to rectify occult lower urinary tract symptoms may be offered, or at least the patient be made aware of the possible sequelae.

Table 98.4. ***Outline of a pragmatic approach to requests for cosmetic vaginal surgery: how should it be managed?***

1. Find out what is *really* troubling the woman
2. Evaluate symptoms from the patient's perspective
   - Concerns about esthetic appearance
   - Functional disorders
   - Specific postpartum problems – physical and psychological
   - Symptomatic prolapse
3. Consider other aspects of the woman's life
   - Overall quality of life and social function
   - Hormonal status
   - Family complete?
4. Consider function of all three pelvic compartments
5. Consider underlying psychosexual problems (female sexual dysfunction) ? 'hidden agenda'
   - Explore body image and sexuality
   - Expectations of future sexual function
6. Examination with prolapse grading
   - Quality of tissues/? atrophic
7. Counseling – to include
   - Discussion about body image and what is 'normal'
   - Reassurance that sexual dysfunction commonly increases with age[22] and after childbirth[23,24] and may be better treated by more conservative measures initially
8. Initial conservative measures
9. Later surgery if appropriate and after realistic preoperative discussion between doctor and patient about likely outcomes

VAGINAL LAXITY

The sensation of vaginal laxity is a commonly reported concern in parous women (Table 98.5)[24] and one of the commonest reasons cited by patients requesting cosmetic vaginal surgery. It is more commonly reported in women who have sustained perineal trauma[23] as a result of a vaginal delivery, than in those who are delivered by cesarean section or with an intact perineum. It is not uncommon for sexual function to alter after the upheaval of childbirth and caring for an infant. Barrett et al.[24] studied 796 women delivered of a live birth in a 6-month period. Sexual problems (e.g. vaginal dryness, painful penetration, pain during sexual intercourse, pain on orgasm, vaginal tightness, vaginal looseness, bleeding/irritation after sex, and loss of sexual desire) increased significantly after the birth. In the first 3 months after delivery 83% of women experienced such problems, declining to

Table 98.5. ***Common complaints associated with vaginal laxity***

- Discomfort and symptoms of prolapse
- Tampons fall out
- Lack of friction during intercourse
- Penis falls out during intercourse
- Vaginal wind[25]
- Bathwater entrapment

64% at 6 months; 89% had resumed some sexual activity within 6 months of the birth. By 6 months there was no association with type of delivery; only the experience of dyspareunia before pregnancy and current breastfeeding were significant risk factors.

Requests for consideration of cosmetic surgery from women who have recently delivered should therefore be treated with particular caution. It commonly takes at least 6 months for the effects of pregnancy-induced progesterone, which relaxes the smooth muscle of the lower genital tract, to resolve. Restoration of normal vaginal health may be delayed further as a result of the hypoestrogenic state caused by breastfeeding. Women are best advised to wait until they have finished breastfeeding and if necessary use topical estrogens before considering any surgical treatment in the postpartum period.

Psychological factors are also extremely important to consider in recently delivered women requesting an opinion on possible surgical correction of perceived 'birth-related' problems. A questionnaire-based study examining the influence of psychological factors[26] (role quality, relationship satisfaction, fatigue, and depression) on women's sexuality after childbirth found that depression was an important predictor of reduced sexual desire and sexual satisfaction during pregnancy, and of reduced frequency of intercourse at 12 weeks postpartum. At 6 months postpartum, the quality of the 'mother role' strongly related to measures of sexuality. Throughout the perinatal period, fatigue impacted strongly on measures of sexuality.

Initial conservative measures for the treatment of vaginal laxity include referral to a specialist physiotherapist for a course of pelvic floor muscle training (PFMT), the use of vaginal cones, correction of any urogenital atrophy present, and lifestyle advice to bring about a reduction in straining and high-impact exertion. Women should be advised that although moderate cardiovascular exercise promotes general health and weight loss, not all exercise is beneficial for improving pelvic floor function.

CONCLUSIONS

All doctors, from whichever specialty, working in the field of reconstructive pelvic surgery should be aware of the likely increase in the numbers of women requesting cosmetic vaginal surgery. Although this reflects a wider public demand for cosmetic surgery generally, there are issues relating to sexual function that are of particular relevance to surgeons operating on the genital tract. It may be necessary to disabuse potential patients of some of the wilder and unsubstantiated claims made for this type of surgery in order that they have realistic and informed expectations. It is vital to take a thorough history on anyone requesting such surgery and to explore in some depth the underlying desire for cosmetic vaginal surgery and what the patient hopes to achieve as a result of the operation. The request may be quite reasonable, but often it is worth trying conservative measures first. It is also important to pick up any underlying sexual problems, as surgery may only make these worse. A multicompartment approach to investigating and treating pelvic floor disorders should always be encouraged.

The almost total lack of good quality evidence in the medical literature on this subject makes advising women accurately on the possible risks and benefits more difficult. Despite these problems, the demand for this type of gynecologic surgery is likely to increase as medicine in the developed world becomes ever more consumer-driven. More research is therefore needed into all aspects of pelvic reconstructive surgery and its association with sexual function.

REFERENCES

1. McIndoe AH. Discussion on treatment of congenital absence of the vagina. Proc R Soc Med 1959;52:952–7.
2. Cali RW, Pratt JH. Congenital absence of the vagina. Long-term results of vaginal reconstruction in 175 cases. Am J Obstet Gynecol 1968;100:752–63.
3. Ashworth MF, Morton KE, Dewhurst J et al. Vaginoplasty using amnion. Obstet Gynecol 1986;67:443–6.
4. Williams AE. Uterovaginal agenesis. Ann R Coll Surg Engl 1976;58:266–72.
5. Creighton SM, Minto CL, Steele SJ. Objective cosmetic and anatomical outcomes at adolescence of feminising surgery for ambiguous genitalia done in childhood. Lancet 2001;358:124–5.
6. Ackard DM, Kearney-Cooke A, Peterson CB. Effect of body image and self-image on women's sexual behaviors. Int J Eat Disord 2000;28(4):422–9.
7. Choi HY, Kim KT. A new method for aesthetic reduction of labia minora (the de-epithelialized reduction of labioplasty). Plast Reconstr Surg 2000;105(1):419–22.
8. Giraldo F, Gonzalez C, de Haro F. Central wedge nymphectomy with a 90-degree Z-plasty for aesthetic reduction of the labia minora. Plast Reconstr Surg 2004;113(6):1820–5.
9. Rouzier R, Louis-Sylvestre C, Paniel BJ, Haddad B. Hypertrophy of labia minora: experience with 163 reductions. Am J Obstet Gynecol 2000;182:35–40.
10. Vassallo BJ, Karram MM. Management of iatrogenic vaginal constriction. Obstet Gynecol 2003;102(3):512–20.
11. Cordeiro PG, Pusic AL, Disa JJ. A classification system and

reconstructive algorithm for acquired vaginal defects. Plast Reconstr Surg 2002;110(4):1058–65.

12. De Filippo RE, Yoo JJ, Atala A. Engineering of vaginal tissue in vivo. Tissue Eng 2003;9(2):301–6.
13. Kahn MA, Stanton SL. Posterior colporrhaphy: its effects on bowel and sexual function. BJOG 1997;104(1):82–6.
14. Weber AM, Walters MD, Piedmonte MR. Sexual function and vaginal anatomy in women before and after surgery for pelvic organ prolapse and urinary incontinence. Am J Obstet Gynecol 2000;182(6):1610–15.
15. Masters WH, Johnson VE Human Sexual Response. Boston: Little, Brown, 1966.
16. Milani R, Salvatore S, Soligo M, Pifarotti P, Meschia M, Cortese M. Functional and anatomical outcome of anterior and posterior vaginal prolapse repair with prolene mesh. BJOG 2005;112(1):107–11.
17. Helstrom L, Nilsson B. Impact of vaginal surgery on sexuality and quality of life in women with urinary incontinence or genital descensus. Acta Obstet Gynecol Scand 2005;84(1):79–84.
18. Tunuguntla HS, Gousse AE. Female sexual dysfunction following vaginal surgery: myth or reality? Curr Urol Rep 2004;5(5):403–11.
19. Sheldon S, Wilkinson S. Female genital mutilation and cosmetic surgery: regulating non-therapeutic body modification. Bioethics 1998;12(4):263–85.
20. Essen B, Johnsdotter S. Female genital mutilation in the West: traditional circumcision versus genital cosmetic surgery. Acta Obstet Gynecol Scand 2004;83(7):611–13.
21. Rogers RG, Kammerer-Doak D, Villarreal A, Coates K, Qualls C. A new instrument to measure sexual function in women with urinary incontinence or pelvic organ prolapse. Am J Obstet Gynecol 2001;184(4):552–8.
22. Hisasue S, Kumamoto Y, Sato Y et al. Prevalence of female sexual dysfunction symptoms and its relationship to quality of life: a Japanese female cohort study. Urology 2005;65(1):143–8.
23. Signorello LB, Harlow BL, Chekos AK, Repke JT. Postpartum sexual functioning and its relationship to perineal trauma: a retrospective cohort study of primiparous women. Am J Obstet Gynecol 2001;184(5):881–8.
24. Barrett G, Pendry E, Peacock J, Victor C, Thakar R, Manyonda I. Women's sexual health after childbirth. BJOG 2000;107(2):186–95.
25. Krissi H, Medina C, Stanton SL. Vaginal wind – a new pelvic symptom. Int Urogynecol J Pelvic Floor Dysfunct 2003;14(6):399–402.
26. DeJudicibus MA, McCabe MP. Psychological factors and the sexuality of pregnant and postpartum women. J Sex Res 2002;39(2):94–103.

Index

Page numbers in *italics* indicate figures or tables.

Pages 1–798 are in Volume 1; pages 799–1384 are in Volume 2.

Pages 1–798 are in Volume 1; pages 799–1384 are in Volume 2.

Pages 1–798 are in Volume 1; pages 799–1384 are in Volume 2.

Pages 1–798 are in Volume 1; pages 799–1384 are in Volume 2.

Pages 1–798 are in Volume 1; pages 799–1384 are in Volume 2.